Integrated Pharmacology

THIRD EDITION

Clive P Page PhD Professor of Pharmacology, Sackler Institute of Pulmonary Pharmacology, Pharmaceutical Sciences Research Division, King's College London, London, UK

Michael J Curtis PhD FBPharmacolS Reader in Pharmacology, Department of Pharmacology and Therapeutics, The Rayne Institute, St Thomas' Hospital, King's College London, UK

Michael J A Walker PhD Emeritus Professor of Pharmacology, Department of Anesthesiology, Pharmacology and Therapeutics, Faculty of Medicine, University of British Columbia, Vancouver, Canada

Brian B Hoffman MD Professor of Medicine, Harvard Medical School, and Chief of Medicine, VA Boston Health Care System, Boston, MA, USA

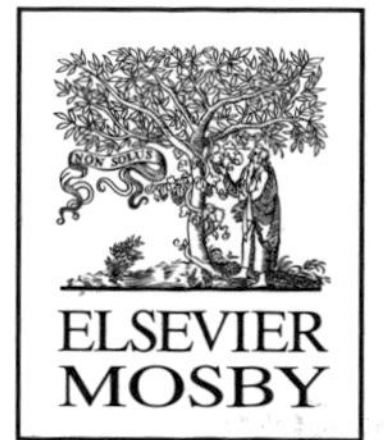

MOSBY
ELSEVIER

MOSBY
An imprint of Elsevier Limited

Second edition 2002
Third edition 2006

ISBN-13: 978-0-323-04080-8
ISBN-10: 0-323-04080-2

British Library Cataloguing in Publication Data
A catalogue record for this book is available from the British Library

Library of Congress Cataloging in Publication Data
A catalog record for this book is available from the Library of Congress

Notice
Medical knowledge is constantly changing. Standard safety precautions must be followed, but as new research and clinical experience broaden our knowledge, changes in treatment and drug therapy may become necessary or appropriate. Readers are advised to check the most current product information provided by the manufacturer of each drug to be administered to verify the recommended dose, the method and duration of administration, and contraindications. It is the responsibility of the practitioner, relying on experience and knowledge of the patient, to determine dosages and the best treatment for each individual patient. Neither the Publisher nor the author assume any liability for any injury and/or damage to persons or property arising from this publication.
The Publisher

Printed in Spain

The Publisher's policy is to use **paper manufactured from sustainable forests**

Last digit is the print number: 9 8 7 6 5 4 3 2 1

Contents

Editorial Advisory Board

Preface

The third Edition of Integrated Pharmacology continues with the unique approach development in the first two editions, presenting drugs and their mechanism of action in the context of the diseases they are used to treat. The Third Edition has been thoroughly revised and updated to comprehensively cover drug action at the molecular, cellular, tissue and organ levels.

The first section deals with the principles of drug action, and introduces concepts of how drugs exert their actions. It offers insights into how our overall knowledge and use of drugs is influenced by a range of factors including history and myth. We have continued to use a system of simple icons to explain the main molecular and cellular actions of drugs in a simple way. These icons are used in subsequent chapters, which deal with drug treatment of diseases within a framework of the body's systems. Each body system chapter addresses the common diseases affecting a system before comprehensively discussing the drug classes and specific drugs used to treat disease. The reader is also introduced to other increasingly important aspects of pharmacology, such as risk-benefit, pharmacoeconomics, and pharmacovigilance. In addition, the relevant background biochemistry, physiology, and pathology are provided for each body system.

Throughout the Third Edition of Integrated Pharmacology beautiful colour illustrations depict the relevant pharmacology in a clear way that enhances understanding and memory. Key facts boxes, tables of adverse actions and drug interactions are used to explain and highlight important issues. All of these illustrations have been redrawn and updated from the first two editions with many new illustrations used to explain new classes of drugs.

Prescribing drugs is the endpoint of many contacts between Health Care professionals and patients. For this reason, it is essential that students acquire a full and detailed understanding of pharmacology integrated with disease. We hope that this Third Edition helps make that understanding easier and will contribute towards training the next generation of physicians and other health care professionals who are faced with a quite bewildering and expanding number of drugs.

The Third Edition of Integrated Pharmacology has been designed for medical students, but will also be useful to other health care professionals, such as dental, nursing, pharmacy, biomedical scientists and other students interested in pharmacology, as it bridges the gap between fundamental mechanisms and the use of drugs to treat human disease.

The Editors hope that the readers of this Third Edition enjoy reading this book as much as we have enjoyed preparing it.

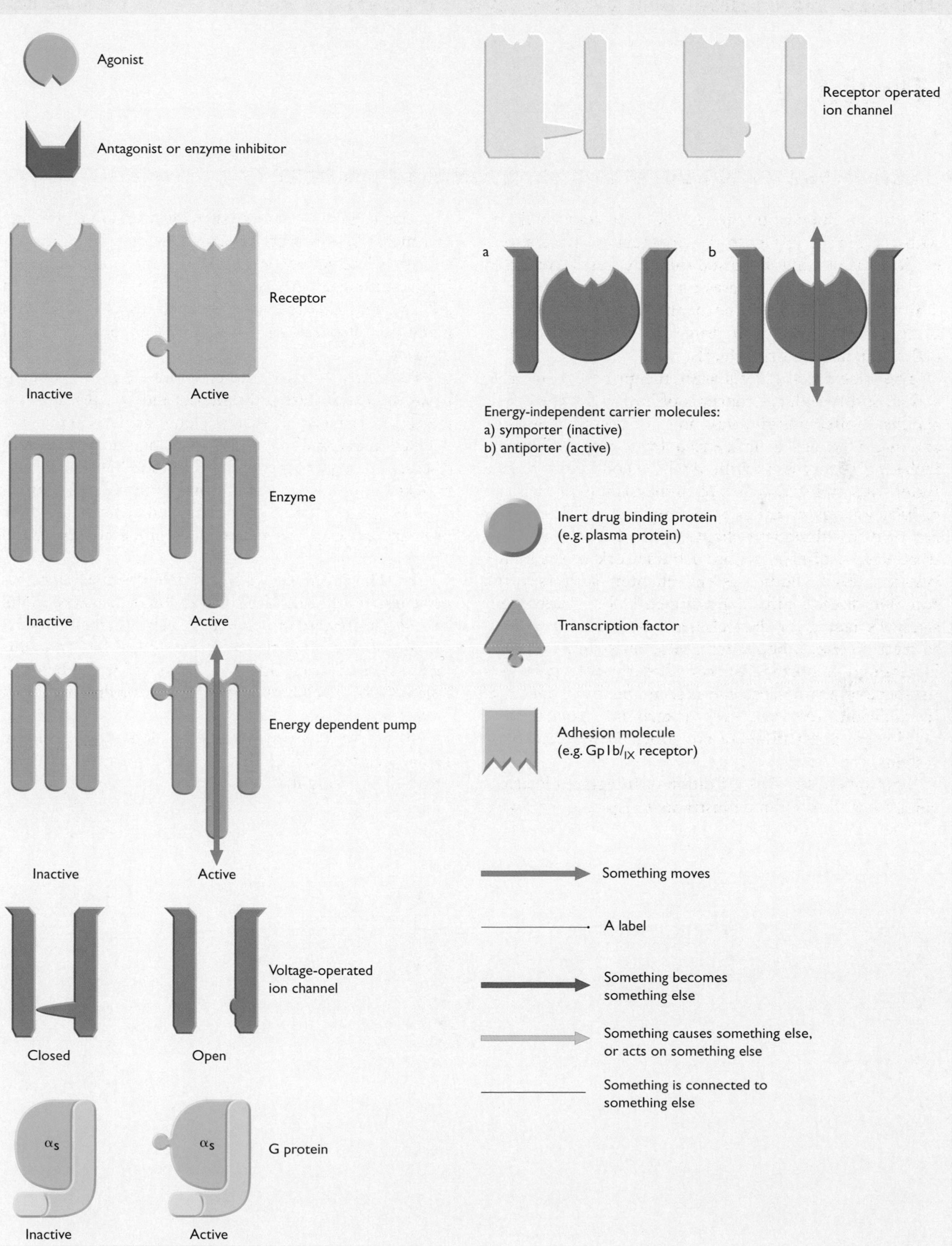

Agonist
Antagonist or enzyme inhibitor
Receptor
Inactive
Active
Enzyme
Inactive
Active
Energy dependent pump
Inactive
Active
Voltage-operated ion channel
Closed
Open
α_s
α_s
G protein
Inactive
Active
Receptor operated ion channel
a
b
Energy-independent carrier molecules:
a) symporter (inactive)
b) antiporter (active)
Inert drug binding protein (e.g. plasma protein)
Transcription factor
Adhesion molecule (e.g. Gp Ib/$_{IX}$ receptor)
Something moves
A label
Something becomes something else
Something causes something else, or acts on something else
Something is connected to something else

1

Principles of Pharmacology

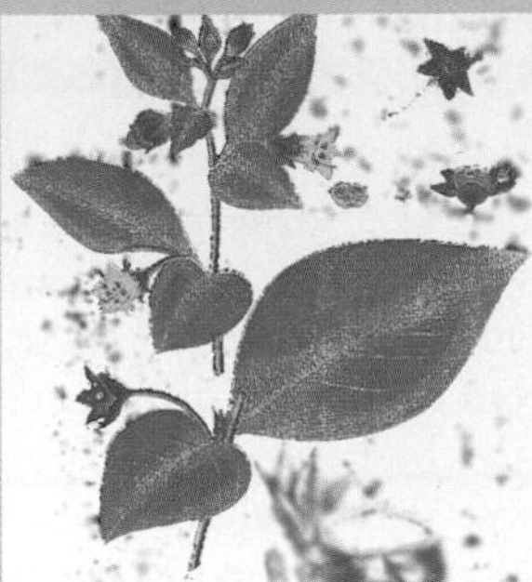

Chapter 1

Introduction

WHAT IS PHARMACOLOGY?

- ***Pharmacology is the science that deals with the actions, mechanism of action, uses, adverse effects and fate of drugs in animals and humans***

The word 'pharmacology' comes from the ancient Greek word for drug, *pharmakon*. It is the study of what biologically active chemical compounds (drugs) do in the body and how the body reacts to them.

The word 'drug' has many meanings but is most commonly used to describe a substance used as a medicine for the treatment of disease. However, the word 'drug' may be used to refer to any biologically active compound which is taken with the intent of producing a change in the body, including:

- Familiar substances such as caffeine, nicotine and alcohol.
- Other chemicals which are abused, such as cannabis, heroin and cocaine.
- Food constituents such as vitamins, minerals and amino acids.
- Cosmetics.

Pharmacology differs from pharmacy, which is a profession that is concerned with the manufacture, preparation and dispensing of drugs.

Pharmacology is concerned with the effects of drugs on living systems or their constituent components such as cells, cell membranes, cell organelles, enzymes and even DNA. As a result, the effects of drugs can be studied at many levels of biologic organization or complexity, ranging from the interaction of drugs with their target molecules in the body (usually proteins), such as enzymes, ion channels or the receptors for neurotransmitters, hormones, etc., to the effect of drugs on human populations. Pharmacologists therefore often identify themselves according to the organizational level at which they study drugs. Thus there are molecular, functional, integrative or clinical pharmacologists. A full understanding of drug action requires integrating information from each of these levels.

A knowledge of pharmacology is essential in the practice of human and veterinary medicine, where drugs are used to treat diseases of humans and animals. The principles of pharmacology also apply to toxicology, where the toxic effects of chemicals (including drugs) are studied. Whether or not a drug is used for therapy, a knowledge of its pharmacology is essential if it is to be used selectively for a defined purpose.

Ideally, all drugs would have selective actions but often they do not. A selective action can be achieved if:

- A relatively high concentration of the drug can be obtained at the target cell, tissue or organ where its action is required.
- The drug's chemical structure is such that it interacts selectively with the discrete target molecule at the location where it is to have its desired effect.

What is pharmacology?

- Pharmacology is the study of the biologic effects of drugs and how they produce such effects
- Drugs are intended to have a selective action but this ideal is seldom achieved
- There is always a risk of adverse effects as well as a benefit connected with using any drug
- A knowledge of pharmacology is essential for using drugs effectively in therapy

Terms used in pharmacology

As with all scientific disciplines, pharmacology has its own vocabulary. This includes terms which cover certain aspects of drug action, such as pharmacodynamics, pharmacokinetics, pharmacotherapeutics, selectivity, selective toxicity, risk–benefit ratio, pharmacoepidemiology, pharmacoeconomics, pharmacogenomics, toxicology, toxins, toxinology, poisons and toxicity (see below).

Pharmacology also has its own terminology to describe the mechanisms by which drugs produce their action. Such terms include agonism, antagonism, inverse agonism, partial agonism and transduction mechanisms. This terminology will be defined in Chapter 2.

Pharmacodynamics and pharmacokinetics

Pharmacodynamics describes the actions of a drug (qualitatively and quantitatively), i.e. what a drug does to the body; this will be discussed further in the chapters based upon body systems. Pharmacokinetics describes the fate of a drug (absorption, distribution, metabolism and excretion), i.e. what the body does to a drug. This will be discussed further in Chapter 4. A knowledge of pharmacodynamics and pharmacokinetics is essential to understand what drugs do, and how they do it.

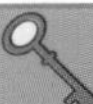

Definitions used in pharmacology

- Pharmacodynamics is the study and measurement of responses to drugs
- Pharmacokinetics is the study of how the body absorbs, distributes, metabolizes and excretes drugs
- Pharmacotherapeutics is the study of the clinical use of drugs to treat diseases
- Pharmacogenetics is the study of how genetics alters responses to drugs
- Pharmacoepidemiology is the study of the effect of drugs on populations
- Pharmacoeconomics is the study of the cost-effectiveness of drug treatments

Pharmacodynamics is the study of how response relates to drug dose or concentration

By examining how the response to a drug varies with dose or concentration (Fig. 1.1), it is possible to plot a 'dose (concentration)–response curve' which provides important pharmacodynamic information: minimal effective dose, the therapeutic dose range, the maximum effect and the drug's potency. Selectivity and safety of a drug can be determined by comparing dose–response curves for therapeutic versus toxic actions.

Pharmacokinetics is the study of how the body absorbs, distributes, metabolizes and excretes drugs

The most common and preferred route of drug administration is by mouth in the form of liquid, tablet or capsule. Drugs in liquid form are immediately available for absorption whereas tablets and capsules must first disintegrate, normally in the stomach, to allow the drug to dissolve in gut fluids. The dissolved drug may cross the intestinal mucosa and so reaches the bloodstream in the portal circulation. Drug dissolved in blood passes through the liver to the heart from where it is distributed via the blood to other parts of the body. It then diffuses out of the blood into the tissues. The total amount of drug presented to a particular region is proportional to the blood flow to that region. The rapidity with which a drug appears in a particular organ is thus dependent on blood flow, and other factors special to that organ. For example, the blood–brain barrier inhibits the entry of many drugs into the brain.

Depending on its chemical nature, the absorbed drug may be metabolized or remain unchanged in the body. Metabolism often converts a drug into less active products (thereby limiting the drug's action). However, some drugs are initially metabolized from a less active (pro-drug) form to a more active metabolite. Most drug metabolism is designed to increase the water solubility of chemicals (i.e. make them more polar), rather than specifically alter their biologic activity, in order to enhance their elimination from the body. The liver is an important site for drug metabolism (see Ch. 4). Excretion occurs primarily via the kidney but may occur by other routes, such as the gut, sweat glands or lungs (see Ch. 4).

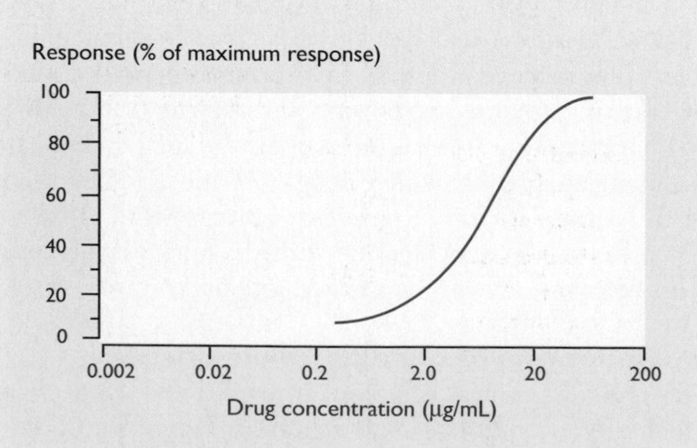

Fig. 1.1 A graph of a dose–response curve. This graph shows that the response to a drug increases with the logarithm to base 10 ($\log_{10}$) of its concentration (dose) in a characteristic S-shaped fashion. At low doses the rate at which a response develops is slow; the response then increases rapidly before reaching a maximum.

Pharmacotherapeutics

Pharmacotherapeutics is the use of drugs to treat diseases. This can be to cure, delay disease progression, alleviate the signs and/or symptoms of a disease, or facilitate other medical interventions, for example:

- Cure of an infection.
- Alleviation of pain and fever during infection.
- Avoidance of stroke by lowering blood pressure.
- Use of insulin in type 1 diabetes mellitus.
- General anesthesia for surgery.

Clearly, a knowledge of pharmacology is essential for the rational use of drugs. A knowledge of the disease being treated, and its pathology, are also required.

Selectivity

A selective drug affects only one target over the therapeutic range (Fig. 1.2). However, if its therapeutic concentration range exceeds the window of selectivity, any drug can produce adverse effects.

The selectivity of a drug depends on:

- The chemical nature of the drug.
- The dose given and the route by which it is administered.
- Special features of the recipient, such as genetic make-up (pharmacogenetics), age and coexisting disease.

Selective toxicity

Selective toxicity is a term applied principally when drugs are used as chemotherapeutic (anti-infective and anti-

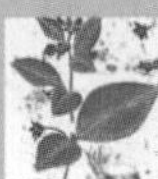

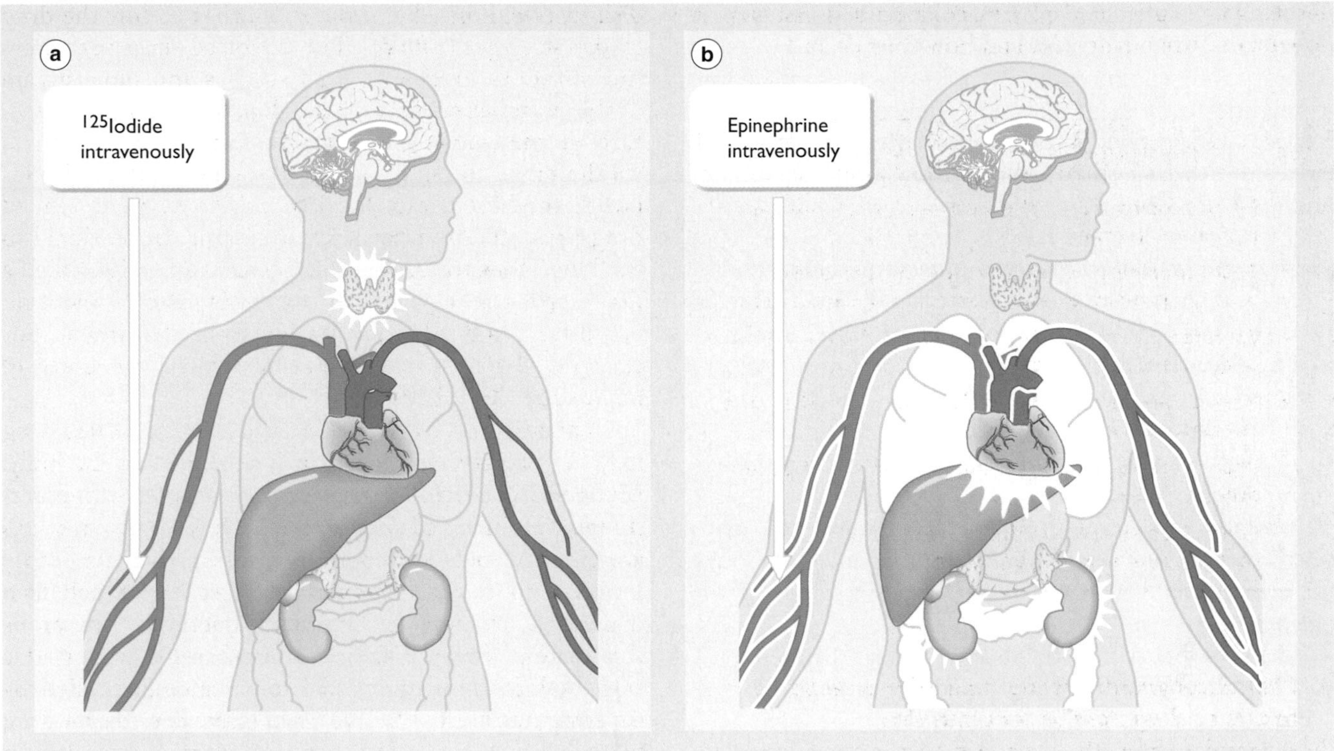

Fig. 1.2 Ideally, all drugs would have selective actions. However, complete selectivity is seldom achieved. (a) ^{125}I (radioactive) is selectively taken up by the iodide uptake system of the thyroid gland. Therefore, radioactivity is high in the thyroid and not elsewhere in the body. (b) Epinephrine, on the other hand, has effects wherever its receptors (adrenoceptors) occur, e.g. in the heart and blood vessels. Adrenoceptors occur throughout the body, and therefore the effects of epinephrine are widespread.

cancer) drugs or pesticides (insecticides or herbicides). The aim is to kill the parasite or unwanted cells but leave the host unharmed. The more closely the target cell resembles the host, the more difficult it is to achieve selective toxicity. Therefore, although drugs can be relatively selective in their actions against bacteria, other drugs are less selective in killing cancer cells rather than normal cells.

Risk–benefit ratio

The phrase 'risk–benefit ratio' is used to describe the adverse effects of a drug in relation to its beneficial effects (Fig. 1.3). The benefits of a drug should be greater than the risks associated with its use. What risk–benefit ratio is acceptable depends on the severity of the disease being treated. A greater risk is acceptable in the treatment of an otherwise fatal disease than in the treatment of a less serious one. All aspects of the use of a drug need to be considered, from basic (e.g. risk of death) to economic (e.g. cost per dose) to determine the risk–benefit ratio for any particular case.

To place risk–benefit ratios in an everyday setting, we must remember that each activity of everyday life, such as driving a car, skiing, flying or swimming, or even taking a

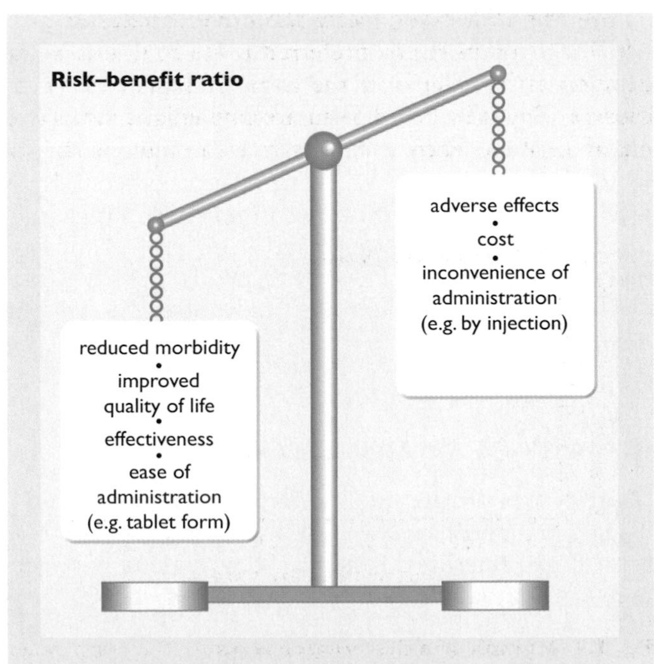

Fig. 1.3 Risk–benefit ratio. The beneficial effects of a drug should outweigh adverse effects. All drugs are capable of producing adverse as well as beneficial effects.

shower, has an associated risk and our perception of these risks may be quite erroneous (see Fig. 3.2 in Ch. 3). Accurate information about the risks of a prescribed drug in relation to those of daily life is needed to keep drug risks in perspective. This is obtained by studying the effects of the drug on large populations (pharmacoepidemiology) (see Ch. 3).

Pharmacoepidemiology and pharmacoeconomics

Pharmacoepidemiology is the study of beneficial and adverse effects of a drug on populations, for example:

- The effect that widespread use of antibiotics in a community has on the type of pneumonia prevalent in that community.
- The influence of use of aspirin on heart attacks in a population.

It is also important to know the financial cost associated with the use of a drug. As a result, the discipline of pharmacoeconomics has evolved. This is the study of the balance of:

- The financial cost of the disease under treatment.
- The true cost of the drug to patients or healthcare providers.

Pharmacoepidemiology is often linked to pharmacoeconomics since determining the financial costs of a drug usually involves studying relevant populations.

Toxicology, toxins, venoms, toxinology, poisons and toxicity

Toxicity is injury or death produced by any substance when it is absorbed by a living organism. Poisons can be synthetic or naturally occurring (toxins and venoms) and poisoning may be produced deliberately or accidentally. The latter is more common in children than adults.

Toxicology is the study of the harmful effects of drugs and other chemicals on humans, animals or plants. The concepts of pharmacodynamics, pharmacokinetics, pharmacoepidemiology and pharmacoeconomics apply to toxicology just as they do to pharmacotherapeutics. The only difference is that the end-points differ: harm is the end-point in toxicology, and benefit in pharmacotherapeutics.

Toxinology is the scientific study of the actions of toxins and venoms.

HISTORY OF PHARMACOLOGY

Magic, medicine and religion intertwined

The roots of pharmacology are entwined with the knowledge of herbal treatments, other potions, and their uses. This knowledge was once the secret of the priest, holy man or shaman in ancient societies, since the effects of such 'cures' and poisons were often viewed as being magical. The person who knew about drugs and potions was respected, and often feared, since intentional poisoning was not unknown.

Ancient and modern pharmacology

- **Ancient civilizations used mixtures of magic, religion and herbal medicines to treat diseases. Drugs were often thought to be magical in their actions**
- **The drugs of antiquity came from plant and animal sources**
- **Knowledge of drugs increased in parallel with knowledge of body function (anatomy, physiology and biochemistry) and chemistry (especially organic chemistry)**
- **Modern drug development depends on intellectual cooperation between academia and industry**

Understanding of drugs evolves in parallel with our understanding of disease

Despite the need to treat disease, knowledge of the mechanisms causing any disease is always limited. If a disease is believed to be caused by gods, spirits or supernatural forces, then its treatment must invoke magic since supernatural causes can only be counteracted by supernatural means. In the past, therefore, drugs were often believed to be magical and, as such, were given magical names such as 'eye of the sun'.

The sources of drugs in ancient times were plants, minerals and animals. A frieze from Mesopotamia dated to the 8th century BC shows priests carrying a goat, mandrake flowers and opium poppyheads. This illustrates the important combination of religion, plants and animals in therapeutics as practiced by ancient peoples. Furthermore, it confirms that the opium poppy was an ancient medicinal plant (Fig. 1.4).

Drug development in ancient civilizations

The earliest written record that specifically mentions drugs is the *Egyptian Medical Papyrus* (translated by Smith) dating from approximately 1600 BC, although it actually deals primarily with surgery and other treatments. The *Ebers Papyrus*, which dates from approximately 1550 BC, also lists some 700 remedies, their preparation and use. Concoctions ranged from the occult, such as the thigh bone of a hanged man, to the familiar, such as preparations containing opium or castor oil. The latter two are still in use some 3500 years later.

Medicine and the use of drugs were evolving in China (as described in the *Shen Nung*) and India (Ayurvedic medicine) in parallel to their evolution in Ancient Egypt, but there was little Western contact with Asia at that time. For example, vaccination was practiced in India in 550 BC, but was only introduced into Western medicine some 2000 years later.

Ancient Greek culture contributed a great deal to the development of pharmacy and drugs. Hippocrates (460–377 BC) wrote on the ethics of medicine as well as on the causes of disease. The Greeks attributed disease to an imbalance of fluids (humors): blood, phlegm, black

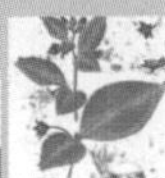

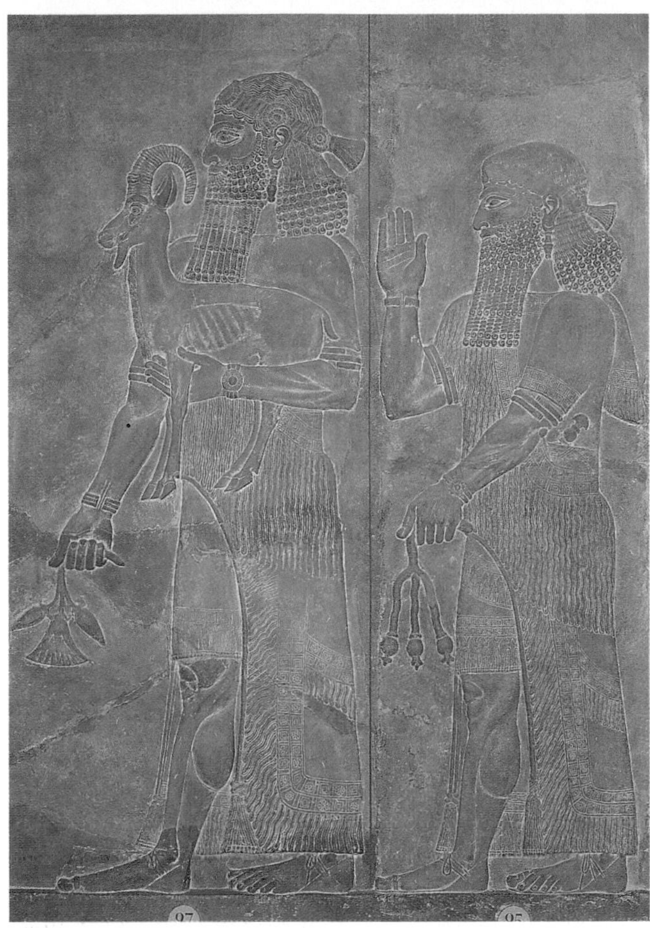

Fig. 1.4 The origins of pharmacology: religion, animals and plants. A frieze from the palace of King Sargon II in Kharasabad, now in the Musée du Louvre, Paris, Antiquités Orientales. (Courtesy of Service de Documentation Photographique de la Réunion des Musées Nationaux, Chateau de Versailles.)

bile and yellow bile. This doctrine was elaborated by Galen (AD 130–201), a Greek physician who practiced in Alexandria and in Rome. Galen's influence on medicines persisted through to the 1500s and can still be seen today in the use of herbal mixtures. The Romans organized and regulated the practice of medicine, including the use of drugs, but contributed little new knowledge to pharmacology. Theophrastus (372–287 BC) listed all that was then known about medicinal plants and Dioscorides (AD 57), Nero's surgeon, used this list as his basis for a compendium of substances used as medicines – materia medica – which described nearly 500 plants, and how to prepare remedies from them.

The Persians preserved Greek views of medicines and later transmitted these to the Arabs. From approximately AD 700 to 1000, the traditions of medicine and of pharmacy were maintained and developed by the Arabs, who regulated the practice of medicine and pharmacy, and established apothecary shops, hospitals and libraries. The Arabs built on the published works of Galen and introduced several new ways of preparing drugs. The

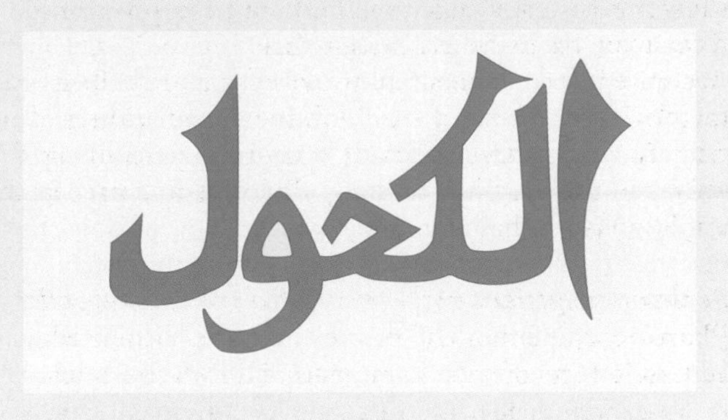

Fig. 1.5 The Arabic word *al-kuhl* or alcohol. It originally referred to one of the first ways of preparing drugs for external use and only later to ethanol and other alcohols.

English word 'alcohol' is from the Arabic word *al-kuhl* (Fig. 1.5). Paradoxically, the original meaning was 'all things very fine' and referred to ground sulfides of lead and antimony used as eye make-up. The Arabs also introduced alchemy to Europe. Alchemy eventually combined Egyptian ideas, astronomy, astrology and Greek natural philosophy with Christian metaphysics, in an attempt to discover the origin and meaning of all things. Alchemy was the parent of chemistry and therefore an important ancestor of modern pharmacology.

Important players in the history of pharmacology

- Dioscorides (AD 57), Greek, compiled a materia medica containing 500 plants and related remedies
- Galen (AD 130–201), a Greek living in Rome, developed a theory of disease, which persisted for hundreds of years
- Paracelsus (1493–1541), itinerant Swiss scholar and alchemist, the 'grandfather of pharmacology'
- Sertürner (1805), German pharmacist, isolated morphine, the first pure drug
- Ehrlich (1909), German pathologist and Nobel prize winner, developed chemotherapy
- Domagk (1935), German pathologist and Nobel prize winner, noticed the antibacterial effect of Prontosil, a prototype of sulfonamides, the first selective antimicrobial agents
- Beyer (1950s), US pharmacologist, instrumental in the development of thiazides, derivatives of sulfonamides, and several other drugs
- Black (1960–1970s), British pharmacologist and Nobel prize winner, invented propranolol and cimetidine

Drug development since the Middle Ages

In Europe in the Middle Ages the practice of medicine and use of drugs were often centered on monasteries.

Many monasteries cultivated herbal gardens to provide a source for their drugs. Prior to the scientific age there was extensive documentation of herbs and their uses in therapy. Unfortunately much of this information became confabulated and confused over time and therefore rendered useless. Interestingly, where people used herbs as poisons for obtaining food, as with arrow poisons, their knowledge base remained intact over the years into modern times.

The 'grandfather' of the science of pharmacology is generally agreed to be Paracelsus, who was born in 1493 in Switzerland. He was the son of a physician, traveled widely in Europe and graduated as a doctor of medicine from Ferrara, Italy. Many of his writings were prescient. For example, he advised against use of the complicated mixtures that were common medications at that time and urged that each drug (or plant) should be used alone. He wrote: 'It is the task of chemistry to produce medicines for the treatment of disease since the vital functions of life are basically chemical in nature .... All things are poisons, for there is nothing without poisonous qualities. It is only the dose which makes a thing a poison'. These statements are still cornerstones of pharmacology today. It is now recognized that drugs are chemicals that alter biologic properties and that their selectivity is a function of the dose of the drug administered.

Evolution of pharmacology depended on the developing sciences of chemistry, pathophysiology, physiology and botany

The evolution of pharmacology depended on the increasing understanding of human physiology and disease processes (pathophysiology), and the development of the scientific method. In the 1600s there were many contributions to the understanding of physiology and diseases, including those of William Harvey (1578–1657), who introduced experimentation to demonstrate the circulation of blood, and Sydenham (1624–1689), who introduced classification into the study of diseases, their causes and their treatment.

Developments in chemistry

The idea of using chemicals as drugs was further suggested by van Helmont (1515–1564), the discoverer of carbonic acid, and who introduced the term 'gas' into chemistry. The theory that an imbalance of body chemicals could cause disease was first proposed by the Dutch physician Sylvius (1614–1672), while the physicist/chemist Boyle (1627–1691) was the first to demonstrate that drugs had an effect when given intravenously as well as by mouth. The activities and thoughts of chemists and physicians became closely linked.

Developments in botany

In the ancient and recent past, most drugs came from plants. For example, the Egyptians used extracts from the opium poppy. Plant use continued and, in the 1640s, cinchona bark, which contains quinine, was introduced into Europe from South America by the Jesuit priests of the Roman Catholic Church. It was used to treat fevers, often caused by malaria, a disease for which quinine is still used. However, one of the problems associated with the use of botanical material as medicines is reliable identification of plants. This was improved by the system of plant classification introduced by the Swedish botanist Linnaeus (1707–1778).

Several Swiss and French botanists such as Schröder (1641) and Lémery (1698) published books on vegetable materia medica. Medieval universities had established botanic gardens to learn more about medicinal plants. The botanic works of Haller (1708–1777), a physician in Berne and Göttingen who combined the study of physiology and botany, were collected into a publication by Vicat in 1776, which in turn was translated into German by Hahnemann, the founder of homeopathy.

William Withering published an important treatise entitled *An Account of the Foxglove and Some of Its Medical Uses* in 1785. In this text he described observations made over a 10-year period on the therapeutic use of extracts of the foxglove (*Digitalis purpurea*) (Fig. 1.6). The principles he laid down at that time for the use of digitalis extracts in the treatment of dropsy (swelling of the ankles and abdomen due to accumulation of extravascular fluid) are largely still valid today, although digoxin, a pure extract of the digitalis plant, is now used.

Isolation of pure compounds

Progress in understanding plants, and the drugs they contain, was aided by the work of the Swedish chemist Carl Wilhelm Scheele (1742–1786). He produced pure chemicals, among them glycerin and malic acid, by crystallization. Scheele's work laid the foundation for the isolation of the first pure drug, morphine, by Sertürner (1783–1841) in 1805. These advances led to pure substances, rather than crude extracts, being isolated and tested for their pharmacologic effects.

Developments in physiology

Understanding how and where drugs act requires a detailed knowledge of how the body functions (i.e. physiology and biochemistry). French physiologists, such as François Magendie (1783–1855), and his pupil Claude Bernard (1813–1878), located certain sites in the body where drugs may act. Claude Bernard demonstrated by 1856 that curare (an extract of a South American jungle dart poison) paralyzed skeletal muscle by acting selectively at the junctions between nerve and muscle.

Developments of concepts in pharmacology

Pharmacology uses physics, chemistry and the biologic sciences to understand what drugs do and how they do it. A few principles are, however, special to and underlie pharmacology, including:

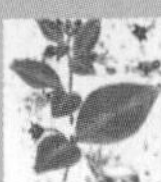

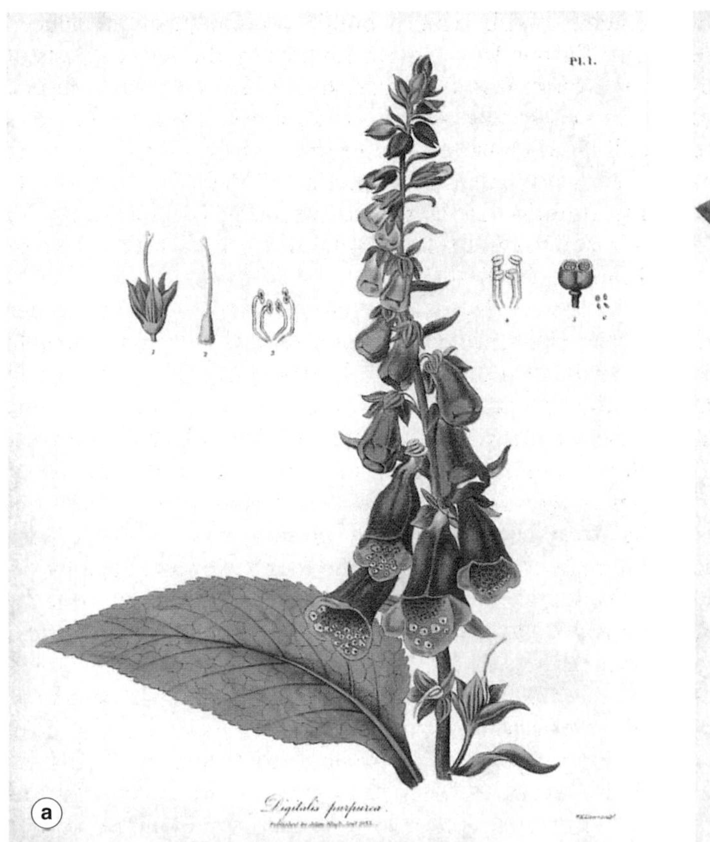

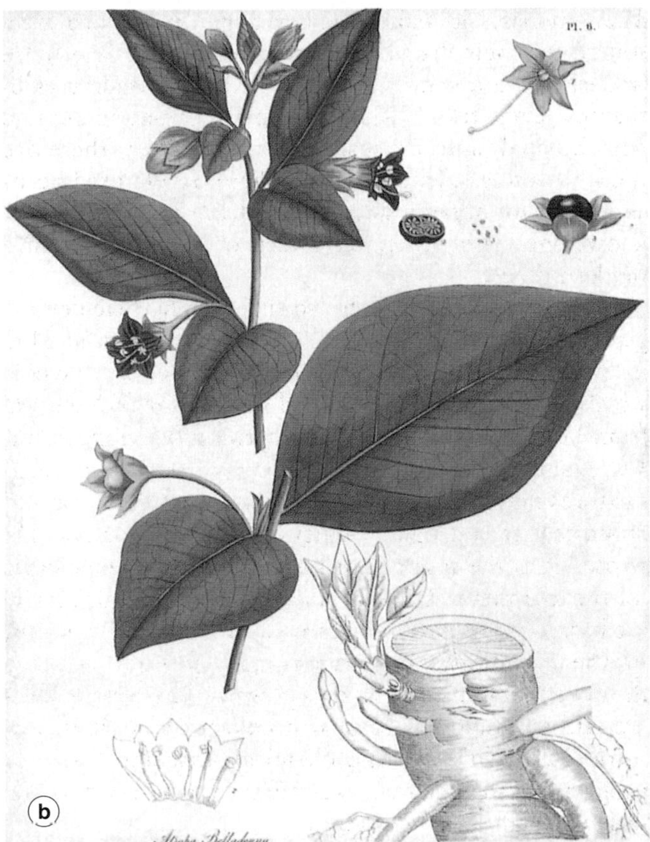

Fig. 1.6 (a) Foxglove and (b) deadly nightshade. These are the plant sources of digoxin and atropine, respectively. (Reproduced from George Graves, *Medicinal Plants*, New York: Crescent Books. Copyright 1990, Bracken Books.)

- The concept first suggested by Felix Fontana (1730–1805) that in plant or other medicinal material there is an active principle that is responsible for its effect.
- The concept of a distinct relationship between the dose of a drug and its effect (see Fig. 1.1). This is attributed to Peter Daries, who postulated it in his doctoral dissertation of 1776, and Paracelsus also made an important contribution to this idea. The dose–response curve is the present day expression of the concept. The mathematical formulation of dose–response curves is derived from the physicochemical mass action construct of Langmuir, which was interpreted for pharmacology by Clarke (1885–1941). The appropriate mathematical analysis for the relationship between dose and response is still evolving (see Ch. 2).
- The concept that structure–activity relationships (SAR) exist for drugs. The study of how chemical alterations to a basic chemical pharmacophore (the minimum chemical structure which gives the pharmacologic effect) could alter the action of a drug began with James Blake (1815–1841). He systematically altered a series of inorganic salts and observed the resulting changes in their pharmacologic effects. Paul Ehrlich (1854–1915) exploited this technique in his search for compounds that would selectively kill invading organisms – the search for a 'magic bullet'.
- The concept that most drugs must first bind to a receptor to produce their actions. This was first proposed by Langley in 1878 and extended by Ehrlich early in the twentieth century.

Modern drug discovery

Interactions between pharmacologic theories developed in academia and the pharmaceutical industry have been highly productive

The beginnings of modern drug discovery were closely allied to the development of the dye industry in Germany. It is from this origin that the modern pharmaceutical industry is derived. Many scientists have contributed to the development of drugs while working in industry. A few selected drugs and individuals are mentioned below.

- Salicylic acid was synthesized from phenol in 1860 by Kolbe and Lautemann.
- Acetylsalicylic acid (aspirin) was synthesized from salicylic acid in 1899 by Dreser.
- Prontosil, a therapeutically inactive dye which is transformed in the body to an antibacterial sulfonamide, was developed by Domagk in 1935.

Other sulfonamides were quickly synthesized following the discovery of Prontosil. This early success gave rise to a series of chemically related drugs developed by the pharmaceutical industry, including acetazolamide (a carbonic anhydrase inhibitor), thiazide diuretics developed by Karl Beyer, followed by sulfonylurea oral hypoglycemic drugs.

At the same time, pharmacology was making headway in the identification and classification of receptors and initiated by Burger and Dale (1910) in industry, and Gaddum (1933) in academia. H_1 receptor antagonists were developed by Bovet (1944), whereas β adrenoceptor antagonists such as propranolol were developed by James Black (circa 1960). Later, around 1970, Black went on to develop H_2 receptor antagonists such as cimetidine for the treatment of peptic ulcer which became, for a time, the biggest selling drug in the world.

Pharmacology is now using molecular biology to develop new drugs. Proving the effectiveness and safety of new drugs, however, still depends on studies involving laboratory animals, individual patients and populations of patients. Thus one of the fascinations of pharmacology is that it spans the spectrum from molecules to the patient. When a chemical is found to affect a particular cellular function, and thereby have therapeutic potential, workers from many scientific disciplines including chemists, biochemists, physiologists, pharmacologists and physicians must cooperate to investigate and develop a new drug.

Continued evolution of the drug discovery process

Drugs save lives and improve the quality of life for millions of people on a global scale. It has been estimated that drug treatments have added 3–5 years to average life expectancy and revolutionized the treatment of many different diseases. However, today's pharmacologists are still faced with the formidable task of finding novel drugs for the treatment of chronic diseases that pose significant health problems, such as cystic fibrosis, Alzheimer's disease, stroke and emphysema. Furthermore, although there are effective medications available for treatment of many diseases caused by microorganisms, resistant strains of such organisms are developing all the time. There is, therefore, a continual need to develop new drugs to treat infection.

It is estimated that, on average, 7–10 years are required to develop a new drug, from the first identification of a novel lead chemical compound through to the successful use in patients of a new medicine, at a cost of US$800 million or more. As pharmacologists are involved in nearly every stage of this discovery and development process, pharmacology is an important branch of medical science.

NAMING AND CLASSIFICATION OF DRUGS

A drug may have several names

A number of ways of naming and classifying drugs have evolved. There is always a need to name drugs unambiguously and to classify them according to a limited set of criteria, but current methods are not especially systematic and, unfortunately, any one drug may have many names:

- Exact or abbreviated chemical name.
- Official generic name.
- Brand or commercial name.

The rules of chemical nomenclature laid down by the IUPAC (International Union of Pure and Applied Chemistry) allow for the exact chemical description of a drug but systematic chemical names are very complex and hard to remember. Abbreviated chemical names are easier to use.

All new drugs are given official abbreviated (generic) names. These are now global, but in the past were national. Pharmaceutical companies also use brand names to describe their drugs, which adds confusion since there can be more than one brand name for a single drug. The generic name for a drug may give clues about the use and structure of the drug and therefore contains elements of classification. The use of the generic name is preferred.

Drugs are classified in many ways

There are many ways to classify drugs:

- Chemical structure.
- Mechanism of action.
- Response produced.

There is no accepted universal method of drug classification in pharmacology.

Ways of classifying drugs

- **Pharmacotherapeutic actions**
- **Pharmacologic actions**
- **Molecular actions**
- **Other factors (source and chemistry)**

Webster's Dictionary defines a drug as 'a substance intended for use in the diagnosis, cure, mitigation, treatment or prevention of disease'. *Collins Dictionary* gives the definition: 'any synthetic or natural chemical substance used in the treatment, prevention or diagnosis of disease' and the *Oxford Dictionary* has a similar definition.

Synonyms for drug include medicine, agent, compound, pharmacologic tool, substance of abuse:

- 'Medicine' is a chemical used to treat diseases (i.e. materia medica), a therapeutically useful drug.
- 'Agent' is a drug that is part of a therapeutic class, e.g. antitubercular or antihypertensive agent.
- 'Compound' is a chemical used for pharmacologic purposes, i.e. a prototype drug.
- 'Pharmacologic tool' is a pharmacologically active chemical used for experimental purposes.
- 'Substances of abuse' are chemicals or drugs used for purposes other than therapeutic purposes.

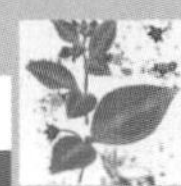

All drugs available on prescription, and many over-the-counter non-herbal drugs, have a generic name, the one which appears in official national pharmacopeias. Pharmacopeias were originally published as source books for materia medica (medical materials) and indicated the animal or plant source of individual drugs, manner of extraction and a chemical or bioassay for determining the concentration of biologic activity. Since most of today's drugs are available in a pure form, modern pharmacopeias are concerned principally with generic drugs. Examples of variations in generic names include norepinephrine or levarterenol in the USA and the World Health Organization (WHO) versus noradrenaline in Europe and the UK; furosemide in the USA versus frusemide in the UK, and cromolyn in the USA versus cromoglycate in the UK.

There is greater harmonization today between the European Union, Japan and the USA in choosing generic names and recent years have seen the increasing use of common roots and name endings constituting a means of classification. Examples include the endings:

- 'olol' for many β adrenoceptor antagonists.
- 'dipine' for the type of Ca^{2+} channel blockers which chemically are dihydropyridines.
- 'tilide' for blockers of the delayed rectifier K^+ channel.

Other examples can be found in Table 1.1.

Brand names are enforced by copyright laws worldwide and are usually catchy, easy to remember and do not constitute a means of classfication.

The generic name should be used in biomedical science and by physicians

When writing orders for drug treatment or prescriptions, use of the generic name causes less confusion and lessens the chance of error. In many countries use of the generic name in a prescription gives the dispensing pharmacist the right to provide the cheapest form of the drug.

In the commercial world, brand names for drugs will never follow a consistent pattern

A potential drug discovered by a pharmaceutical company research team is patented at some time during the discovery and development process. Depending on the country of patenting, this protection (which involves the right to be the sole seller of the drug) will last for a number of years (e.g. 20 years). Drugs still under patent are usually marketed by the patenting manufacturer and will usually have one generic name and one brand name. Once a patent has expired, the generic name remains but different manufacturers may market the drug under their own brand names. The creation of brand names is one of the skills of marketing. Pharmaceutical companies go to great lengths to find euphonious and catchy names for their drugs.

The official drug-naming process generally proceeds as follows. A synthetic drug is first synthesized as a chemical compound with a code name, commonly letters and a number. The letters usually, but not in all cases, indicate the pharmaceutical company concerned. The

Table 1.1 Examples of common endings to official names which indicate the pharmacologic classification of a drug

Ending	Classification	Prototype for class
-olol	β adrenoceptor blocking drug	Propranolol
-caine	Local anaesthetic	Cocaine, procaine
-dipine	Calcium channel blocker of the dihydropyridine type	Nifedipine
-tidine	H_2 histamine receptor antagonist	Cimetidine
-prazole	Proton pump inhibitor	Omeprazole
-quine	Antimalarial drugs	Chloroquine
-ane	Halogenated hydrocarbon general anaesthetics	Halothane
-zosin	α adrenoceptor blockers (not all)	Prazosin
-profen	One class of nonsteroidal antiinflammatory drugs (NSAIDs)	Ibuprofen
-clovir	Antiviral (herpes) drugs	Aciclovir
-mycin	Macrolide/aminoglycoside antibiotics	Erythromycin/streptomycin
-cycline	Tetracycline-derived broad-spectrum antibiotics	Tetracycline
-ium	Competitive neuromuscular blockers	Decamethonium (but the true pharmacologic protoype is *d*-tubocurarine)
-mab	Monoclonal antibodies	Anti-IgE
-zolam, -zepam	Benzodiazepine sedatives	Midazolam, diazepam

number is sometimes just a numeric code, starting at 1 and often exceeding 1 million, or it may reflect somewhat more opaque procedures. There are no universal rules for compound numbering. The vast majority of coded compounds never become drugs and so generic names are only given when a compound is considered to have the potential to be a commercially viable drug. The company usually suggests generic names, but suggestions require approval and ratification by the appropriate national or international nomenclature committee.

Drug names

- **The generic name for a drug is the preferred name**
- **The existence of multiple brand names is confusing**
- **Generic names can vary between countries**
- **The generic name may provide a clue to the pharmacotherapeutic action and/or pharmacotherapeutic classification**

DRUG CLASSIFICATION SYSTEMS

Approaches to classification of drugs have arisen historically from different bases. Current systems are neither exclusive nor hierarchic. Any one drug can be placed in a number of classes. For example, atropine has been classified as:

- A nonselective competitive antagonist at muscarinic receptors, i.e. a muscarinic antagonist, on the basis of its molecular action.
- A parasympathetic antagonist, on the basis of its actions on the autonomic nervous system.
- An atropinic drug, as it is a prototype for the class.
- An antiulcer drug, because one of its pharmacotherapeutic uses is the treatment of peptic ulcer.
- A belladonna alkaloid, as it is a naturally occurring drug from the plant *Atropa belladonna*. (Extracts of *Atropa* were used in medieval times to widen the iris in an attempt to beautify; thus *bella donna* or beautiful lady).

The above provides information about atropine's source, chemical nature, pharmacologic actions, molecular mechanism of action and pharmacotherapeutic use. Even new drugs are still classified in this complex manner and not by means of a universal system, although the IUPHAR (International Union of Pharmacology) and the WHO are currently attempting to provide a universal drug classification system.

The following is an attempt to summarize the present classification systems for drugs, which has some hierarchic features:

- Pharmacotherapeutic class refers to the clinical condition for which a drug is used.
- Pharmacologic class is based on a drug's action. It may also include the type of pharmacologic action produced by the system which is responding to the drug, e.g. excitation, inhibition, block, agonism, antagonism, etc.
- Molecular mechanism of action is a subset of pharmacologic action. However, since this concerns how a drug interacts with its target molecule, it is a class in its own right.
- Chemical nature or source.

According to the above, atropine could be classified as:

- An antimuscarinic for its spasmolytic and antiulcer pharmacotherapeutic actions.
- A muscarinic receptor blocker, for its effects on physiologic processes.
- A competitive antagonist at M_1, M_2 and M_3 receptors, for its molecular mechanism of action.
- Solanaceous (from the plant family Solanaceae — potato, tobacco, deadly nightshade) or atropinic alkaloid, for its chemical nature and biologic sources.

A systematic approach to classification would rely upon agreed definitions of drug actions, these definitions being selective, exclusive, precise and clear-cut, in both pharmacotherapeutic and pharmacologic terms. These prerequisites are rarely met, in either medicine or pharmacology.

Pharmacotherapeutic classification

Pharmacotherapeutic classification can be difficult since the classification of disease is only precise if the pathology is understood, but not otherwise.

Pharmacotherapeutic classifications can be precise

Neuromuscular blockers, for example, is a classification for a drug used almost exclusively for producing skeletal muscle relaxation during surgery.

As an example of how classification by disease can be unambiguous, consider tuberculosis. In this disease, the causative organism is known (*Mycobacterium tuberculosis*) and well understood, and there is no confusion arising from the many possible clinical presentations of this infection. Thus, the classification of a drug as an antitubercular drug is precise for a drug used to treat such infections.

Pharmacotherapeutic classifications can be inconsistent and imprecise

On the other hand, hypertension, characterized by a high blood pressure relative to 'normal' levels, is the symptom of a disease for which the cause is normally not known. As a result, the term 'essential hypertension' is used and so the classification 'antihypertensive drug' reveals only that a drug is, or has been, used to lower blood pressure. This is imprecise

Drug classification based on pharmacotherapeutic use may reveal little about the other actions (pharmacotherapeutic or otherwise) of a drug. Thus it is wrong to assume that drugs within a common pharmacotherapeutic classi-

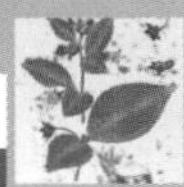

fication share a common mechanism of action or the same adverse effects. However, in some cases drugs in the same pharmacotherapeutic class share similar pharmacologic and molecular mechanisms of action but their effectiveness, toxicity and adverse effects can be very different.

Another example of imprecision is the pharmacotherapeutic classification 'antiarrhythmic' for a drug used to treat arrhythmias (disorders of heart rhythm). Arrhythmias have different anatomic locations, rates, mechanisms and outcomes. Thus, 'antiarrhythmic' only classifies a drug as having been used to treat an arrhythmia and implies nothing else about the drug.

From the above examples, it appears that pharmacotherapeutic classification might be improved by subclassification. For example, the general classification 'antiviral' is useful but a subclassification, based upon the type of virus, is much more helpful. Subclassification is particularly useful for antibacterial and antiparasitic drugs.

It is clear that the pharmacology student must be careful in drawing conclusions from pharmacotherapeutic classifications. In addition, a knowledge of disease conditions, their classification and subclassification is vital for appropriate use of pharmacotherapeutic classifications.

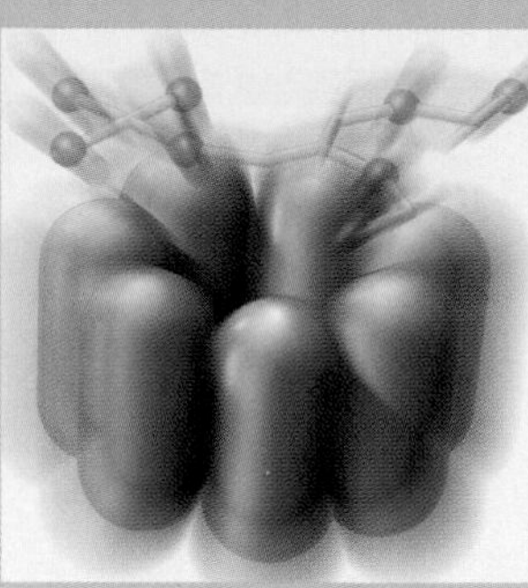

Chapter 2

The General Mechanisms of Drug Action

WHAT DRUGS DO AND HOW THEY DO IT

The purpose of this chapter is to illustrate how the mechanism of action of a drug may be understood by integrating the effects it produces at molecular, cellular, tissue and system levels of biologic function. Consequently, this chapter is subdivided according to these component processes and explains how they are integrated. The main emphasis of the chapter is on drug actions at molecular and cellular levels since the specific actions of drugs on tissue and body systems are considered in each of the systems-based chapters.

Drugs act at four different levels:

- **Molecular**: protein molecules are the immediate targets for most drugs. Action here translates into actions at the next level.
- **Cellular**: biochemical and other components of cells participate in the process of transduction.
- **Tissue**: the function of heart, skin, lungs, etc., is then altered.
- **System**: the function of the cardiovascular, nervous, gastrointestinal system, etc., is then altered.

In order to understand the actions of a drug, it is necessary to know which molecular targets are affected by the drug, the nature of this molecular interaction, the nature of the transduction system (the cellular response), the types of tissue that express the molecular target and the mechanisms by which the tissue influences the body system. In view of this, it is important to consider mechanisms of action of drugs at each of the four levels of complexity.

This can be illustrated with propranolol, a β adrenergic antagonist used to treat several diseases including angina pectoris, a cardiac condition resulting from localized ischemia (i.e. insufficient blood flow) in the heart:

- At the molecular level, propranolol is a competitive and reversible antagonist of the action of epinephrine and norepinephrine on cardiac β adrenoceptors.
- At the cellular level, propranolol prevents β adrenergic agonism from elevating intracellular cyclic adenosine monophosphate (cAMP), initiating protein phosphorylation, Ca^{2+} mobilization and oxidative metabolism.
- At the tissue level, propranolol prevents β adrenergic agonism from increasing the contractile force of the heart and heart rate, i.e. it has negative inotropic and negative chronotropic effects.
- At a system level, propranolol improves cardiovascular function. It reduces the heart's β adrenergic responses to sympathetic nervous system activity, thereby decreasing the requirements for blood flow in heart tissue. This reduced demand for blood flow is useful if blood supply is limited (e.g. in coronary artery disease).

The mechanism of drug action at the four different levels is also illustrated by rifampicin, even though this drug acts on bacterial rather than human tissue. Rifampin is an effective drug in the treatment of tuberculosis:

- At the molecular level, rifampin binds to (and blocks the activity of) ribonucleic acid (RNA) polymerase in the mycobacterium responsible for tuberculosis.
- At the cellular level, rifampin inhibits mycobacterial RNA synthesis and thereby kills the mycobacterium.
- At the tissue level, rifampin prevents damage to lung tissue arising as a result of mycobacterial infection.
- At the system level, rifampin prevents the loss of lung function caused by the mycobacterial infection.

Drugs may be classified on the basis of their molecular, cellular, tissue and system actions

Propranolol is always classified at the molecular level as a β adrenoceptor antagonist. However, its classification at the cellular, tissue and system levels will depend on the condition that is being treated (e.g. angina versus hypertension).

Pharmacologic classification of a drug should include the type of action produced

It is obviously important to classify a drug on the basis of the site at which the drug acts and the type of action it produces. Pharmacology abounds with words used to describe drug actions and these are considered in more detail later in the book. A short discussion is, however, included here with regard to drug classification.

Words used to describe the different types of pharmacologic action often come in pairs: inhibitor and activator, antagonist and agonist, depressant and excitant, direct and indirect. In these examples, each member of the pair is the antithesis of the other. Such terms help to classify the type of pharmacologic action produced by a drug, but are themselves often poorly defined. Furthermore, they are often everyday words and thus liable to be used loosely.

- 'Inhibitor' is used for drugs that prevent or reduce physiologic, biochemical or pharmacologic activity. Inhibition can be considered as happening at the level of enzymes, neuronal, hormonal and autacoid systems; receptors; ion channels and even cell membranes, as well as organs or whole bodies.
- 'Activators' are opposite in actions to inhibitors.

Thus almost any drug can be classified as being either an inhibitor or an activator. One disadvantage is that inhibition in one situation may be activation in another. It is therefore possible to produce excitation at one site by inhibiting at another.

In a sense, the terms 'antagonist' and 'agonist' are related, in that an antagonist prevents an agonist from having its action since agonists are drugs which 'agonize' and thereby produce an action. If the terms are used precisely, both the agonist and antagonist should act on the same receptor. However, the word 'antagonist' can also be used loosely, as with calcium antagonist for a drug which blocks calcium channels.

The terms 'suppressant' and 'excitant' are less precise and describe drugs which respectively decrease and increase activity in a body system, particularly the central nervous system.

Some responses to drugs are produced by a direct action on the tissue concerned, whereas others are produced indirectly, or secondarily to a direct action elsewhere. For example, drugs can relax vascular smooth muscle by a direct action on the muscle itself, or secondarily via the release of a directly acting relaxant, or by inhibiting release or action of a contracting substance. Other examples include the secondary negative effects of β blockers (e.g. propranolol) on cardiac contractility, which prevent the actions of the sympathetic system on the heart. Sympathomimetic amines directly increase heart rate via actions on the pacemaker cells controlling heart rate, whereas atropine can increase heart rate because, as a muscarinic antagonist, it antagonizes the action of parasympathetic nerves (via release of acetylcholine) on the heart.

Responses to drugs can be defined at molecular, cellular, tissue and system levels

Since the mechanism of action of a drug can be defined at four levels of complexity, the responses to a drug can also be defined in the same manner (Table 2.1). Drugs that activate their molecular target are defined as agonists or activators (the exact term depending on the nature of the molecular target). Drugs that prevent or inhibit the actions of agonists or activators, or deactivate a molecular target, are defined as antagonists, blockers or inhibitors. The latter do not directly produce a response at the cellular, tissue and system level, but may do so indirectly by blocking the molecular response to an endogenous or exogenous agonist or activator.

Table 2.1 The four levels of drug action and drug classification

Mechanism	Definition	Response components
Molecular	Interaction with the drug's molecular target	The drug target (e.g. receptor, ion channel, enzyme, carrier molecule)
Cellular	Transduction	The biochemicals linked to the drug target (e.g. ion channel, enzyme, G proteins)
Tissue	An effect on tissue function	Electrogenesis, contraction, secretion, metabolic activity, proliferation
System	An effect on system function	Integrated systems including linked systems (e.g. nervous system, cardiovascular system)

MOLECULAR ACTION OF DRUGS

The target is a molecular entity which contains the bind ing site for a drug. This entity can include membrane proteins for recognition of hormones and neurotransmitters (receptors) and also ion channels, nucleic acids, carrier molecules or enzymes. However, not all drugs act on receptors (see below).

Most drugs must bind to a molecular target in order to produce their actions but there are exceptions, as we will see later on. From the first studies of the effects of drugs on animal tissues in the late nineteenth century, it became evident that many drugs produce specific responses in specific tissues. That is:

- A drug that has profound effects on one type of tissue may have no effect on another type of tissue.
- A drug may have quite different effects on different tissues.

For example, the alkaloid pilocarpine, like the neurotransmitter acetylcholine (see Ch. 8), induces contraction of intestinal smooth muscle but slows heart rate. To account for such differences, Langley (1852–1925) proposed in 1878, on the basis of studies of the effects of the alkaloids pilocarpine and atropine on salivation, that 'there is some "receptor" substance ... with which both are capable of forming compounds ...'. Later, in 1905, when studying the action of nicotine and curare on skeletal muscle, he found that nicotine caused contractions only when applied to certain small regions of the muscle. He concluded that the 'receptive substance' for nicotine was confined to those regions and that curare acted by blocking the combination of nicotine with its receptor.

Paul Ehrlich (1854–1915) appears to have independently developed the receptor concept, starting from the observation that many organic dyes selectively stain

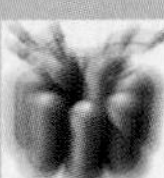

specific cell constituents. In 1885 he proposed that cells have 'side chains' or 'receptors' to which drugs or toxins must attach in order to produce their actions. Ehrlich was very influential in his time and is still remembered for his idea of the 'magic bullet', a chemical compound constructed for its selective toxicity to, for example, an infectious organism, as well as for the synthesis of organic arsenicals that were effective in the treatment of syphilis. In the development of receptor theory, Ehrlich was the first to point out that the rapid reversibility of the actions of alkaloids implied that the 'combination' of such drugs with receptors did not involve strong (covalent) chemical bonds.

Recent developments in molecular biology are rapidly clarifying the nature of drug–receptor binding at the molecular level. Today, a receptor is regarded as a specific molecular entity that acts as the molecular target for a group of related drugs. Since in the past, the binding site was not delineated from the rest of the molecular target, the whole complex is generally described as the receptor.

Molecular drug targets include:

- Hormone and neurotransmitter receptors
- Enzymes
- Carrier molecules (symporters or antiporters)
- Ion channels (ligand-gated or voltage-operated)
- Idiosyncratic targets (metal ions, surfactant proteins, gastrointestinal contents)
- Nucleic acids

Not all drugs have molecular targets

With drugs that target a known enzyme, the molecular target is the enzyme. The receptor for such drugs is that part on the enzyme that binds the drug. While the molecular targets for most drugs are proteins, carbohydrates, lipids and other macromolecules can be targets for drugs. This view of molecular targets is more encompassing than a view in which receptors are only those proteins mediating the actions of neurotransmitters, autacoids and hormones.

Today, receptors are identified and characterized by the techniques of molecular biology. For some types of drugs, actions are easily explained without the need for human molecular targets. These include buffers (antacids) that reduce stomach acidity, bulk laxatives and chelating agents. At the other extreme are agents with obscure mechanisms of action which are characterized by the virtual absence of strict chemical specificity. The prime examples of this are the gaseous and volatile general anesthetics, including the inert gas xenon. For these anesthetics it has been challenging to identify a binding site or a single molecular target. Nevertheless, it is possible that anesthetics owe their pharmacologic effects to actions on a membrane component (e.g. voltage- and ligand-gated ion channels) critical to normal neural function. Such a component would then be the molecular target for anesthetics.

The receptor concept is very important for drugs that mimic or antagonize the actions of hormones, neurohormones, neurotransmitters and autacoids

Drugs (including plant alkaloids such as nicotine, curare and atropine) that mimic or antagonize the effects of neurotransmitters first led Langley to postulate the receptor concept. With such drugs, experimental study of how they act was originally limited to measuring their effects in whole animals and isolated tissues: for example on blood pressure, heart rate, secretion or, commonly, contraction of intestinal, bronchial, vascular or uterine smooth muscle. Such effects have long been recognized as indirect reflections of the interaction of drugs with their receptors. The receptor concept has led to the development of methods using such data to classify drugs in terms of the receptors upon which they act and to develop new drugs targeted to specific receptors.

Classic neurotransmitter or hormone receptors are generally large proteins that contain a site which 'recognizes' drugs and binds them (Fig. 2.1). *This binding site is usually linked to a transduction system*

It has become clear that many receptors are proteins. Such proteins have at least one distinct region to which drugs, both agonists and antagonists, bind. When an agonist binds, it triggers a transduction chain that either directly induces a measurable response, such as opening a channel, or changes the activity of an enzyme that in its turn produces a measurable response. The link between the binding of agonist and transduction can be relatively direct or involve second messengers and a cascade of other proteins. Generally it is not the recognition site that is responsible for transduction but rather, on binding of the drug, there is an allosteric change in the receptor molecule causing other parts of the protein (usually facing the intracellular milieu) to take on catalytic activity. In addition, other parts of a receptor molecule can act

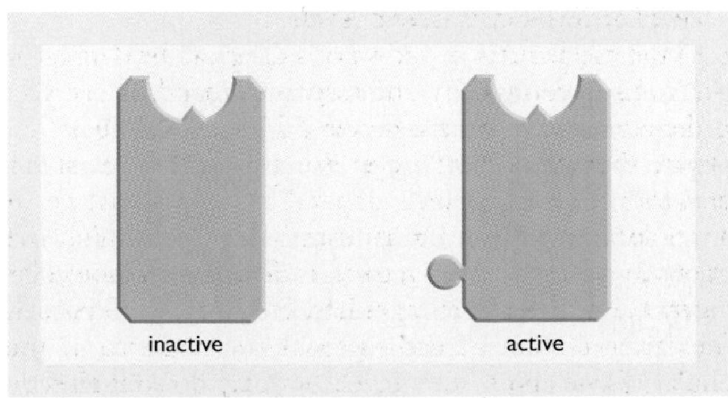

Fig. 2.1 The icon used throughout the text to indicate receptors.

as targets for different types of drugs, inhibitors that are not 'competitive' antagonists.

An active agonist–receptor complex produces a cellular response via 'transduction'

As indicated above, the active agonist–receptor complex initiates transduction either locally at the membrane level or intracellularly. Examples of transduction systems are shown below. It also seems to be generally accepted that, at least in most cases, the combination of an agonist with a receptor must lead to a conformational change in the latter, giving rise to an active drug–receptor complex. This provides the basis for a model in which the different actions of agonists, partial agonists and antagonists can be explained.

Many different classes of drugs may bind with a receptor. Such binding defines a drug as a 'ligand' for a receptor and the consequence of the binding determines whether a drug is an agonist, an antagonist, partial agonist or inverse agonist.

- If the ligand binds to a receptor and produces a molecular response (conformational change in the receptor), with subsequent cellular responses, it is an **agonist**.
- If the ligand binds to a receptor without initiating a molecular response leading to cellular and tissue responses, but competitively denies the agonist access to that receptor, the ligand is considered to be a **competitive antagonist**.
- If the ligand binds to a receptor in a manner that even high concentrations are incapable of producing a sufficient molecular response to cause a maximum cellular response, it is called a **partial agonist**. Consequently, the maximum tissue response to a partial agonist is less than with a 'full' agonist. Thus, a partial agonist can act as an antagonist to a full agonist.
- If the ligand binds to a receptor which, in the absence of the agonist, exists in an activated state and the ligand makes the receptor inactive, the ligand is an **inverse agonist**. The basal level of activation causes a 'background' level of transduction and cellular effects. When an inverse agonist binds to the activated receptor, it inactivates it and therefore inhibits this basal activation.

Tissue responses are not necessarily directly proportional to the molecular responses resulting from an agonist binding to its receptor (see below for details)

Drugs and endogenous substances (hormones and neurotransmitters) that activate receptors are called agonists and the molecular response is the production of the activated state of the receptor, which initiates the cellular response.

Many receptors have endogenous agonists. These are sometimes known as first messengers. This is because the interaction with their molecular target is the first message of intercellular communication (likewise any molecules that participate in the cellular response are known as second messengers).

An agonist that fully activates receptors is known as a full agonist (see the description of partial agonism for further details).

In the absence of agonists, most receptors are in a rested state. However, even in the absence of an agonist, a receptor may convert temporarily, on a random basis, to an activated state. This produces a low-level cellular response. In the absence of an agonist, the rested state is favored. In contrast, the presence of an agonist shifts the equilibrium strongly in favor of the activated state.

The mathematical relationship between agonist concentration (A) and response is defined by binding to the receptor (R), with the response resulting from formation of an agonist–receptor complex (AR) that activates the receptor (R*). Therefore $A + R \rightleftharpoons AR \rightleftharpoons AR^*$. For some receptors, two molecules of agonist have to bind in order to produce activation ($A + A + R \rightleftharpoons AAR \rightleftharpoons AAR^*$). In contrast, for other receptors the reaction is $A + R + R \rightleftharpoons ARR \rightleftharpoons ARR^*$, i.e. binding of an agonist promotes the association of two inactive receptors into an activated homodimer. The mathematical basis of this relationship is discussed in more detail below. For all figures in the book, agonists are indicated by an icon (Fig. 2.2).

In most cells the maximum cellular response to an agonist is achieved when only a small proportion of its receptors are occupied. In other words, the number of receptors is usually much higher than is necessary for obtaining a maximum cellular response. The excess of receptors is usually referred to as 'spare receptors' and is important because spare receptors increase the sensitivity of the cell to small changes in the concentration of agonist (see below).

Partial agonism is the inefficient activation of a receptor

A drug that activates a receptor in a relatively inefficient manner is a partial agonist. Conceptually, a partial agonist is a drug for which each interaction between it and the receptor produces a less than maximal molecular response or randomly produces either a molecular response or no response (a failed molecular response). In either case, the maximum cellular response to the partial agonist is less than the maximum cellular response to a full agonist acting on the same receptor, provided that there are no

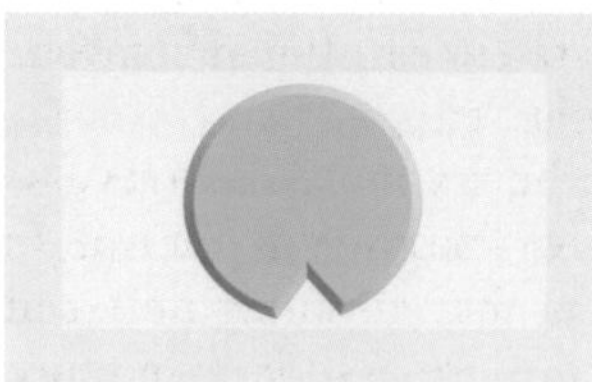

Fig. 2.2 The icon used to indicate an agonist. Note this icon is used throughout the book to indicate drugs that activate all molecular targets, including activators of enzymes.

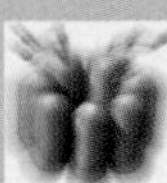

spare receptors. Partial agonists are required to interact with a large proportion of the receptor pool to produce a maximum cellular response, leaving only a small reserve of unoccupied receptors or none at all. If there are many spare receptors, it is possible for a partial agonist to elicit a maximum cellular response, although the partial agonist is said to have less efficacy than a full agonist in that it requires greater occupancy to elicit a maximum cellular response (see below). Most cells have far more receptors than are necessary to evoke a maximum cellular response (spare receptors). Therefore in most systems partial agonists may be capable of eliciting a maximum cellular response similar to that produced by a full agonist, although very high doses may be required.

Inverse agonism is the initiation of an apparent cellular response by the prevention of spontaneous activation of a receptor

The molecular response to an inverse agonist is either:

- Deactivation of the activated receptor, or
- Stabilization of receptors in an inactive conformation.

This is modeled as $R \rightleftharpoons R^*$ and $I + R^* \rightleftharpoons IR$, where R^* is the activated state and I is an inverse agonist.

Antagonism is the prevention of the action of an agonist

Many drugs bind to a receptor and produce a drug–receptor complex that elicits no cellular response. Moreover, the occupancy of the receptor by the antagonist either prevents an agonist from binding or prevents the agonist from evoking a molecular response when it binds to the receptor. Thus, antagonism can result from a variety of different molecular mechanisms. Mathematical descriptions of the effects of different types of antagonists are given below. Briefly, antagonism can be produced by:

- Binding of an antagonist to the same site on the receptor normally occupied by the agonist. The binding of the antagonist denies the agonist occupancy of the site (competitive antagonism).
- Binding of an antagonist to a site different from that normally occupied by the agonist (an allosteric site), resulting in a conformational change of the binding site for the agonist. This either prevents the agonist from binding or prevents the bound agonist from eliciting a molecular response.

An antagonist that binds to its allosteric site only when the agonist is not bound is called a **noncompetitive antagonist**. If the antagonist can bind to its allosteric site even when an agonist is bound, it is called an **uncompetitive antagonist**. The 'site' referred to here is often called a ligand-binding site (where 'ligand' means agonist, antagonist, partial agonist, etc.).

Since antagonist binding can be reversible or irreversible, there are at least six possible types of antagonism, as shown in Table 2.2. The effects that an antagonist can have on the responses to an agonist are described in more detail below. Throughout the text antagonists will be shown using the icon in Fig. 2.3.

Table 2.2 Six possible types of antagonism

	Competitive	Noncompetitive	Uncompetitive
Reversible	+	+	+
Irreversible	+	+	+

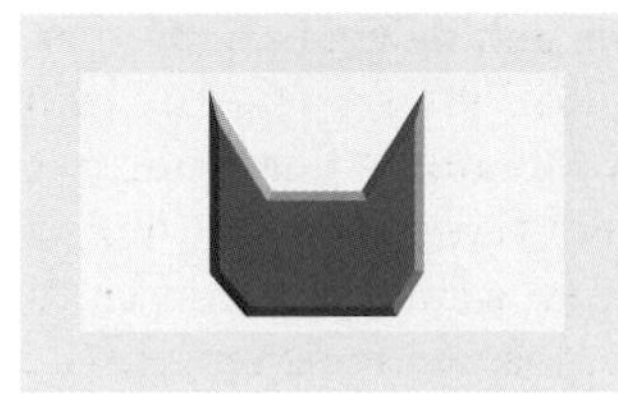

Fig. 2.3 The icon used to indicate an antagonist. Note that this icon is used throughout the book to indicate drugs that block the activity of other molecular targets, such as enzymes (enzyme inhibitors).

Physiologic antagonism is distinct from pharmacologic antagonism

Physiologic (or functional) 'antagonism' is a term that is commonly used but is misleading. It describes the ability of an agonist (rather than an antagonist) to inhibit the response to a second agonist via activation of different receptors that are physically separate. This may occur if the receptors for the two agonists are linked to the same cellular response components, but affect them differently, or are linked to different cellular response components that give rise to opposite tissue responses. A good example is the interaction between norepinephrine and acetylcholine in arterioles. Norepinephrine causes contraction and acetylcholine causes relaxation. It is obviously not helpful to describe norepinephrine as an acetylcholine antagonist, since one could equally describe acetylcholine as a norepinephrine antagonist, thereby rendering the terms 'agonist' and 'antagonist' interchangeable and hence meaningless. The term 'antagonist' is best used to describe a drug that can inhibit the molecular response to an agonist and the term 'functional antagonist' should be avoided.

The quantitative analysis of mechanisms of drug action consists largely of interpreting dose–response curves

The quantitative analysis of drug action is important in the development of new drugs, where the aims are to discover:

- Drugs that are specific in terms of the receptors with which they interact.
- Drugs that are selective by virtue of their interaction with only one subtype of receptor.

Several principles are fundamental to an understanding of drug–receptor binding and dose (concentration)–response curves. These principles, which apply to the majority of drugs used clinically and experimentally, are as follows:

- On any single cell in a tissue there are numerous receptors while most cells express many different types of receptor.
- When a drug is present, drug–receptor complexes are repeatedly and randomly created as the random movement of drug molecules leads to their collision with unoccupied receptors. Drug–receptor complexes are also repeatedly and randomly breaking down, thereby freeing receptors to combine again with the drug.
- Agonist–receptor complexes repeatedly fluctuate between inactive and active conformations (the molecular response). The latter induce biophysical events such as the opening of ion channels or biochemical events such as G protein activation (see page 25) that lead to a tissue response.
- The numbers of receptors expressed on a cell may change in pathologic conditions and with chronic drug administration.

Two useful rules of thumb that may be added to these fundamental principles are:

- Submaximal tissue responses to agonists are proportional to the product of agonist dose (concentration) and the number of available receptors.
- By binding to receptors, antagonists reduce the number of receptors available for agonist binding to an extent that does not depend upon how much agonist is present.

The fundamental principles listed above represent a view of how drugs act in linking empirical observations and experimental results to fundamental chemical and physicochemical events. The quantitative consequences of the theory are in many respects manifested in the binding of radioactively labeled ligands (drugs) to receptors isolated from tissues. As this kind of experiment is relatively easy to perform and understand, it is convenient to consider 'drug-receptor binding' before considering dose–response curves.

Drug–receptor binding

A receptor can be considered as an entity that selectively and specifically binds drugs. For the sake of simplicity, we use here the example of a drug binds selectively only to a single recognition site on the receptor.

The simplest model for reversible drug binding

The simplest possible model for reversible drug binding to a receptor is one in which each molecule of drug (D) can randomly bind to a molecule of receptor (R) in such a way as to form a drug–receptor complex (DR). This complex then breaks down to produce a free molecule of drug and an unoccupied receptor. From the law of mass action, the rate at which new DR complexes are formed is proportional to the concentration of D, i.e. **[D]** and the concentration of free R, i.e. **[R]**. (Square brackets indicate concentration.) At the same time the rate at which the DR complex breaks down to D and R is proportional to the concentration of DR, i.e. **[DR]**.

At equilibrium, the rate at which new DR complexes are formed equals the rate at which DR complexes break down, thus:

$$K_D\,[\mathbf{DR}] = [\mathbf{D}]\,[\mathbf{R}] \qquad \text{(Eqn 2.1)}$$

where K_D is the dissociation constant usually expressed as molar quantity (M = gram molecules/L). The constant K_D depends upon physical factors such as temperature and, most importantly, the chemical nature of the interacting substances. In this simple model, K_D is the ratio of the off and on rate constants for binding. It is worth noting that the same equation applies to more complicated models in which there are multiple conformations of R and DR. In the complex case K_D depends upon all the rate constants needed to describe the system. Nevertheless, regardless of how many conformations of R or DR exist, receptors may be considered in the two forms, R and DR, with K_D **[DR]** = **[D] [R]**. An alternative form of the equation is **[DR]** = **[D] [R]**/K_D.

[DR]+[R] is a constant

Since the total number of receptors is limited, the total concentration of **[DR]** + **[R]** is constant and designated **[R$_t$]**. Therefore:

$$[\mathbf{R_t}] = [\mathbf{R}] + [\mathbf{DR}] = [\mathbf{R}]\,(1 + [\mathbf{D}]/K_D) \qquad \text{(Eqn 2.2)}$$

when **[DR]** is substituted by the term **[R] [D]**/K_D (see above). Further, combining this with K_D **[DR]** = **[D] [R]** gives:

$$[\mathbf{DR}]/[\mathbf{R_t}] = ([\mathbf{D}]/K_D)(1 + [\mathbf{D}]/K_D) \qquad \text{(Eqn 2.3)}$$

with **[DR]**/**[Rt]** being the chance that any one R will at any moment be combined with D.

Semilogarithmic plots are usually used for both binding studies and concentration–response curves

The graph of **[DR]** versus **[D]** for two drugs (A and B with very different K_D values) is shown in Fig. 2.4. It is notable that although both plots show the same initial linear rise with concentration, which gradually flattens to a maximum, it is inconvenient to use the same x-axis for both A and B. In Fig. 2.5 the same information is plotted semilogarithmically, i.e. with **[DR]** versus the log of **[D]** rather than simply **[D]**. Such graphs show that both plots are essentially the same, differing only in their relative positions on the x-axis. Such semilogarithmic plots are now usually used for both binding studies and dose–response.

In a study of binding, receptors are incubated with various concentrations of D, where D is radioactively labeled (usually with ^{3}H), and then rapidly filtered and 'washed' to remove unbound drug. The subsequent count

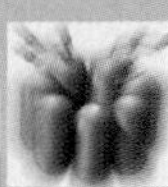

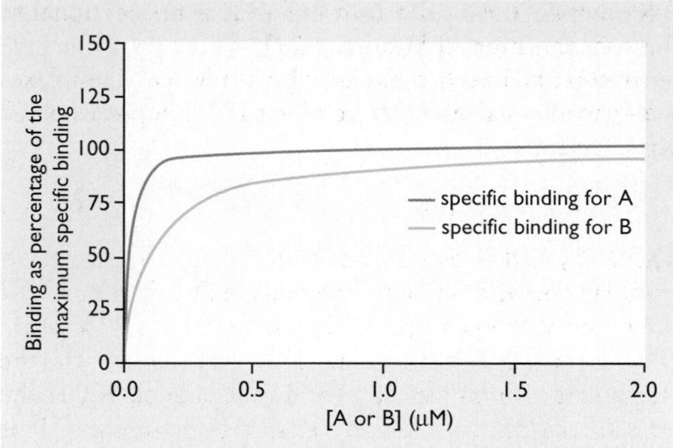

Fig. 2.4 Linear plots for specific and non-specific receptor binding for the two drugs, A and B, which have K_D values of 0.01 (K_A) and 0.1 (K_B) μM, respectively. The *y*-axis is binding (formation of AR or BR) expressed as a percentage of maximum specific binding for A or B, respectively. The *x*-axis is the concentration of A or B. Note the equal spacing on the concentration axis (i.e. it is linear) and that the intercept is 0,0. (μM, micromolar conc.)

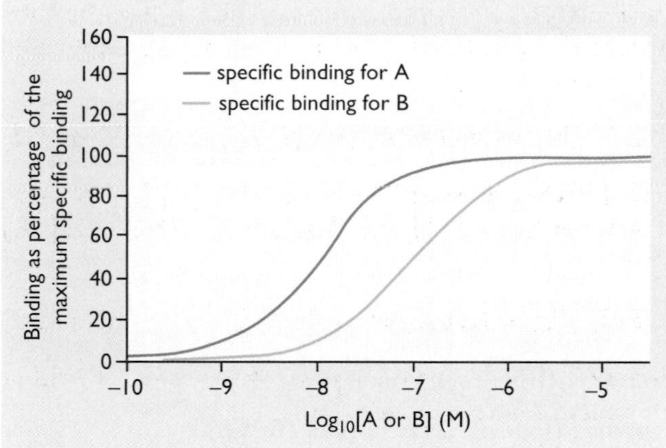

Fig. 2.5 Semilog plot of Fig. 2.4. Higher concentrations of A and B were studied for specific binding with conditions as in Fig. 2.4, with K_A = 0.01 μM and K_B = 0.1 μM. In this figure the *x*-axis is now plotted on a $\log_{10}$ scale over a concentration range from 10^{-10} M to $>10^{-5}$ M, which is a 100 000-fold concentration range. The intercept of the *y*-axis with the *x*-axis is now 0, −10. (M, molar conc.) The affinity is the tendency of a drug to bind to its receptors. This is measured by the K_D. The slope of the binding curve indicates the nature of binding and this simple model has the value of 1 since one molecule of D binds to one molecule of R.

of the retained radioactivity gives the total of how much drug remains. Some of this is, however, simply drug which is non-specifically stuck in the interstices of the filter or between cells or, perhaps, dissolved in the tissue lipid. The effect of non-specific binding is expressed as a percentage of specific binding.

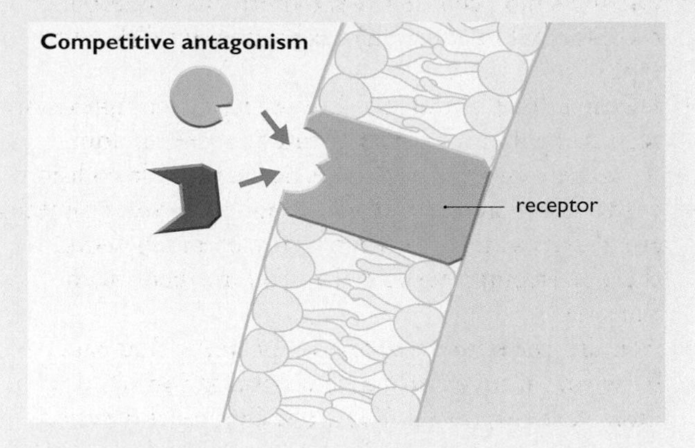

Fig. 2.6 Two different drugs 'competing' for binding to the specific binding site of a receptor.

General model of reversible drug binding to receptors

- **Each molecule of drug (D) can randomly collide with a molecule of receptor (R) in such a way as to form a drug–receptor complex (DR)**
- **The DR complex can then break down at any moment to produce a free molecule of unchanged drug (D) and an unoccupied receptor (R)**
- **At equilibrium, K_D [DR] = [D] [R], where K_D is the dissociation constant (molar)**

Binding studies provide valuable data on drug–receptor interactions

Suppose that a receptor can bind either a molecule of drug (D) or drug (I), but not simultaneously (Fig. 2.6). Receptors can now exist in three forms:

- Free R has a concentration of **[R]**.
- DR has a concentration of **[DR]** = **[R] [D]**/K_D.
- IR has a concentration of **[IR]** = **[R] [I]**/K_I (where K_I is the dissociation constant of IR).

From the above, the following equation can be derived:

$$[R_t] = [R] + [DR] + [IR] \qquad \text{(Eqn 2.4)}$$

where **[R_t]** is the sum of all forms of R. Similar equations can be derived for **[DR]** and **[IR]**. A further series of useful equations can be derived by substitution.

An important feature of such equations is that if **[D]** is high enough, most of the receptors will be bound to drug (DR), despite I being present. Conversely, if **[I]** is high, most of the receptors will be bound to I (IR), despite D being present. Therefore I is said to 'compete' with D and D with I. The competition arises simply because a single receptor cannot bind both D and I simultaneously. Competition is mathematically equivalent to multiplying the dissociation constant by (1 + **c**), where **c** is the concentration of the competitor divided by its dissociation constant (i.e. **c** = **[I]**/K_I). It follows that the effect of any given concentration of competitor is to cause a parallel

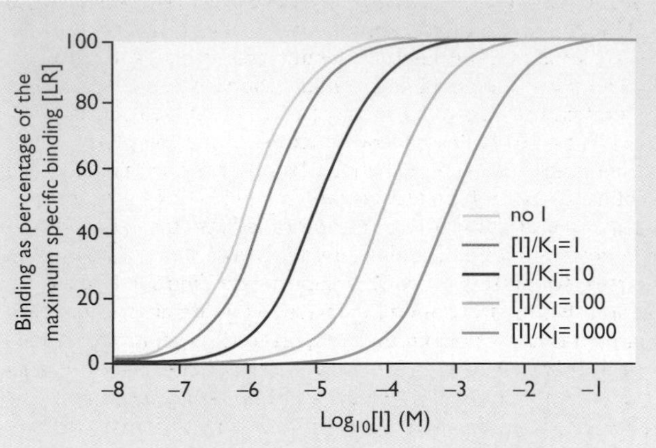

Fig. 2.7 Specific binding of drug (L) in the presence of competitive antagonist (I), present in different concentrations such that [I]/K$_I$ = 1, 10, 100 or 1000. As in Fig. 2.5, this is a semilogarithmic plot in which the *x*-axis is expressed in $\log_{10}$ form. K_I is the dissociation constant for I. Note that the presence of I shifts the concentration-binding graphs for L to the right in a parallel manner. The amount of shift depends upon $[I]/K_I$ with each 10-fold increase causing a log 1.0 (= 10) parallel shift. (M, molar conc.)

shift of the plot of **[DR]** versus log**[D]** (the dose–response curve) to the right on the *x*-axis. The shift will be by a factor log(1 + **c**), where **c** is **[I]**/K_I (Fig. 2.7).

This provides a method for experimentally determining the dissociation constant of a competitive molecule. At any given **[I]**, the dose ratio (DR), which is the ratio of **[D]** values producing the same **[DR]** in the presence and absence of C, is given by:

$$\mathbf{DR} = 1 + [\mathbf{I}]/K_I \qquad \text{(Eqn 2.5)}$$

Rearranging this gives:

$$(\mathbf{DR} - 1)/[\mathbf{I}] = 1/K_I \qquad \text{(Eqn 2.6)}$$

This method is less important in binding studies but of great importance in functional concentration–response studies of agonist/antagonist–receptor interactions where the response to **[DR]** is measured, rather than its binding. Adding a competitive antagonist, I, in the presence of agonist D is equivalent to reducing the agonist concentration by the factor (1 + **[I]**/K_I). This leads to a shift of the response–log[agonist] curve to the right. This shift is analogous to the shifts seen in Fig. 2.7. Therefore, original responses are restored by multiplying agonist doses by the DR, which is equal to 1 + **[I]**/K_I.

Classification of drug receptors

Drugs that act on receptors elicit a wide range of tissue and system responses for two reasons. The first is that different receptors are expressed in different tissues. The other is that different types of receptor have different types of structure and, hence, function. Therefore the cellular responses to receptor activation (transduction) vary considerably according to the structure of the receptor. Based on this there are four types of receptor, referred to as receptor superfamilies (Fig. 2.8), which all have different kinetic characteristics:

- G protein-coupled receptors.
- DNA-coupled receptors.
- Receptors that possess tyrosine kinase activity ('tyrosine kinase receptors').
- Receptor-operated channels (ROCs).

Tyrosine kinase receptors and ROCs are different from the others since they do not require linkage to cellular transduction components to elicit a cellular response when activated by an agonist, meaning that the receptor molecule is more than simply a molecular link between drug and transduction. A tyrosine kinase receptor is actually a membrane-bound enzyme that is 'switched on' by its agonists. An ROC is actually a specialized ion channel that is structurally distinct from the voltage-operated ion channel (VOC, see page 28) in that it is operated by a drug or neurotransmitter binding to a highly stereoselective ligand-binding site instead of a highly specialized voltage sensor region. In an ROC the ligand-binding site and the channel are functionally distinct regions of a single molecule. The ROC is also known as a 'ligand-gated ion channel'. The above classification acknowledges the conventional approach that refers to tyrosine kinases and ROCs as 'receptors'.

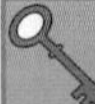

The drug superfamilies

- **Receptor-operated channels (ROCs)**
- **G protein-coupled receptors**
- **Receptors that are enzymes (e.g. tyrosine kinase receptors)**
- **DNA-coupled receptors**

G protein-coupled receptors (GPCR)

G proteins are transduction components (see pages 34 and 35) shown as an icon in Fig. 2.9. G protein-coupled receptors are located in cell membranes and are composed of seven transmembrane helices (I–VII) (Fig. 2.10). In the absence of agonist, the receptor is bound to a G protein that holds the receptor in an inactive conformation. The G protein itself is a complex of three subunits (α, β and γ). In the rested state of the receptor, the three G protein subunits are bound together and guanine nucleotide diphosphate (GDP) is tightly bound to the α subunit of the G protein. Agonist binding to the receptor causes a conformation change in the receptor. This in turn causes a conformation change in the G protein that causes GDP to dissociate from the α subunit. This initiates the sequence of events that constitutes G protein-coupled receptor transduction, which is described in further detail below.

Interestingly, responses mediated by G protein-coupled receptors may wane with time, in spite of the

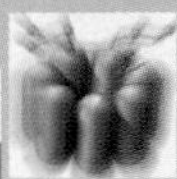

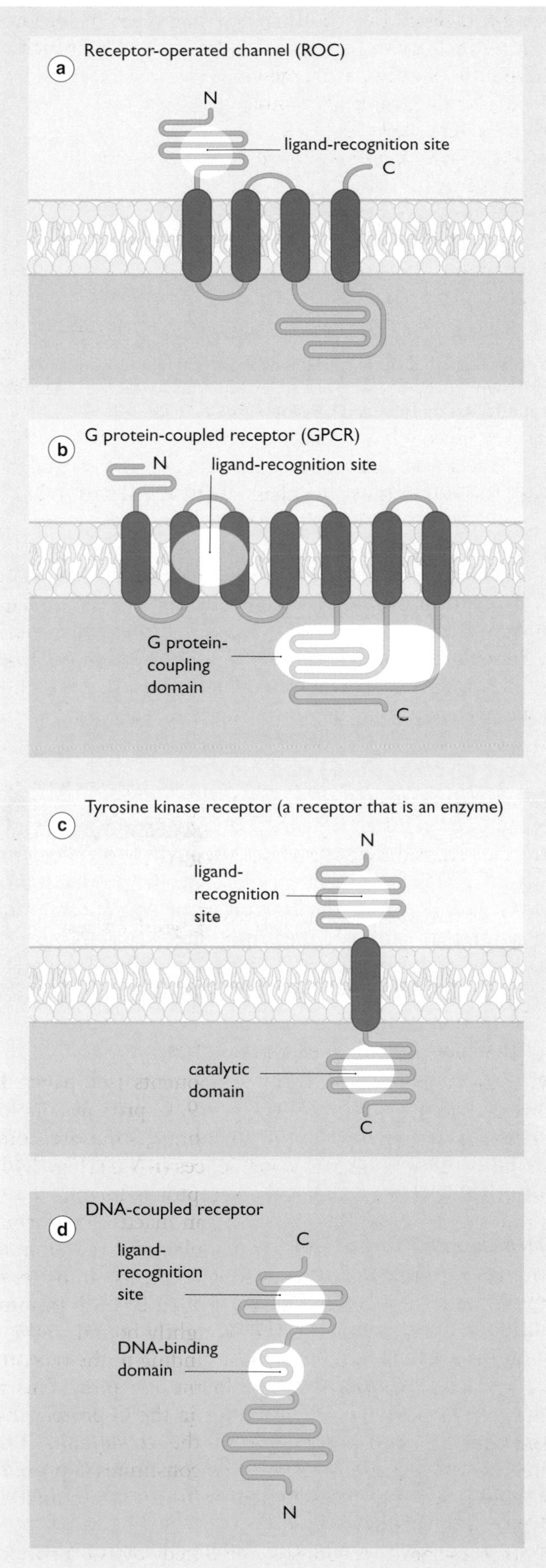

Fig. 2.8 Schematic representation of the general structure of the four hormonal neurotransmitter receptor superfamilies. (a) Receptor-operated channel: an extracellular binding domain is coupled to a hydrophobic α helical region of the protein that forms the membrane-spanning domain. Up to five subunits that have this general structure form a complex surrounding a central ion channel. This is best exemplified by the nicotinic acetylcholine (ACh) receptor (see Fig. 2.14 for more detail). Typically, this type of receptor mediates the very fast action of neurotransmitters. C is the C terminal and N the N terminal of the receptor protein. (b) GPCR: the drug-binding site is found within α helices and a membrane-spanning domain is connected to an intracellular domain that couples to G proteins. This is a typical receptor structure for many hormones and slower-acting neurotransmitter systems that act via G protein-coupled transduction systems (e.g. epinephrine acting on cardiac muscle). The G protein coupling domain is the part of the receptor that interacts with the α subunit of the G protein to facilitate transduction following binding of an agonist to the binding domain. (c) Tyrosine kinase receptors: the receptors for various growth factors and insulin have an extracellular drug-binding site linked directly to an intracellular catalytic domain that has either tyrosine kinase or guanylyl kinase activity when the ligand-binding site is occupied by an appropriate agonist. These tyrosine kinase receptors are enzymes referred to as tyrosine kinase receptors. (d) DNA-coupled receptor: the drug-binding site is linked to a DNA-binding domain as typified by drug receptors for steroid and thyroid hormones. These are defined as DNA-coupled receptors. (Adapted with permission from *Pharmacology*, 3rd edn, by Rang, Dale and Ritter, Churchill Livingstone, 1995.)

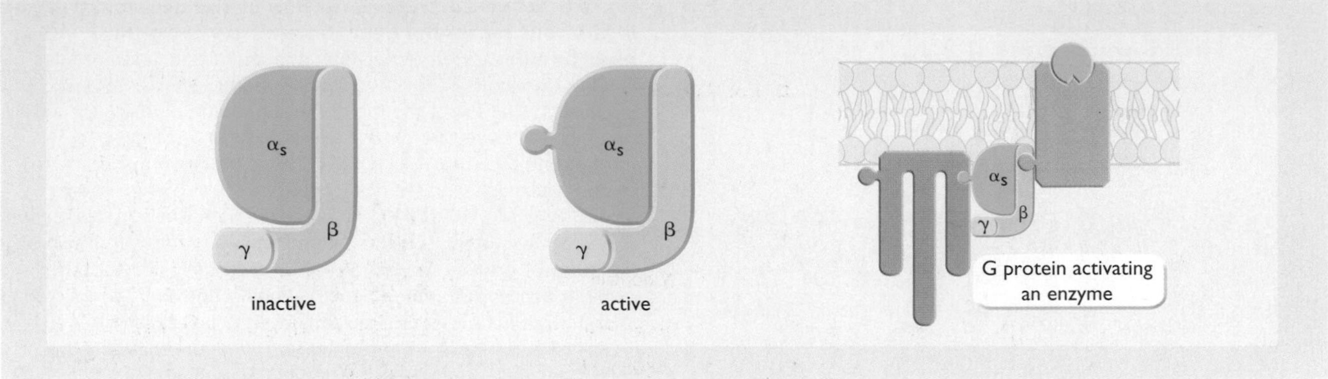

Fig. 2.9 The icon used for the G protein in inactive and active states. Note that the α_s subunit dissociates when the G protein is active (see Fig. 2.11) but, for simplicity, the icon for the active G protein is shown 'intact' but with an 'appendage' (as for 'active' receptors, see Fig. 2.1). Also shown is the role the G protein plays in linking the receptor to the transduction cascade.

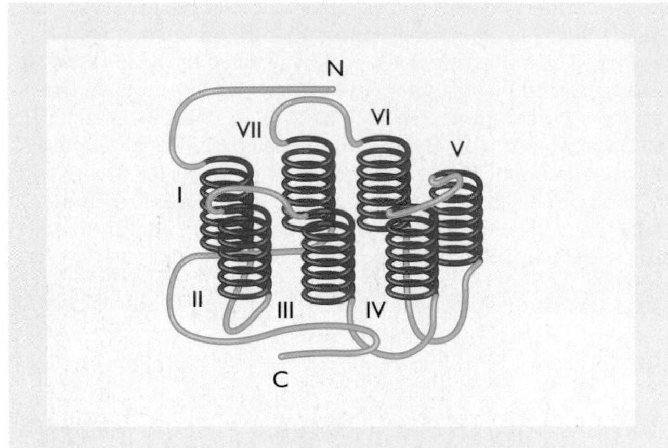

Fig. 2.10 Schematic representation of a G protein-coupled receptor. There are seven transmembrane helices (I–VII).

continued presence of the agonist. This phenomenon has been called desensitization and is described in further detail below.

Cyclic nucleotide-linked transduction

Of the transduction components linked directly to G proteins, the most widely distributed throughout the body is adenylyl cyclase. The cyclic nucleotide cAMP is synthesized from adenosine triphosphate (ATP) by the enzyme adenylyl cyclase. cAMP has diverse biologic actions.

cAMP has effects on energy metabolism, cell differentiation, ion channel function and contractile proteins

cAMP phosphorylates intracellular proteins (many are enzymes) through the action of cAMP-dependent protein kinases. These protein kinases are activated by cAMP and phosphorylate the amino acids serine and threonine, using ATP as a source of phosphate (Fig. 2.11). Phosphorylation results in:

- Activation of hormone-sensitive lipase.
- Inactivation of glycogen synthase.
- Activation of phosphorylase kinase and therefore conversion of inactive phosphorylase to active phosphorylase, which results in increased lipolysis, reduced glycogen synthesis and increased glycogen breakdown.
- Activation of L-type Ca^{2+} channels and sarcoplasmic reticulum in cardiac cells by phosphorylation, so increasing Ca^{2+} currents and Ca^{2+} release, respectively.

Diacyl glycerol (DAG) and inositol 1,4,5-triphosphate (IP3)-linked receptors

Many G proteins activate the DAG-IP_3 pathway. One G protein, termed Gq, stimulates the activity of phospholipase C. This enzyme in turn leads to the production of DAG and IP_3 from the hydrolysis of polyphosphotide inositides. An alternative pathway involves activation of membrane phospholipase A_2 by G proteins, leading to the formation of DAG and phosphatidic acid. These transduction components have a diversity of actions.

IP_3 is not the only inositol phosphate produced in the cell by phospholipase. There is a bewildering array of such compounds, which may have different functions. Inositol (1,3,4,5) tetraphosphate phosphate appears to facilitate the entry of Ca^{2+} into different cellular compartments (see Fig. 2.26).

DNA-coupled receptors

Intracellular receptors that interact with DNA exist for hormones such as retinoic acid, corticosteroids, thyroid hormone and vitamin D. These receptors are mainly composed of nuclear proteins. As a result, agonists have to pass through the cell membranes to reach the receptor. For example, steroids enter a cell and bind with a cytoplasmic receptor, which often has an inhibitory molecule bound to it, such as heat shock protein 90 (HSP90). The molecular response is a receptor conformation change that causes dissociation of the receptor from the inhibitory molecule. The cellular responses to activation of DNA receptors are numerous and varied

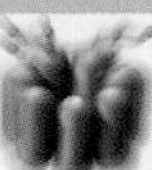

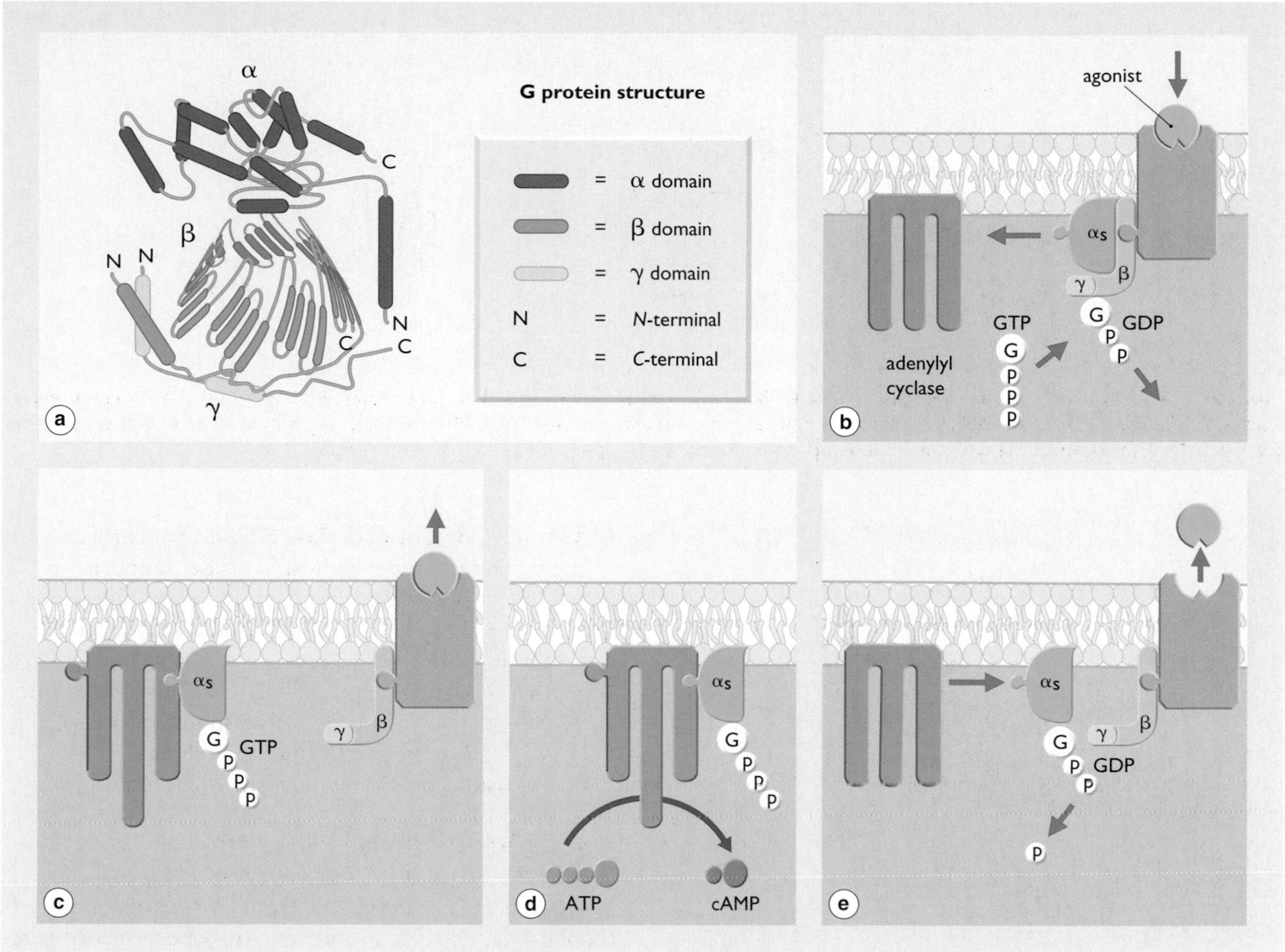

Fig. 2.11 Schematic representation of the activation of a G protein-coupled receptor. (a) The structure has several components. (b) The βγ complex serves to anchor the G protein to the membrane. Agonist binding to a G protein-coupled receptor promotes a conformation change in the receptor which in turn activates the G protein, leading to dissociation of the βγ heterodimer from its associated α subunit; in addition, bound GDP dissociates from the α subunit, leading to binding of GTP to this protein. (c, d) The α-GTP complex subsequently interacts with a target protein (e.g. an enzyme such as adenylyl cyclase or an ion channel). (e) The GTPase activity of the α subunit hydrolyzes the bound GTP to GDP, which allows the α subunit to recombine with the βγ complex.

and are discussed in the section below on transduction; they are shown in Fig. 2.12 (see later chapters for examples).

Receptors that possess tyrosine kinase activity (tyrosine kinase receptors)

Agonist action on tyrosine kinase receptors (Fig. 2.13) is involved in the regulation of growth, cell differentiation and responses to metabolic stimuli. Endogenous agonists include insulin, epidermal growth factors and platelet-derived growth factor. Agonists cause the receptor to change conformation and act as a tyrosine kinase enzyme that phosphorylates tyrosine residues in a wide variety of intracellular molecules.

Receptor-operated channels (ROCs)

ROCs are composed of subunits, each of which has four transmembrane domains. These domains form complexes of varying stoichiometry (Fig. 2.14). There are numerous different types of ROCs. Each possesses, as part of their structure, an extracellular drug-binding site that, when bound to a drug, initiates a conformation change in other parts of the ROC molecule that culminates with the opening of a central ion-selective pore. Passage of ions occurs only when the pore is open (the open 'state'). The molecular configuration of the channel therefore defines the state of the channel.

The simplest model for channel behavior has three recognized states:

- Rested (non-conducting, i.e. closed, but openable in response to an appropriate stimulus).
- Activated (open).
- Inactivated (i.e. closed and unable to open in response to what would be an appropriate stimulus for a rested state channel).

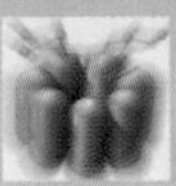

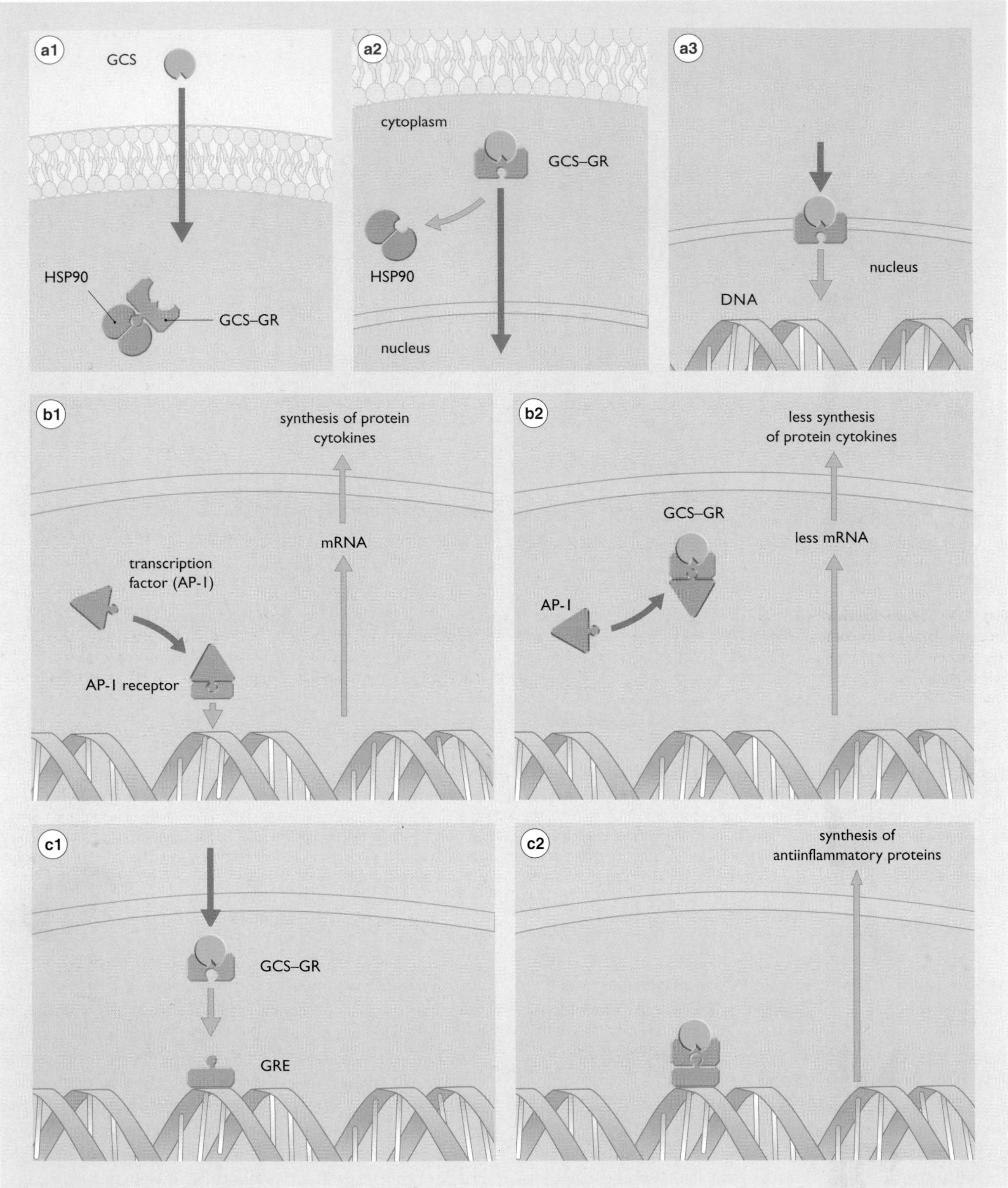

a1
GCS
HSP90
GCS–GR

a2
cytoplasm
GCS–GR
HSP90
nucleus

a3
nucleus
DNA

b1
synthesis of protein cytokines
mRNA
transcription factor (AP-1)
AP-1 receptor

b2
less synthesis of protein cytokines
GCS–GR
less mRNA
AP-1

c1
GCS–GR
GRE

c2
synthesis of antiinflammatory proteins

Fig. 2.12 Example of DNA-linked receptor transduction. Glucocorticosteroids are thought to exert antiinflammatory effects by at least two distinct mechanisms. (a1) Glucocorticosteroids (GCS) cross the cell membrane and bind with receptors located in the cytoplasm (here bound in an inactive form to heat shock protein 90, HSP90). (a2) First stage of transduction: dissociation of the glucocorticosteroid receptor complex (GCS–GR) from HSP90. (a3) Next stage of transduction: translocation of GCS–GR into the cell nucleus. (b1) In some cells, the synthesis of a protein (e.g. pro-inflammatory cytokines) can be initiated by transcription factors acting on their own receptors. (b2) Once in the nucleus, GCS–GR binds to (and 'mops up') the transcription factor (e.g. AP-I), thereby reducing the amount of new protein synthesized. If this protein is a pro-inflammatory mediator (e.g. a cytokine), the net effect is to reduce inflammation. (c1) Alternatively, GCS–GR may bind with a glucocorticosteroid response element (GRE, a receptor on DNA). (c2) Binding of GCS–GR to the GRE stimulates the synthesis of proteins having antiinflammatory actions (e.g. lipocortins).

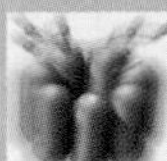

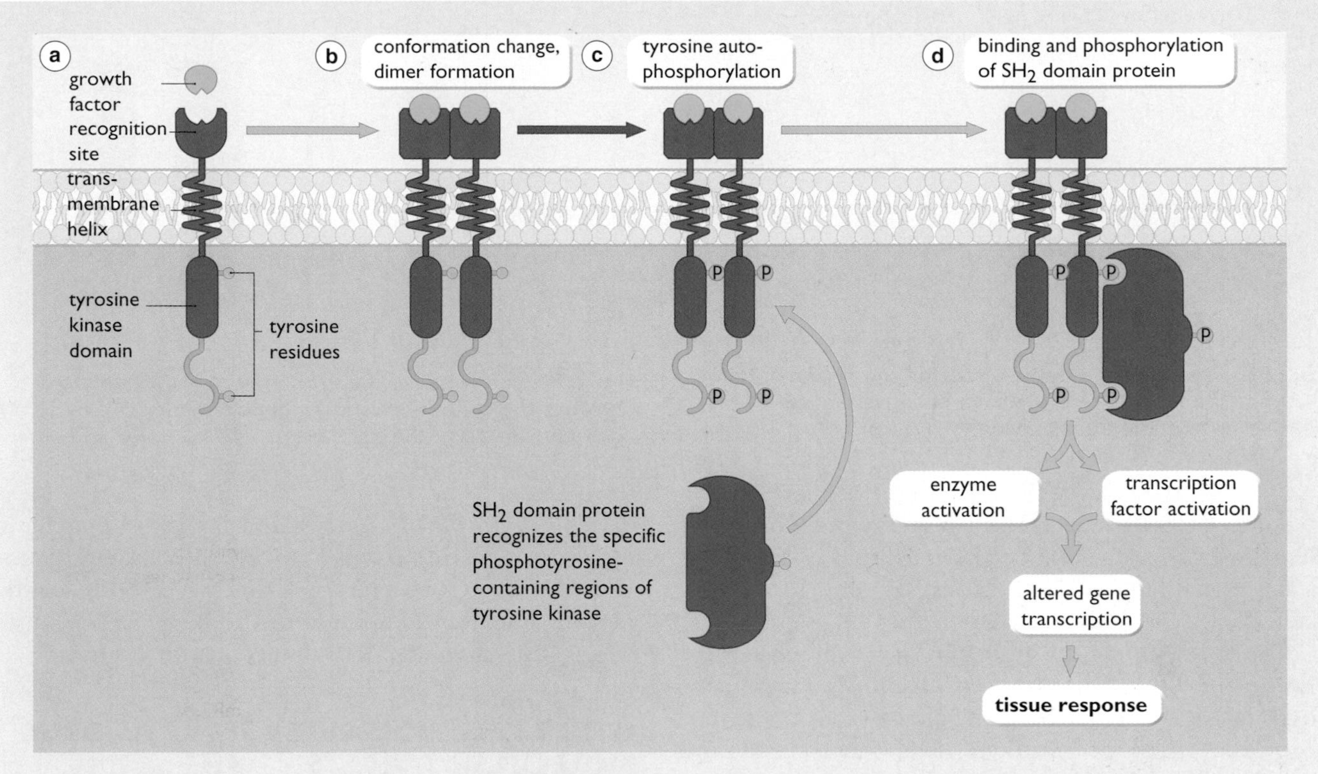

Fig. 2.13 Transduction mechanisms for tyrosine kinase receptors. (a) The binding of a growth factor to the N terminal of the receptor (b) leads to conformational changes resulting in dimer formation. This results in autophosphorylation of the tyrosine residues in the tyrosine kinase domain of the receptor (c). The specific phosphotyrosine-containing regions of the tyrosine kinase domain then bind the SH_2 domain, which results in activation of various intracellular responses leading to the tissue response (d). (Adapted with permission from *Pharmacology*, 3rd edn, by Rang, Dale and Ritter, Churchill Livingstone, 1995.)

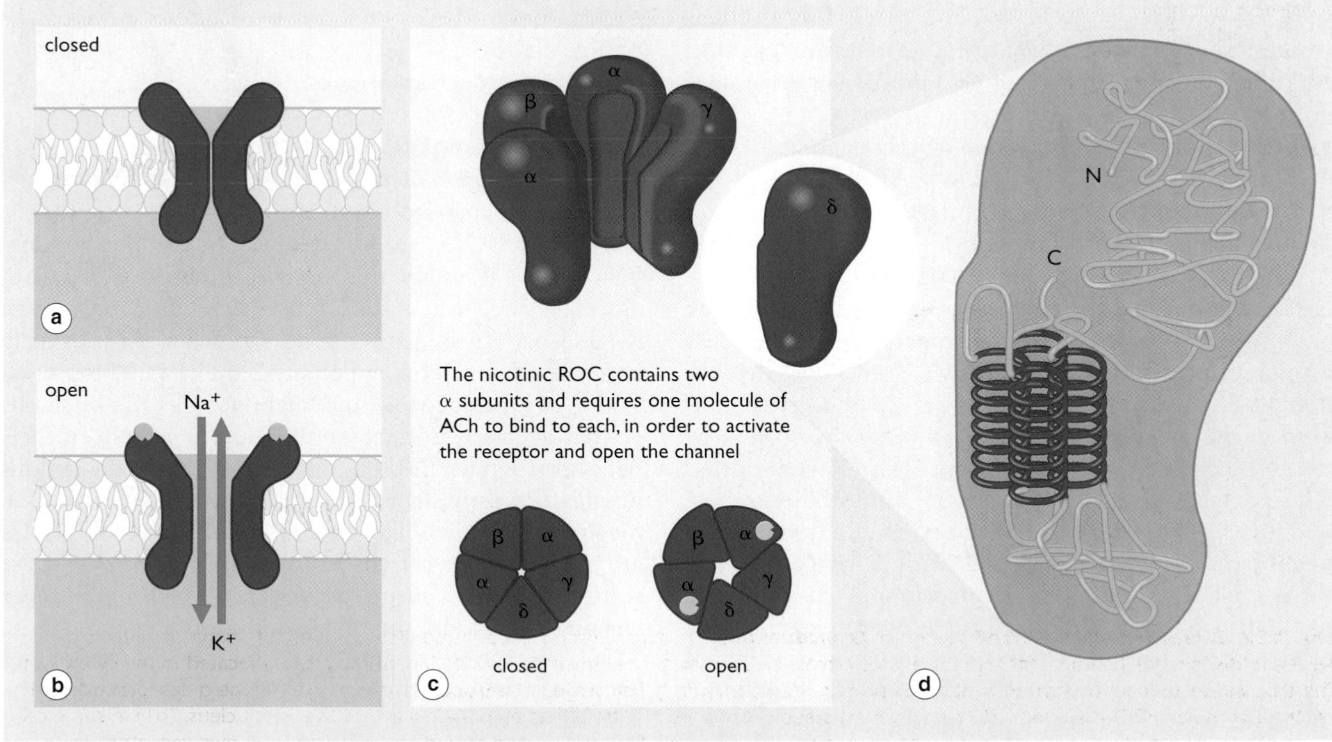

Fig. 2.14 The nicotinic acetylcholine (ACh) receptor-operated channel. The ROC can exist in a closed (a) or open (b) state. The channel consists of five protein subunits (two α, and β, γ and δ), all of which traverse the membrane and surround a central pore (c). ACh binds to the α subunits and the two ACh molecules must bind in order to open the channel (c). The complete structure of a single δ subunit is shown (d). C is the C terminal and N is the N terminal of the protein.

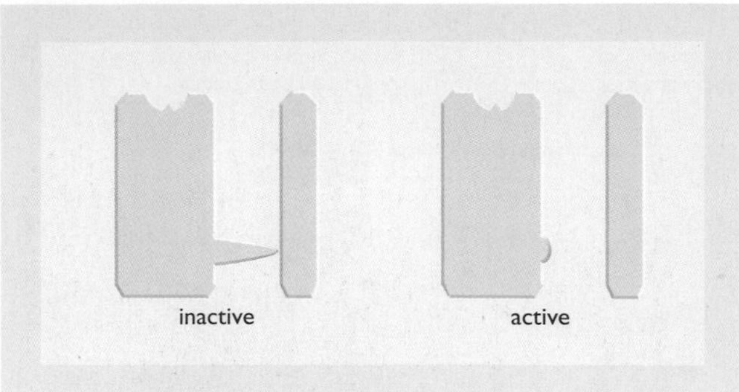

Fig. 2.15 Icon for a receptor-operated ion channel. Note that in certain ROCs the inactive (agonist unbound) state is 'channel open' and the agonist closes the channel.

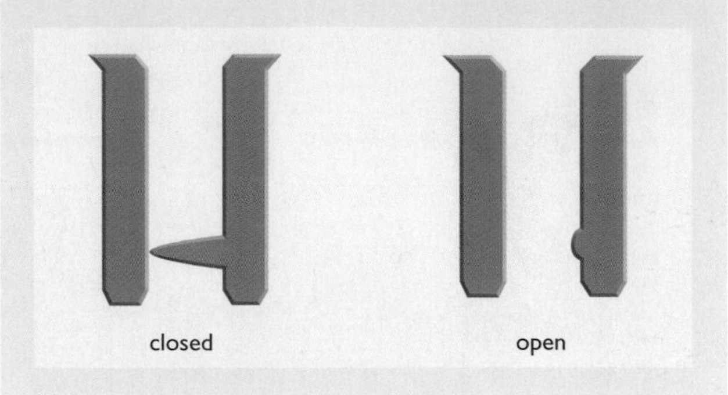

Fig. 2.16 Icon used for a voltage-gated ion channel, showing the channel closed and open. Some VOCs have only one and some two or three or more gates.

Some drugs have a molecular mechanism of action that involves modulation of the transition of the ROC between states (a process known as gating; see also VOCs).

The drug-binding site in an ROC is commonly termed the 'receptor' (that operates the 'channel'). Throughout this book, ROCs are denoted by an icon that is different from receptors for hormone, neurotransmitter and autocoid (Fig. 2.15).

Thus the ROC is conventionally described as a 'receptor' as well as a 'channel' and a 'channel with a receptor site'. Thus, the nicotinic cholinergic 'receptor' is actually an ROC (and, to add to the complexity, this ROC actually possesses two drug-binding sites).

In most cases an ROC agonist opens the channel, whereas an antagonist prevents the agonist from opening the channel and an inverse agonist closes the open channel. ROCs include:

- The nicotinic ROC (activated by acetylcholine).
- The $GABA_A$ ROC (activated by GABA).
- The glycine ROC (activated by glycine).
- The $5\text{-}HT_3$ ROC (activated by 5-hydroxytryptamine).
- The P_{2x} ROC (activated by adenosine).

The nicotinic receptor is part of an ROC that exists as a tetramer with two acetylcholine drug-binding sites on its external lip. Other ROCs show considerable homology with it. When two molecules of acetylcholine bind to the two drug-binding sites, the conformation of the ROC changes so that the channel component opens. This results in a sudden increase in permeability to Na^+ and K^+ ions, which depolarizes the adjacent cell membrane. There are several nicotinic ROC subtypes with small differences in composition, structure and tissue distribution. All are activated by acetylcholine but certain drugs have selectivity for one or other subtype. Some drugs (e.g. hexamethonium) affect ganglionic nicotinic ROCs in preference to the skeletal muscle ROC and others or vice versa (e.g. *d*-tubocurarine).

The $GABA_A$ ROC is a GABA-regulated Cl^- channel with two drug-binding sites, one that binds GABA and another that binds a class of tranquilizer drugs, the benzodiazepines (see Ch. 8). Agonist and antagonist binding to these sites results in a complex range of molecular responses. The $GABA_A$ ROC is found in many places in the central nervous system. Activation of this ROC generally causes hyperpolarization and this inhibits neuronal activity.

OTHER CELL MOLECULES SERVE AS DRUG MOLECULAR TARGETS

The molecular site at which drugs bind is described as its receptor. There are many cellular molecules that have drug receptors. They include:

- Voltage-operated channels.
- Transporters, symporters, antiporters and pumps.
- Enzymes.
- Nucleic acids.
- Structural macromolecules.

Voltage-operated channels (VOCs)

VOCs are modulated by membrane potential (voltage)

VOCs share many properties in common with ROCs. VOCs, like ROCs, are ion channels but are 'gated' only by voltage, although this functional distinction is not absolute since some ROCs have a degree of voltage dependence. If the gating of an ion channel is normally controlled by membrane potential, the channel is classed as a VOC. Endogenous modulation of VOCs by endogenous agents is normally only a minor feature of their behavior – most VOCs have no major endogenous modulators equivalent to acetylcholine (in its role as a nicotinic ROC agonist, for example). However, VOCs are the targets for certain drugs that can alter VOC state shifts or VOC voltage dependence (or simply cause channel block). In this context, different parts of the VOC are acting as molecular targets for exogenous drugs. Throughout this book VOCs are identified by the icon shown in Fig. 2.16.

VOCs constitute a family of molecular targets for drugs because they are structurally and functionally different from ROCs. A VOC drug target therefore possesses one or more drug-binding sites, a voltage sensor

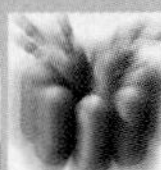

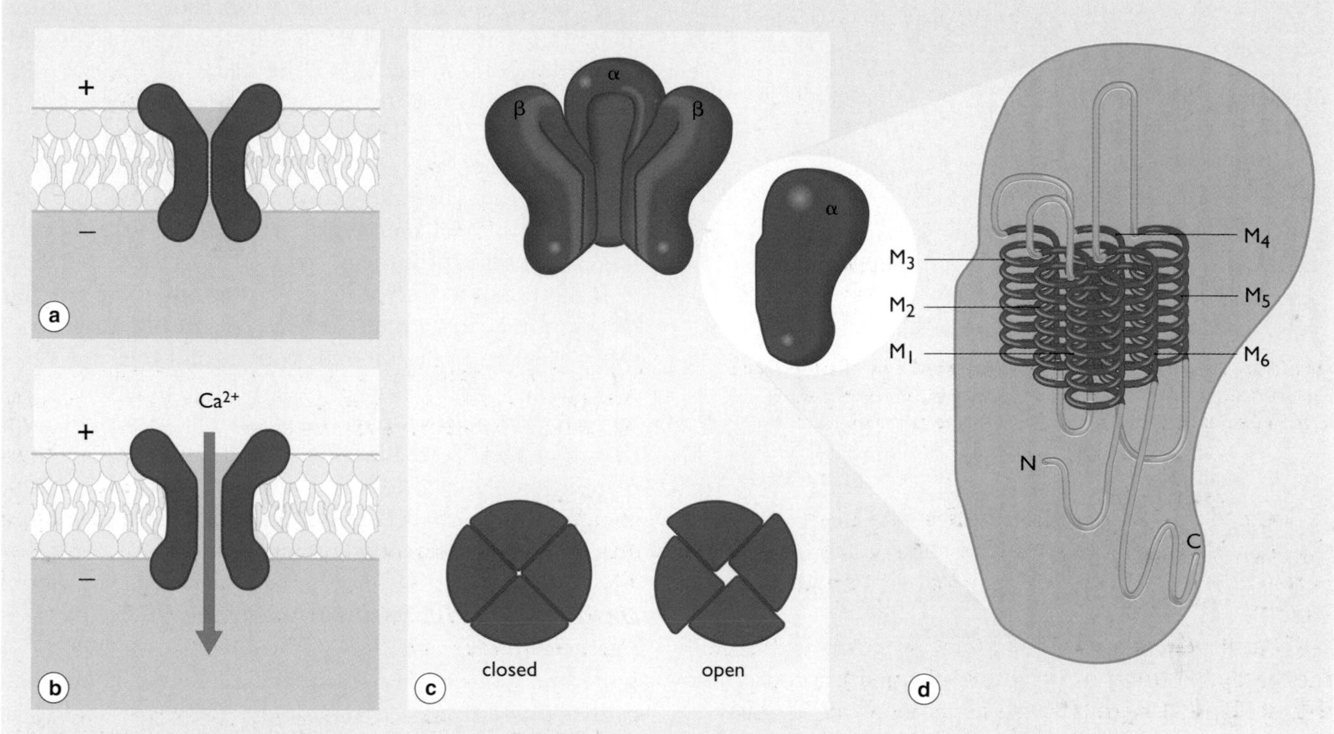

Fig. 2.17 Voltage-gated ion (Ca^{2+}) channel showing structure. (a) The rested channel is closed and ion passage is not possible. (b) When the channel opens, ions move down their concentration and charge gradients. (c) Reorientation of two α and β subunits is responsible for channel opening. (d) The complete structure of one of the α subunits. M_1–M_6 refer to the transmembrane spanning domains of the α subunit. C is the C terminal and N is the N terminal of the protein.

and a gating component. The gating component provides the molecular response and is influenced by both the voltage sensor and the ligand-binding site. The selectivity of VOCs to conduct different ions is determined by specific protein configurations within the channel pore (see Fig. 2.17).

The cardiac Na^+ channel is an example of a VOC

The cardiac Na^+ channel contains at least two voltage-operated gates that cause the VOC to open and close in response to changes in membrane potential (voltage dependence). Thus:

- One gate (the fast gate) opens and closes quickly (in milliseconds).
- The other (the slow gate) opens and closes slowly (in tens of milliseconds).

During diastole, when the membrane potential is negative, the slow gate is open and the fast gate closed. The net effect is that the channel is closed (non-conducting) but, because it can be activated, it is said to be in a 'rested' state (Fig. 2.18). However, if the membrane potential becomes more positive, the fast gate opens very quickly, so both gates are open and the channel becomes conducting and in an 'activated' state. The slow gate then slowly closes in response to the change in membrane potential. As a result, if the membrane potential stays positive, the channel will, with time, become closed again and unable to open in response to any stimulus ('inactivated'). Thus, VOCs that inactivate have the property of 'time dependence'.

Inactivation has an important effect. When the membrane potential repolarizes, the fast gate quickly closes while the slow gate requires further time to open. Thus both gates, and therefore the entire channel, are closed. If the membrane is suddenly depolarized (more positive) under these circumstances, the fast gate, which had rapidly opened before, will open again but the slow gate, which had closed during depolarization, will not open again because it is opened by negative membrane potentials and not by depolarization. The VOC will therefore not open.

If the membrane potential remains negative, the slow gate will open slowly again (characterizing the time dependence of recovery of the channel). A second depolarization will now be able to open the channel again, because the fast gate will open before the slow gate has time to close again.

Certain drugs can bind VOCs and modulate their behavior. Some drugs (notably class I antiarrhythmics, see Ch. 13) can bind to a VOC and change its conformation so that it is fixed in the inactivated state all the while that the drug is bound to it.

The affinity of a drug for its receptor may depend upon the state of the VOC

The apparent affinity of VOC-modulating drugs may depend on membrane potential, which determines the

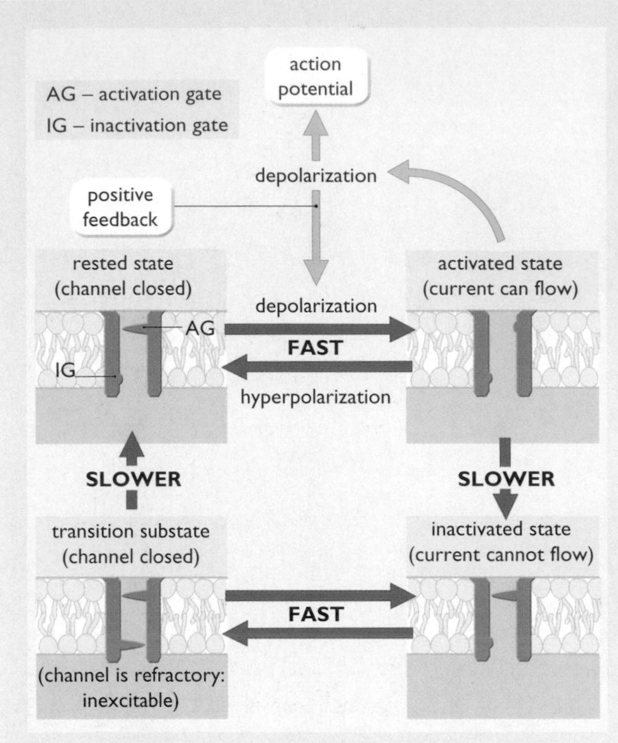

Fig. 2.18 Operation of inward currents in the heart. This is a simplified model showing two gates: one opens on depolarization and closes on hyper (re-)polarization and the other functions in the converse mode. Transition from the rested to activated state, under the influence of depolarization, is fast and elicits a positive feedback. This is the basis of the action potential. Inactivation is time dependent and results from a slower closure of a second gate at positive potentials. When the inactivation gate is closed (in the inactivated and transition substates), the cell is inexcitable. This transition contributes to repolarization. Transition from the slow voltage-dependent opening of the inactivation gate determines the refractory period (the period of inexcitability during the action potential).

state of the VOC and the rate at which it cycles through its different states. This gives rise to the characteristic voltage and frequency dependence seen for the action of some drugs. There are two possible molecular explanations for such behavior:

- The affinity and/or the access of the drug for its receptor are determined by the state of the VOC.
- The access of the drug to its receptor is determined by the state of the VOC.

It is possible to model the action of many VOC-modulating drugs by conceptualizing that the receptor for the drug changes its conformation as the VOC changes state, hence changing the VOC's affinity for the drug. The simplest scenario is one in which a drug can bind to any one of the states of the VOC described above, as shown in Fig. 2.18. A drug therefore will bind to its molecular target preferentially when the VOC is in the rested state, the activated state or the inactive state. A drug whose affinity is greatest for the activated state is therefore referred to as an activated state blocker.

If the receptor is the intracellular or in the intramembrane part of the VOCs, and if the drug reaches this site through the open VOC, the drug will appear to be use-dependent in its action (it requires the opening or 'use' of the VOC). Highly lipid-soluble drugs do not necessarily need an open VOC to access their receptors since they are able to easily move through the lipid bilayer of the cell membrane to access their molecular target. Consequently, their actions are less use-dependent.

It is difficult to discriminate between all of the possible drug binding sites within a VOC. As a result, a variety of terms are used to describe the actions of drugs on VOCs. The terms 'VOC blocker', 'agonist', 'antagonist' and 'negative modulator' have been used to describe drugs that modulate VOC function. The common terms most conventionally used (e.g. Na^+ channel blocker and Ca^{2+} antagonists) do not reflect the exact mechanism by which drugs modulate channel function.

Drug interactions with Na^+-selective VOCs (Na^+ channels)

Different types of Na^+ channels are found in neurons, cardiac muscle and skeletal muscle. They vary slightly in structure and protein composition. Drugs that impair Na^+ channel function are conventionally known as Na^+ channel blockers and, to a certain extent, can be used as experimental tools to discriminate between the role of different types of Na^+ channel in health and disease. For example, tetrodotoxin (a toxin found in puffer fish, some salamanders and one type of octopus) can block neuronal and skeletal muscle Na^+ channels at concentrations as low as 10 nM but the concentration needed to block cardiac muscle Na^+ channels is 10–100 times higher.

Three types of drug that block Na^+-selective VOCs (Na^+ channels) are used therapeutically

Tetrodotoxin, class I antiarrhythmic drugs and local anesthetic drugs block Na^+ channels:

- Tetrodotoxin has a molecular selectivity for neuronal channels. It is a highly charged molecule that does not cross the cell membrane and binds to an extracellular drug binding sites on the VOC.
- Class I antiarrhythmic drugs can be used to treat certain forms of cardiac arrhythmia and bind to an intracellular receptor. There are three types of class I antiarrhythmic (Ia, Ib and Ic), defined according to the relative affinities and kinetics of binding and dissociation (called 'unbinding' in this context) with the VOC in its three states.
- Local anesthetics such as lidocaine and bupivacaine have little selectivity for the neuronal Na^+ channel but when administered locally, they have a preferential effect on sensory nerves (see Ch. 8). Some local anesthetics bind to the neuronal Na^+ channel at an intracellular binding site, meaning that they must cross the cell membrane to block the channel.

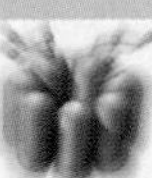

Drug interactions with Ca^{2+}-selective VOCs (Ca^{2+} channels)

At least five types of Ca^{2+} VOC occur in plasma membranes (L, T, N, P, Q) which allow the entry of Ca^{2+} into cells. These VOCs can be found in many different types of tissue. The best characterized and the most important (clinically) is the L (long-lasting) type, found in cardiac and smooth muscle. It opens during depolarization and then inactivates (more slowly than the Na^+ VOC) by voltage-dependent gating. The L-type VOC is blocked by a variety of clinically important drugs, Ca^{2+} channel blockers, known as Ca^{2+} antagonists.

There are three chemical classes of clinically important L-type Ca^{2+} channel blockers

These classes are:

- Benzothiazepine derivatives (e.g. diltiazem).
- Phenethylalkylamines (e.g. verapamil).
- Dihydropyridines (e.g. nifedipine, amlodipine).

All L-type Ca^{2+} channel blockers have selective actions in vascular smooth muscle, but some are more selective than others. For example, the 1,4-dihydropyridines (e.g. nifedipine) show marked selectivity for vascular smooth muscle in comparison with other tissue expressing L channels (notably cardiac tissue). Consequently, lower doses cause vascular smooth muscle relaxation (vasodilation) without impairing cardiac output. This is the basis for the use of nifedipine in the treatment of high blood pressure.

The main reason for this vascular selectivity is that vascular smooth muscle cells undergo sustained periods of depolarization (the basis of vasoconstriction), whereas cardiac tissue is depolarized only transiently (i.e. only during systole). Sustained depolarization maintains a high proportion of L channels in the activated and inactivated states compared with rested state. Nifedipine has relative selectivity for the activated and inactivated state of the L channel and therefore binds relatively slowly during depolarization and dissociates (unbinds) relatively quickly when tissue repolarizes.

Verapamil (a phenethylalkylamine Ca^{2+} blocker) has different characteristics of L channel binding and as a consequence is less vascular selective than the 1,4-dihydropyridines and may block cardiac as well as vascular L channels at high doses. Unlike nifedipine, verapamil is therefore of value in the treatment of cardiac arrhythmias that involve the AV node. This is a good example of how tissue selectivity is determined by subtleties in molecular mechanism of action.

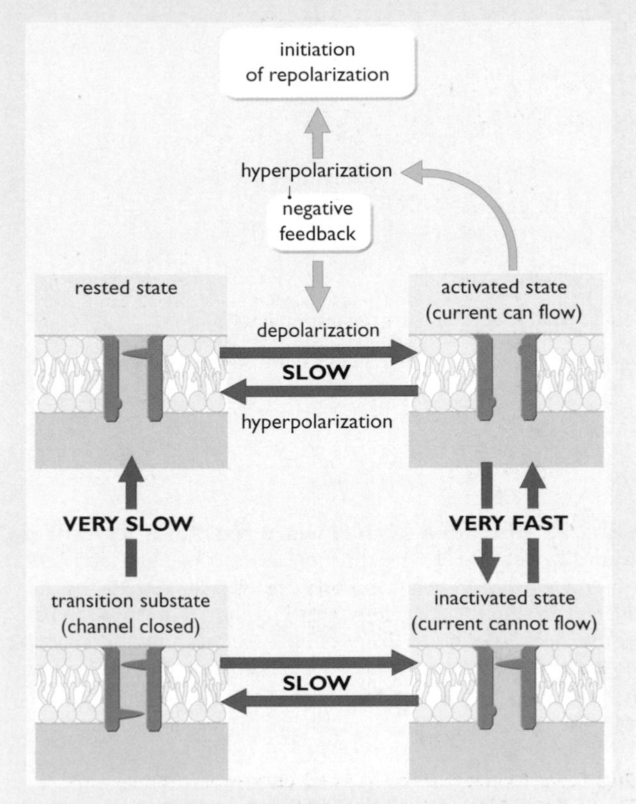

Fig. 2.19 Operation of the rapid delayed rectifier K^+ current (IKr) found in the heart. The channel possesses two gates and can thus cycle between four states. Depolarization shifts the channel state from rested to activated, allowing hyperpolarizing outward current to flow. This has a negative feedback influence on depolarization, thus contributing to the initiation of re-(hyper-)polarization. Time dependence occurs because of slow voltage-dependent transition to an inactivated state. This cycles, via a substate, to the basal state (rested). The relative speed of the state transitions (kinetics) is shown.

Drug interactions with K^+-selective VOCs (K^+ channels)

The opening of VOCs selective for K^+ results in the generation of outward-going (hyperpolarizing) currents. There are many types of K^+ channel and they show great diversity in structure, characteristics of opening and closing, affinity for drugs and expression in different organs and tissues. This has major potential therapeutic implications for targeting of drugs for specific tissues and diseases. At least six different 'families' (with major structural differences) of K^+ channels have been identified and each family contains several members (K^+ channels with minor variations in structure). It is not uncommon for a single type of tissue to express several different K^+ channels (e.g. there are more than 10 different types of K^+ channel in the heart).

The nomenclature for the K^+ currents associated with the different channels is confusing because it is largely determined by the tissue in which the current is observed. For example, the heart has a rapid Ca^{2+}-independent transient outward K^+ current that is called Ito_1 and neuronal tissue has a K^+ current called I_A, but the channel responsible for both currents is actually the same. The nomenclature for K^+ channels is based upon the gene family, protein structure and voltage characteristics (K_v channels).

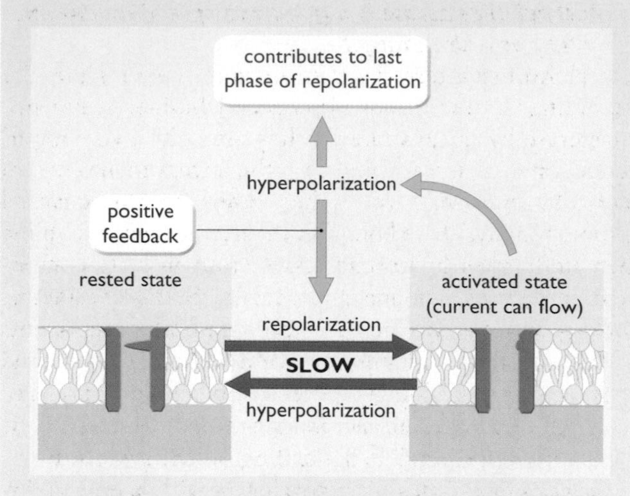

Fig. 2.20 Operation of the inward rectifier K^+ current (I_{K1}) found in the heart. The channel possesses one gate and can thus cycle between two states only. Repolarization shifts the channel to the activated state. The K^+ current that flows causes further repolarization so that a positive feedback ensues. There is no inactivation because there is no second gate that closes after repolarization. However, the outward K^+ current is reduced by intracellular Mg^{2+}.

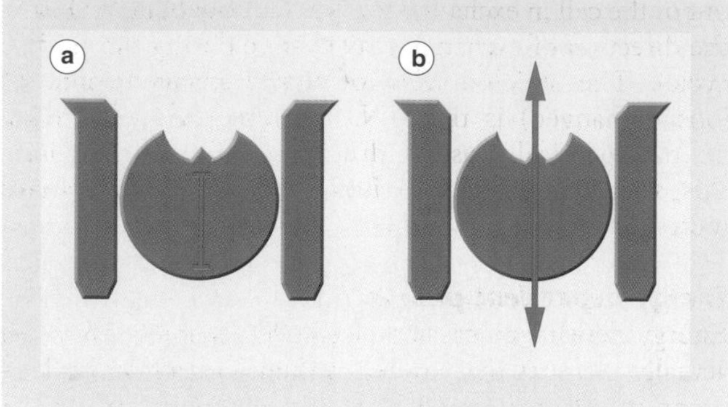

Fig. 2.21 Icon used for an energy-independent carrier molecule (transporter, symporter or antiporter). (a) A transporter or symporter (characterized by unidirectional transport) shown in its inactive state. (b) An antiporter (characterized by two-way transport) shown in its activated state.

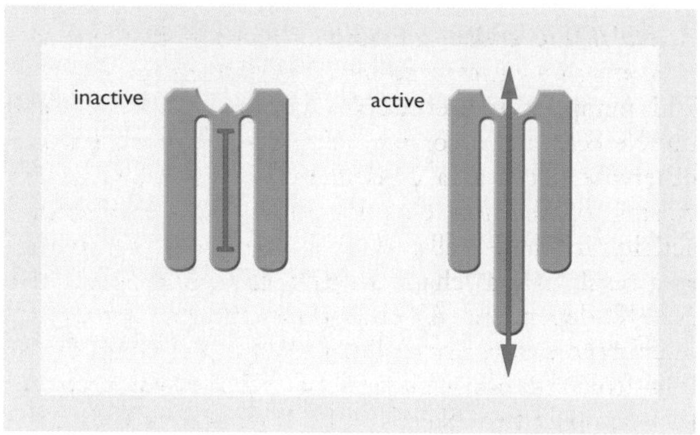

Fig. 2.22 Icon used for a pump, showing the inactive and active states.

K^+ channels and their associated currents vary in their dependence on voltage and time

There are marked differences in dependence on voltage and time between different K^+ currents. For example, the rapid delayed rectifying K^+ current (IK_r) is activated by depolarization and is time dependent (it inactivates), whereas the inwardly rectifying K^+ current (IK_1) is activated by hyperpolarization and shows no time-dependent inactivation (Figs 2.19 and 2.20). In the heart, the mixed properties of the different K^+ channels contribute to the unusual shape of the cardiac action potential.

Other VOCs

Although the majority of the scientific literature on ion channels has focused on cation (Na^+, Ca^{2+} and K^+) channels, it has become apparent that voltage-gated channels exist for anions, for example Cl^-. Cl^- channels are found both peripherally and in the central nervous system (CNS). There are a variety of other ion channels with peculiar characteristics. Some are not selective for a single ion. For example, the channel responsible for the 'funny' current (I_f) in the heart allows the passage of both Na^+ and K^+.

Transporters, symporters, antiporters and pumps

All cells constantly regulate their internal concentrations of ions, as well as molecules such as sugars, nucleic acids and amino acids. Their passage across cell membranes is facilitated by energy-independent carrier molecules (transporters, symporters and antiporters) and by energy-dependent pumps. All are oriented proteins that have one or more sites that bind weakly with one or more passengers (ion or molecule). This binding alters their conformation from a rested to an activated state. The change in conformation translocates the passenger across the membrane. In the case of pumps, the conformation change converts the protein into an enzyme that normally hydrolyzes ATP (the energy dependence of its activity) and ATP hydrolysis is necessary for the pump to translocate its passenger. Pumps and carriers can be molecular targets for certain drugs. Throughout the book, icons are used to indicate energy-independent carriers (Fig. 2.21) and pumps (Fig. 2.22).

Energy-independent transporters, symporters and antiporters

Energy-independent carriers are called transporters (which move one type of ion or molecule in one direction), symporters (which move two or more ions or molecules in one direction) or antiporters (which exchange one or more ions or molecules for one or more other ions or molecules). An example of an antiporter is the Na^+/Ca^{2+} exchanger, which normally extrudes Ca^{2+}

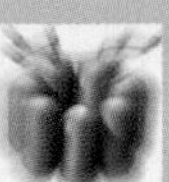

out of the cell in exchange for Na^+ (although, in the heart, the direction of exchange may change during the cardiac cycle). The stoichiometry of this exchanger (ratio of ions exchanged) is three Na^+ to one Ca^{2+}. There are no therapeutically useful drugs that directly modulate this target, although digitalis modulates its activity indirectly.

Energy-dependent pumps

Energy-dependent carriers are called pumps. They are actually enzymes that, owing to their location and orientation in cell membranes, have the ability to translocate ions or other molecules through a central pore as a consequence of conformation changes that take place during the enzymatic hydrolysis of ATP (other enzymes that do not have this property represent another class of drug molecular target and are described below).

Na^+/K^+-dependent adenosine triphosphatase (ATPase) is a well-characterized membrane pump.

This pump acts to prevent Na^+ accumulation in nerve and muscle cells and a corresponding loss of K^+ that would otherwise occur as a consequence of the opening and closing of the ion channels that generate electrical activity in these cells. As Na^+ begins to accumulate as a result of Na^+ channel openings (action potentials), Na^+/K^+-dependent ATPase transfers Na^+ across the membrane to the extracellular fluid in exchange for K^+ ions from the extracellular fluid. The stoichiometry of this pump is two Na^+ for three K^+, meaning that the pump is electrogenic. The energy for this is supplied by the hydrolysis of ATP. This pump is an important molecular target for the heart drug digitalis.

Enzymes

The body contains a large variety of enzymes, each of which is a potential molecular target for drugs.

Drugs can either mimic the enzyme's natural substrate (binding with the enzyme's substrate binding site, also known as its 'active' site) or bind with an allosteric site. Normally such molecular actions result in inhibition of enzyme activity. The icon for enzymes is shown in Fig. 2.23.

Enzyme inhibition has characteristics similar to receptor antagonism

Drugs that bind with an enzyme at the substrate binding site are usually competitive inhibitors (by analogy with drugs that bind receptor in a competitive manner – competitive antagonists). However, other drugs bind to sites separate from the substrate binding site. This can lead to enzyme inhibition via allosteric mechanisms, or by disruption of the enzyme's biochemical integrity which is analogous to non- and uncompetitive receptor antagonism (discussed on page 19 and detailed elsewhere in this chapter).

Acetylcholinesterase is a good example of an enzyme acting as a drug target

Acetylcholinesterase is the enzyme responsible for degrading the neurotransmitter acetylcholine. Acetylcholinesterase has a substrate-binding site with two components, one of which binds to the esteratic moiety of acetylcholine while the other binds to the charged anionic moiety. Once bound to the enzyme, acetylcholine then undergoes hydrolytic dissociation into its component molecules, choline and acetate. Some cholinester analogs of acetylcholine can bind with both components of the substrate-binding site while other analogs bind with only one. In doing so, they inhibit the hydrolysis of acetylcholine. The interaction is competitive and can be reversible or irreversible depending on the inhibitor.

Organophosphates bind covalently with acetylcholinesterase at the esteratic component of the substrate-binding site, resulting in irreversible inhibition. These compounds have been used as nerve gases in chemical warfare and as insecticides (they can be an important cause of accidental poisoning). However, before organophosphates bind covalently there is an initial stage of reversible binding. Antidote drugs (e.g. pralidoxime) can prevent covalent binding during this reversible phase by competing for binding. Their administration (after covalent binding is complete) gives no benefit.

Many anticancer drugs inhibit the activity of enzymes involved in protein and nucleic acid synthesis

Anticancer enzyme inhibitors include:

- Azathioprine, 6-mercaptopurine and 6-thioguanine, which block ribonucleotide synthesis from purines.
- 5-Fluorouracil and methotrexate, which act by blocking deoxyribonucleotides and 2′ deoxythymidylate synthesis.
- Cytarabine, which inhibits DNA polymerase and RNA synthesis.
- Doxorubicin, etoposide, amsacrine and dactinomycin, which inhibit DNA replication and RNA transcription.

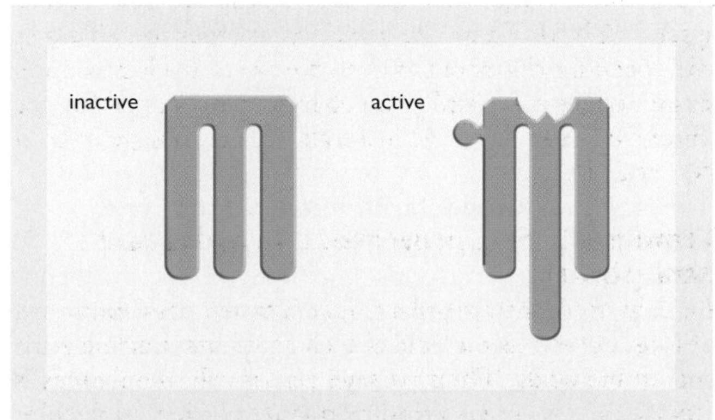

Fig. 2.23 Icon used for an enzyme target showing the inactive and active states.

Nucleic acids

Certain types of anticancer drugs target nucleic acids, i.e. DNA and RNA, to achieve their effects. The cellular response (inhibition of DNA or RNA synthesis) is achieved by a variety of different molecular actions, for example:

- The bleomycins damage DNA and prevent its repair.
- Alkylating agents such as mitomycin and cisplatin cross-link DNA.

Structural macromolecules

Proteins (receptors, channels, symporters, etc.) are the most common molecular targets for drugs that act on cell membranes. However, certain drugs target structural macromolecules that are not linked to transduction components. Therefore, by definition, these drugs alter cell function indirectly by altering cell structure. Moreover, these receptors consist of many repeated chemical motifs that require saturation by an equivalent number of drug molecules for an effect to be achieved. Thus, the typical effective concentration range for drugs that target structural macromolecules is millimolar (10–1000 fold higher than for most other types of drug).

In cell membranes (whether the plasma membrane or intracellular membranes, including those surrounding cellular organelles such as the nucleus and mitochondria), the main structural component is a bilayer of phospholipids with a surrounding coat of glycoproteins. Other structural components include the cytoskeleton (a target for the anticancer drugs colchicine and vinblastine).

Molecular targets not in mammalian cells

Some drugs achieve their therapeutic effect without interacting directly with cells, for example:

- Chelating drugs, which act by binding to certain ions (such as Fe^{2+}, Fe^{3+} and Al^{3+}).
- Surfactants, which alter the surface physical properties of biologic fluids.
- Certain drugs used in the treatment of gastrointestinal disorders, which adsorb substances in the gut and so alter the consistency and transit time of the contents through the gastrointestinal tract, e.g. activated charcoal.
- Osmotic diuretics.
- Antacids.

Targets in or on bacteria, viruses, fungi and parasites

In most cases of infection and infestation, therapeutic drugs act directly on the relevant organism (bacterium, virus, fungus or parasite). The diverse molecular mechanisms of action of such drugs are conceptually identical to those of drugs that act on human tissue (i.e. modulation of receptors, enzymes) and are discussed in detail in Chapter 6.

Summary of the mechanisms of drug action on receptors, ion channels, carriers and enzymes

The mechanisms of drug action on molecular targets are summarized in Fig. 2.24. Examples of molecular targets for drug action are summarized in Table 2.3.

CELLULAR ACTIONS OF DRUGS (TRANSDUCTION)

The majority of molecular targets are linked by various biochemical mechanisms to cellular response components (G proteins, enzymes, ion channels, etc.). The operation of this linkage is known as transduction.

G protein-linked transduction

G proteins are molecules that are linked directly to a specific superfamily of receptors (described on page 25) or are linked indirectly to other drug molecular targets. The activated G proteins initiate (or suppress) many different cascades of cellular events that ultimately affect the function of ion channels, enzymes, DNA and other components of cells. A good example of this is the opening of K^+ channels in cardiac muscle following acetylcholine binding to muscarinic receptors and the increased protein kinase activity following epinephrine binding to β adrenoceptors.

G proteins consist of three subunits, α, β and γ (Fig. 2.25), ***and act as on–off switches for cell signaling***

When an agonist activates a G protein-coupled receptor, a conformational change in the receptor leads to the activation of a G protein. Activation of G proteins involves the release of guanosine diphosphate (GDP) and binding of guanosine triphosphate (GTP) to its α subunit and the dissociation of this subunit from the βγ subunit heterodimer. The α and βγ subunits activate a number of transduction components. The α subunit then hydrolyzes GTP to GDP, which in turn inactivates the α subunit, allowing it to reassociate with the βγ complex, rendering the G protein inactive.

Stimulation or inhibition of G proteins results in modulation of the enzyme system responsible for producing the following other transduction components (sometimes called second messengers):

- Cyclic nucleotides.
- Diacyl glycerol (DAG).
- Inositol phosphates.

For example, following β_2 adrenoceptor agonism, a G protein is activated. This in turn activates adenylyl cyclase, the enzyme that catalyzes the formation of cAMP. Transduction proceeds by cAMP activation, via protein kinases and phosphorylation, of enzymes whose types vary according to tissue.

There are many types of G protein in most cells. The α subtypes define the major properties of a G protein. For example, β adrenoceptors typically interact with G

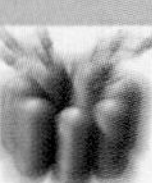

a
Receptors
agonist
transduction mechanisms
antagonist
effect of agonists blocked
b
Enzymes
inhibitor
normal reaction inhibited
false substrate
abnormal metabolite produced
S*
P*
pro-drug
active drug produced from inactive pro-drug
c
Channels
blockers (here of a VOC)
permeation blocked
modulators (here of an ROC)
increased or decreased opening probability
d
Transport carriers
X
antiporter
Y
exchange of ions X and Y across the membrane after binding of activating modulator
symporter
XY
extrusion of ions X and Y after binding of activating modulator

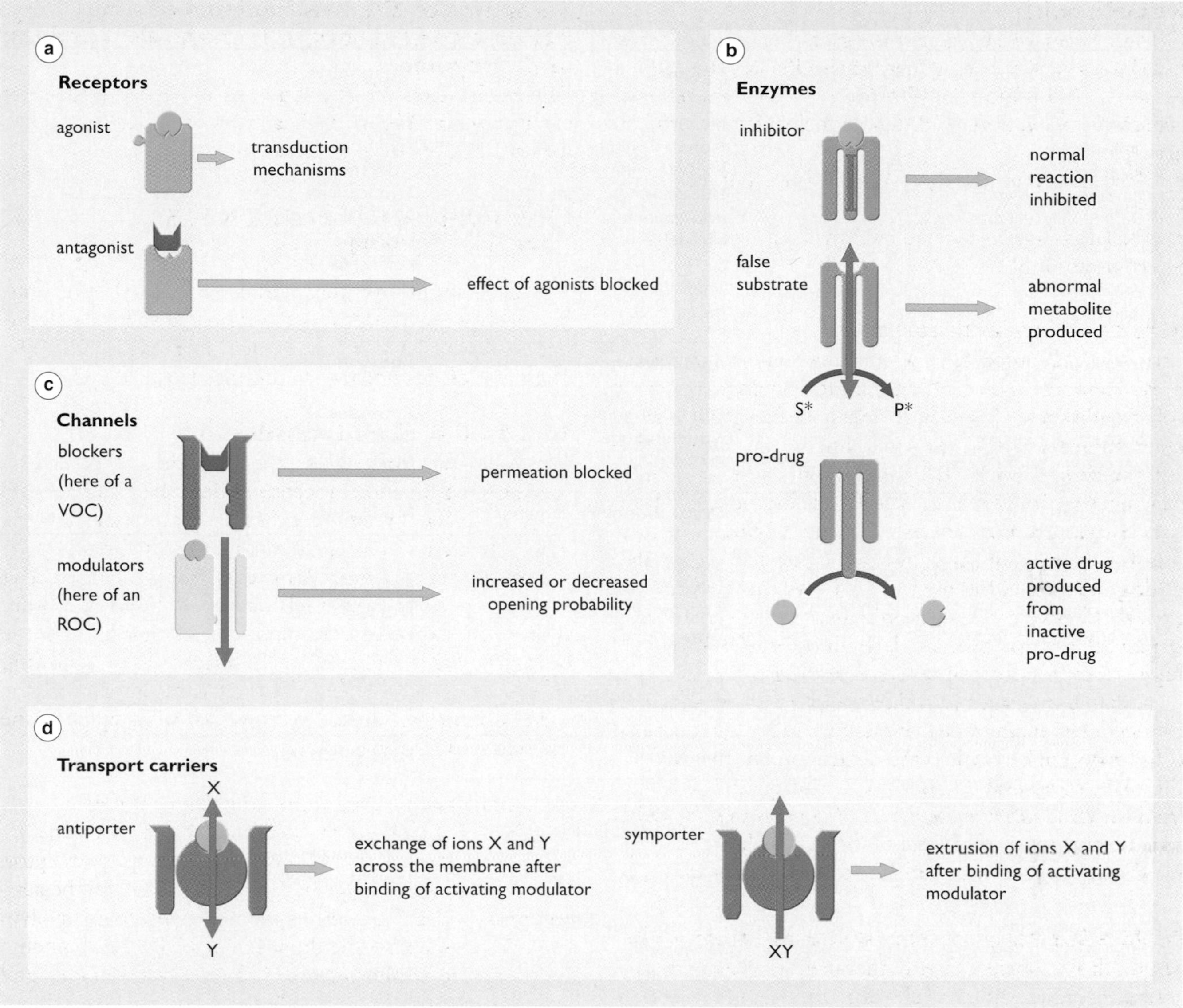

Fig. 2.24 Main molecular targets for drug action. Actions can be broadly divided into four classes. (a) Agonists can bind to receptors to initiate changes in transduction mechanisms, leading to a variety of cellular effects. Antagonists bind to receptors to block the effect of the agonist. (b) Drugs can block the passage of materials across channels or bind to components of the channel proteins to modulate the opening of ion channels. (c) Drugs can interact directly with the action of enzymes via a variety of mechanisms. S* and P* are false substrate and false product, respectively. (d) Drugs can bind to exchange proteins (antiporters) to move ions across the membrane. The direction of ion movement is shown by the direction of the arrow. Here, transporters are shown being activated by drugs but note that some transporters are active at rest and blocked by drugs. X and Y represent ions, which may have a positive or negative charge.

proteins having an α_s subunit which activates adenylyl cyclase.

Ca^{2+}-linked transduction

Mobilization of intracellular Ca^{2+} as a second messenger is the common final link in the chain of events resulting from the production of many transduction components.

Ca^{2+} is involved in transduction in the following processes:

- Smooth muscle contraction.
- Increased rate of contraction and relaxation of cardiac myocytes.
- Secretion of transmitter molecules or glandular secretions.
- Hormone release.
- Cytotoxicity.
- Activation of certain enzymes.

Its mobilization is linked to the activity of other transduction components. Ca^{2+} is stored on the membrane of endoplasmic reticulum of smooth muscle and is released when IP_3 acts on a specific ROC known as the IP_3 receptor.

DAG released by the actions of phospholipase C (and D) directly influences the activity of a membrane-bound protein kinase C, which is the enzyme responsible for

Table 2.3 Examples of molecular targets for drug action

Hormone and neurotransmitter receptors	**Agonists**	**Antagonists**
α_1 adrenoceptor	Norepinephrine	Prazosin
α_2 adrenoceptor	Norepinephrine	Yohimbine
β adrenoceptor	Isoproterenol	Propranolol
Histamine (H_1 receptor)	Histamine	Terfenadine
Histamine (H_2 receptor)	Impromidine	Cimetidine
Opiate (μ-receptor)	Morphine	Naloxone
5-HT_2 receptor	5-HT	Ketanserin
Thrombin	Thrombin	Hirudin
Insulin receptor	Insulin	Not known
Intracellular receptors	**Agonists**	**Antagonists**
Estrogen receptor	Ethinyl estradiol	Tamoxifen†
Progesterone receptor	Norethindrone	Danazol
Glucocorticosteroid receptor	Budesonide	Mifepristone
Ion channels	**Drugs that block channels**	**Modulators**
Voltage-gated Na^+ channels	Lidocaine	
Voltage-gated Ca^{2+} channels	Dihydropyridine	Dihydropyridines
Voltage-gated K^+ channels	4-Aminopyridine	Ibutilide
ATP-sensitive K^+ channels	Glyburide	Lemakalim Sulfonylureas
GABA-gated Cl^- channels	Picrotoxin	Benzodiazepines
Glutamate-gated (NMDA) cation channels	Dizocilpine	Glycine
Enzymes	**Inhibitors**	**False substrates**
Acetylcholinesterase	Neostigmine Organophosphate insecticides	
Choline acetyltransferase		Hemicholinium
Cyclo-oxygenase	Indometacin	Eicosatetraenoic acid
Angiotensin-converting enzyme	Enalapril	
Carbonic anhydrase	Acetazolamide	
HMG-CoA reductase	Simvastatin	
Dopa decarboxylase	Carbidopa	Methyldopa
DNA polymerase	Cytarabine	Cytarabine
Enzymes involved in DNA synthesis	Azathioprine	
Enzymes of blood clotting cascade	Heparin	
Phosphodiesterase	Theophylline	
Carriers	**Inhibitors**	
Choline carrier (nerve terminal)	Hemicholinium	
Norepinephrine uptake 1	Tricyclic antidepressants Cocaine	
5-HT uptake	Fluoxetine	
Renal weak acid transfer	Probenecid	
Na^+ pump	Digitalis	
Na^+/H^+ exchanger	Amiloride	

†Can act as a partial agonist in certain tissues.
GABA, γ-aminobutyric acid; 5-HT, 5-hydroxytryptamine; HMG-CoA, 2-hydroxy-3-methylglutaryl coenzyme A; NMDA, *N*-methyl D-aspartate.
Many of these molecular targets have multiple subtypes or isoforms; these differences may have considerable therapeutic importance in terms of drug specificity

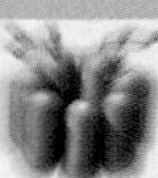

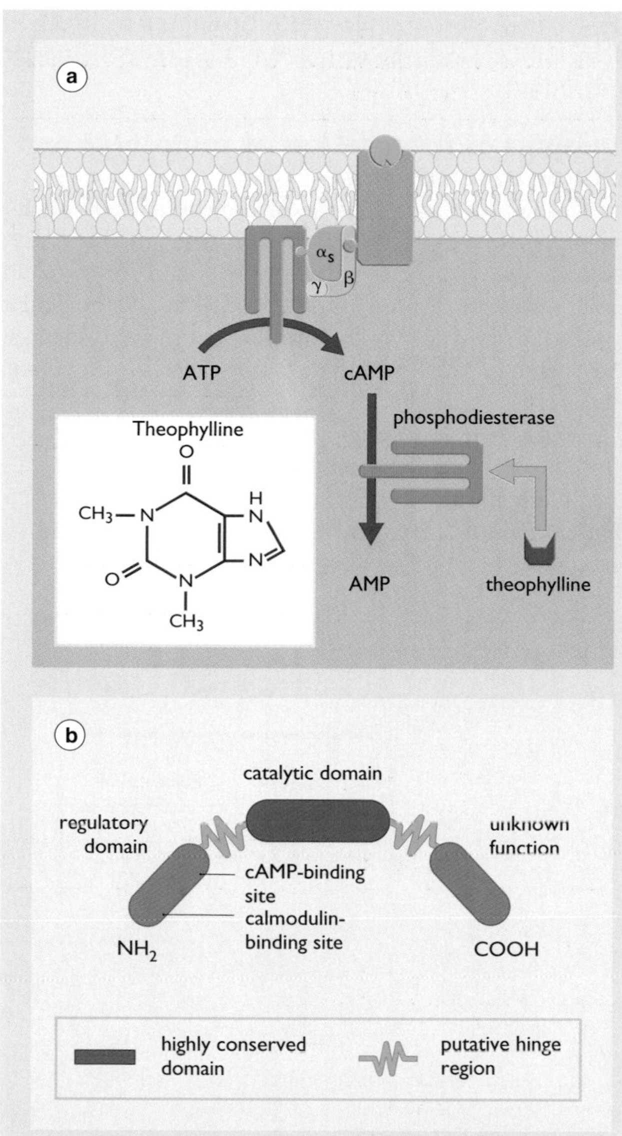

Fig. 2.25 Example of enzyme-initiated transduction. Phosphodiesterase enzymes (a) are involved in the metabolism of the cyclic nucleotides (e.g. cAMP). This family of enzymes is inhibited by theophylline (insert). Inhibition leads to accumulation of cyclic nucleotides within cells (b). Note that cyclic nucleotides accumulate in response to the action of drugs on G protein-linked nucleotide cyclase enzymes.

phosphorylating serine and threonine residues and the subsequent change in activation state of more than 50 different proteins. There are at least six types of protein kinase C, each with its own substrate specificity.

Protein kinase C-linked transduction

Protein kinase C is an important component of transduction in the following processes:

- Modulation of the release of endocrine hormones and neurotransmitters.
- Smooth muscle contraction.
- Inflammation.
- Ion transport.
- Tumor promotion.

> **Actions of important G proteins**
>
> - G_s stimulates adenylyl cyclase and activates Ca^{2+} channels
> - G_i inhibits adenylyl cyclase and activates K^+ channels
> - G_q activates phospholipase C
> - G_o inhibits Ca^{2+} currents
> - G_t stimulates adenylyl cyclase in the eye
> - G_{df} stimulates adenylyl cyclase in the nose
> - βα subunits activate many transduction components

Transduction initiated by DNA-coupled receptors

Activation of DNA-coupled transduction involves a change in protein synthesis. For example, steroids displace HSP90 and the resulting steroid–receptor complex then translocates to the nucleus. Once in the nucleus, the steroid–receptor complex can recognize specific base sequences and activate specific genes. This is a slow process compared with the millisecond responses that are found in other forms of transduction. For example:

- Glucocorticosteroids increase the production of lipocortin, which accounts for some of their actions as antiinflammatory drugs.
- Mineralocorticosteroids increase the production of specific renal transport molecules involved in the renal tubular transport of Na^+ and K^+.

Transduction initiated by receptors with tyrosine kinase activity

The activation of tyrosine kinase receptors allows autophosphorylation of tyrosine residues, which serve as high-affinity sites for a variety of intracellular proteins. The phosphorylated receptor can then act as a platform for other proteins to bind, leading to phosphorylation and the activation of pathways involving a cascade of other protein kinases. Many of the resultant signaling pathways are the same as those initiated by certain G proteins.

Many tyrosine kinase receptors possess binding sites for other proteins involved in signal transduction. One such binding site is termed SH_2. The binding of an inactive enzyme to SH_2 leads to a highly selective activation of the enzyme. Often the activated enzyme is involved in gene transcription. A series of protein kinases, IP_3 and Ca^{2+} may participate in the intermediary stages of transduction. Many growth factors act through this mechanism. There is therefore considerable interest in the possibility of finding drugs that interact with SH_2 or mimic SH_2 activity because they could have profound effects on growth and differentiation and, by implication, cancer, immunologic diseases and other disorders. Proteins involved in tyrosine kinase receptor transduction include the small G protein 'ras'.

Transduction initiated by ROCs

When an ROC initiates transduction, the events are triggered by a change in the membrane potential associated with an increase (or decrease) in the permeability of those ions which pass through the ROC. Thus, transduction begins with the movement of charge. This results in depolarization or hyperpolarization of the membrane. The most common location of an ROC is the plasma membrane but ROCs are also present in mitochondria and other intracellular organelles.

A change in membrane potential can directly modulate tissue function. In skeletal muscle, nicotinic ROC activation depolarizes the end-plate plasma membrane and, subsequently (after action potential generation in the sarcolemma), the sarcoplasmic reticulum, which causes release of Ca^{2+} into the cytoplasm. This triggers muscle contraction.

Examples of integration of molecular and cellular mechanisms

Some examples of integration of molecular and cellular mechanisms are described below and in Fig. 2.26. Characteristically, the speed of transduction and production of the tissue response is determined by the molecular target (receptor) and by the mechanism of transduction. The speed of this determines the onset of the tissue response. For example:

- Interaction of an agonist with an ROC produces rapid (milliseconds) cell hyperpolarization or depolarization.
- Interaction of an agonist with a G protein-coupled receptor may lead to one of many responses on a timescale of seconds.

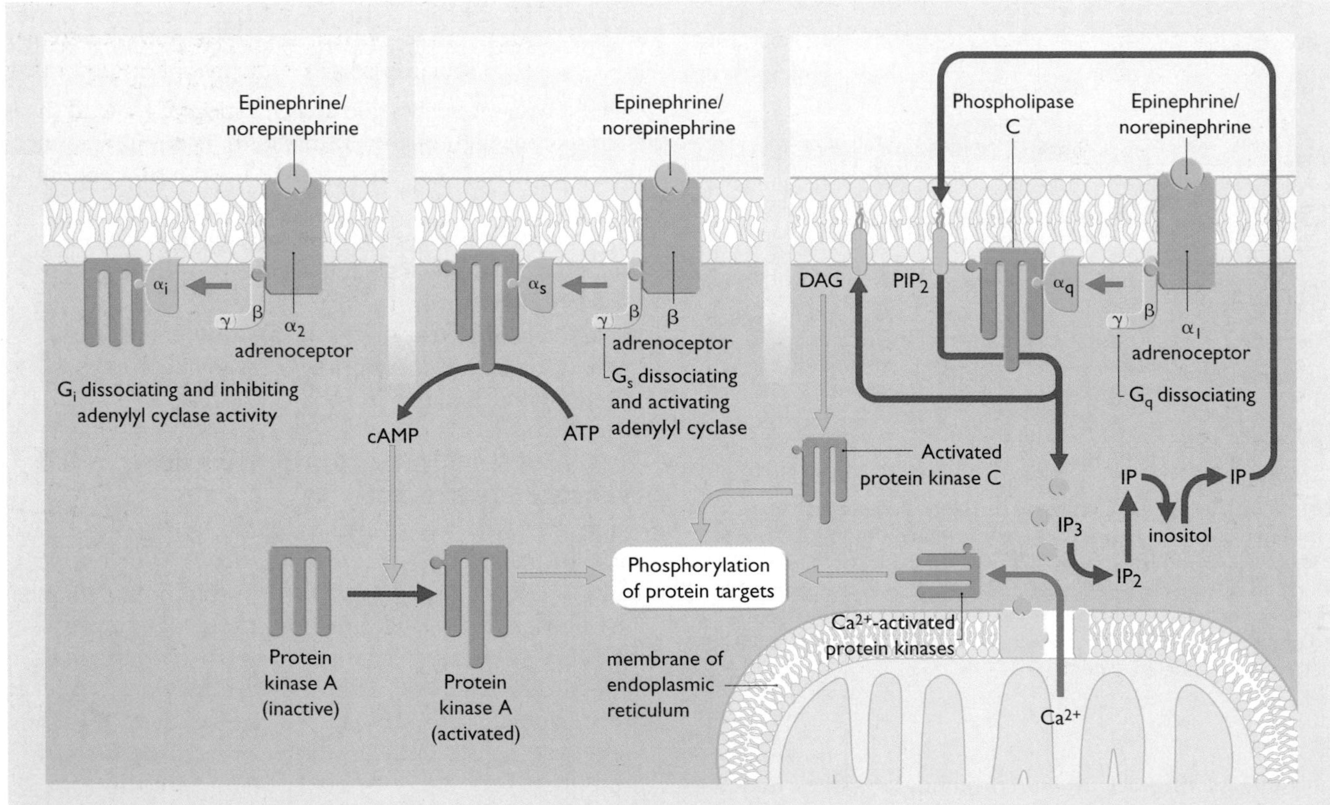

Fig. 2.26 Several types of transduction can lead to phosphorylation of protein targets. cAMP and the phosphatidyl inositol cycle are important transduction components (second messengers). cAMP production increases in response to activation of many G protein-coupled receptors (e.g. α_2 or β_1 receptor activation by epinephrine). The central part of the figure shows this occurring in response to β adrenoceptor agonism. Protein kinases (e.g. protein kinase A), activated by cAMP, are secondary messengers participating in the cellular response. Certain types of agonism (e.g. α_2 adrenoceptor activation) lead to inhibition of cAMP production via activation of inhibitory G proteins (upper left panel of figure). The enzyme phospholipase C (located in the cell membrane) is activated by an agonist to produce the second messengers Ins(1,4,5) P_3 (inositol triphosphate, IP_3) and diacyl glycerol (DAG) (right hand panel). Intracellular IP_3 releases intracellular Ca^{2+}, whereas DAG remains in the membrane where it activates protein kinase C. IP_3 undergoes sequential dephosphorylation by intracellular phosphatases (not shown) to give IP_2, IP and inositol, which can then be incorporated into the membrane to form phosphatidyl inositol (PI) which, via ATP, is phosphorylated in steps to phosphatidyl inositol diphosphate (PIP_2). The recycling of IP_3 and DAG into phosphatidyl inositol is blocked by lithium, which depletes inositol lipids in the brain and is used as a drug in the treatment of manic depression (see Ch. 8).

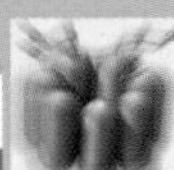

- Interaction of a drug directly with an enzyme may lead to changes on a timescale of minutes.
- Interaction of a drug directly with DNA may lead to altered gene expression and the synthesis of a new protein over a period of hours.

Some examples of the integration between molecular and cellular responses are shown in Figs 2.26 and 2.27.

TISSUE AND SYSTEM ACTIONS OF DRUGS

Drugs have tissue and system actions that result from their molecular and cellular actions. Thus, in the case of some drugs we can now successfully explain their integrated molecular, cellular, tissue and system action. One example is tetrodotoxin, whose molecular action is to block Na^+ VOCs, with a diminishing order of potency in nervous tissue, skeletal muscle and cardiac muscle. Thus we are able to accurately predict tetrodotoxin's actions from cellular to tissue level. Since tetrodotoxin selectively binds to Na^+ VOCs in nerves, low doses block peripheral nerves (sensory, autonomic and motor).

However, it is often difficult to predict tissue and system actions of new drugs on the basis of their molecular and cellular actions. This is because selectivity of action diminishes as one moves from molecular through cellular actions to actions at the tissue and system levels, as a consequence of cells and tissues reacting to the initial effects of the drug (homeostasis). Homeostasis is additionally altered by disease states. Thus we rarely have enough physiologic and pathologic knowledge to be able to predict exactly how molecular and cellular actions of new drugs will translate into tissue and systems actions.

Body systems are complex and under the control of many homeostatic inputs that respond to the initial tissue response and are perturbed by disease. The ultimate system response to any drug (or indeed any other bodily intervention) is therefore difficult to anticipate. Beyond the remit of pharmacology, but of therapeutic relevance, this is also a potentially poignant message for those who predict that diseases may one day be treatable by genetically mutating (and altering the function) of specific individual cell components.

The concept of body systems is useful when considering mechanisms of action of drugs

The division of the body into various systems is somewhat arbitrary and subjective but most pharmacologists accept that a systems approach is useful while recognizing

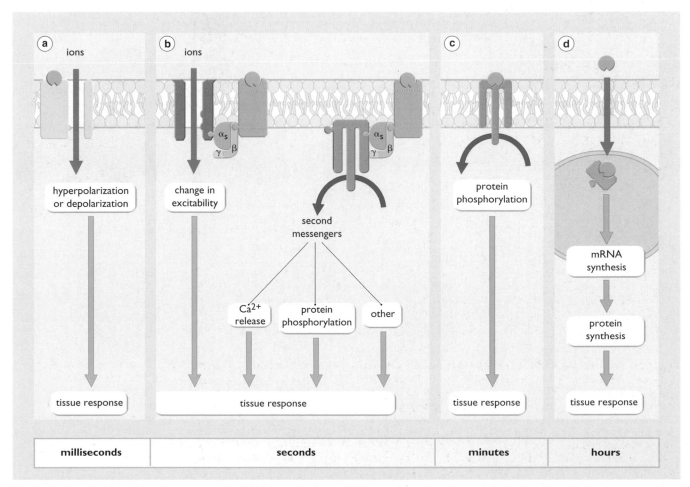

Fig. 2.27 Integration of molecular and cellular mechanisms. (a) Receptor-operated ion channel-linked transduction is very rapid. (b) G protein-linked transduction is rapid. (c) Enzyme- and pump-linked transduction is slow. (d) DNA-linked transduction is very slow.

that the whole body integrates all such systems. It is therefore possible to consider the action of drugs on the CNS separately from their actions on the cardiovascular or endocrine systems.

As an example, the actions of some of the drugs used to treat high blood pressure can be explained solely in terms of their actions on the cardiovascular system (see Ch. 13). Obviously, actions on the cardiovascular system have implications for the rest of the body. However, when examining mechanisms of drug action it is reasonable for the sake of simplicity sometimes to consider only the target system itself and regard all other actions as a consequence of the effects on the target system.

This book is organized on the basis of body systems. Thus Chapters 8–23, inclusive, deal with drug actions on the component systems of the whole body. This 'systems' approach allows the reader to consider drugs from a quasi-pharmacotherapeutic approach since the therapeutic actions of drugs often follow body systems. Furthermore, many medical students now use the problem-based learning approach to study, which is generally systems based.

Previously we have discussed the details of a drug binding to its receptor. We now need to consider how such models translate into the reality of drugs producing effects in cells, tissues, systems and populations.

DOSE–RESPONSE (DR) RELATIONSHIPS

Earlier in this chapter the binding of a drug to a receptor was discussed in terms of a simple mass action type of interaction. It is found that the models developed as a result of these assumptions have their counterpart when we investigate the relationship between response and drug concentration for tissues and organs, or between response and dose for whole animal or human populations. This area of study is generally known as 'dose–response' relationships.

The relationship between the log of the dose (concentration) of an agonist drug and response often resembles a sigmoid curve similar to those shown in Fig. 2.29, which in turn closely resembles the shape of the drug–receptor binding curve shown previously. The effect (E) is a tissue response or, less usually, the inhibition of spontaneous activity (e.g. slowing of heart rate by

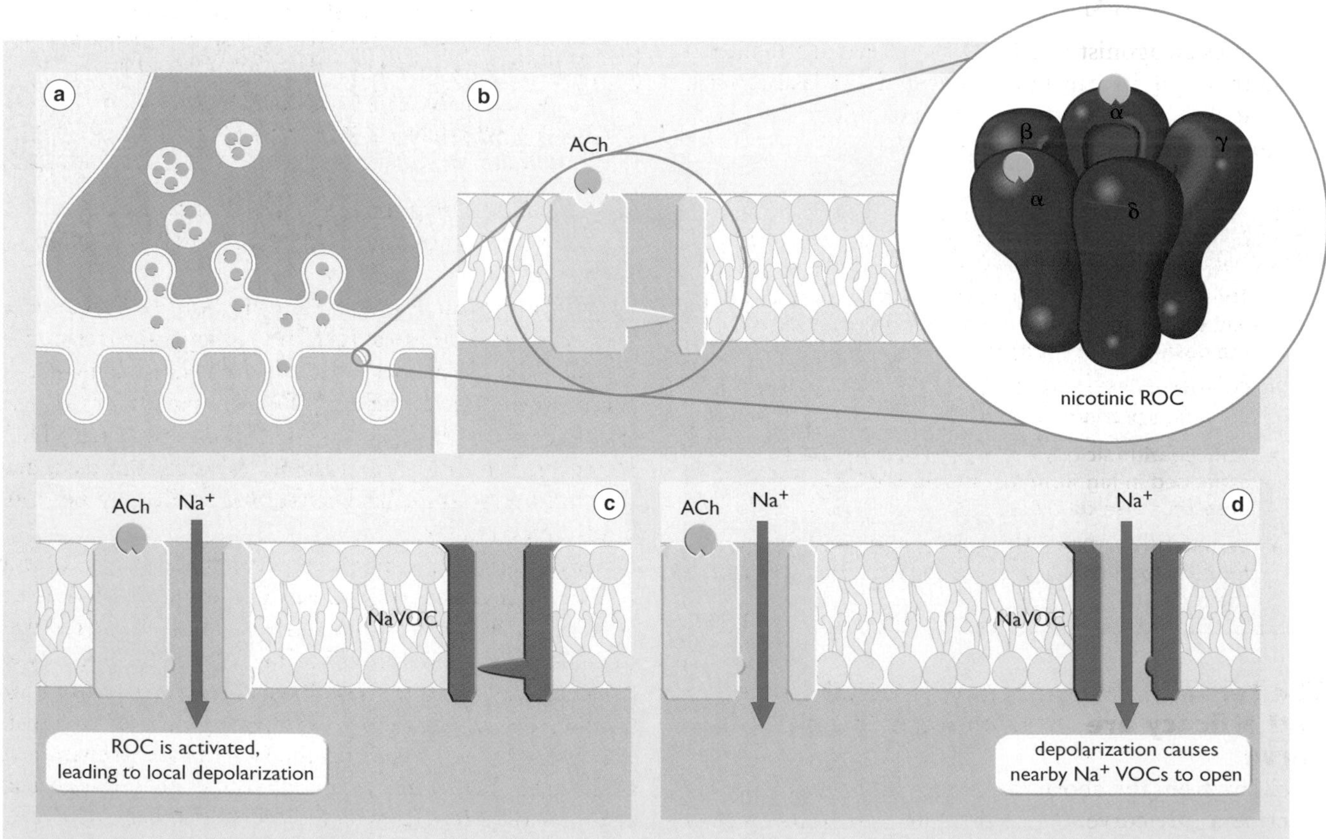

Fig. 2.28 Example of receptor-operated ion channel-linked transduction. (a) In response to an electrical impulse arriving at the nerve ending, vesicles of acetylcholine (ACh) fuse with the membrane of the nerve terminal, resulting in liberation of ACh into the synaptic cleft. (b) ACh binds to receptors on the α subunits of the ROC (insert) leading to opening, allowing an influx of Na^+ and an efflux of K^+, causing local depolarization (c). This depolarization initiates transduction, causing Na VOCs to open in the adjacent regions of the skeletal muscle membrane, producing a further influx of Na^+ and thus triggering widespread depolarization activation of Ca VOC and muscle fiber contraction (d).

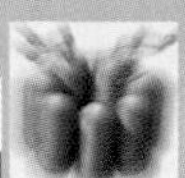

acetylcholine). Below a certain concentration of agonist (**[A]**), **E** is too low to measure but at higher concentrations it becomes appreciable and rises with increasing agonist concentration **[A]** until at sufficiently high concentrations it can no longer be increased by raising **[A]** and asymptotes to a maximum $\mathbf{E_{max}}$. A log (dose)–response curve can be conventionally characterized by three parameters:

- $\mathbf{E_{max}}$ (the maximum possible effect for the agonist).
- The concentration of A at which **E** is 50% of $\mathbf{E_{max}}$ is termed $\mathbf{[A_{50}]}$, for this particular figure of $\mathbf{[ED_{50}]}$, where ED is effective dose or $\mathbf{[EC_{50}]}$ where EC is effective concentration. The EC_{50} is a measure of a drug's 'potency': the lower a drug's EC_{50}, the more potent it is. A drug's potency is in general unrelated to its maximal response. Note that in clinical writings, these concepts may be implicitly intermixed. This parameter locates the central position of the dose-responsive curve on the log dose or log concentration axis.
- The slope parameter (Hill coefficient, h) describes the steepness of the curve. It is obtained by fitting the **E–[A]** curve to another form of the dose–response equation described by the following logistic function:

$$\mathbf{E/E_{max} = [A]^h/([A]^h + A50^h)} \qquad \text{(Eqn 2.7)}$$

Sometimes an agonist which is closely related chemically to another agonist can have a lower E_{max}, despite both drugs acting on the same receptor. For this reason, such an agonist is termed a partial agonist.

Dose (concentration)–response curves

- **The relationship between the response to a drug and drug dose (concentration) is commonly called the dose–response (DR) curve**
- **Quantitative analysis of drug action is dependent upon interpreting dose–response curves**
- **Semilogarithmic graphs (where the dose axis is expressed in log form) are usually used for dose–response curves**
- **Competitive antagonists shift dose–response curves for corresponding agonists in a parallel manner to the right**

The terms slope, potency, intrinsic activity and efficacy are used to describe the DR curve

It follows from the above that three parameters uniquely describe a DR curve. The slope can have values below and above 1.0 but a value of 1.0 is expected with the simplest classical model of A + R $\rightleftharpoons$ AR. The term potency describes the location of the curve on the dose axis but it is important to recognize that ED_{50}, EC_{50} and similar measures of potency are generally not the K_A found by binding studies. Unfortunately, while potency has a distinct meaning it is not always used properly. While it is easy to describe potency and slope there are many difficulties with the maximum response (E_{max}) obtainable with a drug. The term efficacy is used loosely to describe the ability of a drug to produce a desired therapeutic effect. However, pharmacological efficacy (e) is the ability of an agonist to produce a response. Thus an antagonist has an efficacy of zero whereas it is maximum with a full agonist. Partial agonists are intermediate in efficacy. A similar term is intrinsic activity where a full agonist has a value to 1.0. With this measure, partial agonists have value up to 1.0.

Technically, the term 'potency' refers to the A_{50} value. The lower the A_{50}, the less the concentration of drug required to produce 50% of maximum effect and the higher the potency. Thus, maximum $\mathbf{E_{max}}$ is sometimes referred to as intrinsic activity, or efficacy. Therefore, agonist A might be more potent than agonist B even if it falls short of B's maximum effectiveness (i.e. $\mathbf{E_{max}}$ for B is greater than for A).

Definitions

- **Affinity is the tendency to bind receptors**
- **Efficacy is the relationship between receptor occupancy and the ability to initiate a response at the molecular, cellular, tissue or system level**
- **Intrinsic activity is the capacity of a single drug–receptor complex to evoke a response**

The relation between tissue response and concentration of agonist–receptor complex is often non-linear

Since the typical log**[A]** versus response (**E**) curve is similar to the theoretical **[DR]** versus log**[D]** curve, it was assumed that response **E** directly reflects the amount of agonist–receptor complex **[AR]**. In particular, it was assumed that $\mathbf{E/E_{max}}$ was equivalent to $\mathbf{[AR]/[R_t]}$. However, it is now clear that this is rarely the case, and that the relationship between **E** and **[AR]** may be non-linear and complex.

Very often, $\mathbf{E_{max}}$ merely reflects the capacity of the system to produce a response. For example, if A is an agonist which acts on a receptor to lower blood pressure, the maximum possible effect of A would be to lower blood pressure to 0 mmHg. Even when such a limitation to response does not apply, as shown by different agonists with different $\mathbf{E_{max}}$ values in the same tissue preparation, an **E** that is half of $\mathbf{E_{max}}$ is usually obtained with agonists at a value of $\mathbf{[AR]/[R_t]}$ which is much less than 50% of R_t. Such conclusions have been reached because it has been possible to obtain good estimates of the dissociation constants for agonists using the action of irreversible antagonists, as first introduced by R. Furchgott in 1966. Of course, once an agonist's dissociation constant K_A has been obtained, a graph of **E** versus **[A]** can be translated

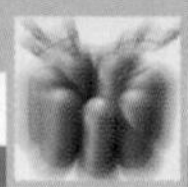

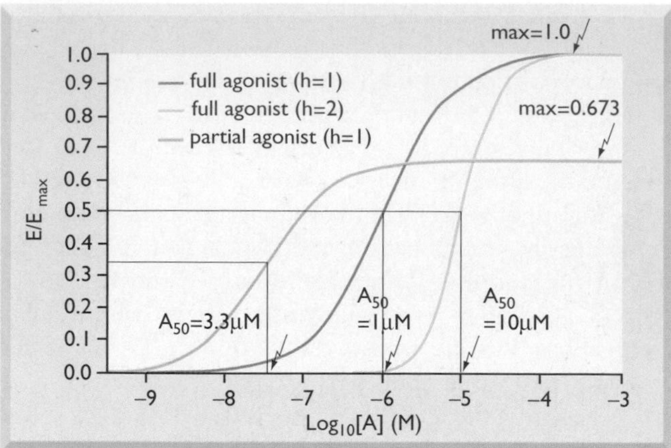

Fig. 2.29 Dose–response curves for different agonists (A) with various values for A_{50}, maxima and slopes (h). Note that the response to agonist on the *y*-axis is in the form E/E_{max}. Three agonists are shown; the higher the A_{50} concentration, the more the curve lies to the right. For full agonists the maximum is the same whereas for partial agonists the maximum is lower. The higher the value of 'h', the steeper the slope of the dose–response curve. (M, molar conc.)

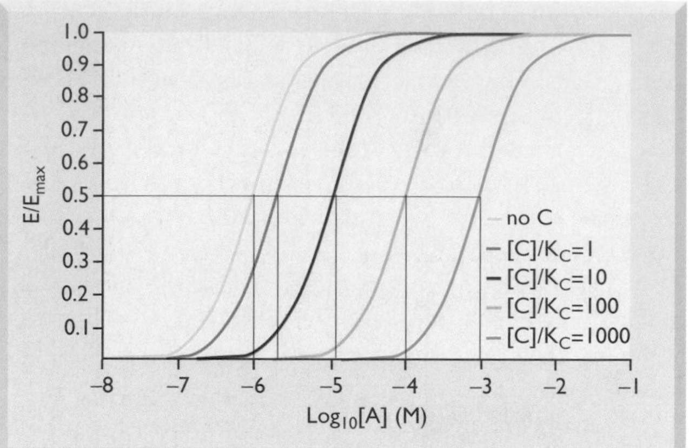

Fig. 2.30 Dose–response curves for an agonist (A) in the presence of competitive antagonist (C), at different concentrations such that $[C]/K_C$ equals 1, 10, 100 or 1000. Compare this figure with Fig. 2.7. Note that the *x*-axes are the same for both figures; however, the *y*-axis here is the ratio of the effects (**E**), produced by different concentrations of agonist, to the maximum effect (E_{max}).

into a graph of **E** versus $[AR]/[R_t]$, yielding information about the transduction system (cellular response) linking **[AR]** to **E**.

Competitive antagonists for endogenous agonists such as neurotransmitters, neurohormones and autacoids

Competitive antagonists shift agonist dose–response curves to the right

As was the case for binding, reversible competitive antagonists produce parallel shifts to the right of plots of **E** (effect or response) versus log**[A]**, where A is an agonist (Fig. 2.30). Such a relationship arises automatically from the equation:

$$[AR] = [R_t]\,[A]/([A] + K_A\,(1 + [C]/K_C)) \qquad \text{(Eqn 2.8)}$$

Whatever the relationship between **E** (effect) and **[AR]**, the inhibitory effect of a competitor (C), at any **[A]**, can always be overcome or nullified by increasing **[A]** by the factor ($1 + [C]/K_C$) which is the dose ratio (**DR**). In other words, inhibition is surmountable at any level of response and E_{max} is not reduced. There is an easy way to check whether experimental results agree with the theory. Since $DR-1 = [C]/K_C$ it follows that:

$$\log(DR - 1) = \log[C] - \log K_C \qquad \text{(Eqn 2.9)}$$

where the latter relationship is known as the Schild plot (Fig. 2.31). In the Schild plot the intercept at $\log_{10}(DR - 1) = 0$ (where $DR = 2$) is the K_C value. By analogy with pH notation, the negative $\log_{10}$ of K_C is known as the pA_2.

Sometimes the equation $(DR - 1) = [C]/K_C$ does not hold for some agonists even though antagonists are clearly competitive in that they produce parallel shifts to the right. Deviations from the equation can be expected

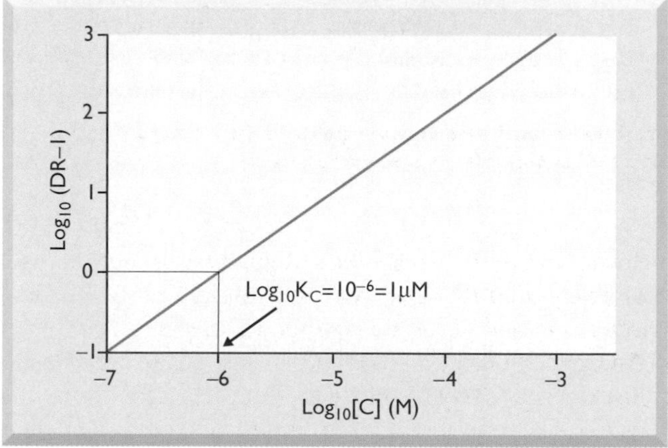

Fig. 2.31 Schild plot for a competitive antagonist (C). In this graph DR is the dose ratio, i.e. the value of A_{50} in the presence of a particular concentration of C divided by A_{50} in the absence of C. The data here are typical of those used to construct a Schild plot. The linear nature of this graph allows for easy estimation of K_C and the slope. Note that a wide range of concentrations of C can be studied.

if the receptor has more than one binding site for agonist and the receptor is in its active form only when two or more agonist molecules are bound. An example of this situation is found with the nicotinic acetylcholine receptor in skeletal muscle.

Not all antagonists are competitive

Not all drugs modify agonist binding in a competitive manner. The simplest reason for this is that a receptor contains more than one drug recognition site and that binding at one site alters the affinity at another. This type of interaction is known as an 'allosteric interaction'. It is characterized in saturation binding experiments by a half-maximal binding value, denoted by D_{50b} (apparent K_D), that can be varied continuously between two limits. At one extreme is the absence of the allosteric agent while at

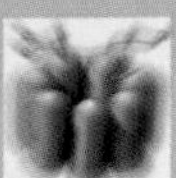

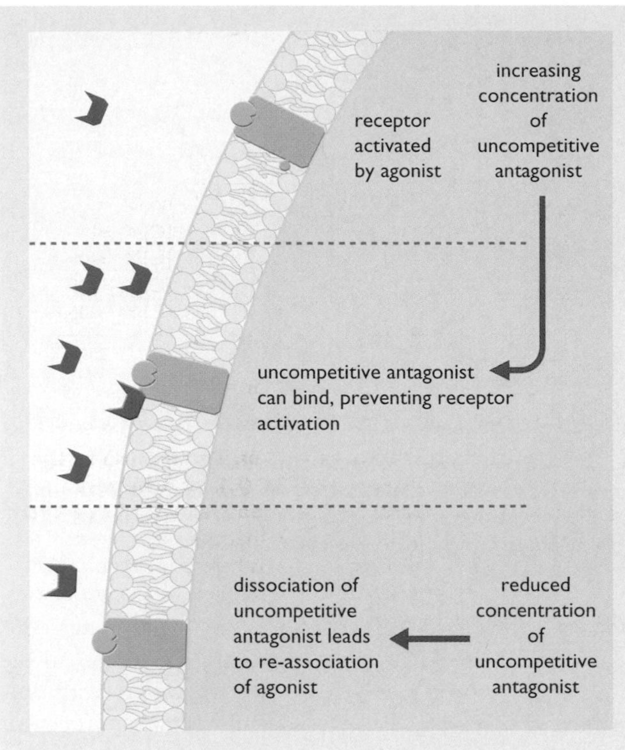

Fig. 2.32 This figure is analogous to Fig. 2.7 but in this case the antagonist is uncompetitive.

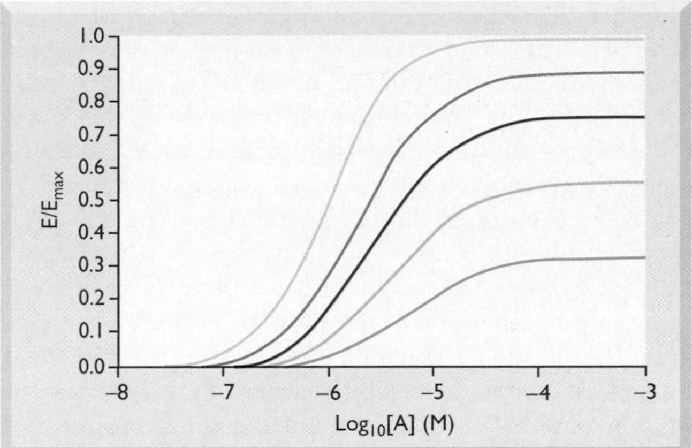

Fig. 2.33 Dose–response curves for an agonist (A) in the presence of different concentrations of a non-competitive antagonist (D). This graph is analogous to that for a competitive antagonist shown in Fig. 2.30. Note the rightward shift of the dose–response curve with increasing concentrations of D and the fall in maximum.

the other extreme virtually all receptors are bound to the allosteric agent. When the antagonist binds in this manner it is said to be non-competitive.

Another theoretical scenario is one where the antagonist can bind only to the drug–receptor (DR) complex. This can occur only if the binding of D causes a change in conformation of the receptor (Fig. 2.32) such that it can now bind the antagonist. In such a case the antagonist may be termed an uncompetitive drug (U). Because of the dynamics of the interaction between drug (D), uncompetitive drug (U) and receptors, the apparent affinity of the receptor for drug D is increased in the presence of U. This essentially occurs because the form DR cannot exist and LUR must first dissociate to form DR and U before breaking down to form free R. So, in effect, D is trapped in the DRU form.

Non-competitive antagonists reduce E_{max}

When an antagonist (D) reduces $\mathbf{E_{max}}$ it is usually (and inaccurately) termed non-competitive (Fig. 2.33). Such antagonism results in marked deviations from the Schild plots for log (**DR**–1) versus log **[D]**, seen with competitive antagonists. A good example of uncompetitive antagonism is ion channel blockade discussed earlier, in which the drug target is the ion channel that has been opened by an agonist.

Many clinically useful drugs are competitive antagonists for endogenous agonists such as neurohormones and autacoids, for example:

- Propranolol (β adrenoceptors).
- Haloperidol (dopamine receptors).
- Naloxone (opioid receptors).
- Phentolamine (α adrenoceptors).
- Cimetidine (histamine H_2 receptors).
- Atropine (muscarinic receptors).
- Curare-like compounds (skeletal muscle nicotinic receptors).

In each of these cases the nature of the antagonism and effectiveness of the compounds (and K_d values) were established using the methods outlined above.

When used clinically, the effects observed with a competitive antagonist actually represent inhibition of responses to an exogenous or endogenous agonist. An example is the depression of endogenous histamine-mediated acid secretion in the stomach by cimetidine. Again, the dose–response curves are characterized by: (i) an $\mathbf{E_{max}}$; (ii) a dose at which effect is half maximum (usually termed EC_{50}); and (iii) a slope parameter (h). As with dose–response curves for agonists, the exact form of such curves depends critically on the transduction system that links the active agonist–receptor complex (AR*) to the tissue response, since for competitive antagonists each concentration of antagonist corresponds to a reduction of **[A]**. Nevertheless, it can be shown that the EC_{50} is generally close to the dissociation constant, K_d multiplied by (1 + **[A]**/$\mathbf{A_{50}}$). That is, the $\mathbf{EC_{50}}$ is much the same, provided that the responses to the agonist are well below the maximum (**[A]**<$\mathbf{A_{50}}$). In general:

- Half-blockade of the agonist effect is associated with at least half-occupancy of receptors.
- Near-maximal effects of the competitive antagonist require that most receptors are bound by the drug.

This contrasts with what is found with most agonists, where near-maximal responses occur with a low receptor occupancy.

When a competitive antagonist is used to block the actions of an endogenous agonist (e.g. a neurotransmitter), it is sometimes found that the EC_{50} is much more than the K_d. The simple explanation for this is that **[A]** at the receptor site is usually high relative to $\mathbf{A_{50}}$. Alternatively, the phenomenon may arise because physiologically **[A]** is far from constant and equilibrium-type equations do not apply.

Dose–response curves for non-competitive antagonists representing inhibition of response to endogenous or exogenous agonist also resemble those shown in Figure 2.30. Since these agents can act by a variety of mechanisms, the only generalization that can be made is that, in contrast to competitive antagonists, the EC_{50} fails to rise in proportion to $1 + \mathbf{[A]/A_{50}}$.

The actions of irreversible antagonists persist

As indicated by their name, irreversible antagonists are characterized by an antagonism that persists despite removal of free antagonist. Generally, irreversible antagonism produced by such a drug is less if a high concentration of agonist is present during incubation with antagonist.

When irreversible antagonists were first developed, their effects on dose–response curves for agonists came as a surprise, since previously, pharmacologists had assumed that drug response was directly proportional to **[AR]**. With irreversible antagonists it became clear that such drugs produced irreversible inhibition of responses to agonists in a manner consistent with the loss of a proportion of available receptors. However, contrary to expectation, despite such losses there was often little or no change in $\mathbf{E_{max}}$. Typical results are illustrated in Figure 2.34, where, at shorter incubation times with an irreversible antagonist, curves are at first shifted in parallel manner with increases in $\mathbf{A_{50}}$ values and no reduction of $\mathbf{E_{max}}$, a pattern similar to that seen with competitive blockade. After a sufficient period of incubation, $\mathbf{E_{max}}$ is reduced while the shifts in $\mathbf{A_{50}}$ are also reduced. The explanation for this phenomenon is that maximal responses normally require the activation of only a small fraction of receptors. The existence of far more receptors than is needed to produce a maximum response is often referred to as 'receptor reserve'.

Receptor reserve implies that the $\mathbf{A_{50}}$ (the value of **[A]** for a half-maximum response) is less than K_A (**[A]** for occupation of 50% of receptors). Thus the ratio $K_A/\mathbf{A_{50}}$ is a reflection of receptor reserve and that reserve varies for agonists acting on the same receptor. Therefore, changes in receptor reserve among closely related analogs of an agonist provide yet another method of characterizing receptors. Receptor reserve is also influenced by the tissue itself; for example, activation of only a few of the available receptors may lead to maximal cellular or tissue responses due to marked amplification of receptor-activated signaling pathways.

The simplest and most generally accepted explanation for differences (of what is technically called 'intrinsic efficacy') between agonists is that only a particular conformation of the AR complex (say, AR*) is 'active' in the sense that it produces a response. Agonists with low intrinsic efficacy ($\mathbf{A_{50}}$ close to K_A and little or no receptor reserve), which include partial agonists, have an AR that is seldom in the form AR*, while agonists with high intrinsic efficacy ($\mathbf{A_{50}} << K_A$) have an AR mostly in the AR* form. Dose–response curves such as those shown in Figure 2.34 contain the information needed to calculate the K_A of an agonist (not shown).

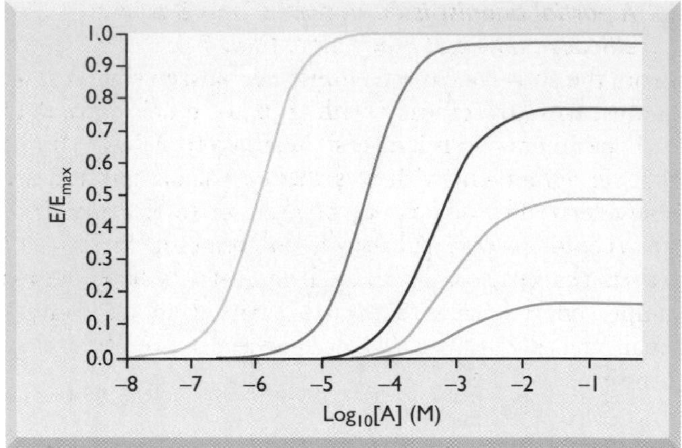

Fig. 2.34 Dose–response curves for an agonist (A) after increasing times of exposure to an irreversible antagonist. The more the curve is shifted to the right, the longer the tissue has been incubated with the irreversible antagonist.

A simple model for efficacy was proposed by Stephenson

The simple model of efficacy introduced by Stephenson is useful for understanding how results such as those in Figure 2.34 can arise. Suppose that AR produces a stimulus (**S**) which is proportional to **[AR]** and that response (**E**) is a function of **S** which is not limitless but saturates, then:

$$\mathbf{S = e[AR]/[R_t]} \qquad \text{(Eqn 2.10)}$$

where **e** is a proportionality constant, called efficacy, that can vary from one agonist to another, and:

$$\mathbf{E = E'S/\ (1 + S)} \qquad \text{(Eqn 2.11)}$$

where **E** is effect and **E′** represents a hypothetical maximum that would occur if **S** could be made infinite. If agonists vary in the fraction (**f**) of AR that is in an active conformation (AR*), **e** will be proportional to **f**. Also, with **e** defined as above, it must be proportional to $\mathbf{[R_t]}$ (or $\mathbf{q[R_t]}$ if some receptors are made inoperable). Intrinsic efficacy is $\mathbf{e/[R_t]}$.

On the basis of this model, agonists may be compared in terms of their relative **e** values, which are the same as relative intrinsic efficacies. The problem here is that the actual values of **e** obtained depend on the particular relationship assumed between **E** and **S**, which might or might not be true of any particular transduction system.

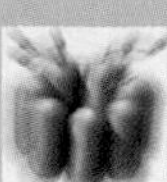

A partial agonist is an agonist of low intrinsic efficacy and e not much more than 1

From the above, a partial agonist can be seen simply as an agonist with low efficacy, with an **e** not much more than 1. Experiments with irreversible antagonists have shown that, in agreement with this theory, partial agonists are characterized by having $\mathbf{A}_{50}$ values close to K_A values and no receptor reserve. As already pointed out, the low **e** of a partial agonist relative to a full agonist may be explained simply on the basis that with a partial agonist only a small fraction of the AR complexes are in the active conformation (AR*).

When a full agonist is present at a high concentration, a partial agonist acts as an antagonist

Since a response to a partial agonist only occurs when receptor occupancy is high, it becomes apparent that partial agonists act as antagonists of full agonists. Therefore, a partial agonist can be used therapeutically to block the effect of an endogenous agonist (e.g. norepinephrine) while at the same time producing a steady low level of receptor activation in the absence of a full agonist. A classic example of partial agonism is seen with certain β blockers (e.g. pindolol) that are partial agonists rather than competitive antagonists. Pindolol becomes an increasingly effective β blocker as sympathetic nerve activity on the heart increases. Thus when sympathetic activity on the heart is low, pindolol can increase heart rate, whereas the effect of sympathetic nerve activity on the heart is blocked by pindolol. A classic β-blocker drug never increases heart rate under any condition.

> **Agonism**
>
> - Agonism is the production of a molecular and cellular response to an interaction between a drug (agonist) and a receptor that activates the receptor. The intrinsic activity of a full agonist is defined as being equal to 1
> - Partial agonism occurs when a drug interacts with a receptor to produce an average of less than 1 unit of molecular response. The average molecular intrinsic activity lies between 0 and 1
> - Antagonism occurs when a drug interacts with a receptor to inhibit the action of an agonist. The molecular intrinsic activity is 0
> - Inverse agonism occurs when a drug interacts with a receptor to reduce its resting level of molecular activity. The molecular intrinsic activity is –1
> - Partial inverse agonism occurs when a drug interacts with a receptor to reduce the resting level of molecular activity. The molecular intrinsic activity lies between 0 and –1

Drug responses change due to desensitization

Responses to drugs are often not fixed and constant over time, even though the concentrations of the drug at its receptor site may have reached steady-state values. In a variety of situations, responses to a drug may wane over time. Many factors lead to a loss in drug effects at an organ or system level, from progression of the disease being treated to physiologic adaptations. When the loss in responsiveness to a drug occurs at the level of the molecular target (e.g. the receptor) it is termed 'desensitization'. Many mechanisms have been found to contribute to desensitization, operating at transcriptional, translational and protein levels of cellular regulation. These mechanisms may operate quickly (seconds to minutes) or relatively slowly, over the course of hours or days.

Mechanisms involved in rapidly developing desensitization have been extensively studied in molecular terms, especially for G protein-coupled receptors and particularly β adrenoceptors. At the cellular level, stimulation of β adrenoceptors with an agonist such as isoproterenol leads to activation of adenylyl cyclase and a brisk rise in intracellular concentrations of the second-messenger cAMP. However, in many cells, the capacity of isoproterenol to activate adenylyl cyclase declines with time, leading to a fall in cAMP concentrations in the cell. Phosphorylation of β adrenoceptors, association of these receptors with other proteins and changes in subcellular localization of the receptors may all contribute to the diminished ability of isoproterenol to activate cAMP accumulation.

Desensitization of β adrenoceptors (and other G protein-coupled receptors) can occur specifically due to the phosphorylation of agonist-bound receptors by a G protein-coupled receptor kinase (GRK). GRKs constitute a family of kinases. GRK2, originally known as βARK kinase, was discovered on account of its capacity to phosphorylate agonist-occupied β adrenoceptors. Agonist occupancy of these receptors leads to binding of a GRK to the receptor and its phosphorylation. This mechanism has been termed 'homologous' desensitization since it specifically involves agonist-occupied receptors. After being phosphorylated, the receptors bind a member of the arrestin protein family, leading to steric hindrance of interaction between receptors and G proteins. The receptors may subsequently be sequestered away from the plasma membrane and move into the cytoplasm. Surprising new information suggests that the internalized receptors may contribute to novel mechanisms of β adrenoceptor signaling.

A second mechanism for receptor desensitization involves second-messenger feedback, which can lead to desensitization of not only agonist-activated receptors but also different classes of receptors expressed in the same cell. This form of desensitization has been termed 'heterologous' desensitization, since the function of multiple types of receptors may simultaneously change after activation of just one receptor type. β adrenoceptors stimulate cAMP accumulation, which leads to activation of protein kinase A; the activated catalytic subunit of protein kinase A can phosphorylate not only β adrenoceptors, impairing their function, but also potentially a number of other receptors in the same cell with appropriate sites for phosphorylation by protein kinase A.

Physiologic antagonism

■ ***Physiologic antagonists oppose the actions of agonists by mechanisms independent of the agonist–receptor interaction***

In an earlier section, antagonist drugs that inhibit the actions of agonists were considered to produce their inhibition by acting in some manner on the same receptors as the agonists. However, drugs may also antagonize the actions of agonists by other mechanisms.

■ ***Drugs can oppose responses to other drugs by acting on different molecular targets***

It often happens that two drugs acting on different receptors have opposing actions at a tissue or organ level. When this occurs, the drugs can be considered to be physiologic or functional antagonists of one another, the former term being preferred. Obvious examples of such physiologic antagonism are epinephrine and acetylcholine, which respectively raise and lower heart rate, and glucagon and insulin, which respectively raise and lower blood glucose levels.

A more subtle example is antagonism of neuromuscular blockade due to a non-depolarizing neuromuscular blocking drug, such as pancuronium, by an anticholinesterase, such as neostigmine. The dose–response curve for neuromuscular block versus dose of pancuronium is shifted by neostigmine in a non-competitive fashion. This occurs because the two drugs act on quite different molecular targets, the nicotinic receptor for pancuronium and the enzyme acetylcholinesterase for neostigmine. Blockade of the activity of the enzyme can do no more than double the height of end-plate potentials and, as a result, an anticholinesterase cannot reverse neuromuscular blockade due to an excessive dose of pancuronium.

MEASURING RESPONSES AND PRACTICAL APPLICATIONS OF DOSE–RESPONSE CURVES

■ ***Responses to drugs are measured in many different ways***

Drugs have their initial actions at a molecular level, for example, by binding to a receptor. This ultimately results in cellular, tissue, organ or body system, whole-body and population responses, all of which can be measured. Biochemical techniques are often used to measure intracellular responses to drugs, whereas the response of whole tissues and organs can be measured using physical (electrical, optical and mechanical) techniques, both in vitro (in glass) and in vivo (in life). For in vitro studies, the tissues and organs are isolated from the body and bathed with suitable physiologic buffers, generally in glass apparatus. When studies are made in intact animals and humans they are referred to as being in vivo.

In the above discussions the terms 'effect' and 'response' have been used synonymously but left undefined because there are innumerable ways in which drugs act and in which their effects can be defined. However, it should always be borne in mind that, if given at sufficiently high concentrations, drugs have many measurable effects that may not be relevant to the desired clinical action of the drug.

Dose–response curves almost always appear similar to those shown in Figures 2.29 and 2.30, the exceptions being those where the drug acts on more than one type of receptor. Below a certain dose or concentration, an effect is undetectable and as the dose is increased the effect increases until a maximum effect is reached. The dose of the agonist at which the effect is half-maximal is usually called the ED_{50}. Similarly, the ED_{10} is the dose producing 10% of maximum response, ED_{25} produces 25%, ED_{75} 75%, etc. If the agonist drug concentration **[A]** is known, the corresponding terms EC_{10}, EC_{25}, EC_{50}, etc., may be used.

The ratio ED_{75}/ED_{25} (or EC_{75}/EC_{25}) provides a simple measure of the steepness of the dose–response curve over the linear portion of the S-shaped dose (concentration)–response curve, which when measured exactly, is 'h', the Hill coefficient (see page 41):

$$\mathbf{E} = \mathbf{E_{max}[A]}^h/(EC_{50}{}^h + \mathbf{[A]}^h) \qquad \text{(Eqn 2.12)}$$

This is another form of the dose–response equation in which **[A]** is drug concentration and h is theoretically expected to be an integer, 1 or 2. It is notable that for drugs with h more than 1 (EC_{75}/EC_{25} less than 9) responses increase steeply with dose, which can be very dangerous. For example, with vapor general anesthetics, the depth of anesthesia may increase alarmingly with only a small increase in concentration of the vapor administered.

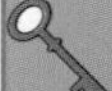

Therapeutic ratio: an experimental index of risk versus benefit

- **The LD_{50} is the dose of a drug that is lethal to 50% of the animals tested**
- **The ED_{50} is the dose of a drug that is effective in 50% of the animals tested**
- **The ratio of LD_{50} to ED_{50} is the therapeutic ratio, an experimental measure of the usefulness of a drug**
- **Other therapeutic indices use non-lethal adverse effects to estimate risk versus benefit**

■ ***Sometimes drug responses are all-or-nothing (quantal) in nature***

In certain contexts the drug response measured is 'quantal' rather than 'graded' in nature (the response either occurs or it does not occur, as in cure or no cure, death or no death). With such quantal data, the response axis for the dose–response curve is expressed as a percentage of people, animals or cells that respond, so it is known as a quantal dose–response curve. The classic quantal dose–response curve is a lethality curve in which

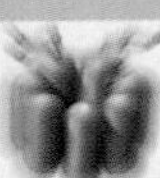

the percentage of animals killed by a drug or poison is plotted for various doses. The dose that is lethal to 50% of animals is known as the LD_{50} (lethal dose 50%). The value of the LD_{50} for a particular drug depends upon the route of administration used and the species in which the drug is tested. The LD_{50} is analogous to the ED_{50} which is the effective dose 50% (the dose which produces a desired effect in 50% of animals).

Drugs are judged according to both their beneficial and adverse effects (risk–benefit ratio)

The 'therapeutic ratio', a classic index of the safety of a drug, is defined experimentally as the ratio LD_{50}/ED_{50}. This index is useful but can be misleading if the log dose–response curve for desired effect is not parallel to the lethality curve (they do not have the same slope 'h'). Some pharmacologists prefer to use ratios such as LD_{25}/ED_{75} or LD_{10}/ED_{90}, reflecting Ehrlich's early suggestion (circa 1900) that a drug is best judged by the ratio between its maximal tolerated dose and its minimal curative dose.

Ratios involving estimation of lethal doses can only be determined using animals. However, other measures of toxicity can be used to estimate risk–benefit ratio clinically. For example, the dose–response curve for beneficial effect can be compared with that for an adverse, but not lethal effect, giving a 'therapeutic index', rather than the classic therapeutic ratio in animal studies too. The desire to reduce the use of animals for lethality testing has led to the increasing use of such indices. At a clinical level it is obviously important to try to compare dose–response curves for beneficial effects with those for adverse effects. Unfortunately the clinical information necessary to calculate reasonable indices is often not available. In the clinic only limited dose–response data can be obtained, since only a limited number of different doses can be given. Ethical considerations prevent further doses being given once an adverse effect has been encountered.

With quantal responses the steepness (h) of the dose–response curve directly reflects the variability in the population being tested. After all, for a lethality curve, if all animals were identical, they would all die at the same dose. There is extensive statistical theory concerning how data of this kind should be treated (such as the use of 'probits') and the reliability of estimates of ED_{50}, LD_{50}, etc. However, quantal results can be fitted to a variant of the standard dose formula:

$$\mathbf{E/E_{max}} = \mathbf{D}^{h} / (LD_{50}{}^{h} + \mathbf{D}^{h}) \quad \text{(Eqn 2.13)}$$

where $\mathbf{D}$ is dose, with $\mathbf{E_{max}}$ = 100% and 'h' the slope coefficient.

Occasionally, what appear to be graded responses in a tissue actually represent hidden quantal responses – what one measures is the sum of responses of many individual cells where each cell responds in an all-or-none fashion. This may sometimes provide an explanation of the steep dose–response curves encountered, for example, when a neuromuscular blocking drug is used to inhibit nerve-induced contractions of skeletal muscle. Here individual neuromuscular junctions in skeletal muscle fibers are either blocked or not blocked by a given concentration of the drug, and single muscle fiber contractions are either present or absent. This contrasts with the situation in smooth muscle where contraction in each fiber is continuously graded with the dose of a drug.

Dose–response relationships are fundamental to the discovery of receptors, development of new drugs and understanding drug actions

In research and drug development, the primary aim is to categorize drugs in terms of the biologic systems with which they interact and to characterize their interactions with molecular targets to test, for example, whether they are agonists, partial agonists, full inverse agonists or competitive, non-competitive or irreversible antagonists. Here, the approach is to measure drug effects on a variety of enzyme systems and tissue preparations that contain molecular targets of different types. Thus a compound may be identified as an H_1 (histamine type 1 receptor) agonist if it acts in the same way as histamine in a preparation that responds to histamine and has its actions inhibited by an H_1 competitive receptor antagonist in a competitive manner. An unidentified active compound in a tissue extract is epinephrine if its potency relative to epinephrine is the same in preparations containing different proportions of adrenoceptors, and appropriate competitive antagonists shift dose–response curves to the unknown agent in the same way as they shift dose–response curves to epinephrine. If a drug or chemical compound has effects that cannot be explained in terms of actions on known receptors, a new receptor may have been discovered and if the compound occurs naturally in tissues, it may be a new autacoid. Historically, such work has led to most of our present understanding of how drugs act, as well as the discovery of endogenous transmitters and their receptors.

It is still common in pharmacologic research to determine the effects of drugs in vitro by measuring specific responses from a smooth muscle preparation such as a piece of intestine, artery, vein, bladder or uterus, etc. Such preparations characteristically respond to a variety of agents by contraction or relaxation, the response being graded with concentration and fairly fast in onset and offset when the drug is added or removed, respectively. It is therefore possible to quickly determine a concentration–response relationship and its alteration by another drug. The use of biochemical drug responses, such as accumulation or turnover of a second messenger, can often be an even more accurate measure of drug action and is essential in cases when the drug being studied acts on molecular targets that are not present in tissue preparations which provide an easily measured physical response.

Identification of novel molecular targets for drugs

Early identification of molecular targets involved in the use of indirect techniques

The introduction of the receptor hypothesis (the notion that a drug interacts with a specific target to initiate its response) in the early part of the twentieth century initiated an interest in the structural and functional identification of molecular targets for drugs. For most of the last century indirect methods were used to identify and understand molecular targets and their function. In particular, the existence of receptor families, and their subtypes, had to be inferred from patterns of responses in a variety of different tissues to a variety of agonists, the inhibition of those responses by reversible and irreversible antagonists and the manipulation of physical conditions, such as temperature. This was very successful in identifying the major known classes of receptors for neurotransmitters and hormones. It was easier to identify the existence of other molecular targets such as enzymes because they possess intrinsic biologic activity.

Molecular biology has been very important in the development of molecular pharmacology

Developments in molecular biology are having major effects on pharmacology. The technique of ligand binding (see earlier) has been important in locating and identifying molecular targets, allowing them to be purified and their amino acid sequence to be revealed. This has facilitated the cloning of genes for the molecular target, allowing the genetic code dictating the amino acid structure to be determined and, by process of comparison, has identified how families of molecular targets are related. Identification of the DNA code for molecular targets allows immediate access to the mRNA carrying the message while ultimately information about the turnover and expression of the molecular target can be inferred. The findings have been remarkably consonant with the classic view of receptors that allow selective binding to drugs. At the same time there has been a growth in our knowledge of intracellular transduction mechanisms for translating the binding of a drug to a receptor into a tissue response. The growth of this collection of knowledge and techniques, known as molecular biology, has initiated a third phase in our understanding of molecular targets and molecular mechanisms of drug action.

The discovery of new drugs

Techniques for discovering new drugs are increasingly (but not exclusively) dependent on the techniques of molecular biology

Pharmacology is the study of what drugs do and how they do it. Consequently, pharmacology is also an important part of the drug discovery process. A lot of new drugs are discovered by pharmaceutical companies who require a constant stream of products in order to ensure their economic survival. The techniques of molecular biology are able to provide in a pure form the target biomolecules with which potential drugs can interact. These molecular targets can then be combined with suitable reporter systems that indicate whether ligands are agonists or antagonists. Because of the large numbers of potential ligands that can be rapidly screened, this type of technique is known as high-throughput screening (HTS). Current HTS can examine up to hundreds of thousands of chemical compounds in one day. This allows millions of compounds, of natural or synthetic origin, to be screened for binding and activation of a host of target molecules. This technique currently works best for hormone and neurotransmitter receptors but is being expanded for enzymes and ion channels, as well as for other molecular targets.

In addition to the large number of existing 'libraries' of ligands, there is a need for rapid methods for synthesizing new and novel compounds. Developments in synthetic organic chemistry, such as combinatorial chemistry, are capable of producing the large number of compounds required to meet the capacity of HTS. In addition, HTS techniques are also being developed to screen potential drugs for desirable pharmacokinetic characteristics.

Combinations of HTS systems, therefore, allow identification of compounds which act on a known molecular target with sufficient potency, selectivity and appropriate pharmacokinetic behavior to suggest they might be given directly to humans to test their pharmacotherapeutic potential.

However, optimism that this approach will provide new drugs for every disease has yet to be justified by results. Why should this be? The reason is that we almost never have a clear understanding of the complete role of the currently available molecular targets in physiology and pathology, and the complexity of the influence of homeostasis on the cellular cascades that they initiate.

Thus, while the molecular biologic approach to pharmacology provides fast routes to drug discovery, reliable assessment of therapeutic potential of new drugs still requires functional analyses of drug actions on isolated tissues, body systems and whole bodies (including animal models of the target disease). After all, the body is an integrated unit in which the whole is considerably more than the sum of the parts. Pharmacology is likewise integrated from molecular to cellular, tissue and system actions and it is this integration that determines the therapeutic (and adverse) effects of drugs.

Clinical responses

Clinical responses to drugs are measured using a wide variety of techniques. These range from simple measurement of physiologic function (heart rate, blood pressure) to cure rates or mortality in populations of patients. In some cases the direct effects of a drug cannot be measured and therefore surrogate measures have to be used (see below). However, since the true aim of drug therapy is to cure or alleviate disease so as to improve

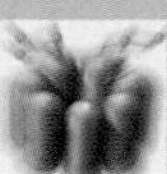

both the quality and duration of life, increasingly attempts are being made to measure such effects directly. As noted previously, large numbers of patients are required to obtain such data and clinical trials of new drugs are now sometimes designed to collect this. In addition, an alternative approach for new drugs entering the market is to monitor all prescriptions (up to some realistic limit) for fatal and adverse events (see next chapter).

Clinically, the use of any drug depends upon knowing the appropriate dose to use, which in turn depends upon dose–response curve data with respect to both desired and undesired (adverse) effects. Dose–response curves for a new drug are first obtained in isolated tissue preparations, then in animals and finally in humans. It may not be possible to define the entire therapeutic dose–response curve in humans on account of greater toxicity as the dose is increased. Generally, such determinations become more difficult and time-consuming the closer one approaches clinical reality. For example, the effect of a drug at a certain dose to diminish pain in people can be assessed using a visual analog pain scale in which a subject indicates the subjective pain experienced on a scale of 0 (no pain) to 10, the maximal imaginable pain. However, the perception of pain varies with people, pain often fluctuates and pain can arise from a variety of pathologic processes. As a result the determination of complete dose–response curves in man for a new analgesic against various kinds of pain would require hundreds of subjects and many person-years of investigator time. This would be impractical. On the other hand, using animals (rats or mice), pain reduction can be measured from the average time animals devote to licking a foot that has been injected by an agent that causes temporary inflammation. To obtain a dose–response relationship in this way may require 100–200 animals and several person-days of observation. This would typically follow 'screens' – simplified dose–response curves obtained with a variety of tissue preparations – to establish the absence of pharmacologic actions that could preclude the clinical use of the drug.

In view of the difficulty in obtaining any true dose–response relationship in humans, recourse is often made to 'surrogate' measures. For example, a chronically elevated blood pressure of unknown cause (primary hypertension) is statistically associated with increased morbidity and mortality. Therefore, the ideal measure of an antihypertensive drug is the extent to which it reduces morbidity and mortality, versus the possibility of adverse effects. However, this would require a prospective clinical trial involving thousands of subjects, followed over many years. The effects of antihypertensive drugs are therefore usually assessed in terms of their effectiveness and potency using the surrogate of blood pressure reduction, something which is fairly easy to measure. A dose–response relationship for true clinical effectiveness has not yet been obtained for most antihypertensives in common use, although increasing attention is being paid to whether they reduce mortality. Interestingly, despite the availability of many different antihypertensive drugs belonging to many different classes, comparatively few have been proven to reduce mortality in patients with essential hypertension.

Population effects

Different people respond in different ways to drugs. As a result, procedures are needed to acquire data regarding the effects of drugs in the population, and experience has shown that data should be gathered according to protocol, rather than during routine care.

Data gathered during phases II and III of clinical trials (Ch. 3) are an important source of information for assessing the effect of drugs in the population; they can be used not only to determine toxicity but also to maximize effectiveness. One major problem associated with information obtained from pre-marketing studies, however, can be a lack of heterogeneity among the pool of patients taking the medication. This problem can be confounded further by differences in the severity of disease between different patients. However, these problems can be partly overcome by designing studies to incorporate a large patient base. Certainly in the long term, a continuous gathering of information about the actions of drugs in the population will serve a useful purpose in optimizing the dose to reduce toxicity and maximize the pharmacotherapeutic benefit (see Ch. 3).

Lifestyle needs to be taken into account when studying the effects of a drug in the population. For example, a patient who is a smoker defines a different population. In effect, this could mean that a physician prescribing a drug may need to shift from the population mean to accommodate individual patients. Therefore, such scenarios play an important role in the decisions that are made by physicians in writing prescriptions.

FURTHER READING

Delmas P, Coste B, Gamper N, Shapiro MS. Phosphoinositide lipid second messengers: new paradigms for calcium channel modulation. *Neuron* 2005; **47**: 179–182.

Felix R. Molecular regulation of voltage-gated Ca^{2+} channels. *J Recept Signal Transduct Res* 2005; **25**: 57–71.

Gainetdinov RR, Premont RT, Bohn LM, Lefkowitz RJ, Caron MG. Desensitization of G protein-coupled receptors and neuronal functions. *Annu Rev Neurosci* 2004; **27**: 107–144.

Gouaux E, Mackinnon R. Principles of selective ion transport in channels and pumps. *Science* 2005; **310**: 1461–1465.

Hawrylyshyn KA, Michelotti GA, Coge F, Guenin SP, Schwinn DA. Update on human alpha1-adrenoceptor subtype signaling and genomic organization. *Trends Pharmacol Sci* 2004; **25**: 449–455.

Kass RS. The channelopathies: novel insights into molecular and genetic mechanisms of human disease. *J Clin Invest* 2005; **115**: 1986–1989.

Lefkowitz RJ, Shenoy SK. Transduction of receptor signals by beta-arrestins. *Science* 2005; **308**: 512–517.

Ray WA. Population-based studies of adverse effects. *New Engl J Med* 2004; **349**: 1592–1594.

Summers RJ, Broxton N, Hutchinson DS, Evans BA. The Janus faces of adrenoceptors: factors controlling the coupling of adrenoceptors to multiple signal transduction pathways. *Clin Exp Pharmacol Physiol* 2004; **31**(11): 822–827.

Thompson MD, Burnham WM, Cole DE. The G protein-coupled receptors: pharmacogenetics and disease. *Crit Rev Clin Lab Sci* 2005; **42**(4): 311–392.

Wray S, Burdyga T, Noble K. Calcium signalling in smooth muscle. *Cell Calcium* 2005; **38**(3–4): 397–407.

USEFUL WEBSITES

http://www.cochrane.org [This is the gateway to Cochrane reviews of the clinical value of drugs as assessed (e.g. by meta analyses) from the results of appropriately conducted clinical trials.]

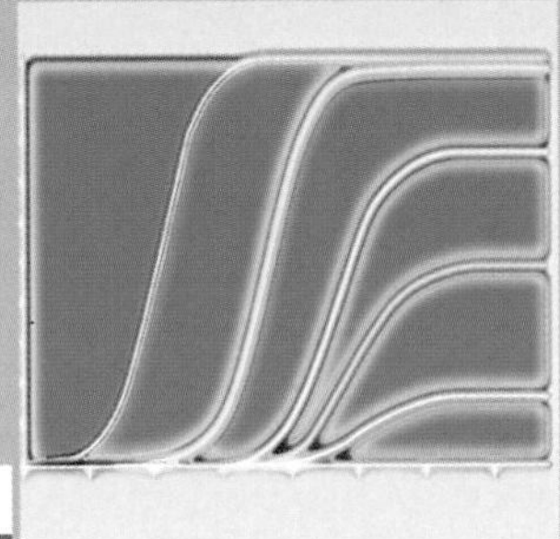

Chapter 3

Evaluation of the Therapeutic Usefulness of Drugs

ISSUES IN DRUG DEVELOPMENT

Drugs can damage health

Drug development and regulation is an assessment of relative risk and benefit. A drug is a chemical used to prevent, investigate or treat disease or to alter physiologic function (Table 3.1) while a medicine is a drug, or a mixture of drugs, combined with pharmacologically inactive substances to make it stable, palatable and useful for therapy. Drugs interact with tissues and organs and alter their function but their effects are not always desirable. Any drug represents a hazard (i.e. has the potential to cause harm). The probability that a drug will cause some specified harm in any given circumstances is the 'risk' that it will cause that harm. This probability can be estimated by experiment or observation or it can be estimated intuitively (see Fig. 3.2 for examples of how risk is perceived).

Drugs are used for many purposes (see Table 3.1).

Drug regulation seeks to ensure efficacy, safety and chemical purity

Most drugs are sold for profit by pharmaceutical companies. Various methods have been developed to test whether a particular drug is effective and safe and most national governments regulate both testing and approval for sale of drugs. Two distinct regulatory steps are generally recognized in this process: approval for clinical testing of a new drug; and approval for sale of a new drug. The main purposes of regulating drug approval are:

- To protect the public because of the conflict of interest between the need for pharmaceutical companies to make a profit and the need of patients for medication that is likely to be of benefit.
- To apply standards of proof of effectiveness and adequate safety, so that practitioners can be assured that a drug has been tested sufficiently.
- To assure that manufacturing processes result in a predictable product with acceptable purity and constant physical properties.
- Regulation is also required to control the public's access to certain drugs, particularly those liable to abuse.

The regulation of drugs began in the United States with the Federal Pure Food and Drug Act 1906. This first drug Act was concerned only with drug purity and was primarily passed in reaction to public disclosures of impurities and carelessness in the preparation of food and medicinal products. Later, the sulfanilamide tragedy led to the establishment of the Food and Drug Administration (FDA). The power of the FDA, and of regulatory authorities around the world, was expanded in the 1960s after the thalidomide tragedy in Europe. Laws were extended to require the demonstration of safety and efficacy in clinical trials prior to allowing the general availability of a new medicine.

As a general approach to evidence-based drug development the new requirements are scientifically sound and sensible. It is important to recognize that, although the rigorous establishment of safety and effectiveness is a worthy goal of drug development and regulation, no system of regulation is guaranteed to prevent all harm that could come from a particular drug. Some effects are too rare to be detected in drug development programs involving only hundreds to thousands of patients. Delaying approval of a drug until tens of thousands of people have been exposed could often result in many patients not getting a beneficial drug.

Drug development and regulation is thus an assessment of relative risk and benefit; quantitation of either is not absolute. Regulation will not prevent all ills resulting from the use of drugs. It can only serve to obtain a certain degree of qualitative and quantitative rigor in establishing the risk and efficacy of a drug. Regulation has also led to a more uniform set of information that is readily available

Table 3.1 Examples of different uses of drugs

To prevent disease (for prophylaxis)	Vaccines, such as pertussis vaccine
	Antimalarial drugs such as chloroquine
To investigate disease	Synthetic adrenocorticotropic hormone (ACTH), to test for adrenal suppression
	Barium sulfate for gastrointestinal radiology
	Ioxaglate for angiographic radiology
To treat disease	
Symptomatic treatment	Acetaminophen for headache
	Metoclopramide for nausea
Specific treatment	Penicillin G to treat streptococcal infection
To alter physiologic function	The oral contraceptive pill

to clinicians who must assess the relative merits of a new drug compared with existing therapeutic agents. Although it is ultimately the responsibility of the prescribing physician or health professional to know what data support the use of a drug in a particular setting and what the risks of such use are, an underlying assumption of regulation is that those authorized to prescribe need assistance in making choices.

Drug testing involves a progression from studies in animals to studies in humans. Since the 1990s, there has been continuing progress in making the requirements for drug development more uniform in the United States, Europe and Japan through harmonizing their different approaches. The International Conference on the Harmonization of Technical Requirements for Registration of Pharmaceuticals for Human Use (ICH guidelines) is an ongoing multinational attempt by authorities in drug development and regulation to evaluate scientific and technical aspects of the process of approving drugs. The effort is officially sanctioned by several bodies, including the European Commission of the European Union, the Ministry of Health and Welfare of Japan, the United States FDA, as well as several international scientific societies. Guidelines have been established and mostly accepted by regulatory authorities for principles of manufacture; methods to evaluate analytic procedures, chemical and physical stability of a product; conduct of preclinical and clinical trials and establishment of safety and effectiveness. Thus regulatory bodies worldwide:

- Set the policy that defines what animal data are sufficient before human studies can start with a new drug.
- Enforce rules of manufacturing and purity for that drug so that the stated contents and amounts of a particular medication are accurate.
- To varying extents, limit what claims can be made about drugs in advertising and for what conditions the drug should be prescribed.

STAGES IN DRUG DEVELOPMENT

Several stages can be defined between the discovery of a new drug and the demonstration of its clinical effectiveness and adequate safety (Fig. 3.1). The initial discovery stage usually involves deciding upon a therapeutic target (disease or condition) or a target molecule such as receptors, enzymes, etc., and then finding a lead chemical compound; that is, a compound with the characteristic actions of the required ideal new drug. In most drug discovery programs nowadays, a particular target molecule is chosen as a critical link in the disease process and small synthetic or natural chemicals are screened to determine whether they target this molecule, and therefore constitute a lead for further attempts to develop better compounds. Obtaining better compounds is an iterative process involving the synthesis of multiple chemical variants of the lead compound. Structure–activity relationship (SAR or QSAR if quantitative)

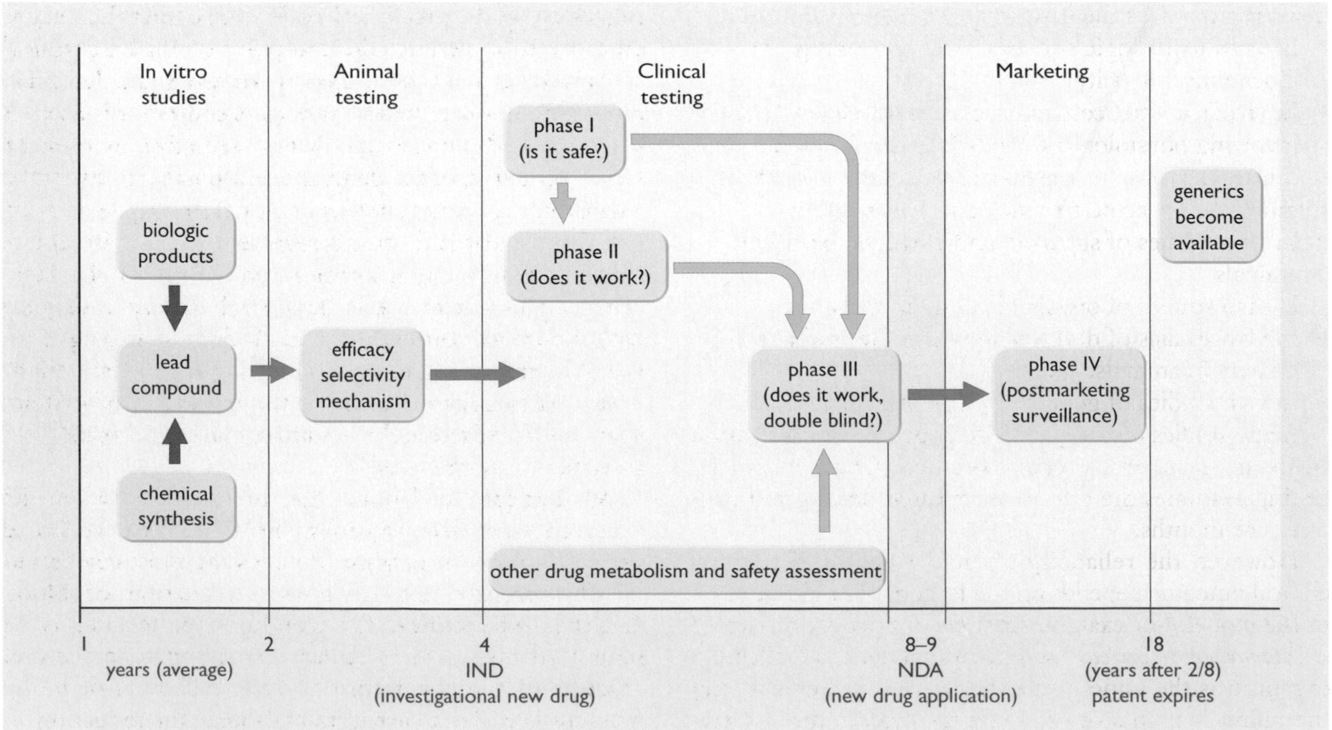

Fig. 3.1 The development and testing process required to bring a drug to market in the USA. Some of the requirements may be different for drugs used in life-threatening diseases. (Adapted with permission from Katzung BG. *Basic and Clinical Pharmacology*, 6th edn. New York: Appleton & Lange.)

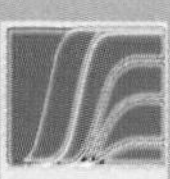

analysis is used to direct the production of new analogs for obtaining the required potency and efficacy.

Some analogs are subjected to extensive pharmacologic and toxicologic studies to identify and characterize the drug candidates sufficiently to gain approval for testing in humans. After a series of clinical trials the data collected are submitted to regulatory authorities to secure approval for marketing the new drug. After approval, experiences with the drug in clinical practice are collected by a variety of methods in an exercise called postmarketing surveillance (see later), an activity which is not as heavily regulated as the procedures that lead to approval.

Animal studies provide the justification for clinical trials

A profile of in vitro and in vivo pharmacologic effects of a drug forms the rationale for considering whether it is likely to have therapeutic value. These data are needed to justify investigating a new drug in humans since, without it, there would be no basis for anticipating either benefit, or an acceptable risk of adverse effects. Preclinical drug development is the name given to in vitro and animal studies that are used to screen for particular molecular actions, test for cellular, tissue and system pharmacologic properties and subsequently (using animal models of human disease) examine potential therapeutic effects. Animal studies also help in deciding the metabolic fate and distribution of a new drug in the body as well as guiding the choice of route of administration. Ultimately, clinical studies cannot proceed unless a drug is shown to be safe. The assessment of possible toxicity of a potential new drug involves the following animal studies:

- In vitro toxicologic studies to test for genetic and biochemical toxicity.
- In vivo acute toxicologic studies in whole animals, involving physiologic systems (e.g. cardiovascular, central nervous and gastrointestinal) and skin and mucosae (for acute irritancy and sensitization).
- In vivo studies of subacute and chronic toxicity in animals.
- In vivo studies of oncogenicity in animals.
- In vivo studies of developmental and reproductive toxicity in animals.
- In vivo studies of genetic toxicity in animals.

Acute studies investigate toxic effects occurring within hours or days of a single exposure. Chronic toxicity testing examines the effects of repeated doses given over weeks or months.

However, the reliability of animal data in predicting clinical outcome depends on the level of clinical relevance of the model. For example, models of pneumonia caused by *Staphylococcus aureus* are quite predictive. The infecting organism is the same in the model, and in humans, and the animal's immunologic defenses against the bacteria and pulmonary pathology are very similar to those in humans. In contrast, animal models of other diseases only indirectly mimic the disease in man and are less predictive. Usually, the ability to develop models in animals is related to a basic understanding of the pathophysiology of a particular disorder. In the above examples, the immediate cause of the pneumonia is known whereas in many diseases the immediate precipitating cause is not known.

Human testing of drugs progresses through a series of clinical trials

Clinical trials begin after sufficient in vitro and animal data have been generated to warrant testing a new drug in humans to ultimately gain the appropriate regulatory approval. The three phases of drug development have been denoted as phase I, phase II and phase III. Phase IV has been defined as postmarketing surveillance and other postapproval clinical studies (see Fig. 3.1).

Phase I comprises the first studies in humans, which are carried out under very close supervision and are usually open label or single blind (see Table 3.2 for terminology) to find the lowest dose that cannot be tolerated because of unacceptable, readily apparent acute toxicity. Further testing is carried out with doses less than this dose. Traditionally, these studies have been carried out in healthy young males but increasingly the latter are being replaced by the type of patients who will eventually use the drug. Initial pharmacokinetic data can also be obtained at this phase.

Phase II studies only begin after the tolerated dose range has been defined and are seen as 'proof of concept' studies. These are carried out in patients for whom the new drug is deemed to have potential benefit. The major purpose is to gather evidence that the drug has the effects suggested by the preclinical evidence, i.e. that the drug is efficacious. Sometimes the end-point of phase II clinical trials is the actual goal of therapy, known as the definitive end-point; at other times a surrogate end-point is used. A surrogate end-point is one that is predictive, or thought to be predictive, of the definitive end-point. For example, a drug that is being tested in heart failure may have as its definitive end-point an improvement in exercise tolerance, or in survival. A surrogate end-point for the same drug may be a decrease in peripheral vascular resistance with improved cardiac output. A drug that might be useful in preventing clotting following angioplasty might have as a surrogate end-point the inhibition of platelet aggregation, whereas the definitive end-point would be a reduction in re-stenosis.

A surrogate end-point has most utility when its occurrence has been rigorously linked to the occurrence of the definitive end-point. Perhaps the most celebrated of all surrogate end-points is a reduction of blood pressure. The reason for treating hypertension is to reduce adverse cardiovascular events and renal failure, sequelae of the hypertension. Thus reduction of blood pressure is really a surrogate end-point for reduction in the consequences of hypertension.

Other purposes of phase II trials are to determine the pharmacokinetic profile of a drug and to relate plasma

Table 3.2 Clinical trial terminology

Term	Definition
Control	The established therapy (or a placebo if there is no established therapy) against which the efficacy of a new drug can be compared
Randomized	Patients entering the trial have an equal probability of receiving the test or control drug so that factors that could affect the outcome, other than the therapy being tested, are equally distributed in the experimental and control groups
Double blind	Neither the health professionals nor the patient know whether the patient is receiving the experimental or control agent, to avoid any bias about which therapy might be better
Single blind	The health professionals know which treatment a patient is receiving, but the patient does not know
Open label	The opposite of double blind. Both health professionals and patients know whether the drug is the experimental or the control drug and the dose that the patient is receiving
Parallel trial	At least two regimens are tested simultaneously, but patients are assigned only one therapy
Crossover trial	Patients receive each therapy in sequence and therefore serve as their own controls. For example, if therapy A is being tested against therapy B, some patients receive A before B and some receive B before A, so that the effect of the drug therapy, and not of the order in which each therapy is given, can be tested
End-point	This is measured to assess a drug's effect (e.g. blood pressure is the end-point for testing an antihypertensive drug, while pain relief is the end-point for testing an analgesic)
Surrogate end-point	An outcome of therapy that predicts the real goal of therapy without being that goal (e.g. reduction in tumor size as a surrogate for survival)

concentrations to effects if possible. The influence of hepatic and renal disease on the elimination of the drug from the body is also investigated and pharmacokinetic and pharmacologic interactions of the new drug with other drugs liable to be coadministered can be explored.

Phase II studies may be single or double blind and may be parallel or crossover in design, with patients being allocated randomly to treatment groups. In ethnically diverse populations, such as exist in the United States, pharmacokinetic studies are sometimes required to elucidate how different ethnic groups metabolize a drug. Ethnic identity is a crude approximation of genetic classification. Perhaps in the future, a more elegant approach to predicting metabolic patterns and clinical outcomes will be employed to classify patients by genetic predisposition to metabolize drugs in particular ways. It may even be possible to predict which genotypes are most likely to benefit from a particular drug or most likely to develop a toxicity. This is referred to as pharmacogenetics.

Phase III trials establish the efficacy and safety of the new drug. Whenever possible, the trials are double blind, randomized and controlled. They are almost always parallel in design. Statistical considerations such as randomization of treatments must underpin the planning of design and size of all clinical trials, but especially phase III trials, so that valid conclusions can be made when the trials are completed. In addition, the population studied in phase III should approximate the target population for the drug. The trials should include patients with a representative range of the manifestations of the disease in question. The distribution of ethnic groups and gender should mirror that in the diseased population. In recent years, more emphasis has been placed on studying pediatric patients as part of the initial application for approval. This is now required in the United States except in instances where such an effort would be absurd, such as in the study of a drug for a disease of the elderly such as Alzheimer's disease.

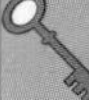

Drug development is a lengthy process

- The time taken from submitting an application for approval to receiving a decision can be 6 months to many years, though 1–2 years is typical
- The process of drug development, from discovery to approval, typically takes from 6 to more than 10 years

DRUG REGULATIONS FOR NEW DRUGS

Drug regulations and approval proceeds by several steps

Although practices vary from country to country, and continent to continent, drug regulations everywhere are aimed to ensure that marketed drugs are safe and effective. However, 'safe' and 'effective' are relative terms and require interpretation. Furthermore, the emphasis placed on either of the two aspects depends upon the intended medical use of an agent. Not unreasonably, toxicity is tolerated for drugs that have beneficial effects in otherwise fatal diseases for which there are few if any cures, for example AIDS and many cancers. However, the safety requirements for an analgesic for mild to moderate pain will be quite different: only minimal and non-medically serious adverse effects would be allowed. Some regulatory bodies give more weight to safety relative to effectiveness than do others. Regulation also seeks to ensure that a drug product has adequate purity and that its chemical and physical characteristics are well described and can be reproduced in each manufactured batch.

As noted above, the process of 'harmonization' is under way to make the regulatory process more uniform, especially between the United States and Europe. Although

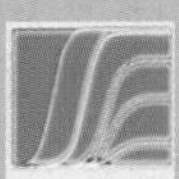

there are differences in the details of the approval process and, indeed, sometimes in the results of the process, the requirements and expectations are much more uniform than they were in the mid to latter third of the twentieth century. While not official policy, the European and US regulatory authorities in fact pay much attention to the activities and decisions of each other.

In the USA, the Food and Drug Administration approves drugs

In the USA a pharmaceutical company submits preclinical data to the Food and Drug Administration (FDA) in a document called an Investigational New Drug (IND) application. The FDA then gives or withholds permission to initiate clinical trials in humans. As clinical trials proceed, the pharmaceutical company keeps the FDA informed of progress and any adverse effect and/or toxicity. When phase III trials are completed, the company submits all preclinical and clinical data to the FDA in a New Drug Application (NDA). The FDA reviews the data and decides whether the data provide adequate documentation of safety and effectiveness to support the use of the drug for a particular disease.

Sometimes, the FDA will seek the advice of independent advisory committees of clinicians and scientists possessing pertinent expertise. This most often occurs when a novel indication is sought, when a first representative of a new class of drugs is being considered, or when the results of a development program are not clear. The committees' deliberations are public events and may be observed by anyone who can get in the door. With or without an advisory committee, if the data so warrant, the FDA will then approve the drug. If the data are not adequate, the FDA will ask for additional clinical trials. Part of the approval process consists of writing a 'label'. The label provides details of the pharmacokinetics, efficacy and toxicity of the drug. In addition, a summary of the main pivotal clinical trials are described.

The FDA also approves the manufacturing process, including the scientific standards for the chemical nature and formulation of the drug. Once an NDA is approved, the company may sell the drug. Although the FDA has the power to approve a drug for marketing for a particular indication or set of indications, it does not have the power to regulate use once such approval is granted. Thus physicians may choose to use a drug for a non-approved indication, so-called 'off-label use'. Often such use is warranted by strong evidence from clinical trials that, for one reason or another, have not been submitted to the FDA. For a drug with one approved indication, the results of clinical trials that would form the basis of an approval for a second indication are publicly available before the approval process runs its course. In these settings, such off-label use of a drug is perfectly reasonable.

A prototypical example of appropriate off-label use was the early employment of propranolol for treating hypertension. This β blocker was initially approved in the United States for angina. However, based on both pharmacologic considerations and clinical observations, it was recognized that propranolol was effective in reducing blood pressure in hypertensive patients. The drug was widely used for this indication for many years before such use was approved. Some off-label use is, however, of dubious merit. It is the responsibility of the physician to know the data and to make judgments about whether the evidence supports expanding the scope of a drug's utility.

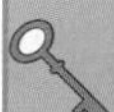

Information provided by the drug 'label' required for FDA approval in the USA

- Data that support the approval
- Pharmacologic actions of the drug
- Indication (approved use) of the drug
- A description of adverse effects
- Instructions on dosing

In Europe, drug approval is regulated by both centralized and decentralized processes aimed at producing more uniform practices across member states of the EU

In Europe the regulation process has changed dramatically since the inception of the European Union (EU), with new procedures replacing the previous country-by-country approval process. As a result the prerequisites for approval have become uniform in the member states.

Once clinical drug development has been completed, a pharmaceutical company can proceed by either a centralized or decentralized (officially called mutual recognition) process, which ultimately results in more uniform practices across all member states. The process chosen by a pharmaceutical company depends on a combination of commercial and political considerations, as well as the kind of molecule being considered.

The centralized EU procedure

Under the EU centralized procedure, applications are submitted to the European Medicines Evaluation Agency (EMEA), which is responsible for administering the regulatory procedures and sending the application to the Committee on Proprietary Medicinal Products (CPMP). The CPMP, composed of representatives of all member states, appoints a rapporteur. The rapporteur is identified with a particular country, and the staff of that country's drug regulatory agency are responsible for the initial review. When the review is complete the rapporteur prepares a report of the data and provides an opinion on whether approval is possible. The reports are then presented to the CPMP. The CPMP may request further information and pose questions that the sponsoring pharmaceutical company must answer. Finally, the CPMP formulates its opinion and a decision is made by majority vote, for or against approval. Approval by this centralized process entitles the pharmaceutical sponsor to sell the product throughout the member states of the EU. The EU 'label' is called the Summary of Product Characteristics, which is uniform in all member states. This label is much less detailed than the label of the United States, the latter presenting more details of the clinical trials that supported the application.

The mutual recognition (decentralized) EU procedure

In the decentralized EU procedure an application is made to one country, a so-called reference member state. The regulatory authority of that state reviews the data and makes a unilateral decision about whether to approve the application or not. If the reference member state approves the application, a report is sent to each of the member states in which the applicant would like to market the drug; these states can either accept the report, and therefore approve the application, or object to the report. In the case of objection, the applicant can choose to forego approval in the rejecting state or to seek arbitration by the CPMP. The CPMP's decision is ultimately binding on all member states. Again, a uniform Summary of Product Characteristics is composed for all states in which the application is accepted.

Although off-label use in Europe is possible, and sometimes occurs, it is much less prevalent than in the United States because payment for drugs in Europe is much more closely tied to the approval process than is payment in the United States.

In Japan, the approval process is carried out under the authority of the Ministry of Health and Welfare, and the Central Pharmaceutical Affairs Council

Initiating clinical trials in Japan requires the approval of the Ministry of Health and Welfare (MHW). An application for approval is sent to the MHW after data have been assembled from clinical trials. The MHW acts as an administrative body and sends the data to the Central Pharmaceutical Affairs Council (CPAC) for review. The CPAC consists of experts in various disciplines such as medicine and pharmaceutical science and recommends a course of action to the MHW, which implements the approval.

In the last few years there have been several internal reviews of the Japanese testing and approval process. The barriers to data from non-Japanese patients have been somewhat penetrated, at least for phase II and phase III studies. Nevertheless, in practice, studies in Japanese patients are required on the grounds that the Japanese are sufficiently biologically and culturally different from the typical European or North American patient for a separate set of trials to be necessary. The underlying principle is the same as that which requires testing in minority ethnic groups versus the dominant population. Traditionally, the Japanese have not relied as heavily on controlled, blinded trials, although this may be changing with the effort towards harmonization.

The United States, the EU and Japan account for by far the most new drug introduction in the world. However, drugs are regulated to one degree or another in most if not all countries. Some of these countries accept the same application made in Europe or the United States. Many of these countries make their own determinations based wholly or in large part on the decisions of the United States and Europe. Some accept these decisions outright, while others remain more independent, using the decisions as a point to consider but by no means regarding them as binding or automatically acceptable.

PHARMACOTHERAPEUTIC DECISION MAKING

Once a drug has been approved for marketing, physicians are then able to prescribe it. Pharmacotherapeutic decisions are among the most difficult decisions in medical practice and are an integral part of medicine.

Why should the patient be treated and with what drug?

The physician's first pharmacotherapeutic task is to decide whether the patient has a condition that would benefit from drug treatment.

If drug treatment is indicated, the physician then needs to consider its benefits versus adverse effects and decide whether the treatment should be prescribed. For example, acne can be treated effectively with the vitamin A derivative isotretinoin but this drug can cause serious adverse effects including liver damage, increases in serum cholesterol concentration and fetal malformation as a result of exposure in utero. It is therefore unsuitable for the treatment of mild acne. The physician also has to consider whether there are alternative treatments. For example, although the antibiotic chloramphenicol is an effective treatment of bacterial pharyngitis, it is avoided because it carries a risk of causing life-threatening bone marrow aplasia, once in 40 000 treatments, and therefore penicillin V (phenoxymethylpenicillin) is preferred.

A most important test of a new drug is how safe it is in clinical use

A new drug is usually given to approximately 1500 patients in premarketing clinical trials. This number of patients is far too small to detect uncommon or rare adverse events. However, increasing the number of patients studied prior to marketing would delay marketing, thereby delaying the use of the potentially beneficial drugs by ill patients.

A useful rule of thumb for gauging the possible occurrence of toxicity is the 'rule of three'. This states that if an event has not been observed in n patients, then it is 95% certain that the true frequency of the event in a larger population of patients lies somewhere between 0 and $3/n$. Therefore, even if there is no fatal reaction to a drug among 1500 patients, the above statistics give a 5%

 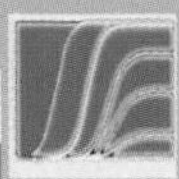

chance it could possibly cause up to one death in 500 treated patients. Caution about safety is particularly important for drugs that do not have greater therapeutic efficacy compared with older, more established drugs.

■ *Phase IV studies involve postmarketing surveillance of treated patients and rely on spontaneous adverse reaction reports*

Postmarketing surveillance is extremely important for ensuring drug safety. Rare and even fairly common adverse effects can be detected only after trials involving very large numbers of patients. Postmarketing surveillance ('pharmacovigilance'), particularly the spontaneous reporting of adverse reactions, is therefore useful and necessary because many more patients receive a drug after it is marketed than during the premarketing phase I–III studies. It is inevitable that some drugs which are licensed subsequently prove to be less safe than is desirable. These drugs can then be removed from the market or their use restricted. Some drugs withdrawn from the market in the United States in the past 5 years are listed in the section below on pharmocovigilance.

The true value of a drug is ultimately determined by cumulative analysis of successive clinical trials (known as meta analysis).

DRUG REGULATIONS RELATING TO ACCESS TO DRUGS

■ *The rules and regulations relating to access to drugs vary between countries, as does the implementation of those rules*

All countries have regulations regarding the possession and prescribing of drugs, but these vary widely between different countries. In some countries the public has ready access to many drugs without needing a prescription. In other countries the sale and release of the same drugs are tightly controlled. This relates not only to which drugs can legally be sold as over-the-counter (OTC) medications, but also to how regulations are applied. For example, vitamins and other herbal remedies are regulated as food products, not drugs, in many countries, including the United States. Thus extravagant and unsubstantiated claims can be made in advertising for herbs that would be illegal for medicinal products. There are, however, laws against adding modern drugs to herbal mixtures (a not uncommon practice).

■ *Many drugs have the potential for abuse and are therefore tightly regulated*

All countries have laws concerning the possession, sales and distribution of drugs that are abused, including narcotics, alcohol and tobacco. The latter two are, after all, also drugs. The drugs most likely to be abused are those with central nervous system (CNS) actions, in particular the opiates (see Ch. 8), nicotine, CNS depressants, such as barbiturates, and psychoactive drugs such as cocaine and lysergic acid diethylamide (LSD). The laws governing these agents vary both within countries (in particular the United States) and between countries. In addition to concerns about health, social acceptance of drug use and other moral concerns also affect policy. Both alcohol and cigarettes (the vehicle for delivering nicotine in a carcinogenic formulation to addicted consumers) have enormous medical and economic costs but their purchase is only restricted on the basis of age. Meanwhile drugs whose possession is illegal, such as heroin, cause a large part of their damage because of unsterile methods of administration and criminal acts to secure illicit supplies. This is not to say that the primary effects of such drugs are benign. They are not.

Nevertheless, some very damaging drugs are tolerated by society, and some are not. Some countries allow addicts to receive drugs on a regular basis at government-controlled centers. In the Netherlands, cannabis is available in limited quantities in commercial establishments, the equivalents of cafés. A law recently passed in California allows for medicinal use of cannabis under defined circumstances. This law is being challenged by the Federal government and is actively being adjudicated in the courts. There is active and lively debate regarding the success, or lack thereof, of the more punitive, legally based restrictions and punishments for drug possession. No matter what overall position one takes on the law, it is clear that both the cause and treatment of abusive self-administration of pharmacologically active agents have medical and psychologic components.

DETECTING ADVERSE DRUG REACTIONS

Adverse drug reactions frequently mimic ordinary diseases. Serious reactions tend to affect:

- Systems in which there is rapid cell multiplication (e.g. the skin, hematopoietic system and lining of the gut).
- Organs in which drugs are detoxified and/or excreted (e.g. the liver and kidneys).

Typical examples of such serious reactions are toxic epidermal necrolysis, aplastic anemia, pseudomembranous colitis, hepatitis and nephritis.

Adverse effects, especially uncommon ones, may be difficult to diagnose and a physician must always consider whether any effect associated with the use of a new drug is actually caused by the drug. However, since a general practitioner might work for a lifetime without seeing a case of aplastic anemia, the detection of both common and uncommon adverse drug reactions requires vigilance on the part of the patient, the physician and others involved in the drug treatment of patients, including the pharmacist and other health professionals.

■ *Adverse reactions to drugs are most easily detected when they are dramatic, differ from natural disease, or are of rapid onset following the start of treatment*

An anaphylactic reaction occurring within minutes of a penicillin injection, characterized by tissue edema, bronchospasm and cardiovascular collapse, is obviously an adverse drug effect. It is much more difficult to detect adverse effects that occur only after a long period of treatment or have an insidious onset. It is even more difficult to detect adverse effects that occur only after the drug has been discontinued. An example of a long-delayed adverse effect is the malignant disease that occurs in about 15% of patients previously treated with cyclophosphamide for lymphomas of childhood.

Adverse effects that mimic naturally occurring disease are more difficult to detect than those with unique features, especially if the adverse effect resembles a common or relatively innocuous disease. The defect of phocomelia is very obvious in its presentation of stunted or missing (seal-like) limbs and is extremely rare; therefore astute clinicians were relatively quick to associate phocomelia with taking thalidomide. In contrast, the increased risk of spina bifida in babies born to women taking the antiepileptic drug sodium valproate during pregnancy could be verified only by carefully designed clinical studies, since spina bifida is not uncommon.

If a specific adverse drug effect has a well-recognized latency to onset, it can be anticipated and therefore detected more easily

In deciding whether an adverse event that occurs with treatment is due to the drug, latency to the onset of the adverse event should be considered. Some adverse effects appear with a well-characterized latency, others less so, while obviously an adverse effect occurring before treatment cannot be due to the drug. Adverse effects may occur with characteristic latencies:

- Just after exposure (e.g. anaphylaxis to penicillin, intense vasodilation and hypotension after an injection of vancomycin – the syndrome known as l'homme rouge or red man syndrome).
- A few days after exposure (e.g. serum sickness induced by snake antitoxins made from horse serum; an ampicillin rash in patients with infectious mononucleosis).
- Only after chronic treatment (e.g. iatrogenic Cushing's syndrome after weeks or months of treatment with oral glucocorticosteroids).
- After cessation of treatment (e.g. withdrawal syndromes from benzodiazepines or 5-hydroxytryptamine reuptake inhibitors).
- In subsequent generations (e.g. phocomelia with thalidomide, retinoid embryopathy).

Certain adverse effects, such as anaphylaxis and bone marrow aplasia, are characteristic for certain drugs.

A drug is more probably the cause of a reversible event if the event disappears after the drug is stopped (de-challenge) and then reappears when the drug is restarted (re-challenge).

A drug is more probably responsible for an adverse effect:

- **If it is well recognized that the adverse effect occurs contemporaneously with the drug**
- **If the adverse effect is recognized as an adverse effect of a class of drugs and the suspect drug resembles this class (e.g. cough is an adverse effect associated with angiotensin-converting enzyme inhibitors)**

An alphabetic classification helps memorize different types of adverse effects due to drugs

The types of adverse effect seen with drugs are listed in Table 3.3. Most fit into an alphabetic scheme, though some may fit into more than one category, and others are difficult to classify. The first two categories are fundamental. Type A (augmented pharmacologic) reactions are easily predicted from the known pharmacologic effects of a drug, while the risk of the reaction depends on dose. Many, such as constipation with opiate analgesic drugs or throbbing headache with nitrate antianginal drugs, are a nuisance rather than a danger.

Type B (bizarre) adverse effects are unpredictable and often severe. Examples include anaphylaxis (which can result in a fatal cardiovascular collapse), renal and hepatic failure and bone marrow suppression. Some of the more important type B reactions are given in Table 3.4.

Some patients are more susceptible than others to adverse effects of a drug

The benefits of any drug treatment must always be weighed against possible harm. Those who are particularly susceptible to adverse effects include the fetus, patients with pre-existing illnesses or genetic enzyme defects, patients who are already taking other drugs and elderly patients.

Pregnant women

Treatment of pregnant women (and women at risk of pregnancy) must take into account the welfare of both fetus and mother. Teratogenic drugs (those that are known to cause malformations to the fetus) must obviously be avoided. However, it is wise to regard all drugs as being potentially teratogenic. Therefore no drug should be prescribed to a pregnant woman, no matter how innocuous it may seem, unless:

- There is a clear need for it and the drug is considered by the professions to be safe to the fetus.
- The mother is so ill that its use is justified even if the fetus might be harmed.

Pre-existing illnesses

Pre-existing illnesses such as liver or kidney disease can exacerbate or precipitate adverse drug effects. As a result of such conditions, a drug may be present in the body in a higher concentration or for a longer period. Reduced metabolism or excretion makes patients more susceptible to type A adverse effects (an augmented pharmacologic

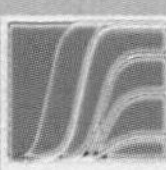

Table 3.3 Alphabetic classification of types of adverse drug effects

Type	Type of effect	Definition	Examples
A	Augmented pharmacologic effects	Adverse effects that are known to occur from the pharmacology of the drug and are dose-related. They are seldom fatal and relatively common	Hypoglycemia due to insulin injection Bradycardia due to β adrenoceptor antagonists Hemorrhage due to anticoagulants
B	Bizarre effects	Adverse effects that occur unpredictably and often have a higher rate of morbidity and mortality. They are uncommon	Anaphylaxis to penicillin Acute hepatic necrosis due to halothane Bone marrow suppression by chloramphenicol
C	Chronic effects	Adverse effects that only occur during prolonged treatment and not with single doses	Iatrogenic Cushing's syndrome with prednisolone Orofacial dyskinesia due to phenothiazine tranquilizers Colonic dysfunction due to laxatives
D	Delayed effects	Adverse effects that occur remote from treatment, either in the children of treated patients or in patients themselves years after treatment	Second cancers in those treated with alkylating agents for Hodgkin's disease Craniofacial malformations in infants whose mothers have taken isotretinoin Clear-cell carcinoma of the vagina in the daughters of women who took diethylstilbestrol during pregnancy
E	End-of-treatment effects	Adverse effects that occur when a drug is stopped, especially when it is stopped suddenly (so-called withdrawal effects)	Unstable angina after β adrenoceptor antagonists are suddenly stopped Adrenocortical insufficiency after glucocorticosteroids such as prednisolone are stopped Withdrawal seizures when anticonvulsants such as phenobarbital or phenytoin are stopped

Table 3.4 Some important type B (bizarre) reactions

Adverse effect	Drug causes
Anaphylaxis	Penicillins and other antibacterial agents Foreign protein such as streptokinase or equine antirattlesnake vaccine Iodinated contrast media in radiology
Anaphylactoid reactions (non-immunologic reactions resembling anaphylaxis but occurring without prior exposure)	Angiotensin-converting enzyme inhibitors (angioedema) Intravenous *N*-acetylcysteine (urticaria and anaphylaxis) The solvent polyethoxylated castor oil
Liver disease (acute hepatic necrosis)	Halogenated anesthetic gases such as chloroform, halothane and enflurane Chlorpromazine, the oral contraceptive pill and floxacillin (intrahepatic cholestasis) Minocycline (chronic active hepatitis)
Kidney disease	Nonsteroidal antiinflammatory drugs (acute interstitial nephritis) Amphotericin (acute tubular necrosis) Angiotensin-converting enzyme inhibitors (vascular renal damage)
Bone marrow damage	The antithyroid drugs carbimazole, methimazole and propylthiouracil Antibacterial agents such as chloramphenicol and co-trimoxazole Antirheumatic drugs such as gold salts and penicillamine

response to a standard dose). The adverse effects of some drugs are also more common in patients with organ failure. For example, the potassium-sparing diuretic amiloride is more likely to cause hyperkalemia in patients with impaired kidneys because K^+ excretion occurs via the kidneys, and therefore their capacity to eliminate K^+ is reduced. In patients with liver disease, the anticoagulant effect of warfarin can be greatly enhanced, because the warfarin is metabolized more slowly and also because the ability of the liver to synthesize clotting factors is impaired.

Pre-existing disease can predispose to adverse effects in other ways. For example, respiratory failure with sedatives such as diazepam is much more likely in patients with chronic obstructive pulmonary disease since their respiratory drive is already reduced.

Genetically determined enzyme defects

As discussed in Chapter 4, the body contains many enzymes that metabolize drugs. Genetically determined deficits in such enzymes can make normally innocuous drug therapy hazardous and sometimes lethal. An example of such a defect is glucose-6-phosphate dehydrogenase (G6PD) deficiency, in its various forms. It is a chromosome X-linked recessive trait and therefore only occurs in males. Oxidants such as aspirin, primaquine and dapsone can cause severe hemolysis in people with this deficiency, which is most common in people of Mediterranean, African or South-East Asian origin.

Drug interactions

Drug interactions are an important clinical problem. They can be classified as:

- Pharmaceutical interactions, in which there is a chemical or physical interaction between two or more drugs before they are absorbed into the body.
- Pharmacokinetic interactions, where one drug alters the concentration of another via an interaction at the level of absorption, metabolism, distribution or elimination.
- Pharmacodynamic interactions, in which the actions of two drugs given together differ from those of either drug given separately.

Pharmaceutical interactions

Pharmaceutical interactions include, for example, the chemical chelation of Fe^{2+} by tetracyclines, which makes both iron sulfate and tetracyclines less effective when given together than when given separately. This is because the concentration available for absorption of one is lowered by the presence of the other. Another example is the precipitation of calcium hydroxide which occurs when calcium gluconate is added to an i.v. infusion of sodium bicarbonate solution.

Pharmacokinetic interactions

Pharmacokinetic interactions are in practice the most important and potentially dangerous of all drug interactions. They include the important interactions that occur between drugs which are metabolized by the cytochrome P-450 (mixed function oxidase) enzyme system (see Ch. 4 for a discussion of this system) and drugs that inhibit it. For example, the anticoagulant warfarin, theophylline (used in the treatment of asthma), and the anti transplant rejection drug ciclosporin are metabolized by cytochrome P-450. These drugs have a low therapeutic index (ratio between therapeutic concentration and toxic concentration; see Ch. 2) and therefore small changes in metabolism can provoke severe type A adverse effects. Drugs that inhibit cytochrome P-450 include the antibacterial agents erythromycin, co-trimoxazole and ciprofloxacin, the antifungal agents ketoconazole and fluconazole and the H_2 receptor antagonist cimetidine.

A small number of drugs can actually induce the production of cytochrome P-450 enzymes and, as a result, reduce the concentration of drugs metabolized by the enzyme system. Such enzyme inducers include the anticonvulsants phenobarbital and carbamazepine and the antituberculous drug rifampicin. Women on oral contraception who take these drugs need to take higher doses of estrogens than normal, otherwise the enhanced estrogen metabolism will leave them unprotected against pregnancy.

Renal excretion of one drug can be influenced by the presence of another: for example, the renal excretion of lithium, which can be inhibited by thiazide diuretics.

Pharmacodynamic interactions

Anticholinergic drugs and levodopa are used to treat Parkinson's disease, with one drug reducing cholinergic activity, and the other increasing dopaminergic activity. Both effects tend to improve the movement disorder, though both can also cause hallucinations and delirium (for a fuller discussion see Ch. 8).

Pharmacovigilance

Since, as discussed earlier in this chapter, far too few patients are normally entered into phase I–III trials to detect relatively rare adverse events, monitoring of possible drug-related side effects continues after marketing approval. This is referred to as pharmacovigilance and it should be recognized that true risk is often very different from perceived risk.

People are generally unable to estimate risk accurately, perceiving new and technical hazards as riskier than they are, while underestimating everyday and familiar hazards. Figure 3.2 illustrates the relationship between perceived risk and actual risk for 41 different causes of death. The 'perceived risk' determines the way people behave and can be manifest in what they say (the 'expressed risk') or what they do (the 'revealed risk'). Patients are sometimes fearful of taking medicines (e.g. after a newspaper article discussing one particularly dramatic case of an adverse effect), but will happily continue smoking even though in smokers the lifetime risk of a fatal illness due to tobacco is about 0.5 (50%). The risks perceived by doctors can also differ markedly from the true risks measured in well-designed studies. (It is interesting to compare this situation with the way we accept the cost–benefit ratio for travel by car. We gladly accept a real risk of death and injury for the benefit of convenient travel.)

Pharmacoepidemiology is the study of the use and effects of drugs in large populations rather than individuals. Pharmacoepidemiology uses the methods of epidemiology and is concerned with all aspects of the risk–benefit ratio for populations using particular drugs. Pharmacovigilance is a branch of pharmacoepidemiology. It is restricted to the epidemiologic study of drug-related

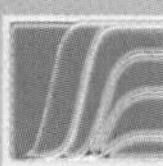

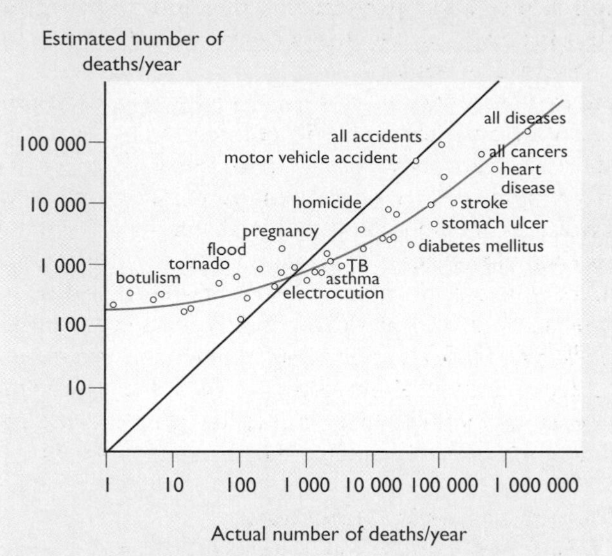

Fig. 3.2 Relationship between perceived frequency and the actual number of deaths/year for 41 causes of death. If the perceived and actual frequencies are equal, the data fall on the straight line. The points and the curved line fitted to them represent the average response. (Adapted with permission from Kahneman D, Slovic P and Tversky A (eds). *Judgment Under Uncertainty: Heuristics and Biases*. Cambridge, Cambridge: University Press; 1982.)

events or adverse drug effects. 'Events' are recorded in the patient's notes during a period of drug monitoring. They may be due to the disease for which the drug is being given, an intercurrent disease or infection, an adverse reaction to the drug being monitored, the activity of a drug being given concomitantly or a drug interaction. An 'event' is something of note that happens in a patient that is not considered an appropriate therapeutic response and is due to the drug. An 'adverse event' is one that is potentially damaging to the patient.

Pharmacovigilance studies can be:

- Hypothesis generating (e.g. to detect unexpected adverse drug effects of a recently marketed drug).
- Hypothesis testing (e.g. to prove whether any suspicions raised about a specific drug are justified).
- Both hypothesis generating and hypothesis testing.

Methods of pharmacovigilance

- **Hypothesis generating: spontaneous adverse drug effect reporting (yellow card in the UK)**
- **Hypothesis generating and testing: prescription event monitoring (green form in the UK)**
- **Hypothesis testing: case–control studies, cohort studies, randomized controlled clinical trials**

Hypothesis-generating studies

It often happens in clinical practice that a patient becomes unwell while taking a medicine and the doctor or pharmacist suspects that the 'adverse event' is due to the drug. In spontaneous reporting schemes, a health professional who suspects an adverse reaction is encouraged to notify a central agency of the suspicion. Such spontaneous reporting has led to the identification of many unexpected adverse drug effects.

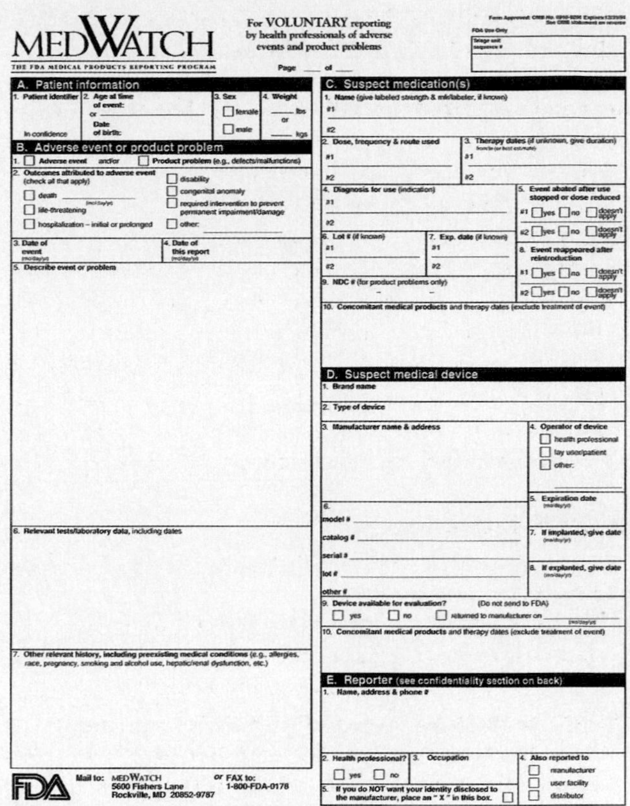

MEDWATCH
THE FDA MEDICAL PRODUCTS REPORTING PROGRAM
For VOLUNTARY reporting by health professionals of adverse events and product problems
Page ___ of ___

A. Patient information
1. Patient identifier 2. Age at time of event: or Date of birth: 3. Sex female male 4. Weight lbs or kgs
In confidence

B. Adverse event or product problem
1. Adverse event and/or Product problem (e.g., defects/malfunctions)
2. Outcomes attributed to adverse event (check all that apply)
death
life-threatening
hospitalization – initial or prolonged
disability
congenital anomaly
required intervention to prevent permanent impairment/damage
other:
3. Date of event
4. Date of this report
5. Describe event or problem
6. Relevant tests/laboratory data, including dates
7. Other relevant history, including preexisting medical conditions (e.g., allergies, race, pregnancy, smoking and alcohol use, hepatic/renal dysfunction, etc.)

C. Suspect medication(s)
1. Name (give labeled strength & mfr/labeler, if known)
2. Dose, frequency & route used
3. Therapy dates (if unknown, give duration)
4. Diagnosis for use (indication)
5. Event abated after use stopped or dose reduced
6. Lot # (if known)
7. Exp. date (if known)
8. Event reappeared after reintroduction
9. NDC # (for product problems only)
10. Concomitant medical products and therapy dates (exclude treatment of event)

D. Suspect medical device
1. Brand name
2. Type of device
3. Manufacturer name & address
4. Operator of device: health professional, lay user/patient, other:
5. Expiration date
6. model # catalog # serial # lot # other #
7. If implanted, give date
8. If explanted, give date
9. Device available for evaluation? (Do not send to FDA) yes no returned to manufacturer on
10. Concomitant medical products and therapy dates (exclude treatment of event)

E. Reporter (see confidentiality section on back)
1. Name, address & phone #
2. Health professional? yes no
3. Occupation
4. Also reported to: manufacturer, user facility, distributor
5. If you do NOT want your identity disclosed to the manufacturer, place an " X " in this box.

FDA
Mail to: MEDWATCH 5600 Fishers Lane Rockville, MD 20852-9787
or FAX to: 1-800-FDA-0178
Submission of a report does not constitute an admission that medical personnel or the product caused or contributed to the event.

Fig. 3.3 The FDA MedWatch reporting card.

This type of system was first introduced in the UK in 1964, as the 'yellow card'. A similar system for the reporting of adverse effects to drugs was established later by the FDA in the USA (Fig. 3.3). Similar systems are found throughout Europe and in most developed countries. All these systems rely on voluntary reporting by the prescriber, or other health professional, if they consider an event to be an adverse effect due to drugs.

The great strengths of these schemes are:

- They are operated for all drugs throughout the whole of the drug's lifetime.
- They are an affordable method of detecting rare adverse effects.

Their main weaknesses are:

- Gross underreporting, since the system is voluntary.
- Bias due to sudden media interest in a particular drug.
- The data provide only a numerator (i.e. the number of reports of each suspected reaction) but do not take into consideration how many patients have actually received the drug.

Nevertheless, these schemes are invaluable and it is essential that physicians fill in such drug report cards.

Table 3.5 Drugs licensed since 1972 and withdrawn in the UK owing to toxicity.

Product	Therapeutic class	Adverse reaction(s)	Type A/B reaction (see Table 3.3)
Aclofenac	NSAID	Anaphylaxis	B
Polidexide	Hypolipidemic	Impurities	–
Nomifensine	Antidepressant	Hemolytic anemia	B
Fenclofenac	NSAID	Epidermal necrolysis	B
Feprazone	NSAID	Nephrotoxicity, GI toxicity	A
Benoxaprofen	NSAID	Photosensitivity, hepatotoxicity	A
Zomepirac	NSAID	Anaphylaxis	B
Indoprofen	NSAID	GI toxicity	A
Zimeldine	Antidepressant	Guillain–Barré syndrome	B
Suprofen	NSAID	Nephrotoxicity	A
Terodiline	Anti-incontinence	Ventricular tachycardia	B
Triazolam	Hypnotic	Psychiatric reactions	A
Temafloxacin	Antibiotic	Multiorgan toxicity	B
Centoxin	Antibiotic	Increased mortality	B
Remoxipride	Neuroleptic	Aplastic anemia	B
Flosequinan	Cardiac failure	Increased mortality	B
Metipranolol	Antiglaucoma	Anterior uveitis	B

The list shows that licensed drugs can be the cause of major unexpected adverse drug reactions and also demonstrates the importance of pharmacovigilance. NSAID, nonsteroidal antiinflammatory drug; GI, gastrointestinal.

Table 3.6 Licensed drugs withdrawn from the United States market 1996–2004

Drug	Use	Problem
Alosetron	Treating irritable bowel syndrome	Ischemic colitis
Phenylpropanolamine	Nasal decongestant	Hemorrhagic stroke
Troglitazone	Oral antidiabetic agent	Toxic to the liver
Cisapride	To increase gut motility	Arrhythmia
Grepafloxacin	Antibacterial	Severe cardiovascular events
Rotavirus vaccine	Protect against rotavirus diarrhea	Intussusception
Astemizole	Nonsedating antihistamine	Arrhythmia
Bromfenac sodium	Nonsteroidal antiinflammatory	Severe hepatic failure
Mibefradil	Antihypertensive and antianginal	Potential for drug interactions
Terfenadine	Nonsedating antihistamine	Arrhythmia
Fenfluramine, dexfenfluramine	Antiobesity agents	Heart valve disease
Chlormezanone	Sedative	Toxic epidermal necrolysis
Rofecoxib	Pain	Increased cardiovascular events
Cerivastatin	Lipid lowering	Rhabdomyolysis

Many of the drugs on the list have been withdrawn voluntarily by the manufacturers. This list shows that licensed drugs can be the cause of major unexpected adverse drug reactions and also demonstrates the importance of pharmacovigilance.

Spontaneous reporting has led to identification of many unexpected adverse effects, resulting in the withdrawal of a number of marketed drugs. Examples of drugs that have been removed from the UK market since 1972 because of adverse events reported under the yellow card system are shown in Table 3.5 and those removed from the US market between 1996 and 2000 are shown in Table 3.6.

Hypothesis-generating and hypothesis-testing studies

Adverse event monitoring related to prescriptions (prescription event monitoring, PEM) is a hypothesis-generating and -testing process

Prescription event monitoring in the UK is an important technique which takes advantage of the way the country's National Health Service system is organized. It provides the denominator that is missing in the above systems. Dispensed prescriptions written by general practitioners are sent to a central Prescription Pricing Authority, which provides confidential copies of all prescriptions for newly introduced drugs that are being monitored to a Drug Safety Research Unit. This Unit then sends a 'green form' questionnaire (Fig. 3.4) to the general practitioner who wrote the original prescription. The green form is sent out 6 or 12 months after the first prescription. This procedure therefore provides the 'exposure data', showing which patients have been exposed to the drug being monitored, while the completed green forms provide the 'outcome data' detailing any events noted during the period of monitoring. The Drug Safety Research Unit can then follow up pregnancies, deaths or

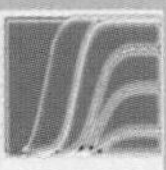

PLEASE REMOVE THIS SECTION OF THE FORM SO THAT THE BOTTOM HALF BECOMES ANONYMOUS.

DRUG SAFETY RESEARCH UNIT
PRESCRIPTION EVENT MONITORING

MEDICAL – IN CONFIDENCE

Dr Ronald D. Mann, MD, FRCP, FRCGP, FRCP(Glas), FFPM.
Bursledon Hall,
Southampton SO31 1AA
Telephone: (01703) 406122/3

We collect **EVENT** data.
An **EVENT** is any new diagnosis, any reason for referral to a consultant or admission to hospital, any unexpected deterioration (or improvement) in a concurrent illness, any suspected drug reaction, or any other complaint which was considered of sufficient importance to enter in the patient's notes.

Example: A broken leg is an **EVENT**.
Please tell us if you suspect an **EVENT** to be an adverse reaction to a drug.

These studies are conducted in accordance with the results of authorative discussions and the International Ethical Guidelines for Biomedical Research Involving Human Subjects prepared by the Council for International Organizations of Medical Sciences (CIOMS) in collaboration with the World Health Organization (WHO), Geneva 1993.

FOLD FOR STORAGE IN NOTES

Ref:

The DSRU is advised by the Drug Safety Research Trust, a registered independent charity (No. 327206) working in co-operation with the University of Southampton. Trustees: Professor D J Finney CBE ScD FRS FRSE, Professor C F George MD FRCP, Sir Gordon Higginson DL FEng, Professor Stephen T Holgate MD DSc FRCP.

PLEASE RETURN THIS HALF OF THE FORM. Ref:

SEX DATE OF BIRTH / /			WAS THIS DRUG EFFECTIVE? Yes ☐ No ☐	
INDICATION FOR PRESCRIBING			PLEASE SPECIFY REASON FOR STOPPING THIS DRUG AND NAME OF DRUG(S) SUBSTITUTED	
DATE PATIENT STARTED THIS DRUG / /			DATE PATIENT STOPPED THIS DRUG / /	
DATE	DOSE mg/day	EVENTS WHILE TAKING THIS DRUG	DATE	EVENTS AFTER STOPPING THIS DRUG
		If there were NO EVENTS ON DRUG please tick this box. ☐		If there were NO EVENTS OFF DRUG please tick this box. ☐

IMPORTANT: PLEASE INDICATE ANY EVENT REPORTED TO CSM OR MANUFACTURER

Fig. 3.4 The data collection segment of the green form used for prescription event monitoring in the UK.

events of special interest by contacting either the prescribing physician or other holders of the patient's medical record. So far 76 drugs have been studied and the average number of patients included in each study (the cohort size) has been about 10 500.

The strengths of the 'green form' method are:

- It provides a numerator (i.e. the number of reports) and a denominator (i.e. the number of patients exposed), both being collected over a precisely known period of observation.
- There is no interference with the physician's decision about which drug to prescribe for each individual patient. This avoids selection biases, which can make data interpretation difficult.

The main weakness of PEM in the UK is that only 50–70% of the green forms are returned. Attempts are now being made to establish PEM outside the UK.

Hypothesis-testing studies

Hypothesis-testing studies are used where previous data have led a specific hypothesis regarding a drug and its adverse effects. The techniques used for this purpose include case–control and cohort studies. A case–control technique will usually be chosen if there are only a few cases of the adverse effect and assembling a sufficiently large cohort of cases would be impossible. However, some pharmacoepidemiologists maintain that the cohort technique provides more accurate results. In this context, a cohort means a group of patients with a common demographic or statistical characteristic.

Case–control studies compare cases of a disease with controls susceptible to but free of the disease

Case–control studies are technically complex but have been successfully used by government agencies and many academic units. The final results compare or relate the risks in the treated cases with the controls. The absolute risk can be determined only in very special circumstances. Great care is needed in accurate diagnosis and in data collection, so that potential biases are minimized or excluded and marginal results are not overinterpreted. Clearly, a fairly small increase in the risk of a common serious condition such as breast cancer may be of far greater public health importance than a relatively large increase in a very uncommon risk, such as primary hepatic carcinoma.

Cohort studies follow up a large group of patients for long enough to assess the outcome of an exposure common to the cohort

Comparative cohort studies include an unexposed control group. Again, potential bias can be a problem but the method, though usually expensive and time-consuming, has the advantage of revealing the absolute risk and not just relative risk.

Randomized controlled trials avoid bias

In randomized controlled trials a group of patients is divided into two in a strictly random order. One group is then exposed and the other is not exposed to the drug, so that the outcomes can be compared. However, although this method is resistant to biases, it has only a limited, but important, role as a pharmacoepidemiologic tool because most serious adverse effects are relatively uncommon. Appropriately large randomized controlled trials are unfortunately unfeasible and expensive.

What are the expected costs and benefits of treatment?

The doctor and, where possible, the patient, have to weigh up:

- The potential benefits of treatment to the patient.
- The risk of adverse effects to that particular patient.
- The health cost entailed if the treatment produces adverse effects.
- The financial cost of the treatment.

Usually, the benefits of treatment are benefits for an individual patient, such as freedom from pain. However, there are circumstances where the benefits accrue to society as a whole. For example, vaccines reduce the prevalence of disease in the community.

The costs fall on:

- The individual, who can suffer adverse effects.
- Society, if the government or insurance schemes pay for expensive drugs.

Recombinant enzymes used to treat the rare hereditary defect in β glucosidase that causes Gaucher's disease cost around US$100 000/year/patient. Lipid-lowering drugs, which can significantly reduce the risk of dying from coronary heart disease for mildly hypercholesterolemic men who have never had a myocardial infarct, are also expensive, costing approximately US$300 000 per life saved. Such expense and limited budgets mean that a decision has to be made whether spending so much money to benefit a single patient is warranted.

Pharmacoeconomics and evidence-based medicine

Increasingly, approval of a new drug does not guarantee acceptance by drug payment agencies, whether they be government health systems or health management organizations. Such organizations require evidence that a new treatment represents an advance on existing treatments or will provide a cost saving. In order to ensure this, such agencies are making greater use of evidence-based medicine; that is, where the value of a particular medication is ascertained by the strictest of scientific requirements. Thus, the type of evidence that represents the gold standard is that obtained from randomized clinical trials, meta-analyses and accumulated reviews such as those provided by the Cochrane Collaboration.

FURTHER READING

Davies DM, Ferner RE, de Glanville H (eds). *Davies's Textbook of Adverse Drug Reactions*, 5th edn. London: Chapman and Hall; 1998. [A textbook of adverse reactions arranged by disease.]

Descotes J. Immunotoxicology: role in the safety assessment of drugs. *Drug Saf* 2005; **28**: 127–136.

Dukes MNG, Aronson JK (eds). *Meyler's Side Effects of Drugs*, 14th edn. Amsterdam: Elsevier; 2000. [A textbook of adverse reactions arranged by drugs.]

Gogerty JH. Preclinical research evaluation. In: Guarino RA (ed.) *New Drug Approval Processes*. New York: Marcel Dekker; 1987, pp. 25–54. [A thoughtful discussion of issues in preclinical research as it bears on clinical drug development.]

Gough S. Post-marketing surveillance: a UK/European perspective. *Curr Med Res Opin* 2005; **21**: 565–570.

Gregson N, Sparrowhawk K, Mauskopf J, Paul J. Pricing medicines: theory and practice, challenges and opportunities. *Nat Rev Drug Discov J* 2005; **4**: 121–130.

Gunawan B, Kaplowitz N. Clinical perspectives on xenobiotic-induced hepatotoxicity. *Drug Metab Rev* 2004; **36**: 301–312.

Haas JF. A problem-oriented approach to safety issues in drug development and beyond. *Drug Saf* 2004; **27**: 555–567.

Japan Pharmaceutical Reference, 3rd edn. Japan Medical Products International; 1993, pp. 14–34. [A description in detail of the requirements for approval for drugs in Japan.]

Mamelok RD. Drug discovery and development. In: Carruthers SG, Hoffman BB, Melman KL, Nielenberg DF (eds). *Clinical Pharmacology*, 4th edn. New York: McGraw-Hill; 2000, pp. 1289–1305. [A more detailed discussion of issues in demonstrating a drug's safety and efficacy.]

Miller P. Role of pharmacoeconomic analysis in R&D decision making: when, where, how? *Pharmacoeconomics* 2005; **23**: 1–12.

Walgren JL, Mitchell MD, Thompson DC. Role of metabolism in drug-induced idiosyncratic hepatotoxicity. *Crit Rev Toxicol* 2005; **35**: 325–361.

Wienkers LC, Heath TG. Predicting in vivo drug interactions from in vitro drug discovery data. *Nat Rev Drug Discov* 2005; **4**: 825–833.

Wilkinson GR. Drug metabolism and variability among patients in drug response. *N Engl J Med* 2005; **352**: 2211–2221.

WEBSITES

http://www.fda.gov/medwatch/index.html [United States Food and Drug Administration.]

http://www.eudra.org.emea.html [European Medicines Evaluation Agency.]

http://www.open.gov.uk/mcahome.htm [United Kingdom Medicines Control Agency.]

http://www.ifpma.org/ich1.html [For ICH guidelines: contains information on the process and details of the guidelines.]

http://www.fda.gov [For FDA: allows access to news about drug regulation, activities of FDA and information on regulations and guidelines issued by FDA.]

www.eudra.org/emea.html [For EMEA: provides information on European regulations, CPMP opinions and deliberations and links to many other relevant websites.]

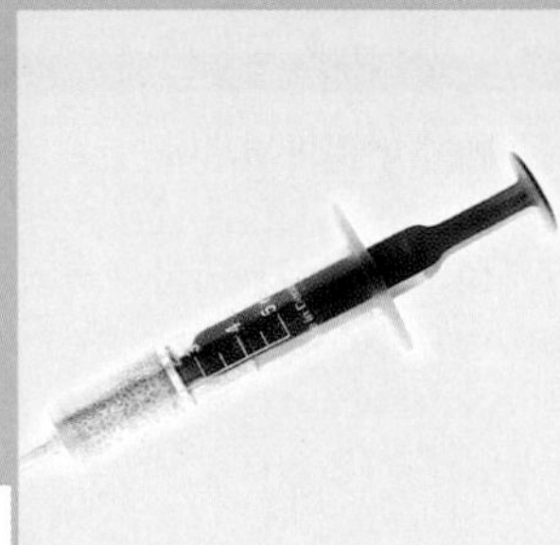

Chapter 4

Pharmacokinetic and Other Factors Influencing Drug Action

Drugs are given by different routes of administration (e.g. oral, intravenous (i.v.) and inhalation). Thus drugs must be in an appropriate form for the particular route (e.g. as a solution for i.v. injection). All drugs, other than those that are designed to act locally (topically) or those directly injected into the bloodstream, are absorbed into the blood from their site of administration.

Drug concentrations in body compartments (blood, tissues, etc.) increase with absorption and distribution and decrease as a result of metabolism and/or excretion. Absorption refers to the processes by which a drug enters the blood from its site of administration. Distribution refers to the processes by which a drug leaves the circulation and enters tissues. Once a drug enters tissues, it is possible for it to enter other cells without using blood as the transport pathway (e.g. by diffusion). Metabolism refers to the processes by which enzymes catalyze the chemical conversion of a drug to more polar forms (metabolites) that are usually more easily excreted from the body. Excretion refers to processes (e.g. renal excretion, etc.) that result in the removal of drug from the body. Alteration of absorption, distribution, metabolism and/or excretion can modify a drug's concentration and therefore its actions.

DRUG DELIVERY

Drugs can be delivered in a variety of forms, including tablets, capsules, solutions, suspensions, modified-release products, injectable solutions, ointments, creams, suppositories and inhalers. In addition, they may be given as pro-drugs (a precursor of the active drug) that make use of the biologic characteristics of the host (i.e. metabolism) to liberate the pharmacologically active substance(s) in the body.

Drug formulation

Depending on the delivery system used, a drug formulation can allow specific tissues to be selectively targeted or systemic absorption of the drug avoided. Thus a drug's formulation and the route of administration determine its absorption and distribution. Some formulations, such as tablets, capsules, solutions and suspensions, are designed only to deliver the drug via the gastrointestinal tract. Solutions and suspensions of drugs are useful for those people who have difficulty in swallowing tablets or capsules.

A strategy for extending the activity of drugs that are rapidly metabolized or excreted from the body is to use a controlled-release formulation that releases the drug slowly during passage through the gastrointestinal tract. Thus the period of delivery is prolonged. Tablets coated with a semipermeable membrane are an example of a controlled-release delivery system (Fig. 4.1). Several other formulation strategies can also be used for similar purposes. Such products include:

- Controlled-release theophylline for the treatment of asthma.
- Controlled-release verapamil for the treatment of hypertension.

Drug absorption through the skin can produce systemic effects

An example of a delivery system for applying drug to the skin, in order to produce systemic actions, is shown in Figure 4.2. The ideal properties for compounds used in this type of delivery system include high potency and a relatively brief persistence in the body. High potency allows for a convenient size of delivery system while brief persistence ensures a prompt termination of drug effect once the delivery system is removed. Examples include:

- Scopolamine (hyoscine) skin patches for the prevention of motion sickness.

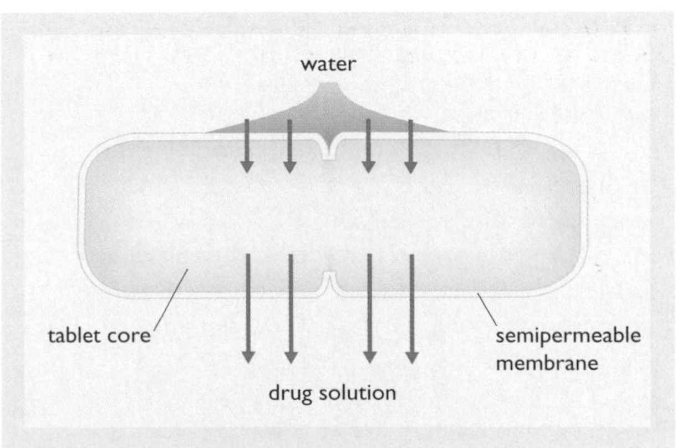

Fig. 4.1 A modified-release tablet. This tablet is coated with a membrane that is selectively permeable to water. Water passes into the core of the tablet and releases the drug solution through small holes in the membrane.

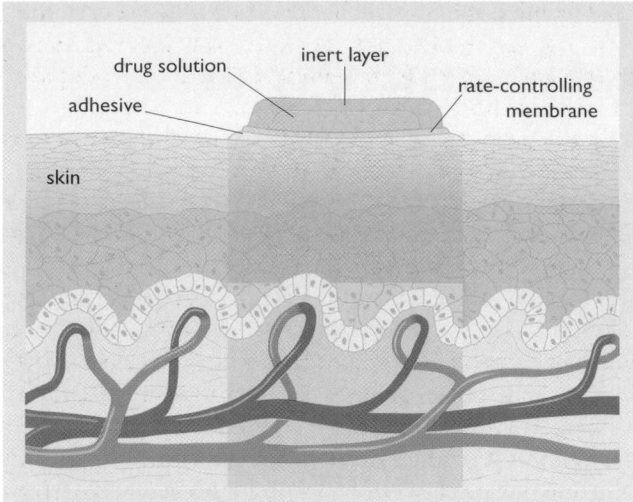

Fig. 4.2 A skin patch drug delivery system. In this system, drug solution diffuses through a membrane to control the amount of drug delivered to the skin for absorption.

- Fentanyl skin patches in the treatment of chronic severe pain.
- Nicotine skin patches to help people trying to stop smoking tobacco.

Topically applied drugs usually produce local therapeutic effects

Topically applied drugs are used in solutions, ointments, creams, suppositories and aerosols. Sites to which they are applied include the eye, ear, skin, nose, mouth, throat, lung, rectum and vagina. Skin and mucous surfaces are relative barriers to systemic absorption of drugs.

Routes for administering drugs

Most drugs are given by mouth – the oral route. A drug absorbed from the upper gastrointestinal tract is exposed to enzymes in the gut wall that can metabolize it. Absorbed drug passes into the portal venous system that carries it to the liver, the major site of drug metabolism. Routes other than the oral route are applicable if:

- A drug is unstable or rapidly inactivated in the gastrointestinal tract.
- The ability of a drug to be absorbed in the gastrointestinal tract is compromised by vomiting or a disease state affecting drug absorption.
- Therapeutic effects that demand local administration and systemic absorption would lead to adverse drug effects (e.g. local anesthesia).

The following routes bypass the gastrointestinal tract and give rapid actions.

The sublingual route

Absorption in the mouth through the buccal or sublingual mucosa means the drug goes directly into the vena cava, thus bypassing exposure to the gastrointestinal tract and immediate exposure to the liver via the portal venous circulation. This route is useful for potent drugs that have an acceptable taste, or where a rapid action is required. A classic example is sublingual nitroglycerin, used to rapidly relieve an acute attack of angina, or to provide prophylaxis against an impending attack.

The cutaneous route

The skin is a formidable barrier to drugs applied to its surface. Indeed, it is challenging to administer drugs by this route in order for them to have systemic effects. Nitroglycerin in a paste formulation is absorbed systemically. Some drugs are available in skin patches; this mode of delivery is possible if the drug is potent (drug content of a patch is quite limited), and if an exipient is available to hasten drug delivery. Due to build-up of a depot of drug in the skin, the onset of drug action may be delayed and the offset of action prolonged when the patch is removed from the skin.

The subcutaneous route

Subcutaneous injection or implantation of a drug provides a slow rate of absorption compared with i.v. and sublingual administration. An example is the subdermal implantation of progestins (e.g. norgestrel) as a method of contraception. In this case the formulation has the advantage of producing a depot of drug under the skin from which it slowly leaches into the circulation, extending the duration of its action.

The parenteral route

The most rapid drug absorption is achieved by injecting it directly into the bloodstream. This is usually accomplished intravenously. On rare occasions, intra-arterial injections are used. Alternative parenteral routes include subcutaneous, intramuscular, topical, epidural and intrathecal routes of injection. Antibiotics are sometimes given intramuscularly and hormones are often administered subcutaneously. Absorption from these sites is usually rapid and drugs bypass the gastrointestinal tract, thereby avoiding its metabolizing enzymes and those in the liver (presystemic metabolism) before reaching the systemic circulation. However, if drug absorption from an injection site is too rapid, it can be slowed by using:

- Formulations that bind the drug and slow its release from the injection site.
- A concomitant second drug in the vehicle so as to reduce blood flow at the injection site (e.g. the use of an α adrenoceptor agonist (vasoconstrictor) with a local anesthetic to prolong local anesthetic action).

The rectal and nasal routes

Drugs can be placed in the rectum as a suppository. The exposure of drug to first-pass metabolism with this route is less than with the oral route because there is a limited portal blood flow system in the lower gastrointestinal tract relative to the upper gastrointestinal tract. However, rectal absorption can be inconsistent.

The nasal mucosa is also a useful site to administer drugs that undergo considerable presystemic elimination (e.g. by first-pass metabolism) when given orally. Nasal sprays can be used to deliver potent drugs for systemic effects (e.g. some hormones and opioid analgesic drugs). However, absorption from the nasal mucosa can be inconsistent.

The inhalation route

Vapors and gases (e.g. general anesthetics) are well absorbed from the lung when inhaled. In addition, if the lung is the target of drug therapy, inhalation is an appropriate method of drug administration, even for powders. Undesirable systemic effects of oral drugs used to treat reversible bronchoconstriction are considerably reduced if a drug is inhaled. The total dose can be reduced and less drug reaches the systemic circulation. Examples of inhaled drugs include glucocorticosteroids and β_2 adrenoceptor agonists for the treatment of asthma. The proportion of a dose that reaches the site of action depends on the ability of the patient to co-ordinate inspiration with triggering of drug release from the delivery canister. Various new technologies are being introduced to facilitate such dosing but, even so, the majority of a dose of powder administered by inhaler is usually swallowed.

FACTORS INFLUENCING DRUG ABSORPTION AND DISTRIBUTION

Absorption

Both chemical and physiologic factors (Table 4.1) can influence drug absorption.

Diffusion of drugs through lipids usually determines their rate of absorption

Most drugs are small organic molecules with a molecular weight less than 1000 that diffuse through biologic membranes in their uncharged form. This is because the major structural component of cell membranes is the lipid bilayer and the uncharged drug form is far more lipid soluble than the charged form. However, some charged molecules are actively transported across membrane barriers (e.g. 5-fluorouracil and levodopa) by special transporter molecules (see Ch. 2).

Since most small molecular weight drugs are either weak acids, bases or amphoteric in nature, the pH of the environment in which the drug is dissolved will determine the fraction available in the non-ionized form that can diffuse across cell membranes. This fraction depends on a drug's chemical nature, pKa and local pH. The pKa of a drug is the pH at which 50% of the drug molecules in solution are ionized and is described by the Henderson–Hasselbalch equation. For acidic (HA) drugs, $HA \rightleftharpoons H^+ + A^-$ where HA is the uncharged form, H^+ a proton and A^- the anionic form. From this relationship the equation $pKa = pH + \log (HA/A^-)$ can be derived. The equation allows the concentration ratio HA/A^- to be calculated at any pH value.

By analogy, for basic (B) molecules $BH^+ \rightleftharpoons B + H^+$ and the equation is $pKa = pH + \log (BH^+/B)$.

The pKa values, and hence fractions of ionized or non-ionized molecules, for different drugs at physiologic pH 7.4 and other pH values show how ionized fractions change with pH for acidic and basic drugs (Fig. 4.3). A useful summary of Figure 4.3 is that a drug will exist in its ionized form when exposed to a pH opposite to its pKa. Therefore, acidic drugs are increasingly ionized with increasing pH (an increasingly basic environment), whereas basic drugs are increasingly ionized with decreasing pH (increasingly acidic environment).

The site at which a drug is administered can alter its rate of absorption

The fraction of dissolved drug in its non-ionized form, and therefore its rate, but not necessarily its extent, of absorption can depend on the pH at the site of delivery. For example, in the stomach, where pH is approximately 2.0, most dissolved acidic drugs will be non-ionized and therefore able to diffuse readily through the stomach lining to the bloodstream. Conversely, many basic drugs will be completely ionized and diffuse only very slowly.

Diffusion of the non-ionized form of a drug across lipid bilayers depends on molecular size and lipid solubility

The diffusion coefficient for a non-ionized molecule in lipid is inversely related to the square root of its molecular weight. This relationship indicates that, if confounding influences are disregarded, smaller molecules diffuse more easily across membranes than larger molecules. However, since most drugs are of low molecular weight (below 1 000), molecular size is rarely the limiting factor in absorption.

Lipid solubility also influences diffusion across membranes. Lipid solubility is measured as a drug's partition coefficient. The partition coefficient reflects solubility in lipid relative to its solubility in water or physiologic

Table 4.1 Important chemical properties and physiologic variables affecting drug absorption through cell membranes, including those of the gastrointestinal tract

Chemical properties	Chemical nature Molecular weight Solubility Lipid partition coefficient (solubility)
Physiologic variables	Gastric motility pH at the absorption site Area of absorbing surface Mesenteric blood flow Presystemic elimination Ingestion with or without food

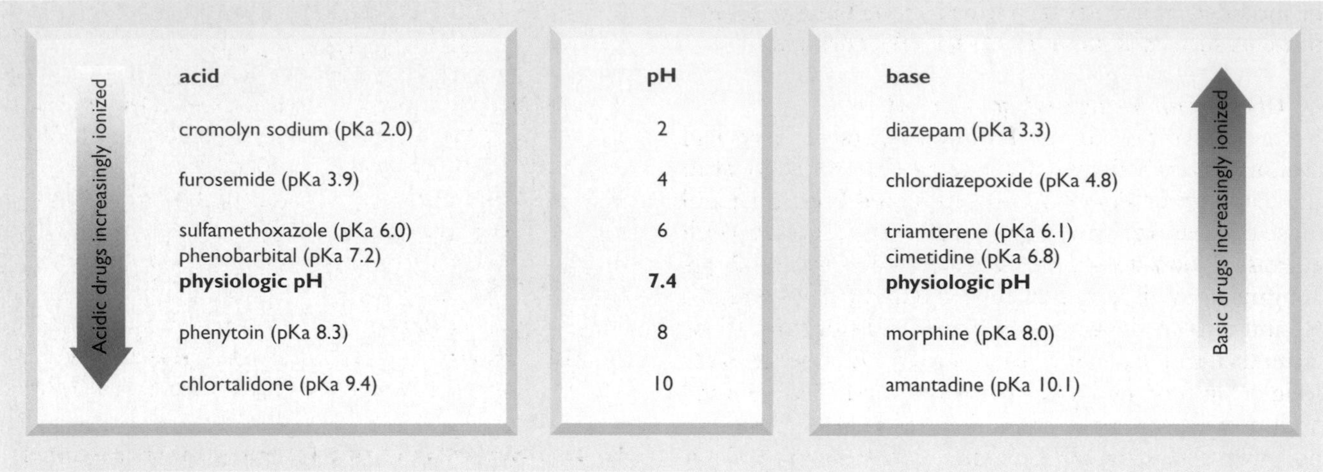

Fig. 4.3 The influence of pKa on the degree of functional group ionization in acidic and basic drugs relative to physiologic pH. The increasing depth of color in the arrows reflects increasing ionization relative to the physiologic pH of 7.4. Thus, for acidic drugs, the more basic the solution (higher pH), the greater is the proportion of drug that is ionized. Conversely, for basic drugs, the more acidic the solution (lower pH), the greater is the proportion ionized. The extent of ionization is calculated from the Henderson–Hasselbalch equation (see text), relating pH and pKa to the fraction ionized.

buffer. Greater lipid solubility is reflected as a larger partition coefficient. The coefficient is determined only for drugs at less than their saturation concentration in both phases. The higher the partition coefficient, the more rapidly a drug can diffuse across a lipid membrane. The therapeutic use of different barbiturates (central nervous system depressants) reflects the importance of partition coefficients. Thus:

- Thiopental, with a pKa of 7.45 and a high partition coefficient (580), is used as a short-acting induction anesthetic by injection, because it rapidly enters brain tissue and therefore quickly induces general anesthesia.
- Phenobarbital, with a similar pKa (7.20) and low partition coefficient (3), is used for the chronic treatment of epilepsy, rather than general anesthesia.

The route of administration can limit drug access to the systemic circulation

As indicated previously, the route of administration can limit drug access to the systemic circulation. For example:

- A drug administered as eyedrops will have primarily local effects, although systemic effects may occur with drugs absorbed via the lacrimal ducts.
- Penicillin G is unstable in the acid environment of the stomach and large oral doses are needed to compensate for drug decomposition at this site.
- Nitroglycerin is administered sublingually to allow rapid systemic absorption and to avoid its presystemic elimination through metabolism in the liver which would occur if given orally.

The rate of drug absorption of an oral dose can be a function of the rate of gastric emptying

The rate of absorption from the gastrointestinal tract can be slowed by retention of an acidic drug in the stomach or hastened by rapid passage of a basic drug into the small intestine. For example, a glass of water ingested together with a drug in an empty stomach will accelerate gastric emptying and hasten passage into the upper intestine with its higher pH and much larger surface area (absorptive surface). Gastric emptying can be accelerated pharmacologically. Metoclopramide increases gastric motility and accelerates gastric emptying. Alternatively, a fatty meal, acid drinks or drugs with anticholinergic effects slow gastric emptying.

Drug absorption in the gastrointestinal tract

- **Many drugs are well absorbed from the gastrointestinal tract**
- **Absorption in the gastrointestinal tract depends on the non-ionized fraction of dissolved drug**
- **Gastric emptying can be accelerated by ingesting the drug with cold water**
- **Basic drugs ingested by mouth are poorly absorbed until they reach the duodenum**
- **Modified-release oral dose forms slow absorption and prolong the duration of drug effect and allow for a more convenient dosage regimen**

Distribution

A drug entering the bloodstream is distributed to different parts of the body at rates depending on various factors, including metabolism, excretion and redistribution in the body. To reach extravascular tissue, a drug must leave the bloodstream. As indicated previously, most commonly used drugs have low molecular weights. As a result, they readily leave the circulation by being filtered through capillaries. However, the rate of filtration may be modified by the extent to which a drug binds to plasma proteins such as albumin or α_1-acid glycoprotein.

Obesity can influence drug distribution

Regardless of the route of administration, a drug will eventually reach tissues at a rate that is proportional to the blood flow (Table 4.2). At rest, blood flow to fat and muscle (measured in ml/kg tissue/min) is similar. With exercise, blood flow rises dramatically in muscle. Drugs accumulate to different extents, and at different rates, in fat and muscle, depending on their lipid solubility. Thus differences in lean:fat tissue ratio for the same body weight can confound dose adjustment on the basis of total body weight for some drugs. Therefore drug doses are not always selected on the basis of total body weight, since the lean:fat ratio will influence plasma levels.

Concentration of free drug in body fluid compartments depends on the pKa of drug and pH of the fluid

At equilibrium, the basis for calculating drug concentrations at a tissue site depends on the principle that the free concentration of non-ionized molecules will be equal on both sides of the cell membrane. Figures 4.4 and 4.5 illustrate the distribution at equilibrium between two biologic environments for an acidic drug (naproxen) and a basic drug (morphine) and demonstrate that:

- Acidic drugs are likely to be concentrated in the circulation.
- Basic drugs concentrate in tissue outside the circulation.

It should be noted that these examples refer only to the unbound fraction of drug dissolved in a specific biologic fluid or tissue and are highly simplified, especially compared to the body as a whole under non-equilibrium conditions.

Binding to plasma proteins contributes to differences in total drug concentrations in different body compartments

Albumin is the most important plasma protein for binding acidic drugs. Competition for the binding sites on albumin can become clinically important for drugs

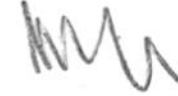

Table 4.2 Total organ blood flow, organ weights and normalized blood flows for various organs in an adult human

Perfusion	Blood flow (mL/min)	Organ mass (kg)	Blood flow (mL/kg/min)
Cardiac output	5400	–	–
Myocardium	250	0.3	833
Liver	1700	2.5	680
Kidney	1000	0.3	3333
CNS	800	1.3	615
Fat	250	10.0	25
Other (muscle, etc.)	1400	55.0	25
Total		69.4	

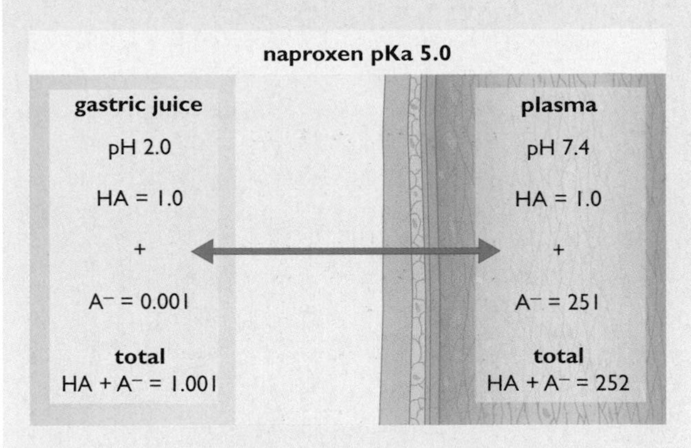

Fig. 4.4 Distribution of an acidic drug. The diagram shows the distribution of naproxen at equilibrium between gastric juice and plasma. This acidic drug is concentrated in plasma.

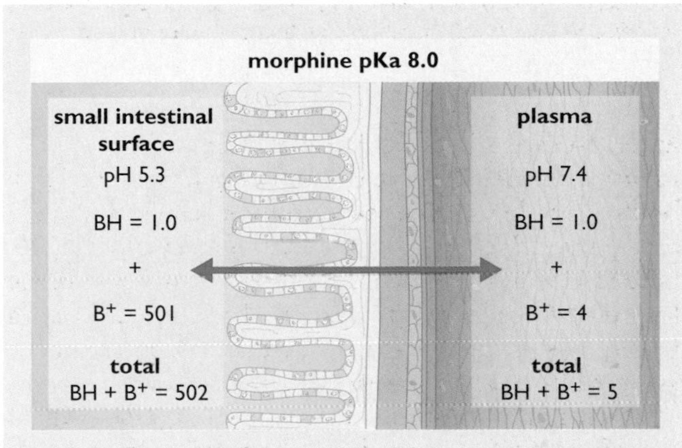

Fig. 4.5 The distribution of a basic drug. The diagram shows the distribution of morphine at equilibrium between the small intestine and plasma. This basic drug is concentrated in the small intestine, as opposed to plasma for the acidic drug in Figure 4.4.

that are more than 80% bound, especially if binding exceeds 90%. In the presence of such a high degree of binding, any small change in the bound fraction will lead to a larger change in the free fraction, i.e. that fraction that exerts pharmacologic effects (Fig. 4.6).

Many basic drugs are bound to a globulin fraction (i.e. α_1-acid glycoprotein). Interpretation of the clinical importance of this interaction is complicated because this protein is an acute-phase reactant in that its concentration fluctuates relatively rapidly and varies widely among people. The concentration of α_1-acid glycoprotein in plasma increases with age, inflammatory conditions and with acute pathologic stress.

In drug overdose, the most appropriate fluid in which to measure the concentration of the drug depends on its chemical characteristics

Drugs that are acidic in nature concentrate in plasma. As a result blood is an appropriate fluid to sample for

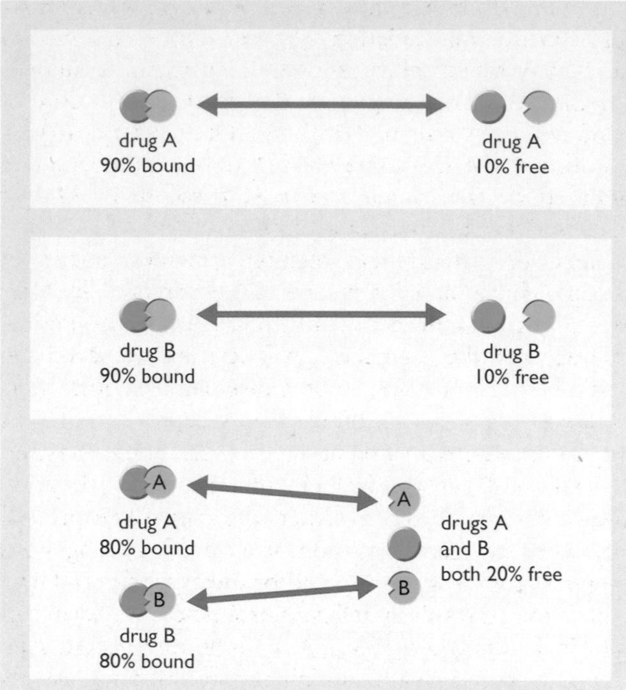

Fig. 4.6 Protein binding and free fraction of drugs. This diagram shows the outcome when one drug (A) is displaced from its protein-binding site by addition of a second drug (B). The change in free fraction is considerable for highly bound drugs.

acidic drugs. On the other hand, the stomach is a suitable sampling site for basic drugs, regardless of the method of drug administration. Diffusion of basic drugs into the stomach results in their almost complete ionization in this environment. If a constant gradient remains, basic drugs concentrate in the stomach until there is distribution equilibrium of the non-ionized fraction. Ingesting bicarbonate to alkalinize the urine can prolong the actions of amphetamine. As a result of such alkalinization, an increasing fraction of urinary amphetamine is in the non-ionized form and as such is readily reabsorbed across the luminal surface of the kidney.

Anatomic and physiologic factors contribute to the differential distribution of drugs

The anatomic and biochemical nature of the blood–brain barrier influences the ability of drugs to enter the brain. Diffusion out of brain capillaries is severely restricted by cellular zonulae; these increase the barrier to drug diffusion into the brain. However, there are five brain regions where this barrier is absent: the pituitary gland, the pineal body, the area postrema, the median eminence and the choroid plexus capillaries. The choroid plexus also contains transporters, which remove charged molecules from the cerebrospinal fluid (CSF). Normally, CSF contains no protein. As a result, the drug concentration in the CSF is similar to the free drug concentration in the blood.

Unless shown otherwise, it is assumed that all drugs cross the placenta, and enter breast milk

Drugs diffuse across the placenta but equilibrium between mother and fetus may be delayed because of the limited placental blood flow from the maternal circulation. Unless proven otherwise, it should be assumed that all drugs cross the placenta, and enter breast milk. The clinical importance of drugs in the placenta and in breast milk must be determined individually for each drug.

The pharmacokinetic space into which a drug distributes is defined as an 'apparent volume of distribution'

The apparent volume of distribution is a calculated space and not an actual anatomic space. Its calculation is based upon the dose administered and the resulting drug concentration in circulating plasma. Some molecules (e.g. ethanol) have an apparent volume of distribution that approximates the total body water (roughly 70% of body weight in non-obese young adults). This might be unexpected since ethanol is lipid soluble and expected to distribute into both water and lipid. Since water is the body's largest space, most ingested ethanol remains in the total body water. Some drugs have apparent volumes of distribution that considerably exceed body weight (Fig. 4.7). Such drugs are usually bases and their high apparent volume of distribution is due to extensive tissue binding. In this situation, almost all of the administered dose will be sequestered outside the circulation. Studies in animals demonstrate that basic drugs are often localized in specific organs of the body (e.g. the concentration of the antiviral drug amantadine in liver, lung and kidney is several times that in blood).

Both the site of action of a drug, and the tissue mass in which it concentrates, are factors to consider when ascribing clinical importance to a drug's localization. The cardiac glycoside digoxin concentrates in muscle and its apparent volume of distribution greatly exceeds body weight. Therefore the dose of digoxin needed to produce therapeutic plasma concentrations depends on the relative muscle weight to total body weight. In addition, it takes several hours to achieve equilibrium between blood and muscle. Thus plasma digoxin concentrations do not readily relate to the therapeutic response if equilibrium has not occurred.

Drug distribution

- **Drug distribution is based on the principle that the non-ionized concentration is the same throughout the body at equilibrium**
- **Charged drug molecules do not easily enter the brain because of the blood–brain barrier, except when the meninges are inflamed**
- **Basic drugs concentrate in the stomach because they are mainly ionized there**

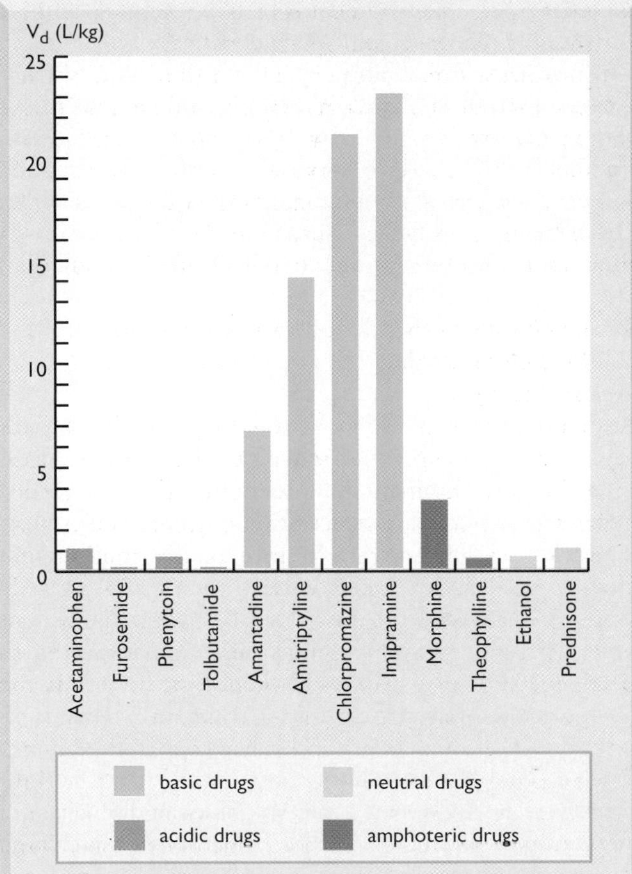

Fig. 4.7 Typical values for the apparent volume of distribution (V_d) for selected drugs. The large V_d values for basic drugs are explained by extensive tissue sequestration.

DRUG METABOLISM

Most drugs are metabolized before being lost from the body. Drug metabolism reactions have been broadly classified into phase 1 and phase 2 processes:

- **Phase 1** reactions are oxidation, reduction and hydrolysis reactions that provide a chemical group to the drug, which increases polarity (and usually water solubility). Such functional groups also provide a site for phase 2 reactions.
- **Phase 2** reactions involve conjugation or synthetic reactions in which a large chemical group is attached. This process also usually increases water solubility and facilitates excretion from the body.

The nature, function and amount of drug-metabolizing enzyme varies among people, resulting in differing rates of drug loss

The drug-metabolizing enzymes have broad substrate specificity but enzyme specificity is relative rather than absolute. This means that one enzyme may catalyze the metabolism of many different drugs and that more than one enzyme isoform may be involved in the metabolism of the same drug. A common metabolic reaction is oxidation. During drug oxidation, a hydroxyl group is added to the drug or a short alkyl group (most commonly methyl) is removed. An example of this is demethylation of theophylline to 1-methylxanthine. The primary enzyme responsible is cytochrome P-4501A2 but the reaction is catalyzed by the cytochrome P-450 isoforms 1A1 and 2D6 also (see later and Table 4.4).

Generally, drug-metabolizing enzymes occur in multiple forms and interindividual differences in their genetic expression can contribute to interindividual differences in drug metabolism. The enzymes have been classified into families, subfamilies and specific gene products. Furthermore, the degree of expression of such enzymes can be regulated at many levels. Some enzymes are expressed constitutively in the sense that they are always present and active. Others are primarily expressed only when triggered by the presence of an exogenous chemical (e.g. drug, poison and/or dietary factors). Gene mutations can result in deficient expression or absence of a particular enzyme isoform. As a result, unexpected drug toxicity may occur with administration of what is usually a safe dose of a drug. Conversely, redundant genetic code may result in multiple copies of a particular drug-metabolizing enzyme. This situation can result in resistance to typical doses due to accelerated metabolism.

The activity of drug-metabolizing enzymes is sometimes increased (induced) or inhibited

Many factors in the diet can influence the activity of drug-metabolizing enzymes, including the protein–carbohydrate ratio, plant foods containing flavonoids (e.g. cruciferous vegetables such as cabbage, mustard and cress) and barbecued foods, high in polycyclic aromatic hydrocarbons from burning charcoal.

Increased enzyme synthesis as a result of the presence of an exogenous chemical is referred to as 'enzyme induction' (Table 4.3). Induction may be due to a combination of changes in nucleic acid transcription as well as translational and post-translational regulation. Induction can be produced by certain drugs, food constituents, alcohol and smoking. When chronically ingested, some drugs (e.g. barbiturates, rifampicin) induce their own metabolism, as well as that for other drugs and

Table 4.3 Examples of enzyme inducers and enzyme inhibitors

Inducers	Inhibitors
Ethanol	Cimetidine
Omeprazole	Erythromycin
Phenobarbital	Grapefruit juice
Rifampicin	Ketoconazole
Smoking	Quinidine

endogenous substances. The tissue site where induction occurs may be determined by the nature of exposure to the chemicals responsible. Smokers induce expression of a particular isoform of the cytochromes P-450, primarily in the lungs and upper intestine.

Sometimes, two drugs will compete for metabolism by the same enzyme, resulting in a decreased rate of metabolism for one or both drugs. This process is referred to as 'enzyme inhibition' (see Table 4.3). One clinically important example of such an inhibition interaction is cardiac arrhythmias, or CNS seizures, produced by theophylline when it is given concurrently with a macrolide-type antibiotic such as erythromycin.

Most tissues have the capability of metabolizing specific drugs

Although the liver is the major site of drug metabolism, most tissues can metabolize specific drugs. Tissue specificity for drug metabolism depends on genetic regulation and expression of drug-metabolizing enzymes in particular tissues. Therefore selective tissue effects may result from a unique drug-metabolizing enzyme reaction at the tissue site of action for a drug. For example, the kidney oxidizes the metabolite sulindac sulfide, the active cyclo-oxygenase inhibitor, back to sulindac, the parent pro-drug, thereby protecting the kidney from impaired function due to inhibition of cyclo-oxygenase by sulindac sulfide.

The loss of drug from plasma (elimination) can follow zero-order or first-order kinetics, or have an intermediate order

Drugs are generally lost from the body by one or a combination of two kinetic processes. In one process, known as zero-order kinetics, the rate of loss of drug from the body (usually plasma) is constant regardless of how much drug is in the plasma. This occurs when the drug elimination processes are saturated. Zero-order kinetics is not common for drug elimination. It can be likened to emptying a bucket (the body) one cup at a time. However, in most cases the concentration of drug is considerably below that required to saturate the body's elimination processes. As a result, the rate of loss of such a drug is proportional to its concentration in plasma (first-order elimination kinetics). The usual parameter used to reflect this process is plasma half-life. First-order kinetics can be likened to emptying a bucket via an open tap at the bottom of the bucket. In this case, the flow of water from the tap will be proportional to the height of the column of water in the bucket. A drug with first-order kinetics can be considered in essence to be removed from the circulation in five half-lives. By two half-lives, 75% of the drug is lost (50% plus half the remaining 50% = 75%), 87.5% in three half-lives, 93.75% in four, etc.

The concept of half-life is, however, inappropriate for drugs with zero-order kinetics (e.g. ethanol) because their rate of elimination does not depend upon plasma concentration, unless the plasma concentration is very low (usually pharmacologically ineffective). The elimination processes for ethanol are effectively saturated at a low concentration. Thus the elimination of ethanol is best described on the basis of the loss of a constant amount of ethanol/unit time (zero-order elimination). The average rate of elimination of ethanol is about 120 mg/kg/h in social (moderate) drinkers. This average elimination rate is equivalent to 150 mg/L plasma/h, a rate equal to the loss of approximately one-half of a standard bottle (350 mL) of beer (5% v/v alcohol) per hour for a 70 kg male.

Some drugs (e.g. aspirin, phenytoin) have elimination characteristics intermediate between zero- and first-order kinetics. With such drugs, once the first-order process is saturated, elimination approximates to zero order. Accordingly, plasma concentrations increase disproportionately to an increased dose since elimination does not increase with dose for zero-order processes. With such drugs it is advisable to monitor plasma concentrations when changing a dose regimen since relatively small changes in dose can lead to a disproportionate increase in plasma concentration and possible toxicity.

Phase 1 metabolism

Oxidation is the most common pathway for phase 1 metabolism. Reduction and hydrolysis, although important, occur less often.

Oxidation

P-450 cytochromes (Table 4.4) are a superfamily of heme protein enzyme isoforms that catalyze oxidative metabolism of many xenobiotics (drugs and other exogenous chemicals).

The process of drug oxidation involves both oxidation and reduction steps (Fig. 4.8). Sites for oxidation vary considerably. They have as a common physical property high lipid solubility.

Most oxidation of drugs is catalyzed by the cytochromes P-450, although other enzymes can be involved to a lesser extent. There are several hundred isoforms of the cytochromes P-450. Some are constitutive (i.e. always present), while others are present only when synthesized in response to appropriate stimuli, usually an exogenous chemical. Substrate specificity is a function of the cyto-

Table 4.4 Examples of cytochrome P-450 families and the isoforms important to oxidative drug metabolism

Family	Isoform	Drug substrate
CYP1	CYP1A2	Theophylline
CYP2	CYP2D6	Codeine
CYP3	CYP3A4	Ciclosporin

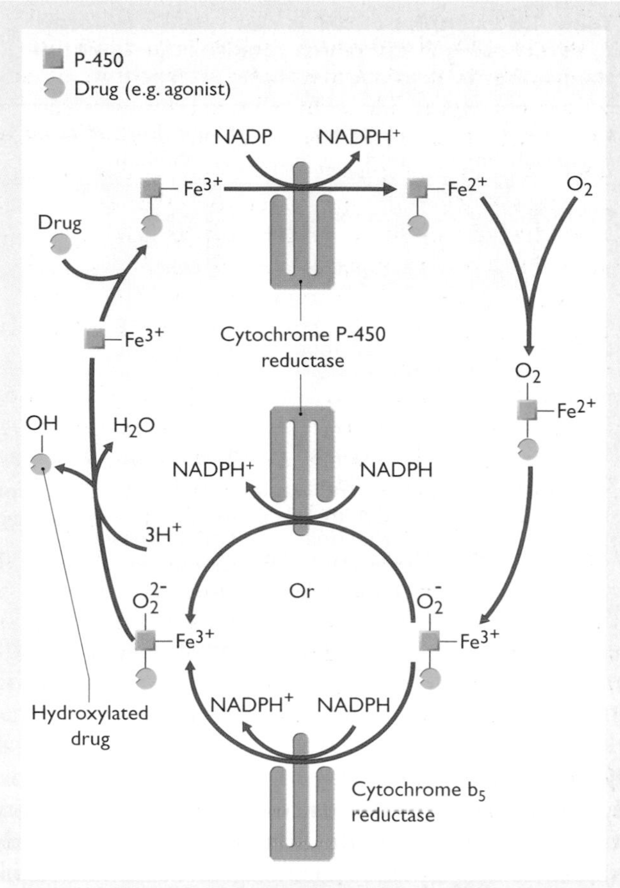

Fig. 4.8 Mechanisms by which the mixed function oxidase system oxidizes a drug. Drug binds to the oxidized form of a specific cytochrome P-450 isoform. This complex then receives a single electron from NADPH via cytochrome P-450 reductase. The reduced complex then reacts with molecular oxygen (O_2) and a second electron is donated either via NADPH and cytochrome P-450 reductase or NADH and cytochrome b_5 reductase. In the process, one atom of oxygen is released as water and the other is incorporated into the drug to produce the hydroxylated metabolite. This metabolic reaction also applies to dealkylation reactions in which short-chain alkyl groups (usually methyl) are removed from a drug and combined with oxygen to yield an aldehyde, which can be further oxidized or reduced.

chrome P-450 isoform, with specificity being relative rather than absolute. As a result, the absence of any particular isoform of cytochromes P-450 does not preclude a particular metabolic reaction. Genes for the cytochrome P-450 superfamily are found on several chromosomes.

A nomenclature for the cytochrome P-450 superfamily has been developed:

- CYP: the capital letters 'CYP' indicate that the isoform is of human origin.
- CYP 'x': where x is an Arabic numeral, used to indicate the isoform family.
- CYP 'x' 'X': subfamilies are designated by another capital letter.
- CYP 'x' 'X' 'x': the final Arabic numeral designates the individual gene product in the subfamily.

Designation of family and subfamily status relates to the degree of homology for the amino acid sequence of various P-450 isoforms. For example, the designation CYP1A2 refers to a human cytochrome P-450 isoform of the first family that is a member of the A subfamily of enzymes and is the second gene product assigned to that subfamily.

Three families of the P-450 cytochromes are important for metabolizing a wide variety of drugs

The three families of cytochromes P-450 that are important in metabolizing drugs are shown in Table 4.4. The CYP3A subfamily has been identified as the major constitutive form in human liver and it contributes to the metabolism of a wide variety of drugs. This subfamily is also expressed in significant amounts in tissues other than liver. The specific isoform CYP3A4 is responsible for intestinal metabolism (presystemic elimination) of many drugs that show poor bioavailability.

The isoform CYP2D6 has been associated with:

- The oxidative metabolism of many drugs, including β adrenoceptor antagonists.
- Demethylation of tricyclic antidepressants.
- Demethylation of codeine to morphine.

Approximately 5–10% of Caucasians are deficient in the phenotypic expression of CYP2D6 as an autosomal recessive trait. Multiple mutations of CYP2D6 have been described. For example, an inability to demethylate codeine to morphine is associated with a lack of analgesic response to codeine.

CYP2E1 is a short-lived isoform induced by chronic alcohol consumption. CYP1A2 is important in the metabolism of theophylline and is induced by flavanoids and polycyclic aromatic hydrocarbons found in some diets. Knowledge of the metabolic constitution of a patient therefore has potential predictive value in determining whether a particular drug therapy is appropriate. Tests for the phenotypic expression of drug-metabolizing enzymes in individuals are expected to be readily available in the future. Such information will be valuable for determining which specific drugs or drug classes should be free of problems with respect to drug oxidation. Caution is advised, however, in interpreting phenotypic expression of a gene product, since the former can be modulated by environmental and physiologic factors.

Cytochrome P-450 enzymes require the presence of the mixed function oxidases

Cytochromes P-450 require molecular oxygen, NADPH cytochrome P-450 reductase and NADPH in order to function. This combination is referred to as the mixed function oxidase system. The cytochrome P-450 isoforms

Drug excretion

- **Renal and fecal excretion are the most important routes for drug elimination**
- **Some drug conjugates are hydrolyzed in the lower gastrointestinal tract back to the parent compound and reabsorbed in a process referred to as enterohepatic circulation, which extends the duration of drug action**
- **For some drugs the fraction of the administered dose excreted unchanged by the kidney depends on the urinary pH**
- **Creatinine clearance can be used to assess renal impairment and indicate whether drug doses need to be reduced if renal excretion is an important component of drug elimination**

Renal excretion

Renal excretion of drugs involves both filtration and secretion. Filtration occurs at the glomerulus of the kidney, secretion along the nephron. The excretion of some drugs is impaired by renal disease. The renal excretion of many drugs correlates with the kidney's ability to excrete creatinine. If it is inconvenient, or impossible, to assess renal function directly by measuring a 24-hour creatinine clearance, renal function can be estimated using the widely accepted algorithm of Cockroft and Gault. These investigators established a relationship between patient age, weight and serum creatinine concentration ($C_{s,cr}$) from which creatinine clearance (Cl_{cr}) by the kidney can be estimated:

$$Cl_{cr}\ (\text{mL/min}) = \frac{[(140 - \text{age}) \times \text{ideal body weight (kg)}]}{[0.8145 \times C_{s,cr}\ (\mu\text{mol/L})]} \qquad \text{(Eqn 4.1)}$$

This equation applies to males. For females, the value for creatinine clearance is multiplied by 0.85.

Although renal creatinine excretion occurs both by filtration and secretion, the fraction excreted by each mechanism changes in favor of secretion as renal function decreases. It is likely that this relationship also applies to all drugs that are filtered and secreted by the kidney.

There are various therapeutic strategies for increasing renal excretion of drugs

By virtue of the relationship between pKa and pH, the pH of the urine will determine the proportion of drug in its ionized state, and therefore the amount of filtered drug that cannot be reabsorbed by diffusion across the luminal surface of the nephron. For example, salicylic acid which is a weak acid (pKa 3.0) is usually mostly metabolized before being excreted into the urine. However, as the urinary pH is increased, a higher fraction of the administered dose is lost in the urine. Indeed, treatment of salicylate intoxication can include alkalinization of the urine with oral or parenteral doses of bicarbonate to increase renal elimination of salicylic acid. This strategy can also be useful in the management of phenobarbital overdose.

Increasing urine flow also increases renal elimination of some drugs, since the contact time with the luminal surface is decreased, thereby reducing the time for reabsorption of non-ionized molecules.

Gastrointestinal excretion

Removal of drugs from the gastrointestinal tract can be accelerated by the use of a polyethylene glycol electrolyte lavage solution. Large volumes of this solution can be ingested, or placed in the gastrointestinal tract through a nasogastric tube, to increase intestinal peristalsis and hasten excretion of unabsorbed drug via the rectum. The decreased transit time through the gastrointestinal tract associated with the induced diarrhea will decrease the absorption of nutrients but in an acute situation this is not clinically important.

Enterohepatic circulation prolongs the pharmacologic effect of some drugs

Some drug conjugates excreted in bile are hydrolyzed in the lower intestine, so releasing the original drug for reabsorption into the bloodstream and in consequence prolong their action. This recycling process is referred to as enterohepatic circulation. Potentially clinically relevant examples include:

- Enterohepatic circulation of the sedative hypnotic drug lorazepam involves hydrolysis of its glucuronide conjugate in the lower intestinal tract.
- The suggestion that failure of oral contraception can be due to inhibition of enterohepatic circulation following antibiotic therapy which removes the bacteria that hydrolyze steroid conjugates from the lower intestine. Thus steroid clearance is enhanced and contraceptive failure is more likely.

Lung excretion

Volatile drugs are excreted via the lungs. This route is only of major importance for the general anesthetics that exist in gaseous or vapor phases. Such anesthetics are administered and lost via the lungs, providing for easily controlled anesthesia by adjusting the anesthetic concentration in the inhaled gas mixture. Excretion via the lung allows for monitoring of the end-tidal concentration of expired anesthetic as a surrogate index of the level of anesthesia. Ethanol is excreted in small amounts by the lung. While this route of elimination is not quantitatively important for ethanol, it provides a non-invasive method for estimating blood ethanol concentrations for legal purposes.

PHARMACOKINETICS

The analysis of the rate of all drug disposition factors (absorption, distribution, metabolism and excretion) is termed pharmacokinetics. The word reflects the rate

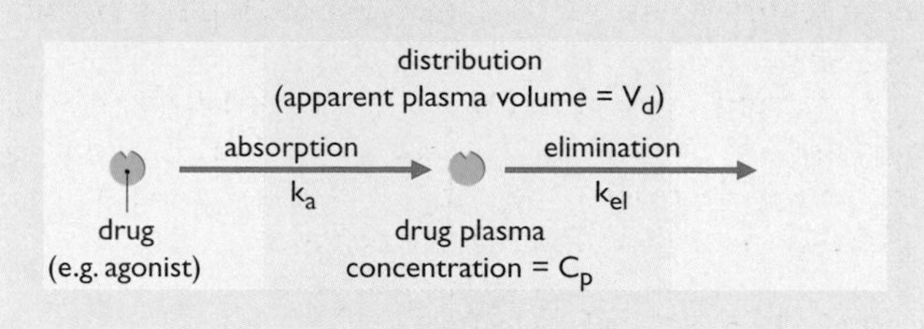

Fig. 4.10 Diagram of the one-compartment open pharmacokinetic model for drug disposition. The plasma concentration of a drug (C_p) is determined by the rate of drug absorption (k_a – rate constant for absorption), the apparent volume of drug distribution (V_d) and rate of drug elimination (k_{el}). When the drug is administered parenterally as a bolus, absorption is instantaneous.

of movement (kinetics) of drugs (pharmaco) into and out of the body.

The one-compartment model

In the simplest model, the body is considered to be a single uniform space (compartment) into which drug is administered and from which it is eliminated (Fig. 4.10). In this model, it is assumed that the administered drug is immediately distributed throughout the space. If elimination is a first-order kinetic process, the elimination rate is proportional to the plasma concentration, resulting in an exponential loss of drug. The mathematical equation for this exponential relationship is:

$$C_t = C_0 \bullet e^{-k_{el}t} \quad \text{(Eqn 4.2)}$$

where C_t is plasma concentration at any time (t), C_0 is the estimated initial plasma concentration at t = 0, k_{el} is the elimination rate constant and e is the base for natural logarithms. By taking the logarithm of plasma concentration, the exponential process is a straight line (Fig. 4.11). The slope of the line in Figure 4.11 is actually $k_{el}/2.303$. Division by 2.303 is because the logarithmic transformation of plasma concentration data was to base 10 rather than to base e. This presentation is used in Figure 4.11 since base 10 is more familiar to pharmacologist. If the initial extrapolated drug concentration (C_0) in the compartment is divided into the administered dose, the theoretical volume needed for the drug dose is described. This space is defined as the apparent volume of distribution (V_d).

While the elimination rate constant tells us how quickly the drug is eliminated, a simple calculation using k_{el} gives the plasma half-life ($t_{1/2}$), a measure that is more commonly used, and better understood. The time for the drug concentration in plasma to decline by 50% is its $t_{1/2}$. Since the decline in logarithmic transformed drug concentration with time is linear, the $t_{1/2}$ will be constant, regardless of drug concentration. The k_{el} of a drug is related to $t_{1/2}$ by the equation:

$$t_{1/2} \times k_{el} = 0.693 \quad \text{(Eqn 4.3)}$$

Since $t_{1/2}$ is related to the V_d, the $t_{1/2}$ value will not always reflect the ability of a body to eliminate a drug. The

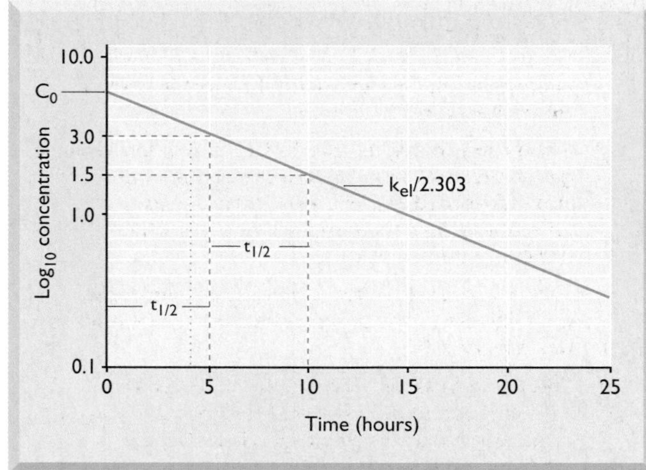

Fig. 4.11 A graph of the log of the plasma drug concentration versus time (hours) with a one-compartment open pharmacokinetic model for drug disposition after an i.v. dose. Extrapolation of the line (slope is k_{el}) to time 'zero' results in an estimate of the initial drug concentration (C_0) in the compartment if distribution were instantaneous. $t_{1/2}$ is the half-life. In this case it has the value of 5.

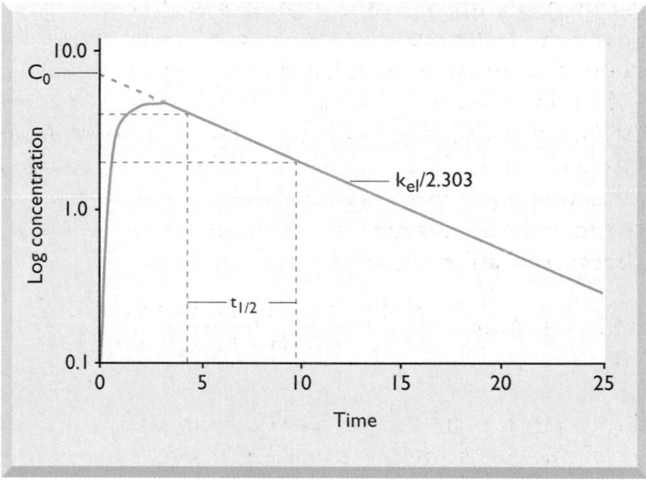

Fig. 4.12 A graph of log plasma drug concentration versus time for a one-compartment open pharmacokinetic model after an oral dose. The shape of the curve should be compared with the straight line in Figure 4.11.

preferred kinetic term that indicates the body's ability to remove a drug from the circulation is plasma clearance (Cl_p), which is equal to $V_d \times K_{el}$. Clearance remains constant for most drugs if the elimination mechanisms are not modified by pathologic and/or physiologic factors.

Figure 4.11 shows the fall in plasma concentration with time when drug is administered intravenously. However, if the drug is given orally, it takes time to be absorpted and the drug disposition curve resembles that shown in Figure 4.12. The shape of the plasma concentration versus time curve reflects the interaction of two first-order processes; both entry (absorption) into and exit (elimination) from single kinetic compartment. Calculation of V_d, $t_{1/2}$, k_{el} and Cl_p is the same as after i.v. dose administration, but some of the derived parameters

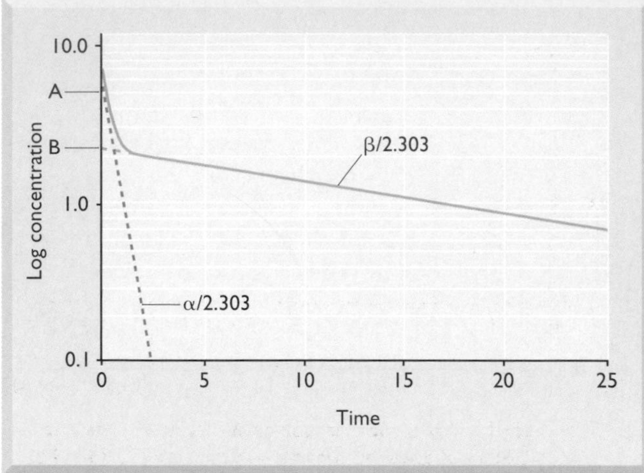

Fig. 4.13 A plot of log plasma drug concentration versus time for a two-compartment open model after an i.v. bolus dose. The terminal disposition rate constant is k_β and not k_{el} and the decreasing plasma concentration with time reflects a more complex relationship between drug distribution and elimination. The initial more rapid decline in circulating drug concentration (α) primarily reflects redistribution of the drug to the peripheral compartment (V_p) (see Fig. 4.14) plus a modest component of elimination. The terminal, apparently linear phase of plasma concentration versus time is a composite of drug elimination buffered by drug returning from V_p to the central compartment in which the drug distributes rapidly (V_c) to decrease the apparent rate of drug removal from the blood plasma. This phase is therefore referred to as the k_β phase. Extrapolation back to time zero provides an intercept (B). The extrapolated values of k_β are subtracted from the observed concentrations of drug at the same time after the dose and the residual values are plotted. A linear regression through these residual data points provides a slope (k_α) and a time zero intercept (A) that reflect drug distribution into V_p. If the discrepancy between k_α and k_{el} is large, a greater error will arise from assuming that a one-compartment model is valid.

(V_d and Cl_p) will increase if there is significant loss of drug before it is absorbed (presystemic drug elimination). This situation occurs because plasma drug concentrations are lowered by presystemic elimination, and estimation of the initial drug concentration (C_0) is therefore lower. This simple model of a single uniform space with first-order kinetics serves remarkably well for the calculation of dosing regimens for most drugs.

The two-compartment model

For some drugs, the plot of the logarithm of plasma concentration versus time results in a curvilinear relationship (Fig. 4.13). To explain such observations, the simple one-compartment model needs to be expanded. The simplest expansion is to consider the body as having two compartments (Fig. 4.14). Intuitively, it can be seen that two linear processes would account for the curvilinear plot in Figure 4.13. These two processes are known as the α and β phases, and are characterized by their respective elimination rate constants (and half-lives). In this model, the terminal linear phase (β) rate constant k_β is not the same as shown in Figure 4.11, k_{el} (one-

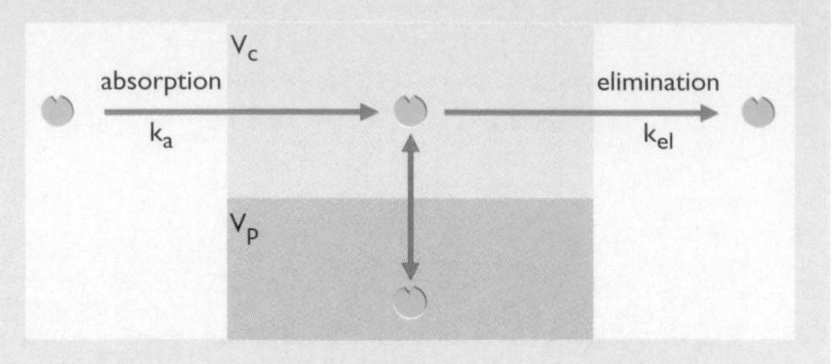

Fig. 4.14 Diagram of the two-compartment open pharmacokinetic model for drug disposition after i.v. dose. With a bolus i.v. dose, k_a is instantaneous and is ignored in solution of the model. When the drug is administered by infusion, k_a is a zero-order constant equal to the rate of drug infusion. There is a central compartment in which the drug distributes rapidly (V_c) and from which drug is eliminated, and a peripheral compartment into which the drug can distribute (V_p) and from which it can return to buffer the changing drug concentration in the central compartment when drug is eliminated (k_{el}, elimination constant).

compartment model). The β phase is a slower rate process than that giving rise to k_{el}. The greater the discrepancy between k_β and k_{el}, the larger the error is in assuming the validity of a one-compartment model. Fortunately, for most drugs, the discrepancy between k_β and k_{el} is not as great as interindividual differences in drug disposition. Therefore, as indicated above, in most cases the one-compartment open model serves as an acceptable clinical approximation for individualization of drug doses.

Obviously, both the one- and two-compartment models are oversimplifications of 'spaces' in the body into which drugs are absorbed and from which they can be metabolized and excreted. When a discrepancy in modeling drug disposition becomes clinically evident for a particular drug, its use has to be learned as a special case so as to account for the more complex disposition–effect relationship. Drugs that undergo dose-dependent disposition (e.g. phenytoin, aspirin) belong to this special category of more complicated relationships between dose, concentration and pharmacologic effects.

Time-course of drug action

- **Clinically it is more important to know the time-course of drug action than the pharmacokinetics of drug concentrations. There may, or may not, be a linear or simple relationship between drug action (effector concentration) and blood concentration**
- **The time required for drug effects to be expressed can be much longer than that for the drug to act at its molecular site since the response systems have their own time constraints**
- **For example, β blockers produce a very rapid slowing of heart rate, whereas the anticoagulant effects of warfarin take days to develop**

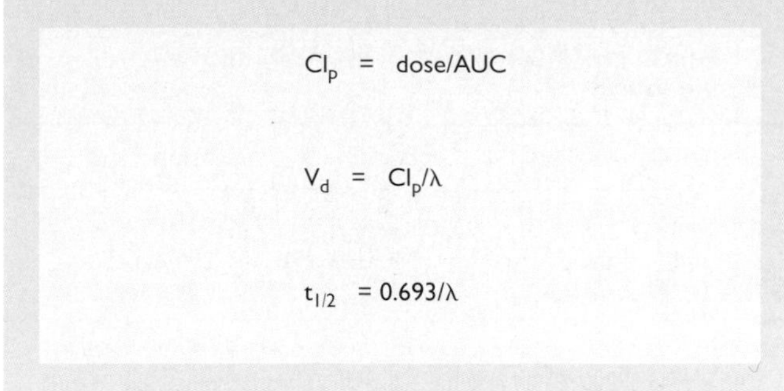

Fig. 4.15 Equations for pharmacokinetic drug disposition for non-compartmental conditions. The terminal disposition constant is renamed λ so that its interpretation is not prejudiced by either of the two models discussed in Figures 4.10–4.14. A new calculation is introduced which is called area under the plasma concentration versus time curve (AUC). Cl_p, plasma clearance; V_d, apparent volume of distribution; λ, terminal disposition rate constant.

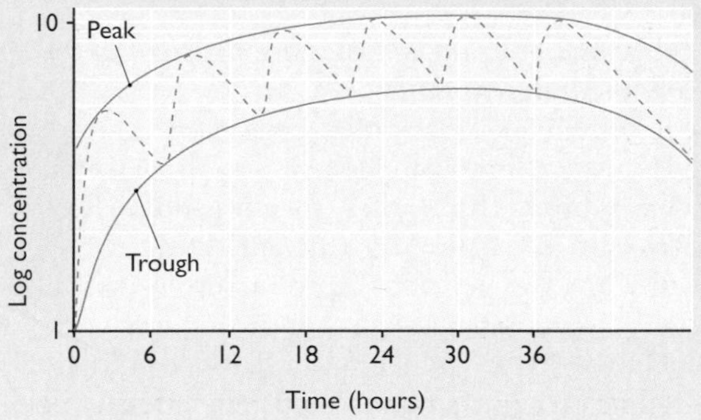

Fig. 4.16 Graph of log plasma concentration versus time for a drug administered by mouth every 6 hours for six doses (*) of 0, 6, 12, 18, 24, 30 when the drug's terminal disposition half-life is 6 hours. The effective steady state occurs 24–30 hours (4–5 half-lives) after starting the drug.

The non-compartmental approach

A non-compartmental approach has been advocated to simplify the determination of pharmacokinetic parameters from which drug doses can be calculated. This approach borrows considerably from the one-compartment open model. The area under the curve (AUC) of plasma concentration versus time is integrated and the calculation of kinetic parameters is performed according to equations presented in Figure 4.15. This method compensates somewhat for the extrapolation of drug concentrations to C_0 in the one-compartment model when no drug has yet been absorbed into the body after an oral dose.

Calculation of dosing

Most drugs are administered chronically. For drugs with first-order elimination, the total amount in the body increases until the amount excreted is equal to the dose administered per unit time, i.e. a steady-state plasma concentration is achieved. The time to steady state for such drugs depends only on the terminal elimination half-life. Simple calculation indicates that 94% and 97% of steady state are achieved after four and five elimination half-lives, respectively. For practical purposes, steady state is assumed to exist at this time (Fig. 4.16). The more frequently a drug dose is administered, the greater will be the amount of drug in the body at steady state, and the less the variation between peak and trough plasma concentrations. The less frequently a drug dose is administered, the lower will be the amount of drug in the body at steady state, and the greater the variation between peak and trough plasma concentrations. If the dose interval is longer than two terminal disposition half-lives, drug accumulation with chronic ingestion is considered to be clinically unimportant.

Pharmacokinetics

- Most drugs are eliminated from the body as a constant fraction of their plasma concentration (first-order process)
- Time to steady state depends only on the rate of drug elimination
- Repeated doses result in significant drug accumulation when ingestion is more frequent than twice the terminal disposition half-life
- Practical time to steady state is 4–5 terminal disposition half-lives
- The amount of a drug in the body at steady state depends on the frequency of ingestion and dose
- The plasma half-life of a drug does not reflect metabolic capacity if the apparent volume of distribution changes

A loading dose of drug can be given to achieve therapeutic drug concentrations rapidly

The loading dose of a drug is calculated on the basis of its V_d and the desired plasma concentration at steady state (C_{ss}):

$$\text{Loading dose (mg/kg)} = V_d\ \text{(L/kg)} \times C_{ss}\ \text{(mg/L)} \quad \text{(Eqn 4.4)}$$

When given intravenously, the loading dose is usually administered by infusion over a short period of time to reduce the risk of adverse effects associated with the presence of very high drug concentrations in the circulation. Maintenance doses are then based upon the Cl_p and the time interval between doses (t):

$$\text{Maintenance dose (mg/kg)} = Cl_p\ \text{(L/kg/h)} \times C_{ss}\ \text{(mg/L)} \times t\ \text{(h)} \quad \text{(Eqn 4.5)}$$

AGE, SEX AND GENETIC BACKGROUND

Age

Drug-metabolizing enzymes are deficient in the fetus and premature infants

The fetus is able to metabolize drugs early in its development but the pattern of expression of drug-metabolizing enzymes differs from that of the adult. Fetal drug metabolism is usually less efficient. Drug-metabolizing enzymes are also deficient in premature versus full-term infants. Drug therapy in premature infants is therefore difficult, particularly when more than a single drug dose is administered. In addition, renal function is not fully developed in these babies and as a result renal drug elimination is impaired (e.g. the diuretic response to loop diuretics).

Children metabolize many drugs more rapidly than adults

A few months after birth, the activity of the oxidative drug-metabolic pathways increases dramatically, such that by 2 years of age children can oxidize many drugs more rapidly than adults. The ability to conjugate drugs with glucuronic acid develops more slowly and at different rates for different isoforms of glucuronosyl transferase. As an example, a greater fraction of an administered dose of acetaminophen is conjugated with sulfate in children than in adults. The frequency of drug administration may have to be altered to compensate for these special characteristics. As children approach puberty, the rate of drug metabolism approaches that of adults.

Changes associated with aging need to be considered when prescribing drugs for the elderly

Some of the changes that occur in the elderly and influence drug treatment include the following:

- Chronic diseases are more common in the elderly and are associated with the use of several drugs in a single individual. As a result, competition between drugs for cytochrome P-450 isoforms is much more likely in the elderly.
- The concentration of serum albumin decreases with age, resulting in a reduced binding capacity for various drugs. This effect can result in saturation of the protein-binding sites for drugs and an increase in the free fraction of drug in the circulation.
- Lean body mass decreases with age and as a result the apparent volume of drug distribution may change for some drugs sufficiently to necessitate dose adjustments.
- Liver weight decreases with age and presystemic drug elimination may be reduced.

The expression of cytochrome P-450 enzyme isoforms appears to change with increasing age. This change is reflected as a reduced capability to oxidize drugs and is seen mainly in elderly males. Available data indicate that induction of drug metabolism can be maintained or impaired in the elderly patient, depending on the drug considered.

Table 4.7 Variations in drug-metabolic pathways in populations of humans of different genetic background

Metabolic reaction	Caucasian	Asian
Acetylation	50% slow	5–10% slow
CYP2D6 oxidation	5–10% deficient	1% deficient
CYP2C18 oxidation	3–5% deficient	20% deficient

Deficiency in one metabolic pathway is not predictive for deficiency in other drug-metabolic pathways in the same population.

Gender

Although some gender differences in drug disposition have been reported (e.g. a lower renal clearance of amantadine in women), the clinical importance of these observations remains to be explored.

Genetic background

Several differences in drug metabolism have been demonstrated for various human groups with preserved differences in genetic background (Table 4.7). Differences with respect to acetylator phenotype and origin have been well documented. There are also differences in the expression of cytochrome P-450 isoforms. These differences sometimes need to be taken into account when drug therapy is considered for patients from such an identified group.

DRUG INTERACTIONS

The concomitant administration of drugs can be either beneficial or problematic in terms of interactions. These interactions can be of a pharmacokinetic and/or pharmacodynamic nature. Examples of beneficial and adverse drug interactions are presented below.

The concurrent use of levodopa and carbidopa for patients with Parkinson's disease produces a favorable drug interaction

Carbidopa inhibits the conversion of levodopa to dopamine, but only in the peripheral tissues, since carbidopa does not cross the blood–brain barrier. As a result, orally administered levodopa is converted to dopamine only after it enters the brain, the site of the desired pharmacologic effect. In this instance, carbidopa eliminates or minimizes systemic adverse effects that would arise from the production of dopamine from levodopa in the periphery.

The hypotensive response of patients receiving a diuretic to treat hypertension can be impaired by concurrent administration of NSAIDs

The renal function of some patients receiving diuretics to treat their hypertension is impaired when concomitant NSAIDs block renal cyclo-oxygenase activity, thus decreasing prostaglandin synthesis in the kidney. Since

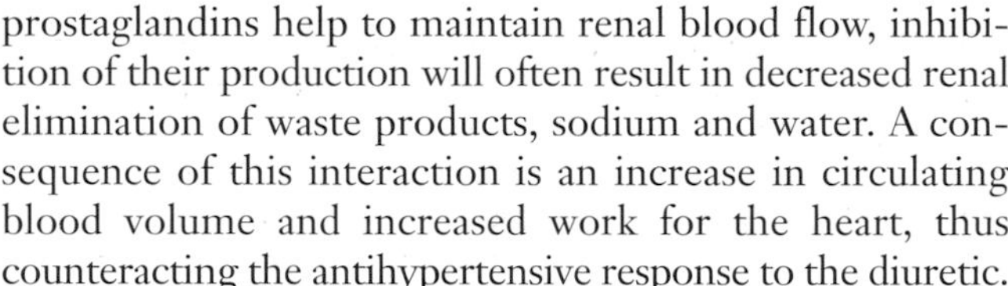

prostaglandins help to maintain renal blood flow, inhibition of their production will often result in decreased renal elimination of waste products, sodium and water. A consequence of this interaction is an increase in circulating blood volume and increased work for the heart, thus counteracting the antihypertensive response to the diuretic.

NSAIDs impair control of coagulation in patients on oral anticoagulant therapy

Two mechanisms contribute to the interaction between anticoagulants and NSAIDs:

- Inhibition of cyclo-oxygenase function by NSAIDs.
- Competitive displacement of oral anticoagulant from plasma protein binding by NSAIDs.

As a result, the anticoagulant effect produced by antagonism of vitamin K is increased by inhibition of platelet cyclo-oxygenase activity and inhibition of platelet aggregation as part of the clotting mechanism. Patients on oral anticoagulants are therefore advised to use acetaminophen for analgesia instead of an NSAID.

Nutrient–drug interactions can interfere with drug efficacy

The iron present in some multivitamin preparations can form complexes with certain chemical groups. For example, the catechol substituent on levodopa complexes with iron, resulting in a decrease in levodopa absorption and decreased drug delivery to the brain. This interaction reduces the efficacy of levodopa in the treatment of Parkinson's disease. Another classic interaction between drugs and nutrients is complex formation of tetracycline antibiotics with Ca^{2+} in milk. This chemical complex results in reduced tetracycline absorption and therefore decreased antimicrobial activity of the antibiotic. In contrast to the first two examples, ingestion of calcium channel blockers with high first-pass elimination together with grapefruit juice will increase the fraction of the administered dose that reaches the peripheral circulation. This results in an enhanced pharmacologic effect. The mechanism involves inhibition of the intestinal drug metabolizing cytochrome P-450 isoform CYP3A4 by grapefruit. This interaction may result in hypotension and other adverse effects associated with high plasma concentrations of calcium channel blocking drugs.

EFFECT OF DISEASE ON DRUG ACTION

The presence of a disease can have a considerable effect on the choice of drug, its disposition and the likelihood of increased interindividual variation in drug responses. In cases of kidney and liver disease, drug doses may have to be reduced in order to prevent toxicity resulting from impaired drug elimination. Usually, the most profound drug–disease interactions occur when the disease process affects organs involved in drug disposition. Some important examples of disease–drug interactions include:

- Cirrhosis and other liver diseases can impair the ability of the liver to metabolize drugs. This effect can lead to unpredictable drug accumulation and toxicity if hepatic impairment is not considered when the drug dose regimen is selected. Interestingly, the reserve capacity for phase 2 metabolic reactions seems to be preserved relative to that for phase 1. Therefore, in the presence of hepatic impairment it can be beneficial to choose a drug that is eliminated primarily by conjugation (phase 2). With respect to dose adjustment, there is as yet no consensus as to which is the best biochemical marker to use as the basis for adjustment. It is not clear that any one biochemical marker of liver function will reflect accurately the changing capacity of the drug-metabolizing enzymes in the diseased liver. If possible, monitoring drug concentrations in patients with liver disease provides the best current approach for adjustment of drug doses.
- In patients with renal disease, prostaglandins help to maintain residual renal function. The use of drugs that inhibit cyclo-oxygenase (e.g. NSAIDs) can lead to a rapid deterioration of residual renal function and consequently impaired drug excretion. Normally, when renal excretion is important for drug elimination, doses are reduced based upon the directly measured or estimated creatinine clearance of the patient.
- Recent data suggest that intestinal CYP3A4 is suppressed in celiac disease, but is restored to normal with a gluten-free diet. Intestinal disease might therefore lead to variability in first-pass elimination of drugs metabolized by this isoform.
- Viral infections appear to suppress hepatic cytochromes P-450, perhaps as a result of interferon induction. A patient with a plasma drug concentration at the upper end of the therapeutic range can therefore suddenly show signs of drug toxicity during a viral infection.
- Achlorhydria (absence of stomach acid) is more common in the elderly. Lack of an acid pH in the stomach may affect the site of absorption of drug formulations with a pH-dependent coating.
- The choice of diuretic for a patient with cardiovascular disease can depend on whether the patient has osteoporosis. Hydrochlorothiazide is a diuretic that does not increase the renal elimination of Ca^{2+} and therefore is advantageous in this type of patient.
- β adrenoceptor antagonists are contraindicated in patients with asthma because these drugs increase bronchoconstriction. This interaction is due to the fact that circulating epinephrine in asthmatics helps to dilate their airways.
- Anticholinergic drugs can increase cognitive impairment in patients with Alzheimer-type dementia.

Variability of drug disposition

- The rate of drug disposition is most likely to be impaired in the very young and the very old
- Radical differences in the genetic expression of drug-metabolizing enzymes complicate the individualization of drug therapy
- Concurrent ingestion of multiple drugs increases the probability of drug interactions owing to the increased likelihood of inducing or inhibiting the drug-metabolizing enzyme systems responsible
- Drug doses should be modified if the patient has a disease that impairs the function of organs with an important role in drug metabolism and/or excretion

FURTHER READING

Benet LZ (ed.) *The Effect of Disease States on Drug Pharmacokinetics.* Washington, DC: American Pharmaceutical Association; 1976. [This classic monograph provides details on how diseases contribute to altered drug disposition.]

Gabardi S, Abramson S. Drug dosing in chronic kidney disease. *Med Clin North Am* 2005; **89**: 649-687.

Gaedigk A. Interethnic differences of drug-metabolizing enzymes. *Int J Clin Pharmacol Ther* 2000; **38**: 61–68. [This review summarizes our current understanding of the role of ethnic origin on the expression of some drug-metabolizing enzymes.]

Johnson MD. Clinically significant drug interactions. What you need to know before writing prescriptions. *Postgrad Med* 1999; **105**: 193–222. [This review provides an indication of the current state of knowledge concerning drug interactions involving cytochrome P-450 isoforms.]

Saito M, Hirata-Koizumi M, Matsumoto M, Urano T, Hasegawa R. Undesirable effects of citrus juice on the pharmacokinetics of drugs: focus on recent studies. *Drug Saf* 2005; **28**: 677–694.

Tang W, Wang RW, Lu AY. Utility of recombinant cytochrome p450 enzymes: a drug metabolism perspective. *Curr Drug Metab* 2005; **6**: 503–517.

Westphal JF, Brogard JM. Drug administration in chronic liver disease. *Drug Saf* 1997; **17**: 47–73.

Wilkinson GR. Drug metabolism and variability among patients in drug response. *N Engl J Med* 2005; **352**: 2211–2221.

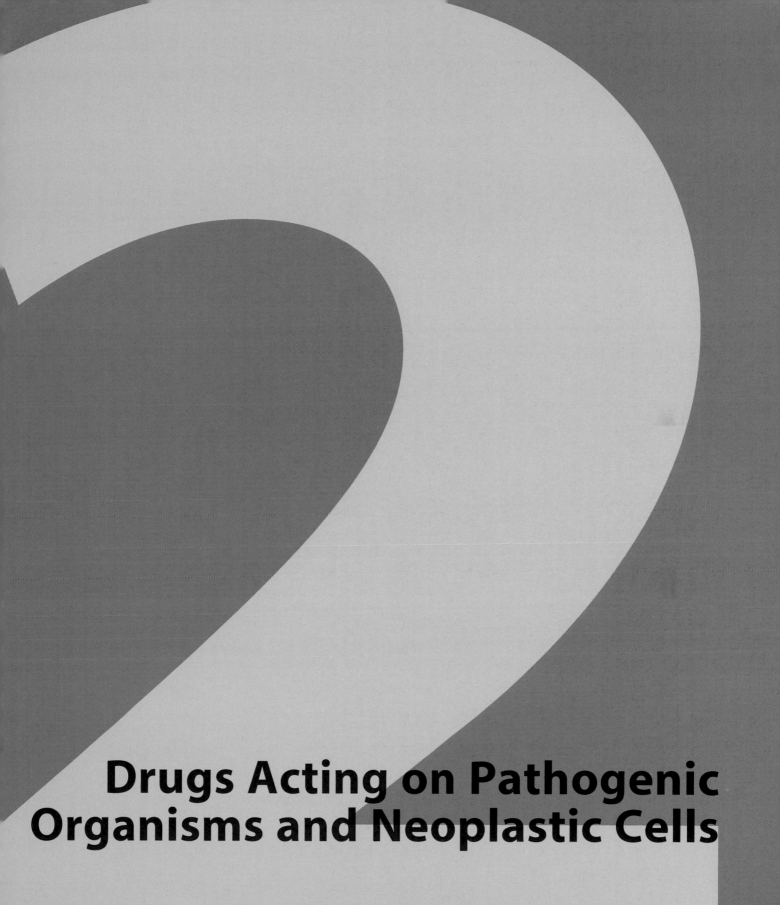

Drugs Acting on Pathogenic Organisms and Neoplastic Cells

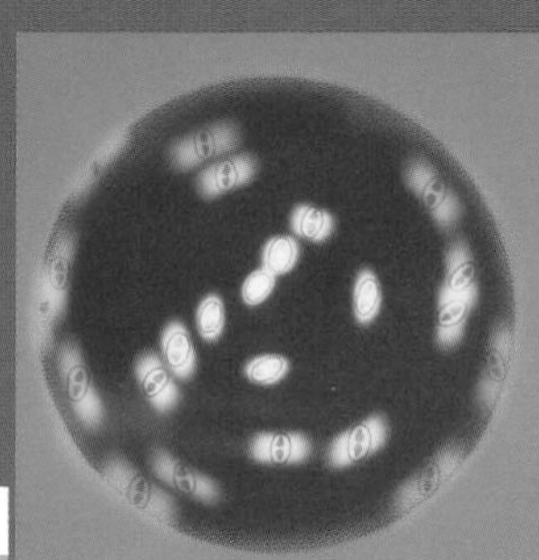

Chapter 5

Introduction to Section 2

This section of the book deals with drugs that act on pathogenic organisms or malignant cells by virtue of selective toxicity for such organisms or cells. These drugs are sufficiently different in their mechanism of action from drugs used to influence the various systems of the body that they may be considered together with respect to their mode of actions and uses. Certain principles can be applied to the use of such drugs.

There exists in viruses, bacteria, parasites and neoplasms of certain molecular processes that provide unique targets to those organisms or cells which are often not found in mammalian tissue. In some cases, viruses, bacteria, parasites and neoplasms contain molecular mechanisms found in mammalian cells, but such mechanisms are often greatly overexpressed when compared with normal mammalian cells. The existence of such differences gives rise to the possibility of selective toxicity. Thus, if a molecular target does not exist in a mammalian cell, then a drug that acts upon that target in viruses, bacteria, parasites or neoplasms, may have relatively limited effects in normal mammalian tissue. In principle it is much more challenging to identify these targets in cancer cells compared to those in microorganisms.

It is important to recognize that drugs designed to selectively kill pathogens or neoplasms are generally not fully effective in the absence of an immune response by the host. The inability to kill all organisms exists despite giving multiple dosing. In the absence of an effective immune system, the disease organism can reappear or even overwhelm the body as exemplified in the multiple reinfections with opportunistic infective organisms in patients with AIDS. Consequently, the efficacy of many of these drugs cannot be determined in the absence of clinical information.

FURTHER READING

Bellenir, K. Infectious diseases sourcebook. Detroit, MI: Omnigraphics, c2004. [Basic consumer health information about infectious diseases old and new, bioterrorism and current research initiatives, with a glossary and directory of resources for more information.]

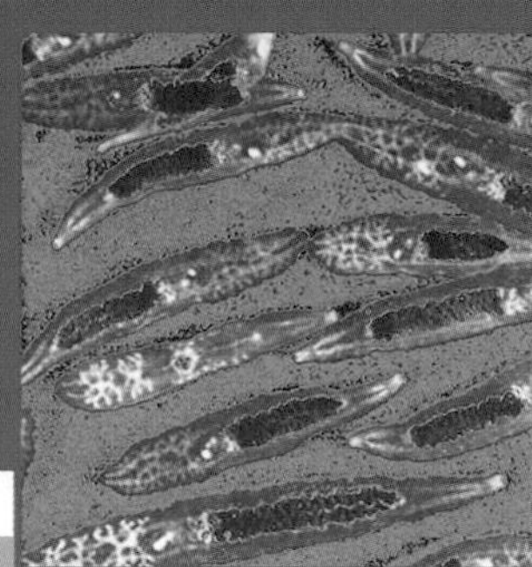

Chapter 6

Drugs Acting on Infectious Organisms

PART 1

DRUGS AND PRIONS

The term prion describes certain proteins which are widely believed to act as infectious agents. Prions have been implicated in mammalian transmissible spongiform encephalopathies (TSEs), including scrapie in sheep, bovine spongiform encephalopathy (BSE) and Creutzfeldt-Jakob disease in humans. In 1996 a new variant of CJD (nv CJD) was described that only affected people under 40 and led to a rapid decline in health. This 'infection' of humans was suggested to be due to consumption of cattle tainted with BSE, raising concerns that some prions could jump species. However, TSEs are comparatively rare diseases that pose a minimal threat to human health, particularly with appropriate health measures in place to prevent tainted meat entering the human food chain. There are currently no drugs that can inhibit prion-mediated neurodegenerative diseases, although recent animal studies have suggested that pentosan polysulfate may have some value in preventing 'infections.'

PART 2

DRUGS AND VIRUSES

BIOLOGY AND DRUG RESPONSIVENESS OF VIRUSES

Viral infections can involve any organ of the body. Most are asymptomatic. Symptomatic infections can range from short, benign illnesses, such as the common cold, to a protracted, potentially lethal infection such as that caused by human immunodeficiency virus, type 1 (HIV-1).

Viruses can be selectively inhibited by drugs

Selective inhibition of viruses by drugs can be achieved in two ways:

- Inhibition of unique steps in pathology for viral replication, such as adsorption of the virus to a cell receptor, penetration, uncoating, assembly, or release (Fig. 6.1).
- Preferential inhibition of steps shared with the host cell, including transcription and translation.

The potential therapeutic efficacy of an antiviral drug can be evaluated in vitro, but this is less predictive than bacterial sensitivity in vitro to drugs. A lack of standardized in vitro testing, and insufficient knowledge of pharmacokinetic–pharmacodynamic relationships, makes it difficult to determine accurately the relationship between drug concentration and antiviral effect.

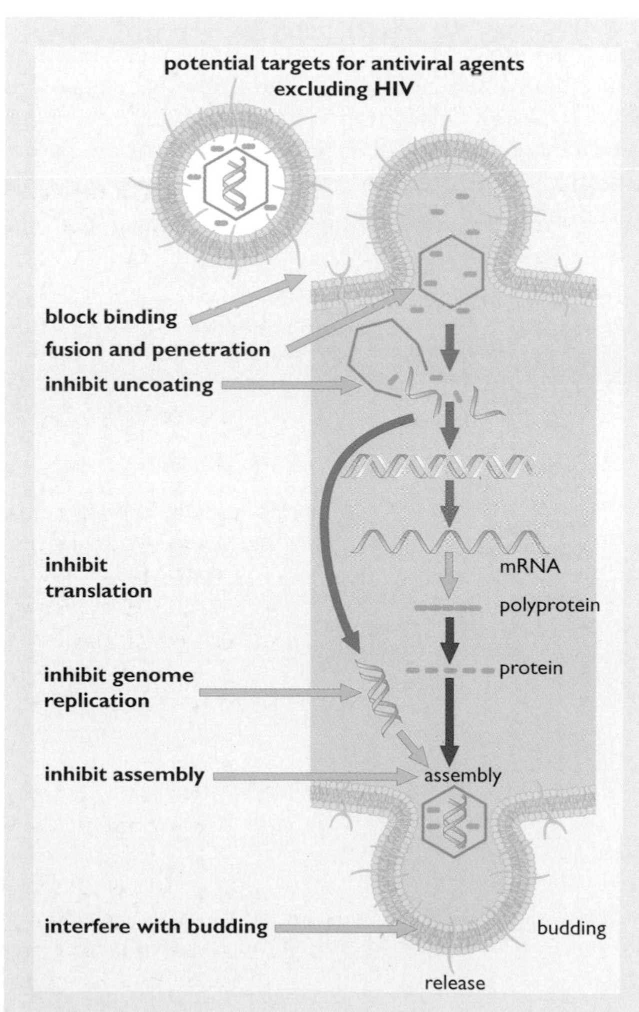

Fig. 6.1 Site of action of antiviral drugs in the non-HIV replicative cycle.

The development of resistance often limits the usefulness of antiviral drugs. Resistance has been reported during therapy with all currently available antiviral drugs except ribavirin, trifluorothymidine, cidofovir and sorivudine. Resistance is due to development of nucleotide mutations but such viruses might still be susceptible to other antiviral drugs acting via a different mechanism of action. The emergence of resistant strains can be minimized by using multiple drugs as in therapy for HIV-1 infection.

Successful antiviral chemotherapy depends upon host immunocompetence

Currently available antiviral drugs are virustatic only.

Symptoms and signs of viral infections are due to a variety of host responses

The response of hosts to viral infections range from acute inflammation (e.g. meningoencephalitis) to hypertrophy and hyperplasia (e.g. warts) and oncogenesis (e.g. human T-cell lymphotropic virus-1 leukemia).

The inflammatory response in cells usually terminates viral replication and leads to recovery from the infection. In patients with an impaired host immune response, viral infections can be associated with a prolonged and more severe illness. Occasionally, the host immune response is pathogenic and causes disease manifestations (e.g. dengue hemorrhagic fever). Rarely, virus replication causes little or no inflammatory reaction, but nevertheless the infection is fatal (e.g. rabies).

Antiviral drugs are effective against some common viral infections

Antiviral chemotherapy is effective in infections caused by:

- Herpes viruses (HSV-1, HSV-2, HHV-8, VZV and CMV).
- Influenza A and B virus.
- Respiratory syncytial virus (RSV).
- Hepatitis B and C viruses (HVB and HVC).
- Papilloma viruses (HPV).
- The arenavirus of Lassa fever.
- Human immunodeficiency virus (HIV-1, HIV-2).

CLASSIFICATION OF ANTIVIRAL DRUGS AND THEIR SITES OF ACTION IN VIRAL REPLICATION

Antiviral drugs can be classified as nucleoside or non-nucleoside drugs according to their sites of action in the viral replicative cycle (see Fig. 6.1). Some of the currently available drugs have more than one site of action (e.g. ribavirin). Some drugs are naturally occurring molecules (e.g. interferons). Antivirals that inhibit viruses other than HIV are presented in Table 6.1 and discussed according to the step in the viral replicative cycle at which they act. These drugs and the viruses against which they are used are presented in Table 6.2. HIV drugs are discussed in more detail later.

Table 6.1 Sites of action of currently available antiviral drugs (other than HIV drugs)

	Currently available drugs	
Viral replicative cycle step	Nucleoside	Non-nucleoside
1. Adsorption		
2. Fusion & penetration		
3. Uncoating		Amantadine Rimantadine
4. Transcription		Interferons
5. Translation		Fomivirsen
6. RNA or DNA replication	Acyclovir Adenine arabinoside (ara-A) Cidofovir Famciclovir Foscarnet Ganciclovir Penciclovir Idoxuridine Ribavirin Sorivudine Trifluorothymidine Valacyclovir	Foscarnet
7. Assembly		
8. Release and budding		Zanamivir Oseltamivir

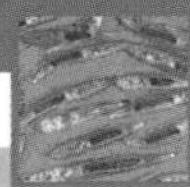

Table 6.2 Drugs used to treat common viral infections other than HIV

Influenza (A, B)	Hepatitis (HBV, HCV)	Human papilloma virus (HPV)	Kaposi (HHV-8)	Cytomegalo-virus (CMV)	Herpesviruses Simplex HSV-1, HSV-2	Varicella-zoster (VZV)
A:	B:	Interferons	Interferons	Cidofovir	Acyclovir	Ara-A
Amantadine	Famciclovir	Cidofovir		Ganciclovir	Valacyclovir	Acyclovir
Rimantadine	Lamivudine			Fomivirsen	Penciclovir	Cidofovir
A & B:	B & C:			Foscarnet	Famciclovir	Famciclovir
Interferons	Interferons			Valganciclovir	Sorivudine	Penciclovir
Ribavirin	C:			Valganciclovir	Foscarnet	Valacyclovir
Zanamivir	Interferons +			Topical:	Ara-A	Sorivudine
Oseltamivir	ribavirin				Trifluorothymidine	Trifluridine
					Idoxuridine	Brivudin
					Trifluridine	
					Brivudin	

INHIBITORS OF UNCOATING

Amantadine and rimantadine are the only antiviral drugs which inhibit viral replication primarily by inhibiting uncoating of the virus. Amantadine was the first drug licensed for the prevention of influenza (1966) and its treatment (1976), followed by rimantadine in 1993.

CHEMISTRY Amantadine and rimantadine are tricyclic 10-carbon ring structures with an amine group on one pole. They are lipophilic and weak bases with a pKa of approximately 10.

MOLECULAR MECHANISM OF ACTION Both amantadine and rimantadine inhibit the replication of all known strains of influenza A viruses in a variety of cells in culture and experimentally infected animals. Influenza B and C viruses are not inhibited.

The two drugs act similarly: they bind inside the ion-channel formed by the M_2 transmembrane protein in the envelope of the virion. Binding creates a steric block (Fig. 6.2), which prevents activation of the H^+ transport function of the channel, which normally acidifies the interior of the virion. The latter is essential for release of the RNA genome from the nucleoprotein complex, a process known as uncoating. Inhibition of uncoating prevents influenza virus replication.

Single nucleotide mutations in the M_2 target site occur readily. These can present drug binding to the target site, confer shared drug resistance on the virion and result in clinical treatment failure. Amantadine- and rimantadine-resistant viral mutants are susceptible to zanamivir and oseltamivir.

Amantadine was discovered serendipitously to possess antiparkinsonian activity (see Ch. 8). Rimantadine has no antiparkinsonian effect.

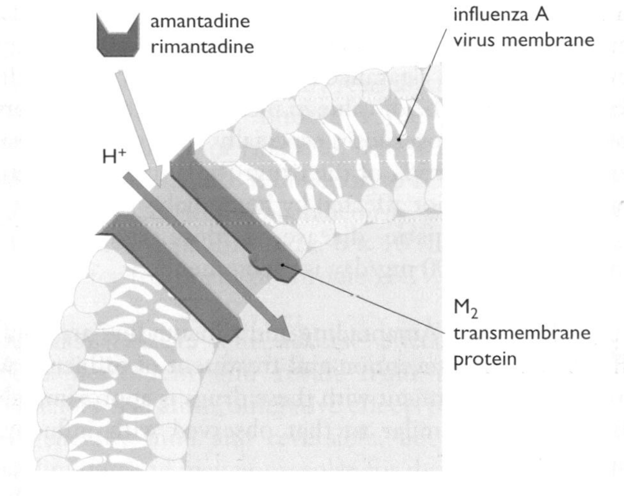

Fig. 6.2 Amantadine and rimantadine bind inside the ion channel formed by the M_2 transmembrane protein formed in the envelope of the virion. This creates a stearic block preventing H^+ transporting and thus uncoating.

PHARMACOKINETICS Table 6.3 shows selected pharmacokinetic characteristics of amantadine and rimantadine in healthy young and old (>65 years) adults.

Amantadine and rimantadine are available only in oral forms. Their pharmacokinetic characteristics relate to their high pKa and lipophilicity, with almost complete ionization in the low pH found in the stomach and slow but relatively complete absorption from intestines. They have large apparent volumes of distribution, which are approximately threefold greater for rimantadine than amantadine. They share similar trough plasma concentrations at steady state (approx 300 mg/L), both are cleared

severe. Delirium and psychosis may occur. Nausea, vomiting and diarrhea occur in up to 50% of patients. Anorexia and weight loss occurs in 25–65% of patients and can necessitate cessation of treatment. Hypo- or hypertension, chest pain and edema have occurred as well as cough, dyspnea and nasal congestion in up to 30% of patients. Proteinuria develops in up to 25% of patients. Serum creatinine increases in up to 10% of patients. Clinically important hyper- and hypothyroidism have been reported, which has been postulated to be due to induction of autoimmune thyroiditis or cross-reactivity of TSH with IFN receptors. Gynecomastia, loss of libido, abortion, skin rash and alopecia have been reported.

ANTIVIRAL DRUGS THAT INHIBIT VIRAL TRANSLATION

Fomivirsen

Fomivirsen is the first antisense therapy drug approved for clinical use in the USA. It is used to suppress eye infections with cytomegalovirus (CMV) strains that are resistant to ganciclovir, cidofovir and foscarnet.

CHEMISTRY Fomivirsen is a 21-nucleotide phosphorothioate antisense molecule that binds to complementary CMV mRNA transcripts which encode proteins that regulate immediate-early gene expression. Fomivirsen inhibits CMV replication by blocking translation.

PHARMACOKINETICS Fomivirsen is administered by intravitreal injection. Details of its pharmacokinetics in the eye are incomplete but it is catabolized over 7 to 10 days by exonucleases.

CLINICAL USES Fomivirsen is approved for the intravitreal treatment of CMV retinitis in AIDS patients who are intolerant of, not responsive to, or have contraindications to, other antiviral treatments.

ADVERSE EFFECTS Iritis, vitritis and increased ocular pressure have been reported in up to 25% of patients. Although fomivirsen is indicated for patients who have not responded to, or are intolerant of cidofovir, there might be an increased risk of ocular inflammation in such patients.

Data on the oncogenicity and carcinogenicity of fomivirsen are not available.

ANTIVIRAL DRUGS THAT INHIBIT RNA OR DNA GENOMIC REPLICATION

Acyclovir

Acyclovir is the prototype antiviral drug in a family of synthetic nucleoside analogs widely used to prevent and treat infections caused by HSV-1 and HSV-2, VZV and CMV. For her work in the discovery and development of acyclovir, Dr Gertrude Elion received the Nobel Prize for Physiology and Medicine in 1988.

Pharmacologic bases for the selective inhibition of herpesvirus replication by acyclovir

- **Selective accumulation (trapping) in infected cells due to avid phosphorylation by herpesvirus thymidine kinase**
- **Preferential affinity of acyclovir triphosphate for viral, rather than cellular DNA polymerase**

CHEMISTRY In addition to acyclovir, the related drugs in this family, which includes valacyclovir, penciclovir, famciclovir, ganciclovir and cidofovir (Fig. 6.3), are all acyclic analogs of nucleosides.

MECHANISM OF ACTION All undergo intracellular phosphorylation to the active triphosphate nucleotide moiety. Acyclovir, penciclovir, and ganciclovir-triphosphate (TP) inhibit herpesvirus replication by competing with deoxyguanosine triphosphate (dGTP) for the viral DNA polymerase, while cidofovir-TP acts as a deoxycytidine TP (dCTP) substitute. In addition, they all interfere with viral DNA replication after incorporation into the elongating herpesvirus DNA chain by causing DNA chain termination. This occurs because absence of the 3′-C, and its OH group, on the acyclic ribose molecule precludes formation of the 3′-5′-phosphodiester linkage for addition of the next nucleotide (Fig. 6.4).

Acyclovir, valacyclovir, penciclovir and famciclovir are discussed together because of their use primarily in patients with HSV and VZV infections. Ganciclovir and cidofovir are considered together because of their utility primarily for management of patients with CMV infection.

Acyclovir is a potent and selective inhibitor of herpes virus DNA replication. The antiviral action of acyclovir is mediated by its triphosphate metabolite, acyclovir-TP (Fig. 6.5). Acyclovir-TP inhibits three steps in the replicative cycle: first, acyclovir-TP competitively inhibits viral DNA polymerase utilization of GTP; second, acyclovir-TP terminates elongation of the HSV DNA strand when incorporated as a guanosine analog substitute (see Fig. 6.4). Third, viral DNA polymerase is inactivated by binding to acyclovir-TP on the DNA primer template. The DNA polymerases of CMV and Epstein-Barr virus (EBV) are less sensitive to the inhibitory effect of acyclovir-TP than those of HSV and VZV, accounting in part for the relative inefficacy of acyclovir in the treatment of CMV and EBV infection. The selective effects of acyclovir-TP on viral rather than host cell DNA replication are due to two factors: first, it is selectively concentrated in virus-infected cells due to the catalytic action of the virus-encoded thymidine kinase enzyme,

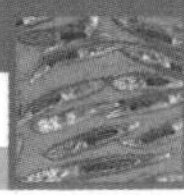

acyclovir penciclovir ganciclovir deoxyguanosine

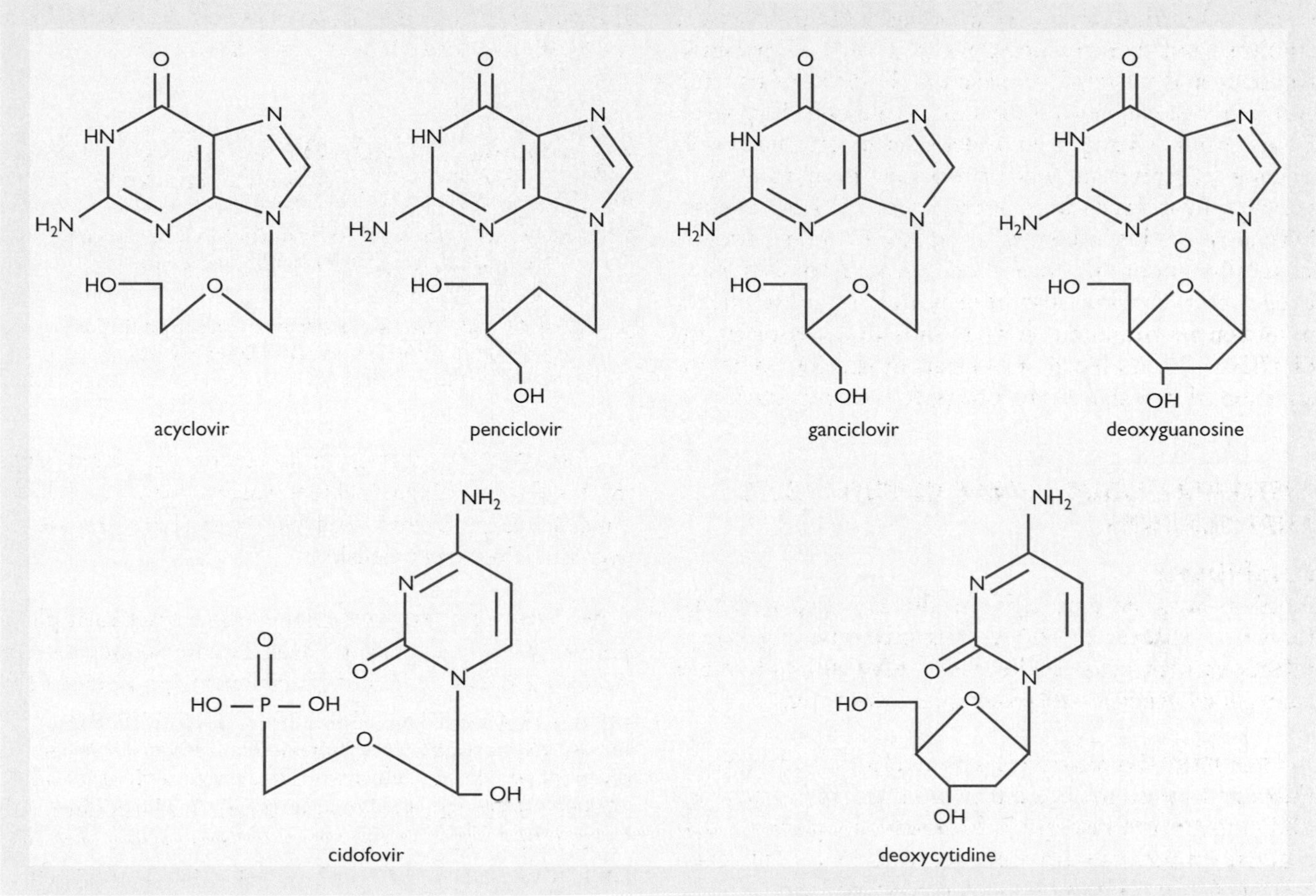

cidofovir deoxycytidine

Fig. 6.3 Structures of deoxyguanosine and deoxycytidine analog inhibitors of herpesvirus DNA replication.

and second, the active antiviral molecule, acyclovir-TP, has a higher affinity for HSV than host cell polymerase.

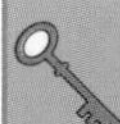

Mechanisms of action of the antiviral actions of acyclovir-TP

- Competitive inhibition of herpesvirus DNA polymerase
- Viral DNA chain termination
- Noncompetitive inhibition of herpesvirus DNA polymerase

PHARMACOKINETICS Acyclovir is marketed as topical 5% cream and ointment, oral tablets and suspension, and in an i.v. form.

Acyclovir is incompletely and slowly absorbed from the gastrointestinal tract (Table 6.5). Its bioavailability is approximately 20% of a 200 mg dose and declines with increasing dose. After i.v. administration, loss of acyclovir is independent of dose and best fits a two-compartment model. Elimination from plasma is first order.

Acyclovir is widely distributed, hence herpesvirus infection in any organ can be effectively treated by oral or i.v. administration. Acyclovir also crosses the placenta at all stages of pregnancy and is secreted into breast milk.

Approximately 80% of acyclovir is excreted unchanged in urine. Acyclovir renal clearance exceeds that of creatinine, indicating that acyclovir is both excreted by glomerular filtration and renal tubular secretion. In anuric patients, clearance is reduced and the elimination half-life increased. Oxidation yields the predominant metabolite, 9-(carboxymethoxy) methyl guanine. Less than 15% of acyclovir is normally metabolized. Dose reduction is recommended when creatinine clearance is reduced. Hemodialysis reduces acyclovir plasma concentration by 60% such that a supplemental dose of 50% of the standard dose is recommended after each hemodialysis treatment. Peritoneal dialysis is much less efficient in removing acyclovir so that no dose supplementation is needed for such patients. No dose reduction is required for patients with hepatic disease.

Topical acyclovir is poorly absorbed into the systemic circulation whether given as the cream or ointment formulation. Acyclovir penetration into the deeper

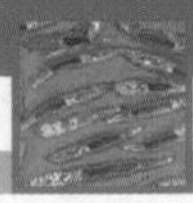

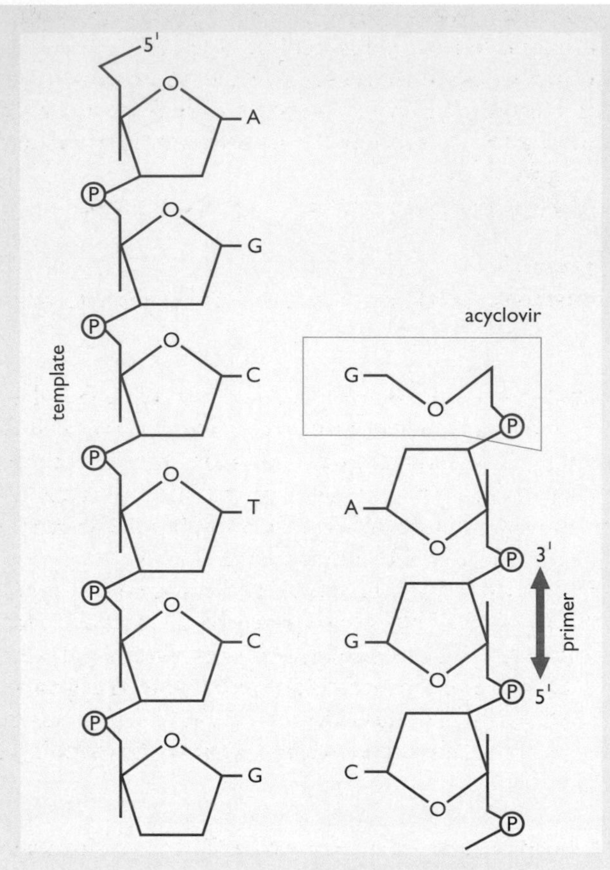

Fig. 6.4 Representation of acyclovir triphosphate termination of DNA chain elongation. Absence of the 3′-C molecule on the acyclic ribose molecule precludes formation of the 3′-5′-phosphodiester linkage needed to allow DNA chain elongation. (Adapted from Elion GB. Mechanism of action and selectivity of acyclovir. *Am J Med* 1982; Acyclovir Symposium: 7–13.)

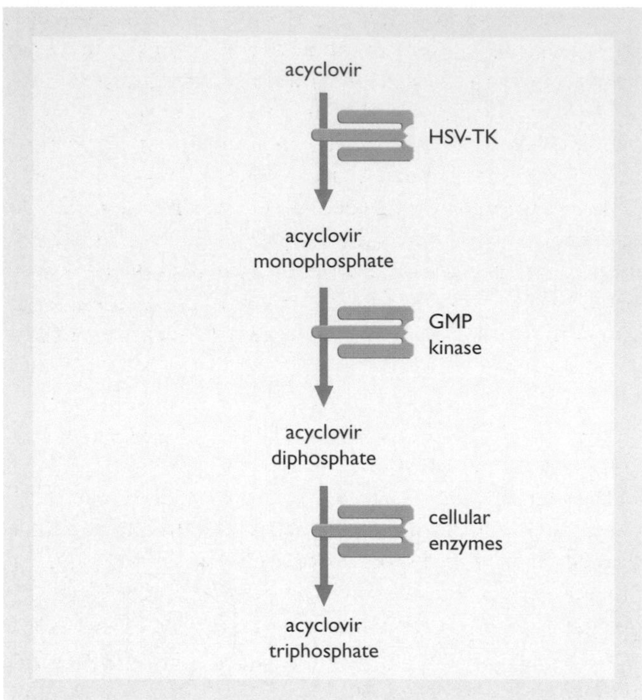

Fig. 6.5 Enzymatic conversion of acyclovir to its mono-, di- and triphosphate forms. Herpes simplex virus thymidine kinase (HSV-TK) catalyzes the formation of acyclovir monophosphate. Cellular kinases convert the monophosphate to the di- and triphosphate forms. Acyclovir triphosphate is the active antiviral moiety. (Adapted from Elion GB. Mechanism of action and selectivity of acyclovir. *Am J Med* 1982; Acyclovir Symposium: 7–13.)

Table 6.5 Selected pharmacokinetic characteristics of oral acyclovir, valacyclovir, penciclovir and famciclovir

Parameter	Acyclovir	Valacyclovir	Penciclovir	Famciclovir
Bioavailability (%)	13–21	54	5	77
Volume of distribution at steady state (Vdss, L/1.73 m^2)	47	47	112	112
Renal clearance (mL/min/1.73 m^2)	250–280	250–280	415–530	415–530
Half-life, mean (range, hours)	3.0 (1.5–6.3)	3.0 (1.5–6.3)	(2.2–2.3)	(2.2–2.3)
Urinary excretion of unchanged drug (%)	80	80	50–60	50–60

layers of the epidermis, where HSV replicates to cause recurrent cold sore and genital herpes, is poor, but greater for cream than ointment. Poor epidermal penetration accounts for part of the relative ineffectiveness of topical acyclovir for treatment of recurrent cold sore and genital HSV infection.

CLINICAL USES Acyclovir inhibits the replication of HSV, VZV, CMV and EBV in infected cells but has no effect on latent infections. Acyclovir is used for prophylaxis and treatment of a wide range of HSV and VZV infections in both immunocompetent and immunocompromised patients. Acyclovir is more effective than placebo in immunocompetent subjects with HSV genital, orolabial, corneal, hand (whitlow) infection, encephalitis and neonatal infection. HSV encephalitis and neonatal HSV infection are treated intravenously. Acyclovir is efficacious in patients with chickenpox and herpes zoster. Acyclovir decreases recurrence of orolabial and genital HSV infection in immunocompetent individuals.

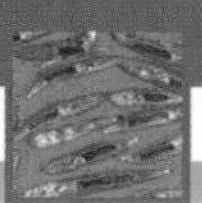

In immunocompromised patients, acyclovir is effective for treatment of mucocutaneous (orolabial and anogenital) HSV infection as well as herpes zoster.

Acyclovir-resistant HSV and VZV strains of virus can develop but usually only after prolonged use of acyclovir and in immunocompromised patients. Resistance arises largely through the selection of strains that do not synthesize thymidine kinase (HSV-TK). Occasionally, strains emerge whose resistance is due to reduced affinity for TK or reduced affinity for viral DNA polymerase. Infections caused by acyclovir-resistant strains respond to i.v. foscarnet.

ADVERSE EFFECTS Acyclovir is well tolerated and safe. Rapid i.v. administration of acyclovir can cause a rise in creatinine due to renal tubular lumen obstruction by acyclovir crystals. Therefore, acyclovir must be administered over 60 min or more. The other dose-related adverse effect of acyclovir is neurotoxicity (lethargy, confusion, tremor, hallucinations, delirium, seizures and coma), particularly in patients with renal insufficiency receiving standard doses of acyclovir intravenously. Nephrotoxic and neurologic side effects are reversible on discontinuation of acyclovir therapy. Extravasation of acyclovir during i.v. administration can cause cellulitis and blistering, probably related to the alkaline pH (9–10) of the drug solution.

Adenine arabinoside

CHEMISTRY AND MECHANISM OF ACTION Adenine arabino-side (Ara-A) is an analog of adenosine that is metabolized by cellular kinases to its triphosphate nucleotide (Ara-A-TP). Ara-A-TP inhibits viral DNA polymerase preferentially and is incorporated into both elongating cellular and viral DNA strands, resulting in chain termination. This antiviral effect is also augmented by its hypoxanthine metabolite, which acts synergistically with the parent molecule. HSV-TK strains resistant to acyclovir are sensitive in vitro to ara-A.

PHARMACOKINETICS Ara-A is poorly absorbed systemically from a 3% ara-A ointment applied to the eye. During i.v. infusion, ara-A is rapidly converted to ara-hypoxanthine by adenosine deaminase. As a result, only the metabolite is measurable in plasma and has a serum half-life of 3–4 hours. Fifty percent of a dose of ara-A is recovered in urine as hypoxanthine arabinoside plus only a very small fraction of the parent drug.

CLINICAL USES Ara-A was the first antiviral drug safe enough to use parenterally for treatment of HSV and VZV infections. Due to its poor aqueous solubility and hence a need for large volumes of i.v. fluid, it has been replaced by acyclovir. However, it continues to be used as a safe and effective topical treatment for HSV keratitis. For HSV keratitis, topical ara-A is as effective as trifluorothymidine and better than idoxuridine.

ADVERSE EFFECT Topical ara-A 3.0% ophthalmic ointment is less toxic than topical idoxuridine.

Intravenous ara-A causes a range of neurotoxic but reversible adverse effects including hallucinations, ataxia, tremor; IFN administered concomitantly may intensify these adverse effects.

Ara-A is mutagenic and carcinogenic in vitro.

Cidofovir

CHEMISTRY Cidofovir is an acyclic phosphonate analog of cytidine.

MECHANISM OF ACTION Cidofovir is phosphorylated to mono- and diphosphate nucleotides by intracellular kinases. The phosphorylated cidofovir metabolite concentrations in infected and uninfected cells are similar. Since cidofovir is itself a phosphonate, cidofovir-DP functions as a TP antiviral drug.

Cidofovir-DP inhibits viral DNA synthesis by both inhibiting viral DNA polymerase and acting as an alternate substrate in competition with the natural substrate, dCTP. Incorporation of cidofovir-DP into the growing viral DNA chain reduces the rate of viral DNA synthesis; incorporation of two consecutive cidofovir-DP terminates chain elongation.

PHARMACOKINETICS Cidofovir-DP has a prolonged intracellular half-life of 13 to 65 hours. A metabolite, cidofovir-phosphate-choline, has a half-life of 87 hours and may serve as an intracellular reservoir of cidofovir-DT. The oral bioavailability of cidofovir is less than 5%. Cidofovir injected intravenously has a terminal half-time of about 2–3 hours. The drug distributes widely, although penetration into CSF and the eye has not been well characterized. Elimination is via the kidney, both by glomerular filtration and renal tubular secretion.

CLINICAL USES It exhibits broad-spectrum inhibitory activity against all human herpesviruses and several other DNA viruses. These include HSV-1 and -2, VZV, CMV, EBV, HHV-6, -7 and -8, and human papilloma virus (HPV) and polyoma and adenoviruses. Cidofovir is approved for i.v. therapy of CMV retinitis in AIDS patients. Cidofovir is administered intravenously once a week for 2 weeks with probenecid (to reduce tubular renal secretion as discussed in Chapter 12) and concomitant i.v. saline hydration. CMV prevents the progression of retinitis in AIDS patients. The therapeutic effect is comparable to that observed with i.v. ganciclovir.

Topical cidofovir may act against HPV skin infections, while intralesional cidofovir may be useful for treatment of laryngeal and respiratory papillomatosis. In vitro studies indicate that cidofovir inhibits replication of papovavirus infection. Thus, i.v. cidofovir may have potential value in the treatment of progressive multifocal leukoencephalopathy, a progressive, fatal opportunistic infection in immunocompromised individuals, particularly those with advanced HIV.

ADVERSE EFFECTS Cidofovir is mutagenic, embryotoxic, gonadotoxic, teratogenic and carcinogenic in animals. In several species, i.v. cidofovir causes dose-dependent nephrotoxicity, which is the principal dose-limiting effect of the drug. Proximal convoluted renal tubular epithelial cell necrosis can be prevented by concurrent probenecid administration and is partially reversible.

Increased serum creatinine has occurred in 10% of i.v. cidofovir recipients and proteinuria in 45%. Ocular hypotony occurs in 12% of treated patients and anterior uveitis or iritis in 7%. Neutropenia occurs in 25% of patients treated with cidofovir.

The nephrotoxic effects of i.v. cidofovir is potentiated by other nephrotoxic drugs. Therefore, the following agents should be avoided during i.v. cidofovir therapy: aminoglycoside antibiotics, pentamidine, amphotericin B, foscarnet, nonsteroidal antiinflammatory drugs (NSAIDs) and ionic, hypertonic radiographic contrast dye.

Famciclovir and penciclovir

Famciclovir, which has no antiviral activity, is the prodrug of penciclovir, a potent and selective inhibitor of herpesviruses comparable to acyclovir.

MECHANISM OF ACTION Penciclovir, like acyclovir, is first phosphorylated to its triphosphate, the antiviral form of the drug. As with acyclovir in herpesvirus-infected cells, the initial monophosphorylation of penciclovir is catalyzed by herpesvirus TK. Penciclovir-TP acts as an alternate substrate for dGTP in the synthesis of viral DNA by viral DNA polymerase. Whereas incorporation of acyclovir-TP immediately causes chain termination, incorporation of penciclovir-TP allows some limited incorporation (3 penciclovir-TP) before chain elongation is arrested. Penciclovir-TP acts as a potent inhibitor of HBV polymerase-reverse transcriptase.

PHARMACOKINETICS Famciclovir is administered orally, and penciclovir as a topical cream. Only 5% of oral penciclovir is absorbed, whereas the oral bioavailability of penciclovir from famciclovir is 77%.

Elimination from plasma is a first-order process with a plasma half-life of 2 hours in people with normal renal function. Penciclovir is 75% excreted into urine and 25% into feces.

In patients with renal dysfunction, penciclovir clearance is reduced, proportional to the reduced renal function. In patients with renal insufficiency the half-life can extend to 10 hours.

CLINICAL USES Famciclovir is used in the treatment of first episode and recurrent genital HSV infection and herpes zoster in immunocompetent and immunocompromised adults. Topical 4% penciclovir cream minimally reduces the duration of recurrent orolabial HSV infection and shortens healing time compared with placebo.

Famciclovir reduces HBV DNA and transaminase levels in patients with chronic HBV infection and appears to be more effective when combined with interferon. Penciclovir-resistant HBV variants have been demonstrated in liver transplant patients receiving chronic famciclovir therapy. Resistance is due to altered DNA polymerase.

Foscarnet

MECHANISM OF ACTION Foscarnet directly inhibits viral DNA polymerase and HIV reverse transcriptase. Unlike nucleoside antiviral drugs, foscarnet does not undergo intracellular metabolism. Foscarnet binds to, and blocks, the pyrophosphate binding site of viral polymerase, thereby inhibiting cleavage of pyrophosphate from deoxyribonucleotide-TP, thus blocking viral DNA synthesis.

PHARMACOKINETICS Oral bioavailability (about 10%) is too low for oral therapy. After i.v. infusion, foscarnet plasma concentration declines triexponentially as first order processes with successive half-lifes of 0.5, 3 and 18 hours. The drug is widely distributed so that i.v. foscarnet is effective therapy for infection of all organs caused by susceptible viruses.

Doses must be reduced progressively with increasing degrees of renal dysfunction, beginning with even minor reductions in creatinine clearance. Foscarnet is not metabolized and no dose adjustment in the presence of liver disease is required.

CLINICAL USES Foscarnet is trisodium phosphonoformate, a pyrophosphate analog which inhibits replication of HSV, VZV, CMV, EBV, and HHV-6 and -8, as well as HIV and HBV. However, its clinical use is limited to CMV and some HSV infections. Intravenous foscarnet is used for treatment of CMV retinitis in AIDS patients and acyclovir-resistant mucocutaneous HSV infections. Compared with i.v. ganciclovir for treatment of CMV retinitis in AIDS patients, foscarnet controls retinitis but also increases survival, presumably due to an antiretroviral effect.

Foscarnet is effective for treatment of ganciclovir-resistant CMV infection plus other CMV infections in HIV patients, particularly gastrointestinal, pulmonary, central nervous system and radicular neurologic infections. Foscarnet may prevent CMV disease in bone marrow transplant recipients but established CMV pneumonia in these patients is unresponsive.

Resistance to foscarnet, demonstrable in vitro, occurs uncommonly during treatment but is associated with clinical treatment failure. Resistance is associated with

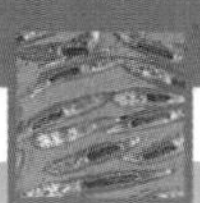

point mutations in the DNA polymerase in herpesviruses and the reverse transcriptase of HIV. Foscarnet-resistant CMV infections may respond to ganciclovir or cidofovir therapy.

ADVERSE EFFECTS Nephrotoxicity, manifest as proteinuria, rising serum creatinine and, occasionally, acute tubular necrosis, is the principal dose-limiting adverse effect of i.v. foscarnet therapy. Approximately 30% of patients show increases in serum creatinine. The incidence of acute renal failure has declined recently, as a result of attention to adequate hydration and dose reductions effected promptly in the face of rising serum creatinine concentration, and avoidance of concomitant nephrotoxic drugs.

Hypo- and hypercalcemia and hypo- and hyperphosphatemia attributed to their chelation with foscarnet deposited in bone, plus hypomagnesia, are reported in 10–44% of patients and necessitate reduced drug. Hypocalcemia may cause paresthesias, tetany and seizures.

CNS adverse effects including headache, irritability and hallucinations occur in up to 10% of subjects. Gastrointestinal adverse effects such as nausea, vomiting and diarrhea are reported in 30–50% of patients. Painful subpreputial ulcers attributed to deposition of urine with foscarnet in high concentration in this area have been described in up to 10% of male patients. Anemia in 20–50% of AIDS patients and granulocytopenia are attributed to myelosuppression.

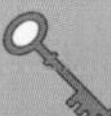

Properties of foscarnet, the only available non-nucleoside herpesvirus inhibitor drug

- Antiviral effect does not require intracellular metabolism
- Directly inhibits herpesvirus DNA polymerase
- Particularly valuable for treating nucleoside-resistant herpes simplex virus, varicella-zoster virus, and cytomegalovirus infection
- Requires i.v. administration
- Causes reversible, but serious, multiple organ toxicity

Ganciclovir

MOLECULAR MECHANISM OF ACTION Ganciclovir is an analog of acyclovir which is equally potent as an inhibitor of HSV, VZV and EBV in vitro. However, it is 10- to 100-fold more active than acyclovir in inhibiting CMV replication in vitro. Ganciclovir acts as its triphosphate as ganciclovir-TP to inhibit viral DNA synthesis. Phosphorylation of ganciclovir within herpesvirus-infected cells is initiated by viral kinases. In HSV- and VZV-infected cells, viral TK catalyzes the initial monophosphorylation step. CMV does not possess a TK enzyme. However, a kinase encoded on the UL97 region of the CMV genome subserves this kinase function. Conversion of ganciclovir-MP to -DP and -TP is by cellular kinases. In uninfected cells, cellular kinases appear to convert ganciclovir to its -TP nucleotide metabolite.

Ganciclovir-TP is a competitive inhibitor of dGTP incorporation into DNA. It preferentially inhibits viral more than host cell DNA polymerase. Incorporation of ganciclovir-TP into viral DNA does not result in obligate chain termination as occurs with acyclovir-TP incorporation. Rather, short subgenomic CMV DNA fragments which cannot be packaged into virions are synthesized. Incorporation of ganciclovir-TP into host cell DNA results in radiomimetic adverse effects on bone marrow, gastrointestinal mucosa and spermatogenesis.

PHARMACOKINETICS Ganciclovir is available as a parenteral formulation for i.v. injection, capsules for oral administration and as a slow-release system for intraocular implantation. A valine ester oral pro-drug of ganciclovir, valganciclovir, has also been developed.

Ganciclovir administered orally is poorly bioavailable. Elimination from plasma is a first-order process. Ganciclovir distributes widely throughout the body so that i.v. therapy can be used to treat CMV disease in any organ. Almost 100% of an administered dose is excreted as unchanged drug in the urine. The plasma half-time in patients with normal renal function is 2 to 4 hours; it increases in direct proportion to declining renal function.

Ganciclovir is 60% bioavailable from valganciclovir. Ganciclovir is marketed as capsules for oral administration. Bioavailability from capsules ranges from 3% to 7%; food increases absorption by 20%. Intravitreal ganciclovir implants release drug at a rate of approximately 1 μg/hour over 5–8 months. They are efficacious for suppression of CMV retinitis in AIDS patients but do not prevent CMV disease in the other eye or extraocular CMV disease.

CLINICAL USES Ganciclovir was the first antiviral drug effective in CMV disease. Ganciclovir is indicated for the treatment and prevention of CMV diseases in immunocompromised patients. These include retinitis in AIDS patients, AIDS-related gastrointestinal and other organ disease and CMV disease in transplant recipients. In immunocompromised transplant patients, CMV primary infection and reactivation of latent infection cause morbidity and mortality and the use of ganciclovir in such patients is warranted. Intravenous ganciclovir reduces the risk of CMV disease in CMV seronegative recipients of heart, liver and lung transplants from CMV seropositive donors.

It is probable that valganciclovir will replace oral and, perhaps, i.v. ganciclovir for some indications.

ADVERSE EFFECTS The vast majority of ganciclovir adverse effects are dose-related. Myelosuppression is the principal dose-related side effect of i.v. ganciclovir therapy with neutropenia observed in about 40% and thrombocytopenia in 15–20% of treated AIDS patients. These effects are usually reversible within 1–2 weeks of discontinuing therapy. Gonadal toxicity, based on preclinical toxicologic studies, is expected after i.v. ganciclovir therapy in both genders but no clear evidence confirming this expectation is currently available. Renal impairment due to obstruction of renal tubules by crystallization of ganciclovir has been reported in 20% of bone marrow transplant patients given i.v. ganciclovir for 4 months. Confusion, abnormal mentation and seizures rarely have been reported. Oral ganciclovir 1000 mg t.i.d. causes diarrhea, nausea and vomiting in 3–13% of recipients compared with 0–7% of recipients of i.v. ganciclovir.

RESISTANCE Ganciclovir resistance associated with CMV treatment failure and in vitro resistance occurs in 8% of CMV isolates from AIDS patients after 3 or more months of continuous therapy. Resistance is mostly due to point mutations in the genome of the UL97 gene and less commonly to point mutations in viral DNA polymerase.

Most resistant isolates retain susceptibility to foscarnet and cidofovir.

Idoxuridine

CHEMISTRY AND MECHANISM OF ACTION Idoxuridine (5-iodo-2′-deoxyuridine) is an analog of thymidine. It resembles acyclovir in being preferentially converted to a monophosphate nucleotide by viral TK with subsequent synthesis of di- and triphosphate nucleotides by cellular kinases. Idoxuridine-TP is incorporated into both viral and mammalian DNA making it more susceptible to breakage, and altered viral proteins may result from faulty transcription, resulting in inhibition of viral replication and adverse effects on rapidly proliferating mammalian cells. Idoxuridine also inhibits DNA polymerase but does not cause chain termination.

Resistance of HSV to idoxuridine develops readily in vitro as well as in patients. Resistance is due to the same mechanisms as mediate acyclovir resistance in HSV.

PHARMACOKINETICS Idoxuridine is poorly absorbed from topical administration. Any idoxuridine absorbed is metabolized to 5-iodouracil, uracil and iodide which are devoid of antiviral activity.

CLINICAL USES Its topical use in treatment of HSV keratitis in 1962 marked the first demonstration of the efficacy of a drug for treatment of a viral infection. Idoxuridine 0.1% ophthalmic solution is administered as one drop onto the cornea every hour during the day and every 2 hours at night. Administration is halved once definite improvement is observed on fluorescein staining. Treatment is continued to a maximum of 21 days to minimize corneal epithelial dystrophy.

ADVERSE EFFECTS Inflammation of the tissues of the eye due to cytotoxic effects of idoxuridine or to allergic reactions can occur. Burning upon instillation, and punctate keratitis, eyelid edema and irritation occur in 2–10% of patients.

Ribavirin

MECHANISM OF ACTION Ribavirin is a guanosine analog with inhibitory activity against several RNA and DNA viruses. Ribavirin is taken up by infected and uninfected cells and phosphorylated by cellular kinases to mono-, di- and triphosphate nucleotides. Ribavirin-MP is a potent inhibitor of inosine monophosphate dehydrogenase. The resulting inhibition blocks synthesis of dGTP and therefore nucleic acid synthesis. Ribavirin-TP can inhibit the RNA polymerase of influenza viruses and inhibit dGTP-dependent 5′-capping of mRNA as well. Additional mechanisms of action probably operate such that ribavirin in vitro inhibits a variety of RNA viruses (ortho- and parmyxo-, arena-, bunya-, RNA tumor, and retroviruses) as well as some DNA viruses (herpes, adeno-, and poxviruses).

PHARMACOKINETICS Ribavirin is effective against a limited number of viral infections when administered intravenously, by mouth and by inhalation as an aerosol.

Oral bioavailability of ribavirin averages 45%. Absorption of ribavirin administered as an aerosol depends on the concentration and duration of exposure and particle size. For lower respiratory tract infections, a special generator is required to produce particles 1–5 μm in diameter that are suspended and do not settle on the walls of the respiratory tract. Such aerosols deliver 70% of inhaled drug to the lungs.

After i.v. injection, ribavirin has half-lifes of 2, 18–36 and 22–64 hours. The apparent volume of distribution at steady state, 650 L (range 380–1140 L), is extremely large and appears to be due to sequestration in erythrocytes (where ribavirin concentration is ninefold greater than in plasma) and perhaps other cells. Ribavirin is eliminated by both hepatic metabolism (65%) and renal excretion (35%). Only 4% of drug is excreted unchanged in urine.

CLINICAL USES It is used as an aerosol in the treatment of severe RSV infection in neonates and infants with associated pulmonary, cardiac and immune deficiency disorders. Oral ribavirin combined with interferon therapy is used for treatment of chronic HCV infection. Intravenous ribavirin reduces mortality in patients with severe Lassa virus infection from 76% to 32%. Ribavirin delivered by aerosol to neonates and infants with RSV lower respiratory infection complicating bronchopulmonary, cardiac or immunodeficiency diseases shortens the

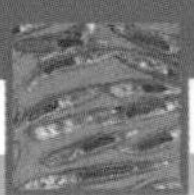

duration of pulmonary RSV shedding and improves selected clinical parameters.

Oral ribavirin in patients with chronic HCV infection does not reduce serum HCV RNA concentration but reversibly reduces fatigue, serum transaminase levels and hepatic inflammation by an unknown mechanism. Concomitant therapy with IFN-α significantly increases the clinical and virologic response so that combined ribavirin–IFN-α is currently the standard treatment for chronic HCV infection.

Ribavirin intravenously or orally reduces mortality in patients with Lassa fever. Intravenous ribavirin reduces mortality and the risk of renal failure in patients with hemorrhagic fever with renal syndrome. The efficacy and safety of i.v. ribavirin for treatment of the hantavirus pulmonary syndrome is under investigation. It is not useful in HIV infections.

ADVERSE EFFECTS Ribavirin accumulation in erythrocytes, which are deficient in triphosphatases, is associated with a shortened erythrocyte lifespan and mild to moderate anemia due to extravascular hemolysis. Hemoglobin falls 20–30 g/L; transfusions and interruption of therapy are rarely required. Aerosolized ribavirin can cause mild conjunctival irritation. Bronchospasm is uncommon even in asthmatics, but airway narrowing due to precipitation of ribavirin on the tracheobronchial mucosa may occur. Anemia is not observed with aerosol therapy.

Ribavirin is not mutagenic in bacteria but may be carcinogenic, embryotoxic and gonadotoxic in animals. Accordingly, ribavirin use is relatively contraindicated for treatment of infection in pregnant patients. Furthermore, pregnant personnel should not be involved in ribavirin aerosol administration.

Sorivudine

MECHANISM OF ACTION Sorivudine is a pyrimidine nucleoside analog that inhibits VZV in vitro at concentrations more than 1000-fold lower than with acyclovir. Sorivudine is active as its triphosphate form following sequential phosphorylation initially mediated by viral thymidine kinase. Sorivudine triphosphate competitively inhibits viral DNA polymerase, but is not incorporated into viral DNA.

PHARMACOKINETICS It is equivalent to acyclovir against HSV-1 but inactive against CMV and HSV-2, the latter being due to the lack of affinity of HSV-2 thymidine kinase for sorivudine. The oral bioavailability of sorivudine is approximately 75%. Most of the drug is eliminated unchanged into the urine.

CLINICAL USES Sorivudine is effective in adults with chickenpox and HIV-1-infected adults with shingles and is used for VZV infections.

ADVERSE EFFECTS Sorivudine is well tolerated, with mild nausea, vomiting and diarrhea, and occasional elevations in hepatic enzymes being observed. Fatal myelosuppression occurred in patients treated concurrently with sorivudine and 5-fluorouracil, probably due to sorivudine inhibition of the metabolism of 5-fluorouracil, which accumulates to myelotoxic levels.

Trifluorothymidine

CHEMISTRY AND MECHANISM OF ACTION Trifluorothymidine (trifluridine or TFT) is a fluorinated analog of thymidine. Structurally, trifluorothymidine differs from idoxuridine in that the iodine atom is replaced by a methyl radical possessing three fluorine atoms. Trifluorothymidine is converted by cellular thymidine kinase to the antiviral metabolite, trifluorothymidine-TP, that is incorporated into both HSV and mammalian cell DNA, as is idoxuridine-TP, which has similar antiviral and cytotoxic effects.

PHARMACOKINETICS Trifluorothymidine enters corneal epithelial cells (like idoxuridine) by diffusion. Little trifluorothymidine is absorbed systemically after topical administration to the eye.

Trifluorothymidine is hydrolyzed to 5-carboxy-2′-deoxyuridine, which has no antiviral activity.

CLINICAL USES A 1.0% ophthalmic solution is 80–95% effective in HSV keratitis, compared with 75–80% for idoxuridine.

ADVERSE EFFECTS See idoxuridine. Trifluorothymidine administered systemically is mutagenic and teratogenic in animals.

Valacyclovir

PHARMACOKINETICS Valacyclovir (VCV) is the L-valyl ester of acyclovir with oral bioavailability three- to fourfold greater than that of acyclovir, independent of dose.

During absorption, valacyclovir undergoes extensive and rapid first-pass metabolism to acyclovir and L-valine. Valacyclovir hydrolysis is mediated by hepatic and possibly intestinal mitochondrial valacyclovir hydrolase.

Only an oral tablet formulation of valacyclovir is marketed. Bioavailability is about 50% of an oral dose and is not affected by food. Acyclovir plasma concentrations over 24 hours after a single oral valacyclovir dose of 1 000 mg are similar to those after an i.v. acyclovir doses of 5 mg/kg q8 h.

The pharmacokinetic characteristics of acyclovir from valacyclovir are identical to those of acyclovir itself (see Table 6.5).

CLINICAL USES The enhanced oral bioavailability of acyclovir produced from valacyclovir has permitted development of regimens that are more effective and more convenient than those using acyclovir. For example, in immunocompetent adults, valacyclovir 1 g t.i.d. was more effective than acyclovir 800 mg five times per day in herpes zoster, as measured by zoster-associated pain or postherpetic neuralgia. It is also approved for once-daily suppression of frequently recurring genital herpes, whereas acyclovir must be ingested at least twice daily.

ADVERSE EFFECTS In patients with advanced HIV infection treated with VCV, thrombotic microangiopathy developed in some recipients whereas none was observed in those receiving acyclovir.

INHIBITORS OF VIRUS RELEASE

Zanamivir and oseltamivir carboxylate (hereafter, oseltamivir) are sialic acid analog inhibitors of influenza neuraminidase that were recently licensed for the prevention and treatment of influenza A and B infection. Their licensure capped five decades of study that began in 1945 with the discovery of enzymatic activity on the surface of influenza viruses that removed virus receptors from the surface of erythrocytes. That enzyme, and those receptors, are now known as neuraminidase and sialic acid, respectively. The design of potent and selective inhibitors of neuraminidase quickly followed delineation of its crystal structure in 1983.

CHEMISTRY Zanamivir and oseltamivir are potent, selective, competitive inhibitors of influenza virus neuraminidase. Other viral and mammalian neuraminidases inhibitors require 80 000 to 1 000 000 times greater concentration for inhibition. The enzymatic site of influenza neuraminidase is highly conserved among influenza A and B viruses, and both drugs inhibit all known subtypes of influenza A virus as well as influenza B. Neither drug is toxic to cells in culture (<10 mM).

MECHANISM OF ACTION Zanamivir and oseltamivir interfere with influenza A and B virus replication by inhibiting viral neuraminidase. Neuraminidase catalyzes the cleavage of the β-ketosidic bond linking a terminal neuraminic acid residue to the adjacent oligosaccharide moiety of sialic acid. Neuraminidase activity is essential for release of daughter virions from infected cells by cleaving terminal sialic acid residues from the cell membrane envelope on the budding virion. Neuraminidase inhibition causes aggregation and clumping of virions at the cell surface resulting from binding of hemagglutinin (protruding from the lipid envelope of virions) to persisting sialic acid residues on adjacent virions.

PHARMACOKINETICS Zanamivir oral biovailability is <5% and so it is administered by oral inhalation as a micronized powder. Of inhaled zanamivir, 80% is deposited in the oropharynx and 10–15%, uniformly, in the lungs; 15–20% of inhaled drug is absorbed. Zanamivir persists in the lower respiratory tract for up to 24 hours. Thus, orally inhaled zanamivir is administered as twice-daily doses for therapy and once-daily doses for prophylaxis.

Oral oseltamivir phosphate is readily absorbed from the intestine and is converted by hepatic esterases to oseltamivir. At least 75% of an oral dose reaches the systemic circulation as oseltamivir. Less than 5% of an oral dose of oseltamivir phosphate is recovered in urine as unchanged drug. Elimination of zanamivir and oseltamivir are first-order processes with similar plasma elimination half-lifes of 1.5–1.8 hours.

Excluding the nervous system, oseltamivir distributes widely throughout the body, such as to the middle ear, where influenza viruses may replicate.

In patients with creatinine clearance less 30 mL/min, oseltamivir doses should be halved even though the drug has little toxic potential. Zanamivir absorption after oral inhalation is so minor that renal function need not be considered during its administration.

CLINICAL USES Both zanamivir and oseltamivir are effective in resolving influenza symptoms. Both reduce the duration and severity of illness by about 25–35% compared with placebo when therapy is initiated within 2 days of onset of symptoms.

Both drugs are 75–80% effective in preventing influenza when compared with placebo. For both prophylaxis and therapy, there are substantial data from studies in healthy adults ill with influenza A virus infection, but fewer data exist on the efficacy of these agents in subjects infected with influenza B virus, or in unhealthy patients, with advanced age, or chronic cardiopulmonary, metabolic or renal disease.

Resistance to both zanamivir and oseltamivir is due to alteration in hemagglutinin or neuraminidase. The former results in amino acid substitutions near the receptor binding site of the hemagglutinin, which reduces affinity for sialic acid, reducing binding and aggregation of daughter virions, even in the presence of neuraminidase inhibitor drugs. The second type of resistance involves amino acid substitutions at positions 119 and 227 that reduce affinity of the drugs for the enzyme and diminished inhibition of neuraminidase activity. In clinical use, zanamivir resistance has not been demonstrated in immunocompetent individuals. Oral oseltamivir therapy has been associated with recovery of resistant viruses in 1–2% of subjects. These levels of emergence of resistance are markedly less than those observed during therapy of patients with influenza with amantadine or rimantadine. Amantadine- and rimantadine-resistant strains are susceptible to neuraminidase inhibitor drugs in vitro.

ADVERSE EFFECTS Orally inhaled zanamivir is well tolerated. However, individual case reports suggest that in individuals with influenza, both with and without underlying bronchopulmonary disease, bronchospastic respiratory distress can be triggered by zanamivir therapy.

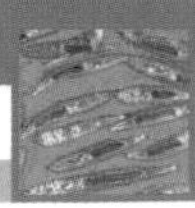

From 5% to 10% more subjects ingesting oseltamivir experience nausea and vomiting compared to placebo.

INHIBITORS OF HIV REPLICATION

The pandemic caused by HIV-1 has led to an intensive search for new antiviral agents to control this disease. Several different classes of drugs demonstrate effectiveness in the treatment of HIV-1 disease:

- Nucleoside reverse transcriptase inhibitors (NRTIs).
- Non-nucleoside reverse transcriptase inhibitors (NNRTIs).
- Protease inhibitors (PIs).
- Antiretroviral fusion inhibitor.

Treatment with antivirals delays the onset of AIDS or death, and leads to improvements in surrogate markers of disease, i.e. CD4-positive T-lymphocyte counts and plasma viral load. Single- and dual-agent regimens are associated with high rates of disease progression and viral resistance to drugs; therefore, three or more drugs are now used concurrently to treat HIV infection. Efforts to induce virus suppression with three antivirals and then maintain the effect with only two drugs have also yielded unacceptably high relapse rates. Generally, drug combinations are chosen from two or more of the currently available classes.

Nucleoside reverse transcriptase inhibitors

Zidovudine (ZDV, AZT), a thymidine analog, is the prototypic nucleoside reverse transcriptase inhibitor (NRTI). It was the first antiviral agent approved for the treatment of HIV infection. It inhibits HIV-1, HIV-2, human T-cell leukemia/lymphoma virus-1, and other mammalian retroviruses.

NRTIs (Table 6.6) share the following characteristics:

- They require intracellular conversion by cellular enzymes to their corresponding triphosphate nucleotides for activation.
- All lose antiretroviral activity through mutations in viral reverse transcriptase resulting in decreased affinity of the enzyme for NRTI. The rate of emergence of resistance and its degree vary with drug type.
- Selectivity is attributable to the greater affinity of NRTI-triphosphate for reverse transcriptase than for host cell DNA polymerases.

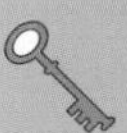

Characteristics of nucleoside reverse transcriptase inhibitors (NRTIs) of HIV-1 replication

- Activated intracellularly by phosphorylation with cellular kinases
- Triphosphate forms competitively inhibit reverse transcriptase
- Incorporation into HIV-1 DNA causes chain termination
- Resistant strains emerge with variable facility

MECHANISM OF ACTION The retrovirus HIV must initially create a proviral DNA copy of its RNA genome in order to replicate. An HIV-specific enzyme, reverse transcriptase (RT), draws from the infected cell's pool of deoxynucleosides (thymidine, guanosine, adenosine, cytidine) for synthesis of the complementary DNA chain. Since NRTIs are dideoxynucleoside analogs and lack a second hydroxyl group, essential for the addition of subsequent bases to the growing DNA strand, their incorporation by RT terminates elongation of DNA chains. They also have a competitive, inhibitory effect on RT itself.

PHARMACOKINETICS The NRTIs are well absorbed orally, although didanosine (ddI) is acid-labile, and must be administered in buffer-containing tablets. The divalent cations in buffer can interfere with the absorption of other medications. However, a newer, enteric-coated preparation of didanosine should not carry the same risk of drug interaction, but might require an empty stomach for absorption.

Elimination of NRTIs from the plasma is rapid, and serum half-lifes vary from 1 hour for stavudine (d4T) to 3 or 4 hours for lamivudine (3TC). However, depletion of intracellular NRTI nucleotides is slower, making extended dosing intervals possible. All NRTIs except abacavir are excreted in urine. Urinary excretion of zidovudine occurs after glucouronidation in the liver. Other NRTIs are excreted unchanged. Dose reductions in renal failure range from 50% for zidovudine, stavudine, and zalcitabine (ddC), to 80–90% for lamivudine and didanosine. NRTI metabolism does not depend on cytochrome P-450s (CYPs). NRTIs are not highly protein bound, and they penetrate the CNS in significant concentrations.

CLINICAL USES In multidrug regimens for HIV, zidovudine can delay disease progression and prolong survival. It has been used successfully in the treatment of HIV-associated dementia. When administered to pregnant women from the second trimester onward, and to their infants for the first 6 weeks postpartum, zidovudine reduces the risk of mother-to-infant HIV transmission by about two-thirds, i.e. from 25% to 8%.

ADVERSE EFFECTS As a class, NRTIs have been rarely associated with hepatic steatosis (fatty liver) and lactic acidosis. These, and other NRTI adverse effects such as myopathy (AZT), neuropathy (d4T, ddC) and pancreatitis (ddI), are thought to arise from inhibition of mitochondrial DNA polymerases and subsequent mitochondrial dysfunction.

Abacavir has been associated with an idiosyncratic 'hypersensitivity reaction.' It most often occurs within the first 6 weeks of treatment (>85%), and includes: fever, rash, sore throat; cough or other respiratory symptoms; nausea, vomiting, or other gastrointestinal symptoms. The drug must be stopped permanently since re-

PI share the following characteristics:

- They bind competitively to the aspartic proteases of HIV-1 and HIV-2, preventing the post-translational breakdown of viral polyprotein into the components required for viral assembly and budding.
- They do not require intracellular activation.
- Marked resistance develops because of an accumulation of mutations with amino acid substitutions at active enzymatic sites and other regions. Viruses with mutated proteases seem less fit than wild-type viruses.

Certain PIs (saquinavir, ritonavir, indinavir, and amprenavir) are peptidomimetic, and structurally fit the cleavage sites of the HIV polyproteins. Others (nelfinavir) are nonpeptidomimetic. Amprenavir is a sulfonamide compound.

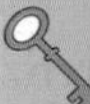

Characteristics of protease inhibitors that inhibit HIV-1 replication

- **Interfere with post-translational processing of HIV-1 precursor proteins**
- **Combination treatment with nucleoside reverse transcriptase inhibitors produces additive antiviral effects**
- **Combination therapy with nucleoside reverse transcriptase inhibitors reduces the occurrence of resistance**
- **Well tolerated**

PHARMACOKINETICS The oral absorption of ritonavir, indinavir, nelfinavir and amprenavir is between 60% and 80%. That of saquinavir is approximately 10%. Cerebrospinal fluid (CSF) penetration is limited, although indinavir may achieve clinically significant concentrations in the CNS.

All PIs are metabolized via CYPs, and important drug interactions occur (Table 6.8).

CLINICAL USES PIs, in combination with NRTIs (and with NNRTIs) are effective inhibitors of HIV-1 and HIV-2 replication. Their use prolongs survival and allow fewer hospitalizations for HIV-infected individuals. In clinical trials, rates of complete suppression of viremia of 80% or better have been achieved for up to 3 years. In clinical practice, results are less impressive, with 1-year rates of the order of 50–60%, possibly because of problems of drug toxicity and adherence to therapy.

ADVERSE EFFECTS The principal side effects of PIs are gastrointestinal, with nausea affecting 3–30% of patients. It is highest for ritonavir and amprenavir. Diarrhea of varying severity occurs in 5–30% of cases and is highest for ritonavir and nelfinavir. Other drug-specific adverse effects are listed in Table 6.9.

Increasingly, a syndrome of lipodystrophy – comprising peripheral fat wasting, central fat accumulation, hyperlipidemias and insulin resistance, in various combinations and proportions – is observed with long-term PI use. Elements of this syndrome can appear in the absence of PI use, and an NRTI-mediated mitochondrial toxicity has been suggested as contributing to the syndrome.

Antiretroviral fusion inhibitor

The fusion inhibitor enfuviritide (T20) was recently introduced for the treatment of HIV. This drug prevents the fusion of the HIV virus with the host cell outer membrane, thereby preventing infection of host cells.

PRINCIPLES OF ANTI-HIV THERAPY

The HIV replication cycle and the various levels that drugs can interfere with this process are shown in Figure 6.6. Approved drugs for the treatment of HIV currently target three steps in this replication process, namely fusion, reverse transcription and proteolytic maturation. Standard anti-HIV therapy now involves so called 'triple therapy,' commonly referred to as 'highly active antiretroviral therapy' (HAART). Such therapy involves the combination of a protease inhibitor or NNRTI with two NRTIs. HAART is, however, often not well tolerated, is expensive and can lead to multidrug resistance if not used correctly. Furthermore, patients do not comply readily with the discipline required to take 'triple therapy.' There is therefore ongoing research looking for novel anti-HIV drugs such as those targeting the third HIV enzyme integrase (see Fig. 6.6). Several integrase inhibitors are in early clinical development.

Table 6.8 Examples of drugs metabolized by CYP enzymes with clinically important adverse interactions when administered concomitantly with antiretroviral protease inhibitor drugs, and alternative drugs

Drug class	Representative drugs	Alternative drugs
Antiarrhythmics*	Amiodarone, propafenone, quinidine, flecainide	(Monitor effects closely)
Antihyperlipidemics	Lovastatin, simvastatin	Atorvastatin, pravastatin
Psychoactive agents*	Bupropion, clozapine, pimozide	SSRIs, haloperidol, respiridone
Benzodiazepines	Midazolam, triazolam, diazepam	Lorazepam, oxazepam
Ergot derivatives	Ergotamine, dihydroergotamine	(Other migraine drugs)

* Principal risk is with concurrent ritonavir use.

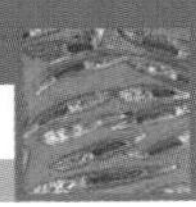

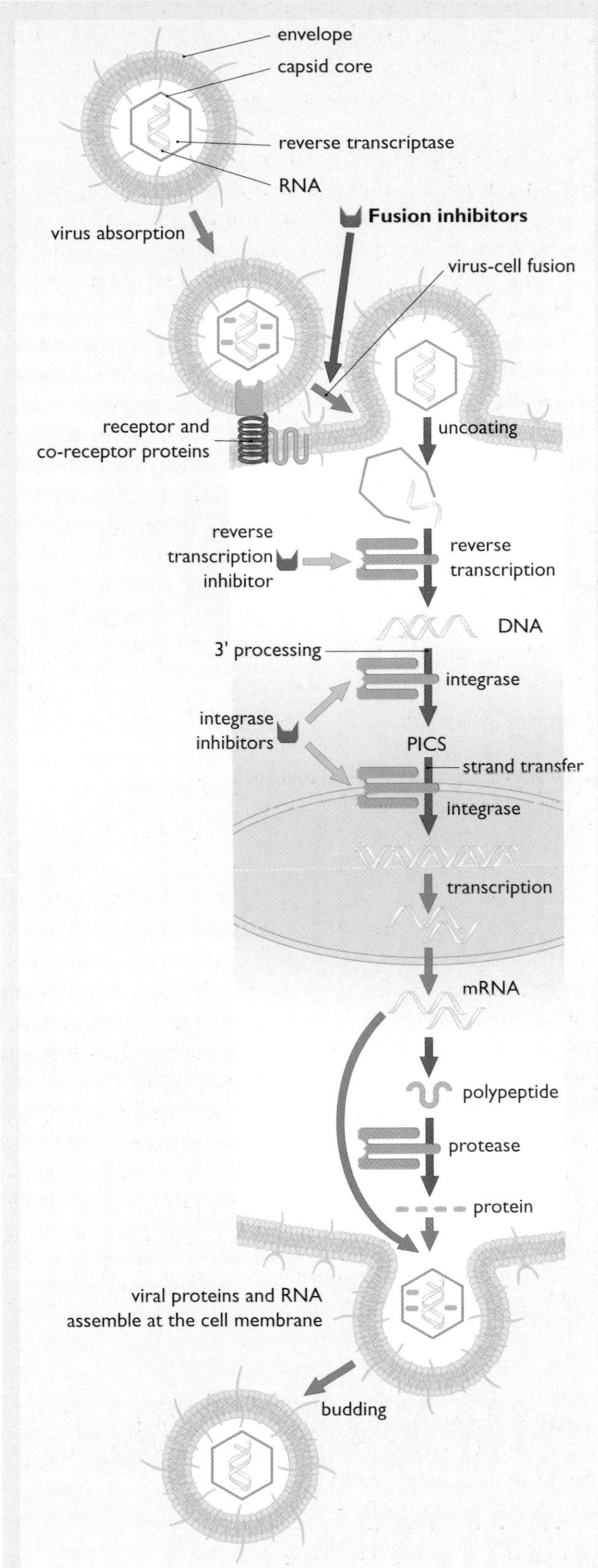

Fig. 6.6 The HIV replication cycle and drug targets. Current antiviral drugs target attachment/fusion of HIV to the host cell outer membrane and the viral enzymes reverse transcriptase or protease. Integrase, the third viral enzyme, catalyzes two steps in the viral replication cycle. First, integrase catalyzes the processing of the 3′-ends of the viral cDNA (3′-processing step); integrase then remains bound in a complex with the viral cDNA ends in the pre-integration complexes (PICs). Following nuclear translocation of the PICs, integrase catalyzes the insertion (strand-transfer-step) of the viral cDNA ends into the host chromosome. (Adapted from Pommier Y, Johnson AA, Marchand C. Integrase inhibitors to treat HIV/AIDS. *Nat Review Drug Discovery* 2004; **4**: 236–248.)

CYTOCHROME P-450 (CYP) INTERACTIONS

All currently available antiretroviral protease inhibitors and NNRTIs are metabolized (oxidized) by the cytochrome-P-450 system (see Ch. 4). These drugs serve both as substrates for this metabolic pathway and as CYP inducers or inhibitors.

The HIV-1 protease inhibitors all function as CYP inhibitors, and the rank order of potency is: ritonavir (most potent), indinavir, lopinavir, nelfinavir, amprenavir, saquinavir. Amongst the NNRTIs, delavirdine is a CYP inhibitor, nevirapine is a CYP inducer and efavirenz has mixed effects. Certain drugs should not therefore be administered concurrently with the protease inhibitors (or other CYP inhibitors) because of the risk of toxic adverse effects related to drug accumulation (Table 6.9). Concurrent use of potent CYP inducers (e.g. rifampin, certain anticonvulsants, dexamethasone) with PIs and NNRTIs should be avoided.

The potent CYP-inhibitory effects of ritonavir have been used therapeutically to block the metabolism of other protease inhibitors, thereby improving PI pharmacokinetics. For example, ritonavir 100 mg administered with indinavir 800 mg, twice daily, increases trough levels fourfold as well as the area under the curve of the latter drug; this reduces the number of pills needed and makes food restrictions unnecessary. Similar effects apply to the proprietary fixed-drug combination of lopinavir–ritonavir. Other pharmacokinetically enhanced combinations which have either proven effective or are currently being evaluated include: saquinavir 400 mg–ritonavir 400 mg b.i.d., indinavir 800 mg–ritonavir 200 mg b.i.d., and amprenavir 600 mg–ritonavir 100 mg b.i.d.

FURTHER READING

Balfour HH. Antiviral drugs. *N Engl J Med* 1999; **340**: 1255–1268.

DeClercq E. Antivirals and antiviral strategies. *Net Rev Microbiol* 2004; **2**: 704–718.

Max B, Sherer R. Management of the adverse effects of antiretroviral therapy and medication adherence. *Clin Infect Dis* 2000; **30**: S96–116. [Review of individual antiretroviral agents and their toxicities.]

Pommier Y, Johnson AA, Marchand C. Integrase inhibitors to treat HIV/AIDS. *Nat Rev Drug Discovery* 2004; **4**: 236–248.

Table 6.9 Protease inhibitor (PI) drugs for the treatment of HIV infection

	Saquinavir	Ritonavir	Indinavir	Nelfinavir	Amprenavir	Lopinavir–ritonavir	Fosamprenavir	Atazanavir
Recommended dose (mg)	SGC 1200 mg t.i.d. HGC*	600 mg b.i.d.	800 mg t.i.d.	750 mg t.i.d. or 1250 mg b.i.d.	1200 mg b.i.d.	400 mg lopinavir/ 100 mg ritonavir b.i.d.		
Oral bioavailability (%)	HGC 4 SGC: not available	Not available	65	20–80	83	Approx. 80	Not available	60%
Effect of food	Increases absorption	Increases absorption	Decreases absorption substantially	Increases absorption	Avoid high-fat, otherwise no effect	Increases absorption (decreases 30–40% if fasting)	No effect	Administer with food only
Serum half-life, hours	1–2	3–5	1.5–2	3.5–5	3.3	5–6	7.7	6.5
Elimination	Hepatic: cytochrome P-450	Hepatic: cytochrome P-450	Hepatic: cytochrome P-450	Hepatic: cytochrome P-450	Hepatic: cytochrome P-450	Hepatic: cytochrome P-450	?	?
Incidence of adverse effects (%)	Elevated hepatic transaminases (2–6)	Circumoral paresthesias (3–6) Taste perversion (5–15) Hypertriglyceridemia (2–8) Elevated hepatic transaminases (5–6)	Nephrolithiasis (3–5) Increased indirect bilirubin (10) Hair, skin, nail changes	(Class effects)	Rash (18 total, 6 severe)	(Class effects)	Hyperglycemia Thirst Frequent urination	Hyperglycemia Thirst Frequent urination

* HGC, hard-gel capsule: use only if combined with cytochrome P-450 inhibitor (e.g. ritonavir); NS, not significant; SGC, soft-gel capsule.

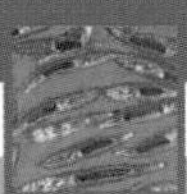

FURTHER READING

Alberti A, Boccato S, Vario A, Benvegnu L. Therapy of acute hepatitis. *Hepatology* 2002; **36**: 195–200.

De Clerq E. Recent highlights in the development of new antiviral drugs. *Curr Opin Microbio* 2005; **5**: 552–560. [Describes recent advances in antiviral drug discoveries.]

Kimberlin D, Rouse D. Clinical practice: Genital herpes. *New Engl J Med* 2004; **350**: 1970–1977 [The how and why of the antiviral treatment of genital herpes.]

Kuritzkes DR. Preventing and managing antiretroviral drug resistance. *AIDS Patient Care* 2004; **18**: 259–273 [A discussion of the techniques used to deal with resistance to antiviral drugs in AIDs patients.]

WEBSITES

http://www.aidsmap.com/about/bhiva/bhivagol.asp BHIVA Writing Committee on behalf of the BHIVA Executive Committee. British HIV Association (BHIVA) guidelines for the treatment of HIV-infected adults with antiretroviral therapy. [British guidelines for the treatment of HIV infection.]

http://www.medscape.com/medscape/HIV/ClinicalMgmt/CM.drug/public/toc-CM.drug.html C, Piscitelli SC. Managing drug–drug interactions in HIV disease. [Review of drug metabolism, including mixed-function oxidases.]

http://hivatis.org/trtgd/ns.html Adult Panel on Clinical Practices for Treatment of HIV Infection (Department of Health and Human Services (DHHS) and the Henry J. Kaiser Family Foundation). Guidelines for the use of antiretroviral agents in HIV-infected adults and adolescents. [The North American guidelines for the treatment of HIV infection.]

http://www/aidsinfo.nih.go/guidelines [Guidelines for the use of antiretroviral drugs for HIV.]

http://www.nlm.nih.gov/medlineplus/viralinfections.html [Provides general information regarding viruses and antiviral drugs.]

http://www.cdc.gov/ncidod/guidelines/guidelines_topic_viral.htm [Provides specific information including treatment options regarding many common viral infections.]

PART 3

DRUGS AND BACTERIA

Bacterial infections are very common and still a significant cause of morbidity and mortality

Bacterial diarrhea is a leading cause of infant mortality worldwide, and tuberculosis a frequent cause of death due to infection. Antibacterial drugs are among the most important therapeutic discoveries of the 20th century and have dramatically changed the course of many bacterial diseases by reducing mortality (e.g. of bacterial meningitis and bacterial endocarditis) and morbidity. On the other hand, antibiotics are now among the most over-prescribed drugs, partly because many of them have excellent safety profiles, which has encouraged inappropriate prescribing, e.g. antibiotics are often wrongly prescribed for viral infections. In addition, some older antibiotics have been used as growth promoters in food animals from which they can enter the human food chain at subtherapeutic doses. As a result, overuse of antibiotics is an important contributor to the growing global problem of antibiotic resistance, particularly the alarming rise is methicillin-resistant staphylococcal infections in both hospitals and the wider community.

Antibacterial drugs can be classified as antibiotics, chemotherapeutic or synthetic drugs or semisynthetic drugs, depending on whether they are:

- Byproducts of microorganisms (antibiotics).
- Entirely synthesized in the laboratory (chemotherapeutic or synthetic drugs).
- A hybrid of the two (semisynthetic drugs).

In practice, the term antibiotic has become synonymous with antibacterial drug, and this more liberal definition of antibiotic is used throughout.

MECHANISM OF ACTION OF ANTIBIOTICS

Ideally, antibiotics block vital functions of bacteria without affecting those of the host cells

Antibiotics are said to possess selective toxicity in that they can disrupt vital functions of bacteria while having no or minimal effects on the cells of the host they have infected. As an example of how selective toxicity occurs, bacteria possess specialized and structured cell walls, whereas mammalian cells have simple cell membranes. Thus, drugs that interfere with the synthesis or integrity of bacterial cell walls are toxic to bacteria, but harmless to the host. Similarly, the prokaryotic bacterial ribosome (70S) is sufficiently different from the eukaryotic ribosome (80S) that the bacterial ribosome provides a good target for antibacterial drugs. Figure 6.7 shows the sites of action of the major classes of antibiotics. As a result of their selective toxicity, many antibiotics have a high therapeutic index (i.e. ratio of toxic to therapeutic dose). Of course, both the innate immune response and the specific immunologic mechanisms aid the clearance of bacterial infections, with antibiotics being prescribed to accelerate this process and prevent overwhelming infections. The use of antibiotics is particularly important in combating infections in patients who are immunocompromised, such as patients with HIV infections or who are neutropenic.

Whether an antibiotic inhibits growth or kills bacteria depends on its concentration

The activity of a given antibiotic against a particular bacterium can be readily measured in the laboratory. By exposing a standard inoculum of a bacterium to a range of concentrations of an antibiotic, the lowest concentration of the drug that inhibits bacterial growth can be determined. This is called the minimum inhibitory concentration (MIC). If the concentration is increased above the MIC, a concentration is eventually reached that will 'kill' the bacterium ('kill' is defined as a 1000-fold ($\log_{10}3.0$) or 99.9% reduction in the number of bacteria in the inoculum). The lowest concentration of antibiotic required to kill the bacterium is defined as the minimum bactericidal concentration (MBC). Generally, the MBC is 2–8 times that of the MIC. The antibiotics in which clinically

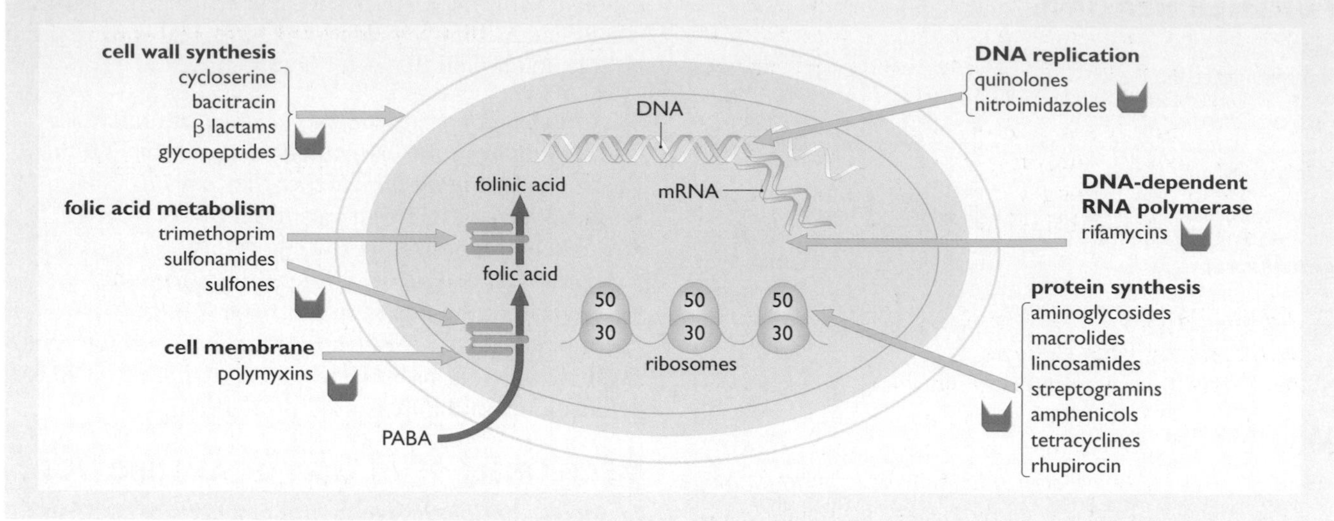

Fig. 6.7 Sites of action of different types of antibiotic agent. (PABA, para-aminobenzoic acid.)

achievable blood concentrations regularly exceed the MBC for common pathogens are classified as bactericidal antibiotics. The antibiotics whose blood concentrations readily exceed the MIC but do not usually exceed the MBC are classified as bacteriostatic antibiotics. However, categorizing antibiotics as predominantly bacteriostatic or bactericidal is an imperfect process since there is a unique relationship between each bacterium and each antibiotic. For instance, while penicillin, which is classically considered a bactericidal antibiotic, is nearly always bactericidal against streptococci it is only bacteriostatic against enterococci. Similarly, chloramphenicol is bacteriostatic against most Enterobacteriaceae, but is bactericidal against most strains of *Haemophilus influenzae*.

Antibiotics may act synergistically, antagonistically, or indifferently

Occasionally, two or more antibiotics are used in combination to treat the same pathogen. In the laboratory it is possible to categorize the antibacterial relationship between two (or more) antibiotics against a particular bacterium as being synergistic, antagonistic, or indifferent. This depends on the effect of the drug combination on the growth of the bacterium compared with that of each drug alone (Fig. 6.8):

- If the combination of drugs markedly increases the antibacterial effect above that of the most active drug, the combination is synergistic, i.e. the effect is greater than additive.
- If the combination results in less inhibition of bacterial growth than the most active drug alone, the combination is antagonistic.
- If the combination is neither synergistic nor antagonistic, it is indifferent.

In practice, most combinations are indifferent. However, important synergistic and antagonistic combinations have been demonstrated clinically.

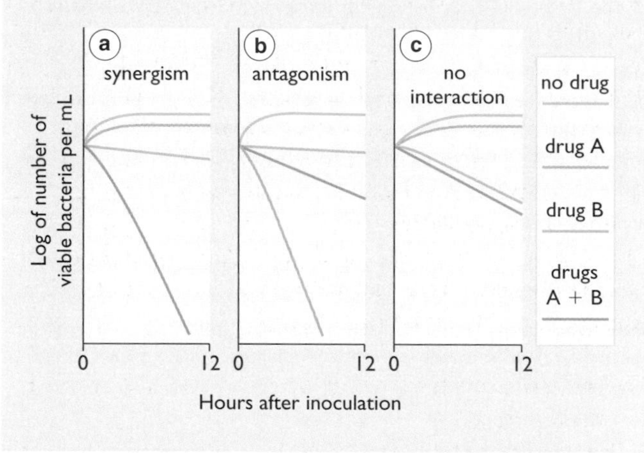

Fig. 6.8 Bacterial growth curves showing synergism, antagonism, and indifference of two antibiotics, A and B, against three different organisms. In (a) the combination is synergistic because it exerts a significantly greater antibacterial effect than the more active drug (B) alone. In (b) the addition of drug B significantly reduces the antibacterial effect of drug A and, therefore, the combination is antagonistic. In (c) the antibacterial activity of the combination is essentially the same as that of the more active drug (B), and the combination is therefore classified as indifferent.

- The success rate of treating enterococcal endocarditis with a combination of penicillin plus aminoglycoside is significantly greater than that using penicillin alone, highlighting the relevance of synergy.
- The combination of penicillin and tetracycline to treat bacterial meningitis is associated with a significantly higher mortality than when penicillin is used alone, an example of antagonism.

Killing by bactericidal drugs can be concentration- or time-dependent

Killing of bacteria by some bactericidal drugs (e.g. aminoglycosides and fluoroquinolones) is concentration-

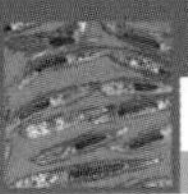

dependent, whereas that by others (e.g. β lactams and glycopeptides) is time-dependent. Concentration-dependent killing implies a greater bactericidal activity with higher concentrations of antibiotic. With time-dependent killing, there is little or no enhancement of bactericidal activity with drug concentrations above the MBC; rather, the killing depends on maintaining the concentration of antibiotic above the MBC for as long as possible.

Normal bacterial replication is often delayed after an antibiotic has been stopped

When bacteria are exposed to an antibiotic at concentrations above the MIC, and the antibiotic is then removed from the medium, bacterial replication often does not resume normally (as if no antibiotic were present) for a variable period of time (usually hours) after removal of the antibiotic. This phenomenon is called the post-antibiotic effect (PAE). The PAE does not occur with all bacterium–drug combinations, but when it does, it is often concentration-dependent. In other words, the higher the concentration of antibiotic to which the bacterium has been exposed, the longer the duration of the PAE. Aminoglycosides and fluoroquinolones consistently demonstrate a PAE against Gram-negative bacteria, whereas β lactams, with the exception of carbapenems, do not. However, β lactams demonstrate a modest PAE against Gram-positive bacteria. Figures 6.9 and 6.10 illustrate concentration- and time-dependent killing of Gram-negative bacteria with PAE occurring in the former, but not the latter.

The PAE provides a rationale for the pulse dosing of antibiotics

Pulse dosing refers to the administration of relatively large doses of antibiotic to produce peak blood concentrations far higher than the MIC or MBC for the causative organism at dosing intervals longer than several serum half-lifes of the drug. For example, crystalline penicillin G has a serum half-life of about 30 minutes and yet it is usually administered every 6 hours (i.e. every 12 half-lifes). This dosing schedule is markedly different from that used with most other drugs, which are generally given no less frequently than every serum half-life. There are several reasons why pulse dosing is effective with antibiotics:

- The therapeutic index of most antibiotics is high and it is often possible to achieve high peak serum concentrations without incurring significant toxicity.
- Some antibiotics demonstrate concentration-dependent killing and therefore it is desirable, and more efficacious, to achieve high peak serum concentrations.
- It is often possible to maintain the serum antibiotic concentration above the MIC of the bacterium for the entire dosing interval despite dosing relatively infrequently with respect to serum half-life (Fig. 6.11).
- Even if the serum antibiotic concentration does fall below the MIC for part of the time between doses, the PAE may prevent bacterial multiplication during this period when serum concentrations fall below the MIC before the next dose (Fig. 6.12).
- Except in highly immunocompromised patients, antibiotics are not the only defense against bacterial infection. The host's immune system plays an active role in combating infection. Indeed, before the discovery of antibiotics many patients survived

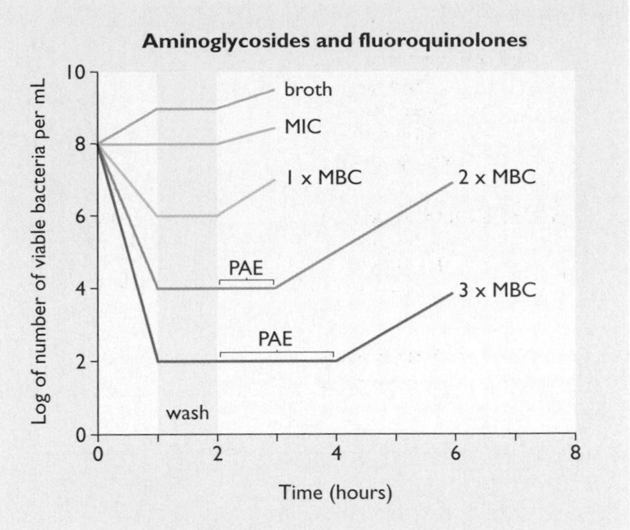

Fig. 6.9 Concentration-dependent bactericidal action and the postantibiotic effect (PAE). Time–kill study in broth containing various concentrations of an antimicrobial drug that shows concentration-dependent bactericidal action. A PAE on the residual organisms is present after washing these organisms and resuspending them in antibiotic-free broth. (MBC, minimum bactericidal concentration; MIC, minimum inhibitory concentration.)

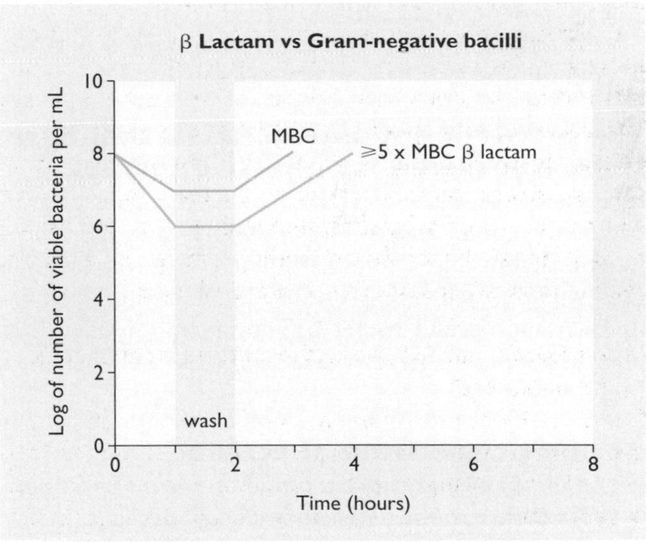

Fig. 6.10 Time-dependent bactericidal action. Time–kill study in broth containing various concentrations of a β lactam that shows time-dependent bactericidal action against a Gram-negative bacillus. There is no postantibiotic effect (PAE) on the residual organisms after washing and resuspending in antibiotic-free broth. (MBC, minimum bactericidal concentration.)

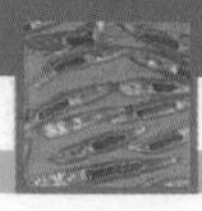

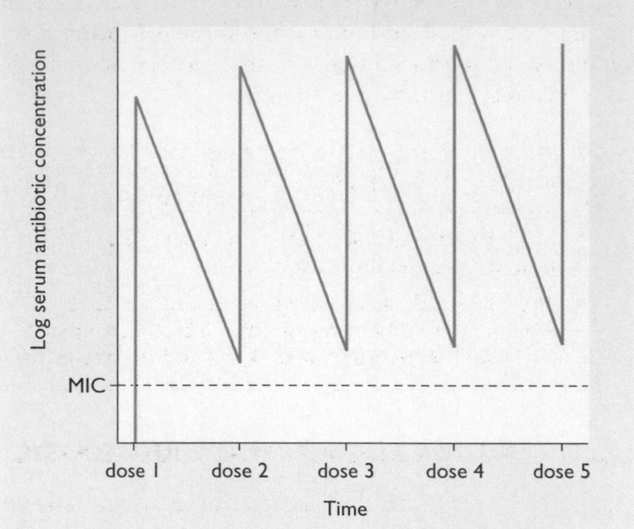

Fig. 6.11 Pulse dosing of an antibiotic. In this example, the antibiotic is very active against the bacteria and the serum antibiotic concentration remains above the minimum inhibitory concentration (MIC) at all times, despite infrequent dosing. Maintaining the serum antibiotic concentration above the MIC at all times is desirable if there is no postantibiotic effect (PAE).

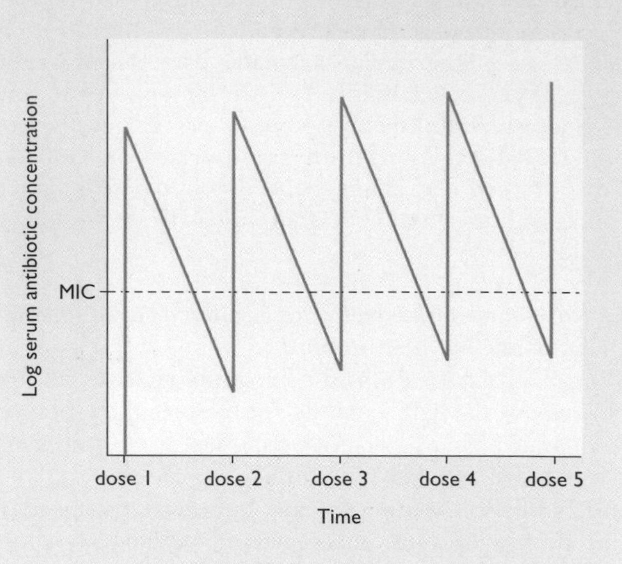

Fig. 6.12 Pulse dosing of an antibiotic. In this example, the peak serum antibiotic concentration following each dose is well above the minimum inhibitory concentration (MIC), but the serum antibiotic concentration falls below the MIC for the latter part of each dosing interval. If there is a postantibiotic effect (PAE), there is no harm in allowing the serum antibiotic concentration to fall below the MIC for a small proportion of the dosing interval.

bacterial infections, although their recovery was generally slower and associated with more complications.

The properties of antibacterials that have to be considered for effective therapy

The choice of antibiotic relates to mechanisms of antibacterial action, effectiveness, toxicity and pharmacokinetic factors. The latter are outlined in various tables in the text after each class of antibiotics. Each antibiotic has its own appropriate routes of administration as well as pharmacokinetic characteristics, and these help define its usefulness.

Antibiotic spectrum of activity

■ ***An antibiotic may have a broad or narrow spectrum of activity against different bacterial species***

Antibiotics that are active against many bacterial species are referred to as broad-spectrum antibiotics, whereas those that are active against only a few species are termed narrow-spectrum antibiotics. However, this distinction is somewhat arbitrary.

Antibiotic resistance

■ ***Antibiotic resistance is classified as either innate or acquired***

Innate bacterial resistance to an antibiotic refers to an intrinsic resistance based on the mechanism of action or other characteristics of the antibiotic. For example, anaerobic bacteria lack the oxygen-dependent transport mechanism that is required for transportation of aminoglycosides into the bacterial cell. Hence, anaerobes are innately resistant to aminoglycosides.

On the other hand, acquired resistance refers to the acquisition of a gene that confers resistance by a bacterium that was not innately resistant. All current antibiotics demonstrate acquired resistance in at least some bacterial species.

The major stimulus for the development of acquired antibiotic resistance is the use of antibiotics themselves. The use of an antibiotic exerts selective evolutionary pressure on bacteria to develop resistance to antibiotics so as to ensure their survival. However, the likelihood of developing specific resistance is dependent upon both the drug and the bacterium involved. In some instances, a single mutation in the bacterial genome is sufficient to result in clinically significant resistance. In others, multiple mutations are needed to produce a phenotypic resistance.

The three main biochemical mechanisms of acquired resistance are as follows:

- Reduced bacterial permeability to an antibiotic(s) resulting from changes in the cell membrane of Gram-negative bacteria (see below).
- The production of bacterial enzymes that change the molecular structure of the antibiotic. These enzymes may be hydrolytic (e.g. β lactamases) or nonhydrolytic (e.g. aminoglycoside-modifying enzymes).
- Alteration in the target for the antibiotic whereby a single mutation in the gene coding for the antibiotic binding site can be sufficient to produce clinically significant drug resistance (e.g. in methicillin-resistant staphylococci).

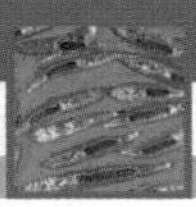

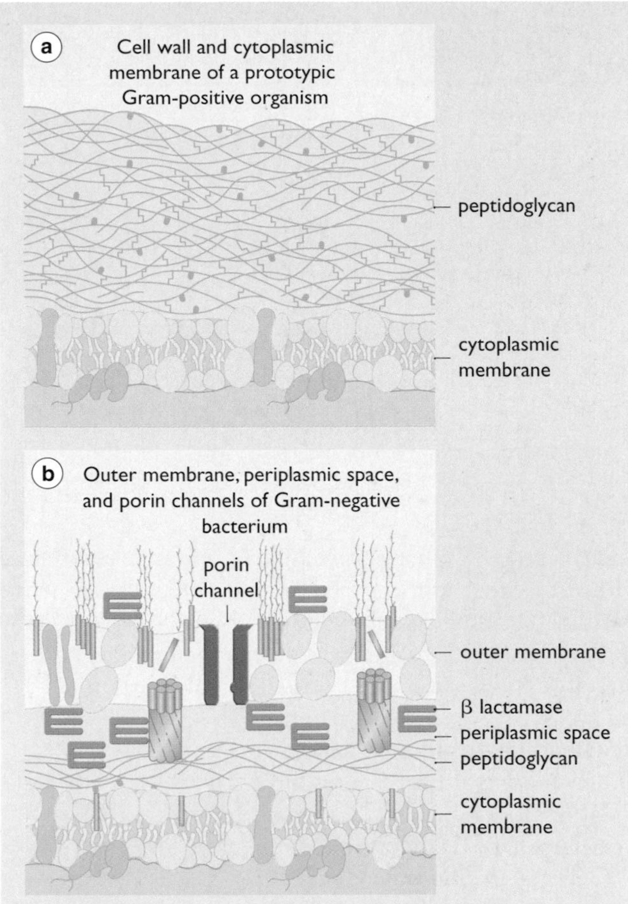

Fig. 6.13 Structure of the bacterial cell wall and membrane. (a) Gram-positive bacterium. (b) Gram negative bacterium. Note that only Gram-negative bacteria possess an outer membrane, which provides an additional obstacle to the entry of antibacterial drugs.

Reduced bacterial permeability

■ ***There are significant cell wall and cell membrane structural differences between Gram-positive and Gram-negative bacteria***

Gram-positive bacteria contain many layers of peptidoglycan beneath which lies the cell membrane. These layers do not present an appreciable barrier to the entry of antibiotics (Fig. 6.13). In contrast, Gram-negative bacteria possess an outer cell membrane that contains copious amounts of lipopolysaccharide, as well as a true cytoplasmic inner membrane. This inner membrane is covered by fewer layers of peptidoglycan than are present in Gram-positive bacteria and is separated from the outer membrane by a periplasmic space. The outer membrane consists of a phospholipid bilayer with aqueous channels formed by outer membrane proteins termed porins. Gram-negative bacteria therefore have a significant barrier to the entry of drugs. Drugs that are lipophilic, or aqueous drugs of low molecular weight, can enter via the porin channels. Changes in the content or composition of porin proteins or in the lipopolysaccharides of the outer membrane can produce antibiotic resistance due to reduced permeability to antibiotics. Mutations leading to alterations in the bacterial cell membrane that lead to decreased permeability to one antibiotic will often result in decreased permeability to other antibiotics and, in consequence, multidrug resistance.

Antibiotic resistance

- **Inappropriate antibiotic use is the major factor leading to antibiotic resistance**
- **The three main mechanisms of antibiotic resistance are (1) reduced bacterial permeability, (2) enzymatic alteration of antibiotics and (3) altered target site**

SELECTING THE APPROPRIATE ANTIBIOTIC

Antibiotics can be used either prophylactically or therapeutically. In either case, the same basic principles apply. Bacterial, host and drug factors must all be considered (Fig. 6.14 and Table 6.10).

Bacterial factors

Antibacterial therapy is effective only for bacterial infections. It is therefore important to restrict the use of antibiotics to those situations where bacterial infection is either known to be present, or is there is a high probability of a bacterial infection. The all-too-common practice of prescribing antibiotics for infections that are probably viral is not only ineffective, but is also costly and increases the emergence of antibiotic resistance.

When making a rational choice of antibiotic it is important to identify the infecting bacterium. If the identity of the infecting organism(s) is not known, as is often the case when antibiotic therapy is started, it is often possible to make an educated and reasonable guess

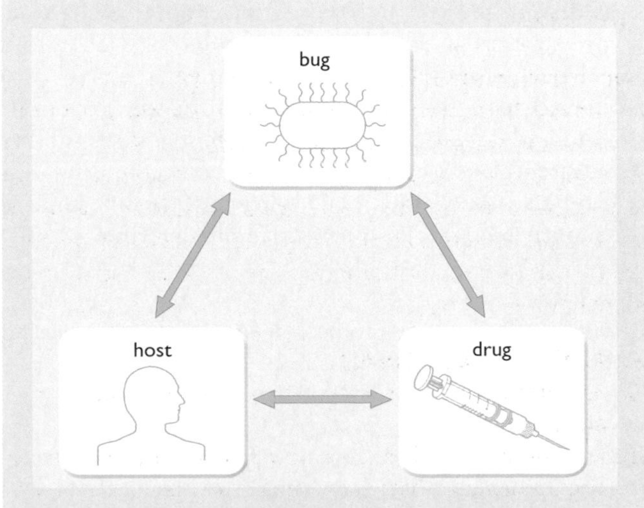

Fig. 6.14 Triangle depicting the classic bidirectional three-way interaction between a microbial pathogen (bug), an antimicrobial agent (drug) and the host, whose immune function is a major determinant of the outcome of an infection.

Table 6.10 The bacterial, host and drug factors that must be considered when selecting an appropriate antibiotic

Bug factors	Host factors	Drug factors
Identity of pathogen(s)[†] Susceptibility of pathogens[†]	Site of infection Allergies Renal function Hepatic function Neutropenia Digestive tract function Other underlying diseases Concomitant medication Pregnancy Desired route of administration	Activity against pathogen(s)[†] Ability to reach the site of infection Potential for drug interactions Available routes of administration Dosing frequency (for outpatients) Taste (for liquid formulations) Stability at different temperatures (for liquid formulations) Cost

[†]Often not known at the start of therapy.

about the likely pathogen(s). Examples of where this is possible include:

- Urinary tract infection in sexually active premenopausal women is due to *Escherichia coli* in approximately 85% of cases.
- Cellulitis of an arm or leg is usually due to either *Streptococcus pyogenes* or *Staphylococcus aureus*.

To make an informed guess about the likely pathogen(s) it is important to know:

- The site of infection.
- Whether the infection is community acquired or nosocomial (hospital acquired).
- Details about the host, including age, underlying illness and/or other predisposing factors.

In certain cases, it is appropriate to start antibiotic therapy without carrying out laboratory studies to identify the pathogen (e.g. in most cases of cellulitis). In cases where the pathogen(s) cannot be reliably predicted, or in patients with severe illness, appropriate specimens should be collected to identify the causative bacteria before starting an antibiotic. A microbiology laboratory can then identify the pathogen(s) and carry out in vitro antibiotic susceptibility testing so that the therapy can be subsequently tailored. Usually, antibiotic susceptibility results require 48–72 hours. Newer disk diffusion and nucleic acid-based tests are improving identification of the nature and antibiotic resistance of bacteria.

Host factors

Many host factors need to be considered before selecting an antibiotic for a given infection.

Site of infection

It is essential that the antibiotic reaches the site of infection at a concentration above the MIC in all cases, and above the MBC in certain infections such as meningitis, endocarditis and osteomyelitis, and in neutropenic patients. Only a few antibiotics are able to enter the central nervous system enough to achieve therapeutic concentrations, i.e. high enough concentrations to treat meningitis or a brain abscess. Urinary tract infections must be treated with drugs that are excreted by the kidney in an active form so that they can act within the urinary tract. Many antibiotics have difficulty penetrating the prostate and are therefore ineffective in chronic bacterial prostatitis.

Other important host factors

Other important host factors include:

- Drug allergies, since certain antibiotics (e.g. β lactams) are relatively allergenic, thus limiting their use in allergic patients.
- Renal and hepatic function, since antibiotics are cleared from the body by either the kidney or the liver.
- Concomitant medications, since some antibiotics are involved in drug interactions.
- Age, since certain antibiotics are contraindicated in neonates (sulfonamides, ceftriaxone), children (tetracyclines and fluoroquinolones) or pregnant women.

A decision must be made about the route of administration

In general, the oral route is preferred. Parenteral therapy is necessary if the digestive tract is nonfunctional, the patient has hypotension, therapeutic drug concentrations are required immediately (e.g. in life-threatening infections), or oral drugs are not absorbed in adequate amounts to achieve therapeutic concentrations at the site of infection. The topical route is appropriate for selected local infections (e.g. bacterial conjunctivitis).

Host factors influencing the choice of an antibiotic

- Site and type of infection
- Renal and hepatic function
- Age
- Drug allergies
- Route of administration

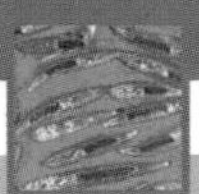

Drug factors

Several important drug factors must be taken into account before selecting an antibiotic

These include:

- Activity against the pathogen(s), though such information may not be known when the treatment needs to be started.
- Ability to reach the site of infection in a therapeutic concentration. This requires knowledge about whether the drug should be bactericidal or bacteriostatic against the known or suspected pathogen, since bactericidal activity is required for certain infections.
- Available routes of administration and whether they are appropriate for the patient.
- Adverse effect profile and whether this could affect underlying illnesses or result in drug interactions.
- Dosing frequency, as compliance of a drug in the outpatient setting is increased with dosing frequencies of two or fewer doses per day.
- When a liquid formulation is required (predominantly in young children), whether the taste is acceptable, as well as whether it is stable at various temperatures. Some antibiotic suspensions require refrigeration to remain stable.
- The cost, recognizing that the true cost of therapy is not merely the cost of the drug itself, but also includes the cost of administration, monitoring, and complications, including treatment failures and the cost of retreatment.

Drug factors influencing the choice of an antibiotic

- Activity against the pathogen
- Ability to reach the site of infection
- Available routes of administration
- Adverse effect profile
- Dosing schedules
- Taste (for oral preparations)
- Cost

MAJOR ANTIBIOTICS

The following sections consider the various major classes of antibiotics as well as other antibiotics that do not easily fit into a particular classification. The classes, in order, are:

- Those inhibiting bacterial cell wall synthesis.
- Those inhibiting bacterial cell membrane function.
- Those that inhibit bacterial DNA synthesis.
- Those that inhibit bacterial RNA synthesis.
- Miscellaneous antibiotics that are not easily classified.
- Those that are used topically.
- Those used to treat myobacterial infections.

In the following, each class is considered as a class and as individuals. The chemical nature of each class is discussed followed by the pharmacology in terms of antibacterial mechanism of action and antibacterial spectrum as well as other pharmacological actions. The therapeutic utility is considered, as are the pharmacokinetic characteristics and the side effects and toxicity.

Antibiotics that inhibit bacterial cell wall synthesis

The unique nature of the bacterial cell wall makes it an obvious target for antibiotics

Unlike other bacteria, mycoplasmas, chlamydiae and rickettsiae lack a cell wall and thus they are innately resistant to antibiotics that inhibit bacterial cell wall synthesis. The two most important classes of antibiotics that inhibit bacterial cell wall synthesis are the β lactams and glycopeptides. Additionally, the topical antibiotic bacitracin and the second-line oral antituberculous drug cycloserine also inhibit bacterial cell wall synthesis.

β Lactams

There are three major classes of β lactams: penicillins, cephalosporins and carbapenems.

β lactam antibiotics possess a four-membered nitrogen-containing β lactam ring with a variety of substituents on the ring. A substituent ring containing sulfur is found in the penicillins, cephalosporins and carbapenems. All interfere with bacterial cell wall synthesis, principally by inhibiting the cross-linkage of the peptide side chains of the bacterial cell wall. The β lactam antibiotics are mainly bactericidal in action and show time-dependent killing. Most are eliminated unchanged by the kidney and so are suitable for treating urinary tract infections. β lactams have a high therapeutic index, with the main adverse event being allergic reactions, most commonly a pruritic erythematous maculopapular rash. Rarely, β lactams cause anaphylaxis. They are considered safe for use during pregnancy.

Four main classes of β lactam antibiotics

- Penicillins
- Cephalosporins
- Carbapenems
- Monobactams

The β lactams are very useful antibiotics whose utility is compromised by the appearance of bacterial resistance. Appropriate use of antibiotics and careful adherence to anti-infection procedures slows the rate of appearance of resistance but will not prevent it entirely because evolutionary pressures are at work and show themselves in the three principal mechanisms of bacterial resistance to β lactams. These are outlined below:

- The most important is enzymatic hydrolysis of the β lactam ring by bacterial β lactamases. This occurs with staphylococci, gonococci, enterobacteriaceae, and *Bacteroides fragilis*. Many isoforms of β lactamases have been found, and these differ in their substrate specificity.
- The second most important mechanism of resistance is alteration of binding sites on penicillin-binding proteins. Alteration in a specific penicillin-binding protein is the principal mechanism of resistance in methicillin-resistant *Staphylococcus aureus* (MRSA), as well as penicillin-resistant pneumococci.
- A third mechanism of resistance is reduced permeability in Gram-negative cell membranes.

PENICILLINS Penicillin was discovered by Alexander Fleming in 1928 as a metabolite of *Penicillium notatum*, from which its name originates. Penicillins consist of a β lactam ring fused to a five-member, sulfur-containing thiazolidine ring. Modification of the side chain at position six of the β lactam ring results in drugs with different antibiotic activity. There are four classes of penicillins: standard penicillins, antistaphylococcal penicillins, aminopenicillins, and antipseudomonal penicillins (Table 6.11).

The commonly used penicillins are benzylpenicillin, known as penicillin G, and phenoxymethylpenicillin, known as penicillin V

Standard penicillins: Penicillin V (Table 6.12) is significantly more stable in the presence of acid than penicillin G and is therefore used for oral administration. Penicillin G is reserved for parenteral therapy.

In addition to crystalline penicillin G, which is used for i.v. therapy, there are two repository forms of penicillin G, which are used exclusively for intramuscular use:

- Aqueous procaine penicillin G (APPG) is a mixture of procaine and penicillin. The procaine delays the absorption of the penicillin, resulting in therapeutic blood concentrations for approximately 12 hours.
- The other repository penicillin is benzathine penicillin G, which contains penicillin G and an ammonium base. Depot injection of benzathine penicillin G produces low but detectable serum concentrations of penicillin G for up to 1 month, and is principally used in the treatment of syphilis, excluding neurosyphilis. It is also used to prevent recurrences of rheumatic fever.

Penicillin remains the drug of choice for streptococcal and meningococcal infections, syphilis, and infections due to *Pasteurella multocida*, although there is some resistance in streptococci, notably *S. pneumoniae*, and meningococci in some parts of the world.

Penicillin is useful in combination with an aminoglycoside in the treatment of infections due to enterococci and *Listeria monocytogenes*. It also remains an important drug in the treatment of dental infections (see Ch. 23), including actinomycosis, since most oral bacteria are susceptible to penicillin.

When penicillin G is given in a large dosage intravenously, cerebrospinal fluid concentrations are adequate for treating neurosyphilis and meningitis due to susceptible strains of *S. pneumoniae* and *Neisseria meningitidis*.

Table 6.11 Classification of penicillins

Standard penicillins	Crystalline penicillin G (i.v.) Penicillin V (p.o.) Aqueous procaine penicillin G (i.m.) Benzathine penicillin G (i.m.)
Antistaphylococcal penicillins	Methicillin (i.v.) Nafcillin (i.v.) Isoxazolyl penicillins (i.v. or p.o.) Oxacillin Cloxacillin Dicloxacillin Floxacillin
Aminopenicillins	Ampicillin (i.v. or p.o.) Amoxicillin (p.o.)
Antipseudomonal penicillins	Carboxypenicillins Carbenicillin (i.v.) Ticarcillin (i.v.) Ureidopenicillins Piperacillin (i.v.) Azlocillin (i.v.) Mezlocillin (i.v.)

The four classes of penicillins are standard penicillins, antistaphylococcal penicillins, aminopenicillins and antipseudomonal penicillins.
i.m., intramuscular; i.v., intravenous; p.o., by mouth.

Antistaphylococcal penicillins are resistant to the actions of staphylococcal β lactamase

Antistaphylococcal penicillins: Most strains of staphylococci mutate to become resistant to standard penicillins as a result of producing penicillinase (β lactamase). Several penicillins have been created that are stable in the presence of the staphylococcal β lactamase. The first of such antistaphylococcal penicillins was methicillin. It is now seldom used because it is associated with a relatively high incidence of allergic interstitial nephritis. Instead, either nafcillin or one of the isoxazolyl penicillins is preferred. The isoxazolyl penicillins are analogs of the parent drug oxacillin in which the substitutions are made by addition of halide (chlorine or fluorine) atoms. The substitution of a chloride for hydrogen gives cloxacillin and dicloxacillin while a fluoride substitution gives flucloxacillin.

Nafcillin and isoxazolyl penicillins are used to treat staphylococcal infections, but are not effective against methicillin-resistant strains. The antimicrobial activity of the four isoxazolyl penicillins is similar, but they differ in their oral absorption, with oxacillin being considerably less well absorbed than the other three. Nafcillin, which

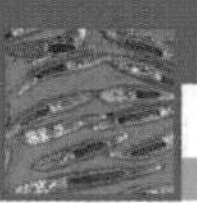

is not an isoxazolyl penicillin, is not well absorbed orally and is reserved for parenteral use (see Table 6.12).

Aminopenicillins have enhanced activity against aerobic Gram-negative bacilli

The addition of an amino group on the penicillin side chain results in aminopenicillins, which have enhanced activity against aerobic Gram-negative bacilli but, unlike standard penicillins, are not metabolized by staphylococcal β lactamase. Aminopenicillins are active against many strains of *E. coli*, *Proteus mirabilis*, and approximately 70% of *H. influenzae* strains. Aminopenicillins are active against some strains of *Salmonella* and *Shigella* species. They are also somewhat more active than penicillin G against enterococci and *L. monocytogenes*, and like penicillin G require the addition of an aminoglycoside to kill bacteria.

The two most important aminopenicillins are ampicillin and amoxicillin. Ampicillin is preferred for i.v. therapy and amoxicillin for oral therapy because of its better oral bioavailability.

Aminopenicillins are used for community-acquired respiratory tract infections because of their activity against *S. pneumoniae* and *H. influenzae*. Amoxicillin can be used to treat uncomplicated urinary tract infections, but trimethoprim–sulfamethoxazole is generally preferred,

Table 6.12 Routes of administration and pharmacokinetics of β lactam antibiotics

Drug	Routes of administration	Oral bioavailability (%)	Clearance route	Serum half-life within normal renal function (hours)	Comments
Standard penicillins					
Penicillin G	i.v., p.o.	20	Renal	0.5	Avoid oral use: acid-labile
Penicillin V	p.o.	65	Renal	0.5	Preferred for oral use
Aminopenicillins					
Ampicillin	i.v., p.o.	40	Renal	1.0	Amoxicillin is preferred for oral use
Amoxicillin	p.o.	80	Renal	1.0	
Antistaphylococcal penicillins					
Nafcillin	i.v., p.o.	35	Hepatic	0.5	Low oral absorption
Oxacillin	i.v., p.o.	30	Mainly renal	0.5	Low oral absorption
Cloxacillin	i.v., p.o.	50	Mainly renal	0.5	Intravenous formulation not in USA
Dicloxacillin	p.o.	60	Mainly renal	0.5	Better oral absorption than oxacillin or nafcillin
Floxacillin	p.o.	70	Mainly renal	0.5	Highest oral absorption
Ureidopenicillins					
Piperacillin	i.v.	Not used	Renal	1.0	Active against *Pseudomonas aeruginosa*
First-generation cephalosporins					
Cefazolin	i.v.	Not used	Renal	1.5	
Cephalexin	p.o.	>95	Renal	1.0	
Second-generation cephalosporins					
Cefuroxime	i.v., p.o.	40	Renal	1.5	Active against *Haemophilus influenzae*
Oral: cefuroxime axetil					
Cefoxitin	i.v.	Not used	Renal	1.0	Active against *Bacteroides fragilis*
Third-generation cephalosporins					
Cefotaxime	i.v.	Not used	Renal	1.5	Has active metabolite
Ceftazidime	i.v.	Not used	Renal	1.5	Active against *Pseudomonas aeruginosa*
Ceftriaxone	i.v.	Not used	Renal and hepatic	7.0	
Carbapenems					
Imipenem–cilastatin	i.v.	Not used	Renal	1.0	Can precipitate seizures
Meropenem	i.v.	Not used	Renal	1.0	Can be used to treat bacterial meningitis

i.v., intravenous; p.o., by mouth.

owing to the latter's greater efficacy. Intravenous ampicillin is often used in conjunction with gentamicin in the treatment of infections due to enterococci and *L. monocytogenes*. Large i.v. doses of ampicillin result in cerebrospinal fluid concentrations adequate to treat meningitis due to susceptible strains of *S. pneumoniae*, *N. meningitidis*, and *H. influenzae*.

Antipseudomonal penicillins are extended-spectrum aminopenicillins

Antipseudomonal penicillins: The antipseudomonal penicillins are best thought of as extended-spectrum aminopenicillins, since they generally possess the same spectrum of activity as aminopenicillins plus additional activity against aerobic Gram-negative bacilli including *Pseudomonas aeruginosa*. They are susceptible to degradation by staphylococcal β lactamase.

There are two subclasses of antipseudomonal penicillins, based on the chemical structure of the side chain: carboxypenicillins (carbenicillin and ticarcillin) and ureidopenicillins (piperacillin, mezlocillin and azlocillin). The ureidopenicillins have generally replaced carboxypenicillins, owing to their broader spectrum of activity and lower sodium content. Piperacillin is also active against anaerobic bacteria, including *B. fragilis*.

The antipseudomonal penicillins are used parenterally in clinical settings where infection due to *P. aeruginosa* has either been confirmed or is suspected.

The routes of administration of penicillins as well as their pharmacokinetic profiles are summarized in Table 6.12 together with the other β lactam antibiotics.

CEPHALOSPORINS Cephalosporins consist of a β lactam ring fused to a six-member sulfur-containing dihydrothiazine ring. Individual cephalosporins are created by side-chain substitutions at position seven of the β lactam ring and position three of the dihydrothiazine ring.

Cephalosporins are traditionally classified as being first-, second-, and third-generation drugs and these differ in their spectrum of action against aerobic Gram-negative bacilli. Activity increases from first to third generation (Table 6.13). However, the antistaphylococcal activity decreases from first to third generation, although there is no loss in antistreptococcal activity. Almost no cephalosporins are degraded by staphylococcal β lactamase and all have activity against aerobic Gram-negative bacilli superior to that of aminopenicillins. Unlike penicillins, cephalosporins are not active against either enterococci or *L. monocytogenes* but, like antistaphylococcal penicillins, they are not active against methicillin-resistant staphylococci.

Although cephalosporins are structurally related to penicillins, there is only approximately 10% cross-allergenicity between the two families of drugs. Accordingly, cephalosporins can often be safely used in individuals with penicillin allergy. In general, cephalosporins should be avoided in patients who have shown IgE-mediated penicillin allergy, but can usually be safely used in patients with non-IgE-mediated adverse reaction to penicillin such as a maculopapular rash.

Table 6.13 Classification of cephalosporins

First generation	Cefadroxil (p.o.), cefazolin, cephalexin (p.o.), cephalothin, cephapirin, cephradine (i.v./p.o.)
Second generation with *Haemophilus influenzae* activity	Cefaclor (p.o.), cefamandole, cefonicid, ceforanide, cefprozil (p.o.), cefuroxime, cefuroxime axetil (p.o.)
Second generation with *Bacteroides fragilis* activity	Cefmetazole, cefotetan, cefoxitin
Third generation	Cefotaxime, ceftriaxone, ceftizoxime, cefoperazone, moxalactam
Third generation with *Pseudomonas aeruginosa* activity	Ceftazidime, cefepime
Oral broad-spectrum	Cefixime, cefpodoxime proxetil

This classification is based on their spectrum of activity against aerobic Gram-negative bacilli, which increases from first to third generation. The drugs are available only parenterally unless indicated otherwise.
i.v., intravenous; p.o., by mouth.

First-generation cephalosporins are useful for skin and soft tissue infections

First-generation cephalosporins are active against streptococci, staphylococci, *E. coli*, *P. mirabilis*, and *Klebsiella pneumoniae* and are useful for skin and soft tissue infections since these are usually due to *Streptococcus pyogenes* and/or *S. aureus*. First-generation cephalosporins are commonly given as prophylaxis against infection following surgical procedures and are also alternatives to penicillins in penicillin-allergic individuals to treat infections that would otherwise be treated with penicillin G, an aminopenicillin, or an antistaphylococcal penicillin. Cefazolin is the most frequently used parenteral agent.

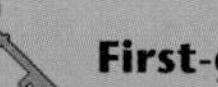

First-generation cephalosporins

- **Are active against streptococci and staphylococci but not enterococci**
- **Are active against most *Escherichia coli*, *Proteus mirabilis*, and *Klebsiella pneumoniae***

There are two subtypes of second-generation cephalosporins

The two subtypes of second-generation cephalosporins are:

- Those with activity against *H. influenzae*.
- Those with activity against *B. fragilis*.

Second-generation cephalosporins are not degraded by β lactamase. However, they do not achieve adequate concentrations in the cerebrospinal fluid to kill *H. influenzae* reliably, unlike third-generation cephalosporins. In other respects, their activity is similar to that of first-generation cephalosporins. These drugs are commonly used in the treatment of community-acquired respiratory tract infections in which either *S. pneumoniae* or *H. influenzae* may be a pathogen (e.g. sinusitis, otitis media, pneumonia). These drugs are also useful for the empiric treatment of a variety of infections in children in which streptococci, *S. aureus* and *H. influenzae* may be pathogens, except for meningitis.

Second-generation cephalosporins with activity against *B. fragilis* are generally used in the treatment of mixed aerobic–anaerobic infections, which although usually intra-abdominal, are occasionally ischemic skin and soft tissue infections, e.g., infected lower limb cutaneous ulcers in people with diabetes mellitus.

Third-generation cephalosporins have marked activity against aerobic Gram-negative bacilli

Compared with first- and second-generation cephalosporins, third-generation cephalosporins have marked activity against aerobic Gram-negative bacilli, particularly Enterobacteriaceae and *H. influenzae*. They are not degraded by β lactamase that can be produced by *H. influenzae* and *N. gonorrhoeae*, and to many of the β lactamases produced by Enterobacteriaceae, with the important exception of the type I chromosome-mediated inducible cephalosporinase, which may be produced by *Enterobacter cloacae*, *E. aerogenes*, *Citrobacter freundii*, *Serratia marcescens* and *P. aeruginosa*. Therefore, it is generally recommended that third-generation cephalosporins are not used as monotherapy for infections due to these pathogens.

In general, third-generation cephalosporins have reduced activity against *S. aureus* compared with first- and second-generation cephalosporins. A few third-generation cephalosporins, particularly ceftazidime, are active against *P. aeruginosa*.

An important property of the third-generation cephalosporins is that they achieve adequate concentrations in cerebrospinal fluid to be bactericidal against Enterobacteriaceae and the three major bacterial meningeal pathogens (i.e. S. *pneumoniae*, N. *meningitidis* and *H. influenzae*).

Third-generation cephalosporins are important drugs for treating bacterial meningitis. They are also useful for treating serious infections such as nosocomial pneumonia due to aerobic Gram-negative bacilli, particularly when treatment with aminoglycosides is contraindicated.

Extended-spectrum cephalosporins are used orally to treat Enterobacteriaceae infections resistant to other oral β lactams

Over the last few years, a variety of orally active extended-spectrum cephalosporins have become available. They are sometimes called oral third-generation cephalosporins, but have considerably less activity against aerobic Gram-negative bacilli than third-generation parenteral cephalosporins. None of the oral agents is active against *P. aeruginosa* and some (cefixime, ceftibuten) are inactive against *S. aureus*. These drugs can provide an oral option for treating infections due to Enterobacteriaceae resistant to other oral β lactams.

The routes of administration of cephalosporins as well as their pharmacokinetic profiles are summarized in Table 6.12 together with the other β lactam antibiotics

CARBAPENEMS Carbapenems structurally are a β lactam ring fused with a five-membered carbon-containing penem ring. The first two carbapenems, imipenem and meropenem, were followed by ertapenem, which was introduced into the USA in 2002.

Carbapenems are β lactams and are antibactericidal via inhibition of bacterial cell wall synthesis

They have the broadest spectrum of all available antibiotics and are stable to most β lactamases. They are active against streptococci, staphylococci, Enterobacteriaceae, *P. aeruginosa*, *Haemophilus* species and anaerobic bacteria, including *B. fragilis*. Carbapenems are also active against many strains of *Enterococcus faecalis*, but not against other species of *Enterococcus*. Like cephalosporins, they are not active against *L. monocytogenes*, or methicillin-resistant staphylococci.

Imipenem is metabolized in the kidney by a human β lactamase called dehydropeptidase-1 to a nephrotoxic metabolite, a specific inhibitor of the renal β lactamase. Cilastatin (an inhibitor of the peptidase) is given in a fixed ratio with imipenem to overcome this problem.

Meropenem and ertapenem are not metabolized by renal dehydropeptidase and therefore do not require concomitant cilastatin. Ertapenem has the longest half-life of the carbapenems and is given daily while imipenem is given every 6 hours and meropenem every 8 hours. Doses are reduced in renal failure because the carbapenems are renally excreted.

The toxicity of carbapenems is equitoxic to other β lactams causing nausea, vomiting and hypersensitivity reactions with a risk of cross-sensitivity with other β lactams.

Imipenem can cause seizures (incidence 0.9%) in susceptible individuals, particularly those with concomitant renal insufficiency. Meropenem, but not imipenem, can be used to treat bacterial meningitis.

Carbapenems are effective in pneumonias, intra-abdominal infections, endocarditis, bacteremia and osteomyelitis. They are particularly useful for treating infections due to bacteria resistant to other antibiotics. Their very broad spectrum of activity results in their use in polymicrobial infections instead of using two or more other antibiotics.

MONOBACTAMS Monobactam is shorthand for monocyclic β lactam antibiotics.

Monobactams consist of a single ring structure, the β lactam ring, attached to a sulfonic acid group.

■ ***The only available monobactam is aztreonam***

Aztreonam is active only against aerobic Gram-negative bacilli including *P. aeruginosa*. Unlike other β lactams, it has no activity against Gram-positive bacteria. Aztreonam also lacks activity against anaerobes and is available only for parenteral use.

A novel property of aztreonam is that it is essentially nonallergenic and can be used in individuals with penicillin and/or cephalosporin allergy.

The routes of administration of carbapenems and monobactams as well as their pharmacokinetic profiles are summarized in Table 6.12 together with the other β lactam antibiotics

β Lactamase inhibitors

Several specific inhibitors of bacterial β lactamases have been developed for clinical use. These are clavulanate, sulbactam and tazobactam. These drugs contain a β lactam ring, but none is clinically useful when used alone. Therefore, none of the β lactamase inhibitors are used as monotherapy. However, they covalently bind to bacterial β lactamase and inactivate it, thus allowing β lactam drugs that would otherwise be destroyed by the β lactamase to exert their antibacterial effect. They are used in fixed-dose combinations with a penicillin (Table 6.14).

The β lactamase inhibitors inhibit most of the important bacterial β lactamases, including those produced by staphylococci, gonococci, *H. influenzae*, *B. fragilis*, and some Enterobacteriaceae. However, they do not inhibit bacterial type I chromosome-mediated inducible cephalosporinase, which can hydrolyze all cephalosporins, including third-generation cephalosporins.

Penicillin–β lactamase inhibitor combinations are useful for polymicrobial infections where the use of a single commercial product (albeit containing two drugs) may obviate the need for two or more agents. In practice, they are most frequently used in the treatment of intra-abdominal infections, bite-wound infections and infected cutaneous ulcers.

Table 6.14 Penicillin–β lactam inhibitor combinations

Amoxicillin–clavulanate (p.o.)
Ampicillin–sulbactam (i.v.)
Ticarcillin–clavulanate (i.v.)
Piperacillin–tazobactam (i.v.)

β lactamase inhibitors are not available for use on their own, but are available in fixed-dose combinations with a penicillin.
i.v., intravenous; p.o., by mouth.

Glycopeptides

■ ***Glycopeptides are high molecular weight drugs consisting of sugars and amino acids (glycopeptides)***

Vancomycin is currently the only glycopeptide available in the US, but teicoplanin is available in parts of Europe. Vancomycin is a predominantly a bactericidal antibiotic that inhibits bacterial cell wall synthesis by covalently binding to the terminal two D-alanine residues at the free carboxyl end of the pentapeptide, thereby sterically hindering the elongation of the peptidoglycan backbone (Fig. 6.15) of bacteria. In contrast to this mechanism of action, β lactams inhibit a later stage of cell wall synthesis by blocking the cross-linkage of pentapeptide side chains. Owing to its high molecular weight, vancomycin is unable to penetrate the cell membrane of Gram-negative bacteria. Therefore, its activity is confined to Gram-positive bacteria.

Vancomycin does not contain a β lactam ring and binds to peptide side chains rather than to penicillin-binding proteins; thus, it is not affected by β lactamase or penicillin-binding proteins As a result, it is useful in the treatment of β lactam-resistant Gram-positive infections. Acquired vancomycin resistance is uncommon, is usually confined to *E. fecium*, and is due to an altered pentapeptide side chain.

THERAPEUTIC INDICATIONS Vancomycin is useful in the treatment of infections caused by streptococci, staphylococci, enterococci, *Corynebacterium jeikeium* and *Clostridium difficile*. It is the drug of choice for infections caused by methicillin-resistant staphylococci and penicillin-resistant pneumococci. Vancomycin is frequently used as an alternative to β lactams in patients with serious β

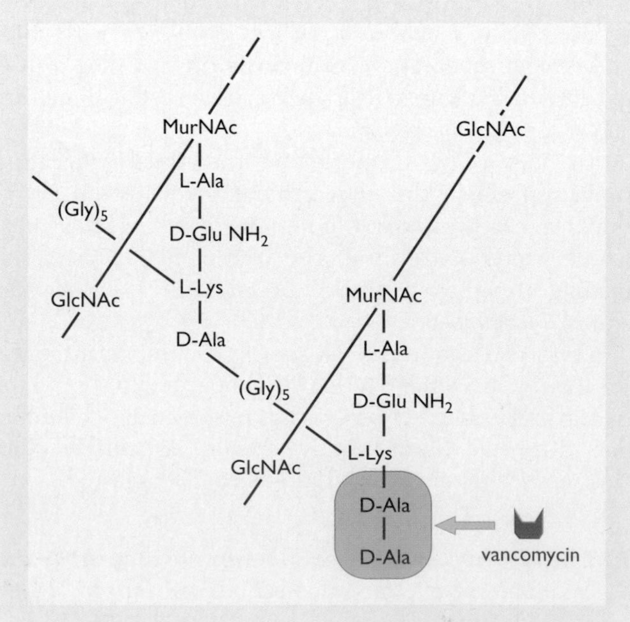

Fig. 6.15 Site of action of vancomycin on the elongating peptidoglycan polymer in bacterial cell walls.

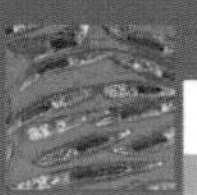

lactam allergy as there is no cross-reactivity between vancomycin and β lactams.

Vancomycin is very effective orally in the treatment of *C. difficile* enteritis since it is poorly absorbed and stays in the intestine. However, metronizadole is usually preferred since it is less expensive.

Vancomycin enters the cerebrospinal fluid to achieve concentrations that are close to the MBC for streptococci and staphylococci, but clinical experience with vancomycin in the treatment of bacterial meningitis is limited. Vancomycin should not, therefore, be used in the treatment of meningitis unless the pathogen is resistant to third-generation cephalosporins and chloramphenicol.

Vancomycin is poorly absorbed from the gastrointestinal tract and is therefore used intravenously for most indications. However, when used as described above, it can be given orally (125–250 mg every 6 hours) to treat intestinal infection due to *C. difficile*.

When infused rapidly, vancomycin causes histamine release from circulating basophils, resulting in an erythematous rash usually confined to the neck and upper trunk. This phenomenon is called the 'red neck' syndrome and can be mistaken for allergy. It is avoided if vancomycin is infused slowly. Vancomycin is excreted unchanged by the kidney.

Other adverse effects include thrombophlebitis at infusion site, chills, fevers, ototoxicity and possibly nephrotoxicity. Monitoring serum levels can be an important guide to avoiding ototoxicity and nephrotoxicity.

Other antibiotics that inhibit bacterial cell membrane functioning

Polymyxin B and polymyxin E (also known as colistimethate) are peptides of high molecular weight that damage the plasma membranes of Gram-negative bacteria, resulting in a bactericidal effect. Due to their considerable toxicity when given systemically, their use is mainly confined to topical therapy of infections due to aerobic Gram-negative bacilli. Colistimethate is used intravenously only to treat serious infections due to aerobic Gram-negative bacilli resistant to all other systemic agents.

Antibiotics that inhibit bacterial protein synthesis

Several major classes of antibiotic act principally by inhibiting bacterial protein synthesis (Fig. 6.16). These drugs exhibit selective toxicity by inhibiting bacterial protein synthesis to a much greater extent than host cell protein synthesis. This is a result of binding to specific

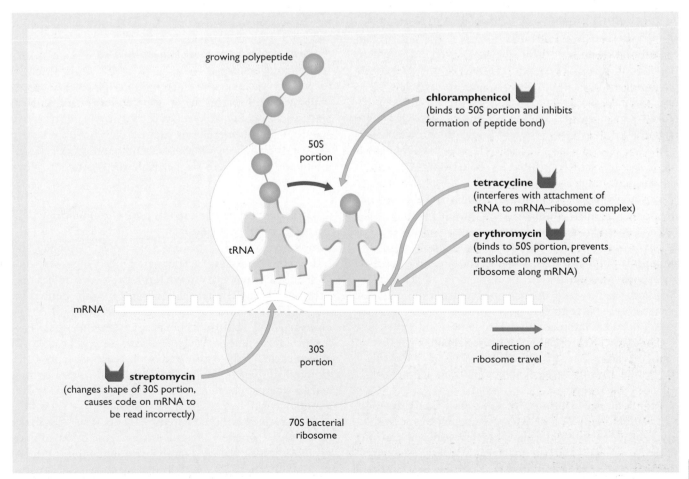

Fig. 6.16 Several classes of antibiotics inhibit bacterial protein synthesis.

Table 6.15 Aminoglycosides currently available in the US, their route of administration and use

Agent	Routes	Comment
Streptomycin	i.m. (i.v.)	For tuberculosis, plague, tularemia, severe brucellosis, some gentamicin-resistant enterococci
Neomycin	p.o.	Used to reduce the load of Enterobacteriaceae in the bowel and to treat hepatic encephalopathy, or with erythromycin as prophylaxis in elective colorectal surgery
Paromomycin	p.o.	For certain intestinal protozoa
Kanamycin	i.v./i.m.	Rarely used, owing to bacterial resistance
Gentamicin	i.v./i.m.	The 'workhorse' aminoglycoside; used for Enterobacteriaceae, *Pseudomonas aeruginosa*, enterococci
Netilmicin	i.v./i.m.	Similar to effect of gentamicin against Enterobacteriaceae and *P. aeruginosa*; poor synergistic activity against enterococci
Tobramycin	i.v./i.m.	Similar to effect of gentamicin against Enterobacteriaceae; more active than gentamicin against *P. aeruginosa*; poor synergistic activity against enterococci
Amikacin	i.v./i.m.	Aminoglycoside least affected by aminoglycoside-modifying enzymes; good activity against Enterobacteriaceae and *P. aeruginosa*; the most active against mycobacteria; poor synergistic activity against enterococci; the most expensive aminoglycoside

i.m., intramuscular; i.v., intravenous; p.o., oral.

bacterial targets. Most of these drugs are predominantly bacteriostatic, except for the aminoglycosides and oxazolidinones, which are bactericidal.

Aminoglycosides

Aminoglycosides have structures in which two or more amino sugars are linked by glycosidic bonds to an aminocyclitol ring. The aminoglycosides currently available in the US are listed in Table 6.15.

Aminoglycosides enter bacteria via an oxygen-dependent transport system, which is not present in anaerobic bacteria, or streptococci. Accordingly, anaerobes and streptococci are innately resistant to aminoglycosides. Once inside bacteria, aminoglycosides bind irreversibly to sites on the ribosome to inhibit protein synthesis. There is also at least one other ill-understood mechanism, which probably contributes to their bactericidal activity.

Aminoglycosides are active against aerobic Gram-negative bacilli, staphylococci and mycobacteria. Although they are not active against enterococci or *L. monocytogenes*, the addition of an aminoglycoside to penicillin G, ampicillin, or vancomycin is often synergistic and usually results in bactericidal activity.

There are two principal mechanisms of acquired bacterial resistance to aminoglycosides:

- Reduced bacterial aminoglycoside permeability caused by alterations in the bacterial cell membrane.
- Production of a variety of enzymes that act on aminoglycosides.

Nonhydrolytic aminoglycoside-modifying enzymes add acetyl, adenyl, or phosphoryl groups to the aminoglycoside thereby rendering them incapable of reaching their target sites on the bacterial ribosome. Each of the aminoglycoside-modifying enzymes has different substrate specificity and may modify only some aminoglycosides. Accordingly, bacteria may be resistant to one aminoglycoside and not to another.

In view of their toxicity, aminoglycosides are used primarily for serious infections due to Enterobacteriaceae and P. *aeruginosa*, usually in a hospital setting. Aminoglycosides are also used in conjunction with penicillin, ampicillin, or vancomycin in the treatment of serious infections due to enterococci and *L. monocytogenes*.

Gentamicin is the most frequently used aminoglycoside

Gentamicin is the most active aminoglycoside against enterococci. Tobramycin is usually more active than gentamicin against *P. aeruginosa*, but is not more active against Enterobacteriaceae, and unlikely to be effective against enterococci. Ophthalmic preparations of gentamicin and tobramycin are available for treatment of eye infections.

Streptomycin can be used as part of a multidrug regimen for tuberculosis

Streptomycin is also the drug of choice in plague and tularemia, although recent evidence suggests that gentamicin is equally effective for these two infections. Streptomycin demonstrates synergy with penicillin, ampicillin, or vancomycin in the treatment of a few enterococcal strains whereas gentamicin does not. Streptomycin plus doxycycline is used to treat brucellosis.

Amikacin is the aminoglycoside least susceptible to aminoglycoside-modifying enzymes and is sometimes active against bacteria that are resistant to other aminoglycosides.

Neomycin is not used parenterally because of its lower efficacy and greater adverse effects than other aminoglycosides. It can be used orally (without systemic effects) to reduce the intestinal Enterobacteriaceae in the treatment of hepatic encephalopathy, or, in combination

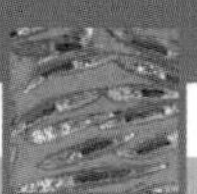

with erythromycin, as a prophylactic regimen to reduce the incidence of wound infection following elective colorectal surgery. Kanamycin is rarely used, owing to acquired resistance.

Paromomycin, which is related to neomycin, is used only orally to treat intestinal protozoal infections.

Aminoglycosides are not absorbed from the digestive tract and must be used parenterally. They are excreted unchanged by the kidney and are suitable for treating urinary tract infections. They do not enter the cerebrospinal fluid to reach adequate therapeutic concentrations, except in neonates.

Aminoglycosides have two major adverse effects

Aminoglycosides can elicit nephrotoxicity and ototoxicity (auditory and vestibular). The risk of these adverse effects is both dose- and duration-dependent. Nephrotoxicity is more common, but is usually mild and reversible. Ototoxicity is often permanent (see Ch. 20). Aminoglycosides elicit more adverse effects than most other antibiotics and must be given parenterally. Owing to their adverse effects, serum aminoglycoside concentrations are often monitored, but adverse effects can occur even with 'ideal' serum concentrations.

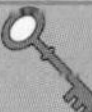

Aminoglycosides

- Are not absorbed orally
- Are active against aerobic Gram-negative bacilli
- Demonstrate concentration-dependent killing
- Cause nephrotoxicity and ototoxicity (their major adverse effects)

Macrolides, lincosamides and streptogramins (MLS antibiotics)

Macrolides, lincosamides and streptogramins (MLS drugs) are chemically unrelated antibiotics that possess similar mechanisms of action, and antimicrobial activity with a similar profile of resistance. They reversibly bind to the 50S ribosomal subunit to block translocation. Although conventionally considered as bacteriostatic antibiotics, they are bactericidal against specific isolates. The principal mechanism of acquired resistance is a specific mutation in the ribosomal ribonucleic acid (RNA) of the 50S ribosomal subunit. Resistance to one member of the MLS class does not necessarily imply resistance to others.

Macrolides have a macrocyclic lactone ring

The prototype macrolide is erythromycin, which is available in different salts. In recent years, newer macrolides have been introduced in the US, including clarithromycin, azithromycin and dirithromycin. Other macrolides are available in Europe and Asia. Macrolides are usually given orally although i.v. forms of erythromycin and azithromycin are available, and erythromycin lotion can be used in the treatment of acne vulgaris. Macrolides are metabolized in the liver and do not penetrate the cerebrospinal fluid sufficiently to achieve therapeutically relevant concentrations.

Erythromycin is active against streptococci, staphylococci, *Bordetella pertussis*, *Corynebacterium diphtheriae*, *Campylobacter jejuni*, *Mycoplasma pneumoniae*, *Ureaplasma urealyticum*, *Legionella species* and *Chlamydia* species. Erythromycin and dirithromycin have limited activity against *H. influenzae*, but both clarithromycin and azithromycin are considerably more effective against this organism. Macrolides are not active against Enterobacteriaceae, *P. aeruginosa*, or *Mycoplasma hominis*.

Macrolides are used primarily to treat respiratory tract infections. They are the alternative to penicillin for treating streptococcal pharyngitis, especially in patients allergic to penicillin.

Marcrolides are the drugs of choice for community-acquired pneumonia as they are active against pneumococci, *M. pneumoniae*, *C. pneumoniae* and *Legionella* species. In cases where infection may be due to *H. influenzae*, clarithromycin or azithromycin are preferred.

Erythromycin is the drug of choice for the treatment of pertussis, legionnaires' disease, *Chlamydia trachomatis* (in pregnancy where tetracyclines are contraindicated) and are equivalent to penicillin in eradicating the carrier state in diphtheria. Erythromycin is equivalent to tetracycline in the treatment of *M. pneumoniae* infections, is used for *C. jejuni* enteritis and is an alternative to β lactams for mild skin and soft tissue infections due to *S. pyogenes* and *S. aureus*.

Clarithromycin and azithromycin are more active than erythromycin against some pathogens

Clarithromycin and azithromycin, but not dirithromycin, are more active than erythromycin against *H. influenzae* and are more appropriate choices for the empiric treatment of respiratory tract infections if *H. influenzae* is a possible pathogen.

Both clarithromycin and azithromycin are active against *Mycobacterium avium* complex, an important pathogen in patients with AIDS. Clarithromycin is useful in the treatment of most other nontuberculous mycobacteria. It is also very active against *Helicobacter pylori* and is routinely used in a multidrug regimen to treat duodenal ulcers caused by *H. pylori*. Azithromycin is active against *C. trachomatis* and is the only drug that can cure *C. trachomatis* urethritis and cervicitis when given in a single dose.

Erythromycin and clarithromycin have a number of interactions with other drugs

Erythromycin elevates serum theophylline concentrations when given concomitantly. In combination with the non-sedating histamine-H_1 antagonists astemizole or terfenadine, or the promotility drug cisapride, erythromycin and clarithromycin is contraindicated as it results in significant prolongation of the QT interval in the electrocardiogram (see Ch. 13). This can result in the torsades de pointes variant of ventricular tachycardia, which can be fatal.

Erythromycin causes gastrointestinal adverse effects

Erythromycin is probably the single most poorly tolerated oral antibiotic, owing to dyspepsia, nausea and vomiting. Independently of its antibiotic activity, it interacts with motilin receptors to increase gastrointestinal motility for the treatment of diabetic gastroparesis. The newer macrolides clarithromycin and azithromycin produce less severe gastrointestinal adverse effects than erythromycin, and may be suitable for individuals who have demonstrated gastrointestinal intolerance to erythromycin.

The routes of administration of macrolides as well as their pharmacokinetic profiles are summarized in Table 6.16.

KETOLIDES (MODIFIED MACROLIDES) Recently, a series of modified macrolides have been synthesized in which the cladinose at position 3 of the macrolactone ring has been replaced by a keto group. These modified macrolides are also known as ketolides. The first agent in this class was telithromycin. The major difference between ketolides and macrolides is that ketolides are much more resistant to the principal mechanism of MLS resistance in *Streptococcus pneumoniae*, so that the majority of macrolide-resistant pneumococci remain susceptible to ketolides. Otherwise, ketolides are similar to the newer macrolides clarithromycin and azithromycin.

LINCOSAMIDES Lincomycin and clindamycin are the two available lincosamides. Lincomycin is named after Lincoln, Nebraska, where it was first isolated from the mold *Streptomyces lincolnensis*. The replacement of a hydroxyl group in lincomycin with a chloride results in clindamycin. Since clindamycin has greater activity and superior oral bioavailability, it has supplanted lincomycin in clinical use.

Clindamycin is active against streptococci, staphylococci and anaerobic bacteria, including *B. fragilis*. It is also active against *Mycoplasma hominis*, but not *M. pneumoniae* or *U. urealyticum*. It has no useful activity against enterococci or aerobic Gram-negative bacilli. Clindamycin is also active against several protozoa. Clindamycin is an important antibiotic in the treatment of anaerobic infections, particularly in mixed aerobic–anaerobic infections where it is usually used in combination with other antibiotics. It can also be used as an alternative to β lactams in people who are allergic to β lactams, particularly if the oral route is appropriate.

Clindamycin can be given either orally or intravenously. There is also a topical solution for the treatment of acne vulgaris and a vaginal cream for the treatment of bacterial vaginosis. Clindamycin is metabolized by the liver and does not penetrate the cerebrospinal fluid.

Clindamycin is associated with a higher risk of *Clostridium difficile* enteritis than other antibiotics.

Streptogramins

Streptogramins consist of a combination of two naturally occurring chemically unrelated groups of molecules, referred to as groups A and B. Pristinamycin is such a combination, which has been available in Europe for many years as an oral antistaphylococcal agent, but it is not available in the US.

Quinupristin–dalfopristin is an i.v. streptogramin consisting of a 30:70 ratio of quinupristin to dalfopristin, which was introduced into clinical use in the late 1990s. This combination is active against staphylococci (including methicillin-resistant staphylococci), streptococci (including penicillin-resistant pneumococci), and *Enterococcus faecium* (but not most *Enterococcus faecalis*). The major clinical indication for quinupristin–dalfopristin is the treatment of infections due to vancomycin-resistant *E. faecium*, and as an alternative to vancomycin in the treatment of infections due to methicillin-resistant staphylococci.

Quinupristin–dalfopristin is rapidly cleared by nonrenal mechanisms, but there is a long postantibiotic effect against *Staphylococcus aureus*, *Streptococcus pneumoniae*

Table 6.16 Route of administration and pharmacokinetics of macrolides, lincosamides and streptogramins

Drug	Routes of administration	Oral bioavailability (%)	Clearance route	Serum half-life with normal renal function (hours)	Comments
Erythromycin	i.v., p.o., topical	25	Hepatic	1.8	Phlebitic i.v. formulation
Clarithromycin	p.o.	5	Hepatic	6	Active metabolite
Azithromycin	i.v., p.o.	35	GI and hepatic	68	Highly concentrated intracellularly
Quinupristin– dalfopristin	i.v.	Not used	Hepatic	8.5	Active against Gram-positive cocci, including phlebitic VRE

i.v., intravenous; p.o., by mouth; GI, gastrointestinal; VRE, vancomycin-resistant enterococci.

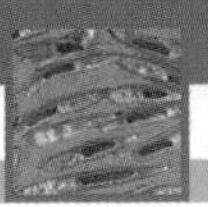

and *E. faecium*, so that twice-daily dosing is clinically effective. Its major adverse effect is an infusion-related phlebitis, which can be avoided if the drug is administered via a central venous catheter.

Clearance is primarily the result of hepatic metabolism and the serum half-life is about 8.5 hours.

Tetracyclines

Tetracyclines are moderately broad-spectrum, primarily bacteriostatic antibiotics that have a nucleus of four fused cyclic rings (Fig. 6.17), hence the name tetracyclines. Different tetracyclines are derived by different substitutions at positions 5, 6 and 7 of the tetracycline nucleus. Tetracyclines reversibly bind to the bacterial 30S ribosomal subunit in such a manner that they block the binding of transfer RNA to the messenger RNA–ribosome complex, preventing the addition of new amino acids to the growing peptide chain (see Fig. 6.16). Acquired tetracycline resistance is usually due to changes in the transport mechanism, resulting in a lack of tetracycline accumulation with bacteria. Since tetracyclines are concentrated intracellularly, they are useful for intracellular infections. Although tetracyclines are active against a wide variety of bacteria, the important organisms against which they are consistently active include chlamydiae, mycoplasmas, spirochetes (including those that cause leptospirosis, Lyme disease and relapsing fever), rickettsial infections, *Legionella* species and *Brucella* species. Tetracyclines, particularly minocycline, are also effective in the treatment of acne vulgaris.

Of the six tetracyclines available in the US, only three are used with any frequency: tetracycline, doxycycline and minocycline.

Tetracycline is a short-acting drug that is usually administered four times daily, whereas both doxycycline and minocycline have longer half-lifes, allowing once- or twice-daily administration.

They are excreted mainly by the kidneys and do not achieve adequate therapeutic concentrations in cerebrospinal fluid. They are usually used orally but i.v. preparations are available, as well as topical formulations for acne vulgaris

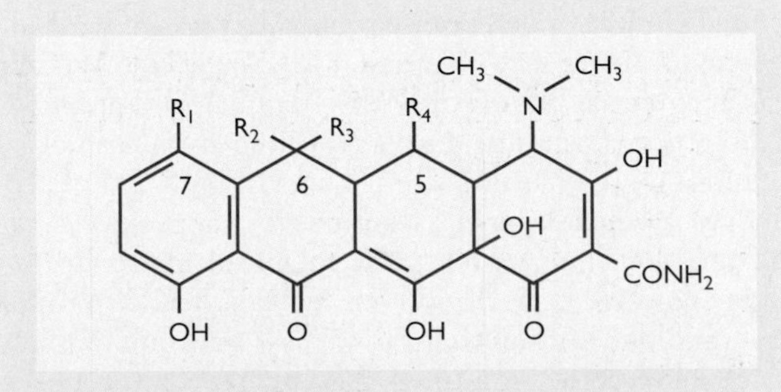

Fig. 6.17 Chemical structure of tetracyclines. Substitutions at positions five, six and seven result in different drugs, including the three common agents: tetracycline, doxycycline and minocycline.

Tetracyclines are chelated by divalent and trivalent cations

Absorption of tetracyclines is markedly decreased when taken orally in conjunction with calcium-, magnesium-, and aluminum-containing antacids, dairy products, calcium supplements, or sucralfate. They have a strong affinity for developing bone and teeth, to which they give a permanent yellow-brown color. They are therefore contraindicated in pregnant and breastfeeding women, as well as in children less than 8 years of age.

The routes of administration of tetracyclines well as their pharmacokinetic profiles are summarized in Table 6.17.

Amphenicols

Chloramphenicol is the only amphenicol available in the US. The related drug, thiamphenicol, is available in parts of Europe. Chloramphenicol is a relatively broad-spectrum, predominantly bacteriostatic antibiotic that reversibly binds to the bacterial 50S ribosomal subunit to prevent the attachment of the amino acid-containing end of transfer RNA to the peptide chain (i.e. it blocks peptidyl transferase) (see Fig. 6.16).

Acquired chloramphenicol resistance results from:

- Reduced bacterial permeability.
- Production of the chloramphenicol-modifying enzyme, chloramphenicol acetyltransferase.

Chloramphenicol is available orally and parenterally and as a topical ophthalmic formulation.

Chloramphenicol enters the cerebrospinal fluid to achieve therapeutically effective concentrations against the three principal bacterial meningeal pathogens (i.e. *S. pneumoniae*, *N. meningitidis* and *H. influenzae*), but not for Enterobacteriaceae. Chloramphenicol accumulates in the brain parenchyma at concentrations useful in the treatment of brain abscess.

Chloramphenicol is seldom used in developed countries, but:

- Is an acceptable alternative for the treatment of bacterial meningitis, particularly in patients with cephalosporin allergies.
- May be used in the treatment of brain abscess or enteric fever, although a variety of *Salmonella* strains around the world are resistant to chloramphenicol.
- Is an alternative to tetracycline in the treatment of Rocky Mountain spotted fever.

Chloramphenicol's main adverse effect is myelosuppression

Choramphenicol exerts a dose-dependent myelosuppression, which is common and reversible. Approximately 1 in 30 000 patients given chloramphenicol develop irreversible aplastic anemia. Although this idiosyncratic reaction is rare it is the major reason why chloramphe-

Table 6.17 Route of administration and pharmacokinetics of tetracycline antibiotics

Drug	Routes of administration	Oral bioavailability (%)	Clearance route	Serum half-life (normal renal function), (hours)	Comments
Tetracycline	p.o.	75	Renal	9	Contraindicated in pregnancy and children <8 years
Doxycycline	i.v., p.o.	95	GI tract	18	Contraindicated in pregnancy and children <8 years
Minocycline	p.o.	95	GI tract	18	Contraindicated in pregnancy and children <8 years Most lipophilic tetracycline

i.v., intravenous; p.o., by mouth; GI, gastrointestinal.

nicol is seldom used. However, chloramphenicol is more widely used in developing countries because of its low price, broad spectrum of activity and efficacy in enteric fevers.

Chloramphenicol is conjugated in the liver to its inactive glucuronide

Neonates have a reduced ability to conjugate chloramphenicol; this sometimes results in high serum chloramphenicol concentrations with resultant toxicity. Such toxicity is manifest as the gray baby syndrome, which is characterized by abdominal distention, vomiting, cyanosis and circulatory collapse. If chloramphenicol must be used in neonates, serum concentrations need to be monitored closely. It is given by oral, i.v. and topical routes. The oral route is associated with 80% bioavailability and clearance is primarily through hepatic metabolism resulting in a half-life of 3 hours.

Oxazolidinones

Oxazolidinones are the newest class of synthetic antibiotics. In 2000, linezolid became the first oxazolidinone to be approved in the USA. It acts by binding to the bacterial 23S ribosomal RNA of the 50S subunit, thus preventing the formation of the 70S initiation complex required for protein synthesis. This inhibition of bacterial protein synthesis is at a very early step, preceding the interaction of transfer RNA and the 30S ribosome with the initiator codon. Currently only linezolid is available for oral or i.v. administration. As a result of its unique mechanism of action, there is no cross-resistance with other classes of antibiotics.

Linezolid is active against most important aerobic Gram-positive cocci, including staphylococci (including methicillin-resistant staphylococci), streptococci (including penicillin-resistant pneumococci) and enterococci – both *E. faecalis* and *E. faecium*, including vancomycin-resistant enterococci. It is bacteriostatic against staphylococci and enterococci, but bactericidal against most streptococci. The spectrum includes most aerobic Gram-positive cocci whereas enteric Gram-negative bacilli and *Pseudomonas* species are not.

In view of its high cost and usefulness, linezolid is best reserved for the treatment of infection due to susceptible Gram-positive cocci, which cannot be treated by other agents. Its principal use in the treatment of vancomycin-resistant enterococci, and as an alternative to vancomycin for methicillin-resistant staphylococci.

The most frequent side effects of linezolid are nausea, vomiting and headaches. A reversible bone marrow suppression can occur; therefore, blood concentrations of linezolid are monitored during prolonged treatment. Linezolid is a reversible inhibitor of monoamine oxidase enzyme (an MAOI); therefore, the usual precautions for this class of drugs apply. Linezolid is rapidly and completely orally bioavailable and has a long serum half-life. The usual dose is 600 mg every 12 hours whether i.v. or oral (serum half-life 5.5 hours). Clearance involves both hepatic and some renal mechanisms.

Antibiotics that inhibit bacterial deoxyribonucleic acid synthesis

Quinolones

The quinolones are synthetic antibiotics based on a nucleus of two fused six-membered rings

The first drug in this class was nalidixic acid. It was of limited clinical value because of its relative inactivity and the rapid emergence of resistance. Since ciprofloxacin was introduced in the 1990s a number of quinolone analogs have been introduced that differ from each other in terms of their antibacterial activity and pharmacokinetics. The addition of a fluorine atom at position six of the quinolone nucleus markedly enhanced activity against Gram-negative bacteria and has led to a new generation of quinolone antibiotics known as fluoroquinolones. Fluoroquinolones inhibit DNA gyrase and topoisomerase IV to an extent that depends upon the bacteria. Quinolones inhibit bacterial deoxyribonucleic acid (DNA) gyrase, the enzyme responsible for supercoiling, nicking and sealing bacterial DNA. Acquired resistance

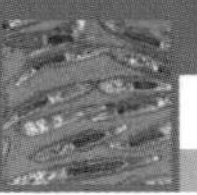

may develop through either decreased permeability or alterations in DNA gyrase.

The first generation of fluoroquinolones includes ciprofloxacin, ofloxacin and norfloxacin. They are active against Gram-negative and a few Gram-positive bacteria. A more recent fluoroquinolone, levofloxacin, has greater activity against Gram-positive and atypical bacteria. Fluoroquinolones are perhaps the best tolerated of all oral antibiotics, but are more expensive than most.

The quinolones are predominantly bactericidal and exhibit concentration-dependent killing. Fluoroquinolones are highly active against aerobic Gram-negative bacilli, including Enterobacteriaceae, *Haemophilus* species, *Moraxella catarrhalis* and, in the case of ciprofloxacin, *P. aeruginosa*. They are active against some mycobacteria, including most strains of *M. tuberculosis*. 'Older' fluoroquinolones, such as norfloxacin and ciprofloxacin, are weakly active against streptococci and staphylococci, and not active against anaerobes. Some of the newer fluoroquinolones (e.g. levofloxacin, gatifloxacin, gemifloxacin and moxifloxacin) have been called 'respiratory fluoroquinolones' because of increased activity against *Streptococcus pneumoniae*, including penicillin-resistant strains. Gatifloxacin and moxifloxacin are also active against anaerobic bacteria.

THERAPEUTIC INDICATIONS Fluoroquinolones are useful in the treatment of infections due to aerobic Gram-negative bacilli that are not susceptible to other drugs. In many instances, they are the only oral drugs active against certain aerobic Gram-negative bacilli, particularly *P. aeruginosa*, where fluoroquinolones can obviate the need for parenteral therapy. Of the currently available drugs, ciprofloxacin is the most active against Gram-negative bacteria and the most commonly used. It is available in oral, parenteral and ophthalmic formulations. The 'respiratory fluoroquinolones' can be used in the treatment of pneumonia, and may be particularly useful in regions where there is a high prevalence of penicillin-resistant *Streptococcus pneumoniae*.

They are renally excreted and have excellent oral bioavailability. They penetrate the prostate in therapeutically useful amounts and are therefore used to treat prostate infections. Although cerebrospinal fluid concentrations appear to be therapeutic, there is very little clinical experience in the use of quinolones for meningitis and their use is not recommended for bacterial meningitis.

Like tetracyclines, fluoroquinolones are chelated by divalent and trivalent cations. Some quinolones, including ciprofloxacin, increase serum concentrations of theophylline when given concomitantly. In addition, as fluoroquinolones cause cystic lesions in the articular cartilage of growing animals, they are relatively contraindicated in children and pregnant women.

The routes of administration of quinolones, as well as their pharmacokinetic profiles, are summarized in Table 6.18.

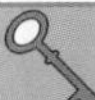

Ciprofloxacin

- The most commonly used fluoroquinolone
- Has excellent oral bioavailability
- Very active against aerobic Gram-negative bacilli
- Not active against anaerobes
- Has only limited activity against streptococci and staphylococci

Nitroimidazoles

Nitroimidazoles are well-absorbed, predominantly bactericidal agents with antimicrobial activity restricted to strict anaerobes and certain protozoa. They can enter most bacteria but only susceptible organisms produce the nitroreductase enzyme that is needed to reduce such nitroimidazoles to short-lived cytotoxic metabolites that bind to DNA and inhibit its synthesis. Aerobic bacteria are innately resistant due to a lack of nitroreductase activity.

Table 6.18 Route of administration and pharmacokinetics of quinolone antibiotics

Drug	Routes of administration	Oral bioavailability (%)	Clearance route	Serum half-life (normal renal function), (hours)	Comments
Norfloxacin	p.o.	40	Renal	3	Used for UTI only
Ciprofloxacin	p.o., i.v.	75	Renal	4	Very active against aerobic Gram-negative bacilli; Weak Gram-positive activity
Levofloxacin	p.o., i.v.	>95	Renal	7	Active against most *Streptococcus pneumoniae*
Gatifloxacin	p.o., i.v.		Renal	8	Broad-spectrum fluoroquinolone
Moxifloxacin	p.o.	85	Hepatic > renal	12	Broad-spectrum fluoroquinolone

i.v., intravenous; p.o., by mouth; UTI, urinary tract infection.

Acquired resistance can develop as a result of:

- Decreased uptake of the drug.
- Decreased nitroreductase production.

Metronidazole is the only nitroimidazole currently licensed in the US

Metronidazole is active against most anaerobic bacteria, but has greatest activity against Gram-negative anaerobes including *B. fragilis*. For the reason given above it has no activity against aerobic bacteria. It is also very effective in the treatment of three important protozoal infections: giardiasis, amebiasis and trichomoniasis.

Metronidazole is useful in the treatment of a variety of anaerobic infections including bacterial vaginosis, which is the most common cause of abnormal vaginal discharge. In bacterial vaginosis, the bacterial flora of the vagina, which is normally dominated by *Lactobacillus* species, becomes replaced by an abnormal polymicrobial flora that is comprised predominantly of anaerobes. Metronidazole is usually considered the drug of choice for *C. difficile* enteritis. In addition to its use against specific microorganisms, metronidazole is useful in hepatic encephalopathy and in Crohn's disease, particularly where there is perianal involvement.

Both oral and i.v. preparations of metronidazole are available, with the oral form having close to 100% bioavailability. A topical formulation is available for the treatment of acne rosacea. Metronidazole achieves therapeutic concentrations in both cerebrospinal fluid and brain parenchyma. It is given orally, i.v. or topically, and is >95% bioavailable. It is cleared mainly by the liver and has a serum half-life of about 10 hours.

Metronidazole should be used with caution in pregnant women

Since metronidazole is mutagenic in bacteria and causes tumors in rodents, it should be used with caution in pregnant women. Its use in the first trimester should be avoided wherever possible. However, there is no evidence to date of human carcinogenicity with metronidazole.

Antibiotics that inhibit bacterial ribonucleic acid synthesis

Rifamycins

Rifamycin antibiotics inhibit bacterial RNA synthesis by inhibiting DNA-dependent RNA polymerase

Acquired resistance to rifamycins is usually due to a mutation in bacterial DNA-dependent RNA polymerase. Two rifamycin derivatives are currently available: rifampin and rifabutin. A third rifamycin, rifapentine, with very long serum half-life, is under development. The rifamycins are all metabolized in the liver and color most body fluids orange, especially urine.

RIFAMPIN Rifampin was originally developed for the treatment of tuberculosis and remains a mainstay of antituberculosis therapy. It is also useful in the treatment of several non-tuberculous mycobacterial infections, particularly *M. leprae* (the cause of leprosy), *M. kansasii* and *M. marinum*.

Rifampin is never used alone for the treatment of mycobacterial infections, because acquired resistance will usually develop. It must be used in combination with at least one other antimycobacterial drug. Rifampin achieves effective therapeutic concentrations in the cerebrospinal fluid adequate to treat tuberculous meningitis.

Rifampin is also active against a number of conventional bacteria, notably staphylococci, *N. meningitidis*, *H. influenzae* and *Legionella pneumophila*. It is also:

- The drug of choice for eliminating the nasal carriage state of *N. meningitidis*, *H. influenzae* type b and *S. aureus*.
- Sometimes used as a second antistaphylococcal agent in combination with a β lactam or vancomycin in the treatment of serious staphylococcal infections, particularly endocarditis and osteomyelitis.
- Sometimes added as a second agent to erythromycin in the treatment of severe legionnaires' disease.

Rifampin is usually used orally, but an i.v. formulation is also available.

Rifampin may cause hepatotoxicity, a 'flu-like' syndrome, or fever (drug fever).

Rifampin is a potent inducer of hepatic microsomal enzymes. As a result, it increases the metabolism of many other drugs including glucocorticosteroids, oral contraceptives, quinidine, phenytoin, barbiturates, theophylline, clarithromycin, ketoconazole, itraconazole, ciclosporin and warfarin.

RIFABUTIN Rifabutin is active against most strains of *M. tuberculosis*, including 30% of the strains that are resistant to rifampin. It is significantly more active than rifampin against *M. avium* complex, and is effective as a single agent in the prevention of M. avium complex bacteremia in patients with AIDS. It is also useful as part of a multidrug combination in the treatment of established *M. avium* complex infection.

Although there is much more clinical experience with rifampin, rifabutin is useful in the treatment of tuberculosis as part of a multidrug regimen.

Rifabutin is available only as an oral formulation.

In comparison with rifampin, rifabutin causes less hepatic microsomal enzyme induction, so the scope for the drug interactions is less than for rifampin.

Rifabutin can cause a reversible uveitis, particularly when it is used in combination with clarithromycin, which is known to increase the serum concentration of both rifabutin and rifabutin's biologically active metabolite. The antifungal drug, fluconazole, as well as the HIV protease inhibitors indinavir and ritonavir, increase serum rifabutin concentrations.

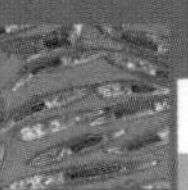

Antifolates

Folates are necessary cofactors in the synthesis of purines, and consequently of DNA

Although mammalian cells can absorb folate, bacteria must synthesize their folate from para-aminobenzoic acid (PABA). The bacterial folate synthetic pathway is outlined in Figure 6.18. This pathway can be blocked at two steps, by inhibition of either dihydropteroate synthetase (DHPS) or dihydrofolate reductase (DHFR).

Sulfonamides

Sulfonamides were developed in the 1930s during the course of investigations into dyes (Prontosil). Over the years, many other drugs were discovered based upon the sulfonamide chemical motif, including antidiabetics and diuretics. The antibacterial sulfonamides compete with PABA for DHPS, thereby inhibiting bacterial folate synthesis (see Fig. 6.18). Their effect is bacteriostatic. Acquired resistance can occur as a result of:

- Decreased permeability to the antibacterial drug.
- Increased PABA production.
- Altered DHPS for which the drugs lack affinity.

In the past, many sulfonamides with various pharmacological and pharmacokinetic profiles were introduced. The use of sulfonamides alone as antibacterial therapy is no longer recommended, owing to the relatively high rates of occurrence of bacterial resistance, and the availability of superior antibiotics. Few laboratories routinely perform susceptibility testing for sulfonamides. However, sulfonamides can be used alone in the treatment of infections due to *Nocardia* species, since the addition of a DHFR antagonist does not improve the activity against these organisms. Ophthalmic preparations of sulfacetamide are useful in the treatment of bacterial conjunctivitis.

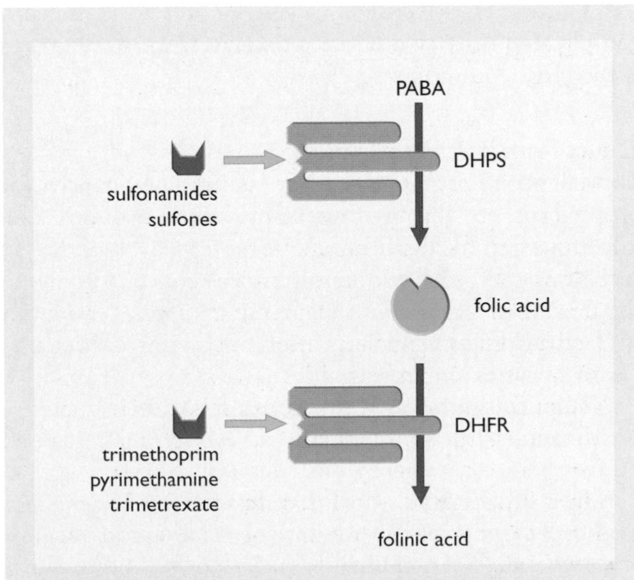

Fig. 6.18 The folate biosynthetic pathway. Sulfonamides and sulfones compete with para-aminobenzoic acid (PABA) for dihydropteroate synthetase (DHPS). Trimethoprim and the antiprotozoal drugs pyrimethamine and trimetrexate inhibit dihydrofolate reductase (DHFR).

Sulfonamides are perhaps the most allergenic of antibiotics

Sulfonamide allergy is most frequently manifest as a diffuse pruritic maculopapular rash. The risk of an allergic reaction with sulfonamides is substantially greater in people with HIV. Rarely, sulfonamides can cause Stevens–Johnson syndrome or toxic epidermal necrolysis, both of which are life-threatening desquamating skin disorders. Of all the drugs that can cause toxic epidermal necrolysis, sulfonamides carry the highest risk.

Sulfones

Sulfones are synthetic agents related to sulfonamides that compete with PABA for DHPS. The only available sulfone is diaminodiphenyl sulfone (DDS), also known as dapsone. Dapsone is active against most strains of *M. leprae*. It is used as part of a multidrug regimen for the treatment of leprosy. It can also be used in the prevention and treatment of *Pneumocystis carinii* pneumonia and in the treatment of some noninfectious skin diseases such as dermatitis herpetiformis.

There is partial cross-allergenicity between sulfonamides and sulfones.

Dihydrofolate reductase inhibitors

Of the three DHFR inhibitors available (i.e. trimethoprim, pyrimethamine and trimetrexate), only trimethoprim is useful for the treatment of bacterial infections. Trimethoprim is a bacteriostatic agent and is active against many Enterobacteriaceae. It is excreted unchanged in the urine and, since it enters the prostate in therapeutic concentrations, it is useful in the treatment of chronic bacterial prostatitis. Trimethoprim can be used alone in the treatment of urinary tract infections and is used in individuals allergic to sulfonamides. Trimethoprim is used mainly in combination with sulfamethoxazole (see below).

Trimethoprim–sulfamethoxazole

Trimethoprim and sulfamethoxazole block two separate steps of the folate biosynthetic pathway (see Fig. 6.18). When used in combination, their antibacterial effects are often synergistic and bactericidal. Both drugs are excreted unchanged by the kidney and because they have similar serum half-lifes, their relative concentrations remain fairly constant. The combination of trimethoprim–sulfamethoxazole is known as co-trimoxazole, and is active against most Enterobacteriaceae, *H. influenzae*, and many strains of streptococci and staphylococci. At concentrations achievable in the urine, co-trimoxazole inhibits many enterococci. Co-trimoxtazole is also very active against *P. carinii*, although it is not active against *P. aeruginosa* or anaerobic bacteria. Co-trimoxtazole does penetrate the cerebrospinal fluid, but there is only limited experience with its use in meningitis, and therefore other agents are preferred for this indication.

Co-trimoxazole is available in both oral and i.v. formulations.

Therapeutic uses of co-trimoxazole:

- It is very important as treatment for urinary tract infections. It is usually the drug of choice for urinary tract infections caused by susceptible bacteria, but can be used to treat infections caused by susceptible organisms at other sites in the body.
- It is the drug of choice for the prevention and treatment of *P. carinii* pneumonia.
- It may be useful for acute exacerbations of chronic bronchitis, shigellosis and enteric fever.

Miscellaneous antibacterial drugs

Both oral and i.v. formulations are used with 85% bioavailability via the oral route. Excretion is primarily renal and the half-life is 1 hour.

Nitrofurantoin

Nitrofurantoin is a synthetic nitrofuran that has been used for 50 years. It is used exclusively for the treatment of urinary tract infections. Its mechanism of action is unknown. It is active against most Enterobacteriaceae and enterococci (including VRE) and, some strains of *Klebsiella* and *Enterobacter* but not *P. aeruginosa*.

Nitrofurantoin is useful in the treatment of urinary tract infections in patients who have allergies and/or intolerance to sulfonamides and β lactams. Trimethoprim alone and fluoroquinolones are alternatives in this setting. Nitrofurantoin should never be used to treat a urinary tract infection if there is any possibility of a concomitant bacteremia, because of its inability to achieve therapeutic serum concentrations.

Nitrofurantoin is administered orally in a dosage of 50 mg four times daily or 100 mg twice daily in those with normal renal function. It is available only as an oral formulation and although it has 45% oral bioavailability most is rapidly metabolized by tissues (half-life, 0.3 hours) and one-third is excreted unchanged in urine. As a result, blood concentrations are very low and insufficient to treat systemic infections. However, urinary and renal concentrations are relatively high and sufficient to treat urinary tract infections Nitrofurantoin's antibacterial activity is reduced in alkaline pH; thus, it should not be used for urinary tract infections due to *Proteus* species since this bacterium contains urease, which converts urea to ammonium and hence alkalinizes the urine.

With prolonged use nitrofurantoin can cause peripheral neuropathy and pulmonary fibrosis. Nausea and vomiting are common side effects, but their incidence is decreased with improved microcrystalline formulations and when given with food. Less frequent adverse reactions include rash, hypersensitivity pneumonitis, peripheral neuropathy, hepatitis, and hemolytic anemia in association with G6PD deficiency.

Daptomycin

Daptomycin is a cyclic lipopeptide (isolated from *Streptomyces roseosporus*) that has a unique antibacterial mechanism of action since it depolarizes the bacterial membrane and causes death of bacteria, i.e. it is bactericidal. It acts against most Gram-positive aerobic bacteria, including resistant species (VRE, MRSA, *S. aureus*, coagulase-negative staphylococci and penicillin-resistant *S. pneumoniae)* and against *S. pyogenes*, *S. agalactiae*, *S. dysgalactiae* and *C. jeikeium*. It demonstrates synergism of antibacterial action with gentamicin. Resistance mechanisms against daptomycin have not been seen, nor has cross-resistance to other antibiotics. Despite such apparent advantages daptomycin has limited use since other antibiotics, e.g. vancomycin and linezolid, are available. Currently, it is used in complicated skin and skin structure infections.

Daptomycin is given i.v. twice daily. The main adverse event seen initially is a reversible skeletal muscle myopathy that affects skeletal muscles and is dose- and concentration-dependent. Reduction in dose is required when renal impairment is present.

Fosfomycin

Fosfomycin is a broad-spectrum antibiotic that inhibits cell wall synthesis and is active against *E. coli* and many other common urinary tract pathogens. It has been used in Europe for many years but currently it is approved in the United States only as a single oral dose for uncomplicated urinary tract infections in women. Diarrhea is the most common side effect.

Topical antimicrobial drugs

Topical antimicrobial drugs are used cutaneously for prophylaxis in the treatment of minor wounds and infections and for eradicating *S. aureus* from the nose. In such uses these drugs give high local concentrations at the treatment site without incurring toxicity.

Bacitracin acts against a variety of Gram-positive and Gram-negative organisms.

Neomycin and polymyxin act against Gram-negative organisms while polymyxin is bactericidal for *P. aeruginosa*.

Silver sulfadiazine is commonly used on burns since it is broad spectrum in its antibacterial actions against *S. aureus* and *P. aeruginosa*.

Mupirocin inhibits bacterial isoleucyl-tRNA synthetase and disrupts protein components of bacterial cell walls. Resistant bacteria have an altered form of the enzyme, although this is rare. It is bactericidal on aerobic Gram-positive cocci, including *S. aureus*, *S. epidermidis*

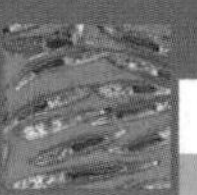

and β hemolytic streptococci. Mupirocin is used to treat impetigo, folliculitis and for treating infected skin injuries and ulcers. It is also used to eradicate *S. aureus* from the nose and to decrease *S. aureus* external infections in other situations. The possible occurrence of resistance should limit its use.

Antimycobacterial drugs

The rifamycins, aminoglycosides, fluoroquinolones, dapsone and the two newer macrolides, clarithromycin and azithromycin, are drugs discussed earlier. They are all used in the treatment of mycobacterial infections. Three additional drugs are used only to treat mycobacterial infections. These are isoniazid, pyrazinamide and ethambutol.

Isoniazid

Isoniazid (isonicotinic acid hydrazine) has an essential role in the treatment of tuberculosis. Mycobacteria, unlike conventional bacteria, have a cell wall that contains large quantities of lipid. One of the most important lipid constituents of mycobacteria is mycolic acid. Isoniazid inhibits the synthesis of mycolic acid and achieves bactericidal activity against *M. tuberculosis*. It has relatively low activity against non-tuberculous mycobacteria.

Isoniazid is a cornerstone drug in the treatment of tuberculosis

In general, the initial treatment of active tuberculosis requires a combination of isoniazid plus rifampin, together with at least one other antimycobacterial drug, until antibiotic susceptibility results are available. Most experts choose to start with four antimycobacterial drugs pending susceptibility results so as to minimize the risk of acquired resistance. In addition, an adjunct in the use of antituberculosis drugs is direct observation of the ingestion of each dose by a healthcare worker. Individuals with positive tuberculin skin tests (indicative of tuberculosis infection), but where activity is not diagnosed, are treated with isoniazid alone (i.e. preventive therapy) to prevent the development of active tuberculosis.

Isoniazid is well absorbed orally and is metabolized in the liver by acetylation. It achieves concentrations in the cerebrospinal fluid sufficient to treat tuberculous meningitis.

Isoniazid causes hepatitis and peripheral neuropathy

Isoniazid has several major adverse effects. It causes hepatitis, the risk of which increases with age, and underlying liver disease. It can also cause a peripheral neuropathy, particularly in malnourished individuals. This peripheral neuropathy can be prevented or reversed by pyridoxine administration. Isoniazid can also cause drug fever.

It increases serum concentrations of phenytoin when these drugs are administered concomitantly.

Pyrazinamide

Pyrazinamide is a synthetic analog of nicotinamide with bactericidal activity against *M. tuberculosis*. It is a prodrug that is converted by pyrazinamidase present in *M. tuberculosis* to pyrazinoic acid, which acts against intracellular organisms. It is commonly used together with isoniazid and rifampin as a first-line drug in tuberculosis but it not useful for other mycobacterial species.

Pyrazinamide is available only as an oral formulation and is metabolized in the liver.

Pyrazinamide can be hepatotoxic and cause hyperuricemia

Pyrazinamide can be hepatotoxic but, curiously, there is no increased hepatotoxicity when a regimen consisting of isoniazid, rifampin and pyrazinamide is used compared with a regimen of isoniazid and rifampin without pyrazinamide. Pyrazinamide also causes hyperuricemia and may rarely cause acute gouty arthritis.

Ethambutol

Ethambutol is active orally and is bacteriostatic against *M. tuberculosis* and several other slow-growing mycobacteria. Its precise mechanism of action is not known, but it is believed to inhibit bacterial RNA synthesis. The kidneys excrete it.

Ethambutol is only ever used in combination with other drugs in the treatment of disease due to *M. tuberculosis* and several nontuberculous mycobacterium species, particularly *M. avium* complex, *M. kansasii* and *M. marinum*.

Ethambutol can cause retrobulbar neuritis

Ethambutol is usually very well tolerated, but retrobulbar neuritis is a unique adverse effect. This is usually manifest first as red-green color blindness, and later as reduced visual acuity. The risk of this is both dose- and time-dependent. Baseline and serial visual acuity and color perception tests should be performed with long-term ethambutol therapy.

Other antitubercular drugs

In cases of multidrug-resistant *M. tuberculosis*, or if there are allergies, intolerance, or contraindications to the use of the main antitubercular drugs, second-line antitubercular drugs may be required. These include:

- Capreomycin and viomycin, parenteral polypeptide antibiotics.
- Ethionamide, an orally active drug chemically related to isoniazid.
- Cycloserine, an orally active drug that inhibits cell wall synthesis but causes considerable CNS toxicity.
- Para-aminosalicylic acid, an oral PABA analog that inhibits DHPS and is similar to sulfonamides and sulfones.
- Clofazimine, an orally active drug, that has a role in the treatment of leprosy.

Antibiotics of choice

The principles involved in the choice of antibiotic selection for particular conditions have all been outlined and discussed in the previous parts of this chapter. It is critical that all factors are considered.

The causal bacterium: its nature and characteristics

- The host: sex (and pregnancy status), age, general and particular health status, liver function, renal function, allergies.
- Drug factors: antibacterial spectrum, resistant organisms, pharmacodynamics (blood concentrations, how high and for how long), pharmacokinetics (metabolism and excretion). As an example, two patients infected with the identical organism may require different antibiotics because of:
  - Differences in the site of infection.
  - Drug allergies.
  - Underlying illness.
  - Concomitant drug therapy.
  - Age.
  - Pregnancy.

In the absence of allergies, pregnancy, other underlying illness and potential drug interactions, there are often accepted antibiotics of choice for common bacterial infections. The appropriate antibiotic choices for selected common pathogens are presented in Table 6.19.

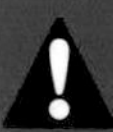

Adverse effects of antibiotics

- **Nearly all can cause *Clostridium difficile* enteritis**
- **Aminoglycosides can cause irreversible aplastic anemia and the gray baby syndrome**
- **Sulfonamides can cause a skin rash, Stevens–Johnson syndrome, and toxic epidermal necrolysis**
- **Tetracycline can discolor the teeth if given to children under 8 years of age**

FURTHER READING

Akins RL, Haase KK. Gram-positive resistance: pathogens, implications, and treatment options: insights from the Society of Infectious Diseases Pharmacists. *Pharmacotherapy* 2005; **25**: 1001–1010.

Boffito M, Acosta E, Burger D et al. Therapeutic drug monitoring and drug–drug interactions involving antiretroviral drugs. *Antivir Ther* 2005; **10**: 469–477.

Bratzler DW, Houck PM. Antimicrobial prophylaxis for surgery: An advisory statement from the National Surgical Infection Prevention Project. *Clin Infect Dis* 2004; **38**: 1706–1715. [Guidelines for the use of antibiotics in surgery.]

Dando TM, Perry CM. Related Enfuvirtide. *Drugs* 2003; **63**: 2755–2766.

Fraaij PL, van Kampen JJ, Burger DM, de Groot R. Pharmacokinetics of antiretroviral therapy in HIV-1-infected children. *Clin Pharmacokinet* 2005; **44**: 935–956.

MacDougall C, Polk RE. Antimicrobial stewardship programs in health care systems. *Clin Microbiol Rev* 2005; **18**: 638–656.

Medical Letter Choice of antibacterial drugs: Treatment guidelines. *Med Let* 2004; **2**: 13–26.

Onyebujoh P, Zumla A, Ribeiro I et al. Treatment of tuberculosis: present status and future prospects. *Bull World Health Organ* 2005; **83**: 857–865 [A world view of the problem of tuberculosis and its treatment with drugs.]

Rom WN, Gray SM eds. Tuberculosis: 2nd Edition. Lippincott, Williams & Wilkins, Philadelphia, 2004 [The definitive and current text on tuberculosis and its treatment with drugs with individual chapters on different antitubercular drugs.]

Shefet D, Robenshtok E, Paul M, Leibovici L. Empirical atypical coverage for inpatients with community-acquired pneumonia: systematic review of randomized controlled trials. *Arch Intern Med* 2005; **165**: 1992–2000.

USEFUL WEBSITES

http://www.cdc.gov/drug resistance/healthcare. [This site is a useful one for obtaining current information regarding resistance to antibiotics.]

http://www.nlm.nih.gov/medlineplus/antibiotics.html [Provides general information regarding bacteria and antibiotic drugs.]

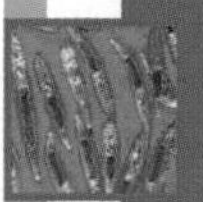

Table 6.19 Drugs of choice and alternatives for selected common bacterial pathogens

Bacterium	Drug(s) of choice	Alternatives	Comments
Streptococcus species	Penicillin	A first-generation cephalosporin Erythromycin Clindamycin Vancomycin	Some strains are penicillin-resistant, especially a growing proportion of *S. pneumoniae* Erythromycin is only for mild infections Vancomycin is only for serious infections Certain fluoroquinolones are active against *S. pneumoniae*
Enterococcus species	Penicillin or ampicillin plus gentamicin	Vancomycin plus gentamicin Quinupristin–dalfopristin Linezolid	There are some strains for which streptomycin is synergistic but gentamicin is not Some strains are resistant to synergy with any aminoglycoside Some strains are resistant to vancomycin (VRE)
Staphylococcus species	An antistaphylococcal penicillin	A first-generation cephalosporin Vancomycin	Vancomycin is required for methicillin-resistant strains Rifampin is occasionally used to eradicate the nasal carriage state
Neisseria meningitidis	Penicillin	A third-generation cephalosporin Chloramphenicol	Rare strains are penicillin-resistant
Neisseria gonorrhoeae	Cefixime	Ciprofloxacin A third-generation cephalosporin	Some strains are fluoroquinolone-resistant (especially in Asia)
Bordetella pertussis	Erythromycin	TMP-SMZ (trimethoprim–sulfamethoxazole)	Other macrolides are also active in vitro
Pasteurella multocida	Penicillin	A first-generation cephalosporin	
Haemophilus influenzae	Aminopenicillin	Cefuroxime A third-generation cephalosporin Chloramphenicol	Approximately 30% are aminopenicillin-resistant; therefore aminopenicillins should not be used empirically in serious infections until susceptibility results are available Rifampin is used to eradicate the nasal carriage state
Enterobacteriaceae in urine	TMP–SMZ	Ciprofloxacin Gentamicin	β Lactams are less effective than TMP–SMZ or fluoroquinolones for the treatment of urinary tract infection
Enterobacteriaceae in cerebrospinal fluid	A third-generation cephalosporin	Meropenem TMP–SMZ	In neonates only, aminoglycosides are equivalent to third-generation cephalosporins Experience with TMP–SMZ in meningitis is limited
Enterobacteriaceae elsewhere (blood, lung, etc.)	Gentamicin or a third-generation cephalosporin or ciprofloxacin	TMP–SMZ Carbapenems	Two-drug therapy is sometimes used in serious infection Monotherapy with a third-generation cephalosporin should be avoided if the pathogen is *Enterobacter cloacae, E. aerogenes, Serratia marcescens* or *Citrobacter freundii*
Pseudomonas aeruginosa	Antipseudomonal penicillin plus aminoglycoside	Ceftazidime Ciprofloxacin A carbapenem	Two-drug therapy recommended except for urinary tract infection
Bacteroides fragilis	Metronidazole or clindamycin	A carbapenem A penicillin β lactamase inhibitor	*B. fragilis* is usually involved in polymicrobial infections; therefore another antibiotic active against Enterobacteriaceae is often required
Mycoplasma pneumoniae	A macrolide (e.g. erythromycin)	A tetracycline	Although tetracyclines are as effective as macrolides, the latter are recommended because of better activity against *Pneumococcus*, which can mimic this infection
Ureaplasma urealyticum	A tetracycline	Erythromycin	A few strains are tetracycline-resistant
Mycoplasma hominis	A tetracycline	Clindamycin	Erythromycin is not active against *M. hominis*
Chlamydia trachomatis	A tetracycline	Azithromycin Erythromycin	Azithromycin is the only therapy effective in a single dose Erythromycin is used in pregnancy
Rickettsial species	A tetracycline	Chloramphenicol	
Listeria monocytogenes	Ampicillin plus gentamicin	Vancomycin plus gentamicin	
Legionella species	A macrolide	A tetracycline A fluoroquinolone	Rifampin is occasionally used as a second agent in severe cases
Clostridium difficile	Metronidazole	Vancomycin (oral)	
Mycobacterium tuberculosis	Isoniazid plus rifampin plus pyrazinamide plus ethambutol	Streptomycin A fluoroquinolone Ethionamide Cycloserine Viomycin Capreomycin	Directly observed therapy (DOT) is recommended Isoniazid is used alone for treatment of latent tubercular infection
Mycobacterium avium complex	Clarithromycin plus ethambutol ± rifabutin	Ciprofloxacin Amikacin	
Mycobacterium leprae	Dapsone plus rifampin ± clofazimine	Clarithromycin	Thalidomide is useful for erythema nodosum leprosum

PART 4

DRUGS AND FUNGI

BIOLOGY OF FUNGI

Fungi differ from higher plants in their structure, reproduction and nutrition. They lack chlorophyll, leaves, true stems, and roots, reproduce by spores, and live as saprophytes or parasites. The method of sexual reproduction of most pathogenic fungi is unknown (i.e. they are Fungi Imperfecti). Fungi that infect skin (dermatophytes) are classified according to their predominant ecologic site (Table 6.20).

Relatively few species of fungi are pathogenic, but when they are, pathogenicity results from:

- Mycotoxin production.
- Allergenicity.
- Tissue invasion.

Zoophilic (see Table 6.20) species tend to cause highly inflammatory skin reactions in humans, whereas anthropophilic species produce mild chronic lesions. The reactions are site-dependent and altered by the host's immune status. Opportunistic fungi are important causes of disease in immunosuppressed patients.

TREATMENT OF FUNGAL INFECTIONS

Most fungi are not affected by antibacterial drugs. There are few specific antifungal drugs and the use of many of these is restricted by their adverse effects.

A diagnosis of systemic fungal infection must be established before starting systemic treatment because many antifungal treatments have significant adverse effects

Certain fungi causing skin lesions, including *Microsporum* (e.g. *M. canis*, *M. audouinii*, *M. distortum*), produce a brilliant green fluorescence under Wood's ultraviolet light, whereas *Trichophyton schoenleinii* causes a paler green fluorescence of infected hair (Fig. 6.19). Wood's light can also be used to diagnose pityriasis versicolor as the scales usually fluoresce yellow.

Superficial skin mycoses can be diagnosed by microscopy and culture of skin scrapings, plucked (not cut) hairs, or nail clippings. Systemic mycoses can be diagnosed by microscopy and culture of pus, exudate, tissue biopsy, feces, urine, sputum, spinal fluid or blood.

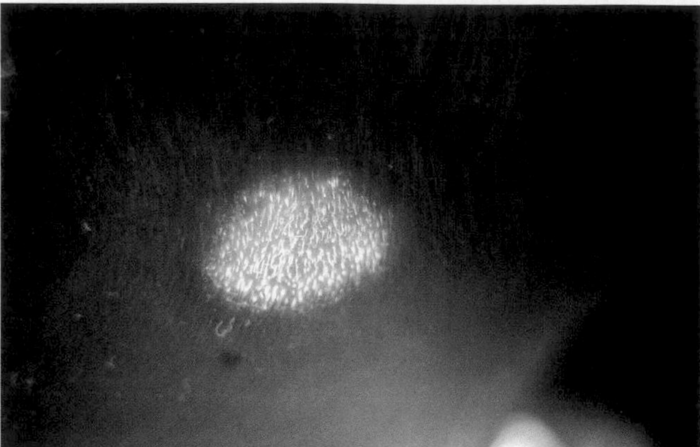

Fig. 6.19 Tinea capitis. Note the characteristic fluorescence under Wood's light. (Courtesy of Dr. Richard Staughton.)

Serologic tests are available mainly in specialist laboratories, and help in the diagnosis of many mycoses (Table 6.21). Skin tests are useful diagnostically only if a patient has recently visited an endemic area for the first time, but may be of value for sporotrichosis and *Aspergillus* hypersensitivity. Positive tests have no diagnostic value in ringworm and candidal infections and are of limited significance in histoplasmosis and coccidioidomycosis.

General measures applied to infected patients

The spread of infection must be minimized (e.g. children should stay away from school until treatment is established (*M. canis*) or until there is no fluorescence and the hair has regrown (anthropophilic species). Topical treatment should be used. Schoolchildren should be screened with Wood's ultraviolet light and scalp massage techniques for early diagnosis and treatment.

Advice regarding the likely source of infection can be given if the species of fungus is known (e.g. treatment of infected pets or prophylactic antifungal dusting powder after swimming).

Table 6.20 Classification of fungi according to site of origin

Origin	Name
Soil	Geophilic
Animals	Zoophilic
Human skin	Anthropophilic

Table 6.21 Availability and usefulness of serologic tests in diagnosing fungal infections

Serologic test useful	Serologic test useful for deep-seated infection	Serologic test useful, but not widely available
Histoplasmosis	Candidiasis	Sporotrichosis
Coccidioidomycosis	Cryptococcosis	Mycetoma
Blastomycosis		Nocardiosis
Aspergillosis (sometimes)		Chromomycosis
		Zygomycosis

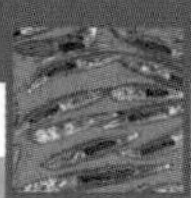

Preventive measures should be taken for patients at high risk (e.g. frequent oral toilet, adequate denture care, and careful attention to drying and ventilation of skin fold areas in the seriously ill can help prevent candidiasis).

Antifungal drugs

The three main classes of antifungal drug are the polyene macrolides, the antifungal azoles and the allylamines (Table 6.22).

Table 6.22 Antifungal medicines and their routes of administration

Drug class	Drug name	Routes of administration
Polyene macrolides	Amphotericin B	T, I, P
	Nystatin	T (O for GI tract only)
	Natamycin	T
	Candicidin	T
Azoles		
Imidazoles	Clotrimazole	T
	Miconazole	T, I
	Ketoconazole	T, O
	Isoconazole	T
	Tioconazole	T
	Econazole	T
	Sulconazole	T
	Terconazole	T
	Oxiconazole	T
	Butoconazole	T
Triazoles	Fluconazole	O
	Itraconazole	O
Allylamines	Naftifine	T
	Terbinafine	T, O
Other	Griseofulvin	O
	Amorolfine	T
	Flucytosine	O

GI, gastrointestinal; I, intravenous; O, oral; P, parenteral; T, topical.

Polyene macrolide antibiotics

AMPHOTERICIN B This antifungal antibiotic is produced by *Streptomyces nodosus*. It binds to ergosterol in the fungal cell membrane (Fig. 6.20) with the formation of 'amphotericin pores' (Fig. 6.21), resulting in a loss of macromolecules and ions from the fungus, and irreversible damage.

Amphotericin is poorly absorbed from the gastrointestinal (GI) tract and is therefore effective orally only for GI fungal infections. Given parenterally, it is highly protein bound (90%) and penetration into body fluids and tissues is poor. Toxicity is common and a test dose should be administered and subsequent administration closely supervised with monitoring of liver and renal function, electrolytes and blood counts. The drug should be administered slowly by infusion to minimize the risk of cardiac arrhythmias. Prophylactic antipyretics or glucocorticosteroids should not be co-administered except to treat anaphylactic reactions, which are rare. The drug is also nephrotoxic and neurotoxic. In addition, pain and thrombophlebitis can occur at the injection site.

Binding to cholesterol (e.g. on red blood cell membranes) may account for some of amphotericin's adverse effects.

Amphotericin is excreted in the urine over several days. Only 2–3% of the blood level is achieved in the cerebrospinal fluid after i.v. injection, so intrathecal (or intracisternal) injection is necessary for fungal meningitis.

Use of amphotericin encapsulated in liposomes reduces its toxicity. It can also be complexed with sodium cholesteryl sulfate. These newer preparations are indicated for severe systemic fungal infections and invasive candidiasis where amphotericin alone is contraindicated due to its renal toxicity.

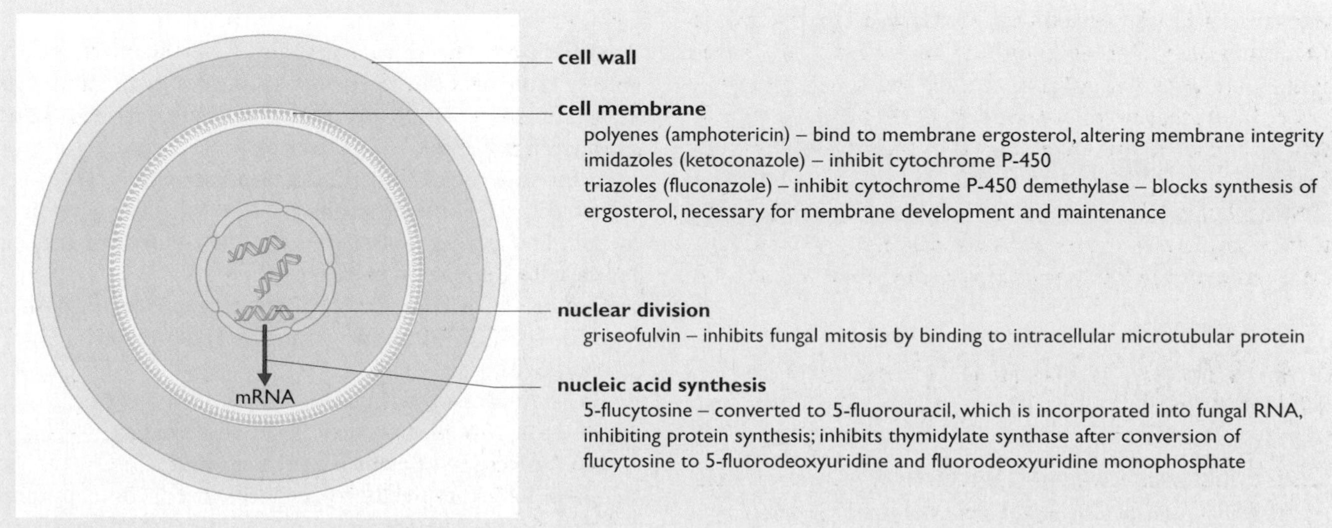

cell wall
cell membrane
polyenes (amphotericin) – bind to membrane ergosterol, altering membrane integrity
imidazoles (ketoconazole) – inhibit cytochrome P-450
triazoles (fluconazole) – inhibit cytochrome P-450 demethylase – blocks synthesis of ergosterol, necessary for membrane development and maintenance
nuclear division
griseofulvin – inhibits fungal mitosis by binding to intracellular microtubular protein
mRNA
nucleic acid synthesis
5-flucytosine – converted to 5-fluorouracil, which is incorporated into fungal RNA, inhibiting protein synthesis; inhibits thymidylate synthase after conversion of flucytosine to 5-fluorodeoxyuridine and fluorodeoxyuridine monophosphate

Fig. 6.20 Sites of action of antifungal drugs. (Adapted from *Human Pharmacology: Molecular to Clinical* by Brody, Larner, Minneman and Neu, Mosby-Year Book Inc., 1994.)

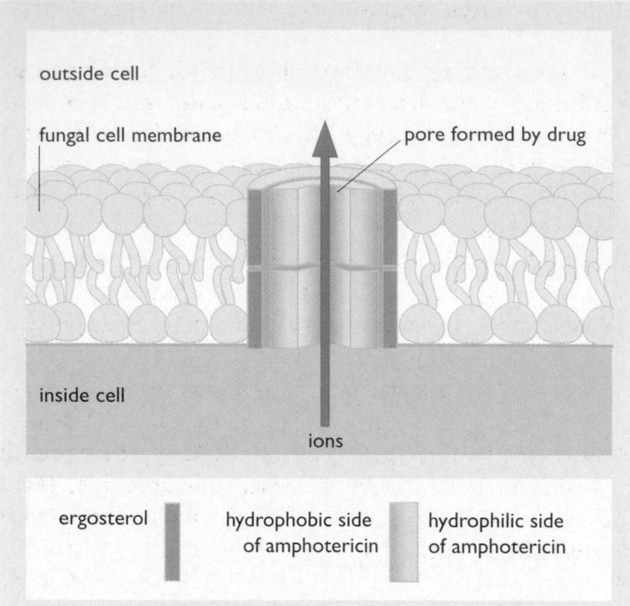

Fig. 6.21 Mechanism of action of polyene antifungal drugs. Binding to ergosterol damages the membrane, with leakage of ions, and leads to irreversible fungal cell damage. (Adapted from *Human Pharmacology: Molecular to Clinical* by Brody, Larner, Minneman and Neu, Mosby-Year Book Inc., 1994.)

Intravenous amphotericin for treatment of systemic fungal infections (see Treatment indications, below) must be given cautiously. An initial dose is administered with careful monitoring, and then a slow infusion, with gradual increases in dose until there is a therapeutic response. Daily treatment often has to be continued for 6–12 weeks. Longer-term treatment, on alternate days, (this is sufficient once a steady state is achieved) is often needed to maintain blood levels.

Amphotericin resistance can develop if the fungus alters the amount of ergosterol in membrane or modifies its structure so that the drug binds less avidly.

Topical amphotericin is used to treat mucosal candidiasis.

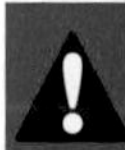

Adverse effects following i.v. infusion of amphotericin

- Fever
- Chills
- Hypotension
- Vomiting
- Dyspnea
- Headaches
- Thrombophlebitis at the site of injection
- Renal toxicity is invariable, but treatment can be continued to a creatinine concentration of 200 mmol/liter

NYSTATIN Nystatin is a polyene macrolide with a similar mechanism of action to amphotericin. It is stable when dry, but quickly disintegrates on contact with water or plasma. It is not absorbed from skin, mucous membranes or the GI tract. Orally administered nystatin is excreted in the feces. It is too toxic for parenteral administration. Its clinical use is limited to topical applications to the skin and mucous membranes (buccal and vaginal), and oral administration to suppress *Candida* in the gut of infants and those with impaired immunity. Resistance to nystatin does not develop in vivo, but some *Candida* species are innately not susceptible.

NATAMYCIN Natamycin is a polyene antifungal agent used as a 5% ophthalmic suspension.

CANDICIDIN Candicidin is a polyene antibiotic used topically for vaginal candidiasis.

Antifungal azoles

Imidazoles and triazoles:

- Inhibit fungal lipid (especially ergosterol) synthesis in cell membranes.
- Interfere with fungal oxidative enzymes (primarily the 14α-demethylase microsomal P-450-dependent enzyme), resulting in accumulation of 14α-methyl sterols, which may disrupt the packing of acyl chains of phospholipids, thereby inhibiting growth, and interfering with membrane-bound enzyme systems (see Fig. 6.20).

Triazoles are more selective for fungi than imidazoles, and cause less endocrine disturbance.

These agents are available mainly for topical use; clotrimazole is too toxic to use systemically. Intravenous miconazole can be used for disseminated mycoses, but is limited by its adverse effects (vomiting, hyponatremia, hyperlipidemia, thrombophlebitis, hematologic disturbances).

KETOCONAZOLE Ketoconazole was the first orally active azole antifungal drug. It is less toxic and less effective than amphotericin. However, it has been associated with fatal hepatotoxicity and should not be used for superficial fungal infections. It is well absorbed, although CSF concentrations are low. It is largely protein bound, and is metabolized by the liver (see Interactions below). Ketoconazole is indicated for:

- Serious chronic resistant mucocutaneous candidiasis (1–2 weeks; 4–10 months for mucocutaneous candidiasis).
- Resistant dermatophyte infections (3–8 weeks).
- Systemic infections, particularly disseminated blastomycosis, but not fungal meningitis.

Liver function needs to be monitored clinically and biochemically. Ketoconazole should be avoided in pregnancy, breastfeeding mothers and patients with porphyria. It has important drug interactions (see below).

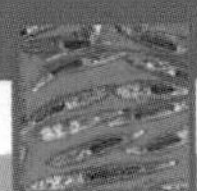

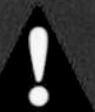

Adverse effects of ketoconazole

- Nausea
- Vomiting
- Photophobia
- Skin rashes
- Hepatotoxicity
- Mild elevation of hepatic enzymes (5–10%)
- Symptomatic hepatitis is rare, but progressive fatal hepatotoxicity is reported with high doses so liver function tests required at regular intervals
- Gynecomastia and reduced libido
- Menstrual irregularities (10% of women)
- High-dose ketoconazole should be avoided in patients with tuberculosis, histoplasmosis, paracoccidioidomycosis and AIDS

FLUCONAZOLE Fluconazole (a bistriazole) is used in the treatment of local and systemic candidiasis and cryptococcal infections. It is more readily absorbed from the GI tract than ketoconazole and penetrates the blood–brain barrier, producing CSF concentrations 50–80% of those in the blood. It is excreted by the kidneys unchanged, so its half-life is considerably prolonged in renal insufficiency.

Skin, genital and mucosal candidiasis; cutaneous dermatophyte infections; pityriasis versicolor and invasive candidiasis can all be treated with fluconazole. It can be used for systemic infections including cryptococcal meningitis, although relapse is common. It has a prophylactic role in immunocompromised patients following cytotoxic chemotherapy or radiotherapy, and in preventing relapse of cryptococcal meningitis in AIDS.

Adverse effects include vomiting, diarrhea and rashes (including Stevens–Johnson syndrome). Thrombocytopenia and transient abnormalities of hepatic function also occur, but there seem to be no effects on the endocrine system. Animal studies suggest that it is teratogenic.

ITRACONAZOLE Itraconazole is a synthetic dioxolane triazole. It is useful in the treatment of oropharyngeal and vulvovaginal candidiasis, pityriasis versicolor, tinea corporis and tinea pedis. It is used for systemic infections such as histoplasmosis and in aspergillosis, candidiasis and cryptococcosis where other antifungal drugs are inappropriate or ineffective.

Absorption from the GI tract is incomplete, but it increases when itraconazole is taken with food. It is 99% protein bound and concentrates in tissues including lung, liver and bone, but has limited CSF penetration. It is excreted by the liver and has one active metabolite, with a half-life of 20–40 hours, which is also excreted by the liver. In neutropenic patients, a loading dose should be given for the first 4 days and a maintenance dose of 400 mg is often required to achieve adequate serum levels.

Itraconazole is generally well tolerated, though nausea, vomiting, headaches, abdominal pain and transient increases in hepatic enzymes can occur. Liver function tests should be monitored in patients with a history of liver disease. Bioavailability may be reduced in patients with renal impairment, and blood levels should be measured in patients with AIDS and neutropenia where absorption can be reduced. The drug should be discontinued if patients develop a peripheral neuropathy.

VARICONAZOLE Variconazole is a recently introduced drug that is more selective for fungal cytochrome P-450 than mammalian CYP-450s. The most frequently reported adverse effects are visual disturbances, fever, rash, which along with elevated liver function tests, led to discontinuation of therapy.

RESISTANCE TO THE AZOLE DRUGS This is rare, but resistant *Candida* strains have been isolated from patients with chronic mucocutaneous candidiasis and AIDS.

IMPORTANT INTERACTIONS OF AZOLE DRUGS These drugs will:

- Increase the phenytoin, oral hypoglycemic, anticoagulant and ciclosporin plasma concentrations (by inhibition of CYP-450).
- Increase simvastatin myotoxicity.

Azole absorption is reduced by antacids, cimetidine or rifampin, and increased by thiazide diuretics. The use of azole drugs together with certain H_1 receptor antagonists or cisapride induces a particular arrhythmia (torsades de pointes).

Allylamines

NAFTIFINE Naftifine is an allylamine naphthalene derivative for topical use. It inhibits the enzyme squalene epoxidase and decreases ergosterol synthesis.

TERBINAFINE Terbinafine is the first orally active allylamine. It prevents ergosterol synthesis by inhibiting squalene epoxidase, resulting in squalene accumulation, which leads to membrane disruption and cell death (Fig. 6.22).

Terbinafine is well absorbed, and is concentrated in the dermis, epidermis and adipose tissue (because it is lipophilic). It is secreted in sebum and appears in the stratum corneum hours after oral administration. It also diffuses from the nail bed, penetrating distal nails within 4 weeks. It is metabolized in the liver and the inactive metabolites are excreted in urine. It is effective mainly against dermatophytes. Clinical trials show impressive clinical and mycologic cure and reduced relapse rates (Table 6.23).

Terbinafine is well tolerated. Nausea, abdominal pain and allergic skin reactions can occur, but are usually mild. Loss of taste has been reported. Terbinafine concentra-

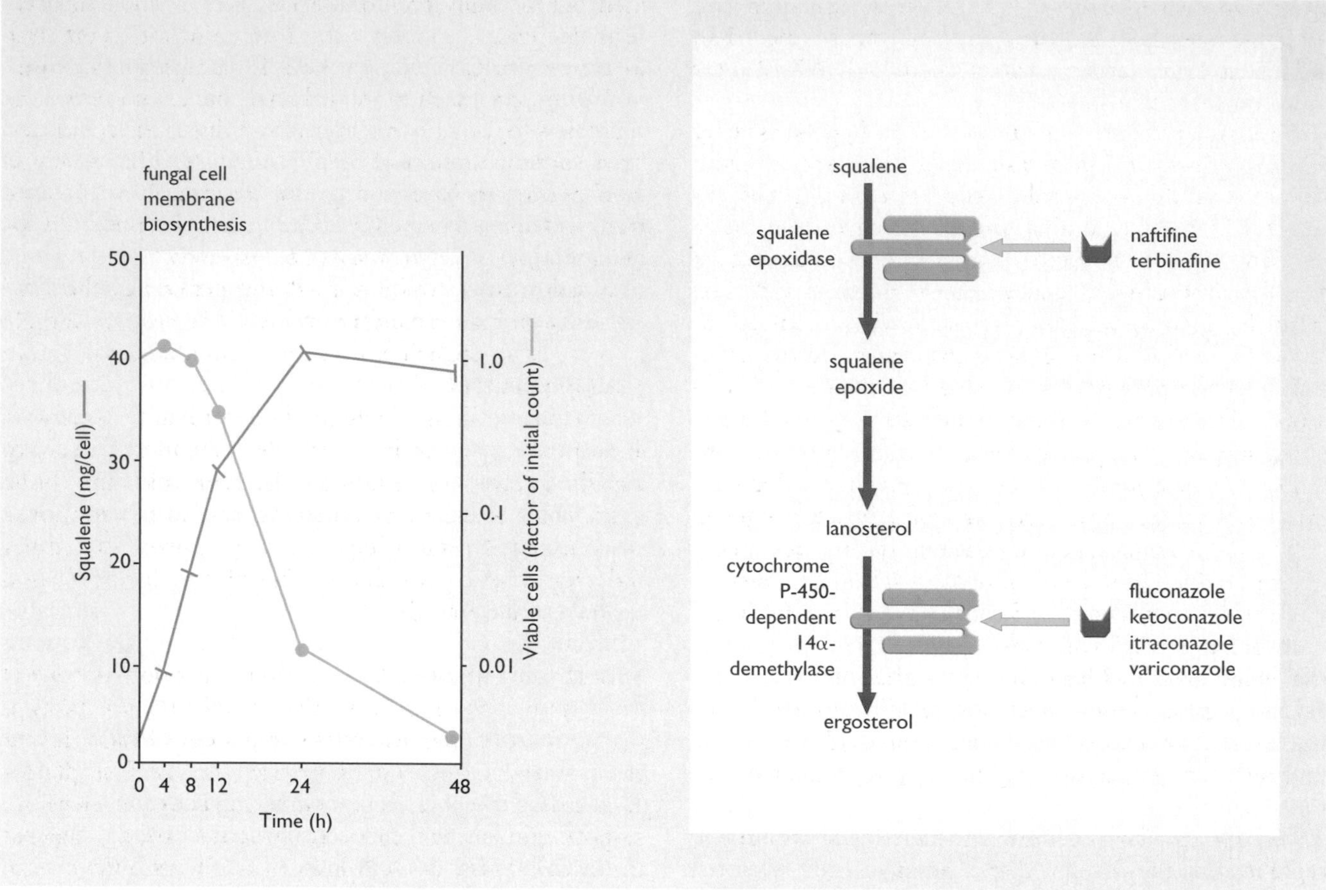

Fig. 6.22 Terbinafine inhibits squalene epoxidase, resulting in the accumulation of squalene in fungal cells. This accumulation of squalene (red line) correlates with cell death (blue line). (Adapted from Ryder NS, *Clin Exp Dermatol* 1989; **14**: 98–100.)

Table 6.23 Effectiveness of terbinafine

Infection	Dosage	Clinical cure (%)	Mycologic cure (%)	Relapse rate (%)
Tinea unguium	250 mg 12 wks		81–88	
Tinea pedis	250 mg 2 wks	87	78	Low 6/52 later
Tinea corporis/cruris	250–500 mg	85	92	80% cure at 3–12 month follow-up
Onychomycosis (hands)	250–500 mg	85	95	
Onychomycosis (toes)	250–500 mg	80	80	
Candidiasis	500 mg 4 wks	70	80	

tions are increased by cimetidine and reduced by co-administration with rifampin.

Other antifungal drugs

GRISEOFULVIN Griseofulvin was the original, orally active, antifungal drug. It is isolated from *Penicillium griseofulvum*. Its mechanism of action is not established, but it probably interferes with fungal microtubule function or nucleic acid synthesis and polymerization. It inhibits dermatophyte growth, but has no effect on the fungi producing deep mycoses, or on *Candida* species. Absorption varies according to the drug preparation used, but microparticle preparations are better absorbed, peaking 1–3 hours after ingestion. Serum concentrations decrease after 30 hours. It is concentrated in actively metabolizing cells of the skin and passes rapidly into fully keratinized cells, reaching the outermost cells in 8 hours, but is not thought to bind firmly to keratin. Since sweat transports griseofulvin in the stratum corneum, excessive sweating can cause rapid clearance from the skin. Griseofulvin is metabolized in the liver to 6-demethyl griseofulvin, which is excreted via the kidneys and perhaps bile.

Although griseofulvin has been largely superseded by the azole drugs in adult practice, it remains the treatment of choice for childhood dermatophyte infections (10 mg/

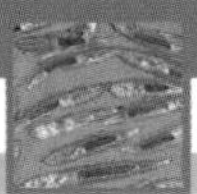

kg in two divided doses). The treatment schedules are prolonged because the drug is fungistatic rather than fungicidal. Long-term relapse rates are high (40–70% for infections of toenails).

Adverse effects are uncommon, but a hypersensitivity reaction with fever, skin rash, leukopenia and a serum sickness-like illness is well recognized. Headaches are common, and irritability and nightmares can be a problem, but usually improve on continuing the drug. If not, the dose can be reduced for a few days and then gradually increased, giving most of the treatment at night. Griseofulvin can cause light sensitivity eruptions and petechial rashes, and has also been associated with urticarial rashes, which improve despite continued treatment. Hepatotoxicity, peripheral neuritis, bone marrow suppression, proteinuria and estrogen-like effects in children have been described. Griseofulvin is teratogenic.

Griseofulvin resistance can develop during treatment.

Griseofulvin interacts with other drugs, including:

- Warfarin, increasing warfarin's metabolism and thus reducing the anticoagulant effect.
- Phenobarbital, with simultaneous oral treatment reducing the blood concentration of griseofulvin.

Griseofulvin exacerbates porphyria, and reportedly precipitates or exacerbates systemic lupus erythematosus.

AMOROLFINE This is a recently introduced antifungal, available as a nail lacquer, that is fungicidal for dermatophytes and has some activity against molds.

FLUCYTOSINE This drug is active orally and interferes with nucleic acid synthesis by inhibiting thymidylate synthetase. It is active only in cells able to transport it into the cell via a cytosine permease and convert flucytosine to 5-fluorouracil. This is then metabolized by fungal uridine monophosphate pyrophosphorylase and can be incorporated into RNA or metabolized to 5-fluorodeoxyuridylic acid, a potent fungal thymidylate synthetase inhibitor. Fungal DNA synthesis is disrupted as a result.

The clinical usefulness of flucytosine is limited by the rapid development of resistance, and this is partly delayed by co-administration of amphotericin B. The proposed mechanisms include loss of the permease for cytosine transport or decreased uridine monophosphate pyrophosphorylase or cytosine deaminase activity.

Flucytosine is well absorbed and penetrates the CSF (60–80% of serum concentrations). It is excreted largely unchanged in the urine, so the dose should be reduced in renal impairment.

Adverse effects include hepatotoxicity (enzyme abnormalities occur in about 5% of patients, but are usually reversible), enterocolitis, hair loss and bone marrow suppression. Blood counts should be monitored weekly. Uracil reduces bone marrow suppression without reducing antifungal efficacy. The plasma concentration should be monitored.

CASPOFUNGIN ACETATE Caspofungin acetate is a novel orally active antifungal drug that inhibits the synthesis of β(1,3)-D-glucon, an essential component of the cell wall of the various species of *Aspergillus* and *Candida*. β(1,3)-D-glucon is not present in mammalian cells and therefore caspofungin acetate provides selective toxicity against these fungal infections. Nonetheless, adverse effects have been reported with this drug, including isolated reports of rash, pruritus and anaphylaxis. Caspofungin acetate has a serum half-life of 9–11 hours and is not adversely influenced by food.

Treatment indications of antifungal drugs

A summary of the effectiveness of antifungal drugs is shown in Table 6.24.

Table 6.24 Treatment indication of antifungal agents

Infection	Amphotericin B	Ketoconazole	Fluconazole	Itraconazole	Terbinafine	Griseofulvin	Flucytosine	Caspofungin
Dermatophytes		x		x	x	x		
Pityrosporum		x		x				
Candidiasis	xC	x	x	x	x	x		x
Aspergillosis	x	x		x		x		x
Blastomycosis	x	x		x				
Coccidioidomycosis	x	x		x				
Cryptococcosis		x	x				x	
Histoplasmosis	x	x		x				
Paracoccidioidomycosis	x	x		x			x	
Chromoblastomycosis								
Sporotrichosis	x			x				
Mucormycosis	x						x	
Torulopsis								
Pseudoallescheriasis		x						
Zygomycosis		x						

C, amphotericin B used in combination with flucytosine.

Table 6.26 Origins and chemical groupings of antiparasitic drugs

Natural origins
- Quinine and quinidine – botanical from *Chincona* sp. – a quinoline derivative
- Artemisinin and related compounds – botanical from *Artemisia* sp. 5-member non-nitrogenous ring
- Ivermectins – from a soil fungus (milbemycin analog)

Antibiotics (antibacterials) – see Drugs and Fungi
- Tetracycline, doxycycline
- Metronidazole, tinidazole, seconidazole, ornidazole, benznidazole
- Clindamycin
- Paromomycin – an aminoglycoside
- Amphotericin B
- Pyrimethamine–sulfadoxine

Organometallo compounds and dyes
- Stibogluconate, meglumine antimoniate
- Arsenicals – melarsen, melarsoprol
- Suramin – from trypan red and blue

Synthetics

N-containing rings
- Quinolines – chloroquine
- Aminoquinolines – primaquine, mefloquine, oxamniquine
- Isoquinoline – praziquantel
- Nitrofuranes – nifurtimox
- Piperazine – piperazine, diethylcarbamazine
- Diaminopyrimidines – pyrantel, oxantel, pyrimethamine

Diamidines
- Pentamidine, diminazene, pentamidine isoethionate
- Acridine
- Quinacrine

Benzimidazoles
- Thiabendazole, mebendazole, albendazole

Organophosphate
- Metrifonate

Other with miscellaneous chemistry
- Atovaquone, eflornithine, diloxanide, proguanil, miltofesine, biotionol, triclabendazole

dyes provided early antiparasitic drugs because of their established ability to bind to parasitic organisms. Some antibacterial drugs have been found to be useful in parasitical infections, sometimes because of similarity of biochemical mechanisms between bacteria and parasites. Thus, there a wide variety of antiparasitic drugs, as shown in Table 6.26.

The process of discovering new antiparasitic drugs has been a mixture of chance, dedicated research and serendipity mixed with political and social factors. Thus, the need to protect troops from malaria in tropical areas led to the creation of many new antimalarial drugs during the 1940s. As the examples in Table 6.26 show, systematic studies around a particular chemical motif led to series of related drugs. Despite the wide variety of types of drugs, one or two of them stand out as having wide utility for may parasites; examples include ivermectin, praziquantel, the benzimidazoles for helminths, metronidazole, eflornithine and chloroquine for protozoans.

In the following, the major parasite infections will be considered in relation to the drugs used to treat those infections. The appropriate pharmacology, pharmacodynamics and pharmacokinetics will be discussed for protozoans and then helminths.

DRUGS AND PROTOZOA

Malaria is the parasite with the greatest mortality and cost to man. It is therefore considered first. In addition, it serves as a good exemplar of the problems associated with the life cycle of the parasite, development of drug resistance and the continuing search for better drugs.

Malaria

Malaria is a protozoan disease that is usually transmitted by a certain species of mosquitoes. Thus, the malaria has two separate hosts, each of which plays a special role in the life cycle of the parasite

Malaria is the most important parasitic disease in tropical medicine. Worldwide, there are 200 million malaria cases each year and 2 million deaths due to malaria. It is endemic in more than 100 countries in Africa, Asia, Oceania, Central and South America, and certain Caribbean islands. Approximately 60% of the world's population live in those countries.

There are four species of malaria parasites (Plasmodia)

Malaria is usually transmitted by anopheline mosquitoes and rarely by congenital transmission, transfusion of infected blood, or the use of contaminated syringes. The four species of plasmodial parasites are:

- *Plasmodium falciparum*, which is widely distributed, results in the most severe infections and accounts for nearly all malaria-related deaths (Fig. 6.23a).
- *P. vivax* is also widespread and is responsible for a more benign form of the disease than *P. malariae* and *P. ovale* (Fig. 6.23b).
- *P. malariae* is also widespread.
- *P. ovale* is confined mainly to Africa.

The four species of malaria

- ***Plasmodium falciparum*** **causes the most severe infection; its resistance to antimalarial drugs is a major problem**
- ***P. vivax*** **causes a more benign disease, as do *P. malariae* and *P. ovale***
- ***P. vivax*** **and *P. ovale* have relapsing forms that are harbored in the liver**
- ***P. ovale*** **is mainly confined to Africa**

The clinical features of infection with malaria depend on the species of the parasite and immunologic status of the host

Acute falciparum malaria is a potentially fatal disease, and non-immune travelers to areas where falciparum malaria

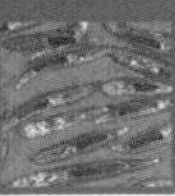

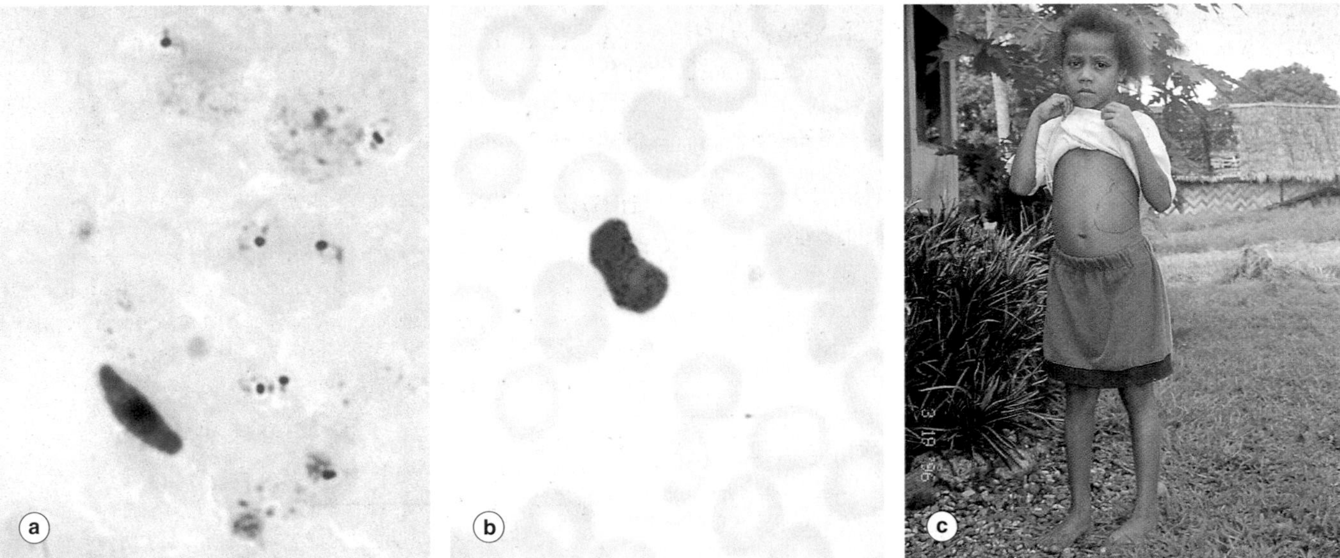

Fig. 6.23 Malaria. (a) *Plasmodium falciparum*, ring forms and a gametocyte stained by Giemsa thick smear. (b) *P. vivax*, a mature trophozoite in an enlarged erythrocyte stained by Giemsa, thin smear. (c) A schoolgirl with anemia and splenomegaly, Vanuatu, the Southwest Pacific.

is endemic risk severe infection. Acute malaria occurs where exposure is limited, or seasonal, and where the collective immunity in the area is relatively low. In these circumstances it can occur as epidemics and affect all age groups. Complications include cerebral malaria, hypoglycemia, pulmonary edema, acute renal failure and massive intravascular hemolysis. Chronic repeated infection often leads to splenomegaly and progressive anemia (see Fig. 6.23c). There is a particularly high risk of death among untreated pregnant women with falciparum malaria, especially where transmission is intermittent. The fetus of such women is inevitably exposed to the effects of placental insufficiency.

Infants born to immune mothers living in holoendemic areas are unlikely to acquire malaria for several months after birth, largely due to passive transfer of maternal antibodies across the placenta. Thereafter, they are subject to severe, recurrent acute attacks that are potentially fatal during infancy and early childhood. From the age of 5 years until adulthood, the severity and frequency of these attacks decrease as immunity develops.

Clinically significant malaria is uncommon among adults (other than pregnant women and immunocompromised individuals) who have always lived in areas of high transmission.

Antimalarial drugs target the different phases of the malaria parasite's life cycle

The malaria parasite's life cycle (Fig. 6.24) includes:

- Sporozoites, which are produced in the mosquito vectors from the sexual forms of the parasite and which migrate to the salivary glands (sporogony).
- Once injected into the human blood stream, the sporozoites rapidly penetrate the parenchymal cells of the liver where they transform and grow into large tissue schizonts containing considerable numbers of merozoites (a process known as exo-red blood cell schizogony).
- The large tissue schizonts begin to rupture after 5–20 days (depending upon species) and the released merozoites then invade circulating red blood cells where they rapidly multiply.
- The host red blood cells eventually rupture, so releasing merozoites, which then invade and destroy more red blood cells in a vicious cycle.
- Some merozoites develop into male and female gametocytes, so the infected human becomes a reservoir of infection for mosquitoes, thus completing the transmission cycle.

The destruction of red blood cells, and subsequent release of the waste products of the parasites, produce the episodic (at intervals of days characteristic for each species of parasite) chills and fever that are so characteristic of the disease. Certain tissue forms of *P. vivax* and *P. ovale* persist in the liver as hypnozoites for months and even years and are responsible for the relapses that are characteristic of these forms of malaria. Hypnozoites are not generated by *P. falciparum* or *P. malariae*. Recrudescence of infections results from persistent blood forms in inadequately treated or untreated patients.

The choice of which drug(s) to treat malaria depends on the species of parasite, drug bioavailability, metabolism, adverse effects and host immunity

Since the effectiveness of a drug against malarial infections is a function of interactions between malaria parasites, antimalarial drugs and human host, the choice of drug depends on:

- Species of infecting parasite and its stage of development. Drug resistance among different

Trichomoniasis

Trichomoniasis is a flagellate protozoan disease caused by *Trichomonas vaginalis*. It is sexually transmitted and the most common protozoan infection in the world. *Trichomonas* species have only a trophozoite stage which is transmitted from host to host. The infection can be asymptomatic in men, but usually causes vaginitis, cystitis and cervicitis in women.

Drug treatment of trichomoniasis is with metronidazole or tinidazole.

Pneumocystosis

Pneumocystosis is caused by *Pneumocystis carinii*. This organism was previously classified as both a protozoan parasite and a fungus. Recently, several studies have reported *P. carinii* as being an organism more closely related to fungi than protozoans. *P. carinii* is a common cause of opportunistic infection in immunocompromised patients with HIV or malnourishment. *P. carinii* pneumonia is a frequent immediate cause of death in AIDS patients.

Drug treatment of pneumocystosis is with high-dose trimethoprim–sulfamethoxazole or pentamidine isethionate. These two drugs have a similar antiprotozoan spectrum and independently inhibit different steps in the protozoan enzymic synthesis of tetrahydrofolic acid (see Drugs and Bacteria in this chapter, above).

Adverse effects of trimethoprim–sulfamethoxazole are common and include nausea, vomiting, glossitis and skin rashes. Hypersensitivity reactions can be severe (e.g. Stevens–Johnson syndrome), while agranulocytosis, aplastic anemia and thrombocytopenic purpura may also occur. Trimethoprim–sulfamethoxazole is contraindicated in people with known hypersensitivity and severe renal dysfunction.

Pentamidine isethionate has an antiprotozoan activity effective (see Trypanosomiasis, above) in *P. carinii* infection. The recommended dose is 4 mg/kg/day for 14 days, either by slow i.v. infusion over at least 60 minutes or by intramuscular injection.

Adverse effects of pentamidine isethionate include nephrotoxicity, which is common and usually completely reversible. Other common adverse effects are hypotension, hypoglycemia and syncope, which occur after rapid i.v. infusion. Pentamidine isethionate is contraindicated in people with known hypersensitivity and severe renal dysfunction.

DRUGS AND HELMINTH INFECTIONS

Helminths are divided into three major groups, nematodes (roundworms), trematodes (flukes) and cestodes (tapeworms). All are metazoans with multicellular structures and specific organs. Most helminths do not replicate in the human host. Very commonly, infections with helminths produce eosinophilia in the host. The relationships and biology of helminths are summarized in Table 6.28.

The eggs of nematodes (roundworms, hookworms, and whipworms) require residence in the soil in order to mature into an infectious phase. As a result, transmission is difficult when high levels of hygiene are practiced. Roundworms (*Ascaris* spp.) are ingested and migrate through the lungs into the intestine. Hookworm parasites

Table 6.28 The helminths responsible for parasitic diseases

	Helminths	
Nematodes	**Trematodes**	**Cestodes**
Intestinal forms ***Intestinal migration*** *Trichurus* *Enterobius* *Trichurus*	**Hermaphrodite forms** *Clonorchis* *Fasciola* *Faciolopsis*	**Species where human is the immediate host** *Taenia* *Echinococcus* *Hymenolepis*
Pulmonary migration *Ascaris* *Ancylostoma* *Necator* *Strongyloides*	**Schistosomic form** *Schistosoma*	**Species where human is not the immediate host** *Taenia solium* (pig) *Diphyllobothrium* (fish)
Tissue forms ***Humans not necessary host*** *Toxocara* (cats and dogs) *Trichinella* *Ancylostoma*	***Human necessary host*** *Wucheria* *Brugia* *Onchocerca* *Loa* *Dracunulus*	

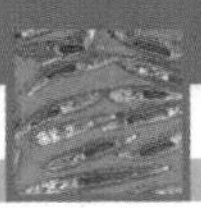

(*Acylostoma duodenale*, *Necator americanus*) enter through the skin while their life cycle includes residence in the lungs, and migration to the intestines. Whipworm (*Trichurus* spp.) is widespread in the tropics.

Drugs and roundworms

Ascariasis

■ *Ascariasis is due to an intestinal nematode acquired from contaminated vegetables and drinking-water*

Ascariasis is caused by *Ascaris lumbricoides* and is the most prevalent helminthic infection in the world. It is acquired by ingesting mature eggs in contaminated vegetables and drinking-water. The adult nematode usually lives in the small intestine. It can migrate to the main bile duct, gall bladder and pancreatic duct, or penetrate the small intestinal wall, resulting in sporadic infection. Clinical manifestations include dull upper abdominal pain, loss of appetite, nausea, vomiting and abdominal distention.

■ *Ascariasis is treated with pyrantel pamoate or piperazine*

Pyrantel pamoate, a broad-spectrum anthelminthic, was first introduced into veterinary medicine but now is the drug of choice for treating ascariasis. Chemically, it has a six-membered nitrogen-containing ring linked via an ethylene bridge to a furan ring. It acts as a depolarizing neuromuscular blocker that opens nonselective cation channels of the nicotininc receptor type so as to produce a depolarizing neuromuscular block in the parasite. It therefore causes a spastic paralysis and slow contracture of the worms. Its actions are antagonized by piperazine (see below).

Pyrantel and its derivatives are also used to treat *Enterobius vermicularis* and hookworm infections, but is inactive against *T. trichiura*. However, its cogener, oxypantel, is active against the latter species.

Since pyrantel pamoate is poorly absorbed from the gastrointestinal tract it can achieve relatively high concentrations in the intestine. Most of the drug is excreted in feces.

Adverse effects (headache, dizziness, rash and fever, and gastrointestinal upset) of pyrantel pamoate are usually rare and relatively mild when it is used at normal doses. It is usually given as a single oral dose of 5–10 mg/kg. At very high doses in animals it can produce neuromuscular blockade.

Piperazine is highly effective against *A. lumbricoides* and *E. vermicularis* infestations. It blocks the neuromuscular junction of the nematode and causes a flaccid paralysis in *A. lumbricoides*. Chemically, it is a simple cyclic secondary amine that produces a flaccid paralysis in these worms by acting as a GABA agonist and increasing chloride conductance (see also ivermectin). Pyrantel pamoate and piperazine have antagonistic effects on each other and should not be used together.

Piperazine is rapidly absorbed after oral administration. Its adverse effects are occasional dizziness and an urticarial reaction. It is contraindicated in people with known hypersensitivity, epilepsy, renal or hepatic disorders.

Hookworm infestation

Hookworm is also one of the most common nematode infestations. It is caused by *Ancylostoma duodenale* (Old World hookworm) or *Necator americanus* (New World hookworm). *A. duodenale* occurs predominantly in temperate zones such as the Mediterranean basin, the Middle East, northern India, China and Japan, while *N. americanus* occurs in the tropical and subtropical areas of Africa, Asia and the Americas. The adult nematodes live in the human intestine as bloodsucking parasites. The life cycles of both are similar, but the penetration sites by infective larvae (filariform) are different. Old World hookworm larvae penetrate the oral mucosa, whereas New World hookworm larvae penetrate the skin. The major symptoms of infestation are related to iron deficiency anemia and loss of plasma proteins.

■ *Hookworm infestation is treated with pyrantel pamoate*

Pyrantel pamoate is more effective against *A. duodenale* than against *N. americanus*. The anthelminthic action of this drug is discussed above. A single dose will decrease the number of nematodes harbored, but complete cure may require several courses of treatment.

Enterobiasis (oxyuriasis, pinworm infection)

Enterobiasis is a worldwide infection caused by *E. vermicularis* and is the most common helminthic infection in the developed countries of the northern hemisphere, especially among schoolchildren. The nematode rarely causes serious complications. The major clinical symptom is pruritus ani.

Enterobiasis is usually treated with pyrantel pamoate.

Strongyloidiasis

Strongyloidiasis (infestation with *Strongyloides stercoralis*) occurs worldwide, particularly in tropical and subtropical areas. The infective form (filariform larvae) can penetrate intact skin causing an itchy erythema at the site of penetration. The larvae are carried in the bloodstream into the lungs. Sputum contaminated with the larvae is swallowed and thus larvae enter the small intestine, penetrate the mucosa, and mature into adult nematodes. The fertilized female discharges partially embryonated eggs which pass in feces. Larvae excreted in the stools may penetrate the mucous membrane of the lower bowel and the anal skin (autoinfection). The host's immune system and the parasite's reproductive mechanisms remain in balance such that neither is seriously affected. If this balance is disrupted, massive numbers of larvae can penetrate into all parts of the body, producing hyperinfestation.

Strongyloidiasis is treated with albendazole or thiabendazole (but not in pregnant women)

Albendazole is a benzimidazole derivative that is highly effective in treating strongyloidiasis nematode infestation and is considered the drug of choice in this infestation. The benzimidazoles, as their name indicates, are derivatives of a bicyclic compound (benzene/imidazole). Three analogs (thiabendazole, mebendazole and albendazole) have been introduced since the 1970s. The latest analog, albendazole, has become the drug of choice of the three. All are versatile anthelminthic drugs, especially for intestinal infestations. Benzimidazoles produce many changes in the biochemistry of parasites including blocking glucose uptake, depleting glycogen stores and decreasing the formation of ATP in susceptible nematodes. It is suggested that they interfere with β tubulin and that resistance involves alterations in the tubulin genes (Fig. 6.28). It has been shown to have vermicidal, ovicidal and larvicidal activity. Less than 5% is absorbed after oral administration. A 3-day course of 400 mg once daily is normally prescribed.

Albendazole is well tolerated by adults and children over 2 years of age, though gastrointestinal discomfort and headache have been reported. It has, however, been shown to be teratogenic and has embryotoxic potential experimentally, and should not therefore be given to pregnant women.

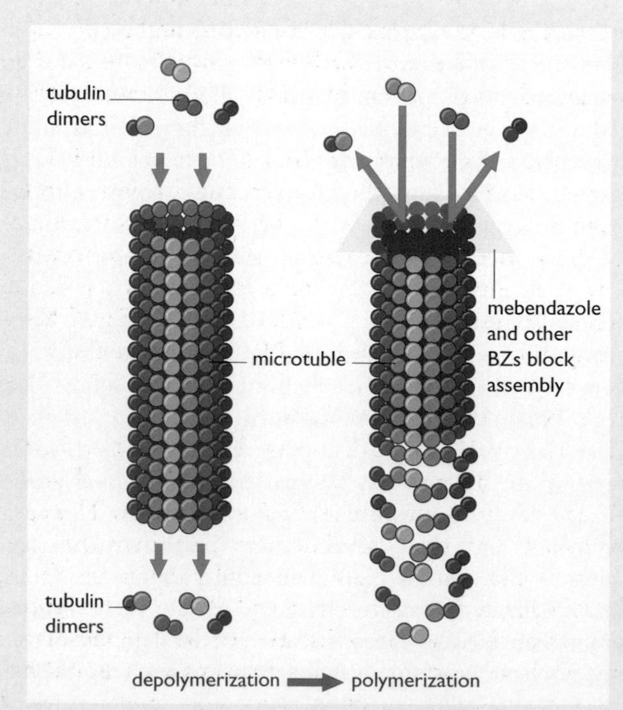

Fig. 6.28 Interaction between the nematode synapse and ivermectin. Potentiation of γ-aminobutyric acid (GABA) results in an influx of Cl^- and motor neuron hyperpolarization. Ivermectin also potentiates GABA release, which may explain its anthelminthic mechanism of action by causing worm paralysis.

Thiabendazole is a benzimidazole derivative that inhibits helminth-specific mitochondrial fumarate reductase systems of various helminths. It is rapidly absorbed from the gastrointestinal tract and treatment with two divided oral doses of 50 mg/kg/day for 3 days is very effective against strongyloidiasis. It should be taken for at least 5 days to treat hyperinfestation of strongyloidiasis.

Thiabendazole is associated with a high incidence of acute adverse effects such as vertigo and gastrointestinal discomfort (e.g. nausea, a loss of appetite and vomiting). It also has a teratogenic and embryotoxic potential experimentally and should not be given to pregnant women. Ivermectin can be used as an alternative drug.

Drugs and nematode larvae

Visceral larva migrans (toxocariasis), angiostrongyliasis and trichinosis are examples of infestation with nematode larvae.

Visceral larva migrans is a syndrome caused by the migration of the larvae of the nematode *Toxocara canis* in the viscera. Most patients are infected with only a small number of larvae and are usually asymptomatic. The infestation is frequently associated with eosinophilia.

Trichinosis is much more common in Europe and America than in Africa and Asia and is caused by the nematode *Trichinella spiralis*. The initial phase of the infestation can cause transient gastrointestinal complaints such as nausea, diarrhea, vomiting and abdominal pain. The phase of muscle invasion by the larvae typically causes the triad of myalgia, palpebral edema and eosinophilia.

Angiostrongyliasis is caused by the nematode *Angiostrongylus cantonensis* in the Asian Pacific area. The major clinical manifestations of cerebral angiostrongyliasis are eosinophilic meningitis with peripheral eosinophilia.

These infestations are all treated by giving oral thiabendazole for at least 1–2 weeks.

Filariasis (Bancroftian filariasis, Brugian filariasis, loiasis)

Bancroftian filariasis and Brugian filariasis are caused by the nematodes *Wuchereria bancrofti* and *Brugia malayi*, respectively, and have different geographic distributions:

- Bancroftian filariasis occurs in central Africa, South America, India and southern China.
- Brugian filariasis is restricted to Indonesia, the Malay peninsula, Vietnam, southern China, central India and Sri Lanka.

Both Bancroftian and Brugian filariasis are referred to as being a lymphatic filariasis since the nematodes locate in the lymphatic system. The infections are diagnosed mainly by detecting microfilariae in peripheral blood.

- Loiasis is caused by the African eye worm (*Loa loa*). It is endemic only to the rainforests of central and west Africa. The major clinical features (fugitive swelling or Calabar swelling) result from the continuous

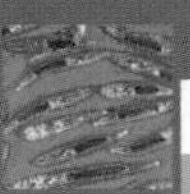

migration of the adult nematodes into subcutaneous tissues.

Diethycarbamazine is used to suppress and cure infestations with the nematodes W. bancrofti, B. malayi *and* Loa loa

Diethylcarbamazine is a diethylcarbamide derivative of piperazine. Its mechanism of action remains obscure. It readily kills the microfilaria but is less active on adult worms. It is only active in vivo. It can kill the microfilariae and the adult nematodes of Bancroftian and Brugian filariasis and loiasis. A total cumulative oral dosage of 72 mg/kg is needed to eliminate *W. bancrofti* infections, but a lower dosage is recommended for treating *B. malayi*. Doses vary depending upon circumstances. It is particularly effective combined with albendazole. It is largely ineffective against complicated lymphatic filariasis.

Diethylcarbamazine is well absorbed orally with a plasma half-life of 2–10 hours depending upon urinary pH, with 50% of the oral dose appearing in urine, especially in acidic urine

Adverse effects of diethylcarbamazine are limited with low doses and disappear with continued therapy. Side effects include anorexia, nausea, headache and vomiting. More importantly, the death of the microfilariae includes early and delayed allergic-type reactions. Diethylcarbamazine appears to be safe during pregnancy.

Onchocerciasis (river blindness)

Onchocerca volvulus is the nematode that causes river blindness and is common in all parts of west and central Africa, particularly along the rivers of the savanna south of the Sahara.

Ivermectin has replaced diethylcarbamazine as the drug of choice to treat onchocerciasis

Ivermectin is a semisynthetic derivative of an avermectin isolated from a soil fungus in the 1970s. β avermectin was used extensively in crop management and for control of nematodes and arthropods in livestock before being used in humans. In the 1990s it was found to be very effective against onchocerciasis (river blindness) and has since be found to be effective against other parasites. It has a very complex multi-ring structure lacking nitrogens. It acts to immobilize *Onchocerca volvulus* by producing a tonic paralysis of its peripheral muscle system. The putative mechanism for this action is illustrated in Fig. 6.29.

Ivermectin is the drug of choice in the treatment of *Onchocerca volvulus* infections and a single oral dose of 0.15–0.20 mg/kg every 6–12 months is sufficient to keep control the disease although not cure it since the adult form of the parasite is not killed. Thus, ivermectin is used for population control of river blindness. It is also effective as single annual doses for lymphatic filariasis (either *W. bancrofti* or *B. malayi*). Albendazole is a useful addition to ivermectin. Ivermectin is also useful for

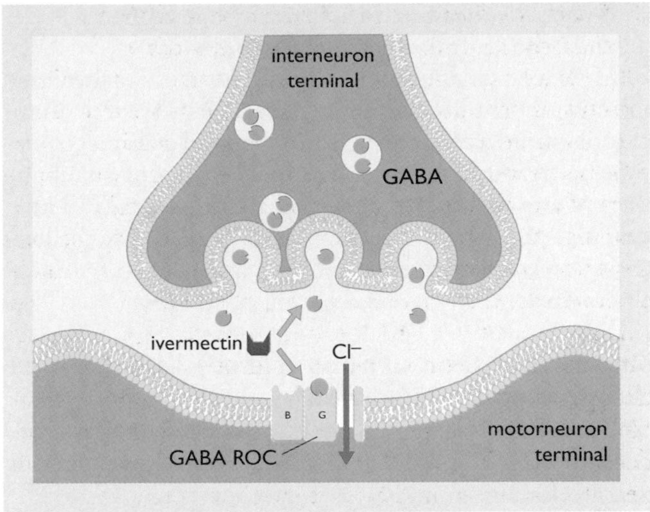

Fig. 6.29 Mechanism of action of mebendazole and other benzimidazoles (BZs). Microtubules are polar, with polymerization continually occurring at one end and depolymerization at the other. These drugs bind with high affinity to a site on the tubulin dimer, so preventing polymerization. Depolymerization leads to complete breakdown of the microtubule. (Adapted from Brody, Larner, Minneman and Neu. *Human Pharmacology Molecular to Clinical*, Mosby-Year Book Inc.; 1994.)

treating intestinal nematodes, and even in the treatment of arthropod infections (head lice and scabies).

Ivermectin concentrations in the blood peak after 4–5 hours. It has a long half-life (60 hours) and a very high volume of distribution. Metabolism is by CYP3A4 and no unchanged drug appears in urine. CNS concentrations are low.

Adverse effects are generally not reported with ivermectin, although a mild ocular irritation, transient nonspecific electrocardiographic changes and somnolence have been reported. Very large doses are toxic to animals. During treatment, an immediate inflammatory reaction occurs as a result from the death of microfilariae. This is usually mild but can be severe (Mazzotti reaction).

Trichuriasis and capillariasis

Trichuriasis (whipworm disease) is distributed worldwide, but is most prevalent in tropical and subtropical areas. It is caused by the nematode *Trichuris trichiura*. The eggs are usually stained with bile, are barrel-shaped, and appear as transparent bipolar mucoid plugs in the feces. These eggs are characteristic and diagnostic features. Patients with mild infection are usually asymptomatic, but may have gastrointestinal symptoms such as abdominal pain, diarrhea, nausea, anorexia, anemia, rectal prolapse, weakness and cachexia.

Intestinal capillariasis is caused by the nematode *Capillaria philippinensis* and is reported in the Philippines, Thailand, Japan and Iran. Symptoms include watery stools, malaise, anorexia, nausea and vomiting.

Both trichuriasis and capillariasis can be treated with albendazole (see above) or mebendazole.

Mebendazole is another benzimidazole derivative that inhibits nematode glucose transport. Its site of action is cytoplasmic microtubules and intestinal cells of nematodes, where it binds to the colchicine receptor on tubulin dimers (see Fig. 6.29). The small amounts absorbed after oral ingestion are extensively metabolized within the liver to inactive moieties, so the drug has selective action on the worm.

Drugs and trematodes (fluke) infestations

Schistosomiasis (bilharziasis)

Schistosomiasis is caused by the trematodes *Schistosoma japonicum*, *S. mansoni* and *S. haematobium* depending on geographic location:

- *S. japonicum* infection is endemic to China, the Philippines, Thailand, Laos and the Indonesian island of Celebes.
- The endemic area for *S. mansoni* includes the Middle East, Africa and South America.
- The endemic area for *S. haematobium* infection includes Africa and the Middle East.

Infected freshwater snails are the intermediate hosts for transmission.

S. japonicum and *S. mansoni* trematodes primarily infest the liver, spleen and gastrointestinal tract, whereas *S. haematobium* affects the genitourinary tract.

Schistosomiasis is treated with praziquantel

Praziquantel is a pyrazinoisoquinoline derivative with a complex piperazine-containing nucleus that has revolutionized treatment of schistosomiasis after its introduction in the 1970s. It has two major effects on the adult schistosome. At the lowest effective concentrations it increases muscular activity in the trematode followed by contraction and spastic paralysis. At slightly higher but still therapeutic concentrations, it causes vacuolization and vesiculation of the tegument of susceptible trematodes (Fig. 6.30) although the exact molecular mechanism remains unknown.

Praziquantel is highly effective against a broad spectrum of trematodes, including all species of schistosomes pathogenic to humans although its use in the USA was restricted to schistosomiasis. It is given various ways, including a dose 50 mg/kg divided into three portions after meals for 2 days that is highly effective. It has orally bioavailable with a peak plasma level in 1–2 hours although there is marked first-pass metabolism. The plasma half-life varies from 1 to 3 hours. There are interaction with CYP-inducing drugs.

Praziquantel is well tolerated and safe when given in one to three doses during the same day for single or mixed infestations with all species of *Schistosoma* trematodes. Adverse effects include abdominal discomfort, nausea, headache and dizziness, and these may occur shortly after administration. Death of parasites can be accompanied by the expected hypersensitivity reactions. This can be dangerous when the eye is infected with the parasite.

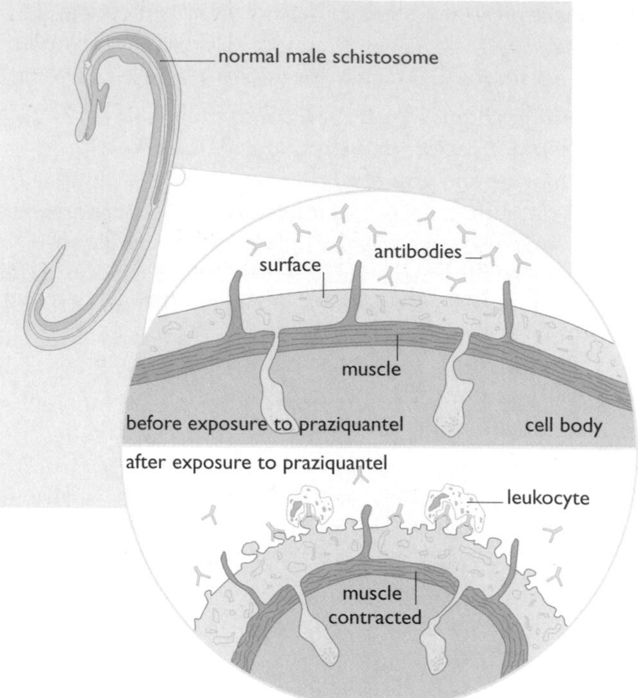

Fig. 6.30 Mechanism of action of praziquantel. Before exposure, the schistosome is unaffected by the numerous antibodies directed towards its surface. Exposure to praziquantel increases membrane permeability to certain monovalent and divalent cations, particularly Ca^{2+}, inducing an influx of Ca^{2+} into the schistosome tegument within 1 to 2 seconds. The resultant change in permeability of the schistosome surface to external ions causes small holes and balloon-like structures to form, making the schistosome vulnerable to antibody-mediated adherence of host leukocytes, thus killing the schistosome. (Adapted from Brody, Larner, Minneman and Neu. *Human Pharmacology Molecular to Clinical*, Mosby-Year Book Inc.; 1994.)

Praziquantel is safe in children, but is preferable to delay treatment of pregnant women until after delivery, though praziquantel has not been reported to be mutagenic, teratogenic or embryotoxic.

Clonorchiasis and opisthorchiasis

Clonorchiasis is caused by the trematode *Clonorchis sinensis* and is endemic to China, Taiwan, Hong Kong, Japan and Korea. Opisthorchiasis is caused by the trematode *Opisthorchis viverrini* and is found in Thailand, Laos and Kampuchea, while *O. felineus* occurs in Russia and Central and Eastern Europe. Most infestations are asymptomatic in the acute stage, but when they occur they can include acute signs and symptoms such as chills, fever, epigastric discomfort, hepatosplenomegaly and eosinophilia. In the chronic stage, patients often have non-specific gastrointestinal symptoms, including nausea, vomiting, a loss of appetite and abdominal pain.

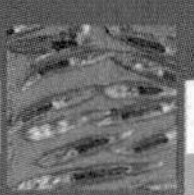

The most frequent complication is recurrent cholangitis. These diseases are also a common cause of pancreatitis.

Clonorchiasis and opisthorchiasis are treated with oral praziquantel, 50–75 mg/kg, divided into three portions, after meals for 2 days.

Paragonimiasis

Paragonimiasis is caused by a lung trematode of a variety of *Paragonimus* species, most commonly *P. westermani*. However, many other pathogenic species have been reported:

- In Asia, *P. skrjabini*, *P. hueitungenesis*, *P. heterotrema*, *P. philippinensis* and *P. miyazakii*.
- In Latin America, *P. kellicotti*, *P. mexicanus*, *P. ecuadoriensis* and *P. calilensis*.
- In Africa, *P. africanus* and *P. uterobilateralis*.

Paragonimiasis is contracted by ingesting infected uncooked crustaceans, which are the second intermediate host of *Paragonimus*. In Japan, the meat of wild boars (the paratenic host of *P. westermani*) is a source of infestation.

The major clinical manifestations of paragonimiasis are pulmonary (e.g. pleural pain, dyspnea, bloody sputum, cough). Complications include pleural effusion, pneumothorax, pulmonary abscess and empyema. Eosinophilia is common. Ectopic migration of the trematodes has been reported in practically all internal organs. The most important complication is cerebral paragonimiasis which is most frequently encountered in children in Japan and Korea.

Paragonimiasis is treated with praziquantel at a daily oral dose of 50–75 mg/kg, divided into three portions for 3 days, or oral bithionol.

Biothionol has a mechanism of action related to inhibition of respiration of the parasite mitochondria. It is used in a dose of 50 mg/kg divided into two or three portions after meals on alternate days for a total of 10–15 doses.

Adverse effects of bithionol are common and are generally mild and transient, but the symptoms are occasionally severe (e.g. anorexic, diarrhea, nausea, vomiting, dizziness, headache and abdominal cramps).

Fascioliasis

Fascioliasis is caused by the trematode *Fasciola hepatica*, *F. gigantica* and other *Fasciola* species (Japanese large liver fluke). It occurs worldwide, is common in cows, goats, and horses, and is endemic in Europe, South and Central America, Africa and Asia. *F. gigantica* has been reported mainly in Africa. After ingestion, these trematodes infect the biliary system of humans. Freshwater plants such as watercress, lettuce and alfalfa, and cow's liver have been reported as sources of infestation. The trematodes are harbored in intrahepatic bile ducts and patients with fascioliasis usually have hepatomegaly, fever and eosinophilia.

Fascioliasis was previously treated with bithionol at a dose of 50 mg/kg divided into three portions after meals on alternate days for a total of 10–15 doses or praziquantel at a dose of 75 mg/kg divided into three portions for 7 days. Recently, triclabendazole, another benzimidazole derivative, has been found to be more effective than bithionol or praziquantel in the treatment of fascioliasis. Triclabendazole is given as a single dose of 10 mg/kg.

Fasciolopsiasis

Fasciolopsiasis is caused by the trematode *Fasciolopsis buski* in endemic areas (eastern China, Taiwan, Thailand, Vietnam, Laos, India and Indonesia). People become infested by eating contaminated aquatic plants, and the trematode then lodges in the duodenum and jejunum. Most infestations are asymptomatic, but clinical signs and symptoms such as fever, eosinophilia, generalized edema, intestinal obstruction and malnutrition can occur in severe cases.

Fasciolopsiasis is treated with praziquantel at a dose of 50–75 mg/kg divided into three portions for 3 days.

Heterophyiasis

Heterophyiasis is caused by the members of the trematode family Heterophyidae (e.g. *Heterophyes heterophyes* and *Metagonimus yokogawai*). *H. heterophyes* is found mainly in Egypt, the Mediterranean basin and Japan. *M. yokogawai* is most common in the Far East and is contracted by eating raw fish. The associated infestations are usually asymptomatic, though severe infestation may produce gastrointestinal signs and symptoms (e.g. colic, abdominal tenderness and diarrhea).

Heterophyiasis is treated with oral praziquantel at a dose of 50 mg/kg divided into three portions for 1–2 days.

Drugs and cestodes

Large intestinal tapeworms (except for Taenia solium)

Taeniasis saginata is caused by the adult cestode *Taenia saginata*, or beef tapeworm, and humans are the definitive hosts. Adult cestodes are harbored in the small intestine. Individual worms are 5–8 m long and are composed of a chain of 1000–2000 proglottides which, when gravid, are expelled in feces. *T. saginata* is distributed worldwide and infestation is common in Ethiopia and in Mexico, and relatively common in South America and East and West Africa. It rarely produces severe clinical features, but must be distinguished from taeniasis caused by *T. solium*.

Diphyllobothriasis infestation is with the adult cestode *Diphyllobothrium latum*, or fish tapeworm. The infestation occurs in most parts of the world (e.g. Europe, the Near East, Siberia, Japan and North America). People become infested from eating poorly cooked fillets of salmon, trout and pike, which are intermediate hosts. The adult cestode is the longest human tapeworm (4–10 m in length). Most patients are asymptomatic, but in Finland some patients with this disease are anemic owing to a lack of vitamin B_{12}.

The above infestations with large cestodes can be treated with praziquantel, niclosamide, or Gastrografin.

PRAZIQUANTEL Before treatment, the patient is given a laxative electrolyte solution (e.g. GoLytely, a polyethylene glycol lavage solution) to reduce the fecal mass. Praziquantel is then given as a single oral dose of 10 mg/kg. Magnesium sulfate is taken 2–3 hours later as a rapid-acting laxative to expel the cestode.

NICLOSAMIDE Niclosamide is a halogenated salicylamide introduced in the 1960s and is no longer approved in the USA. Its anthelminthic action involves stimulation of cestode oxygen uptake at low concentrations and blocking cestode glucose uptake at higher concentrations. When the cestode dies, the scolex is released from the intestinal wall and the worms are digested. With *T. solium* infestations, ova released from the gravid eggs can cause dangerous cysticercosis.

Niclosamide is a cheap, effective and readily available in much of the world. Little is absorbed from the gastrointestinal tract. On the day of treatment, the patient is fasted. The adult dose is 2 g and less is given to children. The tablets should be chewed thoroughly before swallowing and washed down with a little water. Post-treatment purges to expel the worm are not necessary because the scolex and proglottides may be digested as a result of the effect of this drug.

Adverse effects of niclosamide are not severe, though mild gastrointestinal disturbances can occur.

GASTROGRAFIN Gastrografin is a water-soluble contrast material used to reveal the gastrointestinal tract for radiography. It has been shown to have an anthelminthic effect on intestinal cestodes (*T. saginata*, *D. latum*, *Diplogonoporus grandis*) although the mechanism of its anthelminthic action has not been reported. It is given after a laxative solution. Gastrografin (300 ml) is injected through a duodenal tube inserted through the mouth until the tip reaches the duodenal flexure. Under fluoroscopic monitoring, the tapeworms are evident as radiolucent shadows. When the parasites reach the rectum, the patient is encouraged to defecate.

Taeniasis solium and cysticercosis cellulosae

Taenia solium, the pork tapeworm has a worldwide distribution. The adult cestode lives in the human intestine, like *T. saginata* and *D. latum*, possesses 800–900 proglottides and measures 2–3 m in length. The life cycle of *T. solium* is illustrated in Figure 6.31.

Cysticercosis is caused by the larvae of *T. solium* (*Cysticercus cellulosae*), which live subcutaneously in the muscle, orbit and brain. Most cases result from ingestion of food and water contaminated with the eggs of T. *solium*. Taeniasis solium and cysticercosis occur in Latin America, Eastern Europe, India, Pakistan, Indonesia, China and Korea. The clinical manifestations of cerebral cysticercosis depend on the location of the cyst.

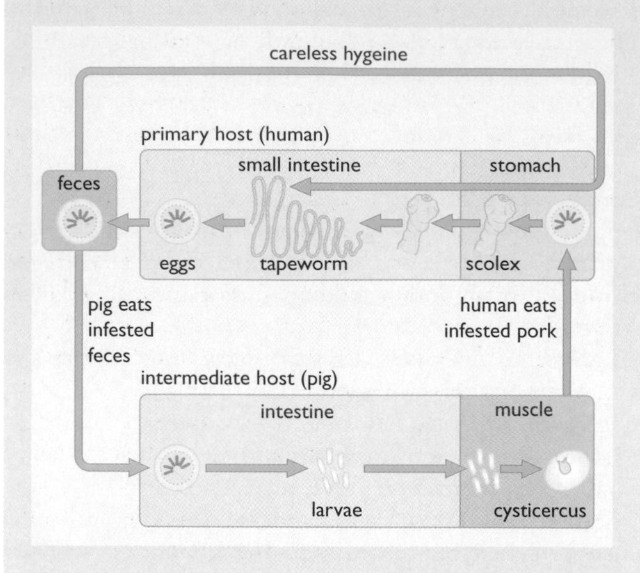

Fig. 6.31 The life cycle of the cestode *Taenia solium* on its journey from pig to man.

■ ***The drugs used to treat taeniasis solium and cysticercosis include Gastrografin, praziquantel and albendazole***

Gastrografin is the drug of choice for taeniasis because it does not damage the cestode. Damage to the cestode releases dangerous live eggs of *T. solium* into the intestinal lumen. The anthelminthic action and dose for therapeutic use of Gastrografin are as above.

Cysticercosis is treated only after Gastrografin to remove the tapeworm. Praziquantel and albendazole are used. Praziquantel is administered in a daily oral dose of 75 mg/kg, divided into three portions, for 7 days. After a further 7 days, it is given again at the same dose. Prednisolone is given throughout the treatment period to prevent or reduce allergic reactions that may result from the destruction of the cysticerci.

Albendazole is used for treating cysticercosis (and hydatid disease, see below). Albendazole is absorbed from the gastrointestinal tract and is rapidly and extensively metabolized in the liver. It is recommended that it be taken on an empty stomach when it is used against intestinal cestodes, but with a fatty meal when used against tissue cestodes. Two 7-day courses of 10–15 mg/kg/day divided into three portions are separated by treatment-free periods of 7 days. Prednisolone is also given throughout treatment to reduce allergic reactions.

Adverse effects of albendazole include transient gastrointestinal discomfort and headache.

Echinococcosis (hydatid disease)

■ ***Echinococcosis is caused by the larval forms of the cestodes* Echinococcus granulosus *and* E. multilocularis*, and is acquired by ingestion***

Echinococcus granulosus is found worldwide and echinococcosis (cystic hydatid disease) occurs in East Africa, the

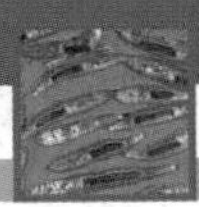

Mediterranean littoral, South America, the Middle East, Australia, India and Russia. *E. multilocularis* is the second most common species. Echinococcosis from *E. multilocularis* (alveolar hydatid disease) occurs in Canada, Central Europe, Siberia, Alaska and northern Japan. The adult cestodes of *E. granulosus* and *E. multilocularis* measure 2–7 mm and 1.2–4.5 mm in length, respectively. The adult cestodes live in the small intestine of a final host (e.g. dog, fox, wolf). Humans are the intermediate hosts, and ingest the eggs excreted by an infested final host. The clinical manifestations depend on the size of the cyst (*E. granulosus*) and the degree of infestation (*E. multilocularis*) in the liver, lung and other organs. Echinococcosis from *E. multilocularis* resembles carcinoma in its ability to metastasize and is frequently fatal.

Surgery is still the treatment of choice for operable cases of echinococcosis. Chemotherapy with oral albendazole can be effective, given as four 30-day courses of 10–15 mg/kg/day divided into three portions separated by treatment-free periods of 15 days.

Hymenolepiasis

Hymenolepiasis is caused by *Hymenolepis nana* (the dwarf tapeworm) and *H. diminuta*. The latter is the smallest cestode in humans. It measures 1–4 cm, and commonly infects children in tropical and subtropical regions. The infestation is acquired by ingesting the worm's eggs contaminating food and water. Autoinfestation and rapid cestode reproduction increase the infestation in malnourished or immunocompromised children, who experience gastrointestinal manifestations including nausea, vomiting, diarrhea and abdominal pain.

H. diminuta is a common parasite of rats and mice that occasionally infests humans. The adult cestode measures 20–60 cm in length. Its life cycle requires an intermediate host (fleas) and a final host (rats and mice). People acquire the infestation by accidentally ingesting infected fleas.

Treatment is with praziquantel administered as a single dose of 10–25 mg/kg. Niclosamide can be used for *H. nana* infestations

Some of the antiparasitic drugs and the diseases for which they are used are summarized in Table 6.29.

Table 6.29 Drugs for the treatment of parasitic infections either as primary, secondary or combination therapy (not all available in the USA)

Drug	Infection(s)	Drug	Infection(s)
Albendazole	Strongyloidiasis Trichuriasis, capillariasis, ascariasis, filariasis,toxocariasis *Taenia solium* and *Cysticercus cellulosae* Echinococcosis (hydatid disease)	Metronidazole Niclosamide	Amebiasis, giardiasis, trichomoniasis Taeniasis saginata, diphyllobothriasis, hymenolepiasis American trypanosomiasis (Chagas' disease)
Amodiaquine	Malaria	Pentamidine isethionate	African trypanosomiasis, pneumocystosis
Antibiotics (clindamycin, tetracycline, doxycycline)	Malaria	Piperazine	Ascariasis (roundworm)
Artemisinin	Malaria	Praziquantel	TREMATODES (schistosomiasis, clonorchiasis, opisthorchiasis, paragonimiasis, fasciolopsiasis) CESTODES (heterophyiasis, taeniasis saginata,diphyllobothriasis, hymenolepiasis)
Atovaquone–proguanil	Malaria		
Benznidazole	American trypanosomiasis (Chagas' disease)	Primaquine	Malaria
Bithionol	Paragonomiasis, fascioliasis	Pyrantel pamoate	NEMATODES (ascariasis (roundworm), hookworms (*Ancylostoma* or *Necator* spp.), Enterobiasis (oxyuriasis, pinworm infection)
Chloroquine	Malaria		
Co-trimoxazole	Malaria		
Dapsone	Malaria		
Dehydroemetine	Amebiasis	Pyrimethamine–sulfadiazine	Malaria, toxoplasmosis
Diethylcarbamazine	Filariasis		
Eflornithine	African trypanosomiasis	Pyronaridine	Malaria
Gastrografin	*Taenia saginata* and *T. solium*	Quinidine	Malaria
Halofantrine	Malaria	Quinine	Malaria
Ivermectin	NEMATODES (onchocerciasis (river blindness), strongyloidiasis dipetalonemiasis)	Sodium stibogluconate Sulfadoxine Sulfalene	Leishmaniasis Malaria Malaria, trypanosomiasis
Mebendazole	Trichuriasis, capillariasis, hookworm, echinococcosis, enterobiasis, ascariasis	Suramin Tafenoquine Thiabendazole	African Malaria Strongyloidiasis, nematode larval infections
Mefloquine	Malaria		
Meglumine antimoniate	Leishmaniasis	Tinidazole	Amebiasis, giardiasis, trichomoniasis
Melarsoprol	African trypanosomiasis	Triclabendazole	Fascioliasis

FURTHER READING

Baird JK. Effectiveness of antimalarial drugs. *N Engl J Med* 2005; **352**: 1565–1577.

Barrett MP, Burchmore RJ, Stich A et al. The trypanosomiases. *Lancet* 2003; **362**: 1469–1480.

Docampo R, Moreno SN. Current chemotherapy of human African trypanosomiasis 2003; **90**(Suppl): 10–13.

Greenwood BM, Bojang K, Whitty CJ, Targett GA. Malaria. *Lancet* 2005; **365**: 1487–1498.

Horton J. Global anthelmintic chemotherapy programs: learning from history. *Trends Parasitol* 2003; **19**: 405–409.

Murray J, Berman C, Davies N, Saravia. Advances in leishmaniasis. *Lancet* **3656**: 1561–1577H.

Olliaro PL, Taylor WR. Antimalarial compounds: from bench to bedside. *J Exp Biol* 2003; **206**: 3753–3759. [A review of antimalarial drugs.]

Petersen E. Malaria chemoprophylaxis: when should we use it and what are the options? *Expert Rev Anti Infect Ther* 2004; **2**: 119–132. [Antimalarial coverage for those not normally exposed to malaria.]

Stanley SL. Amoebiasis. *Lancet* 2003; **361**: 1025–1034. [A comprehensive overview of the use of drugs and for amoebic infections.]

Strickland GT (ed.) *Hunter's Tropical Medicine and Emerging Infectious Diseases*, 8th edn. Philadelphia: W.B. Saunders; 2000. [This textbook describes general aspects of tropical and parasitic diseases and their treatment.]

Upcroft P, Upcroft JA. Drug targets and mechanisms of resistance in the anaerobic protozoa. *Clin Microbiol Rev* 2001; **1**: 150–164.

Wilairatana P, Krudsood S, Treeprasertsuk S, Chalermrut K, Looareesuwan S. The future outlook of antimalarial drugs and recent work on the treatment of malaria. *Arch Med Res* 2002; **33**: 416–421. [Malarial resistance and how to combat it in the future.]

WEBSITES

Van Voorhis, WC, Weller PF. Chapters XXXIV Protozoan infections and XXXV Parasitic infections. In: *ACP Medicine*. Web MD Inc. 2005.

Centers for Disease Control

http://www.cdc.gov/ncidod/srp/drugs/drug-services.html [Information on antiparasitic drugs.]

WHO

http://www.who.int/tdr [Details on the WHO program for tropical diseases.]

http://www.malaria.org/ [This website provides general information about malaria.]

http://www.nlm.nih.gov/medlineplus/parasiticdiseases.html [Provides general information regarding parasites and antiparasitic drugs.]

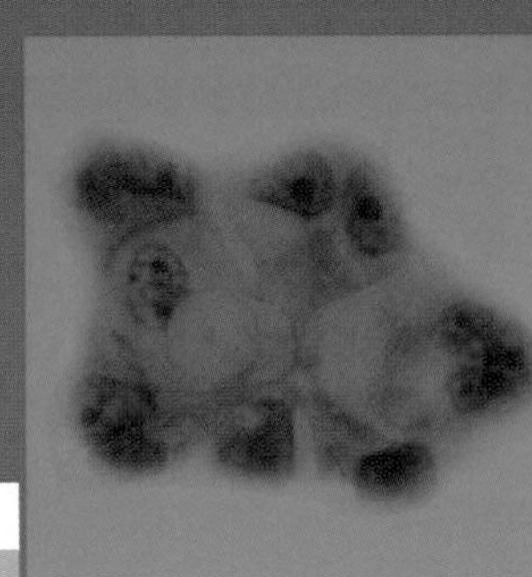

Chapter 7

Drugs and Cancer

Numerous drugs are used for the treatment of cancer. In order to understand the pharmacology of cancer treatment, certain fundamental aspects of the pathophysiology of cancer, and issues relating to its treatment, need to be considered.

CARCINOGENESIS

Cancers are malignant (spreading) tumors. Tumors are neoplastic growths ('new growths') of cells. Benign tumors do not spread or metastasize from their original site. Malignant tumors, which are also known as cancers, spread or metastasize as a result of clonal expansion from a single cell into an increasing mass that invades surrounding normal tissues and spreads throughout the body via the lymphatic system or the blood (hematogenously). The growth of a cancer is known as carcinogenesis or tumorigenesis and is a multi-step process (Fig. 7.1).

Cancer in an individual may be initiated by extrinsic factors (e.g. chemical carcinogens) or by genetic predisposition. For most cancers, there is an apparent interaction between the two. However, the nature and extent of the interaction may vary among individuals. For example, data from twins suggests that genetic factors contribute approximately 42% of the relative risk of prostate cancer, 35% of colorectal cancer and 25% of breast cancer, with a lesser contribution to other types of cancer.

Extrinsic factors that contribute strongly to carcinogenesis include bacteria such as *Helicobacter pylori*, viruses such as Epstein–Barr, human papilloma or hepatitis B and C, fungi, such as those producing aflatoxins, and chemicals such as benzene.

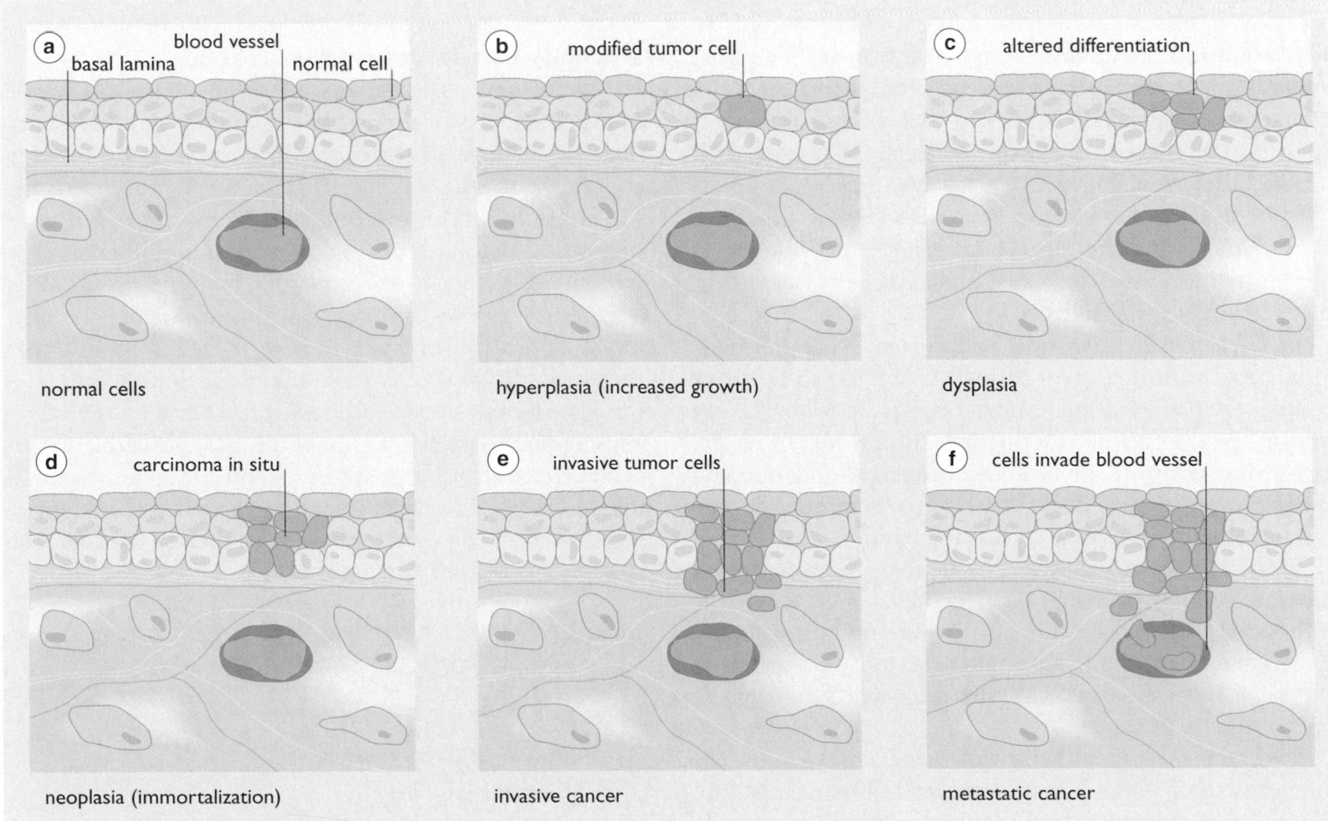

Fig. 7.1 Hypothetical progression from normal to malignant cells.

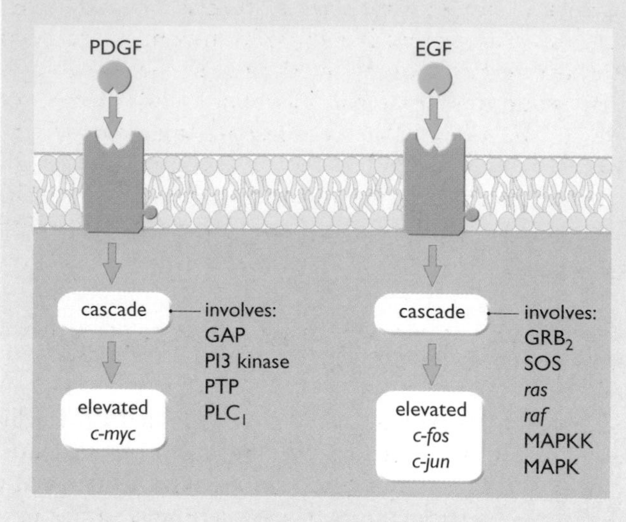

Fig. 7.2 Two schemes showing how extracellular growth factors stimulate cancer cell proliferation. Overexpression of any of these cellular homologs of oncogenes, or a mutation that produces constitutive activation, may contribute to enhanced growth. (EGF, epidermal growth factor; PI3, phosphoinositol-3-kinase; GAP, GTP-ase activating protein; GRB$_2$, G (protein)-related protein B$_2$; MAPK, mitogen-activated protein kinase; MAPKK, mitogen-activated protein kinase kinase; PDGF, platelet-derived growth factor; PLC, phospholipase C; PTP, phosphotyrosine phosphatase; *ras*, *raf*, cellular signal transducers; *c-fos*, *c-jun*, *c-myc*, inducers of DNA synthesis)

Oncogenes are DNA sequences that code for the key proteins involved in carcinogenesis. They were first isolated from viruses that caused cancers in laboratory animals. They are also overexpressed in cancer cells. Oncogenes can code for growth factors and mitogenic factors and, therefore, cancer cells can stimulate their own proliferation (Fig. 7.2).

Functional growth factor receptors can be expressed constitutively on the surface of cancer cells, whereas others are induced (often by chemical triggers released by the cancer cells themselves).

Proliferative pathways in healthy cells are normally linked to antiproliferative pathways, leading to feedback control of proliferation. Some oncogene products can inhibit proliferation. Oncogene mutations or overexpression can shift the balance between stimulation and suppression of proliferation. In carcinogenesis, the balance is shifted in favor of proliferation.

Proliferation in healthy cells is also controlled by a separate set of cancer suppressor genes, which act via the cell cycle. Mutations, or loss of cancer suppressor genes, such as *p53* in the Li–Fraumeni syndrome or *rb* in retinoblastoma, predisposes individuals and families to an increased risk of cancer.

Proliferation in healthy cells is balanced by cell death. The growth of a population of cancer cells is the result of the balance between proliferation and cell death. In healthy cells, apoptosis is an energy-requiring process by which cells undergo a choreographed progression to cell death (programmed death of obsolete or damaged cells). Apoptosis may be the direct result of receptor binding (*Fas* and its ligand in lymphocytes) or release of cytochrome C into the cytoplasm after disruption of the mitochondrial membrane by lethal intracellular events. There are pro-apoptotic proteins, such as Bad and the caspases, which are balanced by antiapoptotic proteins such as bcl-2. Overexpression of bcl-2 may result from oncogene expression and has been associated with transformation of normal cells to cancer.

Loss of normal genomic DNA replication is critical to cancer development

Cancer cells can propagate only when the normal capacity to recognize and repair mutations in the genome is lost. Individuals and families with mutations in DNA repair genes are prone to cancer, for example:

- DNA repair genes that repair mismatched base pairs are mutated in hereditary nonpolyposis colon cancer.
- DNA repair to helicases is absent or defective in xeroderma pigmentosum, a genetic disease characterized by defective repair of damage caused by ultraviolet radiation.

The tumor suppressor gene *p53* may have a crucial role in the cellular response to DNA damage or mutation. Normally, *p53* arrests cells before DNA replication to allow repair to take place, and also initiates apoptosis. Loss of normal *p53* function allows flawed DNA to replicate and thereby facilitates the survival of flawed cells.

Cancer cells are immortalized cells

Every normal cell in the body, except for the germ cells of the gonads, is programmed for a finite number of cell divisions before senescence. This cellular program is contained in the telomere. Telomeres are located at the ends of the chromosome and must pair and align at mitosis. They are produced and maintained by an enzyme, telomerase, in germ cells and embryonic cells. This enzyme loses its function during normal development. A portion of the telomere is therefore lost with each cell division and each telomeric loss serves as a cellular clock. Cancer cells re-express telomerase, which allows them to proliferate indefinitely. Loss of the normal cell cycle controls imposed by *rb* and *p53* genes facilitate the re-emergence of telomerase expression. As many as 95% of cancer cells express telomerase, making this enzyme a potential target for drugs.

Characteristics of cancer

- **Increased proliferation**
- **Loss of regulatory proteins**
- **Genomic instability**
- **Immortalization**

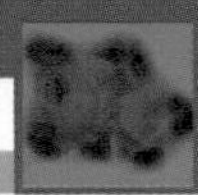

Once established and proliferating, cancer invades through the basement membrane and into adjacent connective tissue

Cancer cells express collagenases, heparanises and plasminogen activators and move through the supporting tissues along the path of least resistance.

Angiogenesis is essential to supply nutrients to the expanding cancer and is stimulated by fibroblast growth factor and vascular endothelial growth factor. Collagen, vitronectin and fibronectin synthesis by the cancer cells promotes cell scaffolding and may aid in cell attachment at sites of metastasis. Many of the essential components of this complex process are also provided by local healthy tissues, which can unwittingly contribute to their own demise. The processes of invasion and metastasis are less important in leukemias and lymphomas as these are diffuse blood cancers.

Invasion and metastasis are often well advanced before clinical symptoms appear and the cancer is detected. Drugs are required once a cancer has spread overtly or microscopically beyond its site of origin.

Expert histologic diagnosis is an essential component of cancer treatment

The histologic diagnosis of some tumors is essential to establish whether the objective of therapy is palliation or cure. For example:

- If a non-Hodgkin's lymphoma (NHL) has a low-grade favorable histologic subtype it is incurable, but its growth is relatively indolent. Treatment is therefore conservative, with one drug rather than aggressive multidrug treatment.
- If an NHL has an intermediate- or high-grade histologic subtype it will be rapidly lethal, but it may be curable using multidrug treatment, whereas single-agent or less intensive regimens have no effect.
- Extensive, even metastatic, small cell lung cancer can be cured with multidrug therapy, but non-small cell lung cancer at the same stage is incurable.
- Histologic typing in acute leukemia to show whether it is lymphoblastic or nonlymphoblastic determines the choice of drugs as well as the outcome.

Staging is the determination of the extent of cancer spread by local invasion and the presence of lymphatic and hematogenous metastases

There are separate staging systems for each histologic type of cancer. They are based upon its clinical and anatomic characteristics. The use of biochemical, cytologic and molecular biologic determinants increases accuracy. Accurate staging serves two purposes:

- It allows comparisons between patients and patient groups for a more accurate evaluation of the effectiveness of a treatment.
- It is a guide for deciding which treatment to use for an individual patient.

Patients with an early stage of cancer and a favorable prognosis may require less intensive treatment (e.g. less extensive surgery and/or avoidance of chemotherapy). This reduces short-term morbidity and long-term adverse effects, which have become apparent as the treatment of cancer has become increasingly effective and more patients, especially children, survive. Long-term consequences of anticancer drugs include infertility, growth retardation and second malignancies.

PRINCIPLES OF CELL PROLIFERATION AND CHEMOTHERAPY

Chemotherapy is the use of drugs to kill or disable cells (in this context, cancer cells). Knowledge of the basic processes of cellular proliferation is essential to permit understanding of the mechanisms of action of anticancer drugs. Healthy cells are in one of the following three stages:

- Actively dividing (cycling).
- Differentiating (dying).
- Dormant (can actively divide if cellular environmental conditions allow).

Four distinct cell cycle phases are recognized: the S, G_1, G_2 and M phases (Fig. 7.3). The activity of replicative enzymes such as thymidine kinase, DNA polymerase, dihydrofolate reductase, ribonucleotide reductase, RNA

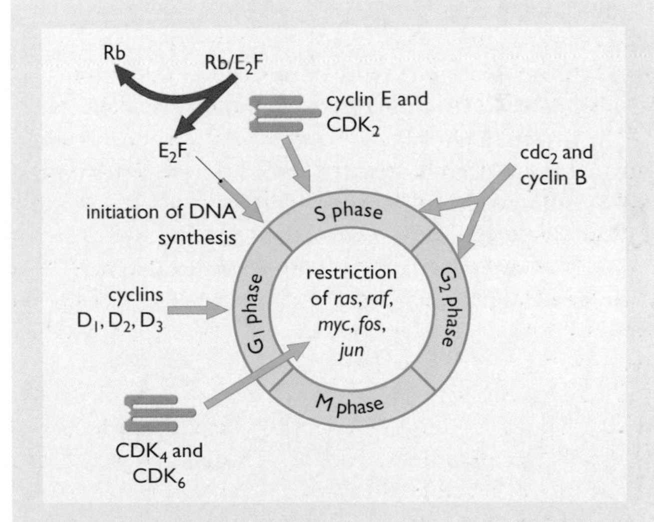

Fig. 7.3 The cell cycle and some of the important regulatory proteins. The S phase refers to the active synthesis of DNA and lasts approximately 12–18 hours. The G_2 phase lasts 1–8 hours and the DNA complement is 4n (twice the normal number of chromosomes). Mitosis (M) lasts about 1–2 hours. The duration of the G_1 phase is variable, and the late G_1 phase is associated with an increase in DNA synthesis enzymes. The complex regulation of the restriction point for the start of S phase involves cyclins and CDKs (cyclin-dependent kinases), which continue to regulate the CDKs through the entire cell cycle. (cdc_2, cell division cycle protein 2, an essential controlling gene for cell cycle progression; *ras, raf, myc, fos, jun*, cellular homologs of viral oncogenes involved in cellular proliferation; Rb, retinoblastoma protein; E_2F, a transcription factor)

polymerase II and topoisomerases I and II is increased during the S phase. Control of a G_2–M checkpoint to allow DNA repair or completion of replicative DNA synthesis is a crucial element in normal cell cycle control. The G_1 phase may be virtually absent, as in embryonic cells, or so prolonged that it produces dormancy (G_0).

Techniques for measuring cell cycles include the use of tritiated thymidine (^{3}H-TdR)-uptake pulse labeling to determine the fraction of cells actually synthesizing DNA. The S phase can also be measured by using a cell sorter to identify chromosome number (i.e. 2n, 4n). These measurements are used clinically in the staging of breast cancer.

Cancer cell populations do not grow in a linear manner with time

The growth of a cancer cell population is best described by Gompertzian kinetics characterized by slow linear growth at the smallest and largest cancer sizes, and exponential growth in between (Fig. 7.4).

Cancer growth retardation and cancer cell loss correlates with cytologic and spatial factors. Proximity to blood vessels and access to oxygen are important determinants of cancer cell viability and growth and therefore have a significant therapeutic impact on:

- Radiation therapy, where oxygen is an essential intermediate.
- Chemotherapy, where many anticancer drugs target multiplying cells.

The dose-limiting toxicity of anticancer drugs on normal tissue is often directly related to rate of growth of tissues

Normal tissues can be divided into different types on the basis of their cell proliferation kinetics:

- Rapidly proliferating tissues (labeling index (LI) >5%) include bone marrow, gut mucosa, reproductive organs and hair follicles.

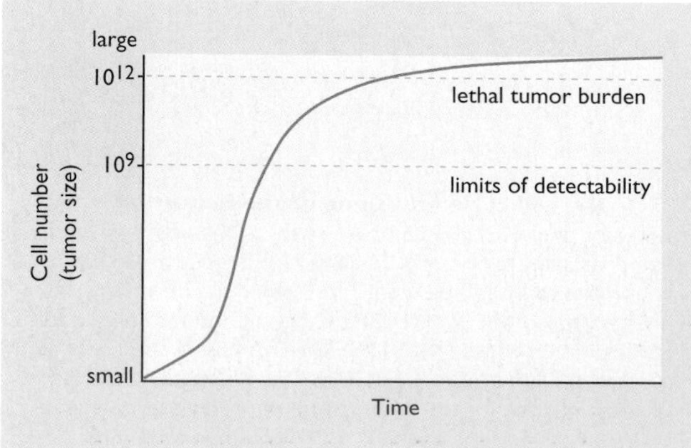

Fig. 7.4 Gompertzian, and not logarithmic, kinetics best describe cancer cell growth. There is a low growth rate in very small and very large tumors, while intermediate-sized tumors grow exponentially.

Table 7.1 Cell kinetics of leukemia and bone marrow

Cell type	Labeling index (%)	Cell cycle time (h)
Acute leukemia	3–12	48–72
Chronic myelogenous leukemia	6–25	48–72
Chronic lymphocytic leukemia	0–1	48–72
Normal myeloblasts	32–75	16–24
Normal myelocytes	18–25	16–24

- Slowly proliferating tissues (LI <1%) include the trachea, bronchial epithelium, liver, kidney and endocrine organs.
- Nonproliferating tissues (in adults) include skeletal muscle, heart muscle, bone and nerve tissue.

The bone marrow is commonly the organ most sensitive to adverse antiproliferative effects of anticancer drugs.

Different cancers have different labeling indexes and doubling times

A comparison of the growth kinetics of normal bone marrow granulocytes and leukemic cells (Table 7.1) shows that the rate of cell proliferation in leukemia is less than in normal bone marrow. However, the cell population in leukemia expands because cell proliferation exceeds cell maturation and death. Solid cancers typically have a much lower fraction of actively growing cells. The LI is 1–5% in slow-growing adenocarcinomas, but up to 30% in Burkitt's lymphoma, testicular carcinoma, Ewing's sarcoma, NHL and subclinical breast cancer.

Doubling times are 30–70 days in Hodgkin's disease, osteosarcoma and fibrosarcoma, while slow-growing adult carcinomas with doubling times longer than 70 days include lung cancer, colon and gastrointestinal cancers and advanced breast cancer. The slower rate of growth results from the presence of many nonproliferating cells and a high rate of cell death.

Several fundamental principles of cancer therapy are determined by cell proliferation kinetics

The log kill hypothesis postulates that a dose of drug kills a constant fraction of cancer cells (related to the log of the number of cells) and not a constant number of cells (Fig. 7.5). This means that a proportion of cells in a cancer can survive a course of treatment by chance without being specifically drug resistant. Therefore, each drug or combination of drugs has a limited cytotoxic capacity. As a result, combination therapy is more likely to provide a cure than single-drug therapy. This is because fractions of fractions of cancer cells survive the treatment, and survivors may be so few that they can readily be dealt with by host defenses allowing a 100% kill rate.

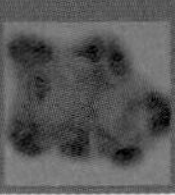

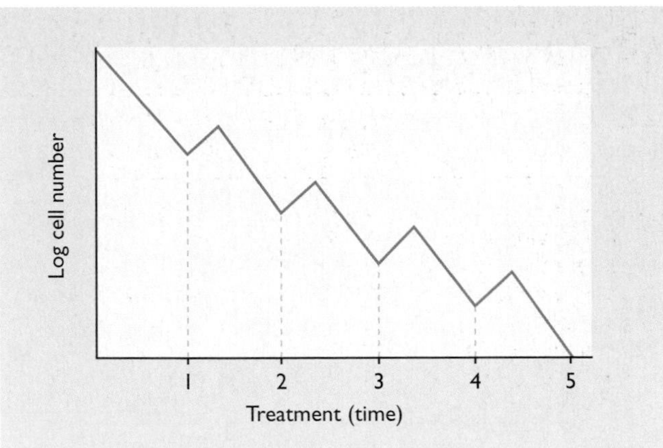

Fig. 7.5 Log kill hypothesis. A drug or drug combination can kill a constant fraction of cancer cells. Certain cells survive each treatment by chance alone and are sensitive to subsequent treatments.

The log kill varies with cell growth rate and so there is a progressive decrease in log kill in the late stages of cancer growth when cells stop cycling. Early recurrences of slow-growing cancers occur because their log kill is small. Late recurrences of rapidly growing tumors may occur despite effective treatment if too few courses of treatment are given. This is referred to as the period of risk.

Some cancer therapies kill cells only during specific phases of the cell cycle

Certain classes of intervention (i.e. anticancer drugs and radiotherapy) show phase-specific lethality.

In cancer therapy there are several characteristic curves of drug dose versus cell survival (Fig. 7.6). In exponential curves, the proportion of surviving cells is exponentially related to the dose of the intervention. As the dose increases, the cell kill increases. Drugs (and other interventions) with this property are not cycle- or stage-specific (i.e. they kill cells anywhere in the cell cycle, even resting cells) and include:

- 5-fluorouracil, cisplatin, glucocorticosteroids, nitrogen mustard and melphalan.
- Radiotherapy.

Cyclophosphamide and other alkylating agents are lethal at all stages of the cell cycle, but have increased lethality in cells at the G_1–S boundary.

Phase-specific survival curves show a plateau with no increase in kill at higher doses. Further kill can be obtained, however, by increasing the exposure time, but not the dose. Drugs producing this type of curve are:

- The antimetabolite cytotoxic drugs such as cytarabine, thioguanine and hydroxyurea, which are active only in the S phase.
- Methotrexate, doxorubicin, epipodophyllotoxin and vinca alkaloids, which have maximum lethal toxicity during the S phase.

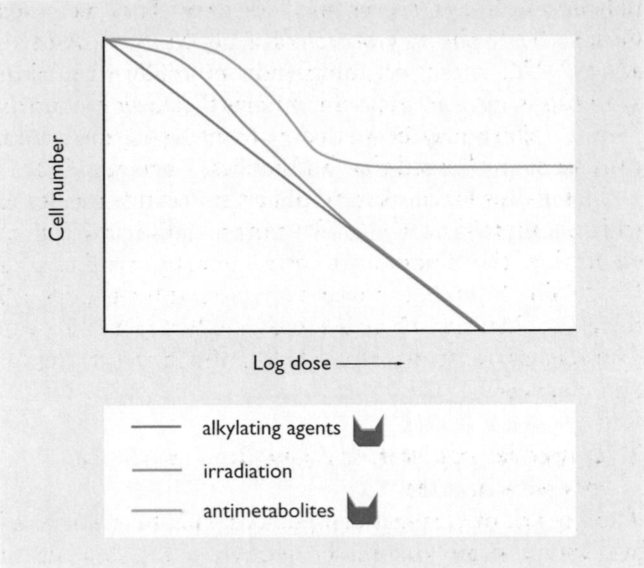

Fig. 7.6 Cycle-specific drug lethality. For noncycle-dependent agents, such as irradiation or alkylating agents, increasing dose produces increasing cell kill. For cycle-specific agents, such as antimetabolites, which kill only actively growing cells, increasing doses have a plateau effect as cell growth slows with chemotherapy. Prolonging the duration of exposure to antimetabolites will increase the cell kill.

- Bleomycin, which has maximum activity in the G_2 and M phases.

Cytotoxic drugs block the cell cycle

All cytotoxic anticancer drugs can interfere with progression of cells through the cell cycle, leading to synchronization and slowing of rapidly proliferating cells. This results in decreased sensitivity to S-phase drugs.

Cytotoxicity is proportional to the total drug exposure

The pharmacokinetics of anticancer drugs can be complex, as cytotoxicity to cancer cells is proportional to the total drug exposure (area under the curve; AUC), and not the peak plasma concentration of drug (Fig. 7.7). The

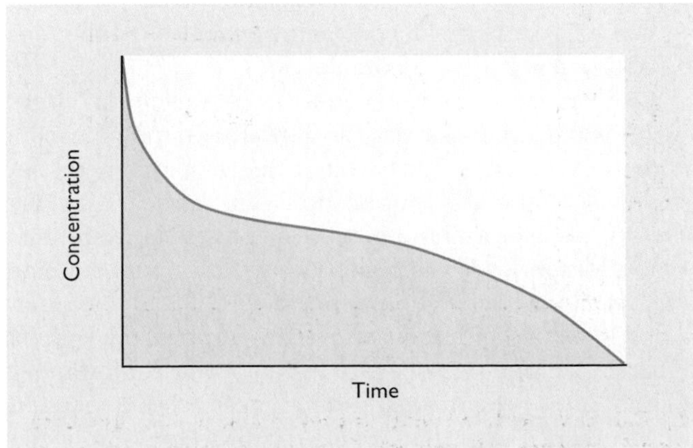

Fig. 7.7 Cytotoxicity is proportional to the total drug exposure or area under the curve (shaded).

drug has first to penetrate into individual cancer cells and then to interact with its molecular target. As this interaction is often reversible, at least initially, a cytotoxic concentration must be maintained at this time. In addition, the number of individual interactions between a drug and target molecules needed to kill a single cell can be enormous. It is estimated that 1 million molecules of cisplatin must bind to the DNA of a single cell to kill it.

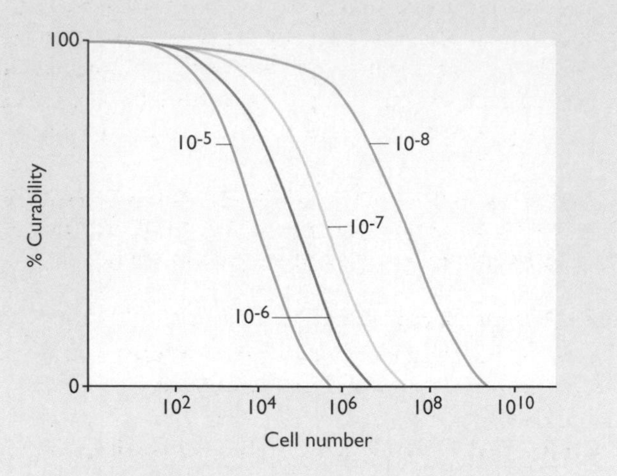

Fig. 7.8 The Goldie–Coldman hypothesis. For an intrinsic rate of mutation to drug resistance, the chances of drug failure (incurability) increase with size of the tumor (10^{-5} to 10^{-8} indicate mutation rate per cell division, i.e. 10^{-5} is one mutation per 100 000 divisions).

Principles of anticancer therapy

- Drugs kill a constant fraction, not a constant number, of cells
- Cells may have discrete periods of vulnerability to cytotoxic drugs
- Cytotoxic drugs slow the progression of cells through the cell cycle
- Cytotoxic drugs are not selectively toxic toward cancer cells
- Cytotoxicity is proportional to total drug exposure

PRINCIPLES OF COMBINATION CHEMOTHERAPY

Combinations of anticancer drugs were introduced because it was found that single drugs did not produce significant remissions or cures (except for the treatment of choriocarcinoma with methotrexate). The log kill hypothesis explains this (see above).

Drugs used for combination therapy should:

- Show some activity when used alone.
- Preferably produce a high fraction of a 'complete response' (defined as a 100% kill of cells in a tumor) rather than a partial response (e.g. less than a 50% kill).
- Have different biochemical mechanisms of action to attack a tumor containing a heterogeneous population of cells.
- Not have similar adverse effects, otherwise the dosage will need to be reduced, resulting in a loss of the added benefit of the combination.

Cancers are heterogeneous in a variety of ways, including drug sensitivity, as a result of their unstable genetic make-up. Cells within a cancer may mutate and this has important implications for anticancer drug therapy as such mutations can lead to resistance to anticancer drugs. Most anticancer drug resistance is innate for the tumor type. It may become clinically apparent when sensitive clones in the cancer are killed and the resistant clones propagate and become dominant. Curability is proportional to the cancer cell number and, in accordance with the Goldie–Coldman hypothesis that there is a greater probability of (drug-resistant) mutations in a larger population of cells (Fig. 7.8).

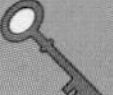

Principles of combination chemotherapy

- Drugs used have individual anticancer actions, nonoverlapping toxicity and different mechanisms of action
- Optimal dose and schedule regimens used
- Shortest possible dosing interval

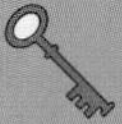

Benefits of combination therapy over single interventions

- Increases maximum cell kill and decreases toxicity
- Kills cells in tumors with heterogeneous cell populations
- Reduces the chances of development of resistant clones

LATE ADVERSE EFFECTS OF CANCER CHEMOTHERAPY

Gonadal dysfunction

The cancer therapies most likely to produce gonadal dysfunction are alkylating agents (and irradiation), and this is dose-related.

About 80% of males with Hodgkin's disease treated with MOPP (mechlorethamine, vincristine, procarbazine and prednisolone) become oligo- or azoospermic, and about 50% recover within 4 years. Procarbazine is the principal culprit.

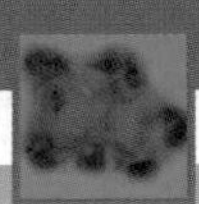

In females treated with MOPP, amenorrhea, vaginal atrophy and endometrial hypoplasia are dose- and age-related. Irreversible changes and menopause due to ovarian failure are more likely with increasing age. Alkylating agents (and irradiation) are the most common causes of such changes.

Gonadal dysfunction is less severe and more reversible in prepubertal children, but boys at puberty appear to be more susceptible than any other patient group.

Carcinogenesis

Carcinogenic chemicals and some drugs can cause cancer. One common factor in their mechanism of action as carcinogenic substances is interaction with DNA.

Testing for environmental and occupational carcinogens involves examining the capacity of an agent to produce mutations in bacteria (Ames test) or to produce sister chromatid exchanges (translocations of genomic sequences from one chromosome to its identical, diploid counterpart) in cultured mammalian cells. However, clinical proof of carcinogenesis is difficult to establish.

Drugs have high, low, or unknown risks of producing cancer. Paradoxically, anticancer drugs are the drugs most commonly associated with drug-induced cancer (Fig. 7.9).

- The alkylating agents are particularly implicated in causing hematopoietic cancer. Those used in low daily doses for prolonged periods are most likely to produce leukemia, characteristically 3–7 years after treatment begins.

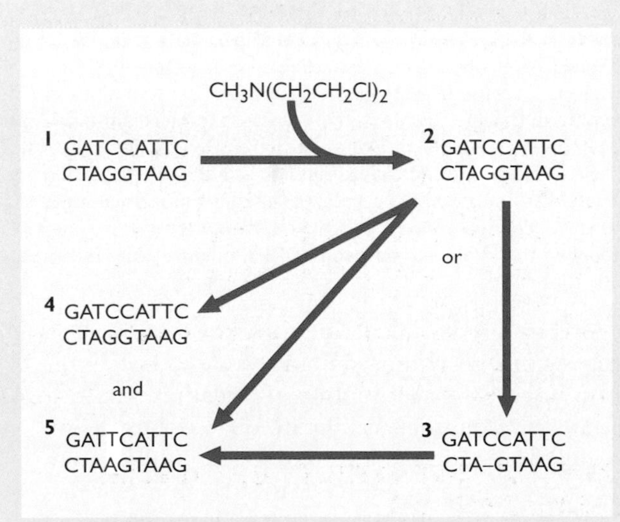

Fig. 7.9 Carcinogenesis or leukemogenesis occurs because drugs, especially the alkylating agents, cause permanent genetic mutations. This is exemplified by the G to A transition shown. (1) Correct base pair sequence (hypothetical). (2) Alkyl adduct binds to guanine (white). (3) Spontaneous loss of the adducted guanine (depurination), producing a strand break. (4) Repair/removal of the alkyl adduct and return to correct base pair sequence. (5) G to A transition producing a mutation. A mutation in a proto-oncogene or tumor suppressor gene would confer a proliferation to that cell and its clonal progeny.

- Ovarian cancer treated with chemotherapy is followed by an approximately 27-fold increase in acute nonlymphocytic leukemia (ANLL).
- Breast cancer treated with melphalan is followed by up to a sevenfold increase in ANLL.
- Myeloma treated with melphalan is followed by an approximately 214-fold increase in ANLL at 50 months (17% of the total incidence) in the population, but there is no increase in ANLL after 20 years of follow-up in patients with breast cancer treated with a combination of cyclophosphamide, methotrexate and 5-fluorouracil (CMF).

An increased incidence of early leukemias (ANLL less than 2 years after treatment) with a different chromosomal translocation at 11q23 has been noted in patients treated with drugs acting on topoisomerase II, such as etoposide and doxorubicin.

Late complications of cancer therapy

- Leukemogenesis/myelodysplasia
- Testicular and ovarian failure
- Secondary cancers

RESISTANCE TO CHEMOTHERAPY

If a cancer is incurable, some fraction of the cancer cells must be resistant to treatment. Resistance that is clinically apparent at the time of initial treatment because the majority of cells in the cancer are resistant is called de novo resistance. If the treatment initially kills non-resistant cells in the cancer, resistance is said to be acquired.

De novo resistance can be de novo genetic (i.e. the cells are initially inherently resistant), or can arise because drugs are unable to reach the target cells because of permeability barriers such as the blood–brain barrier (i.e. the cancer cells reside in pharmacologic 'sanctuaries' as discussed in detail below).

De novo genetic drug resistance is a property of an individual cell and is transferable to its progeny

One widely studied form of genetic resistance involves production of abnormal drug transport mechanisms, resulting in either decreased cellular uptake of anticancer drugs, or increased cellular efflux via the cell membrane. Transporter substrates are primarily natural products such as plant alkaloids, and include anthracyclines, epipodophyllotoxins, vinca alkaloids and paclitaxel. Multiple drug resistance arises from a single mutation or amplification of the *mdr* 1 gene. The *mdr* gene is a member of the functionally diverse ABC transmembrane superfamily of transport proteins and ion channels, including the membrane resistance protein (MRP) and cystic fibrosis genes.

Many drugs are retained in cells after their alteration or activation, for example after the kinase addition of phosphate groups to nucleosides (cytarabine) or polyglutamation of methotrexate. Absent or diminished levels of the relevant enzymes decreases the cellular retention of these drugs and may confer de novo resistance.

Pharmacologic 'sanctuaries' include the inaccessible compartments of the blood–brain barrier and the testes

Pharmacologic 'sanctuaries' can occur in solid cancers because their blood supply and drug diffusion (and therefore access to drug) are limited by the palisading effect (cells piling up in successive rows) that occurs in cancers. Inappropriate local acidosis can also confer resistance. Extracellular acidosis within a tumor will result in ionization of drugs with a low KA (e.g. doxorubicin) and decrease their cross-membrane movement into cells.

Acquired drug resistance never develops in noncancerous cells

Acquired resistance to anticancer drugs is an imprecise term. It fails to distinguish between the unmasking of innate genetic resistance in the initial heterogeneous cancer, which becomes evident only as sensitive cells are killed off, and acquired genetic resistance, which is actually induced by the chemotherapy itself or emerges spontaneously during treatment. Acquired resistance never develops in noncancerous cells and is therefore a property of the unstable mutable genome of transformed cancer cells. In clinical terms, acquired resistance means that the therapeutic ratio (the ratio between the minimum therapeutic and toxic doses) is not constant.

Multiple acquired drug resistance is expressed as a dominant phenotype. Gene transfer can confer drug resistance to cancer cells. The amount of the 170 kDa P-glycoprotein (P-GP170) found on the surface of multiple drug resistant cells correlates with the degree of resistance. The expression of this protein may be increased by oncogenes such as *ras* or mutant *p53*.

Membrane resistance protein is a 190 000 kDa ATP binding plasma membrane protein that can confer acquired multidrug resistance similar to the P-GP170 MDR protein. Decreased uptake due to deletion or altered kinetics of a transport mechanism, as in methotrexate and melphalan resistance, has been described in tissue culture.

An increase in drug metabolism by the cancer cell may produce acquired resistance (Fig. 7.10). Enzymes inactivate many drugs by chemical processes such as oxidation and reduction, and their enhanced activity may inactivate drugs. For example, aldehyde dehydrogenase oxidizes cyclophosphamide to inactive metabolites, and cytidine deaminase inactivates cytarabine.

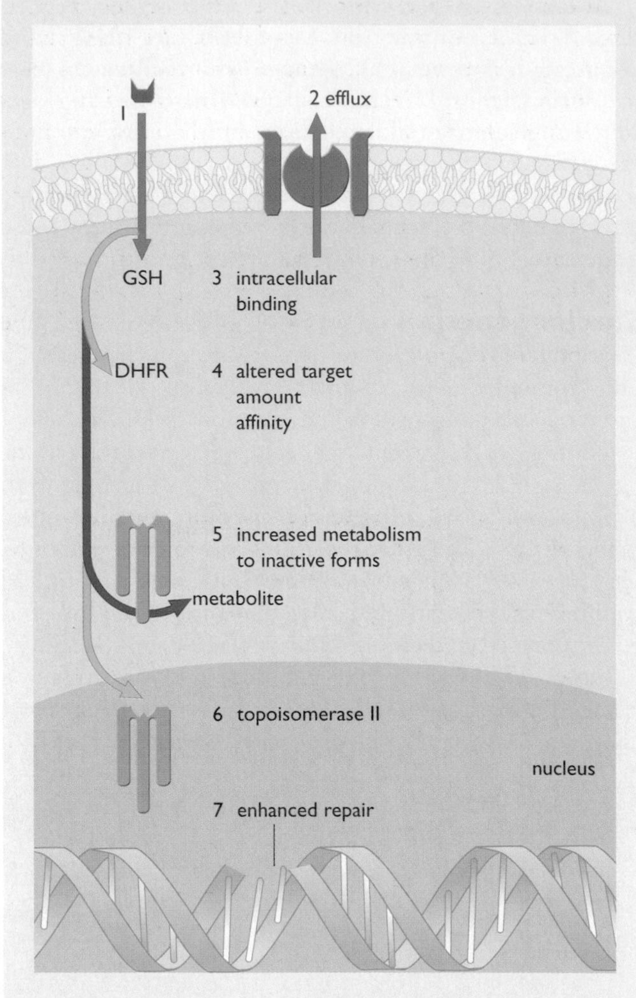

Fig. 7.10 Diagram showing several possible mechanisms of drug resistance. The classical biochemical view. Resistance can occur because of: (1) decreased uptake; (2) rapid efflux via membrane transport proteins; (3) increased intracellular binding to glutathione (GSH); (4) an altered target protein, either an increased amount or decreased binding affinity; (5) inactivation by intracellular detoxifying enzymes; (6) altered topoisomerase II, either a decreased amount or reduced affinity for a drug; and (7) enhanced repair of DNA damage. (DHFR, dihydrofolate reductase)

Altered intracellular concentrations of drug target proteins may result in acquired resistance (see Fig. 7.10):

- An increased concentration of target protein by gene amplification, such as dihydrofolate reductase amplification in methotrexate-resistant cells, may elevate target protein levels to such an extent that they may exceed the capacity for drug uptake and binding to achieve drug concentrations to be effective.
- Decreased topoisomerase concentrations reduce DNA damage and alter cytotoxicity caused by drugs that use topoisomerase I or II as the essential intermediates in producing DNA damage and lethality.
- Compartmentalization of target proteins away from the site of cytotoxic interaction can also produce resistance.

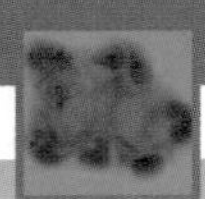

Altered drug target proteins are frequently encountered in highly resistant tumor cell lines. Mutations in the amino acid sequence of drug target proteins may change the active site and decrease or abolish drug binding, as in the case of resistance mediated by mutation of topoisomerase I (camptothecins) and II (etoposide), dihydrofolate reductase (methotrexate) and thymidylate synthetase (5-fluorouracil).

Mutation to a multiple drug resistant phenotype is stepwise. If there are two effective therapies, resistance may be prevented or delayed by alternating the treatments.

Mechanisms of generic resistance to cytotoxic drugs

- Abnormal transport
- Decreased cellular retention
- Increased cellular inactivation (binding/metabolism)
- Altered target protein
- Enhanced repair of DNA damage
- Altered processing

DRUGS DIRECTLY INTERFERING WITH DNA

See Table 7.2.

Alkylating drugs

Paul Ehrlich developed the first rationally designed anticancer drug, methyl nitrosourea, in 1898. Sulfur mustard gas was used as a chemical vesicant on the Western Front in the 1914–1918 war. It caused severe skin burns on contact and pulmonary edema when inhaled. The United States Army developed a derivative, nitrogen mustard, in 1943. When accidental exposure was noted to produce lymphopenia, the agent was administered to patients with malignant lymphoproliferative disorders with resultant partial or complete resolution, albeit transient, of the disease.

Mechlorethamine (nitrogen mustard), melphalan, cyclophosphamide, chlorambucil and ifosfamide are in widespread clinical use. Aziridines, such as thiotepa, epoxides (dibromodulcital) and alkyl alkane sulfonates such as busulfan are less frequently used. The nitrosoureas such as carmustine, lomustine and semustine are highly lipophilic and easily cross the blood–brain barrier and are therefore used to treat brain tumors.

Streptozocin is a monofunctional alkylating agent with no bone marrow toxicity, but it destroys the β cells of the pancreas, causing diabetes mellitus.

Table 7.2 Anticancer drugs

Drugs that interact with DNA ***Direct acting*** Alkylating agents: mechlorethamine hydrochloride, cyclophosphamide, ifosfamide, melphalan, chlorambucil, uracil mustard Nitrosoureas: lomustine, carmustine, streptozocin Miscellaneous: thiotepa, busulfan, dacarbazine (DTIC), pipobroman, procarbazine, cisplatin, carboplatin, altretamine ***Indirect acting*** Anthracyclines: doxorubicin HCl, daunorubicin HCl, idarubicin HCl, epirubicin, mitoxantrone HCl Topoisomerase-acting: etoposide, teniposide, topotecan, irinotecan Miscellaneous: bleomycin, dactinomycin, plicamycin **Antimetabolites** Methotrexate, trimetrexate, fluorouracil, floxuridine, capecitabine, cytarabine, gemcitabine Mercaptopurine, thioguanine, fludarabine, cladribine, pentostatin Hydroxyurea **Drugs that interact with tubulin** Depolymerizing agents: vincristine sulfate, vinblastine sulfate, vinorelbine, estramustine phosphate Polymerizing agents: paclitaxel, docetaxel	**Hormones** Estrogens: diethylstilbestrol, estradiol Antiestrogens: tamoxifen Aromatase inhibitors: anastrozole, letrozole, aminoglutethimide, testolactone Gonadotropin-releasing hormone partial agonists: leuprolide, goserelin Antiandrogens: bicalutamide, flutamide Progestins: medroxyprogesterone acetate, megesterl acetate Androgens **Miscellaneous** Interferons Levamisole HCl Asparaginase Mitotane Phosphotyrosine kinase inhibitors **Radiopharmaceuticals** Sodium iodide (NaI), ^{131}I Sodium phosphate, ^{32}P Strontium nitrate, ^{89}Sr

severe nausea with ethanol via a similar mechanism to disulfuram (see Drugs of Abuse, Ch. 8). Nausea and vomiting are significant. Myelosuppression occurs following oral, but not i.v., administration. Neurologic adverse effects are worse with i.v. therapy owing to higher peak plasma concentrations and include somnolence, confusion, mood changes and paresthesias. This may respond to pyridoxine used as an antidote. Allergic reactions have also been noted. Procarbazine is an alkylating drug in which dose modification may be necessary in patients with hepatic or renal insufficiency.

Dacarbazine
Dacarbazine is a pro-drug that is metabolized in the liver to release a methyldiazonium ion, which is the active alkylating product. It has poor CSF penetration and is therefore of no use for CNS cancers. Its major adverse effects are severe nausea and vomiting. The β half-life is 40 minutes and oral absorption is variable. Fifty percent is excreted in urine and dose modification may be necessary in patients with hepatic or renal insufficiency.

Altretamine
Altretamine (hexamethylmelamine) is a pro-drug that is activated in the liver. It is only available in an oral formulation, although oral absorption is variable. Peak concentrations occur 0.5–1 hours after dosing with two half-lifes, one of 0.5 hours and one of 5–10 hours. It is highly protein bound. Its major adverse effects are nausea and vomiting, and myelosuppression occurs in 50% of all patients. Neurologic adverse effects including mood changes and paresthesias may occur 1–3 months after treatment.

Temozolomide
Temozolomide is a drug that undergoes rapid nonenzymatic conversion at physiologic pH to the reactive compound MTIC, which is cytotoxic via alkylation of DNA. The alkylation induced by MTIC is primarily methylation at 60 and 7N positions on guanine residues. Temozolomide is administered orally to treat brain cancer and the most frequently reported adverse effects with this drug are nausea, vomiting, headaches and fatigue.

Platinum compounds
In 1968, it was observed that passing electric currents through platinum electrodes caused filamentous growth in bacteria, which is a sign of inhibited DNA synthesis. Within 3 years, cisplatin was being evaluated in cancer patients. Cisplatin revolutionized the treatment of testicular cancer, moving cure rates from 5–15% to 70–90% for the metastatic stage of the disease. It is an important component of drug treatment for ovarian, bladder, head and neck and lung cancers.

Cisplatin
Cisplatin (dichloro-diamino-cis platinum II) requires the replacement of Cl^- with water (aquation) for activation (see Fig. 7.12). Activation is slow (2.5 hours) and only the cis enantiomer is therapeutically active as a cytotoxic drug.

MECHANISM OF ACTION Cisplatin binds to guanine in DNA and RNA, and the interaction is stabilized by hydrogen bonding. The molecular mechanism of action is unwinding and shortening of the DNA helix. Although ISCs occur (10% of all adducts), the cellular mechanism of action, cell inactivation, appears to be principally due to the formation of intrastrand links (75–80%). A relationship exists between the number of cross-links, ability to repair cross-links and cytotoxicity.

Resistance to cisplatin may involve a cancer cell DNA repair mechanism similar to that which removes the cyclobutane dimers formed by the interaction of DNA with ultraviolet light.

PHARMACOKINETICS Cisplatin is inactivated in blood and intracellularly by covalent interaction with sulfhydryl groups in glutathione and metallothioneins. Protein binding to tissue, blood cells and plasma proteins also inactivates cisplatin. Cisplatin is filtered by glomeruli and actively secreted in renal proximal convoluted tubules. Approximately 25% of a dose is excreted within 24 hours, and 90% in urine. The α, β and γ half-lifes are 30 minutes, 60 minutes and 24 hours, respectively. Cisplatin is not orally bioavailable.

ADVERSE EFFECTS The major adverse effects of cisplatin is renal toxicity (renal tubular damage and necrosis) similar to that seen with heavy metals. Protective procedures to avoid this include hydration and diuresis. Myelosuppression, usually thrombocytopenia, is less common than with alkylating drugs. If there is adequate renal protection, peripheral neuropathy becomes the dose-limiting adverse effect. Ototoxicity with hearing loss, allergic reactions and severe nausea and vomiting are common. Cisplatin is contraindicated if renal clearance of creatinine in the patient is <60 mL/min.

Carboplatin
Carboplatin is an analog of cisplatin with the same mechanism of action. It was developed to be less nephrotoxic and be less likely to cause vomiting. The intracellular DNA adduct is identical to that formed by cisplatin. Like cisplatin, no metabolism occurs and carboplatin is excreted by the kidneys. Creatinine clearance data enables dosing on a precise AUC (total drug exposure) basis, rather than on a mg/m^2 basis. The half-life of carboplatin is similar to cisplatin. Carboplatin is also myelosuppressive.

Oxaliplatin
Oxaliplatin undergoes nonenzymatic conversion in body fluids to active derivatives via displacement of the labile

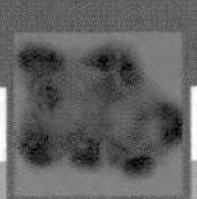

oxalate compound. Several transient reactive species are formed including monoagus and diagus platinum which then covalently bind with DNA. Both inter- and intra-DNA cross-links are formed between the N7 positions of two adjacent guanines, adjacent adenexial guanines and guanines separated by an intervening nucleotide. These cross-links inhibit DNA replication and transcription and occur independently of the stage of the cell cycle. Oxaliplatin has a 391 hour half-life in serum. The most common side effects reported are peripheral sensory neuropathies, fatigues, neutropenia, nauseas, emesis and diarrhea.

DRUGS THAT INDIRECTLY DAMAGE DNA

Anthracyclines

Doxorubicin and daunorubicin have a wide spectrum of usefulness in cancer chemotherapy, which is second only to the usefulness of alkylating drugs. Doxorubicin is effective against:

- Non-Hodgkin's lymphoma.
- Hodgkin's disease.
- Acute leukemias.
- Carcinomas of the breast, lung, stomach and thyroid.
- Sarcomas.

Doxorubicin is used to treat solid tumors and, in leukemia, daunorubicin is sometimes preferred because it causes less mucositis. Doxorubicin is a pro-drug. The active metabolite, idarubicin, is effective against leukemia and is itself used therapeutically since it can be given orally. Anthracyclines have a unique cardiotoxicity. All anthracyclines are quinones capable of generating free radicals. Free-radical quinones cause peroxidation of the cardiac sarcoplasmic reticulum, leading to Ca^{2+}-dependent myocardial necrosis. This adverse effect may be blocked by co-administration of the iron chelator, desrazoxane. Epirubicin is less cardiotoxic than other anthracyclines and is widely used in Europe. It is particularly effective in breast cancer. Anthracycline cardiotoxicity does not depend on the dose.

MECHANISM OF ACTION Anthracyclines and anthracenediones intercalate with DNA and bind avidly to nuclear chromatin, forming a ternary complex of drug intercalated into DNA and topoisomerase II (Top II) to produce strand cleavage. The Top II-mediated mechanism is probably the most important molecular mechanism of action.

Free radical formation leading to cancer cell redox-mediated damage is a second cytotoxic mechanism. All anthracyclines are quinones capable of producing free radicals, which damage membranes, proteins and lipids. Glutathione and catalase can detoxify the free radical quinones, and lack of catalase in cardiac tissue is the basis for anthracycline's apparently selective cardiotoxicity. Complexes of iron and anthracycline bind tightly to cell membranes to cause spontaneous membrane destruction. Recently, activation of a ceramide synthetase pathway that produces apoptotic cell death has been described. The relevance of this to the beneficial effects of these drugs in cancer treatment is not certain.

RESISTANCE Resistance mechanisms to anthracycline include:

- p-Gp 170/*mdr* gene glycoprotein-mediated drug efflux.
- Altered Top II concentrations.
- A mutant topoisomerase II.
- Increased glutathione concentration.
- Increased glutathione peroxidase activity (this enzyme detoxifies free radicals).
- Decreased glucose-6-phosphate dehydrogenase concentration.

PHARMACOKINETICS Anthracyclines and anthracenediones diffuse passively into cells in their non-ionized form. The drugs become charged and are prevented from diffusing into cells if there is extracellular acidification, which is common feature of solid tumors. The long terminal half-life of doxorubicin, 30 hours, makes dosing schedules less important. Prolonged infusions or weekly schedules are less cardiotoxic than monthly bolus injections. Except for idarubicin, all anthracyclines are available only in i.v. formulations. Doxorubicin is a potent radiation sensitizer. Heparin binds the daunosamine sugar and increases clearance. Doxorubicin decreases paclitaxel clearance.

ADVERSE EFFECTS Adverse effects of anthracyclines include myelosuppression, mucositis and stomatitis, especially with doxorubicin, and with continuous infusions rather than bolus doses. Cardiac toxicity, a particular and potentially lethal problem, causes heart failure. Factors increasing the risk of heart failure include pre-existing heart disease, hypertension and cardiac radiation therapy. Cardiac toxicity is a function of peak dose concentrations, and continuous infusions or weekly dosing decrease the risk. Desrazoxane, an iron chelator, decreases cardiotoxicity. Anthracyclines cause extensive and severe soft tissue necrosis if the drug becomes extravascular.

Idarubicin

Idarubicin is effective against acute leukemia and breast cancer. It has the same mechanism of action and resistance as doxorubicin, and its oral bioavailability is 30%. Its effectiveness depends on its metabolism to an active metabolite, 13-epirubicinol.

Idarubicin is less cardiotoxic than doxorubicin.

Valrubian and Epirubicin

Valrubicin and epirubicin are two newer anthracyclines. Valrubicin readily penetrates into cells and arrest cells in

G_2. It does not bind DNA, but some of the intracellular metabolites of valrubicin interfere with DNA topoisomerase II. Epirubicin, in addition to an action of topoisomerase II (via formation of a complex with DNA by intercalation of its planar rings between nucleotide base pairs), also inhibits DNA helicase activity, preventing the enzymatic separation of double-stranded DNA and thereby interfering with replication and transcription. Epirubicin is also involved in oxidation/reduction reactions by generating cytotoxic free radicals.

Mitoxantrone

Mitoxantrone is an anthracenedione that is less cardiotoxic than anthracyclines. Its molecular mechanism of action is interaction with Top II and DNA, resulting in breaks in DNA strands. Mitoxantrone does not generate free radicals. The mechanisms of resistance to mitoxantrone are the same as for doxorubicin.

Adverse effects of mitoxantrone include extravasation injury, alopecia and nausea, and dose-limiting myelosuppression. Overall, the adverse effect profile is much more favorable than that for anthracyclines, especially with respect to cardiotoxicity. However, cardiotoxicity is seen in patients who have previously been treated with doxorubicin. Cardiotoxicity is less frequent, but if it does appear, it is just as severe as with anthracyclines.

Topoisomerase-active drugs

Topoisomerases I and II are nuclear enzymes that cleave one (Top I) or two (Top II) strands of DNA, to allow DNA strand passage to unwind DNA and relieve torsional stress and to decatenate intertwined segments of DNA (Top II only). Top I and/or Top II are necessary for DNA replication and RNA transcription. Top II is necessary for the completion of mitosis. Top II plays a crucial role in the tertiary structure of chromatin. Two isoforms have been isolated. The predominant isoform, Top IIα, is tightly cell cycle-regulated (increased in S phase and increased further in M phase). Top IIα and especially Top I can be elevated in neoplastic cells independently of increased proliferation.

Topoisomerases form a covalent bond with DNA through a tyrosine transester linkage. Topoisomerase-active drugs stabilize this transient intermediate, preventing re-ligation of the DNA strands. The exact molecular mechanism of cytotoxicity is uncertain, since enzyme inhibition is fully reversible. The possible mechanisms of action of these drugs include:

- Inappropriate recombination of topoisomerase-bound DNA strands (sister chromatid exchange; SCE).
- Apoptosis due to unreplicated DNA or unrepaired DNA strand breaks, and/or decreases in mitotic promotion factor (MPF), which is a complex of two proteins, a cyclin and cdc_2 (see Fig. 7.3), a phosphokinase, which phosphorylates other proteins to regulate the passage into mitosis.

Etoposide and teniposide

Etoposide and teniposide are semisynthetic epipodophyllotoxins. They are derivatives of podophyllotoxin, a tubulin-binding extract from the mandrake plant (*Mandragora officinarum*).

MECHANISM OF ACTION The molecular mechanism of action of epipodophyllotoxins is the transient stabilization of a 'cleavable complex' of Top II and DNA, the production of which is reversible after drug withdrawal (Fig. 7.13). Top II is a necessary intermediary since the drugs do not interact directly with DNA. Although the mechanism of cytotoxicity is unclear, there is a linear relationship between drug concentration, double-strand DNA breaks, and cytotoxicity leading to cancer cell death.

RESISTANCE Increased levels of pGp 170 and *mdr* gene amplification/overexpression with enhanced efflux, an enhanced capacity to repair DNA strand breaks, decreased Top II levels (with a collateral increase in Top I) and altered (mutant) topoisomerase II enzymes capable of re-ligating the separated DNA strands, despite the presence of drug, all contribute to drug resistance.

PHARMACOKINETICS Since 95% of these drugs are protein bound, penetration into the CNS (5%) and ascites fluid is poor. Oral absorption (approximately 50%) can be adequate, but marked variability occurs among patients. A divided course of doses spread over many days provides therapeutic efficacy superior to single or weekly doses. Daily oral etoposide for 21 days is significantly more effective than other single drugs.

ADVERSE EFFECTS Adverse effects include myelosuppression, especially neutropenia, which is dose limiting, and oral mucositis. Toxicity depends on the regimen used. A unique form of acute nonlymphocytic leukemia, with a translocation of the AML1 gene at the 11q23 locus, has occurred after treatment with a prolonged and high total cumulative doses of etoposide.

Camptothecin and derivatives

MECHANISM OF ACTION Camptothecin (Fig. 7.14) is an alkaloid derived from a Chinese tree, *Camptotheca accuminata*. It was first introduced in clinical trials in the 1970s, but was then abandoned because it lacked clinical efficacy and caused severe hemorrhagic cystitis. Interest was renewed 15 years later with the discovery that the molecular target of camptothecin is Top I, which is highly expressed in neoplastic tissues. All Top I inhibitors have an intact lactone E ring (see Fig. 7.14). Hydrolysis of the lactone to produce a carboxylate derivative inactivates the drug. Many analogs of camptothecin are now in clinical trials. As S phase-specific drugs, camptothecins have to be present in the cell over a prolonged period.

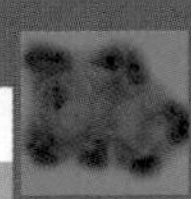

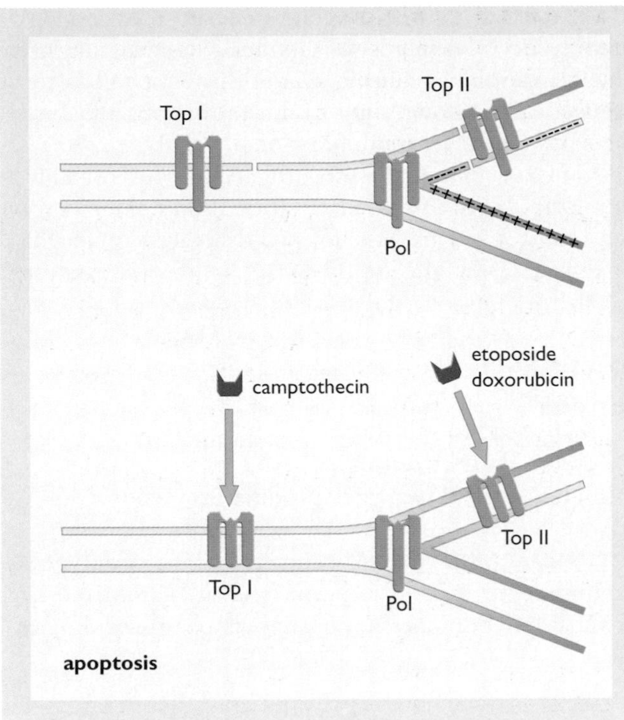

Fig. 7.13 Sites of action of camptothecin and etoposide or doxorubicin. They stabilize the normally transient covalent cleavage in replicating DNA produced by topoisomerase I (Top I) and/or topoisomerase II (Top II), which produces a double-strand DNA break by collision with the DNA replication apparatus of DNA polymerase a (leading strand 5′→3′) and polymerase d (lagging strand 3′→5′) (Pol).

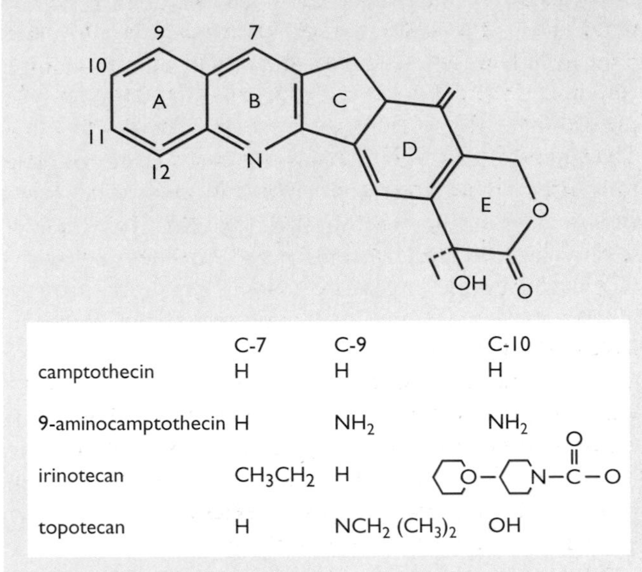

	C-7	C-9	C-10
camptothecin	H	H	H
9-aminocamptothecin	H	NH_2	NH_2
irinotecan	CH_3CH_2	H	O–N–C(=O)–O
topotecan	H	$NCH_2(CH_3)_2$	OH

Fig. 7.14 Chemical structures of the camptothecins, which act on topoisomerase I. The lactone E ring must be intact for topoisomerase I interaction. Substitutions at C-7, -9 and -10 increase water solubility. The C-10 substitution of irinotecan is hydrolyzed to OH. This metabolite, termed SN-38, is 200 times more active than the parent drug.

Common properties of camptothecins include:

- Activity in a wide variety of epithelial cancers.
- A high degree of binding to serum albumin (>80%).
- Severe reversible myelosuppression.
- Marked interpatient variability in pharmacokinetics.
- Significant dose schedule dependency (activation is greater with a divided dose schedule).

Camptothecins have a wide spectrum of activity against solid tumors, including non-small cell lung cancer, small cell lung cancer, and colon, cervical and ovarian cancers. They are also effective against leukemias and lymphomas.

RESISTANCE The mechanisms of resistance to camptothecins include:

- Decreased Top I levels.
- An altered/mutant topoisomerase that cannot bind the drug or one that can re-ligate in the presence of camptothecin.
- Enhanced membrane efflux via p-Gp 170 for water-soluble analogs such as topotecan (see Fig. 7.14), which is a semisynthetic water-soluble camptothecin analog.

Irinotecan (see Fig. 7.14) is a pro-drug and is cleaved by ubiquitous carboxylesterases to a metabolite (SN-38), which is a more effective Top I inhibitor than the parent drug. The protein binding of SN-38 (<60%) is much less than that in most camptothecins. Irinotecan causes a particularly severe diarrhea, which is responsive to octreotide and preventable with high-dose loperamide. Less frequently it causes severe myelosuppression, which is unrelated to serum drug levels but associated with weekly dosing schedules. Conjugation to glucuronides via UDP glycosylases is a major mechanism of metabolism, and enterohepatic recirculation may account for severe adverse effects and plasma pharmacokinetic variability in patients.

Miscellaneous anticancer drugs

Bleomycins

The bleomycins are a family of complex glycopeptides isolated from a *Streptomyces*, which avidly chelate metals. Bleomycin A_2 is the major bleomycin used clinically. Bleomycin is used to treat Hodgkin's disease, NHL and testicular, cervical, head and neck cancers. Its inclusion in regimens for the chemotherapy of germ cell cancers results in an increased cure rate.

MECHANISM OF ACTION All active bleomycins bind reduced iron (Fe^{2+}), and the drug/Fe complex is responsible for producing single- and double-strand DNA breaks that are reflected as DNA chromosomal gaps, deletions and fragments. These result from free-radical formation from Fe^{2+}–bleomycin–oxygen complexes which intercalate between DNA strands. Intercalation of drug into DNA is the initial step, before

Fe^{2+} is oxidized, and oxygen is reduced to the radicals $\cdot O_2^-$ or $\cdot OH$. DNA cleavage occurs after the intercalated bleomycin complex is assembled, and absolutely requires oxygen.

PHARMACOKINETICS Bleomycins are large cationic molecules. They penetrate cell membranes poorly via a bleomycin-binding membrane protein. Internalized bleomycins are either translocated to the nucleus or hydrolyzed by bleomycin hydrolase, a cysteine protease present in normal and malignant cells, but found in decreased concentrations in lung and skin.

ADVERSE EFFECTS Bleomycin adverse effects are confined to the lungs and skin because of the above. Pulmonary adverse effects are the major problem, manifest as subacute or chronic interstitial pneumonitis and, at a later stage, fibrosis.

Dactinomycin

Dactinomycin (actinomycin D) has significant anticancer actions against solid tumors, such as Wilms' tumor, Ewing's tumor, neuroblastoma, rhabdomyosarcoma and choriocarcinoma.

MECHANISM OF ACTION Structurally, dactinomycin is two symmetric polypeptide chains attached to a phenoxazone ring. The molecular mechanism of action is intercalation of the phenoxazone ring perpendicular to the long axis of DNA while the peptide chains lie in the minor groove. This results in inhibition of RNA and protein synthesis by prevention of chain elongation. Dactinomycin enters cells by passive diffusion. Resistance to dactinomycin is associated with increased expression of *p-gP/mdr*.

ADVERSE EFFECTS Adverse effects of dactinomycin include nausea, vomiting, mucosal ulceration, dose-limiting myelosuppression and dermatologic manifestations. Dactinomycin is a severe vesicant and a radiation-sensitizing agent, and can produce severe radiation 'recall injury.'

Mitomycin C

Mitomycin C has significant theoretical appeal because it is selectively toxic to hypoxic cells, and hypoxia is a major feature of solid tumors. Mitomycin C has widespread but limited clinical usefulness in the treatment of a broad range of solid tumors, including those of the gastrointestinal tract, breast, lung, head, neck and bladder, and gynecologic tumors. It is synergistic with 5-fluorouracil and with radiotherapy. Initial trials with mitomycin C alone were disappointing because of severe cumulative bone marrow, pulmonary and renal adverse effects. However, it can be used in conjunction with other drugs using an intermittent dosing schedule which reduces the severity of adverse effects.

MECHANISM OF ACTION The mechanism of action of mitomycin C depends on its bioreductive alkylation under anaerobic, reducing conditions as it needs to be reduced at quinone sites to form the unstable intermediates that react monofunctionally at the guanine 2N position. It is therefore a pro-drug. About 10% of adducts can form ISCs. Free-radical formation under aerobic conditions (a second basis for pro-drug activity) may lead to cancer cell single-strand DNA breaks, or these may result from unsuccessful alkylation repair.

RESISTANCE The mechanisms of resistance to mitomycin C include:

- Decreased bioactivation.
- Increased DNA repair.
- Increased *p-gP/mdr* gene product expression.

PHARMACOKINETICS Mitomycin C is used intravenously since oral absorption is erratic. Impaired liver or renal function does not change its pharmacokinetics.

ANTIMETABOLITES

Amethopterin, an analog of folic acid, has been in use since 1948 when it was first demonstrated that folate antagonists could induce complete (but transient) remissions of childhood acute leukemia. Sidney Farber at the Boston Children's Hospital had noted megaloblastic changes in the bone marrow of children with leukemia and surmised that exacerbating depletion of folate stores could stop the proliferation of leukemic cells. This is an example of rational target selection in cancer therapy, as distinct from the empiric (but invaluable) approach demonstrated with the alkylating agents.

Methotrexate

MECHANISM OF ACTION The molecular mechanism of action of methotrexate is inhibition of the enzyme dihydrofolate reductase.

Folates are one-carbon cofactors in purine and pyrimidine biosynthesis and include:

- Pteridine.
- Para-aminobenzoic acid.
- Glutamate complexes.

Polyglutamates are more efficient cofactors because they are retained longer in the cells. The tetrahydro (reduced) folates are the active forms and the essential role of dihydrofolate reductase is to maintain a supply of reduced folate cofactors. Dihydrofolate and formyl dihydrofolate, which accumulate after inhibition of dihydrofolate reductase, directly inhibit folate-dependent enzymes.

Methotrexate is actively transported via a 5N-methyl tetrahydrofolic acid (reduced folate) system through the cell membrane into the cytoplasm, where it binds and inactivates dihydrofolate. Free methotrexate competes

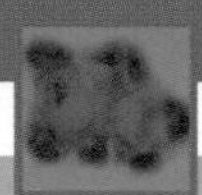

with increased concentrations of dihydrofolate (from decreased thymidylate synthase activity) to inhibit dihydrofolate reductase, resulting in a reduction in the availability of thymidylate synthase.

Methotrexate also has effects on purine synthesis, where 10-formyl dihydrofolate is a necessary cofactor in two steps of de novo purine synthesis. The required intracellular concentration of methotrexate for inhibiting pyrimidine synthesis is 1×10^{-8} M, while that for inhibiting purine synthesis is 1×10^{-7} M. In general, cytotoxicity is directly proportional to the duration of exposure, although increased drug concentrations may overcome resistance and increase cytotoxicity.

RESISTANCE Multiple mechanisms have been described for methotrexate resistance. These include:
- Decreased cellular uptake.
- Decreased affinity of dihydrofolate reductase for methotrexate.
- Increased concentration of dihydrofolate reductase.
- Decreased polyglutamation due to decreased folate polyglutamyl synthase.
- Decreased thymidylate synthesis.

PHARMACOKINETCS Oral absorption of methotrexate is good but variable. Poor absorption accounts for increased relapses in childhood acute lymphocytic leukemia. Methotrexate has three plasma half-lifes (5 minutes, 2–3 hours, 8–10 hours). The latter two are prolonged if there is impaired renal function or fluid accumulation. Re-emergence of methotrexate into the blood from pleural effusions or ascites produces a prolongation of drug exposure, which increases adverse effects. Methotrexate penetration into the CNS is poor, with a plasma:CSF concentration ratio of 31:1. The major mechanisms of metabolism of methotrexate are by intracellular conversion to polyglutamates and 7-hydroxylation in the liver. Elimination is via unchanged drug in urine. Methotrexate doses should be reduced in proportion to any decrease in creatinine clearance in patients with impaired liver function. Special attention should be given to the use of methotrexate in patients with effusions of any kind, and the elderly in whom decreased creatinine clearance, as a result of decreased muscle mass, may occur with a normal serum creatinine (i.e. not as a consequence of impaired liver function).

High doses of methotrexate have been used to overcome the limited transport of methotrexate into cancer cells. Higher intracellular concentrations of methotrexate can partially overcome resistance due to increased dihydrofolate reductase activity or altered dihydrofolate reductase affinity for methotrexate. This increases intracellular polyglutamate formation and so increases the duration of action of methotrexate. The effectiveness of high doses of methotrexate compared with conventional doses is, however, uncertain, and has resulted in folate 'rescue' being required using a reduced folate source, 5-formyl tetrahydrofolic acid (leucovorin). Thymidine and blockade of cell cycle progression with 1-asparaginase have also been used to allow the use of high doses of methotrexate.

ADVERSE EFFECTS Myelosuppression and mucositis are the major adverse effects of methotrexate. CNS damage may be severe when methotrexate is given intrathecally with irradiation and may manifest as one of the following:
- Chemical arachnoiditis, characterized by headache, fever and nuchal rigidity, is the most common and most acute adverse effect. It may be due to additives in the drug diluent (benzoic acid in sterile water).
- Subacute CNS toxicity, which occurs 2–3 weeks after administration and is characterized by motor paralysis, cranial nerve palsy, seizures and coma.
- Chronic demyelinating encephalitis, which produces dementia and spasticity with cortical thinning, enlarged cerebral ventricles and cerebral calcifications.

The latter two adverse effects are sometimes worsened by radiotherapy.

Cirrhosis and portal vein fibrosis result from prolonged oral use. Chemical hepatitis due to methotrexate is reversed by choline administration.

Trimetrexate

Trimetrexate is a methotrexate analog that enters cells by diffusion. It is therefore active against reduced folate-transport mutants and polyglutamation-deficient mutants that are resistant to methotrexate. It is also used to treat *Pneumocystis carinii* pneumonia.

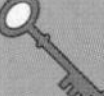

Characteristics of antimetabolites
- Mimic essential cellular 'metabolites'
- Usually effective against actively proliferating cells
- Have common toxicities of myelosuppression and mucositis
- Are teratogenic, but not usually leukemogenic

Pyrimidine analogs

Fluorinated pyrimidines (5-fluorouracil)

5-fluorouracil (Fig. 7.15) was developed by Charles Heidelberger in 1957 on the basis of an observed increased uracil incorporation into rat hepatomas. Despite its long history in the clinic, fluorouracil and its analogs continue to be effective as the optimal scheduling, dosing and usage are continually refined with resultant significantly improved clinical benefits.

MECHANISM OF ACTION 5-fluorouracil is a pro-drug that must be activated (ribosylated, phosphorylated) to 5-fluoro-deoxyuracil monophosphate. The molecular

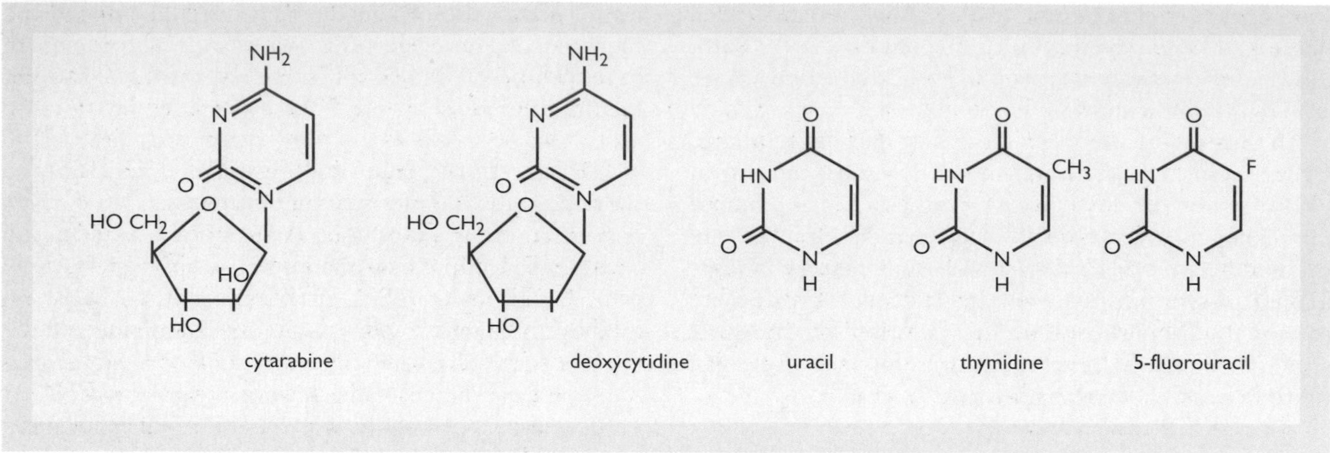

Fig. 7.15 Chemical structures of cytarabine, deoxycytidine, uracil, thymidine and 5-fluorouracil. Like methotrexate, cytarabine and 5-fluorouracil are analogs of nucleotides which are taken up and actuated by normal cellular processes. However, because of a unique feature, they become inhibitors of DNA synthesis rather than building blocks of DNA. There are many potential sites of resistance because of the complex biochemistry involved.

mechanism of action of 5-fluoro-deoxyuracil monophosphate is inhibition of thymidylate synthase (Fig. 7.16). RNA incorporation of 5-fluoro-deoxyuracil monophosphate may account for actions on cancer cells. Thymidine alone cannot reverse all the effects of 5-fluoro-deoxyuracil monophosphate, which also impairs precursor rRNA processing and polyadenylation of nuclear RNA. Incorporation of 5-fluorouracil into DNA also produces base pair mismatching and faulty mRNA transcripts.

5-fluorouracil is rapidly taken up into cells, where a series of phosphorylases and kinases act upon it. Fluorouracil deoxyribose is activated in one additional step by thymidine kinase. Activation is complex and interdependent, with many sites at which resistance can develop.

PHARMACOKINETICS The primary half-life of 5-fluorouracil is 6–20 minutes. 5-fluorouracil is metabolized intracellularly in the liver to nucleotide forms and catabolized to dihydrofluorouracil by the enzyme dihydropyrimidine dehydrogenase (DPD). More than 90% of the drug is metabolized and <5% renally excreted. Oral absorption of 5-fluorouracil is poor as a result of first-pass metabolism in the gut and liver by DPD. An i.v. loading dose rapidly produces steady-state levels. With increasing doses there is nonlinear pharmacokinetic behavior as hepatic metabolism is saturated and total body clearance decreases, producing ever-higher plasma levels. Intra-arterial administration allows selective drug delivery to liver metastases where a first-pass metabolism by the tumor reduces systemic drug levels, and adverse effects.

COMBINATION CHEMOTHERAPY 5-fluorouracil has been used in combination with many drugs in the treatment of solid tumors.

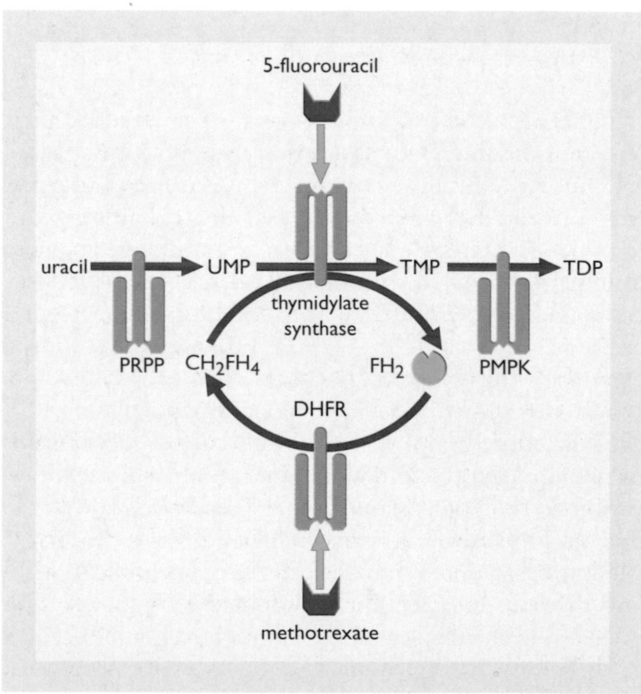

Fig. 7.16 The thymidine pathway showing the inhibition of thymidylate synthase by 5-fluorouracil. Methotrexate and 5-fluorouracil both act to decrease the synthesis of thymidine. (DHFR, dihydrofolate reductase; CH_2FH_4, methylene tetrahydrofolate, the donor of a methyl group to uracil; FH_2, dihydrofolate; PMPK, pyrimidine monophosphate kinase; PRPP, phosphoribosyl pyrophosphatase; TDP, thymidine diphosphate; TMP, thymidine monophosphate; UMP, uracil monophosphate)

Methotrexate increases 5-fluorouracil triphosphate formation and this increases cytotoxicity. Thymidine inhibits 5-fluorouracil degradation and thereby increases its half-life. Infusion of thymidine triphosphate, a feedback inhibitor of ribonucleotide reductase, increases 5-fluorouracil triphosphate incorporation into RNA.

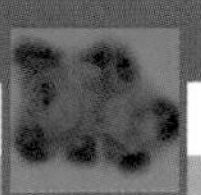

Inhibitors of de novo purine synthesis such as pyrazofurin, L-phosphonoacetyl-l-alanine and allopurinol increase 5-fluorouracil triphosphate production.

Leucovorin increases the inhibition of thymidylate synthase, which requires reduced folate cofactors to form a tight ternary complex with 5-fluorouracil. Leucovorin increases the cytotoxicity in 5-fluorouracil-insensitive tumors by stabilizing the ternary complex, slowing the reversibility of the reaction, and increasing deoxythymidine monophosphate concentrations. Leucovorin doubles the effectiveness of 5-fluorouracil in the treatment of colon and breast cancers. 5-fluorouracil significantly prolongs survival when used in the treatment of locally advanced rectal and pancreatic cancers.

ADVERSE EFFECTS 5-fluorouracil produces reversible myelosuppression, mucositis and diarrhea as its major toxicities. These vary in severity depending on the dose and schedule used and the presence of other drugs. Very prolonged infusions cause palmar erythema and desquamation. Lacrimal duct stenosis and cerebellar ataxia at high doses (due to inhibition of the tricarboxylic acid cycle in the cerebellum) are rarely encountered.

DPD activity is normally distributed in humans. Individuals with activity <5% are at increased risk for severe and even fatal reactions to 5-fluorouracil. DPD saturation kinetics can reduce clearance at higher levels and DPD activity in the gut limits oral absorption. Elevated DPD levels have been identified in certain tumors and the rapid breakdown of 5-fluorouracil in these cells may confer therapeutic resistance.

New developments in fluoropyrimidine chemotherapy

Continuous i.v. infusions of 5-fluorouracil achieve increased activity and decreased toxicity compared with bolus administration, but are technically difficult to obtain. Two other approaches taken are the inhibition of degradative enzymes to prolong exposure to 5-fluorouracil, and the introduction of new orally available drugs.

UFT combines tegafur, a 5-fluorouracil pro-drug, and uracil. Tegafur is converted in the liver to 5-fluorouracil by thymidine/uridine phosphorylase. Uracil is added in a 4:1 ratio as a competitive substrate for DPD to enhance oral absorption and prolong the half-life of 5-fluorouracil. Diarrhea is the dose-limiting toxicity in the 14-day and 28-day schedules, and myelosuppression with the 5-day schedule. UFT has comparable activity to 5-fluorouracil in colorectal cancer and other cancers.

Capecitabine is a pro-drug of 5-fluorouracil that requires a complex activation process. The first step is hydrolysis by carboxylesterases (predominantly in the liver) to form 5´-deoxy-5-fluorocytidine. Cytidine deaminase then removes the C-amine, producing 5´-deoxy-5-fluorouridine. Pyrimidine nucleoside phosphorylase (PNP) produces the actively antineoplastic drug, 5-fluorouracil. PNP has been identified at higher levels in certain tumors and this may confer some selectivity. Oral absorption of capecitabine is rapid and the 6-week b.i.d. dosing schedule produces plasma 5-fluorouracil levels similar to those obtained with i.v. administration of 5-fluorouracil at 300 mg/m^2/day. Hand-foot syndrome, diarrhea and stomatitis are the dose-limiting toxicities.

S1 is an oral 5-fluorouracil preparation of tegafur and 5-chloro-2,4-dihydroxy-pyridine (CDHP) and oxonic acid. CDHP is a DPD inhibitor. Oxonic acid is an inhibitor of orotate phosphoribosyl transferase which decreases 5-fluorouracil conversion to fluorouracil monophosphate (FUMP) and its incorporation into RNA. A 28-day dosing cycle shows promising clinical activity and comparable toxicity to the other oral formulations described above.

Cytarabine

Cytarabine (cytosine arabinoside, also known as ara-C) is a nucleoside analog of cytosine. It is a pro-drug that requires phosphorylation to produce the active monophosphate product, ara-CMP, and subsequently the triphosphate (ara-CTP). The molecular mechanism of action of ara-CMP is ultimately via ara-CTP competition with cytosine triphosphate for DNA polymerases. The resultant incorporation of ara-CTP into DNA produces cytotoxicity which leads to premature DNA chain termination. Resistance to cytarabine correlates with the decreased formation and/or retention of ara-CTP.

PHARMACOKINETICS Cytarabine is deaminated in the intestines, so it cannot be given orally. It is actively transported across cell membranes and rapidly phosphorylated in a stepwise fashion by deoxycytidine kinases to the active triphosphate. Deamination by cytidine deaminase inactivates the drug. The major plasma half-life is 2 hours.

ADVERSE EFFECTS These include myelosuppression, which is dose limiting, severe and reversible. Cholestatic jaundice and mucositis are less common. Cerebellar dysfunction due to a loss of cerebellar Purkinje cells occurs in up to 30% of patients treated with a high-dose regimen >3 g/m^2 for six or more twice-daily doses. This occurs more frequently in elderly patients with renal insufficiency and the syndrome is usually irreversible.

COMBINATION CHEMOTHERAPY Synergism, believed to be due to decreased DNA repair, has been reported with cyclophosphamide, cisplatin, carmustine and thiopurines.

Gemcitabine (2′-2′, difluorodeoxycytidine)

Gemcitabine is a cytidine analog which acts against pancreatic, ovarian, lung and breast carcinomas where cytarabine is inactive. Gemcitabine is 5–8 times more effective in vitro against solid tumors than cytarabine and is similar in that it is deaminated, activated by deoxy-

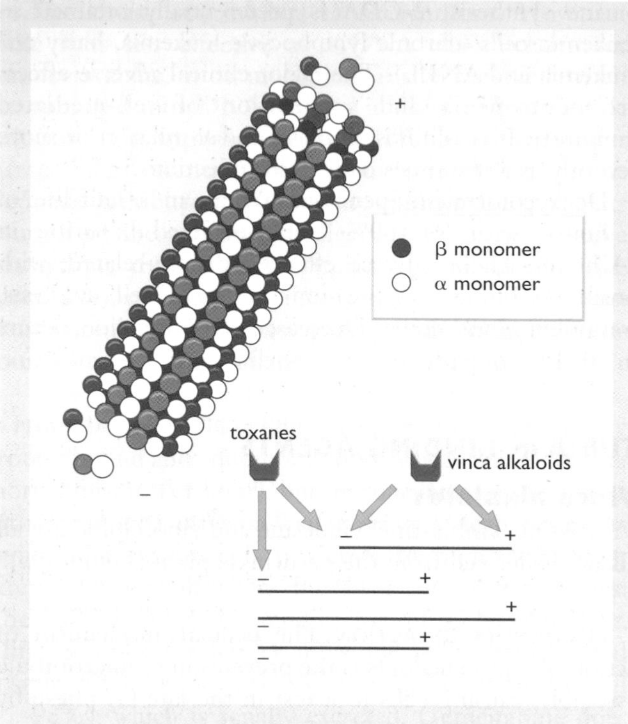

Fig. 7.18 The formation of tubulin polymers and the process of tubulin migration. The polymers are made up of α and β monomers and the process of tubulin migration involves elongation at the (+) end and shortening at the (–) end. Vinca alkaloids decrease the association rate at the (+) end and prevent polymerization of a and b dimers. Toxanes stabilize multimers and prevent dissociation at the (–) end, resulting in increased polymerization. Either of these effects on the dynamic equilibrium is cytotoxic.

vinblastine, with vinorelbine being the least neurotoxic.

- Vinblastine has the most myelotoxic effects, followed by vindesine and then vinorelbine. Vincristine is not myelosuppressive.
- All vinca alkaloids cause mild alopecia, but this is more severe with vinblastine and vindesine than with vincristine and vinorelbine.
- All induce the syndrome of nephrogenic inappropriate antidiuretic hormone action.
- All cause equally severe local extravasation injury.

L-asparaginase decreases vinca alkaloid hepatic metabolism and increases cytotoxicity towards cancer cells, so vinca alkaloids should be given 12–24 hours before L-asparaginase.

Paclitaxel

Paclitaxel is a complex diterpine taxane originally isolated from the bark of the Western yew by Wall and colleagues in 1958. Purification and formulation problems resulted in a 25-year delay before paclitaxel went into clinical trials.

Taxanes enhance all aspects of tubulin polymerization, an action that is the opposite to that of vinca alkaloids, but they are also cytotoxic, emphasizing the dynamic importance of tubulin polymerization as a target for cytotoxic drugs. Taxanes stabilize tubulin polymers and do not prevent polymerization.

A low concentration of paclitaxel increases both the microtubule number and the formation of bundles, changes cell shape, and produces mitotic arrest in actively dividing cells. Altering the microtubul tubulin equilibrium by irreversible polymerization of tubules is the major mechanism for the antineoplastic actions of the taxanes.

PHARMACOKINETICS It is insoluble in water and the only way it may be administered is i.v. in an emulsion, which can induce a severe anaphylactic reaction. Paclitaxel has a biphasic plasma elimination with half-lifes of 20 minutes and 6–8 hours. Paclitaxel is hepatically metabolized by the CYP450 3A4 isoenzyme to inactive products. This produces the potential for interaction with a host of other drugs which share this CYP pathway.

Taxanes act as substrates for multidrug resistance-mediated cellular efflux. At appropriate concentrations Cremophor itself can inhibit the P-gP/mdr efflux pump. Alterations in tubulin itself may reduce or even prevent taxane binding or, in vitro, produce a mutant tubulin that requires a taxane for normal polymerization kinetics.

ADVERSE EFFECTS Anaphylactic reactions due to the solvent Cremophor are frequent but can be controlled by pretreatment with a glucocorticosteroid and an H_1 receptor antagonist. Major adverse effects of paclitaxel are neutropenia and neuropathy, particularly with 24-hour infusions.

Interactions have been reported with several anti-neoplastic drugs. These have occurred only with the prolonged (24-hour) infusions. There is an increased incidence and severity of mucositis when doxorubicin is used before paclitaxel than when paclitaxel is used before doxorubicin.

Docetaxel is derived from the leaves of the European yew. It has similar anticancer properties to paclitaxel, although differences may exist in certain cancers (e.g. breast). There is a decreased incidence of allergic reactions but increased incidence of edema and effusions with docetaxel.

HORMONES

Alteration of hormone levels in the treatment of cancer dates from the nineteenth century. In 1896, Beatson in Edinburgh used bilateral oöphorectomy to alleviate pain from breast cancer metastasized to bone in pre-menopausal women. In 1952, the American surgeon Huggins and colleagues were able to accomplish this in postmenopausal women by bilateral adrenalectomy. In

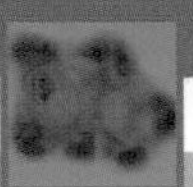

1941, Huggins and Hodges demonstrated regression of prostate cancer metastasis by bilateral orchiectomy or estrogen administration.

Endogenous steroid hormones are ultimately derived via synthetic pathways from cholesterol. Their synthesis in vivo and mechanism of action are described in Ch. 11.

In breast cancer, effective hormonal therapy is dependent on the expression of estrogen receptors (ER) and progesterone receptors (PR) by the tumor cells. Patients with ER-positive tumors are more than fivefold more responsive than ER-negative patients. Quantitative ER/PR analysis (by immunocytochemistry or competitive radiolabeled displacement) is a good guide to prognosis as greater receptor density on tumors increases the probability of response.

A significant body of evidence supports the concept that a substantial portion of the benefit of adjuvant combination chemotherapy in premenopausal women with breast cancer results from chemotherapy-induced menopause.

Estrogen

Knowledge of the role of estrogens as promoters for breast cancer growth dates from observations in the nineteenth century on the effects of menstrual cycle on breast cancer. It is seemingly a paradox that high doses of estrogens can have an anticancer effect. Diethylstilbestrol (DES) produces regressions in breast cancer equivalent to antiestrogens but with significantly more adverse effects, especially venous thromboembolism. The mechanism is uncertain. Proposed mechanisms include the down-regulation of estrogen receptors, direct cytotoxic effects related to perturbations of the cell cycle and effects on chromosome stability. Estrogen therapy of breast cancer is of historical interest only, having been replaced by antiestrogens and aromatase inhibitors. DES is still used, but only in prostate cancer.

DES is well absorbed orally. The initial half-life is 1.5 hours and the terminal half-life is 24 hours. Metabolism occurs through aromatic hydroxylation of the ethyl side chains, the product of which may be carcinogenic. DES is four times more potent than estradiol at suppressing follicle-stimulating hormone. A 1 mg dose produces daily plasma concentrations of 1–2 ng/mL.

Ethinyl estradiol is 20 times more potent than DES. It has a half-life of 24 hours. The metabolism is via glucuronidation. The usual daily dose is 1 mg t.i.d. for breast cancer.

Antiestrogens

TAMOXIFEN Tamoxifen is an important drug in the treatment of breast cancer. It offers significant palliation and tumor regressions in advanced metastatic disease in ER-positive women, provides potentially curative benefit in the adjuvant setting in ER-positive women and has been used to prevent breast cancer in women at high risk for the disease. It is a synthetic triphenyl ethylene.

Tamoxifen has properties of a mixed estrogen antagonist and agonist, i.e. a partial agonist. Tamoxifen blocks estrogen activation of the ER and promotes its tight association, preventing repetitive signaling. This results in decreased transforming growth factor alpha (TGF-α), mid-G_1 arrest, decreased cell proliferation, antagonism of the effect of insulin-like growth factor 1 (IGF-1), and increased TGF-β, an antiproliferative protein. While decreasing breast epithelial proliferation, tamoxifen increases endometrial proliferation, reduces or prevents the mineral loss in bone associated with estrogen withdrawal, and causes a favorable hepatic cholesterol profile seen in menstruating women.

Tamoxifen undergoes hepatic metabolism to 4-hydroxytamoxifen (50-fold more potent in ER affinity than tamoxifen), tamoxifen N-oxide, and N-desmethyltamoxifen (both equipotent as tamoxifen). Tamoxifen has a long half-life such that steady-state levels are achieved only after 4–12 weeks. Elimination is via glucuronide conjugation and biliary excretion. The clinical dose is 20 mg daily. Tamoxifen is continued until progression in advanced disease and for >5 years as an adjuvant. In advanced disease with progression, discontinuing tamoxifen may produce paradoxical tumor regressions. One explanation for this is that imbalances in the intracellular ratio of *cis:trans* species of 4-hydroxytamoxifen may produce estrogenic stimulation, promoting tumor growth.

Tamoxifen has several adverse effects, including a low incidence of endometrial cancers and venous thrombosis. It will produce anovulation in premenopausal women, with resulting menopausal symptoms in some.

Aromatase inhibitors

Postmenopausal women have persistent circulating estrogen levels as a result of conversion of adrenal androstenedione and testosterone to estrone in peripheral tissues. Aromatase is a heme-containing enzyme that hydroxylates steroids at the C-19 position. Aromatase has been assigned to the CYP450 C19 family. In premenopausal women, enzyme aromatase activity in the ovary is stimulated in the theca cells by follicle-stimulating hormone activity, and substrate (androstenedione) levels in granulosa cells are increased by luteinizing hormone (LH) such that estradiol levels increase tenfold at ovulation. In two-thirds of breast cancer patients, there is increased aromatase activity, perhaps responsible for local estrogen levels that may be 4–5-fold higher in transformed versus untransformed cells.

Aminoglutethimide, originally developed as an anticonvulsant, was discovered to inhibit steroid 18-hydroxylation and cleavage of cholesterol side chains, and produced symptoms and signs of glucocorticoid deficiency. This observation was applied to breast cancer to deprive tumor cells of secondary sources of estrogen. Hydrocortisone was co-administered. Approximately one-third of all patients, and 50% of ER-positive patients, respond to aminoglutethimide. Among patients who are already responsive to tamoxifen, 50% responded to aminoglutethimide compared with 25% of non-responders. Rashes, fever and lethargy are major adverse effects. Because of its inhibition of CYP450 hydroxylation, interaction occurs with many other drugs including warfarin and theophylline. The initial half-life of 12 hours is decreased to 7 hours after 6 weeks of therapy because of enzyme induction.

Second- and third-generation aromatase inhibitors have been developed. Suicide drugs compete for and alkylate the aromatase active site. Exemestane is such a drug. It is orally available, and has activity comparable to aminoglutethimide with fewer adverse effects. Anastrozole and letrozole are third-generation nonsteroidal competitive inhibitors of the CYP450 hydroxylation steps. Both show equivalent activity to progestational drugs as second-line therapy with a survival advantage and a superior adverse effect profile. Anastrozole and letrazole are comparable to tamoxifen as first-line therapy, with a lower incidence of venous thromboembolism. Both are available as a single daily oral formulation.

Fulvestrant is an estrogen receptor agonist that binds to the ER in a competitive manner with affinity comparable to that of estradiol and causes the down-regulation of ERs in breast cancer cells. It can be administered orally, i.v. or i.m., and has a very long serum half-life (40 days). The main adverse effects of fulvestrant are nausea, vomiting, headaches, back pain and hot flushes.

Androgens

Androgens have limited use in cancer therapy. Androgen activity in breast cancer is similar to that of estrogens, perhaps for the same mechanistic reasons. Virilizing effects and hepatic toxicity make androgens unacceptable to most patients, especially women. Fluoxymesterone is the most widely used androgen. Danazol has been used in hematology in aplastic anemia and congenital anemias.

Androgen antagonists

Androgen antagonists have a role in the therapy of prostate cancer. Flutamide is a selective androgen antagonist which interferes with activated androgen receptor complex formation in target cells and thus inhibits DNA synthesis in the prostate. The parent drug undergoes extensive hepatic metabolism. The plasma half-life of the major hepatic metabolite is 6 hours. Flutamide is valuable in preventing 'flare,' during the initial testosterone surge induced by gonadotropin partial agonists (see below). Randomized clinical trials have failed to substantiate earlier claims of a survival benefit of flutamide when combined with orchiectomy or gonadotropin partial agonists. A syndrome of 'rebound regression' of progressive prostate cancer growth may be observed following withdrawal of flutamide. The mechanism is uncertain; androgen hyper-responsiveness or mutations in the androgen receptor which utilizes flutamide as a positive effector have been proposed. Bicalutamide has similar activity. Adrenal steroid inhibitors aminoglutethimide and ketoconazole have potential for benefit in refractory cancers.

Progestins

The mechanism of anticancer action of progestins (see Ch. 11) is uncertain. Direct cytotoxicity on cancer cells, suppression of gonadotropin-releasing hormones (FSH, LH and ACTH), decreases in ER levels and production of growth inhibitory factors have been proposed, but scientific evidence for each hypothesis is weak. Therapeutically, progestins are equivalent or nearly so to antiestrogens and aromatase inhibitors.

The progestin medroxyprogesterone acetate is used to treat breast and endometrial cancer. It is usually administered intramuscularly. The α half-life is 1 hour and the β half-life is 4 hours. It is extensively metabolized in the liver; 30–40% is excreted in urine as metabolites.

Megestrol acetate is a synthetic progestin. It is orally available and extensively metabolized in the liver, but 60–80% is excreted in urine, including 10–12% of the parent compound. The half-life is 4 hours.

Progestins have the undesirable effects of weight gain, pedal edema, hirsutism, sweating, hyperventilation and Cushingoid fat distribution. These often cause progestins to be second-line drugs from the perspective of patient preference in spite of their therapeutic level. The increased appetite caused by progestins is widely exploited as treatment for cachexia associated with many cancers.

Luteinizing hormone-releasing hormone agonists and gonadotropin-releasing hormone agonists

Luteinizing hormone-releasing hormone (LHRH) stimulates the release of FSH and luteinizing hormone (LH) and its effect is normally pulsatile (see Ch. 11). The clinically useful LHRH agonists are administered in a formulation to produce a constant release of synthetic peptide, which results in the down-regulation of LHRH receptors and uncoupling of the signal transduction mechanism. This produces desensitization to the gonadotropins with resultant low levels of testosterone in men and estrogen in women. However, there is an initial surge of hormone levels prior to the cessation of sex steroid production. The resultant involution of hormone-sensitive tissues, such as prostate and breast, via apoptosis, is responsible for the anticancer effect.

The oral bioavailability of LHRH agonists is poor because of peptide hydrolysis. Intranasal administration is convenient but again bioavailability is low (1–2%). The most widely used routes of administration are subcutaneous or intramuscular. Native LHRH has good (75–90%) bioavailability. The plasma pharmacokinetics vary depending on the formulation, injection site, volume, blood flow, local proteolysis and antibody

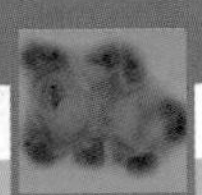

formation. The clinically used compounds are co-polymers of glycides and esterified amides. They degrade and gradually release the active peptides over 28 to 80 days. The potency of the synthetic goserelin is 100 times that of the native LHRH. The α and β half-lifes of native LHRH administered subcutaneously are approximately 5 and 40 minutes. Subcutaneous administration of the synthetic leuprolide produces a half-life of 3 hours, and for subcutaneous goserelin the half-life is 5 hours.

Leuprolide produces responses in men with prostate cancer equivalent to DES or orchidectomy. Premenopausal women treated with goserelin have responses equivalent to those produced by tamoxifen.

Leuprorelin is a newer LHRH analog used to treat prostate cancer, although impotence and decreased libido occur almost universally with 3 months of treating with this drug and 70% of patients experience hot flushes with leuprorelin therapy.

The adverse effects of these releasing hormone agonists are identical with those of castration. Men and women experience loss of libido, hot flashes, losses of muscle mass, weight gain, gastrointestinal disturbances and loss of bone mineral density. Men become impotent; women experience vaginitis, breast atrophy and emotional lability. Due to the partial agonist effects, there may be transient exacerbation of bone pain in patients with osseous disease.

Glucocorticoids

Glucocorticoid hormones have been used in cancer therapy since the 1950s. They are integral components of curative therapy for acute lymphoblastic leukemia, non-Hodgkin's lymphoma and Hodgkin's disease. Glucocorticoids have essential roles in limiting some of the complications of cancer, i.e. intracranial hypertension or spinal cord compression in neurologic complications, and pain and the prevention of allergic reactions (taxanes) and emesis. There are many reports of glucocorticoids producing an increased sense of well-being in patients with terminal cancer. (See Ch. 11 for a complete description.)

MISCELLANEOUS AGENTS USED IN THE TREATMENT OF CANCER

Interferons

Interferons (IFNs) are a family of proteins with chemical, antigenic and biologic variability. The genes that code for IFN-α and -β reside on chromosome 9, have approximately 30% amino acid homology and share a single cell surface receptor. The IFN-α alleles produce proteins with approximately 90% amino acid homology. IFN-γ is located on chromosome 12, has minimal sequence homology with IFN-α and -β and has a unique receptor. There are about 2000 IFN receptors per cell and they are present on every kind of normal and malignant cell type.

The mechanism of action of the IFNs in cancer is not known precisely. Postulated mechanisms include a direct cytostatic effect via the action of 2′-5′-oligoadenylate synthetase (2-5A synthetase, which stimulates the ribonuclease activity of IFNs) on cellular messenger or ribosomal RNAs, prolongation of the cell cycle, or oncogene modulation. Indirect mechanisms of immune activation to increase host defenses possibly include enhanced major histocompatibility complex (MHC) expression and increased tumor-associated antigen expression, Fcγ expression and increased numbers of intercellular adhesion molecules (thereby increasing immune recognition) and the increase in the number and activity of immune effector cells (cytotoxic T cells, helper T cells, natural killer cells and antigen presenting cells). IFN-α has antiangiogenic effects on tumor endothelial cells through inhibition of basic fibroblast growth factor.

The IFNs are proteins and must be given parenterally. IFN-α is given intramuscularly, producing peak plasma concentrations within 4–6 hours. Immunologic activation studies in patients have not conclusively demonstrated a dose–response relationship, perhaps reflecting the individual variability of the response and limited patient numbers. The biologic action of IFN-α may be detected for 24–72 hours. Clinical responses correlate in some studies with the induction of 2-5A synthetase in leukemia, lymphoma, carincoid tumors and breast cancer, suggesting that individuals capable of responding to IFNs may have a better clinical result than non-responders.

The adverse effects of IFN include fever, chills, malaise, myalgia, headache, fatigue, weight loss, anorexia, neutropenia and hepatic transaminase elevation. These acute adverse effects are short-lived (8 hours). With chronic IFN administration, fatigue, anorexia and mental slowing are dose-limiting.

In cancer, the role of IFNs is uncertain. In the adjuvant treatment of melanoma, one large cooperative trial showed a modest (10%) survival advantage but other trials were negative in the same setting. IFNs have shown activity in hairy cell leukemia and chronic lymphocytic leukemia, but have been supplanted by the purine analogs. Similarly, the role of IFNs (with hydroxyurea) in maintaining remissions in chronic myelogenous leukemia will probably be replaced by the *bcr-abl* tyrosine kinase inhibitor, imatinib (see below).

L-ASPARAGINASE L-asparagine is a nonessential amino acid formed by the transamination of L-aspartic acid from glutamine by the enzyme L-asparagine synthetase. The enzyme is present in all tissues but is often lacking in malignant lymphocytes. L-asparaginase, derived from either *E. coli* or *Erwinia*, hydrolyzes asparagine to aspartic acid and ammonia. L-asparaginase has proven anticancer activity in childhood acute lymphocytic leukemia and is a component of standard induction and consolidation therapy.

The mechanism of action is depletion of L-asparagine, leading to the inhibition of protein synthesis. Asparagine donates an amino group in the synthesis of glycine, so depletion of glycine levels may contribute to cytotoxicity.

The affinity for asparagine of the *E. coli* or *Erwinia* enzyme is approximately 1×10^{-5} M, less than the 4×10^{-5} M plasma concentrations achieved in man. This affinity counts for the modest selectivity of this particular enzyme. The agent is given intramuscularly or intravenously; the former produces lower peak levels but may evoke less adverse effects involving the immune system. Clearance is another factor in determining efficacy and the *E. coli* asparaginase has a half-life of 14–22 hours. The half-life falls markedly with antibody production, a significant factor in clinical usage. Levels rise proportionally with increased doses and the remission rate may be higher with doses of 6000 IU/m^2 than 3000 IU/m^2. Asparagine levels may be undetectable for a week after therapy. A recent modification, the addition of polyethylene glycol, increases the half-life of asparginase to 14 days by decreasing clearance without a change in the volume of distribution.

The adverse effects of asparaginase are considerable. Hypersensitivity reactions occur in up to 40% of patients receiving single-agent asparaginase, but in only 20% when it is administered in combination therapy with glucocorticoids and 6-mercaptopurine. The hypersensitivity usually occurs after several doses given in successive cycles. The reaction may be only urticaria, but may be severe with laryngospasm or occasional serum sickness. Fatal reactions occur in <1% of the cases of hypersensitivity reactions. Changing the source of enzyme is the appropriate initial step in reducing hypersensitivity.

Adverse effects can occur as a result of protein synthesis inhibition. Despite prolongation of prothrombin and partial thromboplastin times, clotting, not bleeding, is a more frequent adverse occurrence. Decreases in the anticoagulant proteins antithrombin III, protein C and protein S are responsible. Elevated hepatic transaminase levels occur due to fatty metamorphosis; pancreatitis, and nausea and vomiting also occur. Neurologic complications, with confusion or stupor, may be due to elevated ammonia or to lowered levels of asparagine.

MITOTANE Mitotane, or o,p-DDD0, which chemically is 1,1-dichloro-2-(o-chlorophenyl)-2-(p-chlorophenyl) ethane, is an oral drug which has direct cytotoxic effects on the zona fasciculata and zone glomerulosa of the adrenal gland, and prevents formation of 17-hydroxycorticosteroids. It is biotransformed by the CYP450 system to an acyl chloride which combines with binucleophils in the adrenal cortical cells. The dose is titrated against urinary cortisol/17-hydroxycorticosteroid levels in adrenal cortical cancer. Responses of up to 33% have been observed. Exogenous cortisol and occasionally mineralocorticoids must be given.

IMATINIB Imatinib is 2-phenylaminopyrimidine, a drug that selectively inhibits the *c-abl* tyrosine kinase in cancer cells.

Chronic myelogenous leukemia (CML) has a characteristic chromosomal translocation, 9:22. This places the cellular homologue of the feline Abelson leukemia virus tyrosine kinase downstream from the break point cluster region, *bcr*, and results in the unregulated expression of the fusion p210Bcr-Abl oncogene, which functions as a cytoplasmic protein kinase. Bcr-Abl is necessary and sufficient to produce CML, although additional chromosomal aberrations develop in the later stages of the disease. Imatinib interferes with the binding of ATP to the tyrosine kinase site on *abl*. Imatinib produces hematologic remission in virtually 100% of interferon-refractory patients with the accelerated phase of CML. Nearly 30% of patients have disappearance of the Philadelphia chromosome/9:22 translocation. Imatinib has activity against two tyrosine kinase receptors, c-kit and PGDF (platelet-derived growth factor). C-kit mutations occur in 70% of patients with gastrointestinal stromal tumors (e.g. GIST, a sarcoma arising from the myenteric neurons of Cajal). Imatinib produces significant responses in this otherwise refractory sarcoma.

The usual dose is 400–800 mg/day. Oral absorption is 98%. The peak plasma level after a 400 mg dose is 2.3 μg/mL and the steady state levels, 0.72 μg/mL, exceed the necessary cytotoxic level in plasma. The half-life is 12–18 hours. Seventy percent of a dose is eliminated in feces, 20% unchanged. 13% is excreted in urine, 5% unchanged. The N-desmethylpiperazine metabolite is as active as the parent drug and has a half-life of 40 hours. Metabolism is via CYP450 3A4. This makes for possible interaction with other CYP450 3A4 substrates such as the erythromycins, azole antifungal drugs, ciclosporin and anticonvulsants, such as phenytoin. Adverse effects include elevations of bilirubin/hepatic transaminases (1.5%), rashes and fatigue (each approximately 35%).

RADIOPHARMACEUTICALS

Radiation has been used therapeutically in the treatment of cancer since the early twentieth century. The predominant mode of delivery is by external beam irradiation, the details of which are beyond the scope of this book. Irradiation can also be delivered via soluble chemical isotopes. The potential for more widespread use of radioisotopes has increased with the advent of monoclonal antibody therapy as a method of molecular targeting of specific cell types.

Sodium phosphorous ^{32}P has been used for decades to treat malignant effusions, without reliable benefit. However, ^{32}P is still used in the treatment of polycythemia vera, although its adverse effects, especially its leukemogenic potential, makes it an option in only a small

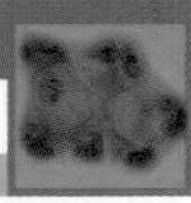

number of patients. ^{32}P is a β-emitter (produces an ionizing electron), with a half-life of 14.3 days. It is taken up into bone as inorganic phosphorous and provides local irradiation. The single dose is 4 mCi, which may be repeated at 3–4-month intervals, up to about 16 mCi as a lifetime dose. The adverse effects of ^{32}P are myelosuppression, some of which is intended, and leukemogenesis.

^{89}Strontium chloride is used for the treatment of painful bony metastases in prostate and breast cancer. Strontium substitutes for calcium in bones. ^{89}Strontium is a β-emitter, with a half-life of 50 days. The half-life in metastatic bone (>50 days) is greater than in normal bone (14 days) and the uptake in metastatic bone is tenfold greater than in normal marrow. The onset of response is 7–12 days, with a peak at 6 weeks, and a duration of 3–12 months. Clearance is into bone. In metastatic bone cancer, 80–90% of the dose remains in bone at 100 days, with renal clearance of the remainder of the dose. In healthy patients, 80% will be cleared by renal (65%) and hepatic (33%) mechanisms. The usual dose is 40 uCi/kg or a fixed dose of 40 miCi. Bone marrow suppression is the major adverse effect and the dosing interval should be 3 months or longer.

^{131}Iodine is used for the treatment of thyroid cancer. Thyroid tissue avidly takes up inorganic iodine and incorporates it into thyroid hormone. After surgery, well-differentiated thyroid cancers with adverse prognostic factors are treated with radioiodine ablation. ^{131}Iodine is a low-energy γ-emitter with a radioactive half-life of 8.0 days. Sodium iodide is rapidly cleared from the blood with half-lifes of 40 minutes, 9 hours and 60 hours. Following ^{131}I treatment, patients require lifelong thyroid hormone replacement owing to radiation damage to healthy thyroid tissue.

^{131}Iodine is a component of the monoclonal antibody tositumomab. ^{131}I-tositumomab is a murine monoclonal antibody directed at the lymphoid cell surface marker CD20 (B1), which is expressed on many transformed lymphocytes in Hodgkin's disease and non-Hodgkin's lymphoma. ^{131}I-tositumomab treatment produces complete or partial regression of refractory diseases in up to 60–90% of patients whose tumors express CD20. The uptake of a 2.5 mg/kg dose is 0.01% per gram of tumor tissue in CD20-positive patients, and 0.002% in CD20-negative patients. ^{131}I-tositumomab has a half-life of 36–48 hours. The dose of irradiation delivered to the tumor is in the order of 10–92 Gy (280–800 mCi), which exceeds the dose to the lung (6.5–30 Gy), bone marrow (1–6.4 Gy) and total body (1–5.7 Gy). Bone marrow suppression is the major adverse effect, but transient pneumonitis has been observed since the lung receives the highest radiation dose of any normal tissue. Adverse reactions to the murine protein include fever, serum sickness, anaphylaxis and the development of tositumomab-neutralizing human antimouse antibodies (HAMA).

Specific cytotoxic drug interactions

- Procarbazine inhibits monoamine oxidase
- Allopurinol inhibits 6-mercaptopurine metabolism
- Barbiturates and cimetidine increase activation of cyclophosphamide
- Cisplatin and doxorubicin enhance paclitaxel toxicity when given before paclitaxel
- Asparaginase inhibits the metabolism of vinca alkaloids

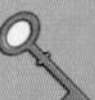

General principles of cancer chemotherapy administration

- Allow for full recovery of myelosuppression before resuming dosing, though this may not apply for aggressive leukemias and lymphomas
- Avoid concomitant administration of platelet-inhibiting drugs
- Avoid drug interactions involving cytochrome P-450 metabolism
- The dose of certain drugs needs adjustment if there is hepatic and renal impairment
- There is no evidence that hematopoietic cytokines given to ameliorate myelosuppression improve outcome, but they markedly increase costs

Epidermal growth factor receptor inhibitors

Although cytotoxic chemotherapy has been the mainstream of cancer treatment over many years, the efficacy of such treatment against most solid tumors is limited and, as described above, is often associated with very significant side effects. This is particularly evident during the treatment of lung cancer, the leading cause of cancer mortality worldwide. Seventy-five percent of lung cancer is non-small cell lung cancer (NSCLC) and use of platinum salts only modestly improves survival and the second-line recommended therapy, docetaxel, is also limited in its usefulness in this condition. The lack of specificity for cancer cells of existing cytotoxic chemotherapy has prompted the development of novel therapies that better differentiate between effects on cancer cells and healthy cells with a result that they have greater efficacy and fewer side effects. One new class of drugs are those that inhibit the activities of cell membrane receptor tyrosine kinases (Fig. 7.19), such as epidermal growth factor receptor (EGFR). This receptor is part of the ERBB receptor family, having four closely related members, EGFR (ERBB1), HER2 (ERBB2), HER3 (ERBB3) and HER4 (ERBB4), that consist of an extracellular ligand-binding domain, a transmembrane domain and an intracellular tyrosine kinase domain (see Fig. 7.19). Binding of EGF to EGFR causes receptor

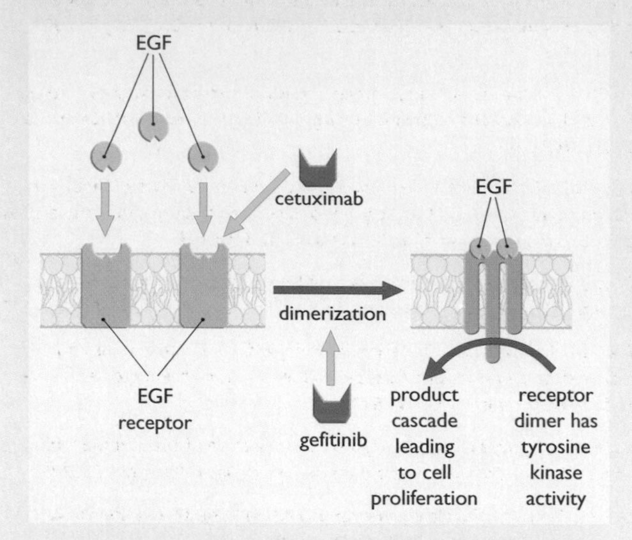

Fig. 7.19 Centuximab, a monoclonal antibody, inhibits EGF binding to its receptor. Gefitinib inhibits the activity of the activated EGF receptor by blocking its ability to dimerize and function as a tyrosine kinase.

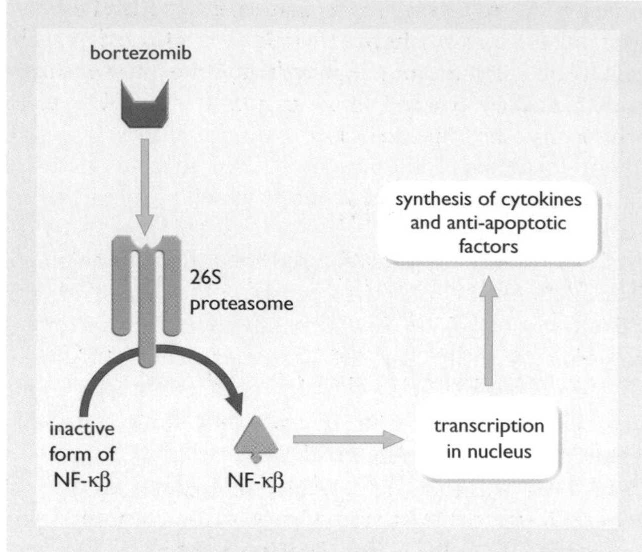

Fig. 7.20 In the intracellular space of the cancer cell, bortezomib inhibits the activity of the 26S proteasome. This protein has enzymic properties and can activate NF-κβ. NF-κβ is a transcription factor that can switch on synthesis of cytokines (some of which stimulate NF-κβ precursor synthesis) and anti-apoptotic factors that contribute to unrestricted cell growth in cancer.

dimerization, which activates the tyrosine kinase activity in the intracellular domain, which in turn leads to receptor autophosphorylation, which initiates the signal transduction cascades involved in cell proliferation. EGFR is expressed in a range of solid tumors (approximately 80% of NSCLCs) and this pathway has been implicated in tumor growth and progression. Several approaches to targeting EGFR have been developed including cetuximab, a monoclonal antibody directed against the extracellular building domain, and gefitinib, an orally active low molecular weight drug that inhibits the intracellular tyrosine kinase domain of the receptor. Gefitinib is now indicated as monotherapy for the treatment of advanced NSCLCs after failure of platinum-based or docetaxel chemotherapy. The most common adverse effects with gefitinib are nausea, vomiting, diarrhea, acne and dry skin.

Cetuximab is a recombinant human/mouse chimeric monoclonal antibody that binds specifically to the EGFR, which blocks the subsequent phosphorylation and activation of receptor-associated kinases, resulting in inhibition of cell growth. It has a serum half-life of 97 hours after infusion and produces an infusion reaction, fever and dermatological toxicity.

Trastuzumab is a recombinant DNA-derived humanized monoclonal antibody directed against ERB-2 which is both cytostatic and cytotoxic. It is used as an infusion for the treatment of breast cancer.

BORTEZOMIB Bortezomib is a reversible inhibitor of the 26S proteasome, a barrel-shaped multiprotein particle found in the nucleus and cytosol of all eukaryotic cells. Proteasomes are involved in destroying proteins marked for degradation following conjugation with ubiquitin and are also involved in the catalysis of proteins involved in the context of the cell cycle, including potentially harmful or abnormal proteins. In multiple myeloma, such abnormal or unfolded proteins are often greatly overexpressed.

Bortezomib is a modified dipeptidyl analog of boronic acid which recognizes the active sites of the proteasome which has these types of catalytic activities: chymotryptic-like, tryptic-like and capsase-like. The boronic acid group forms a complex with the threonine hydroxyl group in the chymotrypsin-like active site, acting as a reversible inhibitor of this activity of the proteasome, thus inhibiting proteolysis (Fig. 7.20). Bortezomib is used to treat multiple myeloma, but only after two other therapies have failed.

Anti-CD20 monoclonal antibodies

CD20 antigen is found on the surface of normal and malignant B cells and monoclonal antibodies directed against this antigen are used to treat B-cell non-Hodgkin's lymphoma. Rituximab and tositumomab are two examples of this class of drug and recently ^{131}I-tositumomab and ^{90y}ibritumomab tiuxetan have been developed which target the killing power of radionuclides to cancer cells.

GnRH receptor antagonists

Abarelix is a novel decapeptide GnRH receptor antagonist used to treat prostate cancer. Androgen ablations have long been used to treat prostate cancer and abarelix has the advantage of lowering testosterone levels, without

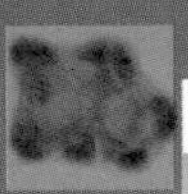

causing a testosterone surge that other approaches such as LHRH agonists have. Abarelix is indicated for the palliative treatment of mean with advanced symptomatic prostate cancer where LHRH therapy is not indicated or who refuse surgical castration.

FURTHER READING

Abraham J, Gulley JL, Allegra CJ. Bethesda handbook of clinical oncology. Philadelphia: Lippincott Williams & Wilkins, 2005. [General information about different types of cancers.]

Adjei AA, Hidalgo M. Intracellular signal transduction pathway proteins as targets for cancer therapy. *J Clin Oncol* 2005; **23**: 5386–5403.

Caponigro F, Basile M, de Rosa V, Normanno N. New drugs in cancer therapy. *Anti-Cancer Drugs* 2005; **16**: 211–221.

Chabner BA, Longo DL. *Cancer Chemotherapy and Biotherapy*, 3rd edn. Philadelphia: Lippincott Williams and Wilkins; 2001. [This is the most comprehensive and current textbook on cancer pharmacology.]

Figg WD, McLeod HL. Handbook of anticancer pharmacokinetics and pharmacodynamics. Totowa, N.J.: Human Press, 2004.

Flescher E. Jasmonates – a new family of anti-cancer agents. *Anti-Cancer Drugs* 2005; **16**: 911–916.

Isoldi MC, Visconti Ma, de Lauro Castrucci AM. Anti-cancer drugs: molecular mechanisms of action. *Mini-Reviews in Medicinal Chemistry* 2005; **5**: 685–695. [A review of the mechanisms of action of anti-cancer drugs.]

Jackman DM, Johnson BE. Small-cell lung cancer. *Lancet* 2005; **21**: 1385–1396.

Lage A, Perez R, Fernandez LE. Therapeutic cancer vaccines: at midway between immunology and pharmacology. *Curr Cancer Drug Targets* 2005; **5**: 611–627.

Lee W, Lockhart AC, Kim RB, Rothenberg ML. Cancer pharmacogenomics: powerful tools in cancer chemotherapy and drug development. *Oncologist* 2005; **10**: 104–111.

Perry MD. *The Chemotherapy Source Book*, 3rd edn. Baltimore: Lipppincott Williams and Wilkins; 2001. [Very good review of cancer pharmacology with guides to the treatment of various malignant diseases.]

Price JT, Thompson EW. Mechanisms of tumour invasion and metastasis: emerging targets for therapy. *Expt Opin on Therap Targets* 2002; **6**: 217–233.

Rau KM, Kang HY, Cha TL, Miller SA, Hung MC. The mechanisms and managements of hormone-therapy resistance in breast and prostate cancers. *Endocr Relat Cancer* 2005; **12**: 511–532.

Scripture CD, Sparreboom A, Figg WD. Modulation of cytochrome P450 activity: implications for cancer therapy. *Lancet Oncol* 2005; **6**: 780–789.

Yao YL, Yang WM. Nuclear proteins: promising targets for cancer drugs. *Curr Cancer Drug Targets* 2005; **5**: 595–610.

WEBSITES

http://www.cancer.gov/cancertopics [This website provides general information regarding cancer treatments.]

http://www.nlm.nih.gov/medlineplus/cancer.html [This website provides general information regarding cancers.]

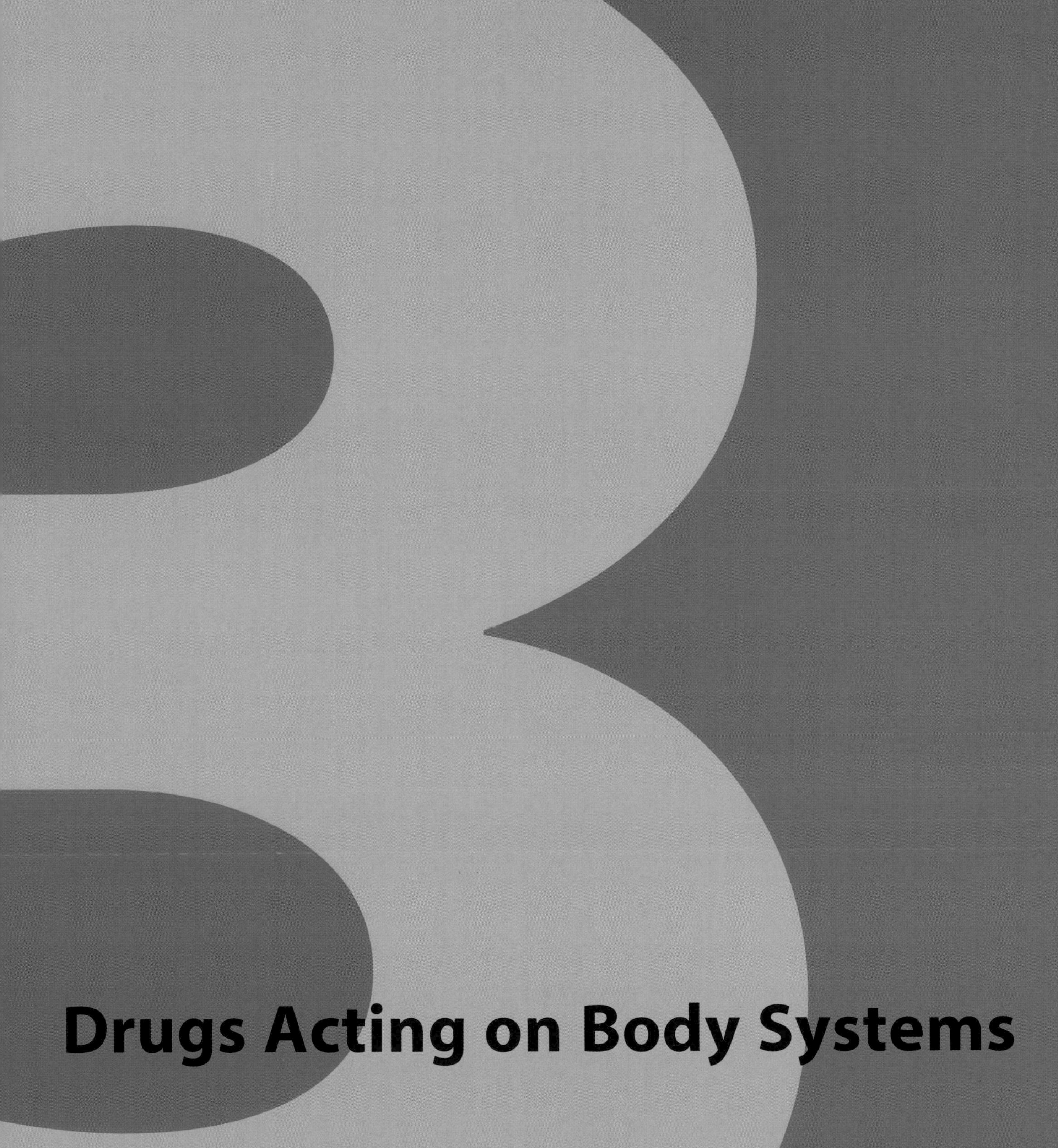

Drugs Acting on Body Systems

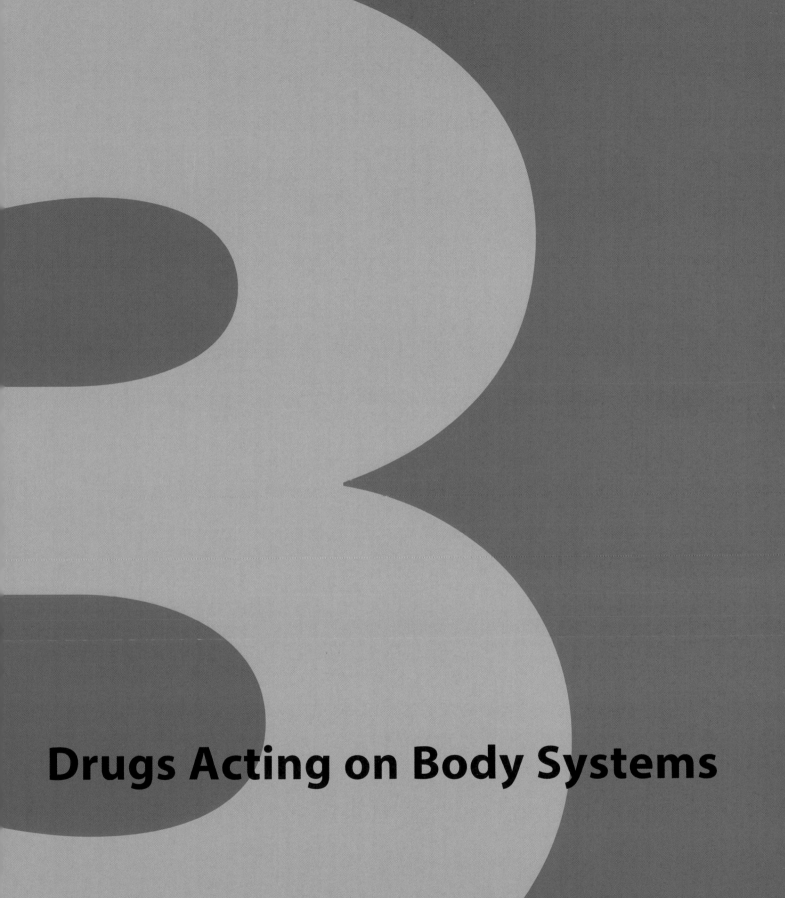

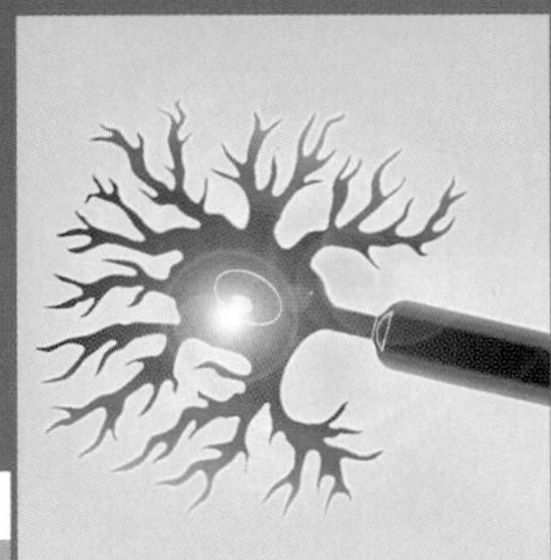

Chapter 8

Drugs and the Nervous System (Peripheral and Central)

GENERAL PHYSIOLOGY OF THE NERVOUS SYSTEM

The nervous system provides conscious or unconscious control of basic motor and sensory activity, as well as emotional and intellectual functions

The nervous system is organized as a hierarchy.

- Afferent fibers passing from peripheral tissues to the spinal cord constitute the part of the peripheral nervous system (PNS) that allows perception of external sensation and body function.
- Efferent neurons from the spinal cord constitute the part of the PNS that regulates the activity of peripheral tissues.
- The central nervous system (CNS) starts at the spinal cord and connects the afferent and efferent neurons of the PNS with the brain, which provides higher processing and executive control (Fig. 8.1).

The neuron is the basic unit of the CNS and PNS

The body contains approximately 10^{10} neurons (nerve cells) of various types. They differ in length and structure, but have four major components (Fig. 8.2):

- The cell body containing the nucleus and structures concerned with basic functioning of the cell.
- The axon, which conducts nerve impulses, in the form of an action potential, from cell body to a distant site, and vice versa.
- Dendrites, which connect neurons with each other and transmit information back to their own cell body.
- Synapses and junctions between nerves and non-neuronal tissue (neuroeffector junction) are the basis of neurochemical communication.

Axons are either long (as in projection neurons such as peripheral motor and sensory nerves) or short (as in interneurons), and most are covered in myelin. In the PNS this covering (myelin sheath) is provided by Schwann cells, while in the CNS it is provided by neuroglia cells (i.e. oligodendrocytes). At the end of an axon there are usually branches that end in axon terminals or boutons that form synapses with other neurons or junctions with non-neuronal tissue. Often, in nervous tissue there is connection with a dendrite from another nerve cell. There are numerous dendrites on most neurons. They have no myelin covering and can be profusely branched. The ends of the axon branches are studded with dendritic spines, the points of synaptic connection. The synapse is therefore the point of connection between neurons. Each neuron may have 1000–10 000 synaptic connections with as many as 1000 other neurons.

The synapse comprises the axon terminal of the presynaptic neuron, the dendrite of the postsynaptic neuron, and the gap between them, the synaptic cleft (Fig. 8.3). The various types of synapses are named according to which two parts of a neuron are connected (i.e. axoaxonic, axodendritic). In addition there are:

- Electrical synapses or gap junctions, which use ions (as electrical currents) as a mode of transmission.
- Conjoint synapses which use both ionic and chemical transmission.

In the case of nerves ending on non-neuronal tissue, this is a neuroeffector junction which relies on chemical transmission. The general actions of drugs at synapses are listed in Table 8.1.

Neurotransmitter release and responses depend on resting membrane and action potentials

The resting membrane potential of a cell is negative owing to preferential distribution of ions and permeability to ions across the cell membrane. The distribution of ions is maintained by membrane ion pumps and ion channels contained in the cell membrane. The principal ions are Na^+, K^+, Ca^{2+} and Cl^- (Fig. 8.4).

The action potential is generated by a massive increase in permeability to Na^+, due to opening of Na^+ channels. The resulting depolarization caused by the action potential in turn opens Ca^{2+} channels (N type) (Fig. 8.5). During the action potential Ca^{2+} enters the cell and initiates neurotransmitter release (Fig. 8.6). The action potential in nerves is followed by a period of hyperpolarization when the neuron is more negatively charged than at rest (Fig. 8.7). This prevents further action potentials and the degree of hyperpolarization has implications for nerve cell excitability.

Neurotransmitters are released in response to an action potential

A neurotransmitter is a molecule synthesized in a neuron and released in response to an action potential. It is then removed or deactivated in the neuron or synaptic cleft.

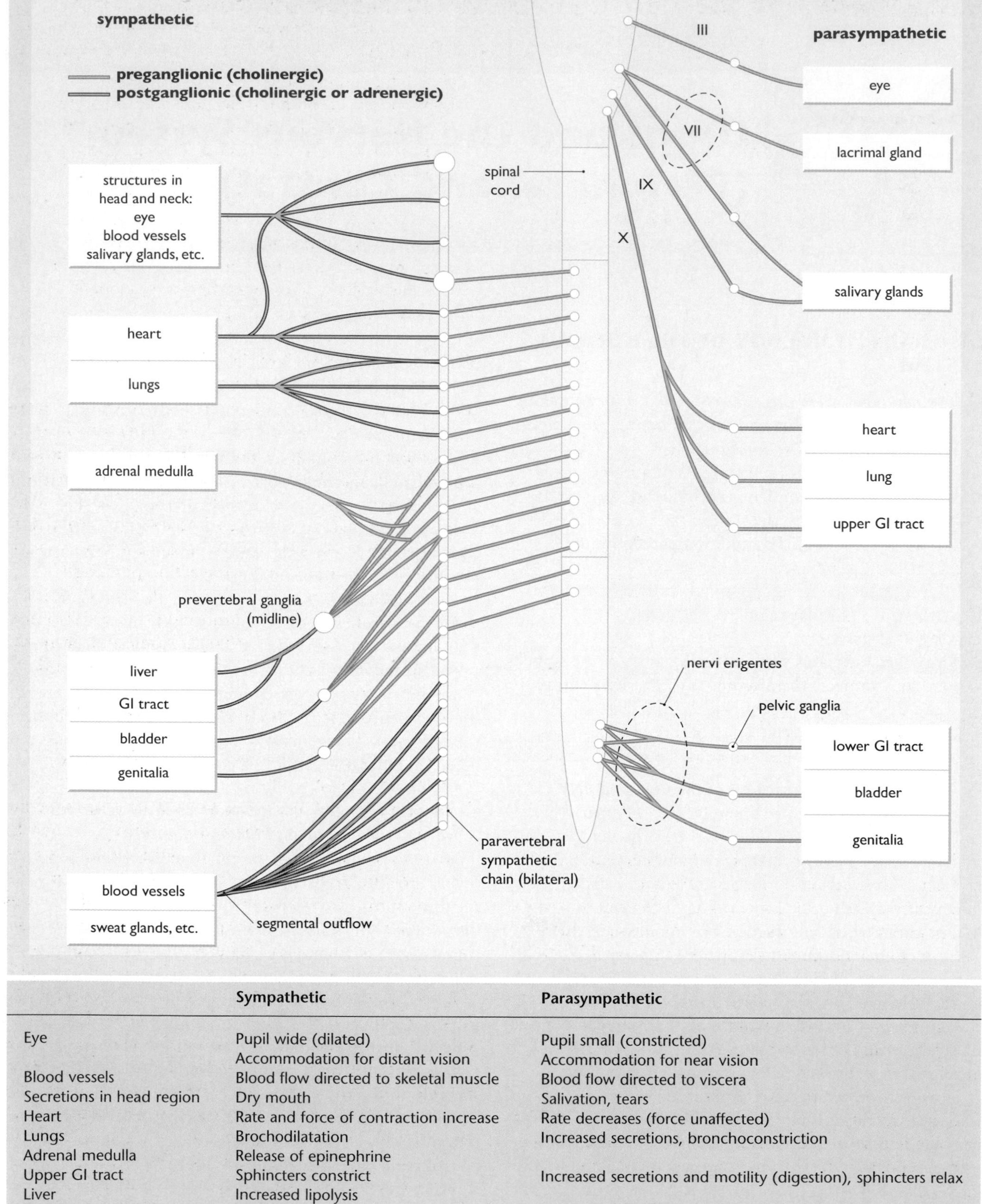

	Sympathetic	Parasympathetic
Eye	Pupil wide (dilated) Accommodation for distant vision	Pupil small (constricted) Accommodation for near vision
Blood vessels	Blood flow directed to skeletal muscle	Blood flow directed to viscera
Secretions in head region	Dry mouth	Salivation, tears
Heart	Rate and force of contraction increase	Rate decreases (force unaffected)
Lungs	Brochodilatation	Increased secretions, bronchoconstriction
Adrenal medulla	Release of epinephrine	
Upper GI tract	Sphincters constrict	Increased secretions and motility (digestion), sphincters relax
Liver	Increased lipolysis	
Bladder	Sphincters constrict	Sphincters relax
Genitalia	Orgasm	Tumescence of erectile tissue
Skin blood vessels	Vasodilatation	
Sweat glands	Activated	

Fig. 8.1 The nervous system is arranged into three main parts. The central nervous system (CNS) controls the activity of the somatic system (which controls skeletal muscle) and the autonomic nervous system. The latter comprises the parasympathetic and sympathetic nerves and both types control smooth muscle function and some glands. Interneurons function independently of the CNS and operate local neuronal regulation of certain tissue functions. (Adapted from Rang H, Dale M, Ritter J. *Pharmacology*, 3rd edn. London: Churchill Livingstone; 1995.)

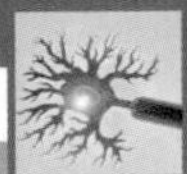

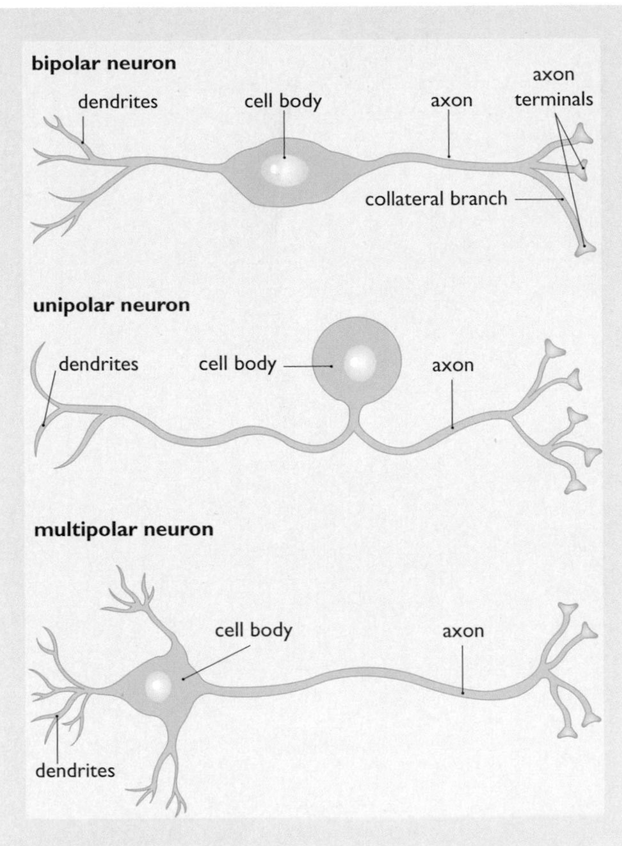

Fig. 8.2 Types of neuron. There are many different types of neuron, which are shaped according to function. Bipolar cells are commonly interneurons, while unipolar cells tend to be sensory neurons, and multipolar cells are often motor neurons.

There are receptors for 300-plus endogenous molecules that act in the nervous system, some of which are referred to as putative since their role as neurotransmitters is not fully established. This is particularly so with endogenous molecules acting in the CNS. Many drugs used to influence the actions of the nervous system exert their effects by altering the function of the receptors for neurotransmitters. The major classes of receptors and transmitters found in the nervous system are listed in Table 8.2.

Receptors are present in the synapse both pre- and postsynaptically. Many presynaptic receptors inhibit further release of the relevant neurotransmitter, though the effect of activating a presynaptic receptor may depend on:

- The number of receptors activated.
- The affinity of the receptor for the transmitter.
- The extent to which the receptor modifies transmitter release.

The two major types of receptor are:

- Those located directly on ion channels such as acetylcholine nicotinic receptors and 5-hydroxytryptamine (5-HT)-3 receptors (both Na^+ and K^+ channels), GABA receptors (Cl^- channels) (Fig. 8.8), and glutamate receptors (*N*-methyl D-aspartate receptors), which are cation channels.
- G protein-coupled receptors, which can exert their effects via second-messenger systems (e.g. by increasing or decreasing concentrations of cAMP; see Ch. 2). For some G protein-coupled receptors, the activated G protein acts directly on an ion channel without the involvement of a second messenger. Other second messengers include Ca^{2+} and metabolities of the membrane component phosphoinositol (see Ch. 2).

Some neurotransmitters inhibit firing of action potentials by hyperpolarizing the neuron

The classic example of a hyperpolarizing neurotransmitter is γ-aminobutyric acid (GABA), which opens Cl^- channels in the cell membrane. These Cl^- channels are examples of ligand-gated ion channels (i.e. ion channels that change in response to a specific chemical) (see Ch. 2). The other general type of ion channel is a voltage-gated ion channel (e.g. the Na^+ and Ca^{2+} ion channels involved in the generation of the action potential).

Neuromodulators are molecules that modulate the response of a neuron to a neurotransmitter, while neurohormones are substances that are released into the blood and have effects on neurons (e.g. cortisol and triiodothyronine).

Major CNS neurotransmitters are shown in Table 8.2.

Functional anatomy of the peripheral nervous system

The peripheral nervous system has two arms, afferent and efferent. Afferent nerves transmit messages generated by physiological receptors (for heat, light, taste, position, blood pressure, blood gases, acidity, stretch) to the CNS for processing in the spinal cord and at higher levels in the brain. The spinal cord and brain integrate the incoming information together with information generally within the higher centers of the brain and sends out messages as action potential to the relevant tissue(s) in the periphery in the efferent arm of the PNS. The efferent arm of the PNS has two major branches. These are the somatic (or motor branch) that innervates skeletal muscle and the autonomic nerves that innervates glands, organs and blood vessels. To some extent, both the somatic and autonomic arms of the PNS have anatomically distinct nerve bundles. Many drugs have an effect (beneficial or adverse) by interacting with the PNS (Fig. 8.9). The major neurotransmitters of the PNS are acetylcholine (ACh) and norepinephrine (NE). The motor nerve fibers arising directly from the spinal cord and brain have ACh as their transmitter at the neuromuscular junction (the term for the neuroeffector junction between nerves and skeletal muscle). ACh is also a major neurotransmitter in the autonomic nervous system (ANS) at all ganglia (parasympathetic and sympathetic; see below) and at the postganglionic neuroeffector

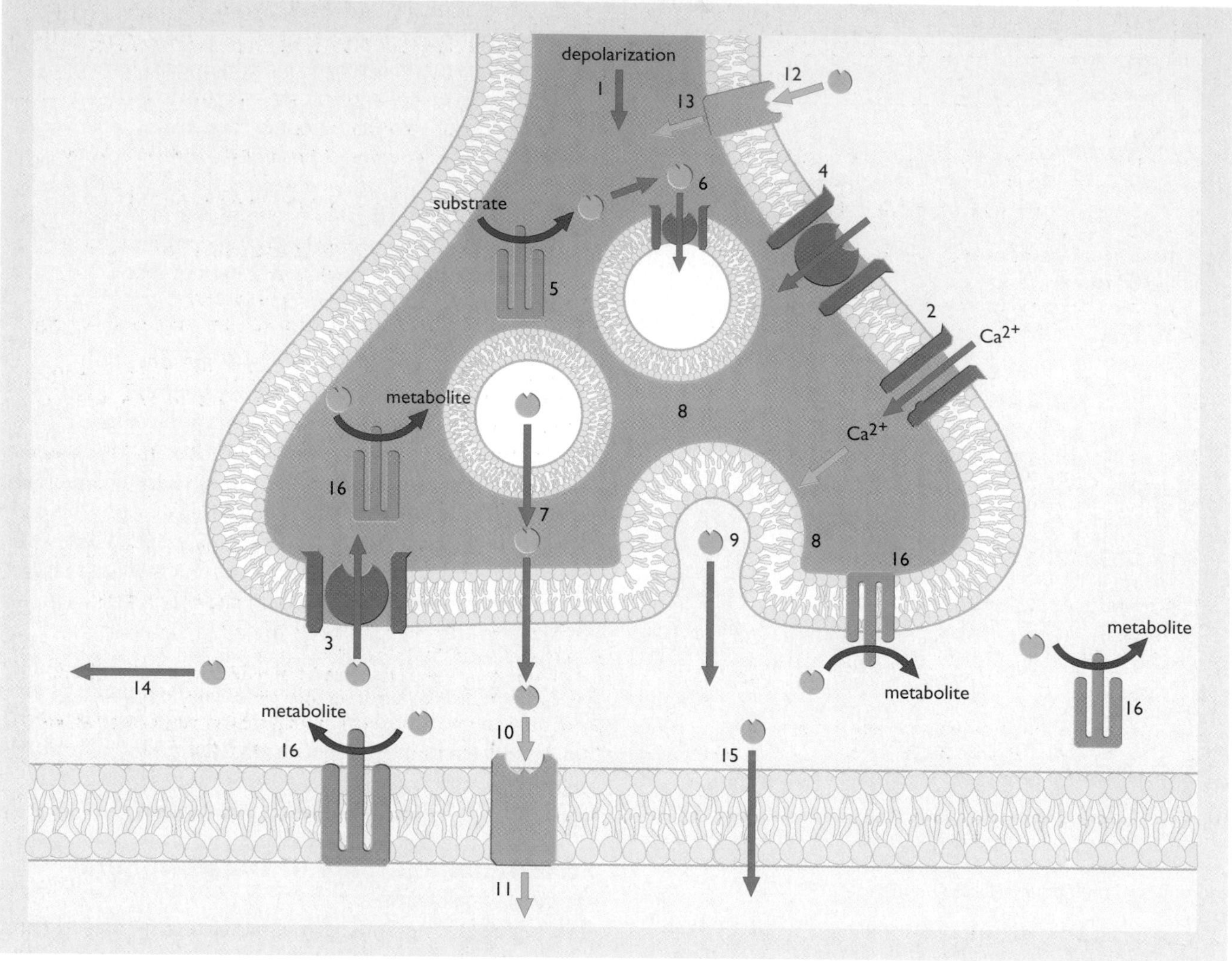

Fig. 8.3 Drug targets in the synapse. The processes shown are described in Table 8.1, in which the number refers to those in this figure.

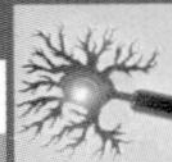

Table 8.1 Targets for drugs acting on neurotransmitters (see Fig. 8.3)

Process	Drug effects examples
1. Nerve action potential	Tetrodotoxin blocks in somatic nerves
2. Calcium entry into depolarized nerve terminal via N-type calcium channels	Neomycin blocks calcium entry into cholinergic nerve terminals
3. Active uptake (or reuptake) of neurotransmitter into nerve terminal	Desipramine blocks 'uptake 1' of norepinephrine in CNS and autonomic nervous system
4. Active uptake of neurotransmitter precursor into nerve terminal	Block of the uptake of choline, the precursor for acetylcholine is not achieved by any therapeutic drugs
5. Synthesis of neurotransmitter	Levodopa stimulates dopamine synthesis in CNS
6. Active uptake of neurotransmitter into storage vesicle	Reserpine blocks uptake of norepinephrine into adrenergic storage vesicles
7. Storage of neurotransmitter in vesicle	β bungarotoxin makes ACh leak from cholinergic storage vesicles
8. Fusion of storage vesicle with neurolemma	Guanethidine blocks fusion of norepinephrine storage vesicle with sympathetic neurolemma
9. Synaptin-dependent exocytosis of neurotransmitter from vesicle	Botulinum toxin inactivates synaptin in cholinergic nerve terminals
10. Activation of postsynaptic receptor	Propranolol blocks activation of β_1 adrenoreceptors by norepinephrine
11. Postsynaptic transduction	Sildenafil enhances nitrenergic transduction by inhibiting degradation of cGMP by PDE-V
12. Activation of presynaptic receptors	Clonidine activates presynaptic α_2 adrenoreceptors leading to inhibition of adrenergic neurotransmission
13. Presynaptic autoinhibitory transduction	No examples of modulators known
14. Diffusion of neurotransmitter or administered drug away from synapse	Epinephrine can cause vasoconstriction which slows diffusion of local anesthetic away from sensory nerve synapse
15. Uptake of neurotransmitter into postsynaptic cell	'Uptake 2' of norepinephrine is inhibited by some corticosteroids
16. Enzymatic inactivation of neurotransmitter in presynaptic or postsynaptic cylosol or cell membrane, or in synaptic space or in blood	Phenelzine inhibits monoamine oxidase B in the CNS

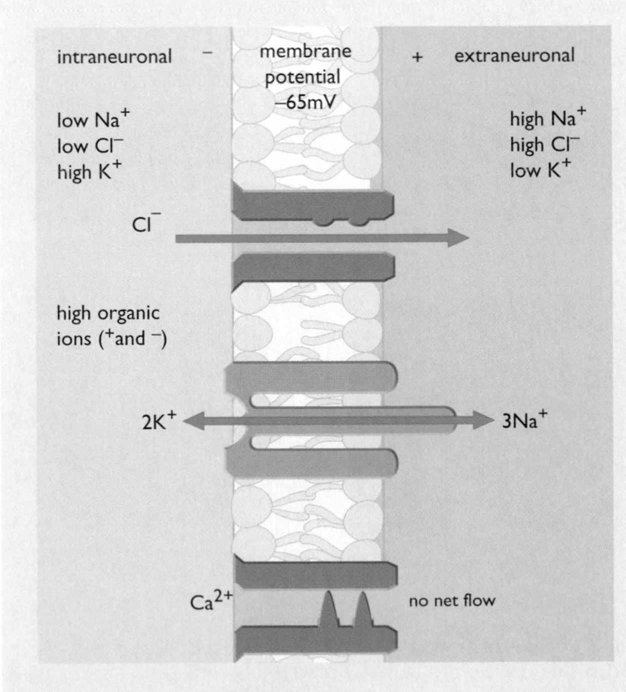

Fig. 8.4 Ion distribution across the neuron membrane at rest. The energy-dependent Na^+/K^+ pump maintains the resting potential by sustaining the Na^+/K^+ concentration gradient across the cell membrane so that the K^+ concentration inside the cell is high. Conversely, the Na^+ concentration outside the cell is high.

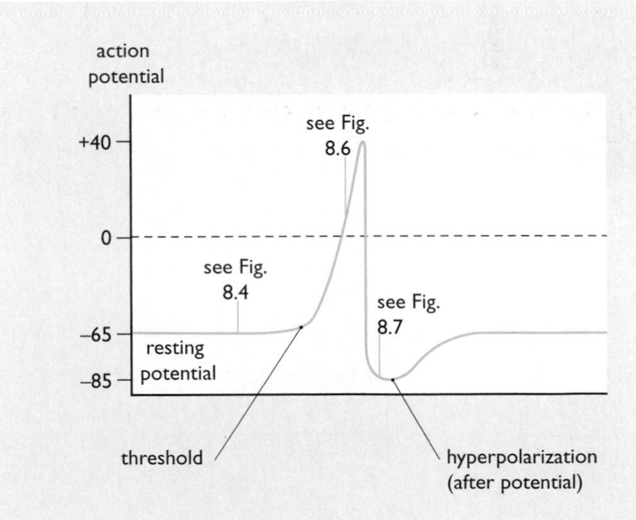

Fig. 8.5 An action potential. This is a brief (0.1–2 msec) wave of reversal of membrane potential (from negative to positive) that moves along the axon away from the cell body.

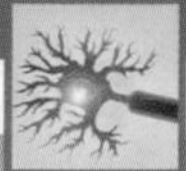

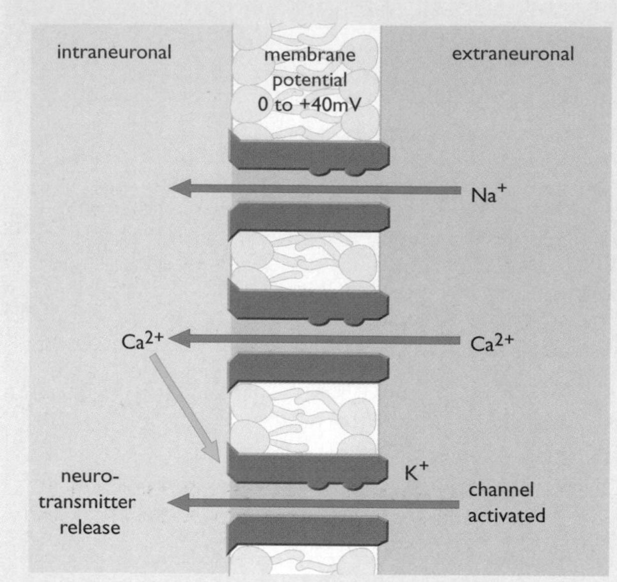

Fig. 8.6 Ion movements during an action potential. An action potential is produced when Na^+ channels open, allowing Na^+ to move along its concentration gradient into the cell. The Ca^{2+} channels then open, allowing Ca^{2+} to enter the cell. Calcium both initiates neurotransmitter release and allows K^+ outflow, which will eventually arrest the action potential.

Table 8.2 Receptor classification for major neurotransmitters

Transmitter	Receptor
Glutamate	NMDA
	Non-NMDA
GABA	$GABA_A$
	$GABA_B$
Glycine	Glycine (strychnine-sensitive)
Acetylcholine	Nicotinic
	Muscarinic
5-HT	$5\text{-}HT_{1a\text{–}d}$
	$5\text{-}HT_2$
	$5\text{-}HT_3$
	$5\text{-}HT_4$
	$5\text{-}HT_5$
	$5\text{-}HT_6$
	$5\text{-}HT_7$
Norepinephrine	α_1
	α_2
	$\beta_{1\text{–}3}$
Dopamine	D_1
	D_2
	D_3
	D_4
	D_5
Cholecystokinin	CCK_A
	CCK_B
Nitric oxide	Activates the enzyme guanylyl cyclase

CCK, cholecystokinin; GABA, γ-aminobutyric acid; 5-HT, 5-hydroxytryptamine; NMDA, *N*-methyl-D-aspartate.

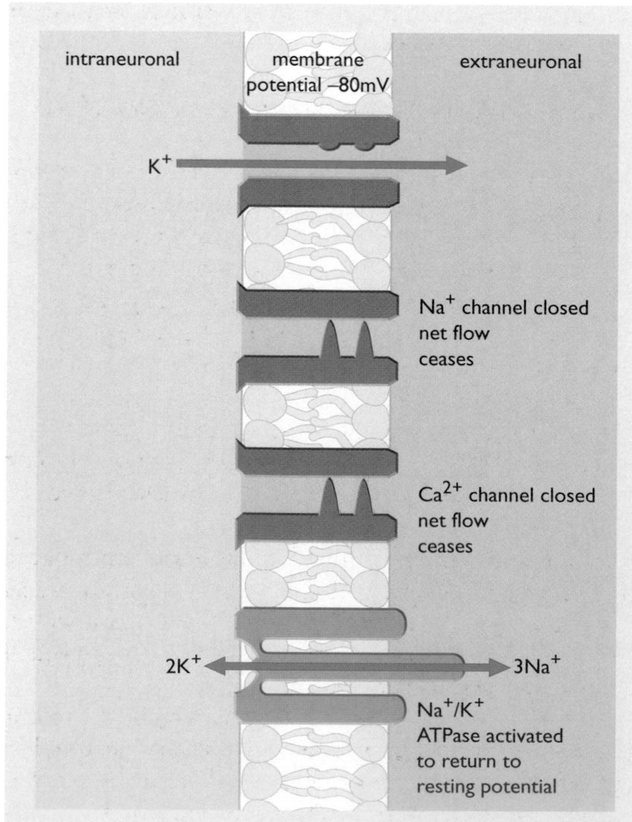

Fig. 8.7 Hyperpolarization. During hyperpolarization, the neuron is more negatively charged than at rest, preventing further action potentials.

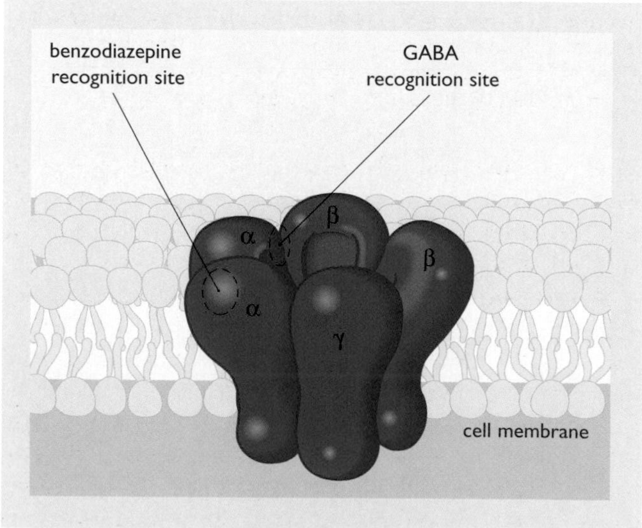

Fig. 8.8 Receptor-operated ionic channels: the γ-aminobutyric acid (GABA) receptor complex. Each subunit is composed of four protein helical strands. Binding of a benzodiazepine or GABA leads to conformational change. The channel opens and Cl^- passes down its concentration gradient.

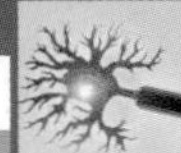

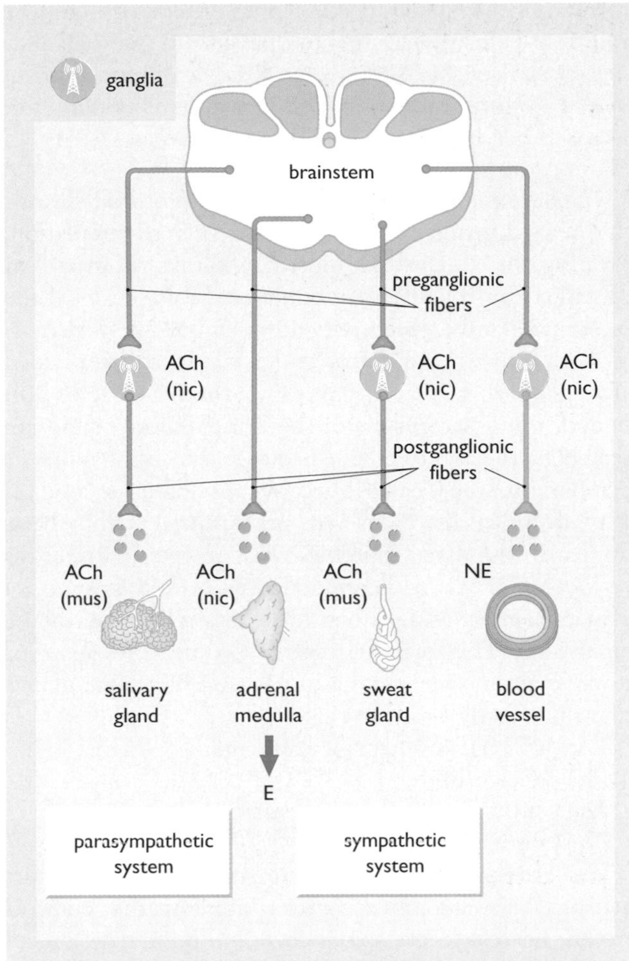

Fig. 8.9 Acetylcholine (ACh) and norepinephrine (NE) are the major neurotransmitters in the peripheral autonomic nervous system. ACh acts on peripheral tissues via two types of receptor, nicotinic (nic) or muscarinic (mus), depending on the tissue. NE acts on peripheral tissues via at least two types of receptors, α and β, depending on the tissue. (E, epinephrine)

junction in parasympathetic nerves. A special case in the ANS is the adrenal medulla, since this gland is a form of specialized ganglion which release epinephrine into the circulation, without an obvious postganglionic fiber.

Knowledge of the ANS innervation and the relative importance of activation or inhibition of this system is very useful in predicting the effects (beneficial or adverse) of drugs that interfere with the ANS. For example, accentuation of the cholinergic system causes profound activation of the gastrointestinal tract, profuse sweating, hypersecretion and bronchospasm in the lungs (symptoms of poisoning with anticholinesterases). Drugs that block nicotinic receptors in ganglia have the most profound effects as they interfere with all ANS activity. This leads to postural hypotension, bradycardia, dry mouth, dry skin, failure of erection and ejaculation, failure of micturation and defecation, an inability to accommodate to near vision in the eye, and mydriasis (enlarged pupils and therefore sensitivity to light). On the other hand, blockade of β receptors generally has no significant effect in healthy people, although it will cause bronchospasm in patients with asthma. Blockade of α receptors can produce hypotension and ejaculatory failure. Drugs which increase the activity in the adrenergic system produce tachycardia, hypertension, tremors, excitability and nervousness. Thus, knowledge of the full physiology of the ANS allows one to predict the actions (beneficial or adverse) of drugs that act upon the ANS. Many classes of drugs coincidentally to their main action have effects on the ANS.

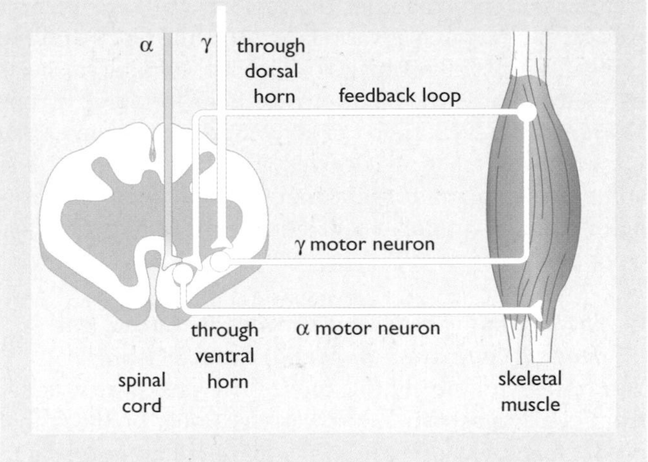

Fig. 8.10 The motor system of the peripheral nervous system. The α and γ neurons provide feedback control of muscle contraction via a loop to the α motor neurons.

Motor neurons innervate muscle fibers or intrafusal muscle spindles (see also p. 205–213)

Motor neurons send their axons to muscle fibers in the periphery. There are two types of motor neuron:

- α motor neurons are large myelinated fibers and form motor units with the muscle fibers they innervate. The number of muscle fibers innervated by each motor fiber varies with the degree of fine motor control. For fine control only a few fibers are innervated.
- γ motor neurons are much smaller than α motor neurons, have limited myelination, and innervate only intrafusal muscle spindles acting as stretch receptors (Fig. 8.10).

Both α and γ fibers are found in the ventral horn of the spinal cord and synapse with the descending motor tracts within the spinal cord. Interneuronal connection within the spinal cord integrates the fine motor control provided by the extrapyramidal system.

Control of skeletal muscle system activity by the motor nervous system is complex and involves intricate CNS regulation. The afferent limb of the system carries information from a variety of sources, including:

- Stretch receptors in the joints and limbs.
- Muscle spindles in the body of skeletal muscles.
- Proprioceptors in joints.
- Labyrinth receptors in the ear.

Information arriving at the CNS from these afferent sources is integrated at various levels of the CNS with the cerebellum playing a major role. The voluntary aspects of skeletal muscle control arise in the cerebral cortex. Within the CNS there is a comprehensive interplay between information derived from the cortex (the voluntary component) and that derived from the cerebellum, midbrain nuclei and spinal cord (the involuntary component).

Efferent motor nerves have myelinated axons and generally one axon supplies one muscle fiber

The efferent limb of the motor nervous system arises from the brainstem and at various levels of the spinal cord. Once they leave the CNS there are no ganglia and the motor nerve axons thus conduct impulses rapidly from the CNS to skeletal muscle. These axons are myelinated and so allow rapid propagation of action potentials along them. Each axon normally innervates a single muscle fiber. Multiple innervated muscles are rare and are found in the muscle spindle and the extraocular muscles of the eye.

Once the axon reaches the skeletal muscle fiber it terminates in a highly discrete region. The axon abuts onto the muscle fiber at the neuromuscular junction, and, at this site, the nerve ending sits within the 'cup' of folded end-plate membrane. Here, ACh mediates its molecular action (activation of nicotinic receptors). This, through a cascade of transduction mechanisms, elicits a system response in skeletal muscle (contraction) (see below).

Sensory neurons originate in peripheral structures and transduce stimuli into action potentials

The endings of sensory neurons in peripheral structures comprise a highly specialized network of physiologic receptors, which transduce stimuli into action potentials. The sensory fibers pass into the spinal cord through the dorsal root (Fig. 8.11). Some fibers synapse at the level of entry into the spinal cord, while others pass to the brainstem before synapsing and passing to the thalamus. The special sensory systems such as vision and hearing have a highly individualized arrangement and are discussed in Chapters 19 and 20, respectively.

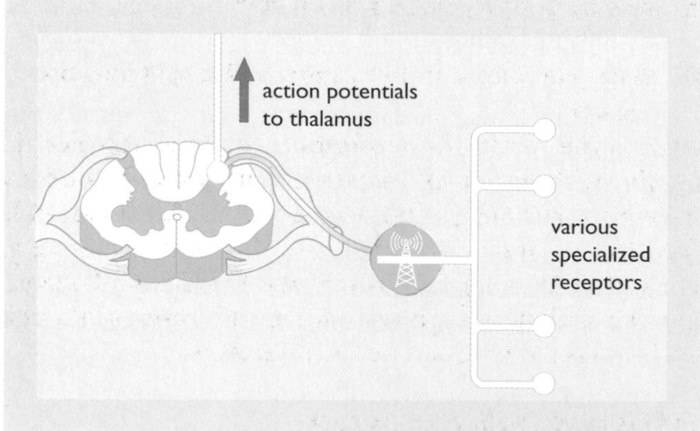

Fig. 8.11 Sensory system of the peripheral nervous system. Sensory neurons originate in peripheral structures and pass into the spinal cord through the dorsal root.

The autonomic nervous system maintains homeostasis

The ANS controls visceral functions such as circulation, digestion and excretion, mostly without voluntary or conscious control. It also modulates the function of the endocrine glands, which regulate metabolism. The ANS has both sensory and motor components, and is divided into sympathetic and parasympathetic systems. In general, the first neurons of the sympathetic system are located in the intermediate horn of the thoracolumbar region of the spinal cord. These synapse with a second set of neurons in the para- or prevertebral sympathetic ganglia. In the parasympathetic system the first neurons are located either in the cranial nerve autonomic nuclei or in the intermediate horn of the sacral region of the spinal cord. They synapse with a second set of neurons either in autonomic ganglia in the case of cranial nerves or in the effecter tissue itself.

The ANS has three major elements:

- The afferent limb.
- The central integrated elements.
- The efferent limb.

The afferent limb carries information from sensors (neuronal physiologic receptors sited at the ends of afferent nerves) to the spinal cord and higher regions of the CNS. Most of this input is then processed within the hypothalamus, and other parts of the lower brain. After processing, appropriate signals pass from the CNS and down the efferent nerves to the effector organs (see Fig. 8.9; see also Fig. 8.1), which are so named because they produce the responses to activity in the CNS.

The efferent part of the ANS is divided into three on the basis of its anatomy and neurotransmitters:

- The parasympathetic (cholinergic) system.
- The sympathetic (adrenergic) system.
- The nonadrenergic and noncholinergic (NANC) system.

A cholinergic system is one in which the neurotransmitter is acetylcholine

Acetylcholine is the neurotransmitter released from presynaptic terminals in the autonomic ganglia and from prejunctional nerve endings at the effector organ. The receptors for acetylcholine are cholinoceptors, which are classified as muscarinic and nicotinic receptors (Table 8.3).

An adrenergic system is one in which the neurotransmitter is norepinephrine

The other major limb of the ANS is the adrenergic system. The nomenclature is an historical accident, as when the system was first described, there was no clear

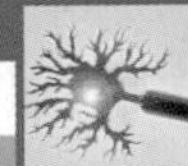

Table 8.3 Acetylcholine receptors and their distribution in the body

Name	Location	Agonists	Antagonists
α_1-nicotinic	Skeletal muscle	Suxamethonium, nicotine, ACh	α-bungarotoxin, pancuronium
α_3-nicotinic	Autonomic ganglia	DMPP, nicotine, ACh	α-conotoxin, dihydro-β-erythroidine
α_4-nicotinic	Neuronal	Tc-2559, ACh	
α_7-nicotinic	Neuronal	Choline, ACh	α-bungarotoxin, α-conotoxin
M_1-muscarinic	Airways, enteric interneurons	ACh	Ipratropium bromide, atropine, pirenzepine
M_2-muscarinic	Neuronal (prejunctional), sinoatrial node	ACh	Ipratropium bromide, atropine, tripitramine
M_3-muscarinic	Bladder, salivary glands, airways, parietal cells	ACh	Atropine, darifenacin

α_2-, α_6-, α_9- and α_{10}-nicotinic and M_4- and M_5-muscarinic receptors are orphans (human expression and or function unknown).

separation between two possible transmitters, namely epinephrine (E) and norepinephrine (NE). It is now known that apart from the special case for the adrenal glands, which secrete epinephrine, the neurotransmitter is always NE.

The ganglionic transmitter for both cholinergic and adrenergic systems is acetylcholine

The efferent nerves for both cholinergic and adrenergic systems arise from the appropriate parts of the brainstem and the spinal cord. These efferent nerves then synapse at ganglia situated throughout the body, with ACh being the major neurotransmitter.

- In the adrenergic system, the ganglia lie mainly in a chain close to the spinal cord, known as the paravertebral sympathetic chain.
- In the cholinergic system, the ganglia are usually situated close to or on their effector organ.

Despite this clear anatomical distinction, both types of ganglia use ACh as the principal ganglionic neurotransmitter acting on nicotinic receptors.

Neurotransmitters can modulate their own release

A further complexity is that neurotransmitters can modulate their own release. Neurotransmitters can act back upon presynaptic receptors on the nerve ending that originally released them, to inhibit their own release.

The NANC system is a third limb of the ANS

In addition to the cholinergic and adrenergic systems, it has been recognized over recent decades that parts of the ANS are neither cholinergic nor adrenergic. This limb of the ANS is therefore known as the NANC system. It is not clear which neurotransmitters act in this limb, although nitric oxide has recently been suggested to be a major neurotransmitter in NANC nerves in various parts of the body, including the penis and the lung (see Fig. 8.1). Nitric oxide is synthesized in nerve endings from the precursor amino acid L-arginine by the enzyme nitric oxide synthase (Fig. 8.12).

An added complication in cholinergic and adrenergic limbs of the ANS is the presence of co-transmitters. These co-transmitters may not serve the primary function of neurotransmission (i.e. passing the neuronal message to effector tissue), but instead have modulator functions. A classic example is adenosine triphosphate (ATP) in blood vessels.

Cholinergic and adrenergic ganglia cannot be differentiated from each other pharmacologically

Both cholinergic and adrenergic ganglia can be considered together since they cannot be differentiated from each other by using drugs, despite having distinct anatomical locations.

The term 'preganglionic fibers' refers to neuronal axons that arise in the CNS and terminate on cell bodies in the ganglia. They are primarily cholinergic. Axons arising from the cell bodies in the ganglia and terminating at the effector tissue are known as postganglionic fibers. Some postganglionic adrenergic fibers have been found to innervate cholinergic ganglia, adding further complexity.

Drugs and ganglionic transmission

Given that transmission in ganglia is primarily cholinergic, it is possible to understand the mechanisms by which drugs may interfere with ganglionic transmission, either to accentuate or to block transmission.

Drugs can interfere with acetylcholine synthesis and storage

ACh is the result of esterification of the amino alcohol choline with acetate. No common drugs or toxins directly inhibit the enzyme (acetylcholine transferase) responsible for this. However, a variety of cholinomimetics (e.g. analogs of choline) can prevent the formation of acetylcholine and its subsequent storage in vesicles, though such drugs are of experimental interest only.

Drugs and choline transport

Release of ACh from nerve terminals requires opening of N-type Ca^{2+} channels, entry of Ca^{2+}, mobilization of vesicles and vesicle fusion with neuronal membranes to

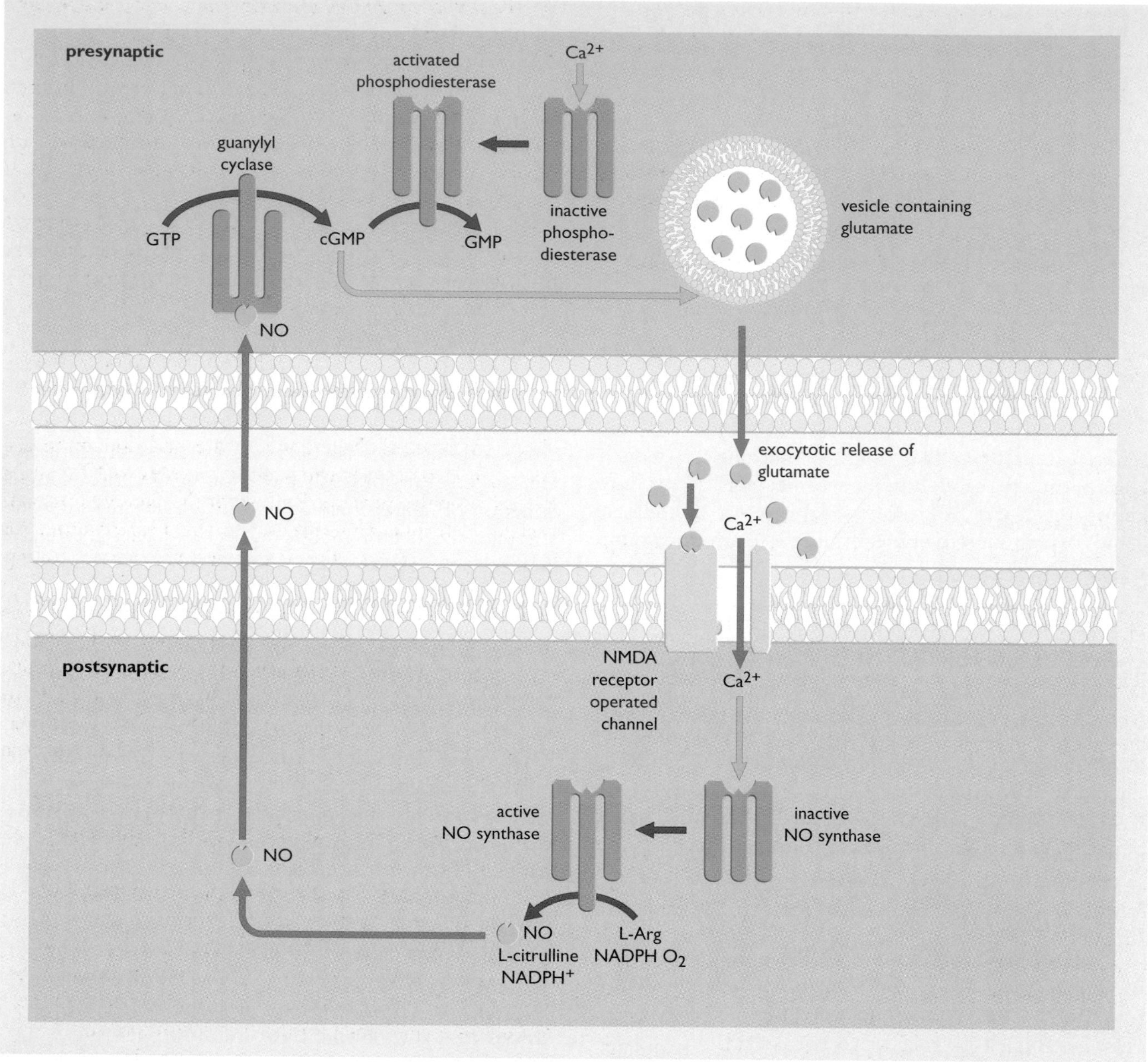

Fig. 8.12 Nitric oxide and glutaminergic neural transmission. In this model, glutamate released from a presynaptic terminal binds to postsynaptic NMDA receptors causing an influx of calcium ions (Ca^{2+}). Alternatively, calcium influx may occur through voltage-gated calcium channels. The increased Ca^{2+} concentration leads to activation of NO synthase, which results in production of nitric oxide (NO). Nitric oxide then diffuses to surrounding tissue, including the presynaptic release terminal, where it binds to and activates guanylate cyclase. This sets into motion a biochemical cascade that results in increased glutamate release from the presynaptic terminal. (Adapted from Holscher C. Nitric oxide, the enigmatic neuronal messenger: its role in synaptic plasticity. *Trends Neurosci* 1997; **20**: 298–303.)

release their contents into the synaptic gap of the ganglia. Once released, ACh can bind to receptors or be metabolized by the enzyme acetylcholinesterase, into its acetate and choline. Choline is taken back up into the cholinergic neuron ending by a special choline transporter. Experimentally, it is possible to interfere with this choline transporter by drugs such as hemicholinium.

Ganglion blockers prevent transmission in the ANS

By blocking transmission in the ANS, ganglion blockers prevent the ANS from participating in body responses.

The first antihypertensive drugs were ganglion blockers, which a molecular mechanism of action of nicotinic receptor antagonism. The nicotinic receptors found in autonomic ganglia are different from those found in skeletal muscle (see below) in that they are preferentially blocked by a group of drugs, e.g. hexamethonium and mecamylamine, which have little effect on nicotinic receptors in the skeletal muscle. Blockade of ganglia with doses sufficient to lower blood pressure resulted in blockade of all other ganglia with the production of an expected variety of signs and symptoms:

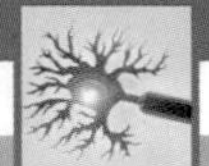

- Inability to accommodate vision for near sight.
- Drying of secretions in the mouth, stomach and eyes.
- Constipation.
- Difficulty with urination.
- Loss of sexual function in the male.
- Orthostatic hypotension.

These symptoms emphasize the importance of resting tone in the ANS in regulating homeostasis in a range of organs. Both parasympathetic and sympathetic ganglia are blocked by ganglion blockers because these drugs are not selective for different ganglia.

Adrenergic nervous system

The adrenergic nervous system innervates many parts of the body, but particularly:

- The gut.
- The heart.
- The lungs.
- Blood vessels.

The adrenergic system innervates some tissues (e.g. the gut and airway smooth muscle) via synapsing at cholinergic ganglia. This means that the role of the adrenergic nervous system in the gut and the lung is to modulate the activity of parasympathetic cholinergic ganglia.

Three closely related catecholamines (NE, epinephrine and dopamine) are found in the PNS and the CNS. Only NE is a major neurotransmitter in the PNS, while dopamine is a major neurotransmitter in the CNS. All three are formed from the same precursor essential amino acid, tyrosine. Tyrosine enters a cascade of enzymes in adrenergic nerve endings (Fig. 8.13). Synthesis stops at NE in noradrenergic neurons or dopamine in dopaminergic neurons. Very little of the tyrosine is metabolized to the N-methyl product of NE (epinephrine) in neurons. However, epinephrine is formed in the adrenal medulla, which is a specialized ANS ganglion lying above the kidney. The outer part (cortex) of the gland is involved in the synthesis of steroid hormones, particularly glucocorticosteroids and mineralocorticoids, whereas epinephrine is synthesized in the center of the gland (medulla). High concentrations of cortisol activate expression of phenylethanolamine N-methyl transferase, the enzyme catalyzing the conversion of NE to epinephrine.

The adrenal medulla is effectively a highly specialized sympathetic ganglion

The adrenal medulla is a ganglion with only a residual postganglionic neuron (see Fig. 8.9). Stimulation by activation of nicotinic receptors on the adrenal medulla results in the release of epinephrine directly into the adrenal medullary veins and then into the vena cava, from where it reaches the heart to be distributed around the body. Epinephrine released in this manner is a circulating hormone, rather than a neurotransmitter.

The initial enzymatic cascade producing epinephrine, norephinephrine and dopamine is the same

Tyrosine is progressively hydroxylated and decarboxylated to produce dopamine. The process can then stop, or can continue with further hydroxylation and methylation to produce NE, where the process can again stop. Further methylation in the adrenal glands results in the production of epinephrine.

The rate-limiting enzyme (a critical control point) in the cascade is tyrosine hydroxylase. Metyrosine is used in the treatment of some cases of pheochromocytoma that is an inhibitor of tyrosine hydroxylase.

Release processes for norephinephrine, epinephrine and dopamine from vesicles is similar to that for acetylcholine

Once synthesized, NE, epinephrine and dopamine are packaged into vesicles where they complex to ATP and a special vesicular protein. Release of the contents of such vesicles is by the same process as for acetylcholine. An action potential at the postganglionic nerve ending results in the opening of N-type Ca^{2+} channels and intracellular flow of Ca^{2+}. The elevation of Ca^{2+} in the nerve ending results in mobilization of the vesicles, which fuse with the membrane of the nerve ending. As a result, the released NE diffuses across the junctional cleft to bind to postjunctional adrenoceptors. The molecular targets for NE are shown in Fig. 8.13. The uses of these drugs are discussed in subsequent chapters.

As with ACh, there is a highly effective system for reusing NE

Once NE has acted upon the postjunctional receptor:

- Some diffuses from the junctional cleft.
- Some acts upon prejunctional receptors on postganglionic nerve endings to inhibit the release of more NE. The presynaptic receptor is the α_2 subtype.
- Most is taken back into the nerve terminal via reuptake that requires a special process involving an NE transporter in the cell membrane. This transporter carries NE back into the nerve ending where it is either metabolized by the enzyme monoamine oxidase (located on mitochondria) or it is repackaged into vesicles.

Thus, as with acetylcholine, there is a highly effective system for reusing the neurotransmitter.

NE escaping from the junctional cleft is exposed to two further metabolic pathways that are less important than reuptake:

- Metabolism by the enzyme catechol-O-methyl transferase.
- Reuptake by the uptake 2 system.

There are two uptake systems for NE. The first, uptake 1, is the physiologically important system that ensures that neurotransmitter is used efficiently and that its time in the junctional cleft is limited. The second, uptake 2, is of doubtful physiologic relevance.

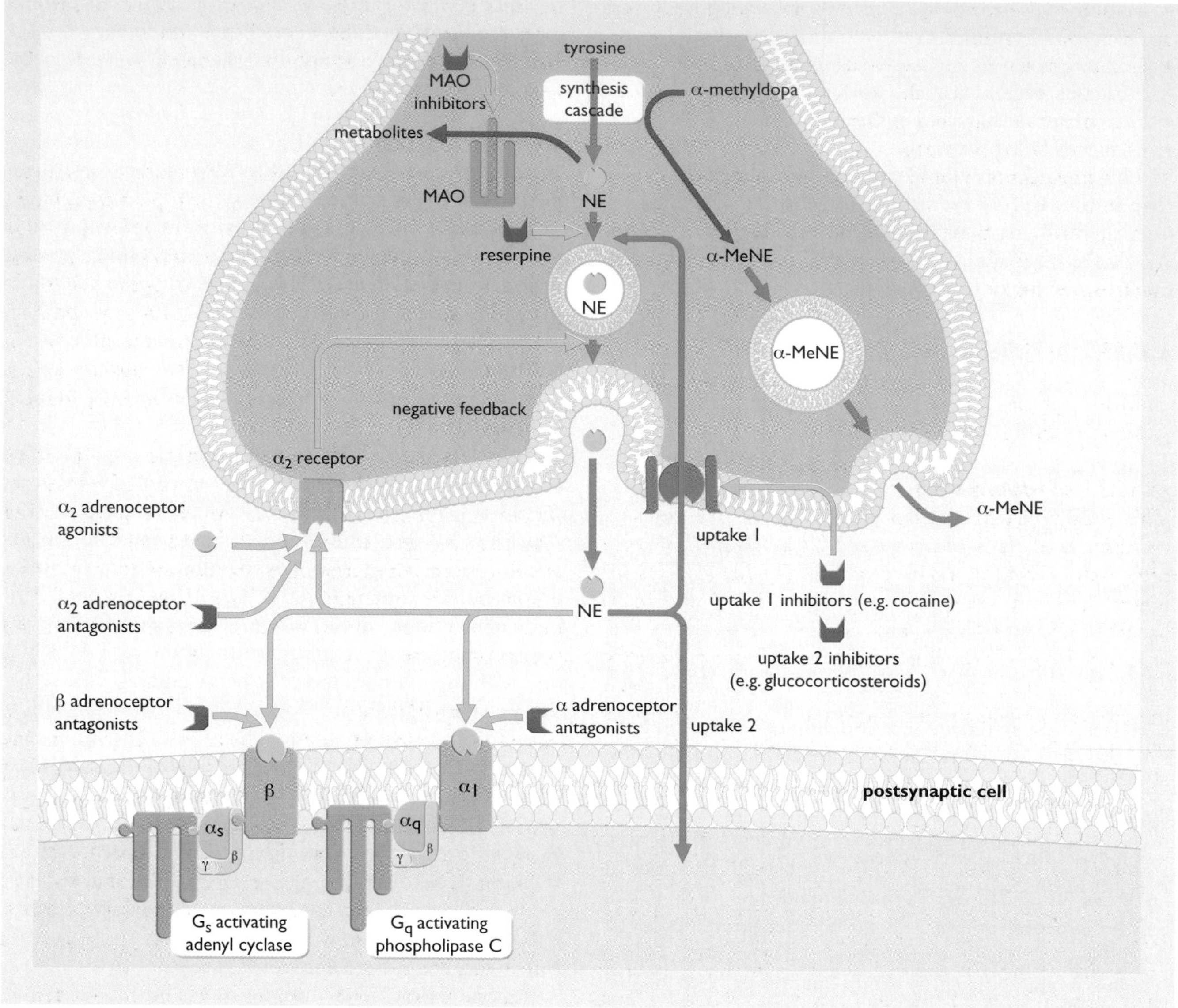

Fig. 8.13 Drug actions on the noradrenergic (sympathetic) nervous system. Drugs may affect synthesis, storage, release, uptake and receptors (MAO, monoamine oxidase; α-MeNE, α-methylnorepinephrine; NE, norepinephrine).

The major action of some drugs is inhibition of the uptake 1 process. Such drugs are therefore known as uptake 1 inhibitors. Uptake 1 inhibition has complex sympathetic nervous system effects.

Cocaine can produce a hyperadrenergic state

The classic uptake 1 inhibitor is cocaine. It extenuates the effects of adrenergic stimulation or injected NE. A cocaine addict therefore has a hyperadrenergic state, both centrally and peripherally. Such a hyperadrenergic state may partly account for the sudden deaths that occurs in some cocaine addicts, which are believed to be due to fatal arrhythmias.

The adrenergic system can be modulated at a number of levels

- By sympathomimetic drugs, which are agonists at pre- and postsynaptic adrenergic receptors.
- By inhibiting uptake 1, or the enzyme monoamine oxidase.
- By interfering with the storage of NE in vesicles.
- By disrupting the process that results in the release of vesicles.

Drugs that reduce NE storage and release reduce activity in the adrenergic system. Therapeutically, this can be advantageous (e.g. in the treatment of hypertension).

Drugs interfering with the adrenergic system innervating blood vessels may cause postural hypotension

One adverse effect of adrenergic neuron blockers is postural hypotension (a dramatic fall in blood pressure on rising to a standing position from a previous sitting or supine position). The fall in blood pressure can be profound and cause dizziness or even fainting. This is because, on standing up, normally there is increased

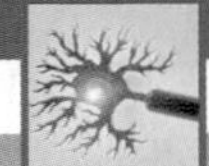

activation of the adrenergic system innervating veins and arteries resulting in:

- Venoconstriction and a squeezing action on capacitance veins, which ensures an adequate venous return to the heart and sufficient cardiac output to maintain blood pressure.
- Vasoconstriction of arteries to help maintain blood pressure.

As a result of these two mechanisms, blood flow in the cerebral arteries is maintained. Impairment of these mechanisms impairs the ability of patients to stand up.

Dysautonomias

Dysautonomias are disorders of the ANS, including familial dysautonomia (Riley–Day syndrome), Shy–Drager syndrome and Horner's syndrome.

Familial dysautonomia

This is an inherited disorder transmitted as an autosomal recessive trait. It is characterized by a complex mixture of symptoms and is more common in Ashkenazi Jewish infants than in other ethnic groups. The disorder is usually present at birth and the child commonly dies during infancy. The major symptoms include an inability to control body temperature and to produce tears, uncontrollable perspiration, hypertension and sometimes postural hypotension, corneal and pain insensitivity, fever and frequent episodes of pneumonia. These symptoms are associated with defects in both the parasympathetic and sympathetic limbs of the ANS as well as defects in some peripheral sensory nerves. Cutaneous nerves contain a decreased number of unmyelinated fibers, the neuronal pathways for pain and temperature sensation. Neurons in the vagus and the glossopharyngeal nerves are typically smaller and reduced in number. Similarly, there appear to be fewer neurons in the cervical and thoracic sympathetic ganglia.

Treatment is symptomatic since there is no cure (Table 8.4). Sedatives (e.g. diazepam) and the phenothiazine drugs (e.g. chlorpromazine) are often used for gastrointestinal and behavioral symptoms. In addition, antibiotics are used for pulmonary infection (see Ch. 14), which is quite common.

Table 8.4 Treatment of dysautonomia

Disorder	Treatment
Familial dysautonomia (Riley–Day syndrome)	1. Symptomatic control with drugs that interfere with the ANS 2. Sedatives 3. Phenothiazines 4. Antibiotics to treat pulmonary infections
Shy–Drager syndrome	Fludrocortisone, phenylephrine and ephedrine to counteract the postural hypotension
Horner's syndrome	Directly and indirectly acting sympathomimetics for preganglionic lesions and directly acting sympathomimetics for postganglionic lesions

Shy-Drager syndrome

This syndrome is also due to ANS failure. It is characterized by a complex mixture of symptoms including severe postural hypotension, urinary incontinence, male erectile dysfunction, akinesia, tremor, muscle rigidity and the inability to sweat. Evidence suggests that the deficiency is due to a loss of preganglionic sympathetic cells from the intermediolateral column of cells in the spinal cord. There is also a CNS motor control involvement with the syndrome, as reflected by akinesia and muscle rigidity.

The most troublesome symptom is postural hypotension, treated with small doses of fludrocortisone (0.1 mg) to increase Na^+ and water retention which may increase the sensitivity of blood vessels to catecholamines. α adrenergic agonists are also used, including phenylephrine and ephedrine. The disadvantage of these drugs is that they tend to produce hypertension when the patient is supine.

Horner's syndrome

Horner's syndrome results from a loss of cervical sympathetic control to the head. It is characterized by miosis due to the loss of pupillary dilation, slight drooping of the eyelids (ptosis), recession of the eyeball (enophthalmos), facial vasodilation and loss of the ability to sweat. These symptoms are often unilateral and may result from an injury or tumor involving either the pre- or postganglionic cervical sympathetic nerves. Lung cancer is a common cause.

The location of the lesion must be clearly defined for effective treatment. For example:

- If the lesion is confined to preganglionic fibers, both directly and indirectly acting sympathomimetics (phenylephrine, ephedrine and cocaine) are effective (e.g. restoration of mydriatic response). This is because their effects are mediated via direct action on the tissue receptor and indirectly by the release of stored NE from the postganglionic nerve terminal, respectively.
- If the lesion is on the postganglionic fiber, only the directly acting sympathomimetics (e.g. phenylephrine) are therapeutically effective. The indirectly acting agents are ineffective because they act on functioning postganglionic fibers.

Physiology of motor nervous system

Neural control of skeletal muscles is accomplished mainly through the somatic motor nerves and afferent influence from sensory receptors present in the muscles (e.g. muscle spindles), tendons (e.g. Golgi tendon organs) and joints (proprioceptors). The main controlling

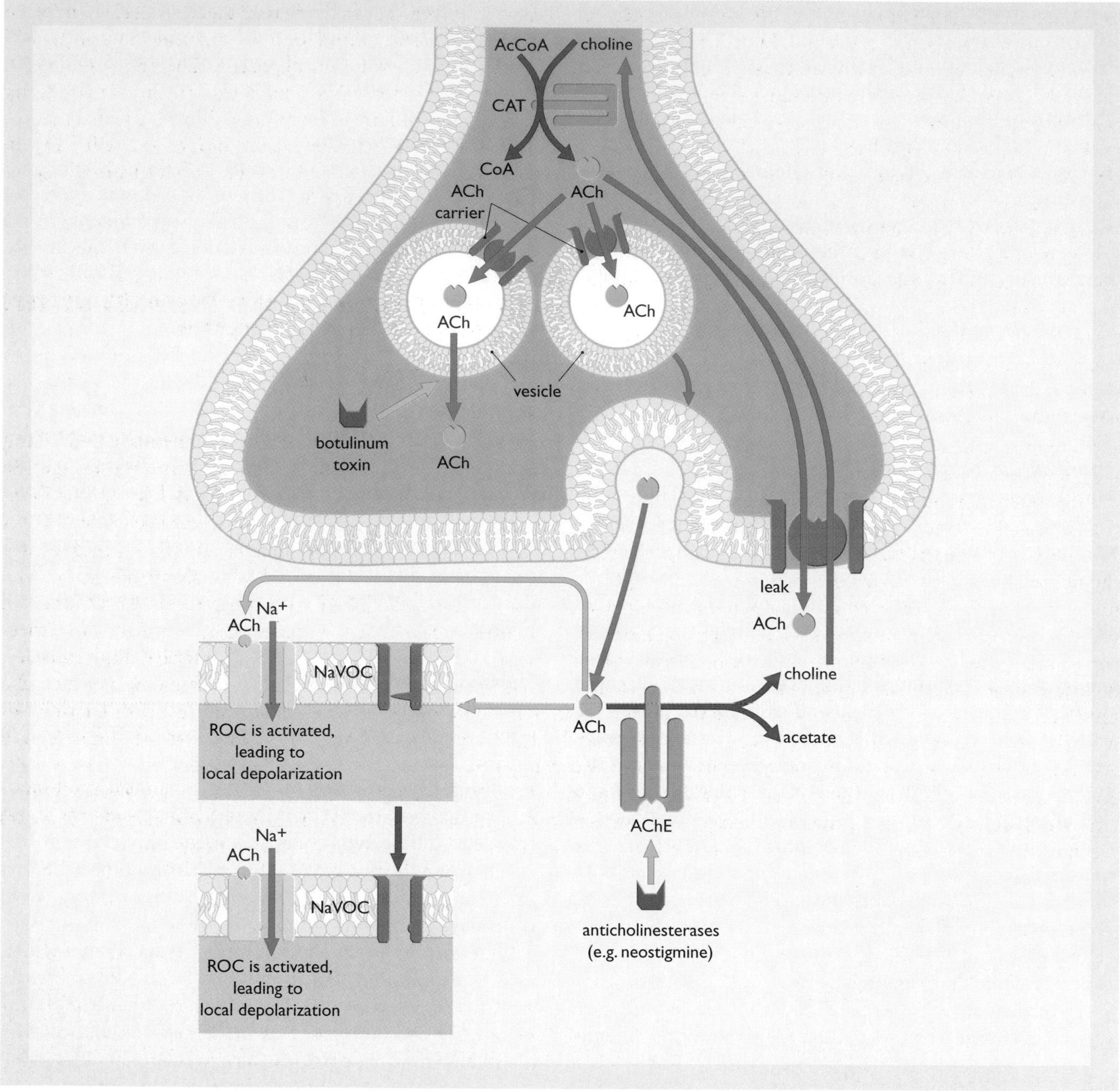

Fig. 8.14 Sites of drug action at a cholinergic motor nerve terminal. Drugs can interfere with cholinergic transmission in a variety of ways, including effects on synthesis, storage, release and uptake, and postjunctional effects. (Adapted with permission from Rang H, Dale M, Ritter J. *Pharmacology*, 3rd edn. London: Churchill Livingstone; 1995.)

influence for somatic nerve activity comes from the motor cortex via the corticospinal tracts (also called pyramidal tracts) to the lower motor neurons (α motor neurons), which is the final neuronal pathway to muscle fibers and their neuromuscular junction.

Physiology of the neuromuscular junction

The physiology of the neuromuscular junction (NMJ) is analogous to that of the cholinergic and adrenergic junctions previously described in the ANS. However, as shown in Figure 8.14, the acetylcholine released from prejunctional nerve fibers acts postjunctionally on nicotinic skeletal muscle receptors. These are similar to nicotinic ganglionic receptors, but differ in their drug sensitivity phenotype and genotype. Furthermore, the skeletal muscle NMJ is such that the nerve ending is engulfed in a particular structure on skeletal muscle known as the skeletal muscle end plate. The cell membrane of this region consists of mainly nicotinic receptors and acetylcholinesterase. The end-plate region does not contain actin and myosin filaments. The nicotinic skeletal muscle receptor is an integral part of

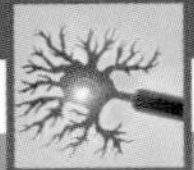

the ACh gated ion channel that is selectively permeable to Na^+ and K^+ ions (see Fig. 8.8 and Table 8.3 for example of nicotinic receptors). Two of these skeletal muscle nicotinic receptors have to simultaneously bind ACh if the ion channel is to open. The increased permeability to both K^+ and Na^+ resulting from the simultaneous opening of many channels results in depolarization of the end-plate membrane. This depolarization spreads electrically to the surrounding skeletal muscle membrane where it opens voltage-gated Na^+ channels and initiates an action potential leading to release of Ca^{2+} from the sarcoplasmic reticulum and activation of actin/myosin interaction and contraction. The neuromuscular junction has a large safety reserve in as much that there is an excess of nicotinic receptors such that, providing there are enough ACh vesicles, a contraction always occurs once an actual action potential arrives at the junction.

The process of initiating a contraction in a single muscle fiber is as follows: an action potential invading the prejunctional nerve ending initiates the opening of N-type Ca^{2+} channels and the entry of a Ca^{2+} wave into the nerve ending that results in a fusion of an appropriate number of vesicles, each containing a large number of ACh, molecules. The junctional cleft therefore receives very many molecules of ACh, which rapidly diffuse to the nicotinic receptors, where approximately 90% of them bind. This results in the generation of an action potential in the skeletal muscle membrane. As the ACh comes off the receptor it is generally hydrolyzed by the nearby acetylcholinesterase. Thus, very few of the ACh molecules have the chance to rebind to nicotinic receptors. By such mechanisms, many discrete and unambiguous commands can be given to individual skeletal muscle fibers to contract. Excess stimulation of nicotinic receptors will induce such a profound depolarization of the end plate that voltage-gated Na^+ channels in the surrounding membrane will remain inactivated. This is the mechanism responsible for depolarization block (see Ch. 21 on anesthesia for further details on the pharmacology of neuromuscular blockers).

PATHOPHYSIOLOGY AND DISEASES OF THE PERIPHERAL MOTOR SYSTEM

Skeletal muscle disorders

Myasthenia gravis

Myasthenia gravis is a rare autoimmune disease affecting the NMJ (Fig. 8.15). Characteristic symptoms are skeletal muscle weakness and fatigability after a brief period of repeated activity with recovery after a short period of rest. However, adequate muscle strength may not always return after rest in patients in whom the disease has progressed to a crisis level. About 85% of myasthenic patients experience generalized weakness involving the eyelids, extraocular muscles, limb muscles, diaphragm and neck extensor muscles. Sometimes the weakness is localized to eyelids and extraocular muscles (15% of patients) and is manifested by the characteristic appearance of drooping eyelids (ptosis).

Myasthenia gravis occurs at about 100 cases/million of the US population and usually in women under 50 years of age, or in men over 60 years of age.

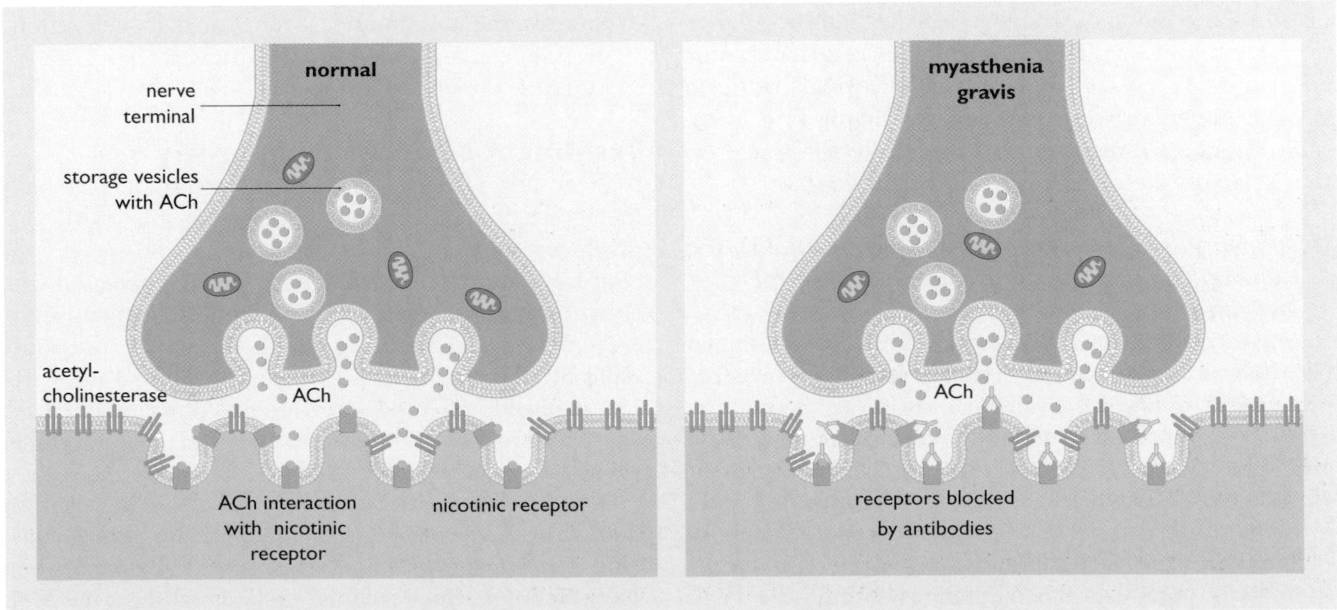

Fig. 8.15 Neurotransmitter release and its interaction with nicotinic receptors at the neuromuscular junction (NMJ). In myasthenia gravis the nicotinic receptors are blocked by antibodies, preventing interaction between the neurotransmitter and the receptor (ACh, acetylcholine).

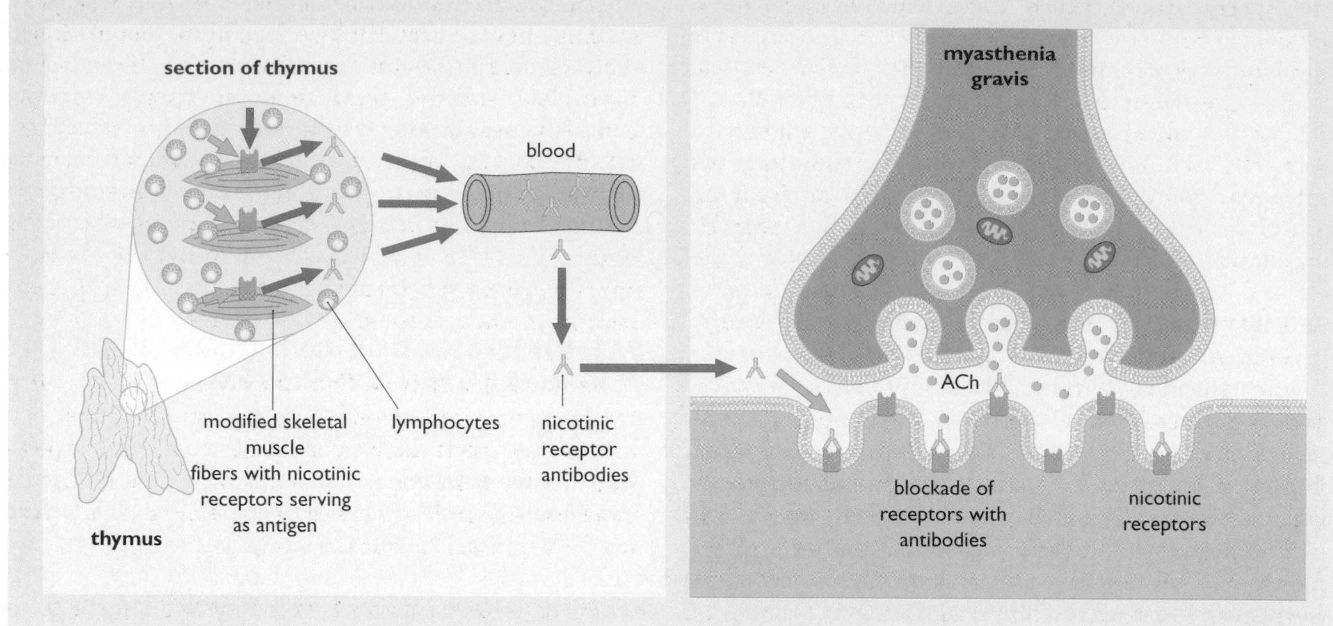

Fig. 8.16 Postulated source of antigen and antibody production in myasthenia gravis. A diagrammatic representation of a section of the thymus gland containing modified muscle cells with nicotinic receptors on the surface. It is suggested that this gland may be the source of the antigen that serves as a template for the production of nicotinic antibodies in myasthenic patients. These antibodies block the nicotinic receptors at the neuromuscular junction and prevent interaction between the neurotransmitter and the nicotinic receptors (see Fig. 8.18) (ACh, acetylcholine).

The pathophysiologic features of myasthenia gravis result from a deficit in the number of nicotinic cholinergic receptors at the NMJ

The population of nicotinic cholinergic receptors at myasthenic muscle end plates is only about one-third of that at normal muscle end plates. The receptor deficit is linked to an immunologic response involving the thymus gland, since muscle strength usually improves after thymectomy in myasthenic patients. Nicotinic receptor antibodies are present in serum of myasthenic patients and the antigen may be located in the thymus (Fig. 8.16), since cholinergic receptors have been demonstrated on the surface of muscle-like cells in the thymus.

In myasthenia gravis, neurally induced skeletal muscle contraction is inadequate for sustained physical activities

In myasthenia gravis, contraction cannot be sustained because the number of neurotransmitter–receptor interactions is lower than normal, owing to the number of available functioning nicotinic receptors at the muscle end plate being reduced due to occupancy with antibodies (see Fig. 8.16). Failure of transmission occurs in many muscle fibers because of this reduced number of neurotransmitter–receptor interactions. This means that action potentials can be generated only in a small proportion of the muscle fibers. Contraction is therefore likely to fail after a brief period of muscle activity. However, this failure can be prevented by enhancing the number of cholinergic neurotransmitter–receptor interactions.

Effective drug treatment of myasthenia gravis enhances the number of cholinergic transmitter–receptor interactions

Treatment of myasthenia gravis involves procedures that:

- Increase the neuromuscular junctional concentration of ACh (e.g. anticholinesterase drugs).
- Suppress the immune response.

Treatment of myasthenia gravis

ACh is not effective as a drug because it is rapidly metabolized by acetylcholinesterase at the NMJ and produces adverse muscarinic effects. However, the concentration of ACh at the NMJ can be increased with anticholinesterase drugs, which inhibit the metabolism of ACh. The peak effects of anticholinesterase drugs are typically obtained promptly during the initial phases of treatment but, after weeks or months of treatment, such drugs often lose their effectiveness. It then becomes necessary to add other drugs.

The cholinesterase enzyme, which is inhibited by these drugs, exists in two structurally related isoenzymes. One is acetylcholinesterase (which specifically metabolizes acetylcholine), which is found predominantly at the NMJ (and at other cholinergic neuroeffector junctions). The other species is a family of esterases called pseudocholinesterase or butyrylcholinesterase (the substrates are

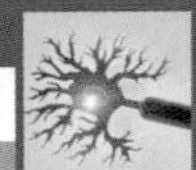

non-specific esters), which is found mainly in the blood plasma. These two species of enzyme have two major binding sites (esteratic and anionic) for which the anticholinesterase drugs compete with acetylcholine to inhibit its metabolism. The drugs that inhibit the acetylcholinesterase enzyme can be grouped into two categories based on the site and stability of the interaction with the enzyme, e.g. reversible and irreversible inhibitors.

Carbamates are reversible anticholinesterases widely used in the treatment of myasthenia gravis

The carbamates, particularly neostigmine and pyridostigmine, reversibly inhibit acetylcholinesterase by binding at its anionic and esteratic sites. During the period of inhibition (3–6 hours), ACh concentration increases at the NMJ and as a result there are repeated interactions with the reduced number of nicotinic cholinergic receptors. This leads to improved muscle contraction in the myasthenic patient. Both drugs are given orally, but pyridostigmine has a greater bioavailability and longer duration of action (half-life 4 hours) than neostigmine (half-life 2 hours) which is incompletely absorbed.

Grip strength and lung vital capacity are usually used for monitoring the improvement in muscle strength produced by anticholinesterase drugs

An ultra-short acting anticholinesterase edrophonium chloride is used for the monitoring and diagnosis of myasthenia gravis. This monitoring procedure is a precautionary measure to prevent excessive dosing, which may decrease muscle strength by ACh-induced depolarization blockade of nicotinic cholinergic receptors at the NMJ of patients with myasthenia gravis. To produce its effect, edrophonium chloride competes with acetylcholine for reversible binding at the anionic site of acetylcholinesterase. Improvement in muscle strength with edrophonium chloride lasts for about 5 minutes when the drug is given intravenously. However, despite the short duration of action of edrophonium chloride, atropine should be available to counter muscarinic side effects due to any accumulation of acetylcholine.

Longer-acting anticholinesterase drugs

Longer-acting (i.e. longer than 3–8 hours) anticholinesterase drugs such as ambenonium are also used to treat myasthenia gravis. This drug acts similarly to the carbamates. However, the organophosphates are irreversibly long-acting anticholinesterases and they are not used clinically because of difficulty in controlling the dose in relation to a patient's need. This difficulty is due to the irreversible binding of this category of drug to the esteratic site of acetylcholinesterase. Organophosphate anticholinesterases are used primarily as insecticides (e.g. parathion, malathion) and as biologic weapons (e.g. tabun, sarin). Occasionally, echothiophate is used to treat some forms of glaucoma.

ADVERSE EFFECTS These result from the widespread accumulation of acetylcholine leading to stimulation of muscarinic receptors on many tissues. The effects include abdominal cramps, increased salivation, increased bronchial secretions, miosis and bradycardia. These effects can be controlled with muscarinic receptor antagonists such as atropine, but this is not usually given as it is preferable not to mask the appearance of the muscarinic effects, which are indicative of excessive anticholinesterase treatment. However, most patients become tolerant to these adverse effects.

DRUG INTERACTIONS The effectiveness of the anticholinesterases is diminished and the symptoms of myasthenia gravis are worsened if the patient is exposed to either tubocurarine (a nondepolarizing neuromuscular blocker) or an aminoglycoside antibiotic, which interferes with neuromuscular transmission.

DRUGS THAT SUPPRESS THE IMMUNE RESPONSE IN MYASTHENIA GRAVIS Since the effectiveness of anticholinesterase treatment often diminishes within weeks or months, additional therapeutic measures are used. These include oral use of immunosuppressant drugs such as the glucocorticosteroids, which are indicated if muscle strength is inadequate.

Glucocorticosteroids

The mechanism of action of glucocorticosteroids is discussed in greater depth in Chapter 9. Glucocorticosteroids are used in the treatment of myasthenia gravis because they inhibit the synthesis of antibodies to nicotinic cholinergic receptors at the NMJ (Table 8.5). Prednisolone or prednisone are the usual orally active glucocorticosteroids used for this indication. Their use leads to an increase in the number of available nicotinic cholinergic receptors for interaction with ACh, and as a consequence muscle strength improves in myasthenic patients. It has been suggested that the beneficial effects of prednisolone may be partly due to increased synthesis

Table 8.5 Drugs used for the treatment of myasthenia gravis

Drug	Major effect
Anticholinesterases (e.g. neostigmine, pyridostigmine, ambenonium)	Increase acetylcholine concentration at the neuromuscular junction
Glucocorticosteroids (e.g. prednisolone, prednisone)	Inhibit the synthesis of nicotinic receptor antibody
Azathioprine	Inhibits the synthesis of nicotinic receptor antibody
Ciclosporin	Inhibits the synthesis of nicotinic receptor antibody

of ACh receptors, which would also improve neuromuscular transmission in myasthenia gravis, partly due to the suppression of antibody formation.

In the early stages of treatment with prednisolone, muscle weakness may increase; therefore, patients should be hospitalized when it is first used. Alternatively, the risk can be minimized by starting therapy with a combination of an anticholinesterase and a small dose of prednisolone (20 mg). As the muscle strength improves, the glucocorticosteroid dose can be gradually increased while the anticholinesterase dose is simultaneously reduced until the glucocorticosteroid alone produces a desirable level of muscle strength. However, since glucocorticosteroid treatment of myasthenia gravis is often long term, an alternate-day treatment regimen is preferred to reduce the risk of adverse effects. With this regimen, maximum therapeutic benefits are obtained within 6–12 months.

Azathioprine

Azathioprine (see also Chs 7 and 9) is used as an alternative to prednisolone in advanced myasthenia gravis not responding adequately to glucocorticosteroid therapy (see Table 8.5). Azathioprine suppresses nicotinic cholinergic receptor antibody synthesis by inhibiting B-lymphocyte proliferation. Also, its effectiveness may be due to the metabolite 6-mercaptopurine, which inhibits DNA synthesis (see Ch. 7). However, its therapeutic effectiveness develops slowly, taking up to 1 year to produce satisfactory clinical responses.

MAJOR ADVERSE EFFECTS OF AZATHIOPRINE These include a reaction similar to influenza, nausea and vomiting, dermatitis, bone marrow depression and hepatotoxicity. Many of these adverse effects may develop into serious toxicity if azathioprine is used in combination with either 6-mercaptopurine or allopurinol.

Ciclosporin

Ciclosporin is another immunosuppressant drug used in the treatment of myasthenia gravis (see Table 8.5). Its effectiveness is due to inhibition of the synthesis of nicotinic cholinergic receptor antibody by blocking the activation of T-helper cells (see Ch. 9). The therapeutic benefits of ciclosporine are obtained within 1–2 months.

MAJOR ADVERSE EFFECTS These include renal toxicity, hepatotoxicity, hypertension and tremor (see Ch. 7).

Other approaches to the treatment of myasthenia gravis

Surgical removal of the thymus is sometimes used in an attempt to reverse the antigenic stimulation for the production of antibodies to the nicotinic cholinergic receptors at the NMJ. This surgical procedure is not recommended for children below the age of puberty because of the need to preserve the role of the thymus in the developing immune system.

Plasmapheresis can be used to remove ACh nicotinic receptor antibodies from the circulation, but only as short-term therapy in patients who are experiencing a myasthenic crisis (i.e. exacerbation of symptoms of the disease). The therapeutic effectiveness of this procedure occurs within days but only lasts for a few weeks.

Spasticity

Spasticity is a hypertonic skeletal muscle contraction. It often occurs as a symptom of neurologic disorders such as cerebral palsy, multiple sclerosis and stroke. The causes of hypertonia in muscles are:

- Excessive tendon (stretch) reflexes driven by increased γ neuron activity and triggered by excitation of muscle spindles.
- Flexor muscle spasms, which are due to clonus produced by a volley of discharge from spindle afferents onto several lower motor neurons (α motor neurons).

Spasticity is treated with drugs that reduce excessive afferent stimulation of α motor neurons innervating the skeletal muscles

Drugs that reduce excessive afferent stimulation of the α motor neurons (Fig. 8.17) are preferable to neuromuscular blockers for treating spasticity because they are more selective. In comparison with these drugs, neuromuscular blockers produce relaxation by disrupting both normal muscle tone and increased tone due to spasm of any etiology.

Baclofen

Baclofen is a chlorophenyl analog of the CNS inhibitory neurotransmitter GABA. It was designed as a source of GABA that readily crosses the blood–brain barrier.

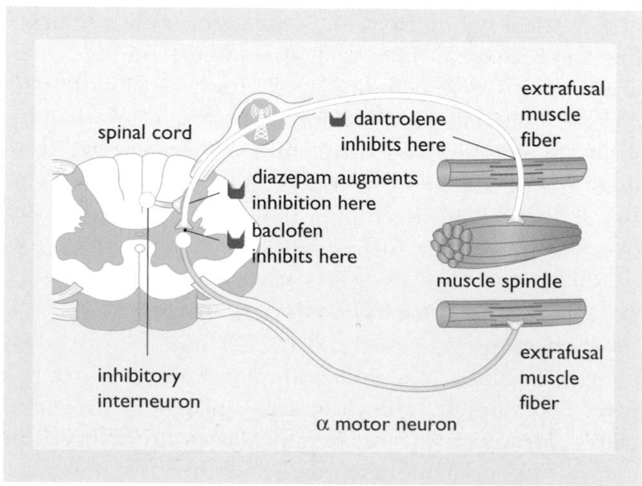

Fig. 8.17 The neuronal pathway that contributes to the development of clonus in spasticity is inhibited by diazepam and baclofen. Stretching the muscle activates the IA afferents from the muscle spindle and sends a flood of impulses to the α motor neuron, triggering contraction of the muscle. This relieves the tension on the spindle and terminates activity in the afferents. However, when the muscle relaxes, the tension on the spindle returns because the sensitivity of the reflex is increased in spasticity and the cycle of events is repeated, giving rise to clonus.

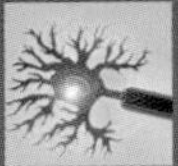

Baclofen is most useful for reducing flexor and extensor spasms. These effects are produced at the level of the spinal cord, but are not associated with any interference with voluntary muscle power or normal tendon reflexes.

Baclofen inhibits afferent input to the α motor neurons via interaction with presynaptic $GABA_B$ receptors on the afferent nerve terminals and associated interneurons. It is believed that the binding of baclofen with $GABA_B$ receptors (coupled to a G protein) reduces Ca^{2+} influx into the afferent nerve. Thus, less neurotransmitter is released for activating the α motor neurons, which become less active and less susceptible to the cycle of events that sustain spasticity.

■ ***Baclofen is effective for spasticity due to spinal cord lesions and multiple sclerosis, but is ineffective for spasticity due to stroke and other cerebral lesions***

Baclofen is usually given orally and is rapidly absorbed from the gut. It has a plasma half-life of 3–4 hours and approximately 35% is excreted unchanged by the kidneys and in feces.

MAJOR ADVERSE EFFECTS These include drowsiness (less than with diazepam), motor incoordination, mental confusion, nausea and hypotension (especially after overdose). An overdose may produce seizures, and therefore is not recommended for patients with epilepsy. Furthermore, baclofen should be withdrawn gradually at the termination of treatment after prolonged use because sudden withdrawal can cause hallucinations, anxiety and tachycardia.

Diazepam

■ ***Diazepam is effective for treatment of spasticity associated with spinal cord lesions, but is less effective than baclofen, especially against flexor spasm***

Diazepam is a benzodiazepine (see below). It is useful in the treatment of spasticity because it reduces muscle tone by depressing polysynaptic and monosynaptic reflexes. These reflexes help to maintain muscle spasticity. Although this action of diazepam occurs at both spinal and supraspinal levels, the spinal level is the important site of action in reducing spasticity. To produce this effect in the spinal cord, diazepam binds to benzodiazepine receptors in the $GABA_A$ receptor complex on afferent nerve terminals that synapse with α motor neurons (see Fig. 8.17). It therefore increases presynaptic inhibition mediated by GABA which increases $C1^-$ influx following interaction with $GABA_A$ receptors (Table 8.6). Diazepam can be given orally or intravenously. Its half-life is about 60 hours to which the active metabolite nordiazepam contributes.

■ ***Diazepam causes dose-dependent drowsiness as a side effect***

Dantrolene

Unlike baclofen and diazepam, dantrolene relieves spasticity by a direct action on skeletal muscle (see Table 8.6).

Dantrolene is a hydantoin derivative that not only relieves skeletal muscle spasticity but also produces muscle weakness, which limits its clinical usefulness. Its mechanism of action involves inhibition of skeletal muscle excitation–contraction coupling. It decreases the amount of Ca^{2+} released from the sarcoplasmic reticulum and therefore reduces the link between excitation and contraction, resulting in a reduction in tension generated by the muscle. Dantrolene's pharmacological activity relates to this action in that it reduces skeletal muscle contractions in experimental and clinical settings.

■ ***Dantrolene is used to relieve the spasticity of paraplegia and hemiplegia***

Dantrolene is also used to treat malignant hyperthermia, a condition that can occur during general anesthesia, and relates to excessive intracellular Ca^{2+} accumulation. Dantrolene is usually given orally, but it is not completely absorbed. It has a half-life of 9 hours and it is metabolized by the liver.

MAJOR ADVERSE EFFECTS OF DANTROLENE These include muscle weakness and sedation, and sometimes hepatotoxicity. It is contraindicated in patients with either respiratory muscle weakness or liver disease. Also, it is recommended that regular liver function tests should be carried out.

Table 8.6 Drugs used for treatment of spasticity

Drugs	Mechanism of action
Baclofen	Inhibits flexor and extensor muscle spasm via $GABA_B$ receptor-mediated blockade of afferent stimulation of the α motor neuron
Diazepam	$GABA_A$ receptor-mediated presynaptic inhibition of afferent stimulation of the α motor neuron
Dantrolene	Inhibition of skeletal muscle excitation–contraction coupling by decreasing Ca^{2+} released from the sarcoplasmic reticulum

GABA, γ-aminobutyric acid.

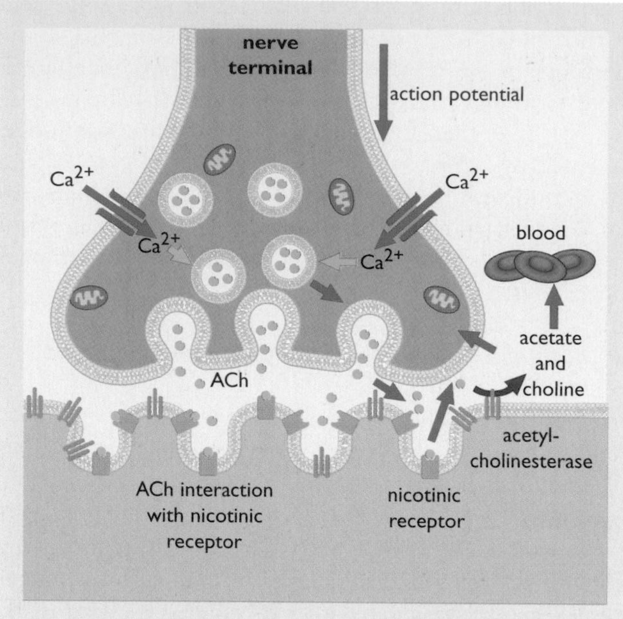

Figure 8.18 Action potential-induced release of the neurotransmitter acetylcholine (ACh) and its metabolism at the neuromuscular junction.

Movement disorders resulting from defects in muscle excitability

Although many movement disorders are attributed to defects in the basal ganglia, some disorders result from impairment of neuromuscular transmission and skeletal muscle excitability (e.g. Lambert–Eaton syndrome, McCardle syndrome, congenital myotonia and tetany).

Lambert–Eaton syndrome (myasthenia syndrome)

Lambert-Eaton syndrome is associated with some cancers, especially lung cancer. This syndrome occurs more frequently in males aged 50–60 years. As the NMJ is the site of the defect, it resembles myasthenia gravis in terms of symptoms of fatigability and depressed limb reflexes. However, the symptoms differ from those in myasthenia gravis because the weakness, which particularly affects the limb muscles, does not respond to anticholinesterase drugs. This is because the Lambert–Eaton syndrome results from disrupted coupling between nerve terminal excitation and ACh release at the NMJ. In some patients this is associated with autoantibodies against neuronal voltage-gated Ca^{2+} channels. It appears that voltage-gated Ca^{2+} channels are expressed in the tissue of small cell lung cancer, and act as the antigen leading to the development of Ca^{2+} channel antibodies found in Lambert–Eaton syndrome. Treatment of this syndrome involves increasing the release of neurotransmitter at the NMJ by:

- Physical exercise to improve muscle power.
- Ca^{2+} salts, which could be beneficial because of the role Ca^{2+} plays in the release of neurotransmitters from nerve terminals (Fig. 8.18 and Table 8.7).

Table 8.7 Treatment of movement disorders due to defects in muscle excitability

Disorder	Treatment
Lambert-Eaton syndrome	Ca^{2+} salts, physical exercise
McCardle syndrome	Large doses of glucose, injection of epinephrine or glucagon
Congenital myotonia	Membrane stabilizers such as quinine and phenytoin
Tetany	Normalize plasma Ca^{2+}

- 3,4-diaminopyridine, which increases neurotransmitter release by blocking K^+ conductance at the nerve terminals. 3,4-diaminopyridine is a simple pyridine analog that is capable of blocking a variety of voltage-dependent Ca^{2+} channels, with some selectivity for one type of K^+ channel compared with another. This type of drug is used experimentally but has limited clinical use because of the widespread adverse effects associated with inhibiting a variety of voltage-gated K^+ channels. This gives rise to a wide range of side effects, the major one of which is CNS stimulation. This drug is given orally about 4 to 5 times daily.

McCardle syndrome

The main symptoms of this syndrome are disabling weakness, muscle pain, and stiffness after a brief period of exercise. These symptoms are produced because skeletal muscles fail to relax, owing to inadequate production of ATP, which is necessary for Ca^{2+} sequestration in the sarcoplasmic reticulum that terminates contraction. The underlying cause of inadequate ATP production is an inability to liberate glucose from glycogen. This is due to an inherited deficiency of glycogen phosphorylase in skeletal muscles. These patients have only a limited supply of ATP from blood glucose and fatty acids available for muscle activity. This results in only brief periods of normal skeletal muscle activity being possible. These patients do not show the typical increase in blood lactate and pyruvate after exercise.

Treatment of the syndrome includes the administration of large doses of glucose or the injection of epinephrine or glucagon to increase glucose release from the liver (see Table 8.7).

Congenital myotonia

Congenital myotonia is an inherited disorder characterized by violent muscle spasm due to irritability of the skeletal or muscle fiber membrane. The irritability is due to a structural defect in the muscle fiber membrane that renders the fiber hyperexcitable and therefore easily re-excited by afterpotentials.

This disease is treated with quinidine or phenytoin given orally to reduce the frequency and severity of the spasm. These drugs block Na^+ and other voltage-

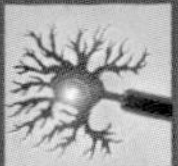

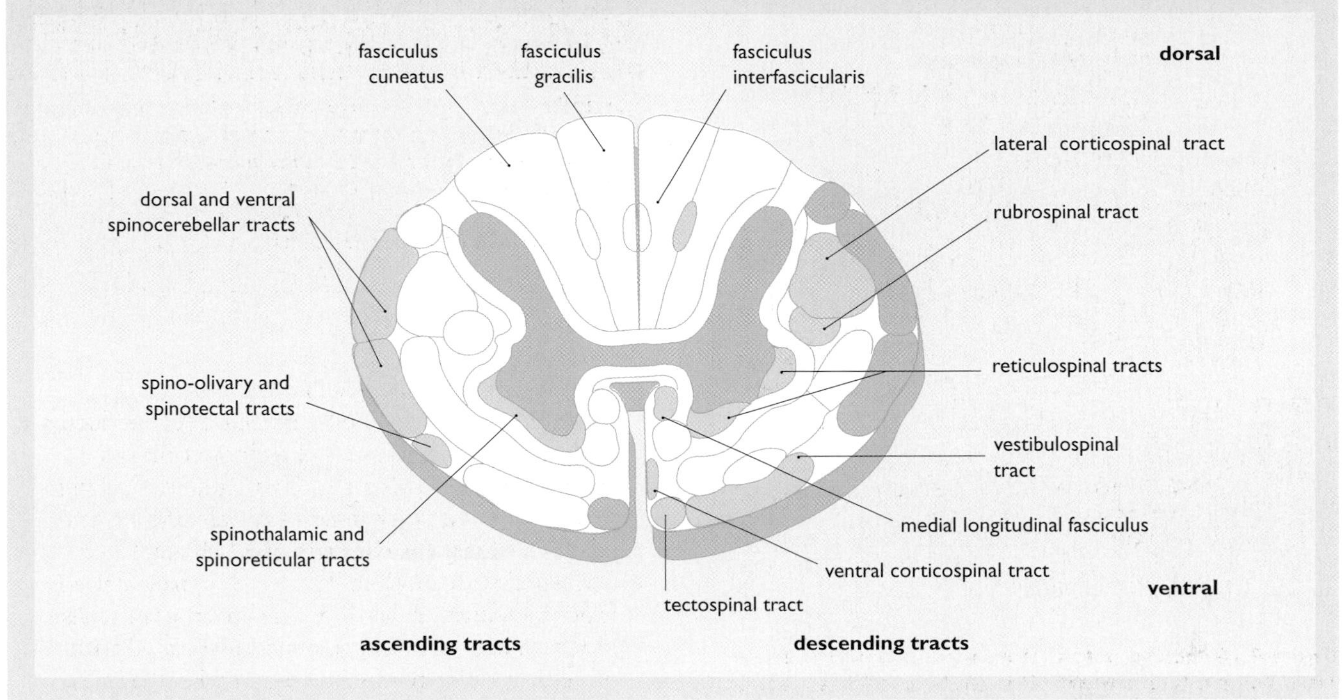

Fig. 8.19 The spinal cord at the midcervical level, showing the major tracts of the spinal white matter.

dependent ion channels. They are often used in the treatment of epilepsy and arrhythmias and are described in detail below and in Chapter 13.

Tetany

Tetany is characterized by widespread muscular twitching, together with persistent contraction of muscles in the hands and feet, resulting in painful cramps. The major cause of tetany is hypocalcemia, which increases excitability of the somatic nerves. It is suggested that low extracellular Ca^{2+} increases the excitability of somatic nerves and causes repetitive firing, leading to persistent muscle contraction. This is also caused by tetanus toxins.

Tetany is treated with Ca^{2+} salts (e.g. Ca^{2+} gluconate) to restore extracellular Ca^{2+} concentrations.

FUNCTIONAL ANATOMY OF THE CENTRAL NERVOUS SYSTEM

The spinal cord is part of the CNS and consists of ascending and descending tracts passing information between the brain and the PNS. The tracts are interconnected at various levels by short interneurons, which allow a degree of integration and control of motor function and sensory input at a spinal level (Fig. 8.19).

The medulla oblongata is directly continuous with the spinal cord and is the first part of the brainstem (Fig. 8.20a). It also contains the nuclei for cranial nerves V, IX, X, XI and XII, and is where motor fibers and some sensory fibers cross.

The pons lies between the medulla and midbrain. It can be viewed as a relay station between the cerebellum, the brain and the PNS. It contains the nuclei for cranial nerves V, VI, VII and VIII, and motor nuclei in the pontine reticular formation that participate in postural, cardiovascular and respiratory control (Fig. 8.20b).

The cerebellum lies posterior to the pons (Fig. 8.21), and has incoming and outgoing connections, with sensory and motor tracts ascending and descending the spinal cord. It is the largest motor structure in the brain. Although its function is not entirely clear, the multiplicity of its connections allows the cerebellum to exert fine control over motor functioning and to act as a center for integrating sensory and motor information in order to perform complex tasks.

Above the pons lies the midbrain (mesencephalon). This is the most primitive part of the human brain and ends in two huge fiber bundles which form the cerebral peduncles, carrying fibers to and from the thalamus and cerebral hemispheres. It also contains the superior (visual) and inferior (auditory) colliculi (see Figs 8.20c, 8.20d), the nuclei for cranial nerves III and IV, two motor nuclei, the red nucleus and the substantia nigra, which links and acts as a relay between the basal ganglia and the motor system (see Fig. 8.20c).

The diencephalon, the central core of the cerebrum, consists of the hypothalamus, subthalamus, epithalamus and thalamus (Fig. 8.22).

- The hypothalamus subserves many homeostatic functions such as regulation of the ANS and the

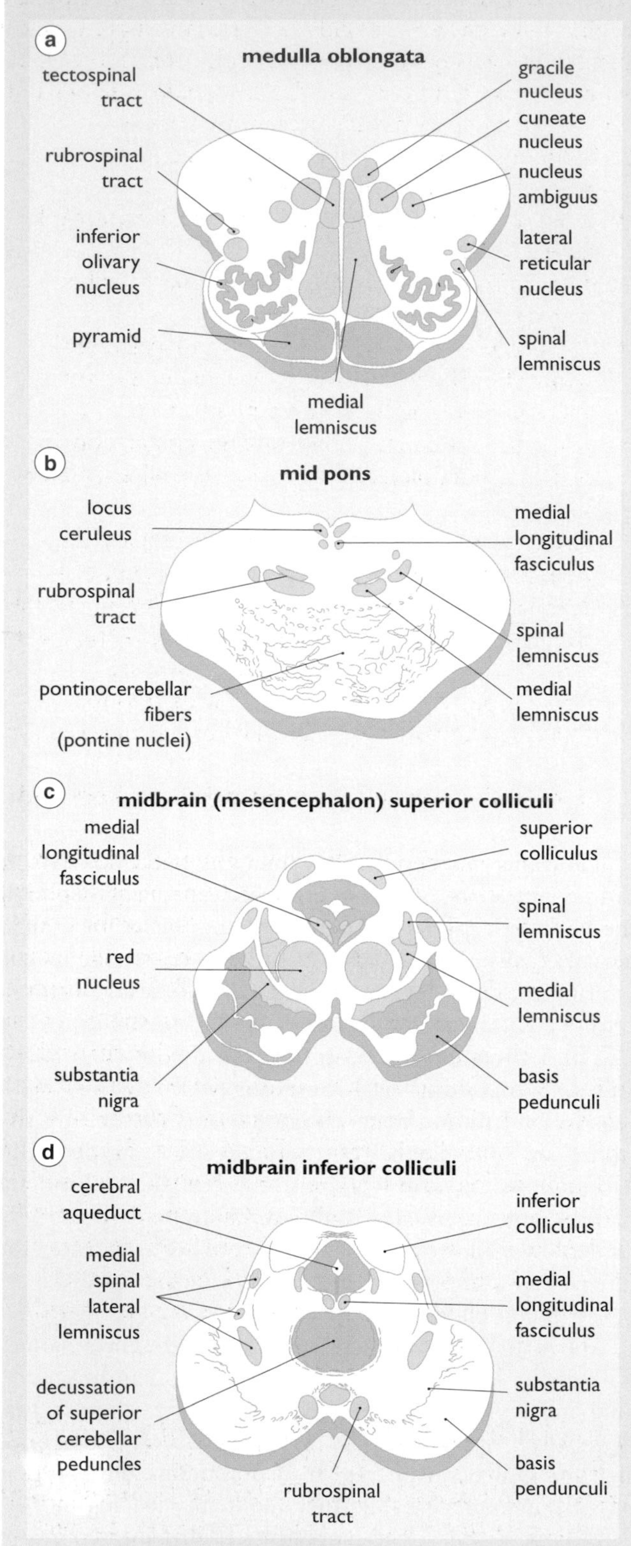

Fig. 8.20 The medulla oblongata, pons and midbrain. (a) The medulla oblongata is the first part of the brainstem and motor fibers and some sensory fibers cross here. (b) The pons lies between the medulla and midbrain. It can be considered as a relay station between the cerebellum, the brain and the peripheral nervous system. (c) The midbrain superior colliculi allow tracking of visual stimuli. (d) The midbrain inferior colliculi provide selective attention to auditory stimuli.

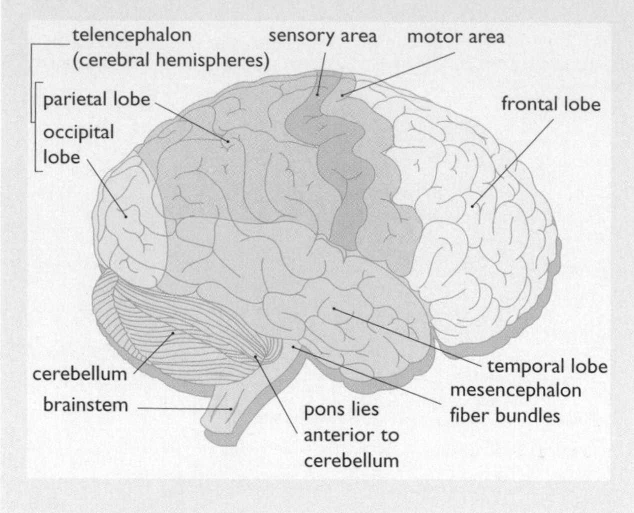

Fig. 8.21 A lateral view of the brain.

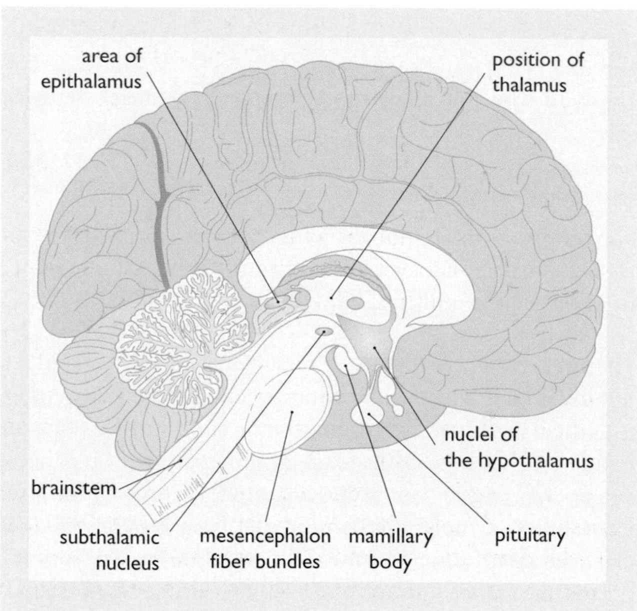

Fig. 8.22 The diencephalon. This consists of the hypothalamus, subthalamus, epithalamus and the thalamus.

endocrine system via the pituitary. It also has a role in the control of basic drives such as those involved in hunger, thirst, threat, sex and fatigue.

- The subthalamus is involved in motor function and has connections to the basal ganglia, the red nucleus and the substantia nigra.
- The epithalamus consists of the habenular nuclei and the pineal gland. The habenular nuclei are the center for the integration of olfactory, visceral and somatic afferent pathways, and are connected to the reticular formation. The function of the pineal gland is unclear, but it contains high concentrations of melatonin and 5-HT. It may have a role in circadian rhythm regulation.

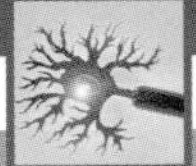

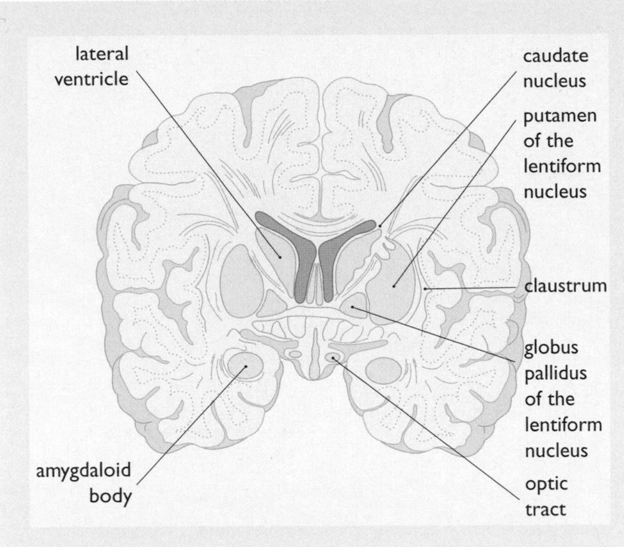

Fig. 8.23 Basal ganglia. The bilaterally represented masses of gray matter form deep structures. The corpus striatum consists of the caudate nucleus and the lentiform nucleus, which are separated by the internal capsule except at the anterior–inferior aspect of the caudate nucleus where the head of the caudate is continuous with the putamen of the lentiform nucleus. The lentiform nucleus consists of the putamen and the globus pallidus.

- The thalamus is the largest part of the diencephalon and is closely related both functionally and anatomically to the cerebral cortices. Almost all fibers passing to the cerebral hemispheres pass through and synapse within the thalamus. It has outgoing connections with virtually every part of the cerebrum and its function is most likely to be integration of incoming sensory information via its interconnected nuclei. The information is then passed to the cerebral cortex for interpretation.

Basal ganglia is a collective term given to bilateral masses of deeply sited gray matter (Fig. 8.23). Basal ganglia have afferent and efferent connections with the cerebral cortex, the thalamus, subthalamus and brainstem, and they are thought to control motor function by an effect on the cerebral hemispheres.

The cerebral hemispheres form the telencephalon. Consciousness and the ability to adapt and react to changing circumstances result from the complexity and size of the right and left hemispheres. The ability to use complex methods of communication is also provided by the telencephalon. These capabilities lead to the capacity for abstract thought and therefore the ability to learn and profit not only from our own experiences but also those of others, and to generate hypotheses. This higher functioning leads to the development of a rich emotional life and therefore the risk of profound mental illness.

Certain functions are associated more with some areas of the cerebral hemispheres than others

The cerebral hemispheres can be divided into the frontal, temporal, parietal and occipital cortices (see Fig. 8.21). The precise location of any particular function within the brain is not known, possibly because no single function resides exclusively in any one particular area. However, as with the lower parts of the CNS, certain functions are associated more with some areas than others:

- Voluntary motor function is subserved by the precentral gyrus of the frontal lobe.
- Sensory function lies in the postcentral gyrus of the parietal lobe.
- Part of the dominant frontal lobe appears to have a primary role in speech.
- Part of the frontal lobes bilaterally appear to be involved in the formation of personality, higher reasoning and intellectual functioning.
- The temporal lobes provide a large proportion of memory function and integration as well as auditory centers.
- The parietal lobes appear to have a complex integrating function for sensory, motor and, to a lesser extent, emotional functioning. They also allow planning and initiation of complex actions and have a crucial role in topographic, object and word recognition and their association with emotion.
- The occipital cortices receive and process visual input.

The limbic system has a crucial role in memory and emotion

The limbic system is a collection of connected structures in the cerebrum, including a variety of deep structures such as the amygdala, selected areas of the cerebral cortex such as the cingulate, and segments of other structures such as the hypothalamus (Table 8.8; Fig. 8.24). The basic component of the limbic system is the Papez circuit. In this loop the hippocampus transmits information through the fornices to the mamillary bodies of the hypothalamus, which transmit to the anterior nucleus of the thalamus via the mamillothalamic tracts. Information is then sent via the internal capsule back to the hippocampus. The precise functions of the limbic system remain unclear, but lesions of specific parts of the various loops lead to:

- Amnesia, which is associated with lesions of the mamillary bodies in Korsakoff's syndrome, or with lesions of the temporal lobes.

Table 8.8 The major components of the limbic system

• Regions of the limbic cortex (cingulate, parahippocampal gyrus, entorrhinal cortex)
• Hippocampal formation (dentate gyrus, hippocampus)
• Amygdala (basolateral complex, centromedial complex, parts of the stria terminalis and the hypothalamus)
• Nucleus accumbens
• Mamillary bodies
• Anterior and dorsomedial nuclei of the thalamus (some authors also include other cortical regions including the orbitofrontal area, the temporal poles and the insula)

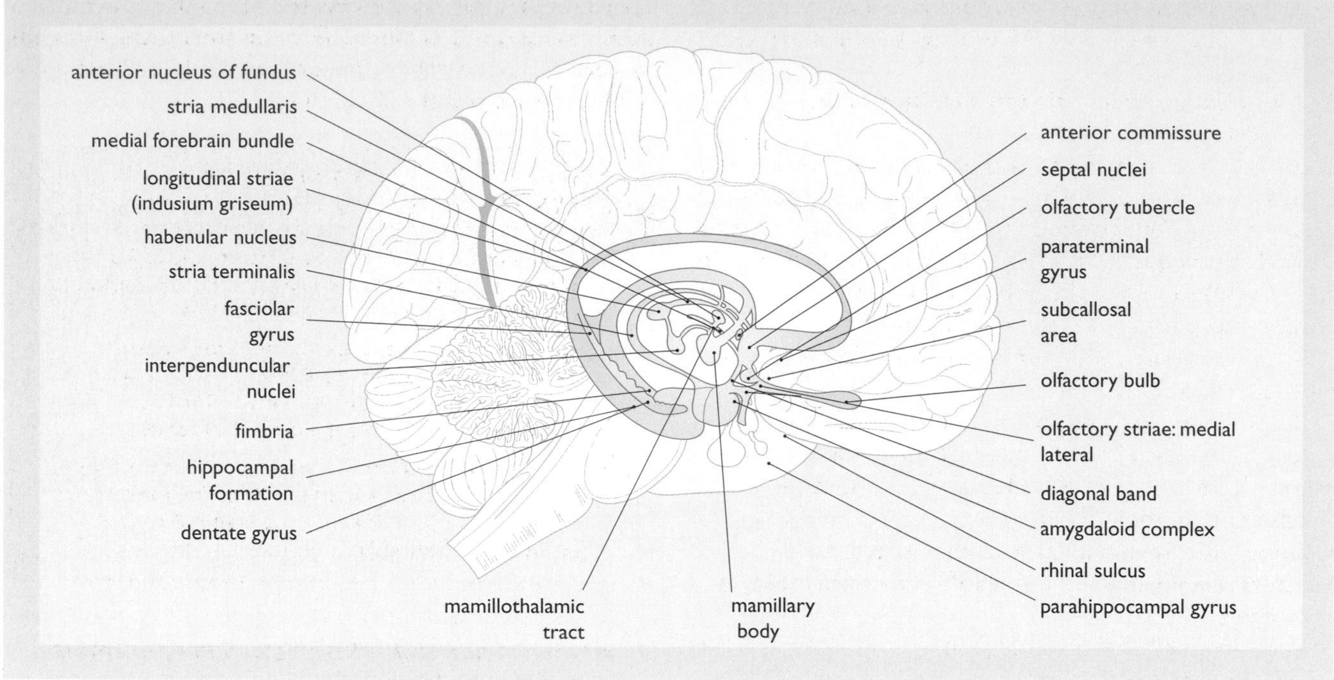

Fig. 8.24 The anatomic relations of the amygdala, the hippocampus and other components of the limbic system.

- Placidity, which is associated with lesions of the amygdala.
- Rage, which is associated with lesions of the posterior hypothalamus.

The symptoms of hallucinations and delusions in psychiatric patients may result from limbic system dysfunction.

The reticular formation has a non-specific alerting function and contributes to motor, sensory (pain) and autonomic functions

The reticular formation is a network of neurons with diffuse dendritic connections that occupies the midline of the brainstem and extends upwards from the substantia intermedia of the spinal cord to the intralaminar nuclei of the thalamus. It is loosely organized into three longitudinal nuclear columns (i.e. median, medial and lateral), which are each subdivided into three ventrocaudally (mesencephalic, pontine and medullary).

The reticular formation has input from ascending sensory neurons, the cerebellum, the basal ganglia, the hypothalamus and the cerebral cortex. There are outputs to the hypothalamus, the thalamus and the spinal cord.

The non-specific alerting function of the reticular formation appears to be related to the ascending reticulo-thalamocortical pathway (ascending reticular activating system). The reticular formation also makes contributions to motor, sensory (pain) and autonomic functions, especially affecting respiration and vasomotor function.

FUNCTIONAL NEUROCHEMISTRY OF THE NERVOUS SYSTEM

The neurotransmitters listed in Table 8.2 and Table 8.9 are found within specific regions of the nervous system and together with the complex anatomic arrangement provide for the sophisticated function of the human brain.

Glutamate is the major excitatory neurotransmitter in the CNS

Glutamate is an amino acid and acts on *N*-methyl-D-aspartate (NMDA) and non-NMDA receptors. It is the primary neurotransmitter in thalamocortical, pyramidal cell and corticostriatal projections, and is an important neurotransmitter in the hippocampus. It has been suggested that since some drugs that act on NMDA

Table 8.9 Classification of the major central nervous system peptide neurotransmitters

Family	Examples
Opioid	Endorphins, enkephalins, dynorphins
Neurohypophyseal	Vasopressin, oxytocin
Tachykinins	Substance P, neurokinin
Gastrins	Gastrin, cholecystokinin
Others	Neuropeptide Y, substance P, neurotensin, galanin

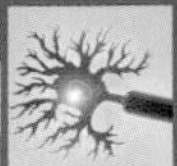

receptors produce psychotic symptoms, abnormalities of the glutamate system may underlie psychotic illnesses.

GABA is the major inhibitory neurotransmitter in the nervous system

GABA is an amino acid and acts primarily on $GABA_A$ and $GABA_B$ receptors. $GABA_A$ receptors are the most common and are present on 40% of neurons. The cortical distribution of $GABA_A$ is illustrated in Figure 8.25. $GABA_A$ is a receptor-operated Cl^- channel, while $GABA_B$ receptors are coupled to G proteins.

Benzodiazepines and most anticonvulsants act via actions on GABA receptors:

- Benzodiazepines bind to specific benzodiazepine receptors located on a subunit of the GABA receptor complex to enhance the effects of GABA, thereby acting as neuromodulators.
- Some anticonvulsants have similar effects to benzodiazepines, but most act directly on the GABA receptor.

Abnormalities of the GABA system are thought to be associated with anxiety disorders, and recent work has suggested a role for GABA in the etiology of schizophrenia.

Glycine is a 'requisite neurotransmitter' for glutamate action

Glycine must be present for glutamate to have it's actions. It also acts on its own receptor-operated Cl^- channel and is inhibitory for neural function.

ACh is a central as well as a peripheral neurotransmitter

ACh acts as a neurotransmitter in the CNS as well as in the periphery, as described previously.

Centrally, the primary ACh-containing nucleus is the nucleus basalis of Meynert, which is situated in the basal forebrain and has projections to the cerebral cortex and limbic systems. Cholinergic fibers in the reticular system project to the cerebral cortex, the limbic system, the hypothalamus and the thalamus.

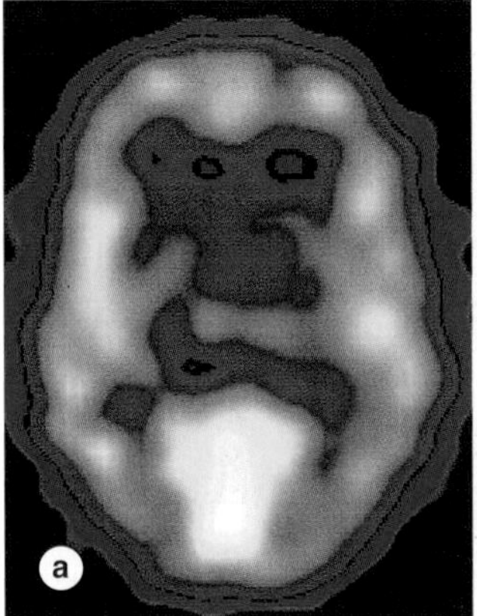

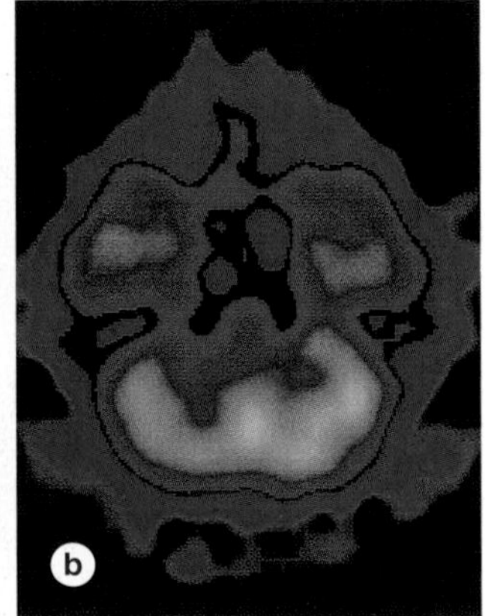

Fig. 8.25 The cortical distribution of $GABA_A$ receptor complexes. This is shown using a radioactively labeled benzodiazepine analog lomazenil and single-photon emission tomography (SPET). The brightest areas have the highest density of receptors. (a) An image at the level of the midoccipital cortex. (b) The image at the level of the cerebellum.

> **Acetylcholine, Parkinson's disease and Alzheimer's dementia**
>
> - The symptoms of Parkinson's disease result from a defect in the balance between acetylcholine and dopamine's actions in the basal ganglia
> - Anticholinergic medication is used to treat the parkinsonian-like adverse effects associated with the use of antipsychotic medications and in the treatment of idiopathic Parkinson's disease
> - Nicotinic and muscarinic agonists as well as drugs that enhance endogenous acetylcholine function appear to be beneficial in the treatment of Alzheimer's dementia

More than nine distinct 5-HT (serotonin) receptors have been identified

The $5\text{-}HT_{1A}$, $5\text{-}HT_{2B}$, $5\text{-}HT_{2C}$, and $5\text{-}HT_3$ subtypes of 5-HT receptors have been the most extensively studied. The major site of serotonergic cell bodies is in the area of the upper pons and midbrain. The classic areas for 5-HT-containing neurons are the median and dorsal raphe nuclei. Neurons from the raphe nuclei project to the basal ganglia and various parts of the limbic system, and have a wide distribution throughout the cerebral cortices in addition to cerebellar connections (Fig. 8.26).

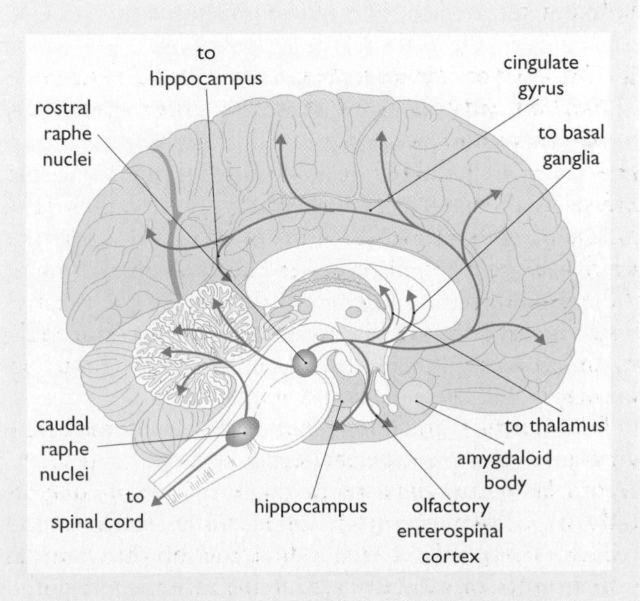

Fig. 8.26 5-hydroxytryptamine (5-HT) pathways. 5-HT-containing neurons are found in the median and dorsal raphe nuclei, the caudal locus ceruleus, the area postrema and the interpeduncular area.

All 5-HT receptors identified so far are G protein-coupled receptors, except the 5-HT_3 subtype, which is located on a receptor-operated Na^+/K^+ channel.

5-HT is synthesized from tryptophan by tryptophan hydroxylase, and the supply of tryptophan is the rate-limiting step in its synthesis. 5-HT is primarily metabolized by monoamine oxidase-A to 5-hydroxyindoleacetic acid (5-HIAA).

5-hydroxytryptamine, depression and anxiety

- **Most antidepressant drugs inhibit the uptake of 5-HT from the synaptic cleft**
- **Buspirone is a partial agonist of presynaptic 5-HT_{1A} receptors and is an effective treatment of anxiety and depression**
- **5-HT_{2A} and 5-HT_{2C} receptors play a role in depressive illnesses, the negative symptoms of schizophrenia and protection against the long-term sequelae of neuroleptics**
- **There is a relative increase in the number of 5-HT_{2A} receptors in the frontal cortices of suicidal patients**
- **5-HT_{2A} receptor antagonists have been used to treat negative symptom schizophrenia with some success**
- **Antipsychotics acting as selective 5-HT_{2A} receptor antagonists (atypical antipsychotics) are a more effective treatment of negative symptom schizophrenia than typical antipsychotics and produce fewer adverse motor effects at a similar level of dopamine blockade**
- **5-HT3 receptor antagonists are used in the treatment of nausea**

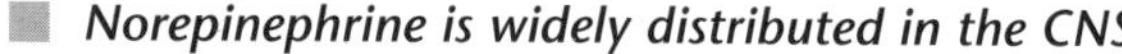

Norepinephrine is widely distributed in the CNS

Norepinephrine acts as a neurotransmitter in the CNS as well as in the ANS (as described above). NE acts in several types of adrenoceptor, α_1, α_2, β_{1-3}. The majority of NE-containing neurons in the CNS are located in the locus ceruleus in the pons/midbrain. Their projections to other areas of the brain are shown in Figure 8.27 (see also Figs 8.20b, 8.20c for orientation).

In general in the CNS:

- Postsynaptic α_1 receptors are linked to stimulation of phosphoinositol turnover.
- α_2 receptors inhibit the formation of cAMP.
- β receptors stimulate the formation of cAMP.

Five types of dopamine receptor (D_1–D_5) have been identified in the human nervous system

D_1 and D_5 receptors stimulate the formation of cAMP by activating a stimulatory G protein, while D_2, D_3, and D_4 receptors inhibit the formation of cAMP by activating an inhibitory G protein. D_2 receptors are more ubiquitous than D_3 and D_4 receptors. D_3 receptors are primarily located in the nucleus accumbens (one of the septal nuclei in the limbic system) and D_4 receptors are particularly concentrated in the medial frontal cortex.

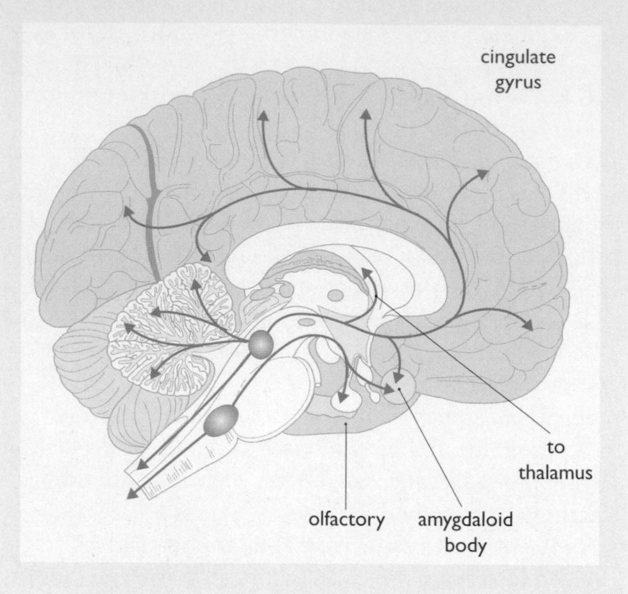

Fig. 8.27 Norepinephrine pathways. Most of the NE-containing neurons in the central nervous system are located in the locus ceruleus in the pons and midbrain. These neurons project through the medial forebrain bundle to the limbic system, cerebral cortices, the thalamus and the hypothalamus. A second group of NE-containing neurons in the ventral tegmental area have projections to the hypothalamus and amygdala.

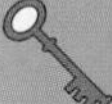

Norepinephrine and affective and anxiety disorders

- **NE is thought to play a crucial role in affective disorders, and to a lesser extent in anxiety disorders**
- **Abnormalities of NE-containing neurons are incorporated as part of the monoamine theory of depression**
- **Most traditional tricyclic antidepressants inhibit the uptake of NE from the synaptic cleft and thereby increase the availability of synaptic NE**
- **Monoamine oxidase inhibitors inhibit the breakdown of NE**
- **It is thought that the antidepressant effect of NE manipulation is mediated by a down-regulation in postsynaptic β receptors**

There are a variety of dopaminergic pathways or tracts (Fig. 8.28):

- The nigrostriatal tract projects from the substantia nigra in the midbrain to the corpus striatum, and has a role in motor control.
- The mesolimbic/mesocortical tract has cell bodies in the ventral tegmental area adjacent to the substantia nigra and projects to the limbic system and neocortex in addition to the striatum. It supplies fibers to the

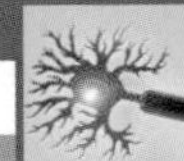

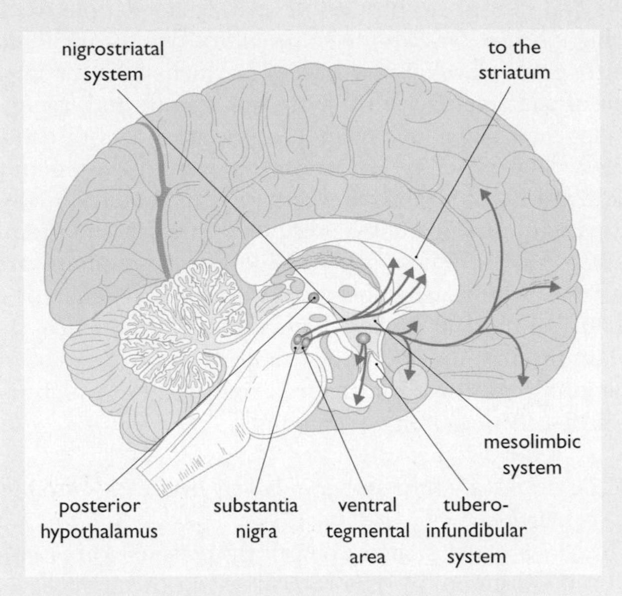

Fig. 8.28 Dopamine pathways. These tracts include the nigrostriatal tract, the mesolimbic/mesocortical tract and the tuberoinfundibular tract.

medial surface of the frontal lobes and to the parahippocampus and cingulate cortex.

- The third major pathway is the tuberoinfundibular tract. The cell bodies reside in the arcuate nucleus and periventricular area of the hypothalamus, and they project to the infundibulum and the anterior pituitary. Dopamine inhibits the release of prolactin within this tract.

Dopamine is synthesized as part of the common pathway for catecholamines (see above), and it is metabolized by two enzymes: MAO-B, which is intraneuronal, and catechol-*O*-methyl transferase (COMT), which is extraneuronal. The primary metabolite of dopamine is homovanillic acid (HVA).

D_2 receptors were considered to be the most important dopamine receptor involved in psychosis, since the potency of antipsychotic medications correlate with their affinity for D_2 receptors. However, the advent of atypical antipsychotics, with equal efficacy but a relatively low potency at the D_2 receptor, raises the possibility that other subtypes of the dopamine receptors may have a more important role in the etiology and treatment of psychosis.

Chronic blockade of dopamine receptors leads to their up-regulation, which may contribute to movement disorders seen with long-term neuroleptic therapy.

There is evidence that the mesolimbic and mesocortical pathways play an important role in the regulation of behavior governed by positive reinforcers (rewards), and these findings may lead to the development of novel medications for the treatments of addictions.

Dopamine, Parkinson's disease and psychosis

- **Idiopathic Parkinson's disease results from degeneration of cells in the substantia nigra**
- **Parkinsonian-type effects seen with typical antipsychotics (e.g. haloperidol, chlorpromazine) result from blocking of dopamine receptors within the nigrostriatal tract**
- **Antipsychotic medications are thought to exert their beneficial effects via actions on the mesolimbic and mesocortical tract**
- **The inhibitory drive of prolactin release is removed by dopamine receptor blockade within the tuberoinfundibular tract by antipsychotics and leads to prolactinemia**

Peptide neurotransmitters

There may be as many as 300 different peptide neurotransmitters in the brain

A peptide has fewer than 100 amino acids. The best-characterized neuropeptides are listed in Table 8.9. Often these peptides are synthesized as part of much larger molecules termed preprohormones. These are cleaved in the neuronal cytoplasm to prohormones, which are then taken up into vesicles. Within vesicles the prohormones are further cleaved into the neuroactive peptides. Most peptide neurotransmitters coexist with other neurotransmitters.

Opioids are thought to regulate stress, pain and mood

The three endogenous opioid groups in Table 8.9 (i.e. endorphins, enkephalins and dynorphins) are synthesized from larger precursor molecules. Enkephalin is found in noradrenergic and serotonergic neurons. Opioids act on three types of receptors:

- μ, where their action is to decrease production of cAMP and increase K^+ conductance.
- δ, where they have a similar action to that on μ receptors.
- κ, where their action is to decrease K^+ conductance.

The neurohypophysial neuroactive peptides vasopressin and oxytocin may be involved in mood regulation

The two neurohypophysial hormones vasopressin and oxytocin are synthesized in the hypothalamus and released in the posterior pituitary. There are three receptors for vasopressin and its actions are mediated either by changes in membrane phospholipids or by increasing cAMP.

Tachykinins include substance P and neurokinin

Substance P is a primary neurotransmitter in most primary afferent sensory neurons and is present in the nigrostriatal tract. It is associated with ACh and

5-HT and has been implicated in Huntington's chorea, Alzheimer's dementia and affective disorders.

Cholecystokinin may have a role in schizophrenia, panic disorder, eating disorders and some movement disorders

Cholecystokinin (CCK) is coexistent in neurons with dopamine and GABA. It acts on two receptor subtypes, CCK-A and CCK-B receptors. The signal transduction mechanisms of the B receptor are not yet understood, but the A subtype acts via an effect on membrane phospholipids.

Neurotensin may have a role in schizophrenia

Neurotensin is coexistent in neurons with NE and dopamine. It acts on G protein-coupled high-affinity receptors present in dopamine-rich areas and the enterorhinal cortex implicated in schizophrenia.

PATHOPHYSIOLOGY AND DISEASES OF THE CENTRAL NERVOUS SYSTEM

Psychosis

Psychosis describes a mental state characterized by a loss of touch with reality. The patient may describe a variety of abnormalities of perception, thought and ideas. Psychosis is not a specific illness and psychotic symptoms may occur in depression and other mood disorders and in medical conditions that interfere with brain function. Psychotic illnesses include schizophrenia, schizoaffective disorder, delusional disorders and some depressive and manic illnesses. The most prevalent psychotic illness that includes all the cardinal psychotic symptoms is schizophrenia.

Schizophrenia

Schizophrenia is a psychotic illness characterized by multiple symptoms affecting thought, perceptions, emotion and volition. Its incidence in industrialized countries is approximately 15 new cases/100 000 population/year. Its prevalence is 0.5–1%, rising to 2.8% in some areas (e.g. northern Sweden).

Schizophrenia characteristically develops in people aged 15–45 years, but it may occur before puberty or be delayed until the seventh or eighth decade. The typical age of onset for males is 23–28 years and for females, 28–32 years. There is an increased rate among people living in inner cities and those from lower social classes, and in immigrant populations. This appears to be because patients 'drift' down the social ladder into inner cities or overseas as part of their illness during the time before onset of symptoms or admission to hospital.

Florid symptoms of schizophrenia include delusions, hallucinations, abnormal thought processes and passivity

The premorbid personality is often described as emotionally and socially detached. Such people have few friends, are often cold and aloof, and engage in solitary occupations. Their behavior may be eccentric and they are indifferent to praise or criticism. People with schizophrenia slowly become more withdrawn and introverted, develop new interests, which are sometimes out of character, and drift away from family and friends. They may begin to fail in their occupation or school work. The onset of overt schizophrenia is commonly slow and insidious, taking weeks to years, but eventually, often with an apparently precipitating event, the symptoms of florid illness appear. The florid symptoms are variable, but usually include delusions, hallucinations, abnormal thought processes and passivity experiences. In addition there may be formal thought disorder, a flat or inappropriate affect and abnormal motor signs, which are usually called catatonic symptoms.

Delusions are false personal beliefs held with absolute conviction

The beliefs of delusions are outside the person's normal culture or subculture in spite of what everyone else believes and evidence to the contrary. They dominate the individual's viewpoint and behavior. Delusional disorders are disorders in which delusions are prominent and hallucinations and abnormal thought phenomena are vague or absent.

Hallucinations are false perceptions in the absence of a real external stimulus

Hallucinations are perceived as having the same quality as real perceptions and are not subject to conscious manipulation. Hallucinations in schizophrenia are equally varied and may involve any of the sensory modalities. The most common are auditory hallucinations in the form of voices. They occur in 60–70% of patients diagnosed with schizophrenia. Visual hallucinations occur in about 10% of patients, but should raise the suspicion of an organic disorder. Olfactory hallucinations are more common in temporal lobe epilepsy (TLE) than schizophrenia, and tactile hallucinations are probably experienced more frequently than reported by patients. No one type of hallucination is specific to schizophrenia, but the duration and intensity is probably more important diagnostically.

Thought alienation and disordered thought are common in schizophrenia

Disorders of thought possession in schizophrenia are described as thought alienation. The patient has the experience that his thoughts are under the control of an outside agency or that others are participating in his thinking. Disorders of the form of thought are also characteristic, and as a result the speech is difficult to follow or incoherent and follows no logical sequence.

Catatonic symptoms can occur in any form of schizophrenia

Catatonic symptoms form part of a subtype of schizophrenia. However, these, mainly motor, symptoms can occur in any form of schizophrenia. They include:

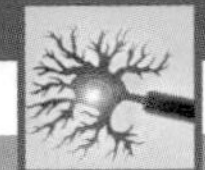

- Ambitendence (alternation between opposite movements).
- Echopraxia (automatic imitation of another person's movements).
- Stereotypies (repeated regular fixed parts of movement, or speech, that are not goal-directed).
- Negativism (motiveless resistance to instructions and attempts to be moved or doing the opposite of what is asked).
- Posturing (adoption of an inappropriate or bizarre bodily posture continuously for a substantial period of time).
- Waxy flexibility (the limbs can be 'molded' into a position and remain fixed for long periods of time).

The differential diagnosis of acute schizophrenia includes other psychotic illnesses and organic disorders

The differential diagnosis of acute schizophrenia includes other psychotic illnesses such as schizophreniform disorder, schizoaffective disorder, bipolar affective disorder, paranoid psychosis and psychotic depression. Certain organic causes must be excluded, including drug/substance-induced psychosis, early dementia, some forms of epilepsy, endocrine causes, infections, metabolic disorders, systemic lupus erythematosus (SLE) and the long-term sequelae of head injury.

Fifty to 65% of patients with acute schizophrenia develop chronic schizophrenia

Symptoms in acute schizophrenia are generally termed the positive symptoms of schizophrenia and are characteristic of the acute phase of the illness. In chronic schizophrenia some florid (positive) symptoms may remain, but the predominant negative symptoms are:

- Poverty of speech (a restriction in the amount of spontaneous speech and in the information contained in speech; alogia).
- Flattening of affect (a restriction in the experience and expression of emotion).
- Anhedonia–asociality (an inability to experience pleasure, few social contacts and social withdrawal).
- Avolition–apathy (reduced drive, energy and interest).
- Attention impairment (an inattentiveness at work and interviews).

Some of these symptoms may also occur as part of a florid psychotic episode. Their presence is associated with a poor prognosis, a poor response to neuroleptics, poor premorbid adjustment, cognitive impairment and atrophic changes seen in a computed tomography (CT) scan.

Once schizophrenia is diagnosed there are four main outcomes:

- The illness resolves completely, with or without treatment, and never recurs (pattern A, 10–20% of patients).
- The illness recurs repeatedly with full recovery every time (pattern B, 30–35% of patients).
- The illness recurs repeatedly, but recovery is incomplete and a persistent defective state develops, becoming more pronounced with each successive relapse (pattern C, 30–35% of patients).
- The illness pursues a downhill course from the onset (pattern D, 10–20% of patients).

There is some debate about the impact of treatments for acute schizophrenia on the long-term course and prognosis of the illness. Approximately 55% of people with schizophrenia now live and work normally. Factors contributing to a poor prognosis include an early onset, an insidious onset, a lack of a prominent affective component, a lack of clear precipitants, a family history of schizophrenia, poor premorbid personality, confusion or perplexity, low IQ, low social class, social isolation and a previous psychiatric history. The converse of these factors usually points to a better prognosis.

The tendency to develop schizophrenia is genetically transmitted

Although the mode of transmission remains obscure, it appears to be polygenic. Twin studies indicate that the genetic contribution to schizophrenia is approximately 50%.

The neurotransmitters dopamine, 5-HT, GABA and glutamate may be involved in schizophrenia

Many hypotheses have been put forward to explain schizophrenia at the level of neurotransmitters in the brain. The potential pivotal role of excess dopamine in various brain regions has received considerable attention. Although many antipsychotic drugs block dopamine receptors, particularly D_2 and D_2-like receptors, there is little support from current research for a primary receptor-based dopaminergic abnormality in schizophrenia. Recently, however, it has become increasingly clear that people with schizophrenia may release too much dopamine. The precise implications of this are not yet clear. Other neurotransmitters that may have a role in schizophrenia include 5-HT, GABA and glutamate.

Treatment of schizophrenia and other psychotic illnesses involves the use of antipsychotic neuroleptics

Chlorpromazine and other antipsychotics produce a general improvement in all the acute symptoms of schizophrenia, but their efficacy in negative schizophrenia and their ability to affect the course and prognosis of schizophrenia is less clear. The therapeutic effect of these 'typical' antipsychotic drugs was thought purely to be related to their ability to block dopamine (primarily D_2) receptors (Fig. 8.29). However, the development of newer 'atypical' antipsychotic drugs (e.g. clozapine, olanzapine, quetiapine), which have lower affinity for the D_2 receptor, but are still clinically effective, has challenged this simple hypothesis.

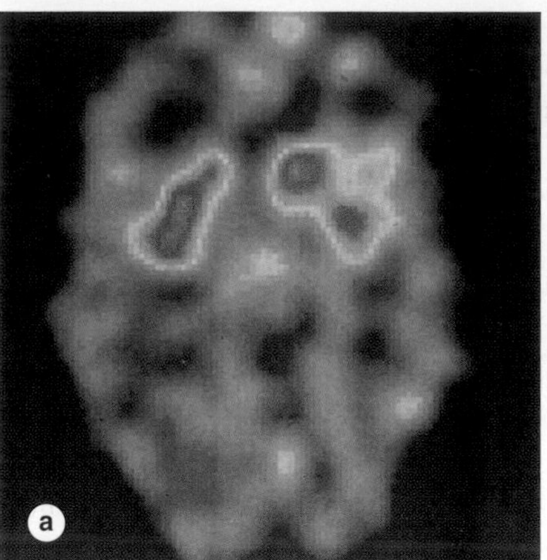

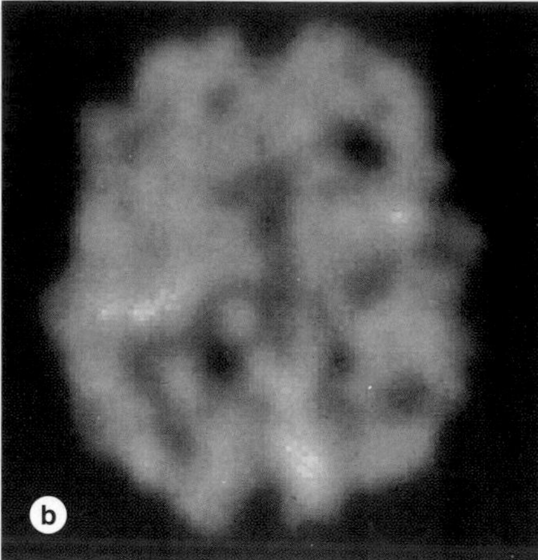

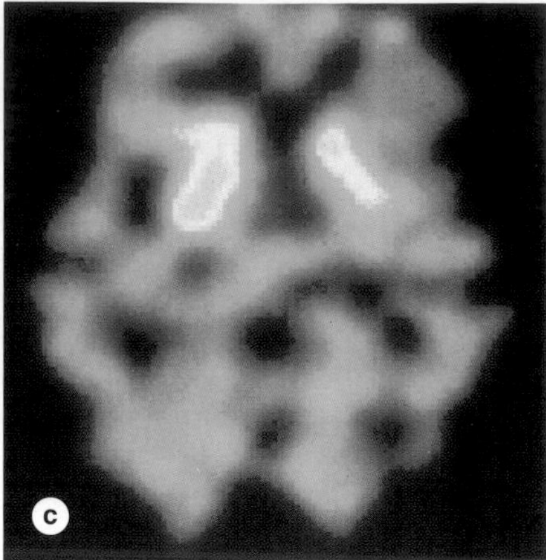

Fig. 8.29 The cerebral distribution of dopamine receptors in treated and untreated schizophrenia. Single-photon emission computed tomography (SPECT) scans acquired using the dopamine D_2 ligand I [^{123}I]-iodobenzamine. (a) Striatal dopamine receptors in an untreated schizophrenic patient. (b) Complete blockade of the receptors shown in (a) with a typical antipsychotic. (c) Partial blockade of the receptors shown in (a) with an equally effective dose of clozapine, an atypical antipsychotic. (Courtesy of the Institute of Nuclear Medicine, Middlesex Hospital, London, UK.)

Psychotic illness is usually first treated with an oral antipsychotic such as chlorpromazine (sedating), trifluoperazine or haloperidol

Doses of antipsychotic are titrated against symptoms for a period of 4–6 weeks, which is the time considered necessary for an adequate trial. Some advocate using the atypical antipsychotics as first-line drugs because they cause fewer adverse motor side effects at therapeutic doses. If medication is effective it may then be given as a depot preparation if the patient is poorly compliant, or oral treatment can be continued. If the medication is ineffective, an alternative class of typical antipsychotic should be tried. If the medication is still ineffective, the medication should be changed to an atypical antipsychotic such as clozapine. Approximately 35% of patients do not respond to classic antipsychotics.

The general consensus is that all acute episodes of schizophrenia should be treated with an antipsychotic and that the medication should be continued for 1–2 years before being cautiously withdrawn.

Most patients require maintenance therapy after an acute psychotic episode

Generally, the lowest possible dose of antipsychotic should be used for maintenance therapy. In chronic schizophrenia, antipsychotics are used to prevent further acute episodes. Although most studies show a much higher relapse rate for patients whose medication is discontinued, some studies have failed to show a drug/placebo difference. Approximately 16–25% of patients relapse despite the use of medication.

Antipsychotic (neuroleptic) drugs

Antipsychotic drugs are not a homogeneous pharmacological class of drugs. There are various classes (Table 8.10). Typical antipsychotics cause catalepsy in animals via D_2 receptor blockade. Atypical antipsychotics do not, when administered at therapeutic doses. Phenothiazines typically include:

- Drugs with aliphatic side chains such as chlorpromazine.

Table 8.10 The classes of antipsychotic drugs

Type	Class	Examples
Typical antipsychotics	Phenothiazines	Chlorpromazine, thioridazine, trifluoperazine
	Butyrophenones	Haloperidol and droperidol
	Thioxanthenes	Flupenthixol and zuclopenthixol
	Diphenylbutylpiperidines	Pimozide
Atypical antipsychotics	Dibenzodiazepines	Clozapine
	Benzixasoles	Risperidone
	Thienobenzodiazepines	Olanzapine
	Dibenzothiazepines	Quetiapine
	Imidazolidinones	Sertindole
	Benzothiazolylpiperazines	Ziprasidone
	Substituted benzamides	Sulpiride and amisulpride (NB: sulpiride considered by some to be a typical antipsychotic)

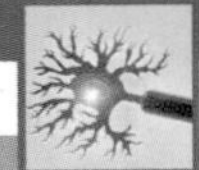

- Drugs with piperidine chains such as thioridazine.
- Drugs with piperazine side chains such as trifluoperazine and fluphenazine.

Other classes of antipsychotic include:

- The thioxanthenes (e.g. flupenthixol and zuclopenthixol).
- The butyrophenones (e.g. haloperidol and droperidol).
- The diphenylbutylpiperidines (e.g. pimozide).
- The substituted benzamides (e.g. sulpiride and amisulpride).
- The dibenzodiazepines (e.g. clozapine).
- The benzixasoles (e.g. risperidone).
- The thienobenzodiazepines (e.g. olanzapine).
- The dibenzothiazepines (e.g. quetiapine).
- The imidazolidinones (e.g. sertindole).

ADVERSE EFFECTS OF ANTIPSYCHOTICS Acute neurologic adverse effects due to D_2 receptor blockade include acute dystonia characterized by fixed muscle postures with spasm and include clenched jaw muscles, protruding tongue, opisthotonos, torticollis, and oculogyric crisis (mouth open, head back, eyes staring upwards). It occurs within hours to days and is most common in young males. It is treated immediately with anticholinergic drugs (procyclidine 5–10 mg or benztropine intramuscularly or intravenously). The response is dramatic.

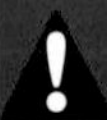

Adverse effects of antipsychotics

- Acute neurologic effects: acute dystonia, akathisia, parkinsonism
- Chronic neurologic effects: tardive dyskinesia, tardive dystonia
- Neuroendocrine effects: amenorrhea, galactorrhea, infertility
- Idiosyncratic: neuroleptic malignant syndrome
- Anticholinergic: dry mouth, blurred vision, constipation, urinary retention, ejaculatory failure
- Antihistaminergic: sedation
- Antiadrenergic: hypotension, arrhythmia
- Miscellaneous: photosensitivity, heat sensitivity, cholestatic jaundice, retinal pigmentation

Medium-term neurologic adverse effects due to D_2 blockade include akathisia and parkinsonism.

Akathisia is a motor restlessness, generally lower limb, accompanied by an inner feeling of restlessness. It is usually very distressing to the patient. Treatment primarily involves reducing the drug dose.

Parkinsonism is due to blockade of D_2 receptors in the basal ganglia. The symptoms appear after a few days to weeks and treatment involves anticholinergic drugs (e.g. procyclidine, orphenadrine), reduction of the neuroleptic dose, or switching to an atypical antipsychotic that is less likely to produce extrapyramidal symptoms (EPS).

Chronic neurologic adverse effects due to D_2 blockade are tardive dyskinesia and tardive dystonia.

Tardive dyskinesia usually manifests as orofacial dyskinesia, lip smacking and tongue rotating. Tardive dystonia appears as choreoathetoid movements of the head, neck and trunk after months to years of drug treatment. There is an increased risk of tardive dyskinesia in older patients, females, the edentulous and patients with organic brain damage. Approximately 20% of patients who are taking typical antipsychotics long term develop tardive dyskinesia, but there is no clear relationship to duration, dose, or class of antipsychotic used. There is no effective treatment, so prevention by limiting the use of neuroleptics and early recognition of symptoms are important. Increasing the dose may temporarily alleviate the symptoms, while reducing the dose may worsen them. Clozapine has been shown to improve these symptoms. Newer atypical antipsychotics may be less likely to induce tardive dyskinesia.

Neuroendocrine adverse effects due to D_2 blockade include hyperprolactinemia due to reduction of negative feedback on the anterior pituitary. High serum concentrations of prolactin can produce galactorrhea, amenorrhea and infertility in some patients.

Neuroleptic malignant syndrome (NMS) is the most life-threatening adverse effect of neuroleptic use. It is thought to be due to deranged dopaminergic function, but the precise pathophysiology is unknown. Symptoms include hyperthermia, muscle rigidity, autonomic instability, and fluctuating consciousness. It is an idiosyncratic reaction that appears from a few days to weeks after beginning treatment, but can occur at any time. Mortality is 20% if untreated. Immediate treatment is:

- Bromocriptine (a D_1/D_2 agonist) to reverse dopamine blockade.
- Dantrolene (a skeletal muscle relaxant) for muscular rigidity.
- Dehydration and hyperthermia are managed with supportive treatment.

Renal failure from rhabdomyolysis is the major complication and cause of mortality. NMS can recur on reintroducing antipsychotics. It is therefore recommended to wait at least 2 months before reintroduction and to use a drug of a different class, at the lowest recommended dose. Conventional antipsychotics often have anticholinergic side effects, which include a dry mouth (hypersalivation with clozapine), difficulty urinating or retention, constipation and blurred vision. Profound muscarinic blockade may produce a toxic confusional state.

Sedative adverse effects of antipsychotics may involve the antagonism of histamine-1 (H_1) receptors by these drugs.

ADVERSE EFFECTS DUE TO α ADRENOCEPTOR BLOCKADE Many neuroleptics have the capacity to block α adrenoceptors, and this may contribute to postural hypotension.

Adverse effects possibly due to immune reactions include urticaria, dermatitis, rashes, dermal photosensitivity and a gray/blue/purple skin tinge, which may be autoimmune responses. These are more commonly seen with the phenothiazines, as are the conjunctival, corneolenticular and retinal pigmentation, which are sometimes reported. Cholestatic jaundice due to a hypersensitivity reaction is a rare adverse effect of chlorpromazine. Weight gain is common.

Adverse effects related to individual drugs include neutropenia with clozapine and sudden death secondary to a cardiac arrhythmia with pimozide. It has therefore been recommended that all patients have an ECG before starting pimozide and that it should not be used in patients with a known arrhythmia or a prolonged QT interval. Recently droperidol and thioridazine have been withdrawn from regular clinical use due to prolongation of the QT interval.

Atypical antipsychotics

CLOZAPINE has been used since the 1960s for treatment of schizophrenia, but its use has become restricted (see below) due to several deaths from neutropenia. Clozapine has a low affinity for the D_2 receptor and a higher affinity for D_1 and D_4 receptors. The low incidence of extrapyramidal adverse effects associated with its use is thought to be due to its low activity at the D_2 receptor. Clozapine is an antagonist at the 5-HT_{2A} receptor and this may possibly underlie its clinical efficacy in improving negative symptoms. Clozapine is effective over a range of doses; this is because it has quite variable pharmacokinetics. Plasma levels of clozapine above 350–420 µg/L are a better predictor of response.

Clozapine is restricted in its use because it can cause a fatal neutropenia

In the UK and US, clozapine can be used only if a patient:

- Is unresponsive to two other neuroleptics.
- Has tardive dyskinesia or severe EPS.

Careful monitoring, especially of the formed elements in blood, is mandatory. Each patient has to be registered and the drug can be dispensed only after the white cell count has been found to be normal. A white cell count is then performed every week for 18 weeks, and regularly thereafter. The frequency of testing varies by country. Clozapine is contraindicated in patients with a history of neutropenia. The risk of neutropenia is 1–2% and it is usually reversible.

Other adverse effects of clozapine include hypersalivation, sedation, weight gain, tachycardia and hypotension.

OLANZAPINE is pharmacologically similar to clozapine. It is an antagonist at a wide range of receptors with a higher affinity for D_2 and 5-HT_{2A} receptors than clozapine but a lower affinity for D_1 receptors. Acutely, olanzapine is efficacious for positive and secondary negative symptoms and slightly superior to haloperidol for overall improvement. Olanzapine may also be effective for the primary negative symptoms of schizophrenia. Olanzapine does not cause neutropenia, but otherwise it shares a similar side-effect profile to clozapine, with weight gain and sedation, the most common side effects. EPS are rare at therapeutic doses. The dose range is up to 20 mg, the minimal effective dose recommended is 10 mg. EPS are increasingly seen above doses of 25–30 mg.

QUETIAPINE has a similar receptor binding profile to clozapine with lower affinity for all receptors and little affinity for muscarinic receptors. Quetiapine is effective in acute-phase treatment of positive and negative symptoms. Its efficacy is similar to 'classical' antipsychotics. The rates of EPS with quetiapine are similar to those seen in placebo-treated groups and significantly lower than with 'classical' antipsychotic comparator groups. The most common side effects demonstrated by quetiapine are somnolence and postural hypotension. Quetiapine has less potential for weight gain than clozapine and olanzapine and does not increase serum prolactin. The dose range is 300–750 mg. The lowest dose at which quetiapine produces EPS is not known.

RISPERIDONE, as with clozapine, has a high affinity for 5-HT_{2A} receptors and an affinity for D_2 receptors similar to most 'classic' antipsychotics. It is at least as effective as haloperidol for positive symptoms and may be more effective for negative symptoms. At higher doses, adverse effects include the extrapyramidal effects of tremor, rigidity and restlessness, but these occur less frequently than with 'classic' antipsychotics, at doses of less than 6 mg of risperidone. At doses above 8 mg per day EPS rates are similar to that observed with equivalent doses of haloperidol.

AMISULPRIDE, in contrast to all of the other atypical antipsychotics, is only a potent antagonist at the dopamine D_2 and D_3 receptors. It has a similar efficacy to haloperidol and at low doses (50–300 mg) may have a unique effect in patients with only negative symptoms. The dose range used in acute schizophrenia, in contrast, is between 400 and 800 mg per day. Amisulpride has a lower incidence of EPS, at doses below 800 mg per day, than haloperidol. Amisulpride causes less weight gain than other atypical antipsychotics but does increase plasma prolactin.

SERTINDOLE binds to 5-HT and dopamine receptors similar to risperidone, but is also a potent antagonist at adrenoceptor. Sertindole has been withdrawn from routine use due to prolongation of the QT interval.

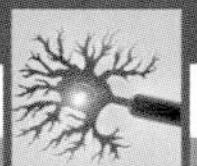

ZIPRASIDONE has a high affinity for the 5-HT_{2A} and the D_2 receptors similar to risperidone and sertindole, with a slightly higher 5-HT_{2A}/D_2 receptor affinity ratio. It is an agonist at the 5-HT_{1A} receptor. Ziprasidone also has high affinity for D_3 and moderate affinity for D_4 receptors. It exhibits weak serotonin and noradrenergic reuptake inhibition. Ziprasidone again is as efficacious as haloperidol in acute and chronic schizophrenia. It appears to have relatively low levels of side effects. These may include somnolence, headache and mild weight gain.

Two new drugs have recently been introduced for the treatment of schizophrenia: aripiprazole, an orally active D_2 receptor agonist, and zotepine, which has multiple pharmacological actions including dopamine receptor antagonism, 5-HT receptor antagonism and inhibition of adrenergic neurotransmitter uptake.

Affective disorders

The primary affective disorders are major depressive disorder and bipolar affective disorder.

Major depressive disorder

Major depressive disorder has a lifetime prevalence of approximately 9–15%, perhaps as high as 20% in women. The mean age of onset is 35–40 years, although onset can be at any age. There is no correlation with socioeconomic status.

The etiology of major depressive disorder is not clear

Life events (e.g. loss of job, moving house) and environmental stress are associated with an increased risk of a depressive disorder, but the precise causal relationship is unclear. It may involve neurochemical changes in the CNS in reaction to stress. There is evidence that major depression also has a genetic component, although the evidence for this is not as strong as for schizophrenia. Concordance rates, however, are similar in twin studies. There appears to be a genetic factor of approximately 50% in the causation of depression.

Putative neurohormonal and neurochemical causes for depression have received considerable attention. The hypothalamic–pituitary–adrenal axis, which controls much of the body's hormonal equilibrium, has been particularly implicated. It has long been noted that depressed patients have a raised baseline cortisol concentration and that cortisol is not suppressed in response to dexamethasone in approximately 50% of depressed subjects. Fast feedback mechanisms have suggested that the cortisol receptors in the hippocampi of depressed subjects are abnormal. Non-specific abnormalities have also been noted in thyroid hormone and growth hormone responses.

The most widely accepted neurochemical theory of depression involves the biogenic amines, NE, 5-HT (serotonin) and dopamine

The original hypothesis of depression suggested that it was due to a functional deficit of a transmitter amine (e.g. NE, dopamine, 5-HT), partly because tricyclic antidepressants (TCA) and monoamine oxidase inhibitors (MAOI) facilitated neurotransmission in aminergic neuron systems and were effective treatments. It was also known that drugs that depleted amine stores (e.g. reserpine) could cause depression. Increased numbers of 5-HT receptors in the brains of people who have committed suicide have been attributed to a low 5-HT concentration while low levels of 5-HT metabolites is a relatively consistent finding in studies of cerebrospinal fluid (CSF) in depressed patients. Work in animal models has shown that all effective antidepressants decrease the sensitivity to β adrenoceptors and 5-HT_{2A} agonists. The delay in treatment response coincides with the time taken for these receptors to down-regulate. It is therefore possible that biogenic amine receptors and not their levels are related to depression.

The dopaminergic system may also be involved in the etiology, since reducing central dopamine concentrations can lead to depression and drugs that increase the central dopamine concentration improve depression.

Other systems that may be involved in depression include the GABA system and neuropeptide systems, particularly vasopressin and endogenous opiates. Second-messenger systems may also have a crucial role in the efficacy of some treatments.

Evidence for the monoamine hypothesis of depression

- **Drugs that deplete monoamines induce depression**
- **Most antidepressant drugs enhance monoaminergic transmission in the synapses**
- **Concentrations of monoamines and their metabolites are reduced in the cerebrospinal fluid of depressed patients**
- **In postmortem studies, the most consistent finding is elevation in cortical 5-HT_2 binding**

The cardinal symptoms of depression are usually divided into emotional/cognitive and biologic symptoms

In order to make a diagnosis of a major depressive disorder, symptoms must have been consistently present for at least 2 weeks. Emotional/cognitive symptoms include sadness and misery, decreased pleasure in life, hopelessness, guilt and worthlessness, slowed thinking and speech, and suicidal ideation. Symptoms vary throughout the day, but are characteristically worse in the morning. Symptoms include low energy and fatigue, apathy and poor concentration, a change in appetite (usually decreased, with weight loss), a change in sleep pattern, classically with early morning wakening (a change in sleep pattern when the sufferer wakes very early in the morning and cannot return to sleep), low libido and diurnal variation of mood.

Major depressive disorders are classified as psychotic depression if accompanied by delusions and hallucinations. These are usually consistent with the mood and therefore negative in content.

The differential diagnosis of major depression involves consideration of a variety of psychiatric, drug-induced and medical conditions

The differential diagnosis of major depression includes the depressive phase of bipolar affective disorder, minor depressive disorder, adjustment reaction with depressed mood, anxiety disorders, dementia and dysthymia. Abuse of alcohol, barbiturates, benzodiazepines, cocaine or amphetamines can produce a depressive syndrome. Certain prescription drugs (e.g. some antihypertensives, especially reserpine, some antibiotics and analgesics, steroids, cimetidine and some anticonvulsants) can worsen or cause depression. Many illnesses are associated with a depressive syndrome, including Parkinson's disease, cerebrovascular disease, Cushing's and Addison's diseases, parathyroid disorders, thyroid disorders and porphyria.

Sixty-five percent of depressive episodes last 4–6 weeks, provided that the patient is given appropriate treatment

The remaining 35% of depressive episodes have a longer course despite appropriate treatment. Untreated depressive illnesses tend to last 6–13 months. Most depressive illnesses relapse at some time, 65% within 5 years.

Antidepressants

The molecular mechanisms of action of drugs used to treat depression are listed in Table 8.11.

Most antidepressants are metabolized by the cytochrome P-450 enzyme system. Some antidepressants, i.e. the selective serotonin reuptake inhibitors (SSRIs), are potent inhibitors of specific P-450 enzymes. These may result in pharmacokinetic interactions with other drug classes that influence P-450s. A summary of this and other relevant pharmacokinetic data is in Table 8.12.

Tricyclic antidepressants and related drugs

Tricyclic antidepressants (TCAs) are an effective therapy for depression, but their adverse effects can reduce patient compliance and acceptability.

All TCAs act by preventing 5-HT and NE uptake into the presynaptic terminal from the synaptic cleft. The potency of different tricyclic antidepressants for blocking uptake varies. Some also block dopamine uptake. All TCAs also have some affinity for H_1 and muscarinic receptors and for α_1 and α_2 adrenoceptors.

Overdose of TCAs are relatively dangerous due to cardiac arrhythmias.

The choice of TCA usually depends on the degree of sedation considered necessary:

- Clomipramine is the TCA of choice for obsessive–compulsive disorder.
- Trimipramine is the TCA of choice for agitated states.

Some TCAs produce pharmacologically active metabolites (e.g. amitriptyline is metabolized to nortriptyline, imipramine is metabolized to desipramine). Trazodone is a triazolopyridine derivative and is not strictly a tricyclic. It is less anticholinergic and cardiotoxic. Although it is quite sedative it is commonly used in the elderly and may be the antidepressant of choice in epilepsy.

ADVERSE EFFECTS Adverse effects of tricyclic antidepressants due to muscarinic blockade include dry mouth, constipation, urinary retention, tachycardia and blurred vision. α_1 adrenoceptor antagonism may cause postural hypotension, while H_1 receptor antagonism leads to sedation. Alterations in serotonergic function lead to sexual dysfunction, including loss of libido and anorgasmia. Generally, tolerance develops to the anticholinergic adverse effects within 2 weeks. These can be minimized by gradually increasing the dose.

Table 8.11 Mechanism of action of drugs used to treat depression

Mechanism of action	Examples
Non-specific blockers of monoamine uptake	Tricyclic antidepressants (amitriptyline, imipramine, nortriptyline, clomipramine, lofepramine)
Selective serotonin reuptake inhibitors (SSRIs)	Fluoxetine, paroxetine, sertraline, citalopram
Serotonin and norepinephrine reuptake inhibitors (SNRIs)	Venlafaxine
Noradrenergic and specific serotonergic antidepressant (NaSSA)	Mirtazapine
Selective norepinephrine reuptake inhibitor (NARI)	Reboxetine
Noncompetitive, nonselective, irreversible blockers of MAO_A and MAO_B	Monoamine oxidase inhibitors, (MAOIs) (phenelzine, tranylcypromine)
Reversible inhibitors of MAO_A (RIMAs)	Moclobemide, brofaromine

Table 8.12 Pharmacokinetic considerations with antidepressants

Drug	Class	Half-life (hours)	Daily doses	Cytochrome P-450 metabolism	Potential interactions	Active metabolites	Route of administration/ formulation
Amitriptyline	TCA	8–24	75–150 mg o.d.		Other sedatives (i.e. alcohol, benzodiazepines (BDZs), antipsychotics), also sympathomimetics, cimetidine	Nortriptyline	Available as liquid
Imipramine	TCA	4–18	75–200 mg o.d.		Other sedatives (i.e. alcohol, benzodiazepines (BDZs), antipsychotics), also sympathomimetics, cimetidine	Desipramine	Available as liquid
Nortriptyline	TCA	18–96	75–150 mg o.d.		Other sedatives (i.e. alcohol, benzodiazepines (BDZs), antipsychotics), also sympathomimetics, cimetidine		
Clomipramine	TCA	17–28	50–250 mg o.d.		Other sedatives (i.e. alcohol, benzodiazepines (BDZs), antipsychotics), also sympathomimetics, cimetidine		Available as liquid and as i.v. forms
Lofepramine	TCA	1.5–6	70–210 mg/ day b.d. or t.d.s.		Other sedatives (i.e. alcohol, benzodiazepines (BDZs), antipsychotics), also sympathomimetics, cimetidine	Desipramine	Available as liquid
Fluoxetine	SSRI	24–140	20–60 mg o.d.	Inhibits: CYP2D6+++ CYPIA2+ CYP3A4+	MAOIs contraindicated. Increases plasma levels of TCAs, BDZs and clozapine. No alcohol potentiation	Norfluoxetine	Available as liquid
Paroxetine	SSRI	24	20–60 mg o.d.	Inhibits: CYP2D6++	MAOIs contraindicated. Increases plasma levels of TCAs, BDZs and clozapine. No alcohol potentiation		Available as liquid
Sertraline	SSRI	24–26	50–150 mg o.d.	Inhibits: CYP2D6+++	MAOIs contraindicated. Increases plasma levels of TCAs, BDZs and clozapine. No alcohol potentiation & care with alcohol		
Citalopram	SSRI	33	20–60 mg o.d.	Inhibits: CYP2D6+	MAOIs contraindicated only		
Nefazodone	5-HT$_{2A}$ antagonist & weak SNRI	2–4	200–600 mg/ day b.d.	Inhibits: CYP2D6+ CYP3A4+++	MAOIs contraindicated. Increases plasma levels of haloperidol, carbamazepine and digoxin		
Venlafaxine	SNRI	5–11	75–375 mg/ day o.d. or b.d.	Inhibits: CYP2D6+	MAOIs contraindicated		*O*-desmethyl-venlafaxine
Mirtazapine	NaSSA	20–40	15–45 mg o.d.	Inhibits: CYP2D6+/- CYP1A2+/- CYP3A4+/-	MAOIs contraindicated, potentiates other sedatives and alcohol		
Reboxetine	NARI	13	8–12 mg/ day as b.d.	Inhibits: CYP2D6+/- CYP3A4+/-	MAOIs contraindicated. No alcohol potentiation		
Phenelzine	MAOI	1.5	45–90 mg/ day as t.d.s.		See text: tyramine reaction common and severe		
Moclobemide	RIMA	1–2	300–600 mg/ day as b.d.		See text: tyramine reaction rare, avoid meperidine, sympathomimetics, SSRIs and L-dopa		

MAOI, monoamine oxidase inhibitor; NARI, norepinephrine reuptake inhibitor; NaSSA, noradrenergic and specific serotonergic antidepressant; RIMA, reversible inhibitor of MAOIA; SNRI, serotonin and norepinephrine reuptake inhibitor; SSRI, selective serotonin reuptake inhibitor; +++, strong inhibition; ++ moderate inhibition; +, weak inhibition; +/–, equivocal inhibition not clinically relevant. (Adapted from the South London and Maudsley NHS Trust 2001 Prescribing Guidelines, 6th edn.)

CONTRAINDICATIONS These include prostatism, narrow angle glaucoma, recent myocardial infarction, and heart block. Care is needed if the patient has:

- Heart disease (because TCAs increase the risk of conduction abnormalities).
- Epilepsy (because TCAs lower the seizure threshold).

DRUG INTERACTIONS TCAs potentiate the effects of alcohol, other anticholinergic drugs, epinephrine and NE. A fatal interaction can occur with lidocaine in local anesthetic preparations.

Selective serotonin (5-hydroxytryptamine) reuptake inhibitors

MECHANISM OF ACTION After release from nerve terminals, serotonin activates various subtypes of serotonin receptors on nerve cells. Serotonin is inactivated by several mechanisms. The two primary mechanisms are metabolism by monoamine oxidase (MAO) to the major inactive metabolite 5-HIAA and reuptake of the transmitter into serotonergic nerve endings (Fig. 8.30). This latter important pathway is a useful target for antidepressant drugs.

Reuptake of serotonin into nerve endings requires a specific transporter expressed on nerve endings. The serotonin transporter is a member of a gene family of neurotransmitter transporters. Transporters for serotonin, as well as for NE, dopamine, glycine and GABA, have been identified. The overall structure of these transporters involves proteins with 12 membrane-spanning domains with *N*-glycosylation sites that are likely to be important for transporter function. There is homology between these transporters and transporters for nutrients such as glucose. The expression of the serotonin transporter has been localized primarily to serotonergic nerves. The specificity with which this transporter is expressed in nerve cells and the selectivity with which it moves serotonin across cell membranes is of major importance in the function of serotonergic nerves. It should be emphasized that the serotonin transporter, as well as transporters for dopamine and NE, is quite distinct from the vesicular monoamine transporters that concentrate transmitters such as NE into synaptic granules. Those transporters are inhibited by drugs such as reserpine (see Ch. 3).

Serotonin transporters belong to a class of Na^+/Cl^- coupled transporters. Overexpression of this transporter, as well as very extensive experimentation in serotonergic neuronal preparations, has led to the discovery and development of a novel class of therapeutic agents with high specificity for potent inhibition of serotonin reuptake into nerves and only minimal effects on

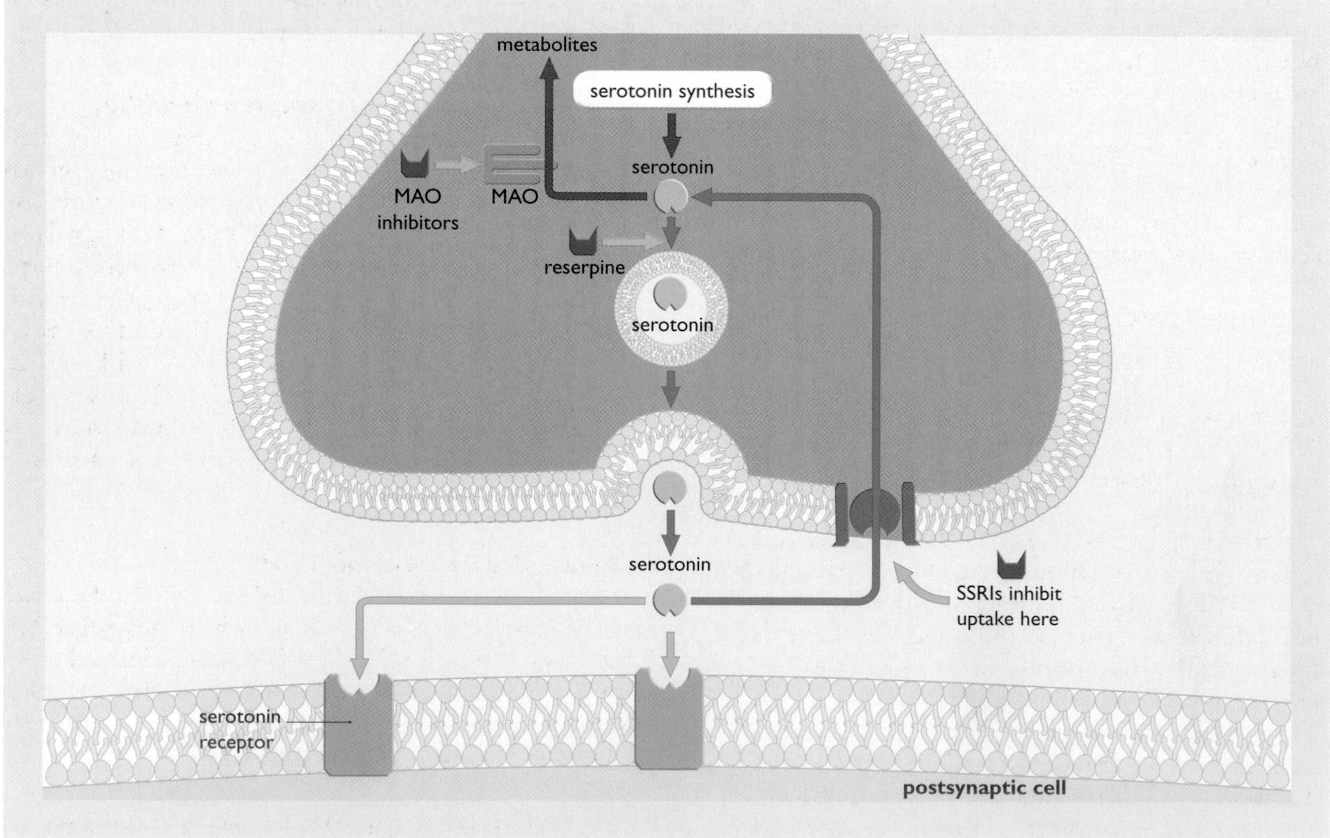

Fig. 8.30 Site of action of selective serotonin reuptake inhibitors (SSRIs) and monoamine oxidase (MAO) inhibitors. Reserpine leads to depletion of serotonin.

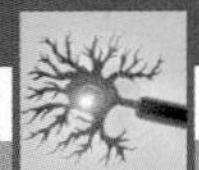

reuptake of other neurotransmitters or on other related drug targets. These SSRIs are efficacious in the treatment of depression. Some of these drugs also inhibit reuptake of NE. In some animal models SSRIs have been found to change expression of β adrenoceptors and serotonin receptor subtypes in the brain. The potential clinical significance of these differences between SSRIs in terms of specificity and on effects on receptor expression in the brain is not known.

SSRIs have efficacy in the treatment of depression similar to that of TCAs. In addition, they have the following clinical advantages:

- No anticholinergic activity, thus increasing patient acceptability.
- Lack of toxicity in overdose – a major reason for their use.
- Do not induce cardiac arrhythmias and are therefore the drugs of choice in patients also suffering from heart disease.

SSRIs act by inhibiting the uptake of 5-HT from the synaptic cleft and have only minor effects on noradrenergic uptake. Nefazodone is often classified as an SSRI, but may have more effect on NE uptake. Thus, it is better thought of as an SNRI. It is also a potent 5-HT_{2A} receptor antagonist. This may underlie its effects in improving sleep and its low level of sexual side effects.

The most potent SSRI is citalopram, followed in descending order by paroxetine, fluoxetine, sertraline and fluvoxamine. The half-life of fluoxetine (active metabolite, 7–9 days) means that it may take longer to reach steady-state concentrations but may be prescribed on alternate days. The half-lifes of the other SSRIs vary from 15 to 24 hours.

The newest SSRI is escalitalopram which has an 80% bioavailability and a half-life of 29 hours. Duloxetine has also recently been introduced and has mixed SSRI activity and adrenergic uptake inhibitory activity.

ADVERSE EFFECTS Adverse effects of SSRIs include nausea, diarrhea, insomnia, anxiety and agitation due to their effect on 5-HT receptors throughout the body. Sexual dysfunction may also occur. The adverse effect profile of nefazodone is similar to that of other SSRIs, but the associated incidence of sexual dysfunction may be lower.

CONTRAINDICATIONS AND INTERACTIONS Contraindications and interactions are few, but SSRIs should not be used with MAOIs since the combination is likely to produce a serotonergic syndrome, which can be fatal. Care should be taken when prescribing SSRIs concurrently with lithium for similar reasons.

Serotonin (5-hydroxytryptamine) and norepinephrine reuptake inhibitors (SNRIs)

The only drug currently in this new class of antidepressants is venlafaxine, a phenethylamine bicyclic derivative. Its half-life is approximately 5 hours and it has an active metabolite with a half-life of 10 hours.

The pharmacologic effects of venlafaxine are similar to those of the TCAs, but it has fewer adverse effects because it has little affinity for cholinergic, histamine or adrenoceptors. Its adverse effects are similar to those of SSRIs, but occur with a lower frequency. Drug interactions are similar to those of SSRIs, though extra care must be taken with patients with increased blood pressure since venlafaxine increases blood pressure.

Noradrenergic and specific serotonergic antidepressant

Mirtazapine is the only drug in this class (NaSSA) and it is pharmacologically unique. Mirtazapine enhances noradrenergic transmission by blocking α_2 autoreceptors, thereby increasing norepinephrine release. It also increases 5-HT neuronal activity by acting on the noradrenergic α_2-heteroreceptors on serotonergic neuronal cell bodies to increase synaptic serotonin. It is also an antagonist at 5-HT_{2A} and 5-HT_3 receptors. It has affinity for muscarinic receptors (but greater than venlafaxine). It also has relatively high affinity for H_1 receptors. Thus, mirtazapine causes less nausea, less headache and less anxiety than 'pure' SSRIs since it blocks the 5-HT receptors which mediate these side effects. However, probably due to the H_1 receptor antagonism, mirtazapine's side effects include increased appetite and weight gain, drowsiness and sedation. These occur in 14–37% of patients treated with mirtazapine and are greater at initiation of therapy.

Selective norepinephrine reuptake inhibitor

Reboxetine is currently the only drug in this class, although the TCAs desipramine and nortriptyline are effectively selective noradrenaline reuptake inhibitors (NARIs). These drugs selectively block the reuptake of norepinephrine with little or no effect on serotonergic reuptake and are said to be better for depression with marked psychomotor retardation. Reboxetine has a better side-effect profile than the TCAs with relative selectivity for norepinephrine reuptake. The side effects of reboxetine include dry mouth, constipation and insomnia. The incidence of impotence and decreased libido increases at higher doses.

Monoamine oxidase inhibitors

Monoamine oxidase inhibitors (MAOIs) block the action of MAO-A and MAO-B, enzymes which metabolize NE, dopamine and 5-HT. MAO-A is primarily located in the gut and preferentially breaks down 5-HT and NE, while MAO-B is primarily located in the brain. MAO-A inhibitors are used to treat depression.

ADVERSE EFFECTS Gut MAO-A breaks down tyramine in food. Tyramine in the circulation releases NE, causing sudden and potentially fatal rise in blood pressure.

Patients on MAOIs must avoid foods rich in tyramine. These include:

- Cheese, especially mature varieties.
- Degraded protein such as chicken liver, hung game, pickled herring and pâté.
- Yeast and protein extracts.
- Beer.
- Chianti red wine.
- Broad bean pods.
- Green banana skins.

Drug preparations containing amines to be avoided include:

- Opiates (e.g. meperidine).
- Sympathomimetics, which are often included in cough and cold remedies, nose drops and laxatives bought over the counter.
- SSRIs.
- Levodopa.
- Some H_1 receptor antagonists.

The above restrictions last for at least 2 weeks after discontinuing MAOIs since MAO blockade is irreversible and requires new enzyme synthesis to restore function. After ingesting such food or drugs, patients on MAOIs usually experience flushing and a pounding headache. This may progress to a fatal hypertensive crisis. This so-called 'cheese reaction' is the most important adverse effect of MAOIs.

Other rare adverse effects of MAOIs include hepatotoxicity (especially with phenelzine) and a theoretic risk of precipitating psychosis by increasing the availability of dopamine.

Because of the dietary and drug restrictions, MAOIs are largely reserved for treatment of depression in those resistant to other antidepressants and treatment

Phenelzine has traditionally had a role in treating atypical nonbiologic depression with pronounced anxiety and hypochondriac symptoms. It has also been used in the treatment of phobias and panic disorder.

The three irreversible MAOIs currently available are:

- Phenelzine, which is the most common.
- Tranylcypromine, which has amine uptake and amphetamine-like activity.
- Isocarboxazid, which is now rarely used.

Moclobemide, a newer MAOI, reversibly inhibits MAO-A

Moclobemide carries the risk of an interaction with tyramine resulting in raised blood pressure if high levels of tyramine are consumed (e.g. more than 50 g of mature cheese), but in general no dietary restrictions are required. The likelihood of an interaction with tyramine is reduced if moclobemide is taken after a meal. Although the clinical efficacy of moclobemide is probably similar to that of other antidepressants (i.e. TCAs and SSRIs), it is not recommended as a first-line treatment.

The adverse effects of moclobemide include insomnia, nausea, agitation and confusion. Drug interactions include interactions with cimetidine, meperidine and SSRIs, and moclobemide should be used with caution with TCAs as all these combinations may lead to a 'cheese reaction.'

Depression is usually treated with an antidepressant

The choice of antidepressant depends on:

- The clinical characteristics of the patient's illness.
- The drug's adverse effect profile.
- The danger of overdose.
- Previous treatments.

Generally, if there are no medical contraindications (e.g. heart disorders) and there is no or little risk of suicide, a TCA can be used. The TCA chosen will depend on whether sedation is required. The newer antidepressants (SSRIs, SNRIs, NaSSAs, etc.) are increasingly used as first-line treatments because of better tolerability. If there are medical contraindications, or suicide is a risk, or the patient has previously not tolerated the anticholinergic adverse effects of TCAs, then a newer antidepressant should be used.

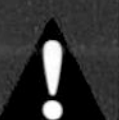

Adverse effects of antidepressants

- **Tricyclics: blurred vision, dry mouth, constipation, urinary retention, mania, hypotension, arrhythmias**
- **Serotonin and NE reuptake inhibitors (SNRIs): sedation, mania**
- **Selective serotonin reuptake inhibitors (SSRIs): nausea, vomiting, dry mouth, agitation**
- **Monoamine oxidase inhibitors (MAOIs): as for tricyclics plus sympathetic crisis with dietary tyramine**
- **Reversible inhibitors of monoamine oxidase (RIMAs): mild agitation**

Bipolar affective disorder

Bipolar affective disorder (BPAD) is characterized by swings in mood from mania (or hypomania) to depression. There is a high concordance rate for BPAD (ranging from 33% to 90%) in monozygotic twins. Family studies indicate an 18-fold increased risk for BPAD, and a tenfold increased risk for major depression, in the first-degree relatives of affected probands. The neurochemical basis for BPAD is unclear.

BPAD is characterized by episodes of depression and mania with periods of normality in between

The cycle of depressive and manic episodes in BPAD may take months or years, but may occur over days or weeks. There is no typical sequence of episodes.

Mania and hypomania are distinguished according to their severity and duration:

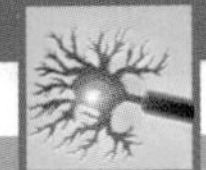

- A manic episode usually lasts longer than a week, significantly impairs social and occupational functioning and may be accompanied by psychotic phenomena such as delusions and hallucinations.
- Hypomania is, by definition, not accompanied by psychotic features.

For ease of explanation, both mania and hypomania are here considered to be a manic episode. The signs of a manic episode include an elevated mood, increased motor activity, accelerated thoughts and speech, irritability, decreased sleep, increased or decreased appetite, distractability, grandiose ideas, and delusions and hallucinations, usually of a grandiose nature. Features normally considered typical of schizophrenia occur in approximately 10% of patients. Patients with the severest form of manic episode may exhaust themselves, or carry out dangerous plans based on their grandiose ideas.

Depressive episodes in BPAD are clinically identical to depression in the absence of manic episodes. Patients may experience several episodes of depression in sequence, or several episodes of mania.

BPAD is treated with a combination of mood stabilizers, antipsychotics and antidepressants.

Mood stabilizers

Lithium

Lithium is the most widely used mood stabilizer:

- It is used in the prevention of relapse in manic depressive (bipolar) and recurrent unipolar (i.e. no mania) depressive disorders.
- It is an effective treatment in acute mania.
- It is used sometimes in resistant depression to augment antidepressant activity.

Lithium inhibits the scavenging pathway that captures inositol for the resynthesis of polyphosphoinositides. Since the entry of inositol into the brain is relatively poor, this action of lithium may diminish the concentrations of lipids important in signal transduction in the brain (see Ch. 3).

Renal and thyroid function must be checked before starting lithium

Owing to adverse effects and contraindications (see below), before starting therapy, renal (urea, creatinine, electrolytes) and thyroid function must be checked. Once treatment is started, plasma lithium concentration should be monitored (every 5 days) with dose increases until the concentration is 0.6–1.0 mmol/L. During maintenance, lithium concentrations should be determined along with renal function every 2–3 months. Thyroid function should be determined every 6 months.

ADVERSE EFFECTS In the early stages of lithium therapy, patients commonly complain of thirst, nausea, loose stools, fine tremor and polyuria, but these often disappear with continued therapy. Other adverse effects include weight gain, edema and acne. A possible long-term adverse effect can be diabetes insipidus leading to polydipsia. This occurs because lithium inhibits vasopressin action in the kidney (see Ch. 12), leading to obligate water loss. Goiter and, less commonly, frank hypothyroidism can occur due to impaired release of thyroid hormone from the thyroid gland.

The first signs of lithium toxicity, occurring at plasma lithium concentrations of 1.5–2.0 mmol/L, are anorexia, vomiting, diarrhea, coarse tremor, ataxia, dysarthria, confusion and sleepiness. Later signs, when the plasma lithium concentration is higher than 2.0 mmol/L, are impaired consciousness, nystagmus, muscle twitching, hyper-reflexia and convulsions. Coma and death occur at higher concentrations. At the first signs of toxicity the plasma lithium concentration should be measured urgently and, if high, the lithium should be stopped and efforts made to increase lithium elimination, possibly including hemodialysis.

Interactions between lithium and other drugs are common, often leading to a rise in plasma lithium concentration. Such interacting drugs include:

- Antipsychotics (especially haloperidol), which increase neurotoxicity.
- NSAIDs, except aspirin, which increase plasma lithium concentration by decreasing excretion.
- Diuretics (especially thiazides), which increase plasma lithium concentration by decreasing excretion.
- Cardioactive drugs (digoxin, angiotensin-converting enzyme inhibitors), which increase the risk of neurotoxicity, possibly secondary to membrane effects.

Carbamazepine

Carbamazepine may be as effective as lithium in preventing relapses in BPAD and in the treatment of acute mania. It is commonly indicated for rapid cycling bipolar illness.

Carbamazepine shares with lithium a mechanism of action possibly mediated via effects on second-messenger systems. Carbamazepine also inhibits calcium influx through the NMDA and $GABA_B$ receptors. Furthermore, carbamazepine treatment leads to a sodium channel-mediated membrane stabilization and potentiation of α_2 adrenoceptors.

At the start of therapy, carbamazepine induces its own catabolic enzymes in the liver; plasma concentrations therefore should be monitored to establish a maintenance dose.

Adverse effects of carbamazepine include drowsiness, diplopia, nausea, ataxia, rashes and headache. Hematologic disturbances include agranulocytosis and leukopenia, and patients therefore should be warned about fever and infections as these may indicate agranulocytosis and should be investigated. It is advised that the plasma carbamazepine concentration is measured and a full blood count obtained every 2 weeks for the first 2 months of treatment.

Acute carbamazepine toxicity includes diplopia, ataxia, hyper-reflexia, clonus, tremor and sedation.

Interactions between carbamazepine and other drugs include:

- Lithium, with the potential for CNS adverse effects of carbamazepine and carbamazepine toxicity despite 'normal' plasma carbamazepine concentrations. It must be noted, however, that combinations of lithium and carbamazepine may be more effective than either drug alone.
- Antipsychotics, resulting in drowsiness and ataxia.
- TCAs, decreasing the plasma TCA concentration as a result of enzyme inductions by carbamazepine.
- MAOIs, precipitating the cheese reaction.

Carbamazepine is an enzyme inducer (see Ch. 4) and therefore affects the plasma concentrations of many drugs metabolized in the liver.

Valproate sodium and divalproex sodium

Valproate (an antipsychotic drug) is an effective mood stabilizer and can be used as a first-line treatment or as an adjunct in refractory cases. Divalproex sodium is a mixture of valproate sodium and valproic acid that improves bioavailability and tolerability. The active moiety remains valproate. The mechanism of action of valproate is not fully understood. It is known to enhance the synthesis, turnover and release of GABA. It also inhibits Ca^{2+} influx via NMDA receptor activation. Perhaps related to these two actions, valproate enhances serotonergic function and reduces dopaminergic function.

Adverse effects of valproate sodium include gastrointestinal effects (nausea, vomiting, diarrhea), CNS effects (sedation, ataxia, dysarthria, tremor) and hepatic effects (persistent elevation of liver transaminases). It may also cause hair loss. A rare adverse effect is hepatotoxicity leading to death.

New antiepileptics for the treatment of bipolar affective disorder

Although all new antiepileptics are potential treatments for bipolar affective disorder, only lamotrigine is superior or equal to existing treatments. Lamotrigine is thought to inhibit neuronal kindling. It inhibits sodium currents by selectively binding to the inactivated state of the sodium channel and subsequently suppresses the release of the excitatory amino acid glutamate. Early data suggest that it is well tolerated in bipolar affective disorder and may have a role in treating the depressive phase of the illness.

Anxiety disorders

Anxiety is common. Psychologic symptoms include a diffuse, unpleasant and vague feeling of apprehension that is often accompanied by physical symptoms of autonomic arousal such as headache, perspiration, palpitations, 'upset stomach' ('butterflies'), tightness in the chest and, in some people, restlessness. Anxiety warns of impending danger, and enables the individual to take measures to deal with a threat that is usually unknown, internal, vague or conflictual (with stimulatory opposite emotions, e.g. excitement and guilt) in origin. This is in contrast to fear, which is a response to a threat that is known, external, definite or nonconflictual in origin.

Anxiety is a common symptom in a variety of distinct mental illnesses and is a predominant symptom in phobias, panic disorder and obsessive–compulsive disorder. Other anxiety disorders include generalized anxiety disorder, post-traumatic stress disorder and hysterical conversion reactions.

The two neurotransmitters most implicated in the etiology of anxiety disorders are GABA and 5-HT

Norepinephrine also has a role, particularly in panic disorder. There have been no conclusive studies to confirm the role of these neurotransmitters, but functional imaging of benzodiazepine receptors in the brain has shown differences in receptor binding in the temporal lobes between patients with panic disorder and normal subjects. Benzodiazepines act on the GABA receptor complex.

Anxiety disorders are treated with anxiolytics and antidepressants.

Anxiolytics

Benzodiazepines

Benzodiazepines (Table 8.13) act by potentiating the action of GABA, the primary inhibitory neurotransmitter in the CNS. The benzodiazepine receptor lies within the $GABA_A$ receptor complex, and benzodiazepines enhance inhibitory activity (Fig. 8.31). Benzodiazepines reduce anxiety, and the duration of their action will be determined to some extent by their half-lifes (see below).

Adverse effects of benzodiazepines include dependence and a potential for abuse. Generally, tolerance to its actions develops within 14 days and its efficacy then declines. Sudden cessation after long-term use can result in a withdrawal syndrome characterized by insomnia, anxiety, tremor, loss of appetite, tinnitus and perceptual disturbances. Controlled benzodiazepine withdrawal is performed by switching to an equivalent dose of a benzodiazepine with a long half-life (e.g. diazepam) and reducing the dose gradually by approximately one-eighth every 2 weeks. This process may take many weeks to 1 year, depending on the severity of tolerance.

The most common adverse effects with benzodiazepines are drowsiness, ataxia and reduced psychomotor performance. Care should be taken when driving or operating machinery. These effects can become more marked after a few weeks because the long half-life of some benzodiazepines leads to accumulation of drug. Disinhibition with aggression may occur, but is rare and more likely to be seen with short-acting benzodiazepines (i.e. midazolam).

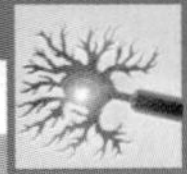

Table 8.13 Mechanism of action of drugs used to treat anxiety

Drug	Mechanism of action	Use
Anxiolytics		
Benzodiazepines (diazepam, alprazolam)	Act on GABA receptors	Short-term treatment of anxiety
Buspirone	Acts on 5-HT_{1A} receptor	May be effective in generalized anxiety disorder
Autonomic suppression		
Propranolol	Acts by inhibiting β adrenoceptors	Useful for some social/performance anxiety disorders
Antidepressants		
Imipramine	Tricyclic antidepressant	Most studied biologic treatment in panic disorder
Phenelzine, moclobemide	MAOIs	Useful for social phobia and panic, may also be useful for PTSD
Fluoxetine, sertraline	SSRIs	Proven efficacy in OCD and panic disorder

GABA, γ-aminobutyric acid; 5-HT_{1A}, 5-hydroxytryptamine-1A; MAOIs, monoamine oxidase inhibitors; OCD, obsessive–compulsive disorder; PTSD, post-traumatic stress disorder; SSRIs, selective serotonin reuptake inhibitors.

Half-lifes of benzodiazepines

- **Diazepam: 14–70 hours (one metabolite is active for up to 200 hours)**
- **Nitrazepam: 15–30 hours**
- **Lorazepam: 8–24 hours**
- **Temazepam: 3–25 hours**
- **Oxazepam: 3–25 hours**

Benzodiazepines are indicated only for short-term relief of severe, disabling or unacceptably distressing anxiety

Severe anxiety may occur alone or in association with insomnia or be a short-term psychosomatic, organic or psychotic illness. Diazepam (5–20 mg/day) is the most commonly prescribed anxiolytic. The use of benzodiazepines to treat short-term 'mild' anxiety is inappropriate since dependence and withdrawal are more problematic with benzodiazepines prescribed as anxiolytics than with those prescribed as hypnotics. Alprazolam is effective for panic attacks.

Azapirones

Buspirone is the first of a new class of drugs, termed azapirones, that act to reduce 5-HT neurotransmission via a partial agonist action at 5-HT_{1A} receptors. 5-HT_{1A} receptors are inhibitory presynaptic receptors and their activation results in decreased firing of 5-HT neurons. Buspirone does not act at the GABA–benzodiazepine receptor complex and cannot therefore be used to ameliorate the benzodiazepine withdrawal syndrome. It is not an hypnotic.

Adverse effects of buspirone include nervousness, dizziness, headache and lightheadedness.

Buspirone is indicated for the short-term management of generalized anxiety disorder

The anxiolytic effect of buspirone gradually evolves over 1–3 weeks. In contrast to benzodiazepines, buspirone does not cause significant sedation or cognitive impairment and carries only a minimal risk of dependence and withdrawal. It does not potentiate the sedative effects of alcohol.

β adrenoceptor antagonists

β adrenoceptor antagonists such as propranolol reduce heart rate and other manifestations of excess β adrenoceptor (sympathetic activity).

Propranolol:

- May ease the somatic manifestations of an anxiety characterized by marked sympathetic autonomic arousal (e.g. palpitations and tremor).
- Is useful for social phobia and acts by reducing the symptoms of autonomic arousal, thereby preventing amplification of the sufferer's anxiety.
- Reduces performance anxiety in musicians for whom fine motor control may be critical.

Antidepressants

Certain antidepressants have specific applications in particular anxiety disorders:

- Imipramine produces a beneficial effect in 60–70% of patients with panic disorder. Generally, the dose used is higher than that for depression and the therapy must be continued for longer before a response is seen.
- MAOIs are used in several anxiety disorders including panic disorder, agoraphobia, social phobia and post-traumatic stress disorder. These are beneficial over and above regular TCAs.

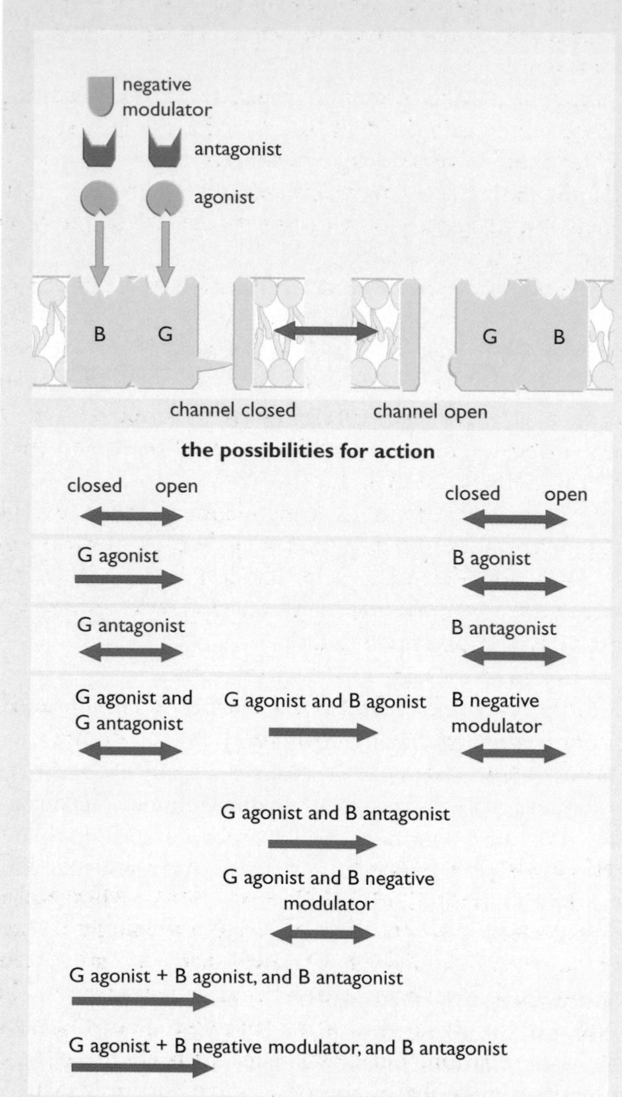

Fig. 8.31 Benzodiazepine agonist and antagonist activity and modulation of γ-aminobutyric acid (GABA) agonist and antagonist activity. A Cl^- channel, part of a receptor-operated channel (ROC), exists in open to closed states. This ROC has two distinct ligand-recognition sites, a GABA site (G) and a benzodiazepine site (B). Equilibrium between closed and open states of the Cl^- channel is altered by GABA agonism. Neither benzodiazepine agonism or antagonism alone affect channel opening. However, GABA agonist-induced channel opening is facilitated by concomitant benzodiazepine agonism. This potentiation is blocked by a benzodiazepine antagonist. In addition, benzodiazepine negative modulators reduce the ability of GABA to open the channel, and benzodiazepine antagonists can block the effect of negative modulators. The G and B ligand-recognition sites presumably interact allosterically, with the B site functioning as a modulator of the G site.

- SSRIs, especially fluoxetine and the TCA clomipramine, are most effective in the treatment of obsessive–compulsive disorder. Doses, however, are higher than those used for depression while the therapeutic effect may take 1–3 months to become fully apparent.

Patients often present with a mixed picture of anxiety and depression (agitated depression). Antidepressants are then indicated, and generally a more sedative one is used.

Eating disorders

The two well-defined eating disorders are anorexia nervosa and bulimia nervosa. There is considerable overlap between the two disorders with patients moving from one to the other. Treatment is almost purely with psychotherapy, though these disorders are often accompanied by depression, which may need drug treatment.

Epilepsy

Epilepsy is characterized by recurrent unprovoked seizures, where a seizure is a particular behavior produced by an altered neurologic function resulting from paroxysmal discharges of neurons in the cerebral cortex. Seizures are sometimes called fits. Approximately 10% of the US population experiences one or more seizures during their lifetime, and epilepsy will develop in approximately 1.5% of the population. Behavior during a seizure varies from immobility, and slight twitching of a digit, to violent tonic–clonic movements or even purposeful activity, depending on the type of epilepsy.

The cellular mechanisms of epilepsy are not known, but may involve altered GABA metabolism.

Appropriate drug treatment depends on the nature of the epilepsy

A diagnosis of epilepsy is made from the patient's history, the nature of the seizure (Table 8.14) and the electroencephalographic (EEG) pattern.

Table 8.14 Classification of epileptic seizures

Partial (focal, local) seizures
Simple partial seizures (consciousness not impaired) (motor signs, somatosensory or special sensory signs, psychic symptoms)
Complex partial seizures (consciousness impaired) (simple partial onset followed by impaired consciousness, consciousness impaired at onset)
Partial seizures evolving to generalized seizures (tonic, clonic, or tonic–clonic)
Simple partial seizures evolving to generalized seizures
Complex partial seizures evolving to generalized seizures
Simple partial seizures evolving to complex partial seizures evolving to generalized seizures
Generalized seizures (convulsive or nonconvulsive)
Typical absence seizures (brief stare, eye flickering, no motion)
Atypical absence seizures (associated with movement)
Myoclonic seizures
Clonic seizures
Tonic seizures
Tonic–clonic seizures
Atonic seizures

From the Commission on Classification and Terminology of the International League Against Epilepsy.

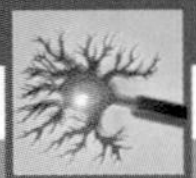

Partial or focal seizures arise from a restricted region of the cerebral cortex. The resulting effect depends on the involved region of brain and can be sensory (including visual disturbances) or motor in nature. The motor behavior can be quite purposeful. Consciousness is variable and usually there is no memory of the seizure.

Generalized seizures are convulsive or nonconvulsive and range from a blank stare to a generalized tonic–clonic seizure:

- Absence seizures are the most common nonconvulsive seizure. They occur most often in children and can be confused with daydreaming.
- Myoclonic seizures are rapid symmetric arrhythmic jerks of the extremities or body.
- Tonic seizures are characterized by stiffening of body and limbs and can produce fractures.
- Atonic seizures involve loss of muscle tone and can cause a fall.
- A generalized tonic–clonic seizure (grand mal seizure) starts with increased muscle tone (stiffening), which is followed by clonic movements lasting a few minutes. This may be accompanied by vocalization, cyanosis and incontinence of urine and/or feces. The seizure is followed by confusion and fatigue.

Seizures can be classified into different epileptic syndromes based on:

- Seizure type.
- Other clinical features such as age at onset.
- Anatomic location.
- Etiology (e.g. fever).

Status epilepticus describes a state of continuous seizures.

Drug treatment can control, but not cure, 60–90% of recurrences of seizures and treatment is therefore long term

The aim of drug treatment is to control seizures without producing adverse drug effects, but this is not always accomplished. Partial seizures are controlled in only approximately 45% of cases despite optimal medical treatment. The appropriate drug depends on the nature of the epilepsy (Table 8.15).

Table 8.15 Drugs used for epilepsy

Seizure type	Primary drugs	Secondary drugs
Partial and/or generalized tonic–clonic seizures	Carbamazepine, phenytoin	Phenobarbital, primidone, valproate
Absence seizures	Ethosuximide, valproate	Clonazepam
Myoclonic seizures	Valproate	Primidone

Treatment should always be initiated with a single drug and its use optimized before adding a second drug

Optimization of drug therapy usually involves increasing the dose of a single drug until toxicity appears. The incidence of adverse drug effects has been reported as 22% in patients on monotherapy, 34% for two antiepileptic drugs and 44% with three drugs. A single drug is therefore preferable.

The pharmacokinetic properties and adverse effects of an antiepileptic drug must be known to obtain its maximum therapeutic benefit. Monitoring of blood concentrations is useful with phenytoin in particular because of its zero-order pharmacokinetics and a relationship between its blood concentration, therapeutic and toxic effects (see Ch. 4).

The adverse effects of antiepileptic drugs must be considered when starting treatment because such drugs are used for extensive (even lifelong) periods. Drug interactions (see Ch. 4) with antiepileptic drugs are particularly important because:

- Antiepileptic drugs are used long term.
- There are small differences between therapeutic and potentially toxic blood concentrations for several antiepileptic drugs.

Antiepileptic drugs

BARBITURATES (PHENOBARBITAL AND PRIMIDONE)

Phenobarbital was the first effective antiepileptic drug, and despite the availability of newer drugs it is still useful against tonic–clonic seizures. It is also inexpensive. The antiepileptic dose is limited because phenobarbital produces sedation, but this lessens with continued use. Sometimes phenobarbital produces excitement instead of sedation in children. Primidone is a structural analog of phenobarbital and is converted to phenobarbital in the body.

The cellular mechanism of action of barbiturates probably involves synaptic inhibition by enhancing the effects of GABA. Phenobarbital and other barbiturates are suggested to act at $GABA_A$ receptors.

Not all barbiturates are used as antiepileptic drugs because of excess sedation at antiepileptic doses. It is not known why phenobarbital is less sedative.

Phenobarbital is an inducer of cytochrome P-450 and so it is involved in drug interactions (see Ch. 4). Its plasma half-life is 100 hours.

Phenytoin

Phenytoin (diphenylhydantoin) is used in the treatment of tonic–clonic seizures. At a molecular level it slows the rate of recovery of Na^+ channels from inactivation, thereby reducing neuron excitability. This may be responsible for its antiepileptic activity. The use of phenytoin is complicated by its characteristic toxicities, zero-order pharmacokinetics and the necessity for long-term administration. Zero-order pharmacokinetics implies that when blood concentrations of phenytoin approach those that will saturate the enzymes that metabolize phenytoin, a small increase in dose can cause a disproportionately large increase in plasma concentration with resulting toxicity. This can be partly prevented by measuring plasma phenytoin concentrations.

Adverse effects of phenytoin may be dose- or nondose-related:

- The dose-related adverse effects of phenytoin relate to the cerebellovestibular system – blurred vision, ataxia, hyperactivity and confusion. Gastrointestinal disturbances also occur.
- Other adverse effects include skin rashes, gingival hyperplasia, lymphadenomas and hirsutism. Phenytoin is also considered teratogenic.

DRUG INTERACTIONS Phenytoin is an enzyme inducer and is liable to produce drug interactions with isoniazid, warfarin, chloramphenicol, erythromycin and cimetidine.

Carbamazepine

Carbamazepine is chemically related to TCAs. Its antiepileptic activity is similar to that of phenytoin, but it is also used for pain such as with trigeminal neuralgia, and in the treatment of manic depressive illness. Like phenytoin, it blocks Na^+ channels and this may be involved in its antiepileptic activity. Serum concentrations of carbamazepine are not clearly related to its therapeutic effects.

Carbamazepine is an inducer of enzymes, including its own metabolizing enzymes. Its plasma half-life is therefore shortened by chronic administration.

Adverse effects of carbamazepine include drowsiness, vertigo and ataxia. It is probably as teratogenic as phenytoin.

Valproate sodium

Valproate sodium is useful in reducing the frequency of tonic–clonic and, particularly, absence seizures. Like phenytoin and carbamazepine it interacts with Na^+ channels. It also increases the GABA content of the brain when given long term. Blood concentrations of valproate sodium do not correlate well with therapeutic effects.

Adverse effects of valproate sodium include gastrointestinal upset and, more importantly, hepatic failure. Hepatic toxicity appears to be more common when valproate is used with another antiepileptic drug. Liver function tests do not predict subsequent liver toxicity.

Ethosuximide

Ethosuximide is the agent of choice for absence seizures. It is believed to act by inhibiting low-threshold Ca^{2+} currents (T-currents) in the thalamus, which is currently thought to be the origin of absence seizures. Plasma ethosuximide concentrations do not correlate well with therapeutic effectiveness.

Adverse effects of ethosuximide include gastrointestinal upset, drowsiness, lethargy, euphoria, urticarial skin lesions and, most importantly, leukopenia, and rarely bone marrow depression.

Benzodiazepines

Clonazepam is useful for absence and myoclonic seizures while diazepam and lorazepam are effective in the management of status epilepticus (continuous seizures). The benzodiazepines enhance GABA-induced increases in Cl^- conductance and this is probably involved in their antiepileptic activity.

The common adverse effect of the benzodiazepines is sedation. Since intravenous (i.v.) diazepam can depress respiration, resuscitation equipment should be available when treating status epilepticus. Repeated seizures can damage the brain and can be life-threatening, so status epilepticus should be controlled.

Newer antiepileptic drugs

The exact role of the newer antiepileptic drugs, gabapentin and lamotrigine, in the treatment of seizures remains to be defined.

GABAPENTIN Gabapentin is a highly lipid-soluble molecule and has been designed to mimic GABA in the CNS. It is useful add-on therapy for patients with partial seizures and is relatively free from adverse effects other than somnolence, dizziness and fatigue.

LAMOTRIGINE Lamotrigine is intended for use in partial seizures and acts on Na^+ channels. Reported adverse effects are dizziness, ataxia, blurred vision and gastrointestinal upset.

Lamotrigine is metabolized by glucuronidation in the liver, and concomitant administration of phenytoin, carbamazepine or phenobarbital decreases the serum half-life of lamotrigine from 24 to 15 hours, presumably by inducing increased hepatic glucuronidation of lamotrigine. In contrast, sodium valproate inhibits lamotrigine metabolism and increases the half-life of lamotrigine to 60 hours.

Other new antiepileptic drugs include the GABA receptor agonist zonisamide, although the exact mechanism of action of this drug in reducing seizures is not clear. It has a long plasma half-life (approx 15 hours) and the most commonly observed adverse effects include somnolence, anorexia, dizziness, headache, nausea and irritability. The Na^+ channel blocker oxcarbazepine has also recently been introduced for the treatment of epilepsy, as have fosphenytoin, the GABA uptake inhibitor tiagabine and levetiracetam, although the precise mechanism of action of the latter drug remains unidentified.

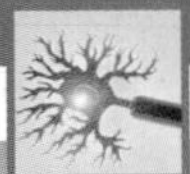

Sleep disorders

Normal sleep

Normal sleep is characterized by patterns of electrical activity that can be recorded on an EEG. On the basis of this record, sleep is separated into five stages. Stages 1–4 are periods of nonrapid eye movement (NREM) sleep, while stage 5 is the period of rapid eye movement (REM) sleep (Fig. 8.32).

- Stage 1 makes up 5% of total sleep and is the lightest sleep.
- Stage 2 makes up 45% of sleep and is characterized on the EEG by 'sleep spindle' waveforms.
- Stages 3 and 4 are the deepest stages of sleep and make up 12% and 13% of total sleep, respectively. These stages are often classified together on the basis of the EEG as slow-wave sleep or δ wave sleep.
- Stage 5 (REM) sleep makes up 25% of sleep and the EEG record shows low-voltage random saw-toothed waves.

The time between the onset of sleep and the initiation of the first portion of REM sleep is termed REM latency and is usually 90 minutes. NREM is a generally restful state with a regular low blood pressure and heart and respiratory rate. Restless movements are made during these stages and dreaming is lucid and purposeful. Body muscle tone is drastically reduced during REM sleep and the subject is still. However, the blood pressure, heart and respiratory rate are all raised, partial or full penile erections occur, and dreams are abstract and surreal.

The central control of sleep is complex and involves:

- Serotonergic neurons in the raphe nuclei.
- Noradrenergic neurons in the locus ceruleus.
- ACh-containing neurons within the pontine raphe nuclei, which have a central role in the production of REM sleep.

The sleep-wave pattern may be governed by melatonin secreted by the pineal gland, which is in turn controlled by the hypothalamus. It is hypothesized that sleep's on/off switch is situated in the hypothalamus as part of a neuronal circuit connecting the hypothalamus with the reticular activating system.

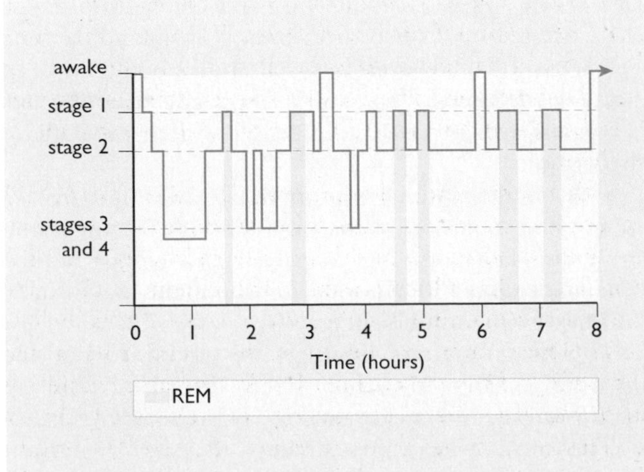

Fig. 8.32 A normal sleep cycle. This shows the normal stages of sleep (REM, rapid eye movement).

The normal length of sleep required by an adult is 6–9 hours per night. Deprivation of REM sleep causes irritability and lethargy and a subsequent rebound in REM sleep. Prolonged total sleep deprivation can lead to death.

A variety of sleep abnormalities have been noted in psychiatric illness:

- In depression there is a marked decrease in REM latency and an increase in REM sleep.
- Alzheimer's dementia leads to a decrease in REM and slow-wave sleep.

Various drugs alter sleep patterns:

- Benzodiazepines, and to a lesser extent antidepressants, reduce REM sleep.
- Drugs that increase dopamine release (e.g. amphetamine) increase wakefulness.

Insomnia

Insomnia is a common and non-specific disorder and may be reported by 40–50% of people at any given time. Of these cases:

- 30–35% are due to psychiatric illness.
- 15–20% are psychophysiologic or primary.
- 10–15% are due to alcohol or drugs.
- 10–15% are due to periodic limb movement disorder.
- 5–10% are due to sleep apnea.
- 5–10% are due to medical illness.

Among those seeking treatment, the female:male ratio is 2:1 with a preponderance of cases in lower socio-economic groups.

The prognosis, etiology and treatment of insomnia depend upon the underlying cause

A history should be taken to define the problem (e.g. initial or middle insomnia or early awakening). Is it due to a physical cause (e.g. pain or a cough)? Is it due to environmental factors such as noise?

In many cases, education in 'sleep hygiene' (e.g. reducing caffeine intake, changing sleep habits or pain relief) is more appropriate than a sedative drug. Early morning wakening is one of the biologic features of depression; an antidepressant might therefore be appropriate. Generally, treatment should be for the underlying cause. Insomnia without an obvious underlying cause is known as primary or psychophysiologic. Severe psychophysiologic (primary) insomnia is treated with hypnotics.

Hypnotics

Benzodiazepines

Benzodiazepines act by potentiating GABA-ergic neuro-transmission to enhance inhibitory activity.

Benzodiazepines induce sleep, and their duration of action is determined to some extent by their pharmacokinetics.

■ ***Benzodiazepines should be used as hypnotics only for severe, disabling or extremely distressing insomnia, and preferably for only 1 week***

Benzodiazepines should never be used as hypnotics for more than 3 weeks, and should not be used for chronic insomnia.

Other drugs for insomnia

Chloral hydrate is generally used only in the elderly. Zopiclone, zaleplon and zolpidem are nonbenzodiazepine hypnotics, but bind to particular subtypes of the benzodiazepine receptor. They are rapidly acting, with a short pharmacokinetic half-life of approximately 2 hours and minimal hangover effects. Long-term use is not recommended and they should not be used for more than 4 weeks.

Narcoleptic syndrome

The narcoleptic syndrome is a relative rare disorder that occurs in 20–160 adults per 100 000. It is excessive daytime sleepiness and cataplexy (a sudden loss of muscle tone in response to emotional stimuli such as laughter, pain and fear). Cataplexy affects the jaw, neck, legs or whole body, leading to collapse. Associated symptoms include sleep paralysis, which is an inability to move any muscles on awakening while apparently conscious. This occurs in 40% of narcoleptics and can last several minutes. Short-duration sleep paralysis lasting seconds can be a normal phenomenon, as can pre-sleep dreaming (sometimes called hypnagogic hallucinations), which occurs in 30% of people with narcolepsy.

Attacks of sleep can occur at any time of the day and cannot be avoided. They usually start in the late teens, and almost invariably before 30 years of age. The attacks may progress in severity and frequency, or reach a plateau. Spontaneous remission is rare.

The night-time sleep pattern is disrupted, with a markedly reduced REM latency and sleep-onset REM occurring within 10 minutes after the onset of sleep.

■ ***Narcolepsy is treated with CNS stimulants***

The first management strategy in narcolepsy is to encourage the patient to have regular daytime naps and sometimes this can almost abolish the sleep attacks. However, most patients require medication.

CNS stimulants used to treat narcolepsy

Methylphenidate hydrochloride and amphetamine

Both methylphenidate hydrochloride and amphetamine are indirectly acting sympathomimetics. Their primary effect is to cause the release of catecholamines from presynaptic neurons. They also inhibit catecholamine reuptake. These actions lead to stimulation of many adrenergic brain regions, including the ascending reticular activating system and the striatum.

Adverse effects of methylphenidate and amphetamine include anxiety, irritability, insomnia, dysphoria and increased blood pressure and heart rate. Long-term effects include a delusional disorder similar to schizophrenia. Overdose leads to psychosis, cardiovascular symptoms and seizures.

Modafinil

Modafinil is a centrally acting stimulant. It is an effective treatment of excessive daytime sleepiness (EDS). It may reduce attacks and improve performance in narcolepsy with a better adverse effect profile and less addictive potential than the sympathomimetics. Its mechanism of action is not clear, but it is as an agonist at α_1 adrenoceptors.

Other drugs used in the treatment of narcolepsy

These include:

- The MAO_B inhibitor selegiline.
- Anticholinergic drugs to treat cataplexy.
- SSRIs (e.g. fluoxetine) and SNRIs (e.g. venlafaxine) to improve cataplexy.
- Dopamine receptor antagonists (e.g. sodium oxybate).

Sleep apnea

This disorder has been recently recognized and is characterized by disturbed sleep at night and excessive daytime sleepiness. Its prevalence is not yet known, but it appears to be relatively common, particularly in the obese and the elderly. Periods of apnea are more likely and lengthened by alcohol.

There is little pharmacologic treatment at this time although modafinil may help in patients who do not respond to continuous positive airway pressure therapy.

Periodic limb movement disorder

Like sleep apnea, periodic limb movement disorder is characterized by disturbed night-time sleep and daytime sleepiness. It is, however, less well understood than sleep apnea or narcolepsy. Up to 30% of patients over 60 years of age and as many as 10% of people with insomnia have this disorder.

The night-time symptoms typically involve a stereotypic extension of the big toes with flexion of the ankle and knee, leading to partial awakening. If they occur more than 30 times during the night they usually lead to daytime somnolence.

The prognosis and etiology are unknown, but the disorder occurs in other sleep disorders, and in parkinsonism, and is worsened by TCAs and MAOIs.

The most effective treatments to date have been clobazam, clonazepam, selegiline (a MAO_B inhibitor, see above) and levodopa (the dopamine precursor used in Parkinson's disease).

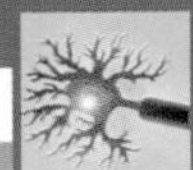

Circadian rhythm disorders

These are an important group of sleep disorders that affect most people at one time or another. The sufferer has by definition a sleep–wake cycle out of step with his or her environment, resulting in impaired social or occupational functioning.

The most common reasons for this disorder include:

- Shift working, and particularly reversing shifts to opposite sides of the day/night.
- Jet lag, in which the sufferer has traveled east or west across more than one time zone.
- Delayed sleep phase syndrome, which affects adolescents, particularly males. In this syndrome the sleep onset and awakening times steadily advance by 1–2 hours/day until the sufferer is out of synchrony with the environment.

Circadian rhythm disorders are usually self-limiting. However, re-establishment of a normal sleep–wake pattern with a hypnotic and with bright light exposure may be helpful. Melatonin is a hormone secreted by the pineal gland and is involved in the sleep–wake cycle experimentally. It is available over the counter and may have some uses in re-establishing a normal sleep–wake cycle in delayed sleep phase syndrome and jet lag.

Dementia

Dementia is defined as a global impairment of higher cortical functions, including memory, the capacity to solve the problems of day-to-day living, the performance of learned perceptual–motor skills (e.g. playing an instrument), the correct use of social skills, and control of emotional reactions, in the absence of gross clouding of consciousness. The condition is often irreversible and progressive. A short definition of dementia is 'an acquired global impairment of intellect, memory and personality, but without an impairment of consciousness.'

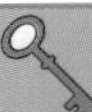

Common causes of dementia

- Alzheimer's disease
- Vascular (multi-infarct dementia)
- Pick's disease
- Dementia of parkinsonism
- Huntington's disease
- Creutzfeldt–Jakob disease

Senile dementia of the Alzheimer's type (Alzheimer's disease)

Alzheimer's disease (AD) is the most common cause of dementia, accounting for 50–60% of all cases. It is a senile and presenile (i.e. onset before 65 years of age) dementia with women affected twice as often as men after the age of 70, but equally at younger ages. The average duration of the disease is 5–10 years and is increasing as general health improves.

Signs of AD are progressive global memory loss, parietal lobe function abnormalities of spatial orientation, deteriorating social skills, loss of drive, initiative and intellect, depression, anxiety, aggression, emotional lability, unconcern, agitation and disruption of the sleep–wake cycle.

Drug treatments for Alzheimer's dementia target the cholinergic system and inflammation

Pharmacologic treatments for AD are still being developed and several approaches (Table 8.16) are in use:

- Combined NMDA antagonists and glutamate release inhibition (memantine hydrochloride).
- An ACh precursor such as lecithin choline, but while this has been shown to increase CNS ACh concentrations in the rat, there has been no demonstrable improvement in cognition in patients with AD.
- Drugs that enhance the release of ACh from rat cortical slices such as hydergine (ergoloid mesylates), but to date there have not yet been any trials of these drugs in humans.
- Cholinesterase inhibitors such as tacrine, donepezil, rivastigmine, galantamine and velnacrine, which are significantly better than placebo at increasing short-term memory, selective attention, language abilities and praxis functions in AD. However, the clinical benefits are generally quite modest with only about a 10% improvement.

Adverse effects of tacrine and velnacrine include abdominal cramps, nausea, polyuria and diarrhea. Serious adverse effects have been noted with tacrine, including a persistent rise in liver transaminases in 15–30% of patients, as well as severe liver toxicity. This is thought to be due to a mild drug-induced dose-dependent hepatic inflammation. The more recently introduced anticholinesterase inhibitors donepezil, rivastigmine and galantamine are better tolerated than tacrine and velnacrine but still exhibit side effects such as nausea, vomiting and diarrhea. These are worse at higher doses and during a rapid titration.

Table 8.16 Treatment strategies for Alzheimer's dementia

Strategy	Drug
Drugs that increase ACh concentrations in synapses or stimulate brain cholinergic receptors directly using a precursor	Lecithin
ACh release enhancers	Hydergine
Cholinesterase inhibitors	Tacrine, velnacrine, donepezil, rivastigmine, galantamine

Vascular dementia (multi-infarct dementia)

Multi-infarct dementia (MID) is traditionally thought to be the second most common dementia, and accounts for 15–30% of all cases of dementia. Although some experts believe that diffuse Lewy body disease is more common, this remains to be confirmed. MID can coexist with other degenerative dementias and this accounts for 15% of all dementias.

MID is more common in men and in people with a high risk of cardiovascular problems. The onset is usually relatively acute and the progression is typically stepwise as each infarct occurs. The site and extent of the infarcts determines the cognitive deficits. Neurologic signs are generally more common than in AD.

The typical clinical features of MID include an abrupt onset, emotional incontinence, stepwise deterioration, a history of hypertension, a fluctuating course, a history of strokes, nocturnal confusion, atherosclerosis, relative preservation of personality, depression, focal neurologic symptoms and signs, somatic complaints and patchy cognitive deficits.

Pharmacologic treatments for MID are based on attempts to reduce the risk of further cerebral infarction

Hypertension should be treated with appropriate antihypertensives (see Ch. 13), and any coexisting conditions that predispose to emboli formation (e.g. cardiac arrhythmias, cardiac valve disease) should be treated. Daily enteric-coated aspirin is indicated for any patient suspected of suffering from MID, because of its antithrombotic activity (see Ch. 10). If there are coexistent features of AD, a therapeutic trial of cholinergic medication (see above) may be prescribed.

Parkinson's disease

Parkinson's disease is a neurologic disorder characterized by impaired voluntary movements. Voluntary movements are controlled centrally by neuronal pathways that travel in the pyramidal (corticospinal) tracts from the motor cortex and down the spinal cord to the lower motor neurons (α motor neurons). The lower motor neurons directly control the activity of voluntary muscles. Although these are the main neuronal pathways, neuronal inputs from other sources also exert some influence on the pyramidal pathways. These subsidiary pathways provide the extrapyramidal influence, which smoothes voluntary movements. One major extrapyramidal source is the basal ganglia (caudate nucleus, putamen and pallidum), and disease of these structures (e.g. Parkinson's disease) affects the smooth execution of voluntary movements.

Parkinson's disease is characterized by the major symptoms of:

- Bradykinesia (i.e. slow initiation of movements).
- Tremor at rest involving the hands in 'pill-rolling' movements.
- Muscle rigidity, reflected as resistance to passive limb movements.
- Abnormal posture (Fig. 8.33).

The signs displayed by parkinsonian patients include:

- A characteristic shuffling gait.
- A blank facial expression.
- Speech impairment.
- An inability to perform skilled tasks.

The disease occurs more frequently in the elderly and gets progressively worse with time unless it is treated.

Parkinsonism is usually idiopathic, but can be induced by neuroleptics

Although there is usually no identifiable underlying cause of Parkinson's disease, it is associated with loss of dopaminergic neurons in the basal ganglia and it has been suggested that it may be caused by an environmental toxin. For example, in primates, 1-methyl-4-phenyl-1,2,3,6-tetrahydropyridine (MPTP), a chemical contaminant produced in the illegal synthesis of a heroin analog, causes irreversible damage to the nigrostriatal dopaminergic pathway and leads to the development of symptoms similar to idiopathic Parkinson's disease seen in humans. It appears that a metabolite (MPP^+) produced from MPTP by MAO_B is responsible, and MAO_B inhibitors (e.g. selegiline) can prevent the damage produced by MPTP.

Parkinsonism can be induced by drugs that block striatal dopaminergic receptors (e.g. neuroleptics such as chlorpromazine). Indeed, when such drugs are used in the treatment of schizophrenia, a parkinsonian-like syndrome can occur as an adverse effect. Similarly, drugs such as reserpine, which deplete the nigrostriatal nerves of dopamine, also produce a parkinsonian-like syndrome.

At postmortem, the brains of parkinsonian patients contain a substantially reduced concentration of dopamine (less than 10% of normal) in the corpus striatum and substantia nigra.

Striatal cholinergic hyperactivity is also associated with the development of Parkinson's disease. Usually, the activity of this neuronal pathway is opposed by the dopaminergic pathway that projects from the substantia nigra (Fig. 8.34).

Treatment of Parkinson's disease involves enhancing striatal dopaminergic activity and inhibiting striatal cholinergic muscarinic activity

Treatment of Parkinson's disease is based on correcting the imbalance at the basal ganglia between the dopaminergic and cholinergic systems. Two major groups of drugs are used:

- Drugs that increase dopaminergic activity between the substantia nigra and the corpus striatum.
- Drugs that inhibit striatal cholinergic muscarinic activity.

Tissues rich in dopamine (e.g. chromaffin cells from the adrenal medulla) have been surgically implanted into

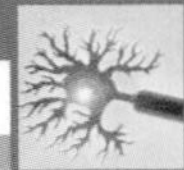

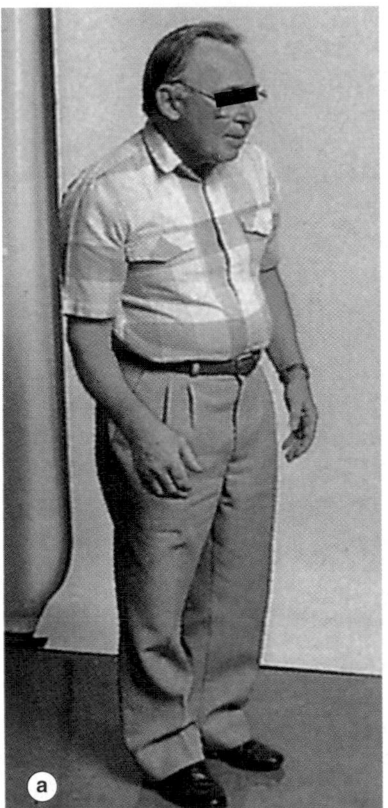

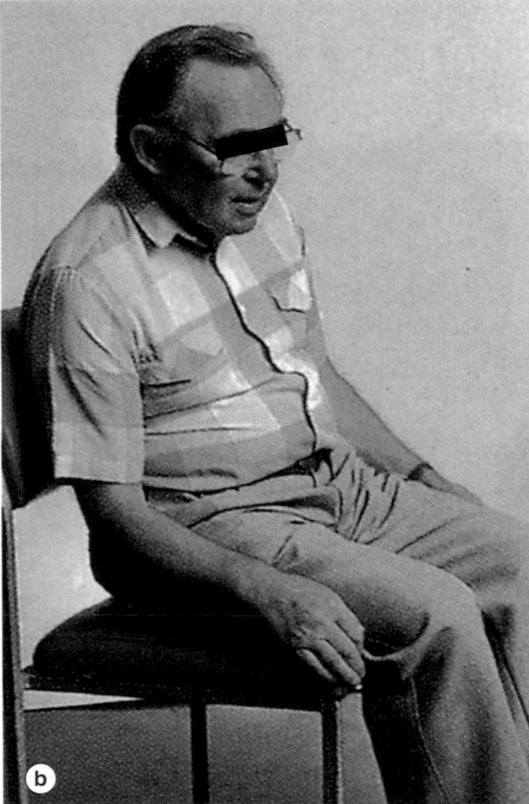

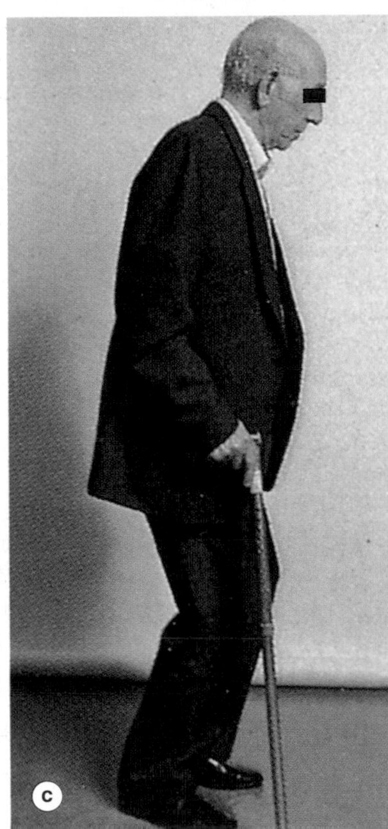

Fig. 8.33 Parkinson's disease. Posture and gait can give important clues to neurologic diagnosis. (Courtesy of Dr. R. Capildeo)

the corpus striatum to improve dopaminergic activity, but the clinical effectiveness of such procedures is uncertain. Gene therapy to increase striatal dopamine content by transfecting the tyrosine hydroxylase gene to the corpus striatum to enhance the rate of synthesis of dopamine has also been considered.

Drugs that increase dopaminergic activity

Levodopa (L-dopa)

Levodopa is used instead of dopamine (the latter does not cross the blood–brain barrier) to increase the dopamine content of the striatum. L-dopa is a precursor from which dopamine is produced by decarboxylation (Fig. 8.35). Levodopa crosses the blood–brain barrier, undergoes decarboxylation, and increases the content of releasable dopamine to oppose excessive striatal cholinergic activity and restores balance between the two systems.

Levodopa is rapidly absorbed from the small intestine by an active transport system for aromatic amino acids. Its absorption can be impaired by dietary aromatic amino acids, and by gastric juice hyperacidity, delayed gastric emptying and the presence of food. Peak plasma concentrations are reached 1–2 hours after an oral dose. The plasma half-life is only 1–3 hours, owing to extensive metabolism in the wall of the intestine (Fig. 8.36). Levodopa is also metabolized in the blood and peripheral tissues and only about 1% of the administered dose enters the brain. Dopamine is the major peripheral product of levodopa metabolism and it is responsible for most of the peripheral adverse effects of L-dopa. Other metabolic products include HVA and 3,4-dihydroxyphenylacetic acid (see Fig. 8.35). The extensive peripheral metabolism of levodopa means that large doses have to be given to produce therapeutic effects in the brain, but such doses produce many adverse effects (see below).

Peripheral adverse effects of levodopa can be reduced by combining it with a peripheral dopa decarboxylase inhibitor or by co-administering domperidone or selegiline

These effects can be reduced by combining levodopa with a peripheral dopa decarboxylase inhibitor such as carbidopa or benserazide. Both reduce the peripheral metabolism of levodopa so that it can be used at lower doses. Neither carbidopa nor benserazide cross the blood–brain barrier; consequently, they block levodopa metabolism only in the periphery. However, this drug combination not only maximizes the therapeutic effectiveness of levodopa but also increases the unwanted central effects of dopamine. Additionally, pyridoxine (vitamin B_6), which usually exacerbates peripheral metabolism of levodopa, does not interfere with the therapeutic effectiveness of the drug combination.

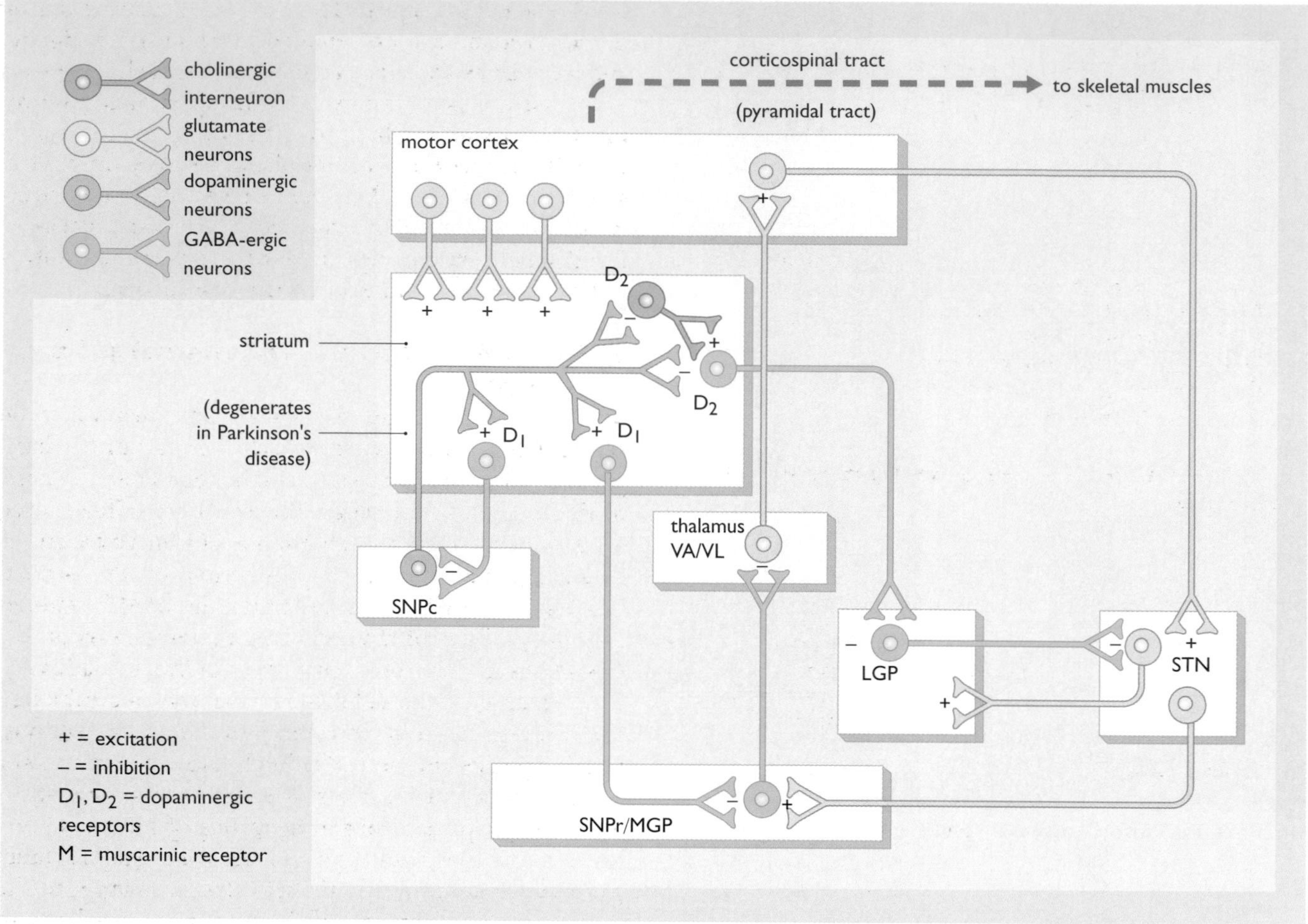

cholinergic interneuron
glutamate neurons
dopaminergic neurons
GABA-ergic neurons
corticospinal tract
(pyramidal tract)
to skeletal muscles
motor cortex
striatum
(degenerates in Parkinson's disease)
D_2
D_1
thalamus VA/VL
SNPc
LGP
STN
SNPr/MGP
+ = excitation
– = inhibition
D_1, D_2 = dopaminergic receptors
M = muscarinic receptor

Fig. 8.34 The basal ganglia systems involved in Parkinson's disease. In Parkinson's disease, inhibitory dopaminergic activity of the extrapyramidal pathway from the substantia nigra pars compacta (SNPc) to striatal GABA-ergic neurons is depleted (20–40%), usually through neurodegeneration. This results in unopposed cholinergic excitation of the striatal GABA-ergic neurons leading to the pathologic features of Parkinson's disease. Normally, two neuronal pathways from the basal ganglia regulate thalamic feedback input to the motor cortex for smooth execution of movement. Both pathways are activated by glutamate neurons from the motor cortex. The direct pathway consists of striatal GABA-ergic neurons which send inhibitory activity to the substantia nigra pars reticulata (SNPr) and the medial globus pallidus (MGP) leading to disinhibition of the output from these sites to the thalamus and thus allowing thalamic feedback input to the motor cortex. The indirect pathway also consists of another group of striatal GABA-ergic neurons which send inhibitory activity to the lateral globus pallidus (LGP), to prevent it from inhibiting excitatory neuronal output from the subthalamic nucleus (STN) to the SNPr and MGP. Excitation of the latter sites leads to inhibition of the thalamic feedback input to the motor cortex and interferes with the smooth execution of movement. The relative activity of these two pathways is regulated by dopaminergic neuronal activity from the SNPc to the striatum. ACh is found in interneurons that exist in the indirect pathway. VA and VL are ventroanterior and ventrolateral thalamic nuclei.

Some of the peripheral adverse effects of levodopa can also be decreased by co-administration of the dopaminergic D_2 antagonist domperidone, which does not cross the blood–brain barrier. Alternatively, selegiline, an MAOI that selectively blocks MAO_B, can be used to inhibit dopamine metabolism selectively in the brain. MAO_B is the predominant MAO isoform responsible for metabolizing dopamine in the brain (MAO_A predominates in the periphery). Unlike the nonselective MAOIs, selegiline does not inhibit the peripheral metabolism of tyramine and thereby induce the 'cheese reaction' (see above). Although selegiline is used mainly with levodopa to prolong and increase central dopaminergic effects, this drug can be used alone in the early stages of parkinsonism to slow the progressive loss of dopaminergic neurons in the basal ganglia.

Other therapeutic approaches to increasing central levodopa include catechol-*O*-methyl transferase (COMT) inhibitors (e.g. entacapone, tolcapone). These drugs prevent the metabolism of levodopa to 3-*O*-methyldopa. This effect is produced peripherally by both drugs and centrally by tolcapone, which crosses the blood–brain barrier.

EFFECTS OF LEVODOPA DURING TREATMENT When levodopa is first given, parkinsonian symptoms of rigidity,

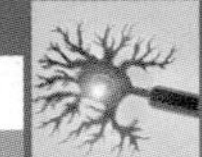

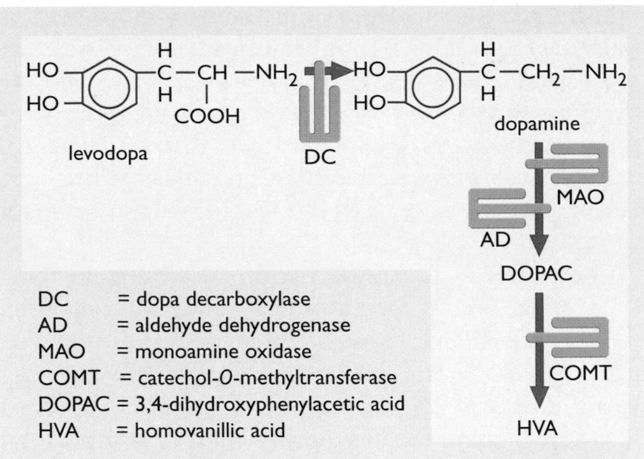

Fig. 8.35 Conversion of levodopa to dopamine and other metabolites.

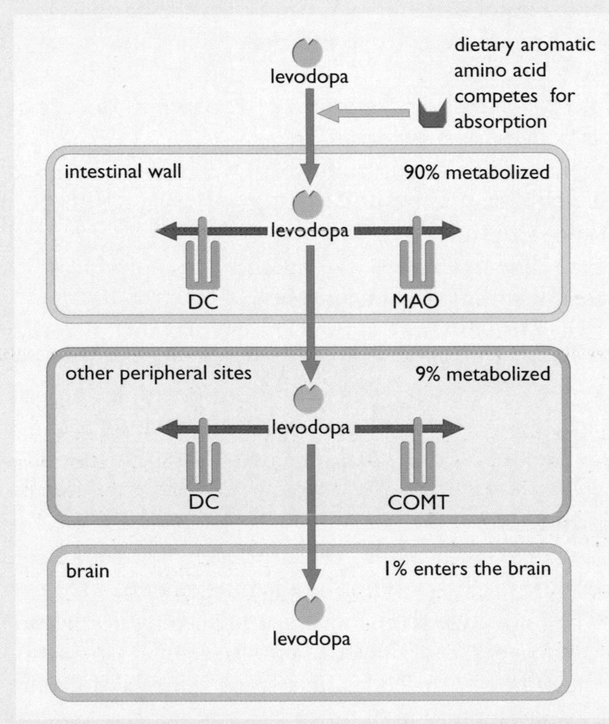

Fig. 8.36 Percentage of levodopa entering the brain after oral administration. There is extensive metabolism in the wall of the intestine by dopa decarboxylase (DC) and to a lesser extent by monoamine oxidase (MAO). Levodopa is also metabolized in blood and peripheral tissue by catechol-*O*-methyltransferase (COMT) and DC. The extent of peripheral metabolism is of the order of 99%, leaving only about 1% of the administered levodopa to enter the brain and produce therapeutic effects.

bradykinesia and motor functions, as well as facial expression, speech and handwriting, usually improve. However, its effectiveness decreases after several years of treatment, possibly due to a progressive loss of dopaminergic neurons with time.

The beneficial effects of levodopa can fluctuate during therapy, leading to a worsening of symptoms (e.g. rigidity and bradykinesia). This phenomenon, termed the 'on–off effect' (see below), results in difficulty initiating movement, even while walking or attempting to rise from a chair. The mechanism of this phenomenon is not understood, but it occurs when the plasma levodopa concentration is falling. More frequent, but lower, doses of levodopa may reduce its occurrence, as does the addition of bromocriptine with lower doses of levodopa.

The beneficial effects of levodopa are mainly through D_2 receptors

The D_2 receptors are distributed postsynaptically on striatal GABA-ergic neurons that form part of the basal ganglia indirect pathway which regulates thalamic feedback input to the motor cortex. At the cellular level, activation of D_2 receptors inhibits adenylyl cyclase and as a consequence decreases production of the second messenger, cAMP. This reduction in cAMP opposes excitatory effects of the cholinergic interneurons on the GABA-ergic neurons (of the indirect pathway). Consequently, these GABA-ergic neurons are inhibited and prevented from activating the indirect pathway, which opposes thalamic feedback input to the motor cortex. There is evidence that D_1 receptors are distributed postsynaptically on another group of striatal GABA-ergic neurons that form part of the basal ganglia direct pathway which facilitates thalamic feedback input to the motor cortex. Activation of these D_1 receptors leads to stimulation of adenylyl cyclase and increased cAMP that activates the basal ganglia direct pathway and as a consequence facilitates thalamic feedback input to the motor cortex (see Fig. 8.34).

As a result of these actions, dopamine re-establishes regulatory control on the neuronal output from the basal ganglia to the thalamus (see Fig. 8.34), which sends appropriate feedback nerve impulses to the motor cortex for smooth execution of movement and alleviation of the symptoms of Parkinson's disease.

Adverse effects of levodopa include:

- Nausea, vomiting and anorexia.
- Hypotension and cardiac arrhythmias.
- Abnormal involuntary movements (dyskinesias).
- The 'on–off' effect.
- Behavioral changes.

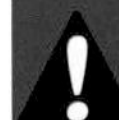

Adverse effects of levodopa

- **Involuntary movements**
- **'On–off' effect**
- **Nausea**
- **Hypotension**
- **Some cardiac arrhythmias**

Nausea, vomiting and anorexia result from stimulation of dopaminergic receptors in the chemoreceptor trigger zone of the area postrema. They are reduced by either domperidone or a dopa decarboxylase inhibitor (e.g. carbidopa) given with levodopa.

The cardiac effects of levodopa are usually tachycardia or extrasystoles, both due to increased catecholamine stimulation following the excessive peripheral metabolism of levodopa. Although the explanation for the hypotension is uncertain, there is evidence that central interference with sympathetic activity may be involved. However, the hypotension diminishes with continued levodopa treatment in many patients.

Dyskinesias develop after long-term treatment with levodopa. These involve mainly the face and limbs and are more common when levodopa is used in combination with a dopa decarboxylase inhibitor or when other measures are taken to increase central dopamine. The abnormal movements can be reduced by lowering the doses of levodopa and thereby reducing the central dopamine concentration, but rigidity may reappear.

The 'on–off' effect is manifested as rapid fluctuations in clinical features, varying from increased mobility and general improvement to increased rigidity and a general deterioration in the patient's ability to perform voluntary movements. This effect occurs suddenly and for short periods lasting from a few minutes to a few hours. At present, there is no cogent explanation for the effect, but similar worsening can occur when the plasma levodopa concentration falls (see above).

Behavioral changes include insomnia, confusion and other effects that are commonly seen in schizophrenia. Schizophrenia is attributed to increased dopaminergic activity in the mesolimbic area of the brain and can be controlled with a neuroleptic such as clozapine.

Another dopamine agonist, melevdopa, has also been introduced for the treatment of Parkinson's disease, as has the orally active D_3 receptor agonist pramipexole.

Bromocriptine

Bromocriptine is one of a group of drugs derived from ergot alkaloids that includes pergolide and lisuride maleate.

It is used in the treatment of Parkinson's disease as a dopamine agonist at D_2 receptors in the corpus striatum. However, it also activates other central D_2 receptor sites (e.g. in the anterior pituitary gland) and D_1 receptors. Members of the ergot alkaloid group can also be used in the treatment of hyperprolactinemia and to suppress growth hormone release in acromegaly (see Ch. 11).

Bromocriptine is often added to levodopa in the treatment of Parkinson's disease when levodopa alone does not adequately control the symptoms or when patients experience severe 'on–off' episodes. Usually, the combination consists of submaximal doses of levodopa and bromocriptine, but occasionally full doses of bromocriptine alone. Good results are obtained with both regimens and the incidence of involuntary movements is reduced. However, it has not been clearly established that bromocriptine is effective in patients who have become refractory to levodopa. The plasma half-life of bromocriptine (6–8 hours) is longer than that of levodopa, although peak plasma concentrations of both drugs are reached over the same period (1–3 hours) following oral administration.

Adverse effects of bromocriptine are similar to those of levodopa, except that in some patients hypotension can be severe enough to cause fainting, especially with the first dose. It is therefore recommended that before starting full treatment with bromocriptine patients should be tested for susceptibility to the hypotensive effect by using a 1 mg test dose of the drug after a meal and with the patient lying in bed. Other unwanted effects include visual and auditory hallucinations and erythromelalgia involving the feet and hands. Dyskinesia occurs much less frequently than with levodopa, perhaps because the agonist effect at the D_2 receptor in the striatum is greater than the partial agonist effect at the D_1 receptor at this site.

Pergolide relieves symptoms of Parkinson's disease as effectively as bromocriptine

Both pergolide and lisuride are D_2 agonists. Pergolide relieves the symptoms of Parkinson's disease as effectively as bromocriptine.

Pergolide is also a D_1 agonist that produces less nausea, vomiting and hypotension.

Other recently introduced D_2 agonists include cabergoline (an ergot derivative), ropinirole and pramipexole. They are recommended in combination with levodopa to reduce 'on–off' effects, and motor fluctuations, and to allow the use of lower maintenance doses of levodopa.

Amantadine

Amantadine is used in the treatment of Parkinson's disease. It increases central dopamine release. However, it is less effective than the dopamine receptor agonists, possibly because of its different mechanism of action, which is thought to be facilitation of neuronal dopamine release and inhibition of its uptake into nerves. A modest anticholinergic effect may also contribute to its therapeutic effectiveness. However, based on its dopaminergic mechanism of action, it is expected that the effectiveness of amantadine would be brief, since there is progressive degeneration of the nigrostriatal dopaminergic neurons through which amantadine produces its therapeutic effects in Parkinson's disease. Amantadine is therefore only of short-term benefit, since most of its effectiveness is lost within 6 months of initiating treatment. Nevertheless, addition of amantadine to the levodopa regimen leads to synergistic effects and improvements in therapy.

Amantadine is usually given orally and is well absorbed from the gastrointestinal tract. Its plasma half-life is 2–4 hours, but it accumulates during renal impairment since it is excreted unchanged in the urine.

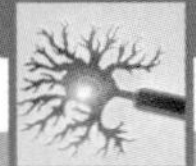

Adverse effects of amantadine are similar to, but less severe than, those of levodopa. They include hallucinations, confusion, nightmares and anorexia. Prolonged use of amantadine may lead to development of livedo reticularis believed to be due to catecholamine-induced vasoconstriction in the lower extremities.

Drug therapy of parkinsonism

- Drugs are used to restore nigrostriatal dopaminergic activity or to inhibit striatal cholinergic overactivity
- Levodopa (L-dopa), a precursor of dopamine, is the major drug used. It can cross the blood–brain barrier and is converted to dopamine centrally
- The effectiveness of levodopa lasts for only about 2 years because its central conversion to dopamine gradually diminishes, owing to progressive degeneration of the dopaminergic neurons
- The therapeutic benefits of levodopa are maximized by giving it in combination with a peripheral dopa decarboxylase inhibitor (e.g. carbidopa) or a selective monoamine oxidase-B (MAO_B) inhibitor (e.g. selegiline) or a catechol-*O*-methyltransferase (COMT) inhibitor
- Peripheral adverse effects of levodopa can be prevented by combining it with domperidone, a peripheral dopamine antagonist
- Bromocriptine (a dopamine agonist), amantadine (which increases dopamine release) and the anticholinergic drugs (e.g. trihexyphenidyl hydrochloride and benztropine mesylate) are also used to treat Parkinson's disease
- The anticholinergic drugs are more effective in controlling tremor than other symptoms of the disease

Drugs that inhibit striatal cholinergic activity

Inhibition of striatal cholinergic activity is useful for treating Parkinson's disease. The drugs most commonly used are muscarinic antagonists since striatal cholinergic excitation opposes dopaminergic inhibition of striatal GABA-ergic nerve activity (see Fig. 8.34). Their major function in the treatment of Parkinson's disease is to reduce the excessive striatal cholinergic activity that characterizes the disease.

The prototype of this group of drugs is trihexyphenidyl hydrochloride. Others include benztropine mesylate, biperiden, orphenadrine hydrochloride (which is also an H_1 receptor antagonist) and procyclidine hydrochloride. As a group, their therapeutic effectiveness is less than levodopa, and tremor is reduced more than the rigidity and bradykinesia. They also reduce the excessive salivation associated with Parkinson's disease. These drugs are given orally. There is no major difference in the therapeutic effectiveness among members of the group.

The expected peripheral anticholinergic adverse effects (i.e. dry mouth, blurred vision, urinary retention and constipation) are common. More often, patients experience a variety of CNS adverse effects, including mental confusion, delusions, hallucinations, drowsiness and mood changes. Since parkinsonism can worsen when these drugs are discontinued, any termination of treatment should be gradual.

Huntington's disease

Like Parkinson's disease, Huntington's disease is a movement disorder associated with defects in the basal ganglia and related structures. However, unlike Parkinson's disease, it is a hyperkinetic disorder characterized by excessive and abnormal movements. The movements are involuntary, irregular and jerky; different groups of muscles of the face, trunk and neck are involved. The disorder is also characterized by progressive dementia.

Huntington's disease is hereditary and often appears during adult life. The symptoms are associated with biochemical defects in the basal ganglia that in many ways are the mirror image of the defects in Parkinson's disease. For example, increased concentrations of dopamine are found in the putamen of patients with Huntington's disease at postmortem. Reduced glutamic acid decarboxylase (an enzyme that synthesizes GABA) and choline acetyltransferase activities correlate with the production of deficient levels of GABA and ACh in the basal ganglia. It is thought that these deficiencies reduce the inhibitory influence (via striatal GABA neurons) on the nigrostriatal dopaminergic neurons (see Fig. 8.34) and lead to the dopaminergic hyperactivity associated with Huntington's disease. Further evidence for this pathophysiologic process is provided by the observations that the symptoms of Huntington's disease are suppressed by drugs that block dopamine receptors and worsened by drugs that increase basal ganglia dopaminergic activity.

Treatment of Huntington's disease involves the use of drugs to reduce basal ganglia dopaminergic activity

Drugs that deplete central dopamine stores by blocking entry into the neuronal storage vesicles include reserpine (given in small doses of 0.25 mg daily; no longer used in the UK) and tetrabenazine. The adverse effects of these drugs include hypotension, depression, sedation and gastrointestinal disturbances. These effects occur less frequently with tetrabenazine than with reserpine.

Drugs that reduce dopaminergic activity by blocking the receptors include phenothiazines (e.g. perphenazine) and butyrophenones (e.g. haloperidol), which are neuroleptics. The major adverse effects associated with their use include restlessness and parkinsonism.

Migraine and headache

Migraine is a common condition affecting 5% of men and 15% of women. It is a familial disorder in which two major syndromes have been identified: firstly, classic migraine (migraine with aura); secondly, common migraine (migraine without aura). Migraine is characterized by periodic, often unilateral pounding pulsatile headaches, that often begin in childhood. It is exacerbated by physical activity and/or emotional stress. Accompanying symptoms include phonophobia, photophobia, nausea and vomiting. The classic view of migraine is that it results from complex vascular factors, in particular distention and excessive pulsation of branches of the external carotid artery.

The treatment of migraine has two goals: treatment of acute attacks, and prophylaxis of future attacks.

Treatment of an acute attack should be initiated during the neurologic (visual) prodrome, or if this is absent, at the very start of the headache. Treatment of mild to moderate headaches is with an NSAID, acetaminophen or propoxyphene. Codeine or oxycodone can be combined with aspirin or acetaminophen, caffeine and butalbital, but only for short periods since the combination can cause dependence. For severe attacks, ergot alkaloids (ergotamine tartrate or dihydroergotamine; DHE) are used. Ergotamine is an a adrenergic agonist with affinity for 5-HT_1, receptors, stimulation of which leads to vasoconstriction. These drugs are administered subcutaneously or intramuscularly and re-administered 30–60 minutes later if necessary. Ergotamine is contraindicated in patients with coronary artery or peripheral vascular disease. A single dose of the H_1 receptor antagonist promethazine or the dopamine agonist metoclopramide helps relax the patient and reduce the nausea and vomiting. A single dose of sumatriptan, a highly selective 5-HT_{1D} agonist is effective in the treatment of migraine. It is well tolerated and administered orally (100 mg), although it is not as effective as when administered subcutaneously. Sumatriptan is not used for prophylaxis. Other 5-HT_{1D} agonists used to treat migraine include zolmitriptan (which can also be administered as a nasal spray), naratriptan, almotriptan, rizatriptan, eletriptan and frovatriptan. Further details about these drugs are given in Chapter 9.

In patients with frequent migraine attacks, efforts at prophylactic prevention are important and considerable success has been obtained with the β adrenoceptor antagonists propranolol or altenolol. In patients who do not tolerate these drugs, a calcium channel blocker such as verapamil or nifedipine can be used. The monoamine oxidise inhibitor phenelzine is sometimes useful. Methysergide can also be used to prevent migraine attacks, as can the NSAIDs ketoprofen and tolfenamic acid.

Cluster headaches are another type of headache having a characteristic 'cluster pattern' which occur predominantly in young adult men. Cluster headache is usually treated with a single dose of ergotamine. Subcutaneous DHE or sumatriptan can also be used.

STROKE

Stroke is one of the leading causes of death in the Western world and may be the most important disease causing long-term disability. The management of strokes has changed considerably as it is now possible to intervene and ameliorate neurologic deficits in many patients if treatment is initiated quickly after symptoms develop. In view of these developments, stroke needs to be viewed in the same context as acute myocardial infarction where public education has influenced people to go quickly to emergency medical departments.

The initial diagnosis of stroke is primarily clinical and will not be discussed here. The major distinction between ischemic and hemorrhagic stroke must be made quickly as the early treatment and therapies aimed at secondary prevention are quite different for these two disorders. Computed tomography (CT) of the brain, or possibly magnetic resonance imaging (MRI) in some cases, may be the most useful way to make this demarcation even if the clinical presentation seems straightforward. Ischemic stroke is usually caused by occlusion of a cerebral artery. The clinical deficits found in the early stage of ischemic stroke are due to the local death of neuronal cell function; at this stage, the loss of function may be reversible if cerebral blood flow can be restored. The time window for this opportunity is not clear. Once this is exceeded, the damage will progress to an irreversible stage associated with neuronal cell death. Thrombolytic therapy is appropriate in many patients with ischemic stroke whereas it is contraindicated in patients with hemorrhages.

Thrombolytic therapy for acute strokes

Systematic reviews of many controlled trials have demonstrated benefit from thrombolytic therapy, especially in decreasing neurologic deficits and dependency when evaluated after 3–6 months. Although thrombolytic therapy with tissue plasminogen activator (TPA), streptokinase or urokinase can cause intracranial bleeding, the efficacy more than outweighs this risk. Moreover, for patients with an ischemic stroke treated within 3 hours of onset, the risk of intracranial bleeding is less and the benefits are greater. These results of clinical trials highlight the importance of emergency treatment of ischemic stroke. While further information is necessary in order to characterize the use of TPA in patients with concomitant diseases such as diabetes and hypertension, current evidence favors implementing TPA therapy at an early time. This therapy is generally contraindicated in patients taking anticoagulants or having clotting disorders or low platelet counts. The use of TPA in thrombotic states is described in Chapter 10.

There may be a small benefit in using aspirin in the early phases of acute stroke. The potential benefits of anticoagulants during acute stroke are not established.

Stroke prophylaxis

Aspirin has a well-established benefit in preventing stroke, especially in patients who have had a transient ischemic attack (TIA) or have carotid atherosclerosis.

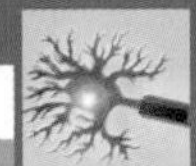

Aspirin and other antiplatelet drugs are discussed in Chapter 10.

Anticoagulation with warfarin has established benefit in preventing stroke in patients with atrial fibrillation. The use and therapeutic monitoring of warfarin is discussed in Chapter 10.

DRUGS AND INFECTIONS OF THE CENTRAL NERVOUS SYSTEM

Infections occur in every part of the CNS and include:

- Meningitis (inflammation of the meninges).
- Radiculitis (inflammation of the spinal nerve roots).
- Myelitis (inflammation of the spinal cord).
- Encephalitis (inflammation of the brain).
- Brain abscess (a localized collection of pus).

In addition, new imaging techniques such as MRI have revealed that many regions of the CNS show dynamic fluctuating inflammatory processes in currently unnamed CNS syndromes. The cause of these lesions is unknown, but could be a virus or other infectious agent.

The CNS is protected by the skull, spinal column and meningeal membranes, but infectious agents gain access:

- Through any breach in the CNS protection (e.g. a skull fracture).
- Via the blood (e.g. septicemia with subsequent abscess formation).
- Via the nerves (e.g. rabies virus).
- By uncertain means (e.g. herpes simplex virus; HSV).

The local immune response of the CNS to infection varies with site and infecting organism. The degree and nature of the tissue response to different microbial agents is therefore quite diverse.

Organisms that infect the CNS range from helminthic parasites (e.g. *Trichinella spiralis*, a nematode), to fungi and bacteria (e.g. *Coccidioides immitis* and *Mycobacterium tuberculosis*), to viruses (e.g. HSV) and subviral proteins (e.g. prions in Creutzfeldt–Jakob disease and bovine spongiform encephalitis; BSE).

Diagnosis of CNS infection is based on the patient's history, physical examination and laboratory tests

Signs and symptoms vary and depend on the site affected. They include fever, irritability to the extent of convulsions, altered mentation, altered motor function, and lassitude, drowsiness, or coma. Abscesses and parasitic cysts, as space-occupying lesions, can produce symptoms and signs resulting from pressure on, or destruction of, adjacent structures (e.g. visual field defects due to pressure on, or destruction of, the optic nerve).

Examination of the CSF can be helpful:

- An increased initial pressure and an increased concentration of CSF protein suggests infection.
- Microscopy reveals increased leukocytes (bacterial infection), increased lymphocytes (viral infection) or increased eosinophils (parasitic infection).
- A Gram stain may demonstrate meningococcus (*Neisseria meningitidis*) or *Streptococcus pneumoniae* and India-ink staining reveals some fungal infections.
- Biochemical examination may reveal the presence of viruses or parasites or their corresponding antibodies.
- Special CNS scanning techniques such as computerized axial tomography (CAT) or MRI also help in the diagnosis, especially of an abscess or other space-occupying lesion.

Whenever bacteria enter the bloodstream (septicemia) there is a possibility that a cerebral abscess will develop. Although rare, this can occur after staphylococcal skin infections.

Encephalitis can occur without inflammation of the meninges and vice versa, but they often occur together. Meningeal irritation is due to either an infection or the presence of an inflammation-inducing substance in the CSF (e.g. blood). The particular symptoms and signs of meningeal irritation are:

- A stiff neck.
- Pain on neck flexion.
- Pain accompanying limitation of passive straight leg raising.

These physical findings should always lead to further investigations.

Use of drugs to control or eliminate CNS infections

The responsible organism must be identified and the drug most likely to be selectively toxic to the invading organism chosen. This drug must reach the site of infection at adequate concentrations. It must therefore cross the blood–brain barrier at an adequate rate and there have access to the infected site (i.e. abscesses must be surgically treated in addition to any pharmacologic treatment).

Drugs are also used in CNS infections to control responses to infection

Such responses include seizures, treated with antiepileptic drugs, and allergic and other immunologic responses treated with glucocorticosteroids (see Ch. 11).

Antibiotics and antiviral agents do not readily penetrate into the CNS

The relative concentration of penicillin G in the CSF compared with that in the serum is 5%, ampicillin 15%, nafcillin 5%, vancomycin 10%, chloramphenicol 30%, gentamicin 20%, cefotaxime 15%, ceftriaxone 5% and ceftazidime 20%. Antibiotics and antivirals are discussed in more details in Chapter 6.

The question of whether antibiotics should be given directly into the CSF has not been satisfactorily answered, but the mortality rate of children with meningitis due to Gram-negative bacilli increases when gentamicin is injected into the cerebral ventricles. This suggests that injecting antibiotics into the CSF carries considerable risk.

Viral meningitis and encephalitis

Almost any virus can cause encephalitis (accompanied by varying degrees of meningeal inflammation), including rubeola or mumps virus, a variety of herpes viruses, HSV types 1 and 2, Epstein–Barr virus (EBV), cytomegalovirus (CMV), varicella-zoster virus (VZV), Coxsackie virus and human immunodeficiency virus (HIV) (see Ch. 6).

Treatment involves the use of the appropriate antiviral drug, if such exists, and i.v. administration of drug is almost always required:

- Acyclovir is the drug of choice for treating encephalitis due to HSV-1. Its use has reduced the mortality rate from 80% to 20%.
- Ara-A or foscarnet is used for acyclovir-resistant HSV-1 encephalitis.
- Sorivudine is selective for VZV infections.
- Ganciclovir is useful for CMV encephalitis, but is used with care because of bone marrow toxicity and, since it is excreted primarily by the kidneys, renal function should be monitored.

The treatment of cerebral disease in patients with HIV is evolving and involves decisions as to whether HIV or some other agent is causing the problem (see fungal and parasitic infections below).

Several viruses that cause encephalitis (e.g. the virus causing eastern equine encephalitis) are not susceptible to antiviral drugs.

Bacterial meningitis and encephalitis

The bacterium most likely to produce meningitis varies with the age of the patient. The commonest causal bacteria of meningitis are:

- Gram-negative bacilli and group B streptococci in neonates less than 1 month old.
- *Haemophilus influenzae*, *N. meningitidis* and *S. pneumoniae* in children aged 1 month to 15 years.
- *N. meningitidis*, *S. pneumoniae* and staphylococci in adults (i.e. those over 15 years of age).

Bacterial CNS infections must be diagnosed as soon as possible so that specific antibiotics can be used. The CSF should be cultured to identify bacteria with appropriate antibiotic sensitivity tests.

If the etiology of a CNS infection is unknown but believed to be bacterial, the initial antibiotics listed in Table 8.17 are used. If the bacterial etiology is known, the currently recommended antibiotics of choice for beginning therapy are used (Table 8.18).

CNS tuberculosis and syphilis

Mycobacterium tuberculosis and *Treponema pallidum*, the cause of tuberculosis and syphilis, respectively, are important causes of CNS infections.

M. tuberculosis can infect the CNS and cause meningitis, tuberculous abscesses or widespread miliary tuberculosis in the brain and spinal cord. All these are serious diseases and require appropriate antibiotics (see Ch. 6).

Table 8.17 Initial antibiotic therapy for meningitis or encephalitis if the etiology is unknown but believed to be bacterial

Patient group	Antibiotics
Neonates less than 1 month old	Ampicillin plus either gentamicin or ceftriaxone or cefotaxime
Children aged 1 month to 15 years	Ampicillin plus either chloramphenicol or ceftriaxone or cefotaxime
Adults (i.e. those over 15 years of age)	Ampicillin or penicillin G
Immunocompromised adults	Ampicillin plus ceftriaxone or cefotaxime plus gentamicin
Postcraniotomy patients	Nafcillin plus ceftriaxone or cefotaxime plus gentamicin

Table 8.18 Currently recommended initial antibiotic therapy for bacterial meningitis or encephalitis if the bacterial etiology is known

Bacterial cause	Antibiotic
S. pneumoniae, streptococcus A and B, *Listeria monocytogenes*, *N. meningitidis*	Penicillin G
H. influenzae (β lactamase negative)	Ampicillin
Methicillin-sensitive *Staphylococcus aureus*	Nafcillin
Methicillin-resistant *S. aureus*	Vancomycin
H. influenzae (β lactamase positive)	Cefotaxime or ceftriaxone
Escherichia coli, *Klebsiella*, and *Proteus*	Cefotaxime or ceftriaxone with gentamicin
Pseudomonas aeruginosa	Gentamicin plus ceftazidime

Syphilitic meningitis and neurosyphilis are manifestations of infection with *T. pallidum* during secondary and tertiary syphilis. Neurosyphilis is often accompanied by changes in mental status and can be mistaken for other forms of mental illness. During tertiary syphilis, syphilitic gummas (areas of focal degeneration of brain tissue similar to abscesses) may form in the CNS. All stages of syphilis should be treated with penicillin as soon as they are diagnosed; even gummas are reduced by penicillin treatment.

Fungal CNS infections

Various fungi can cause meningitis and/or focal lesions in the brain and spinal cord, particularly in immunocompromised patients (e.g. in people with AIDS or those on anticancer or immunosuppressant drugs). Such fungi include *C. immitis* and *Histoplasma capsulatum* (see Ch. 6). These organisms resemble *M. tuberculosis* in that they are inhaled, and the resulting disease usually involves the lungs, but may involve the CNS. The CSF contains complement-fixing antibody in 95% of cases of

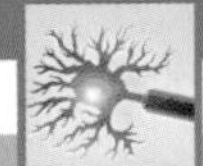

coccidioidomycosis, and the demonstration of such antibodies justifies starting antifungal therapy. In approximately 50% of cases *C. immitis* can be found on microscopic examination of CSF. Complement-fixing antibodies are less common in histoplasmosis and its diagnosis depends on isolating *H. capsulatum* in culture.

Treatment of both coccidioidomycosis and histoplasmosis is difficult, but centers on amphotericin B.

Protozoal CNS infections

MALARIA Worldwide, cerebral malaria resulting from infection by *Plasmodium falciparum* (see Ch. 6) is probably the most serious and common CNS infection. There are approximately two million deaths due to malaria each year. African children with cerebral malaria account for about half a million of these deaths. The death rate of cerebral malaria is approximately 20% despite the best current treatment, which involves i.v. quinine (or quinidine) or *Artemisia* derivatives such as artemether.

TOXOPLASMOSIS CNS infections with *Toxoplasma gondii* can occur in immunosuppressed patients. If immunosuppression has a cause other than AIDS, 2–5% of CNS infections are due to this agent, but in patients with AIDS, the incidence rises to 25–80%. In these conditions, there are often cerebral lesions, which are best detected by MRI. Motor weakness, hemiparesis and convulsions can occur, depending on the location of the lesions.

The drugs of choice for treating toxoplasmosis are pyrimethamine plus a sulfonamide. However, bone marrow depression due to the antifolate activity of pyrimethamine can be a problem. Another antifolate trimethoprim is of little value in this disease. The macrolide antibiotic clarithromycin may be of use.

Helminthic CNS infections

Three helminths can infect the CNS: *Trichinella spiralis*, *Taenia solium* and *Echninococcus granulosis*. The first two are ingested in infected inadequately cooked pork or game (e.g. bear). *E. granulosis* is harbored by dogs and the eggs are excreted in the feces from where they can then be ingested by humans. Once in the intestine, all three parasites can be transported in the blood to the brain where they produce space-occupying cerebral lesions shown by CAT or MRI scans. The neurologic signs they produce will depend on the location of the lesions.

Trichinosis involving the CNS is definitively diagnosed by identifying the larvae in the CSF. It is usually treated with prednisone to suppress the CNS immune response to the nematode, which is often accompanied by marked eosinophilia in the CSF. Mebendazole is given to suppress the parasite.

T. solium cysticerci (larvae) develop in the brain. The definitive diagnosis is obtained by biopsy of one of the cystic lesions. Drug treatment involves glucocorticosteroids to suppress immune responses, plus albendazole or praziquantel.

Echinocollal cysts usually develop in the liver or lungs but, if they rupture, eggs can then be carried to the brain, where new cystic lesions develop. Such cysts are often detected by CAT or MRI scan. Surgical removal of the cyst is the definitive therapy, but the cyst must not be ruptured, otherwise eggs will be spread elsewhere by the blood. Giving albendazole during the surgery may reduce the risk of spreading the infection.

Multiple sclerosis

Multiple sclerosis is a chronic inflammatory condition of the CNS. Interferon β has been shown to reduce the severity and frequency of relapses. It is administered once daily or on alternate days by injection, but can produce 'flu-like' adverse effects such as chills and muscle ache. Recently, glatiramer acetate has been introduced to treat relapses of multiple sclerosis, which is thought to act by an agonist action at IL-4, IL-6 and IL-10 receptors. Additionally, a number of α_4 integrin antagonists such as natalizumab are in later-stage clinical development for the treatment of multiple sclerosis (Fig. 8.37). However, while this pharmacologic approach appears to show promise, trials with natalizumab have been stopped due to a number of fatalities from a rare leukoencephalopathy.

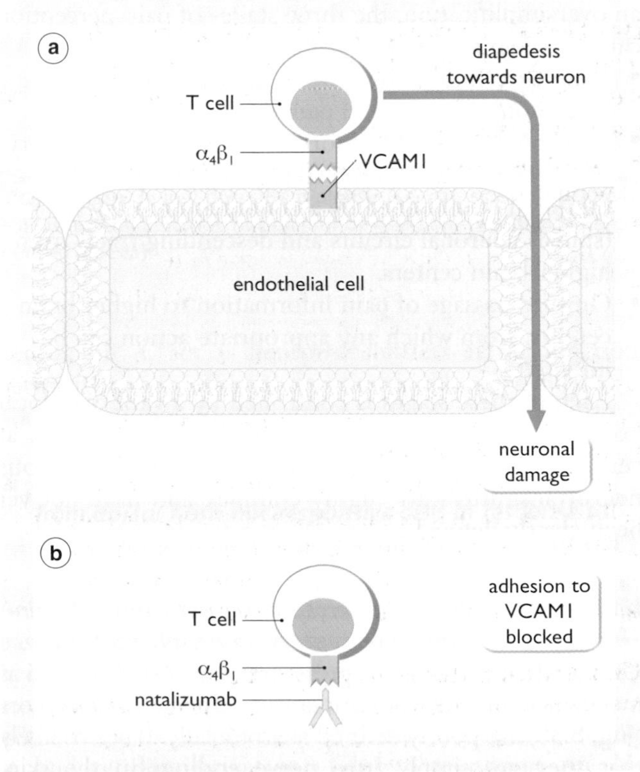

Fig. 8.37. Multiple sclerosis (a) The $\alpha_4\beta_1$ integrin binding to the VCAM1 adhesion molecule, which triggers T-cell diapedesis and consequently autoimmune damage to the underlying neuron. (b) The antibody natalizumab is shown binding to $\alpha_4\beta_1$ thereby blocking T-cell adhesion and the cascade leading to autoimmune neuronal damage and progression of multiple sclerosis.

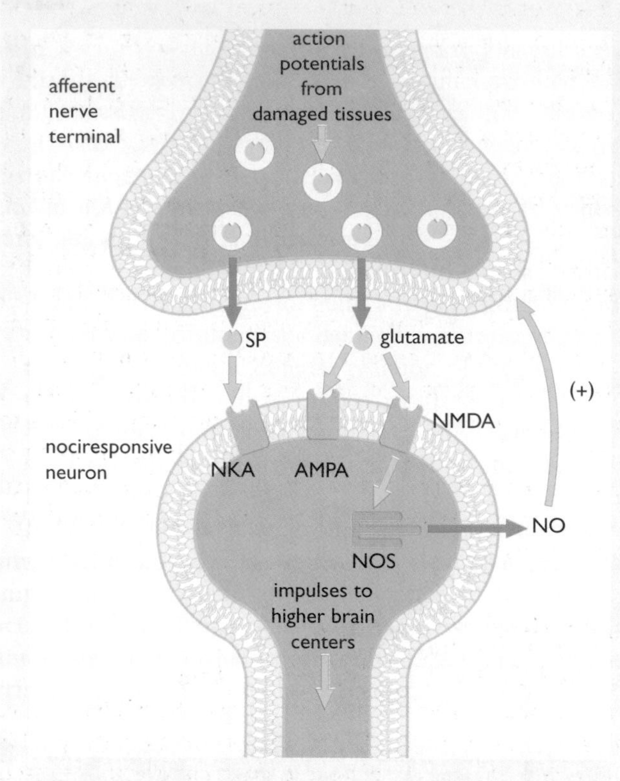

Fig. 8.40 Mechanism of pain perception. Activation of peripheral nociceptors in damaged, diseased, or inflamed tissues by a range of algesic and hyperalgesic chemical mediators stimulates Aδ and C sensory afferent nerves, which terminate in the superficial laminae (I and II) and lamina V of the spinal cord. Nitric oxide (NO) is the retrograde transmitter, increasing substance P (SP) and glutamate release to cause 'wind up' (AMPA, 2-amino-3, 3-hydroxy-5-methylisooxazol-4-yl propionic acid; NKA, neurokinin A; NMDA, *N*-methyl-D-aspartate receptors; NOS, nitric oxide synthase).

An additional important role for glutamate acting on NMDA receptors located on the spinal nociresponsive neurons is in the induction of spinal 'wind up.' 'Wind up' is an electrophysiologic phenomenon analogous to 'long-term potentiation' in other brain areas. It can be defined as an increase in amplitude of membrane depolarization in spinal nociresponsive neurons, following repetitive stimulation of their C fiber input by painful stimuli applied to a peripheral tissue. 'Wind up' might account for why pain (e.g. inadvertently hitting a thumb with a hammer) not only provokes instantaneous pain (carried by Aδ fibers) but also causes a dull and throbbing painful sensation in the damaged region minutes or even hours later. Such secondary pain reaction is triggered by the formation of proinflammatory algesic mediators such as BK and histamine in the damaged tissue, in this case the thumb. As inflammation occurs, the resulting activation of nociceptors results in a barrage of impulses along sensory C fibers, gradually 'winding up' nociresponsive neurons in the spinal cord. Ultimately, a situation is reached where normally innocuous stimuli, such as lightly brushing the thumb, or applying an adhesive plaster, can cause tenderness and pain (i.e. hyperalgesia). Spinal 'wind up' may explain why acute pain sometimes converts to chronic pain spontaneously and for no good physiologic reason. The cellular mechanism of this 'wind up' is now believed to involve the following steps:

- Activation of NMDA receptors by glutamate, either on the nociresponsive neuron itself or on adjacent neurons.
- Opening of NMDA-linked Ca^{2+} channels in these neurons.
- Activation of Ca^{2+}–calmodulin-dependent nitric oxide synthase (NOS) to yield nitric oxide (NO).

NO is a freely diffusible and highly lipid-soluble mediator and rapidly passes retrogradely to the primary afferent nerve terminal to increase efflux of glutamate (and perhaps also substance P). In this way, the initial release of even a very small amount of glutamate from sensory C fiber terminals is able to trigger the efflux of larger and larger quantities of glutamate, enhancing depolarization of nociresponsive neurons and ultimately completing the 'wind up' process. It might therefore be predicted that breaking this 'circle' by administering NOS inhibitors such as L-N^G-nitro-arginine methyl ester (L-NAME) in experimental animals will relieve pain. Whether such drugs will be effective for chronic pain awaits the identification of novel NOS inhibitors, with fewer adverse effects, that can be studied in humans.

The electric activity of spinal nociresponsive neurons is 'fine tuned' by neurotransmitters released from spinal neurons and major supraspinal descending nerve bundles

Local control over spinal cord pain sensitivity is provided by opioid peptides, particularly met-enkephalin and β-endorphin, and perhaps to a lesser extent leu-enkephalin and dynorphin. Each of these peptides is located within the neurons of laminae I and II of the dorsal spinal cord and provides analgesia by agonism of specific opioid receptors (i.e. μ, δ and κ).

Intrathecally applied opioids (e.g. morphine) are analgesic, indicating a spinal site of action, but systemically administered opioids also influence pain perception at higher brain centers. The mechanism of action of opioids at the spinal cord involves inhibition of the release of substance P and glutamate from C-fiber terminals, although the cellular mechanism for this is not clear.

Opioid receptors have been cloned. The μ, δ, κ_1 and κ_2 receptors belong to the G protein-coupled family of receptor proteins

Activation of opioid receptors results in various cellular consequences, including inhibition of adenylyl cyclase, causing a reduction in intracellular cAMP concentrations. This fall in neuronal cAMP was believed to account entirely for the analgesic effect of opioids, but recent studies indicate that other cellular mechanisms are also important, including:

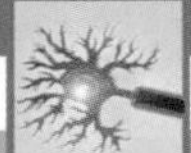

- K^+ channels opening to cause hyperpolarization of the nociresponsive neuron, thereby reducing excitability.
- Blocking the opening of voltage-gated Ca^{2+} channels to inhibit glutamate and substance P release from primary afferent terminals.

Other neurotransmitters that play a role include GABA, which has also been detected by mapping the synthetic enzyme glutamic acid decarboxylase (GAD) in the dorsal spinal cord. Like opioids, GABA, acting on $GABA_B$ receptors located presynaptically on primary afferent nerve fibers, is believed to reduce the release of glutamate and substance P. In this way, baclofen, which is a $GABA_B$ agonist, produces behavioral antinociception in experimental animals.

The third step in pain perception is the onward passage of pain information to higher brain centers

The plethora of excitatory and inhibitory neuronal inputs acting on nociresponsive neurons in the dorsal spinal cord highlights the major importance of these neurons in transferring information from nociceptors in the tissues to the brain. This function underlies the 'gate control' theory of pain put forward by Melzack and Wall in the mid-1960s. According to this theory, nociresponsive neurons in laminae I and II act as intelligent 'gatekeepers' between damaged tissues and the brain. The information they receive is modified by both spinal and supraspinal influences before being transmitted as a 'package' of knowledge about the painful stimulus to higher centers. The ascending nociceptive pathways involved in this final stage of the process travel in the ventrolateral and dorsolateral funiculi of the spinal cord and terminate mainly in the thalamus and reticular formation. Further ascending tracts terminate in the cerebral cortex and limbic systems where the cognitive and emotional aspects of pain are coordinated.

Testing analgesic drugs

A wide variety of procedures are available to assess analgesic drugs. Tests used in human volunteers include:

- Application of a tourniquet to the upper arm and measuring the length of time a volunteer can bear the resulting ischemia-induced discomfort. This is probably the best-characterized human model of pain.
- Application of radiant heat or pressure to skin.
- Electric shock stimulation of skin or tooth pulp.
- Cold pressor tests in which the arm or hand is placed in ice-cold water and the time to removal recorded.
- Blister base.

A variety of measures can be used to quantify perception of the level of pain

Objective measurement of pain is difficult. Experimental subjects are therefore required to express an opinion on their perception of levels of pain. This is commonly obtained using a sliding scale, which can either be verbal (e.g. 0 for no pain to 10 for worst possible pain) or visual (e.g. placing a mark on a 10-cm line graded from no pain to the worst possible pain). Occasionally, such a system cannot be used. For example, assessing pain in young children is difficult, using such scales. The children can then be asked to draw a face that can be graded between a happy face to indicate no pain and a sad face to indicate intense pain. Clearly, all these measurements are highly subjective, and properly trained personnel and rigorous statistical evaluation of the results are needed to avoid misleading or biased conclusions. Furthermore, the personality of the individual and other factors, such as the nature of the environment in which testing takes place and the general attitude of the investigator, can markedly affect the response of individuals to pain. There is therefore a need for randomization, allocating subjects to control and test groups. Despite these problems, however, each of the tests described above has been used with varying degrees of success to demonstrate drug-induced analgesia.

Drug therapy of pain

Nonsteroidal antiinflammatory drugs

Nonsteroidal antiinflammatory drugs (NSAIDs) inhibit the synthesis of hyperalgesic and proinflammatory PGs and form a chemically disparate group of drugs discussed in Chapter 9. Pharmacologically, NSAIDs exhibit mild analgesic activity in addition to their antiinflammatory and antipyretic activity described in Chapter 9. Tissue damage (associated with, for example, inflammation) and the accompanying plasma membrane distortion activate phospholipase A_2 enzyme activity, which cleaves free arachidonic acid from its binding sites in membrane phospholipids and renders it susceptible to attack by cyclooxygenase (COX or PGH synthase). All NSAIDs inhibit the COX enzymes and this effect underlies their analgesic activity. Two separate isoforms of COX have been identified:

- COX-1 is a constitutive (constantly present) enzyme found in a wide variety of cells throughout the body. It maintains the formation of PGs involved in 'housekeeping' (i.e. control of vascular flow through individual organs, regulation of platelet aggregation, etc.).
- COX-2 is synthesized de novo in inflammatory cells, such as neutrophils and mast cells, following exposure to stimuli such as bacterial endotoxins and/or cytokines (e.g. tumor necrosis factor (TNF) and interleukin-1β). It is responsible for generating PGs at the site of inflammation and/or tissue damage.

The majority of available NSAIDs show little or no selectivity as inhibitors of the two COX isoforms. Some compounds such as meloxicam and nimesulide have been reported to exhibit some preference for inhibiting the COX-2 enzyme although the selectivity of these compounds vis-à-vis COX-1 is not great. More recently, highly selective COX-2 inhibitors (celecoxib, precoxib and rofecoxib) have become available, although rofecoxib has recently been voluntarily withdrawn by the manufacturer because of an increased risk of unwanted cardiovascular events (see also Ch. 9). Both of these compounds are several orders of magnitude more potent as COX-2 versus COX-1 inhibitors, and exhibit potent antiinflammatory and analgesic activity. An added advantage is that these compounds appear to be associated with markedly reduced gastrointestinal side effects (a consequence of COX-1 inhibition) than do the classical NSAIDs.

Aspirin is the archetypal NSAID and was first used clinically in 1899. It acts by covalently modifying serine residues in both COX-1 (serine 530) and COX-2 (serine 516), effectively preventing further prostanoid biosynthesis. Over the last three decades numerous other NSAIDs have been developed. These are probably best classified according to their chemical structure. On this basis they can be divided into: (1) salicylic acids (e.g. aspirin along with diflunisal, olsalazine and sodium salicylate); (2) p-aminophenol derivatives, notably acetaminophen; (3) indole acids such as indomethacin and sulindac; (4) arylacetic acids such as tolmetin and ketorolac, and arylpropionic acids such as the widely used ibuprofen, as well as flurbiprofen, naproxen and ketoprofen; (5) anthranolic acids, including mefenamic acid; and (6) enolic acids such as piroxicam and tenoxicam. Unlike aspirin, most of these newer compounds bind reversibly to COX-1 and COX-2 isoforms. For the treatment of pain, NSAIDs are generally given orally and the analgesic activity is likely to persist for approximately 6–8 hours, although the effect of some NSAIDs such as piroxicam, lornoxicam and phenylbutazone (withdrawn several years ago) can last much longer (i.e. 12 hours to several days).

NSAIDs provide an effective pain-relieving strategy for mild to moderate pain such as:

- Pain associated with an inflammatory component (e.g. gout, rheumatoid arthritis, osteoarthritis, toothache, ultraviolet light-induced sunburn).
- The pain of cancer metastases, injury (e.g. bone fractures, surgical procedures), and some types of headache, which are also associated with an inflammatory reaction.
- Dysmenorrhea, which results from increased uterine PG formation.

In this respect, the most commonly used analgesic NSAIDs are aspirin and the various salicylates. In the clinical setting there is usually very little to choose between the various NSAID classes. However, some NSAIDs (e.g. acetaminophen and ketorolac) are good analgesics but have relatively weak antiinflammatory activity. Acetaminophen is a relatively weak inhibitor of COX enzymes and its precise mechanism of action in controlling pain remains something of a mystery. However, it should be noted that NSAIDs are generally not effective against severe pain (particularly that of visceral origin) for which opioids are much better. Also, the maximal degree of pain relief available with NSAIDs is less than that provided by opioids.

Adverse effects of NSAIDs include gastric blood loss and ulceration, particularly with aspirin. This is less prevalent with other NSAIDs such as ibuprofen. Inhibited gastric formation of PGE_2 and PGI_2, which are vasodilating and cytoprotective, is important in the development of this adverse effect. Replacement therapy with synthetic PG (e.g. 15-methyl PGE_2) is available if gastric damage presents a major problem. NSAIDs also inhibit platelet aggregation and accelerate bleeding time as a result of inhibiting platelet formation of thromboxane A_2 (TxA_2), which is vasoconstricting and pro-aggregatory. Other adverse effects include dizziness, headache, and water and sodium chloride retention (all adverse effects of piroxicam). Finally, large doses of aspirin (1000–1500 mg/day) and other NSAIDs can cause auditory and visual disturbances accompanied by fever and changes in blood pH, and sometimes coma.

Adverse effects of nonsteroidal antiinflammatory drugs

- **Gastric bleeding and ulceration**
- **Reduced platelet aggregation**

Opioids

All opioid drugs, whether naturally occurring such as morphine, or chemically synthesized, bind with specific opioid receptors to produce their pharmacologic effects. Three major classes of opioid receptors are μ, δ and κ. A fourth opioid receptor (σ) was suggested, but a variety of other nonopioid drugs also appear to act as ligands at this site so it is doubtful whether this receptor should now be considered a true opioid receptor. Further subclassification of some opioid receptors (e.g. into μ_1 and μ_2) is possible, but the pharmacologic and clinical significance of this remains unclear. Drugs bind to opioid receptors as either full agonists (e.g. morphine and methadone), partial agonists, mixed agonists (full agonist on one opioid receptor, but partial agonist on another, e.g. pentazocine and butorphanol), or antagonists, such as naloxone and naltrexone (see Ch. 3 for definitions). Presently available opioids (with major opioid receptor target shown in brackets) include morphine ($\mu > \kappa$), methadone (μ), etorphine and bremazocine (μ, δ and κ), levorphanol (μ and κ), fentanyl (μ) and sufentanil (mainly μ).

Opioids are used for moderate to severe pain, particularly for postoperative or cancer-related pain

Opioids are less effective against nerve pain (neuropathic pain) such as trigeminal neuralgia or phantom limb pain. In addition to analgesic effects, opioid drugs have a variety of other actions in the CNS, not all of which are beneficial. For example, opioids cause euphoria accompanied by a general sense of peace and contentment, which accounts for the addictive nature of such drugs by addicts (see below). This calming activity undoubtedly

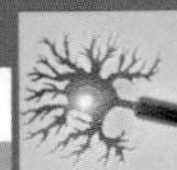

contributes to their analgesic efficacy by helping relieve the anxiety and distress associated with pain. This can be important in the treatment of acute myocardial infarction and congestive heart failure, for example. Morphine-induced euphoria appears to be mediated by activation of μ and/or κ receptors, presumably within the limbic system.

Opioid analgesics are administered systematically (orally, intramuscularly or subcutaneously) or directly into the spinal cord (intrathecally). Usually a loading dose is given, followed by maintenance dosing to ensure steady-state plasma concentrations.

TOLERANCE AND DEPENDENCE Tolerance to the analgesic effect of opioids develops rapidly and can often be detected within 12–24 hours of administration. As a result, larger and larger doses of the drug are needed to achieve the same clinical effect, leading to an increased severity and incidence of adverse effects. Physical dependence may develop and is characterized by a definite abstinence syndrome following drug withdrawal. This syndrome comprises a complex mixture of irritable and sometimes aggressive behavior, coupled with extremely unpleasant autonomic symptoms such as fever, sweating, yawning and papillary dilation (see below).

ADVERSE EFFECTS OF OPIOIDS These limit the dose that can be given and the level of analgesia attained. All adverse effects are a direct consequence of opioid receptor activation and relate largely to the preponderance of opioid receptors in the medulla and peripheral nervous system. Such actions can be inhibited by opioid receptor antagonists such as naloxone. The most serious adverse effect is probably respiratory depression, which results from reduced sensitivity of the medullary respiratory centers to carbon dioxide. Respiratory depression is the most common cause of death from opioid overdose. Another common adverse effect is constipation due to reduction in lower gastrointestinal smooth muscle tone resulting in decreased propulsion. Other adverse effects include pupillary constriction (miosis) and vomiting via an action on the CTZ in the medulla. The antitussive activity of opioids is an adverse effect that has been exploited clinically and, as a result, codeine and dextromethorphan are frequently included in proprietary cough medicines (see Ch. 14).

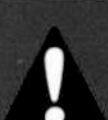

Adverse effects of opioid drugs

- Respiratory depression (μ, δ and κ receptors)
- Constipation (variable, μ and κ receptors)
- Nausea and vomiting
- Pupillary constriction (μ/δ receptors)
- Rapid development of tolerance
- Physical dependence and abstinence syndrome

Pharmacologic adjuncts to analgesia

BENZODIAZEPINES Severe pain leads to emotional distress, and therefore drug therapy of the associated anxiety is frequently considered to be helpful. The benzodiazepines, diazepam and lorazepam are usually the drugs of choice, providing effective anxiolytic cover over a long period, coupled with a mild amnesic effect, which, although beneficial in some patients, can cause distress and confusion, particularly in older patients.

NITROUS OXIDE (N_2O) (see Ch. 15) The anesthetic gas is analgesic in its own right for acutely painful procedures of short duration (e.g. dental procedures, childbirth). The analgesia it provides when inhaled (sometimes as a 50% mixture in air, i.e. Entonox) is rapid in both onset and offset.

KETAMINE (see Ch. 21) This was originally introduced as a dissociative anesthetic but is a useful short-term analgesic, although unpleasant adverse effects such as delirium and bizarre hallucinations limit its widespread use.

Opioids and NSAIDs are the mainstay of pain relief, but cannot be considered to be 'ideal' analgesics

Both opioids and NSAIDs are relatively effective against different types of pain, but the relatively high incidence of adverse effects and other problems associated with their clinical use means that neither group can be considered to be the 'ideal' analgesic. It is hoped that the continually improving understanding of the physiologic basis of pain will ultimately be translated into the development of more powerful and safer analgesic drugs.

DRUGS OF ABUSE

Since drugs that act on the CNS can have profound effects on emotions, mood and behavior it is not surprising that such drugs are used for such actions in a nontherapeutic setting. This nontherapeutic use of drugs is generally categorized as being abuse of those drugs. Such a term is widely understood and can be used effectively, despite the fact that a more precise term might be 'substance abuse,' since common substances such as gasoline and solvents are sometimes inhaled for their pharmacologic effect. Furthermore, substances such as ethanol, caffeine and nicotine, in all their forms, are not generally regarded by the public as being drugs in the therapeutic use of that term. Since such substances are taken for the effect that they produce in the human brain there is no need, pharmacologically speaking, to separate such substances from drugs of abuse. It could be even speculated that the excessive intake of food in general or of particular types of foods is abuse in much the same way as drug abuse. The common theme of such use, or overuse, is an attempt by the taker to achieve some form of psychologic reward.

Each of the drugs of abuse is used for its own particular purpose, and whatever that is, it appears to involve mechanisms that are common to other mammals. Thus, drugs of abuse will, with the use of the appropriate experimental paradigm, produce an analogous pattern of abuse in other species as well as man.

All of the drugs and substances that are taken for non-therapeutic reasons have their own profile with respect to various properties. The most important of these are the pharmacologic actions of the drug in question. Drugs that are abused have a wide variety of pharmacologic actions that can be very loosely divided into at least four categories: depressant, stimulant (excitant), opioid and hallucinogenic. Drugs in the first category are recognized to reduce activity in the CNS to the point, in the case of drugs such as barbiturates and general anesthetics, of coma and death. The term depressant is, of course, not exact or very descriptive. Stimulant drugs on the other hand induce alertness, excitement and euphoria and presumably are taken for such reasons. Opioid drugs are agonists at opioid receptors and produce a mix of actions in that, in addition to producing euphoria, they also have depressant actions. Hallucinogenic drugs produce altered perception, especially with respect to time and space, i.e. hallucinations. Dissociative anesthetics, besides producing anesthesia, also produce hallucinations.

The extent, onset and duration of the above effects are very dependent upon the route of administration and pharmacokinetic properties of the drug. Thus, in order to achieve the greatest effect most rapidly, use is made of the i.v. route. An alternative to this is nasal administration (especially cocaine and nicotine) where absorption into the circulation is very rapid and avoids first-pass metabolism in the liver. An analogous route is by inhalation into the lungs in the form of smoke and this is used especially for nicotine, cannabis and opiates. The oral route, while being the easiest, is often not the favorite one since it involves an unavoidable delay between ingestion and effect.

There are many classes of drugs that are abused. Many of these affect the CNS and can induce tolerance and dependence. This is best illustrated by the opioids.

Opioids

Opioids are well known as drugs of dependence and have been, and are commonly abused in many societies with economic and social consequences. In many countries an extensive illegal economy exists for producing and marketing drugs of abuse and this is particularly the case for opioids, as well as for cocaine, marihuana and recreational drugs such as 'ecstasy.' In the case of the opioids the starting point is opium produced organically from the poppy *Papaver somniferum*. The opiate latex is collected from the seed pod and then variously treated for local use or export. A relatively simple chemical process converts the main alkaloid, morphine, to heroin. The latter is the choice for those whose preferred route of administration is i.v. injection.

Abusers of opioids can show tolerance and psychologic dependence to opiate effects and in addition show withdrawal when opioids are discontinued after regular use. Tolerance, or more correctly, physiologic dependence occurs when the same dose shows lesser effects upon repeated administration or, alternatively, larger and larger doses are needed to produce the same effect. The mechanisms underlying tolerance to opiates appear to involve adaptation to the continued presence of the drug. This adaptation is neuroadaptive in the sense that up- and down-regulation of receptors and neurotransmission occurs in an attempt to maintain normal function. In animal experiments, physiologic dependence or tolerance can be seen to develop within hours.

Psychological dependence is seen when a drug is used repeatedly because it provides a psychological reward of some kind, whether of pleasure or freedom from pain and anxiety. This rewarding effect relates to the main pharmacologic actions of the drug. There are elements of habit formation with any psychological dependence such that there may be very little difference between an ingrained habit and psychological dependence to a drug.

The signs and symptoms of withdrawal are often opposite in nature to the acute pharmacologic effects of the drug. With stimulants the withdrawal syndrome is often depression, while for depressants the withdrawal syndrome is marked by excitation. In addition, some of the changes seen upon withdrawal are compounded by autonomic responses to the accompanying stress.

Depending upon the particular opiate and as a result of its pharmacologic actions and pharmacokinetics, tolerance, psychological dependence and withdrawal can be pronounced or limited. For such reasons both morphine and heroin produce marked physiologic and psychological dependence and withdrawal whereas methadone produces much less. Much of these differences can be attributed to pharmacokinetic factors, namely the slower excretion of methadone. Drugs that are slowly eliminated from the body generally show less withdrawal effects.

When considering drugs of abuse there is a need to consider the dangers to society associated with abuse of that drug, as well as dangers to the individual abuser. The opiate abuser generally does not constitute an immediate problem to society since the acute pharmacologic effects of opiates lead to social withdrawal and inactivity. In the longer term, the abuser incurs a social cost in terms of criminal activity related to obtaining illegal drugs and in terms of interpersonal relationships. The pharmacologic and toxicological harmful effects of opiates include confusion and, in severe cases, respiratory depression. More importantly, the mode of taking the drug carries a great risk when dirty needles and solutions are used to inject heroin (or other drugs). The risk of AIDS is very high in addicts who inject drugs.

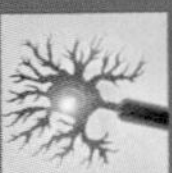

TREATMENT The primary treatment for heroin and morphine abuse is substitution with methadone, an orally active opiate receptor agonist, and withdrawal symptoms are limited since it is eliminated slowly from the body. Supportive and symptomatic therapy is an important component in treating opiate abuse.

A summary of opioid abuse is provided below:

- Analogs: morphine, heroin, fentanyl, methadone.
- Routes: oral, smoked, parenteral, particularly i.v.
- Type of action: depressant.
- Desired psychological actions: euphoria, analgesia, relaxation.
- Pharmacologic actions/effects of overdose: confusion, respiratory depression.
- Psychological dependence: marked and develops rapidly if the i.v. route is used.
- Tolerance: very marked.
- Withdrawal symptoms: can be severe but generally not fatal, includes shaking, tremors, diarrhea, dysphoria, sleep disturbance.
- Note: methadone has slower metabolism and produces less marked effects; therefore, it is used as morphine and heroin opiate replacement.

The properties of other classes of drugs of abuse are summarized below.

Cocaine ('coke')

- Analogs: none.
- Route: oral (South America), nasal, smoked, i.v.
- Type of action: stimulant.
- Desired psychological actions: highly rewarding for euphoria and arousal.
- Pharmacologic actions/effects of overdose: psychosis, cardiovascular death (arrhythmias and hypertensive crisis), tissue damage at site of application or injection. Fetal damage.
- Psychological dependence: strong, particularly for i.v. form.
- Tolerance: limited.
- Withdrawal symptoms: depression, dysphoria, sleep disturbance.

Amphetamines

- Analogs: methamphetamine (ecstasy).
- Routes: oral, or sometimes parenteral.
- Type of action: stimulant.
- Desired psychological actions: euphoria, arousal and increased state of wakefulness.
- Pharmacologic actions/effects of overdose: psychosis, cardiovascular death (arrhythmias and hypertensive crisis), hyperthermia.
- Psychological dependence: strong but 'rush' not so apparent as with cocaine.
- Tolerance: limited.
- Withdrawal symptoms: depression, dysphoria, sleep disturbance.

Nicotine

- Analogs: none.
- Forms of use: smoked tobacco in cigarettes, cigars, pipe; intranasally as snuff; chewing tobacco (buccal cavity); transdermal patches; and chewing gum for treating nicotine addiction.
- Type of action: stimulant.
- Desired psychological actions: some euphoria, relaxation and increased concentration.
- Pharmacologic actions/effects of overdose: due to stimulation of nicotinic receptors. Overdose occurs with accidental poisoning since nicotine insecticides are absorbed through the skin and cause death from cardiovascular accidents and neuromuscular blockade. Smoking, snuff and oral administration associated with cancer (principally in lungs and oral cavity): smoking specifically results in emphysema, bronchitis and cough.
- Psychological dependence: can be surprisingly strong.
- Tolerance: limited.
- Withdrawal symptoms: irritability, weight gain with increased appetite, headache.

Caffeine

- Analogs: none for abuse but theophylline used therapeutically.
- Forms of use: chiefly, orally ingested as drinks (coffee, tea, cocoa, chocolate, cola and some other soft drinks).
- Type of action: stimulant.
- Desired psychological actions: increased alertness and concentration.
- Pharmacologic actions/effects of overdose: anxiety, tremors, arrhythmias and convulsions in children.
- Psychological dependence: very limited.
- Tolerance: limited.
- Withdrawal symptoms: limited.

Barbiturates

- Analogs: large number exist but relatively few abused.
- Route: usually oral.
- Type of action: depressant.
- Desired psychological actions: sedation.
- Pharmacologic actions/effects of overdose: sedation, confusion, coma, respiratory depression resulting in death.

Benzodiazepines

- Analogs: large number.
- Pharmacologic actions/effects of overdose: coma and death due to respiratory depression.
- Withdrawal symptoms: potentially the most lethal of all drugs: convulsions, tremors, shakes.

Ethanol ('alcohols')

- Analogs: by far the most important is ethanol but other low molecular weight alcohols are also abused, especially methanol. Can be treated with disulfiram, which provides a powerful deterrent for alcoholics to

Table 18.9 Tryptans used in the treatment of migraine

Drug Name	Routes of Administration	Half Life	Metabolism
Sumatriptan	Oral, Nasal, and Subcutaneous. Time to peak concentration is ~1–2 hours after oral or nasaladministration and within ~15 minutes after subcutaneous injection	3 hours	metabolized predominantly by monoamine oxidase (the MAO-A isoenzyme)
Almotriptan	Oral	3 hours	metabolized extensively by cytochrome P450 3A4 isoenzyme
Eletriptan HBr	Oral	4 hours	metabolized extensively by cytochrome P450 3A4 isoenzyme
Frovatriptan	Oral	26 hours	cytochrome P450 1A2 appears to be the principal enzyme involved in the metabolism of frovatriptan.
Naratriptan	Oral	6 hours	metabolized by a wide range of cytochrome P450 isoenzymes. About 50% of the drug is eliminated in the urine
Rizatriptan	Oral	2 hours	metabolized predominantly by monoamine oxidase (the MAO-A isoenzyme)
Zolmitriptan	Oral and nasal	3 hours	metabolized by a wide range of cytochrome P450 isoenzymes and has an active *N*-desmethyl metabolite with a half life similar to the parent drug

abstain from alcohol ingestion. When alcohol is taken by a patient taking disufiram, the alcohol and disulfiram react to form acetaldehyde, a toxic substance producing a throbbing headache, nausea and palpitations.
- Route: oral.
- Type of action: depressant.
- Desired psychological actions: euphoria, release of inhibitions, increased sociability.
- Pharmacologic actions/effects of overdose: excitement, confusion, ataxia, and coma and death with acute overdose. Chronic abuse leads to hypertension, and cardiac, brain and liver pathology. Damaging to the fetus (fetal alcohol syndrome).
- Psychological dependence: moderate to severe.
- Tolerance: limited.
- Withdrawal symptoms: can be fatal, convulsions, seizures, hallucinations (pink elephants).

Phencyclidine ('dissociative anesthetics')
- Analogs: ketamine
- Type of action: hallucinations.

Solvents
- Analogs: gasoline, glue and other solvents.
- Route: inhalation.
- Type of action: depressant.

LSD ('hallucinogens')
- Analogs: LSD principally, also mescaline, cohabe, peyote.
- Route: oral or snuff for some analogs.
- Type of action: hallucinogen.
- Desired psychological actions: hallucinations and disturbances of perception of space and time.
- Pharmacologic actions/effects of overdose: psychosis and 'flashbacks.'
- Psychological dependence: limited.
- Tolerance: limited.
- Withdrawal symptoms: very rare, probably reflecting infrequent pattern of use.

Cannabinoids
- Analogs: cannabinoid alkaloids from *Cannabis sativa*, principally delta-9-tetrahydrocannabinoid (Δ^9THC).
- Route: oral (cookies) or smoked.
- Type of action: weak hallucinogen.
- Desired psychological actions: relaxation, euphoria, disturbance of perception of time and space, pleasurable effects are to some extent learned.
- Effect of overdose: not conspicuous.
- Psychological dependence: moderate.
- Tolerance: moderate or weak.
- Withdrawal symptoms: limited, sleep disturbance, anxiety.

FURTHER READING

Kedar NP. Can we prevent Parkinson's and Alzheimer's disease? *J Postgrad Med* 2003; **49**: 236–245.

Pinna A, Wardas J, Simola N, Morelli M. New therapies for the treatment of Parkinson's disease: adenosine A2A receptor antagonists. *Life Sci* 2005; **77**: 3259–3267.

Robert E Hales, Stuart C, Yudofsky. Essentials of clinical psychiatry. Washington, DC: American Psychiatric Pub., c2004.

Sadock BJ, Kaplan & Sadocks's concise textbook of clinical psychiatry/ Benjamin James Sadock, Virginia Alcott Sadock. Philadelphia: Lippincott Williams & Wilkins, 2004.

WEBSITES

http://www.merek.com/mrkshared/mmanual/sections.jsp [Merck Manual.]

http://www.psychiatryonline.com/resourceToc.aspx?resourceID=5 [Free online textbook.]

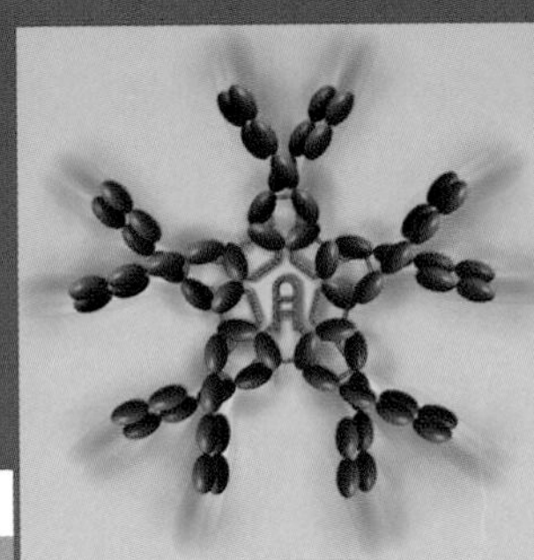

Chapter 9

Autacoids, Drugs and the Inflammatory and Immune Responses

This chapter considers the pharmacology of substances that function as 'signaling molecules' and mediate local cellular and tissue responses to physiologic needs, tissue injury or activation of the immune system by external stimuli or autoimmune mechanisms. Injury produces a variety of substances that initiate and sustain inflammatory responses and which also activate and moderate the repair process. These substances are termed 'autacoids' and, as with neurotransmission, the inflammatory and immune responses are tightly regulated under physiologic conditions (homeostasis), but can be inappropriately activated or underactivated, leading to diseases. In many ways the pharmacology of these substances resembles that of the neurotransmitters in that drugs are available that will modulate their release or secretion, or mimic or block their actions so as to favorably influence a particular disease state. Similarly, activation of the immune system causes the synthesis and release of a large variety of endogenous substances that control the recruitment and activation of all of the various cells involved in mediating immune responses (Fig. 9.1).

The term autacoid was originally introduced to describe small molecular weight compounds that are derived from amino acids found to be involved in tissue injury and immune responses, and included substances such as histamine, 5-HT(serotonin) and later eicosanoids (a term used to describe products of fatty acid metabolism, primarily metabolism of arachidonic acid). The term 'autacoid' is also used to describe polypeptides and proteins involved in the immune and inflammatory responses such as bradykinin, endothelin and the growing family of cytokines and chemokines. The term was coined to indicate that such substances are, in a sense, the body's own pharmacologic regulators of the immune and inflammatory response, often acting close to their sites of release or synthesis. However, it was quickly recognized that this term covered substances that were not like classic hormones or neurotransmitters, even though some of these substances have their actions remote from their site of release or synthesis and in the case of histamine and 5-HT, the classic autacoids, both are also neurotransmitters within the central nervous system (CNS) and the peripheral nervous system (PNS). In this chapter, however, we only consider the actions unrelated to the actions of these substances as neurotransmitters.

While the number of substances that can regulate the inflammatory and immune response now runs into hundreds, this chapter will only deal with those systems and mediators that can be manipulated by drugs that have clinical utility discussed in this and subsequent chapters.

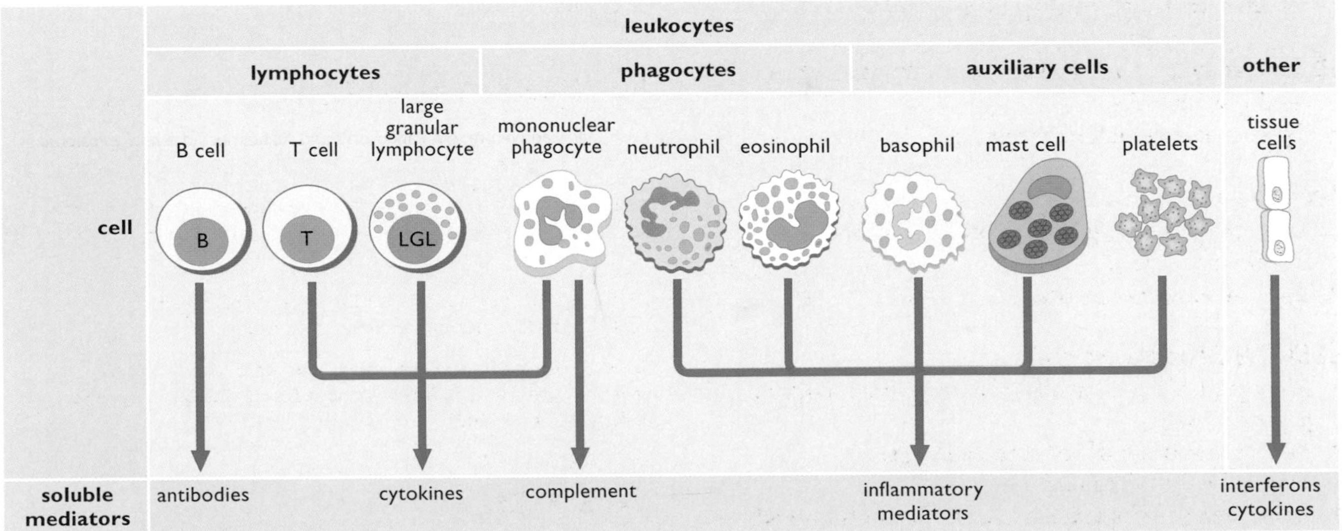

Fig. 9.1 The principal components of the immune and inflammatory system. Complement is made primarily by the liver, although there is some synthesis by mononuclear phagocytes. Each cell produces and secretes only a particular set of cytokines or inflammatory mediators.

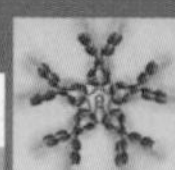

PHYSIOLOGY OF THE IMMUNE SYSTEM

The immune system and the inflammatory response are involved in the defense against invading organisms and responses to injury. However, inappropriate activation of these systems results in a wide range of inflammatory disorders. Inflammation is characterized by a number of features:

- Vasodilation leading to redness.
- Increased vascular permeability leading to swelling of tissues (edema).
- Pain
- Recruitment of leukocytes into tissues.
- When inflammation occurs chronically, this can lead to alterations in tissue function.

The physiology of the inflammatory response and injury share certain characteristics in that the responses they mediate have the common aim of allowing the body to respond to invasion by organisms, stress or damage by adjusting local blood flow at the site of injury and allowing recruitment of leukocytes and other blood elements into the area of injury. These serve a number of functions including the initiation of pain, presumably in an attempt to reduce the degree of injury, changing the local milieu so as to dilute any damaging agents and to recruit leukocytes to kill organisms. In addition, many autacoids released in response to injury or infection induce increased vascular permeability leading to edema, and initiate processes of repair and tissue protection, which if inappropriate or chronic may lead to altered tissue function.

A key additional feature of the immune response is the ability of lymphocytes to recognize foreign proteins (antigens) which can be surface proteins on pathogens or, in some people, otherwise innocuous proteins (such as grass pollen or animal dander) which are responsible for inducing allergic responses (see below). Lymphocytes are derived from bone marrow stem cells. T lymphocytes then develop in the thymus, while B lymphocytes develop in the bone marrow (see Fig. 9.1).

T cells have T-cell antigen receptors (TCRs) on their cell surfaces

T cells specifically recognize antigens in association with the major histocompatibility complexes (MHCs) (HLA antigens) on antigen-presenting cells (APCs) such as macrophages and dendritic cells. When T cells are activated by an antigen through a TCR they produce soluble proteins, called cytokines, which signal to T cells, B cells, monocytes/macrophages and other cells (Fig. 9.2).

T cells are classified into two subsets:

- CD4-positive (CD4+) T cells, which interact with B cells and help them to proliferate, differentiate and produce antibody. They are therefore called helper T (TH) cells. TH cells can be subdivided further into TH_1 and TH_2, based on the profile of cytokines which they release (Fig. 9.3).
- CD8-positive (CD8+) T cells, which destroy host cells that have become infected by viruses or other intracellular pathogens. This kind of action is called cytotoxicity and these T cells are therefore called cytotoxic T (Tc) cells.

B cells use surface immunoglobulins as their antigen receptors

B cells specifically recognize a particular antigen and, when stimulated by an interaction between surface

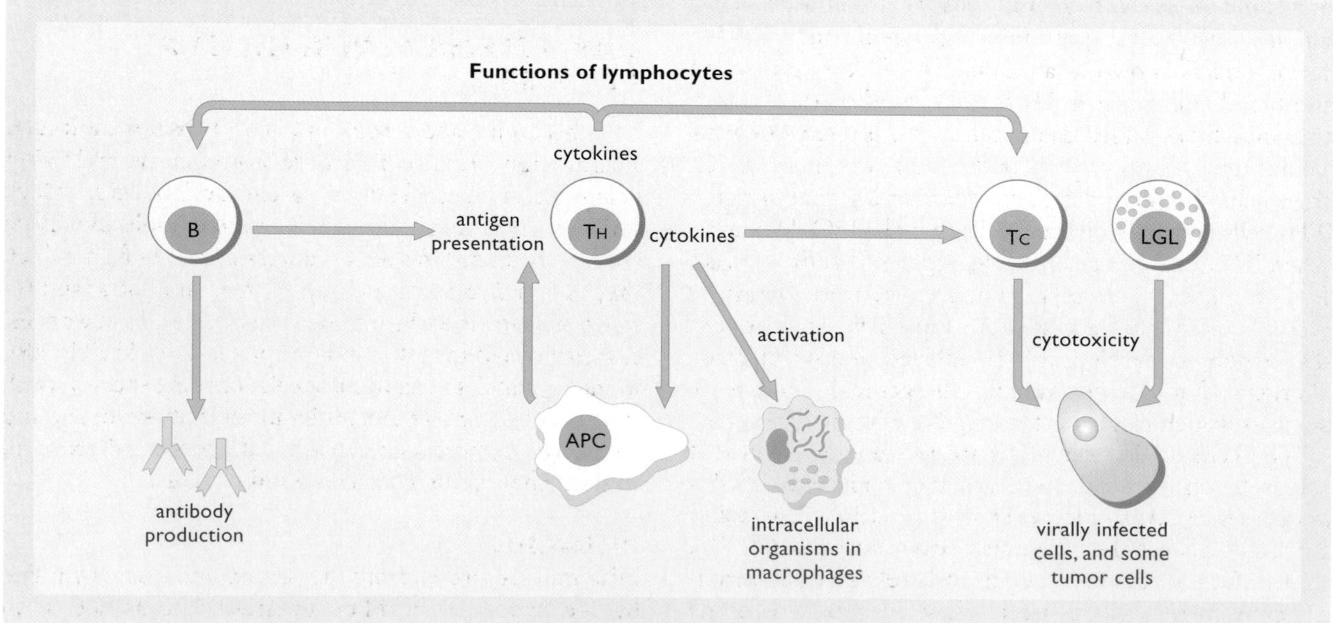

Fig. 9.2 Functions of B cells and T cells. B cells produce antibodies, while T-helper (TH) cells are stimulated by antigen-presenting cells (APCs) and B cells to produce cytokines, which control immune responses. Macrophages are activated to kill intracellular microorganisms. Cytotoxic T (Tc) cells and large granular lymphocytes (LGL) recognize and kill target host cells.

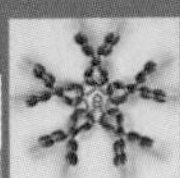

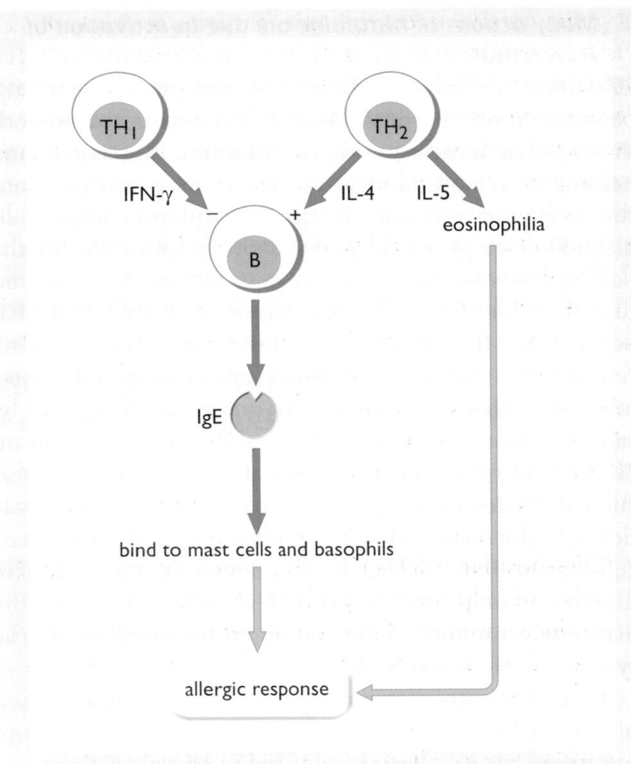

Fig. 9.3 CD4-positive (CD4+) T cells are divided into TH_1 and TH_2 based on the profile of cytokines they release. TH_1 cells release IFN-γ which can inhibit the ability of B cells to make immunoglobulin E, the antibody that is central to the induction of allergic responses. Meanwhile, TH_2 lymphocytes release both IL-4, which is a necessary co-factor for the induction of IgE synthesis by B cells, and IL-5, which is a powerful chemoattractant for eosinophils that characterize the allergic responses.

immunoglobulin and the specific antigen, they proliferate and differentiate into plasma cells, which produce large amounts of the receptor immunoglobulin in a soluble form. This is known as an antibody, which is present in the blood and tissue fluids and can bind to the antigen that initially activated the B cells. The presence of antibodies activates other parts of the immune system, which then help eliminate the pathogen carrying that antigen. TH_1 cells normally direct B cells to make IgG. However, when TH_2 cells make IL-4, this signals B cells to make IgE, the antibody thought to be important in allergic or atopic conditions. People with atopy have an inherited disposition to develop IgE to inhaled and/or ingested allergens that are not usually allergenic in nonatopic subjects, which can lead to a range of allergic diseases.

The hemostatic system is a special category in that it serves to limit blood loss, although activation of this system also leads to the generation of various 'autacoids' that can influence the inflammatory response (see Ch. 10).

All of these responses require the release of autacoids either from the cells in which they are stored or by de novo synthesis. The local control of blood flow is very important in the whole process and it is not surprising to find that a whole host of autacoids and transmitters, for example histamine, serotonin (5-HT), nitric oxide, thromboxane A_2, prostaglandins, bradykinin and endothelin, serve to locally regulate blood flow. The pain associated with tissue injury involves not only the direct stimulation of afferent nerves via activation of receptors on sensory nerves but also involves a variety of endogenous local transmitters that can of themselves initiate pain and also change the receipt of the pain message by changing the responsiveness of pain fibers. Such an algesic action accentuates and exaggerates pain and is termed hyperalgesia (see Ch. 8).

In addition to physical injury of tissue being a prime cause of inflammation, activation of immune mechanisms is also an important cause. The immune system serves to protect the body from invasion by foreign organisms. The term foreign organism covers a variety of substances from nonbiological material in the form of particles to parasites, bacteria, viruses and even foreign proteins. In order to deal with such 'invaders,' the body has to recognize self from non-self so as to define what is foreign and therefore has to be attacked and removed. In autoimmune conditions, unfortunately, the immune system loses the ability to properly differentiate between self and non-self and thereby begins to attack the body's own proteins with disastrous results.

Therefore, the immune system has a number of roles to play. The first of these is to be able to correctly recognize self from non-self, the second is to initiate a memory or recognition process for non-self that is linked to and capable of activating appropriate responses designed to inactivate and remove the invading non-self. Responses have to include the appropriate messages to recruit, activate and generate all of the various and appropriate components of the immune system.

LOW MOLECULAR WEIGHT AMINE AUTACOIDS

Both histamine and serotonin (5-HT) are low molecular weight amine autacoids that are stored in the body after being synthesized from a parent amino acid, which involves decarboxylation of the parent molecule. Both amines are stored in special vesicles in nerves from which they are released to subserve their neurotransmitter function. However, histamine is also stored in mast cells, enterochromaffin cells and in platelets. 5-HT is also found in platelets and in mast cells of some species. Both substances share commonalities in their physiological and pathological roles but remain sufficiently different to warrant their being considered individually.

Histamine

Histamine is formed from the parent amino acid histidine by the action of histidine decarboxylase as shown in Figure 9.4. No clinically useful drugs affect the synthesis of histamine, but certain drugs cause the release of histamine from mast cells as a side effect, including

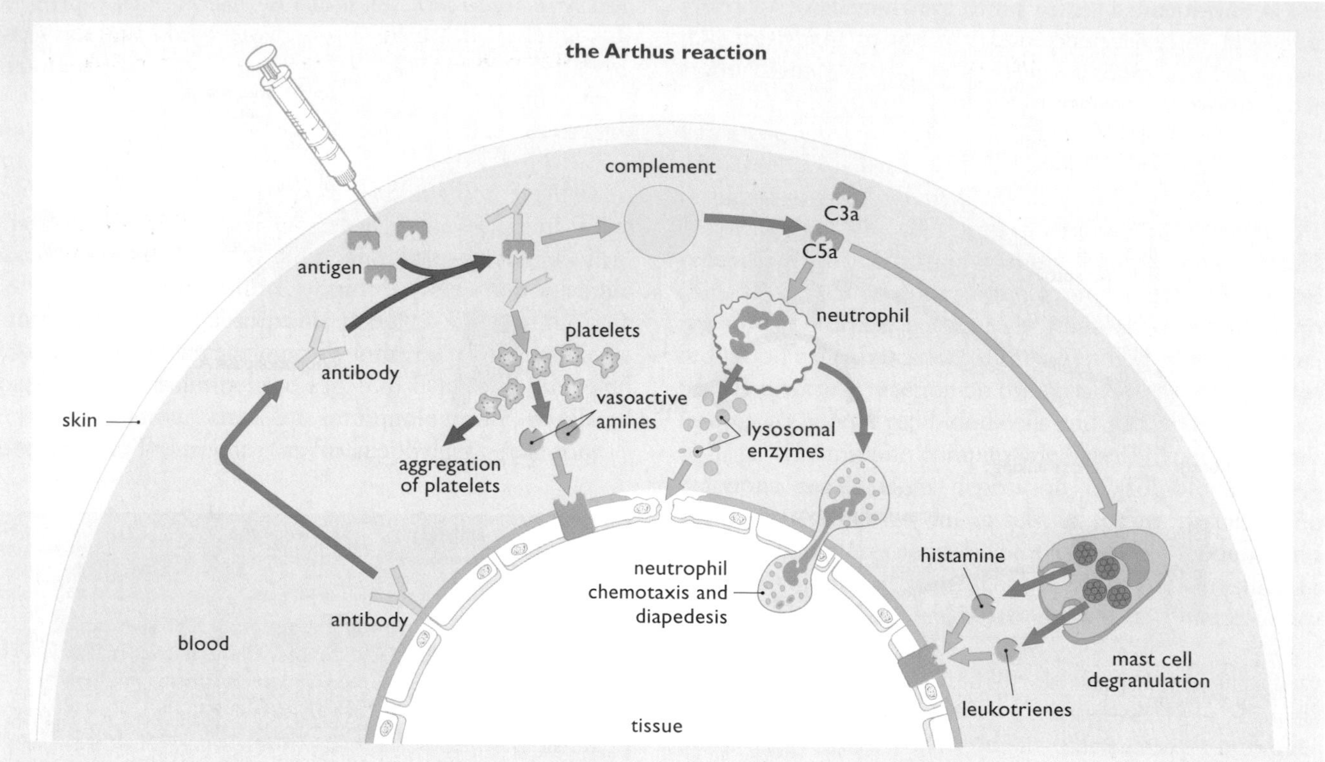

Fig. 9.8 Mechanism of type III hypersensitivity reactions. Antigen injected intradermally combines with specific antibody from the blood to form immune complexes. The complexes activate complement and act on platelets, which release vasoactive amines. Immune complexes also induce macrophages to release tumor necrosis factor (TNF) and interleukin-1 (IL-1) (not shown). Complement C3a and C5a fragments cause mast cell degranulation and attract neutrophils into the tissue. Mast cell products, including histamine and leukotrienes, increase blood flow and capillary permeability. The inflammatory reaction is potentiated by lysosomal enzymes released from the polymorphs. Furthermore, C3b deposited on the complexes opsonizes them for phagocytosis. The Arthus reaction can be seen in patients with precipitating antibodies (e.g. those with extrinsic allergic alveolitis associated with farmer's lung disease).

Table 9.3 H_1 receptor antagonists

Class	Drugs	Duration of action (hours)	Side effects
Ethylenediamines	Pyrilamine	4–6	Gastrointestinal symptoms and weak CNS effects
	Tripelennamine	4–6	
Ethanolamines	Diphenhydramine	4–6	Strong anticholinergic and sedative effects
	Dimenhydrinate	4–6	
	Clemastine	12–24	
Alkylamines	Chlorpheniramine	4–6	Relatively weak sedative effects and CNS excitement
	Dexchlorpheniramine	4–6	
	Triprolidine	4–6	
Piperazines	Meclizine	12–24	Weak sedative effects
	Cyclizine	4–6	
	Hydroxyzine	6–24	
Phenothiazines	Promethazine	4–6	Anticholinergic effects
	Trimeprazine	4–6	
New derivatives	Cyproheptadine	6–8	†QT prolongation and torsade de pointes
	Loratadine*	24	
	Cetirizine*	12–24	

* Crosses the blood–brain barrier relatively less readily, and therefore induces less sedation. Causes dangerous arrhythmias, especially in combination with macrolide, antibiotics, ketoconazole and itraconazole.

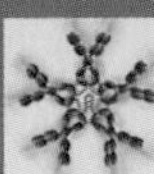

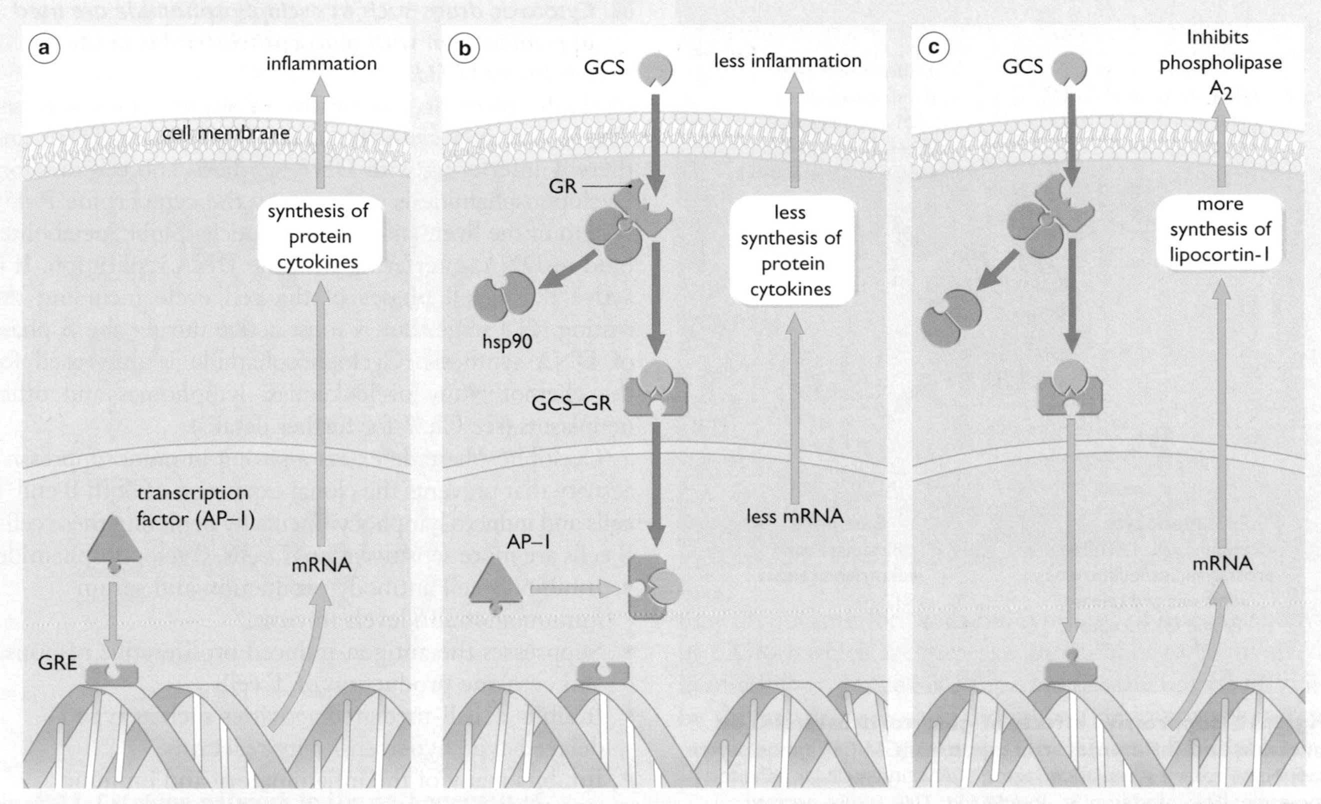

Fig. 9.9 Effect of glucocorticosteroids on gene transcription. (a) Transcription factors (e.g. AP-1) bind to receptors on DNA to bring about mRNA synthesis. This then leads to the synthesis of new proteins (e.g. cytokines) which are released by the cell to cause inflammation. (b) Glucocorticosteroids (GCSs) bind to cytosolic glucocorticosteroid receptors (GR), which are normally associated with two molecules of a 90 kDa heat shock protein (hsp90). The GCS–GR complex translocates to the nucleus and binds to glucocorticosteroid response elements (GRE) in the promoter sequences of target genes. (c) This leads to increased transcription of new proteins (e.g. lipocortin-1), or decreased transcription of proteins via binding to transcription factors (e.g. AP-1), resulting in reduced synthesis of inflammatory products (i.e. cytokines, neurokinin 1 (NK1) receptors, inducible nitric oxide synthase (NOS), cyclooxygenase-2, endothelin-1, phospholipase A_2 [PLA_2]).

and inducing local vasoconstriction. The mechanism of action of glucocorticoids as antiinflammatory drugs is complex:

- They induce synthesis of a polypeptide which inhibits phospholipase A_2, a key enzyme in the production of inflammatory mediators, including prostaglandins, leukotrienes and platelet-activating factor (PAF) (see Fig. 9.5).
- They interact with 'glucocorticosteroid response elements' in inflammatory cells, which are believed to neutralize the transcription factors for the synthesis of cytokines such as interleukin (IL)-5 and tumor necrosis factor (TNF)-α (Fig. 9.9).
- They are unique in having the ability to resolve established inflammatory responses in the airways, though the mechanism responsible for this is not clear.

These drugs can be used topically in the treatment of allergic rhinitis, allergic asthma and atopic skin diseases (see Chs 8, 14 and 18, respectively), and can also be used orally and intravenously. However, oral glucocorticosteroids have systemic adverse effects and can cause suppression of the hypothalamic–pituitary axis. Chronic use can lead to a variety of serious adverse effects, including stunting of growth in children (see Ch. 11).

MECHANISM OF ACTIONS OF DRUGS USED FOR AUTOIMMUNE DISEASES

Systemic lupus erythematosus

Systemic lupus erythematosus (SLE) is an autoimmune disease that occurs predominantly in young women and is characterized by the production of autoantibodies, especially anti-DNA antibodies. It is discussed in more detail in Chapter 12.

Glucocorticosteroids have a profound inhibitory effect on many cells in the immune system

The immunosuppressive effects of glucocorticosteroids in relation to the treatment of autoimmune diseases such as SLE are summarized in Figure 9.10. They suppress the proliferative responses of T cells to antigens and mitogens by inhibiting the synthesis of IL-2; in vivo, delayed type IV hypersensitivity reactions with antigens

Table 9.5 Disease-modifying antirheumatic drugs used in treatment of rheumatoid arthritis

Drug	Usual dose	Plasma half-life	Elimination	Time to benefits	Side effects
Injectable gold salts	25–50 mg i.m., every 2–4 weeks	25 days	70% renal	3–6 months	Rash, stomatitis, myelosuppression, thrombocytopenia, proteinuria, interstitial pneumonia
Oral gold	3 mg oral daily, or twice daily	17–25 days	60% renal	4–6 months	Same as injectable gold but less frequent, plus frequent diarrhea
D-penicillamine	250–750 mg oral daily	2 hours	Liver	3–6 months	Rash, stomatitis, dysgeusia, proteinuria, myelosuppression, autoimmune diseases
Hydroxychloroquine	200 mg oral twice daily	40 days	60% renal	2–4 months	Rash, diarrhea, retinal toxicity
Sulfasalazine	1000 mg oral twice or 3 times daily	4 hours	Liver	1–2 months	Rash, myelosuppression, gastrointestinal intolerance
Methotrexate	7.5–15 mg oral per week	8–10 hours	80% renal	1–2 months	Gastrointestinal symptoms, stomatitis, rash, alopecia, myelosuppression, interstitial pneumonia
Azathioprine	50–150 mg oral daily	0.2 hours	Metabolized in the liver, the metabolites secreted to urine	2–3 months	Myelosuppression, hepatotoxicity, infections, gastrointestinal symptoms
Leflunomide	20 mg oral daily after 100 mg oral for 3 days	11–18 days	43% renal 48% feces	1–2 months	Diarrhea, alopecia, liver dysfunction, rash, fetal death, teratogenic effect

i.m., intramuscular.

drugs actually retard the development of bone erosions in the joints.

Gold salts are used in the treatment of RA, but have limited efficacy alone. Approximately 20–35% of patients treated with the intramuscular preparation show a significant response, which is maximal at 6–12 months. This remission is sustained in about 50% of the responders. A 5-year follow-up revealed no difference between treated and untreated patients when gold salt therapy was used alone.

Gold salts act mainly to inhibit monocyte and macrophage function. They reduce the migration, phagocytosis and expression of Fc and CR3 receptors in macrophages as well as accessory cell function, as indicated by the suppression of lymphocyte blastogenesis. They may also inhibit aggregation of γ globulin and induce complement C1 inactivation.

The adverse effects of gold salts include rashes, leukocytopenias and proteinuria (see Table 9.5). Oral gold salt therapy is less effective when used alone, but is easier to administer than the parenteral courses of gold salt therapy and has fewer adverse effects.

D-penicillamine is also used in the treatment of RA. Although its mechanism of action remains unknown, it has immunomodulatory effects in vitro, the most important of which may be inhibition of TH cell function. Its adverse effects include gastrointestinal intolerance, skin rash, nephrotoxicity and elicitation of autoantibodies with associated autoimmune diseases.

Hydroxychloroquine can also control the symptoms of RA, but its mechanism of action in the therapy of RA is unknown. It may inhibit the release of prostaglandins or lysosomal enzymes, inhibit lymphocyte proliferation and immunoglobulin production by interfering with IL-1 production by macrophages, or alter the processing and presentation of peptide antigen in the macrophage. Hydroxychloroquine is principally used as a basal agent for attenuating a mild inflammatory process or stabilizing a remission. It should be discontinued if the patient fails to show any improvement after 6 months.

The adverse effects of hydroxychloroquine include dermatitis, myopathy and corneal opacity, which is usually reversible. Irreversible retinal degeneration can occur and is a cause for concern, but is not common at the doses currently used. Nonetheless, ophthalmologic examination is required every 6 months during treatment.

Sulfasalazine may reduce the rate of progression of erosions in RA. Its adverse effects include gastric symptoms, neutropenia, hemolysis, hepatitis and rash.

Methotrexate is another immunosuppressive drug that is useful in the treatment of RA. It is a folic acid antagonist and is given in a single oral low dose (7.5–15 mg) once a week. This treatment of RA is discussed in more detail in Chapter 12. Methotrexate inhibits cell division by competitively binding dihydrofolate reductase, resulting in decreased thymidine and purine nucleotide synthesis. Its action is therefore cell-cycle specific, destroying cells during the S phase of DNA synthesis but

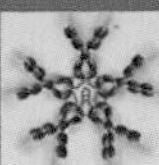

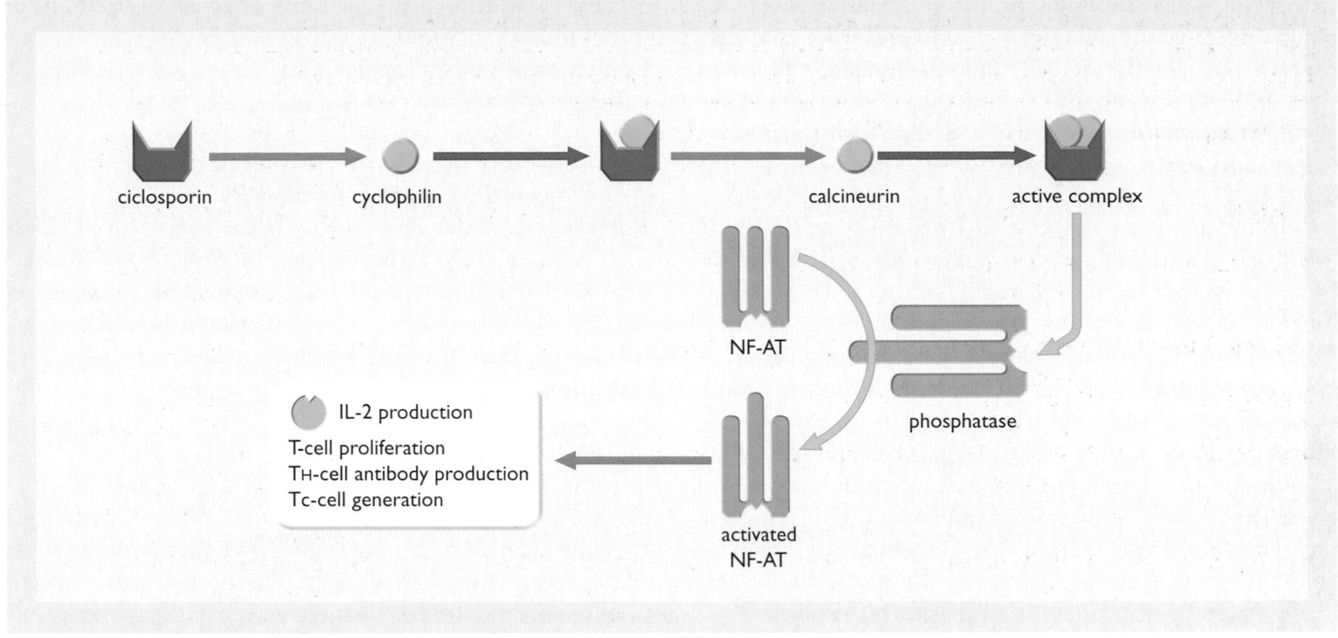

Fig. 9.12 Mechanism of action of ciclosporin. The drug forms a complex with cyclophilin and calcineurin inside T cells. The complex inhibits a phosphatase responsible for activating NF-AT. As a consequence, NF-AT-mediated processes are inhibited.

having little to no effect on resting cells. Methotrexate suppresses primary and secondary antibody responses in vivo, but few effects have been observed on pre-existing delayed-type hypersensitivity reactions.

The effect of weekly low-dose methotrexate may be anti-inflammatory and not immunosuppressive. Methotrexate significantly reduces the generation of the 5-lipoxygenase pathway products by leukocytes, and may also decrease IL-1 production by macrophages.

The major adverse effects of methotrexate include bone marrow suppression (leukopenia and thrombocytopenia), increased appearance of opportunistic infections, and hepatotoxicity with fibrosis. Liver fibrosis is most common in those who have a cumulative dosage of 1.5 g, in those receiving the drug daily, and in those with pre-existing liver disease, alcoholism or diabetes mellitus. Other adverse effects include interstitial pneumonitis, gastrointestinal upset, stomatitis with oral ulcerations, dermatitis, osteoporotic fractures and fetal malformation. Unlike other cytotoxic drugs, methotrexate is not associated with an increased risk of malignancy.

Azathioprine is another immunosuppressive drug used for RA. Azathioprine is pro-drug of 6-mercaptopurine (6-MP) and transformed to 6-MP in the liver. The metabolites of 6-MP block purine synthesis, cause DNA damage and have cytotoxic actions. Azathioprine suppresses T cell-mediated immune response including delayed-type hypersensitivities to a greater degree than antibody production. Adverse effects of azathioprine include bone marrow suppression and an increased risk of malignancy. The immunosuppressive effects and adverse effects of azathioprine are milder than those of cyclophosphamide. The effects of azathioprine are amplified by allopurinol, an inhibitor of xanthine oxidase that also inactivates 6-MP.

Leflunomide is a newly developed selective inhibitor of de novo pyrimidine synthesis. Unlike other proliferating cell types, lymphocytes cannot undergo cell division when the pathway for the de novo synthesis of pyrimidines is blocked. Thus, leflunomide selectively suppresses lymphocyte proliferation. Leflunomide is similar to both sulfasalazine and methotrexate in efficacy for RA. Adverse effects of leflunomide include diarrhea, liver dysfunction, alopecia and rash. This drug is contraindicated in pregnant women because of teratogenicity.

Glucocorticosteroids can be used in the treatment of RA

This is discussed in more detail in Chapter 15.

CICLOSPORIN AND T-CELL SUPPRESSION Ciclosporin has a selective inhibitory effect on T cells by inhibiting the TCR-mediated signal transduction pathway. It specifically binds to its cytoplasmic binding protein, cyclophilin, and this complex then binds to calcineurin, inhibiting phosphatase activity and therefore the nuclear translocation of the nuclear factor of activated T cells (NF-AT) (Fig. 9.12). Ciclosporin inhibits IL-2 production, T-cell proliferation, TH-cell activity for antibody production and Tc cell generation, and so could have a beneficial effect on autoantibody production and immune complex-mediated diseases. Ciclosporin has therefore been used to treat autoimmune diseases, though most available data are for RA. A clinical improvement is generally observed, but the adverse effects of ciclosporin, as well as the flares that occur after ciclosporin is discontinued, may limit its use. Ciclosporin is also an effective therapy for ocular Behçet's disease, psoriasis, atopic dermatitis, aplastic anemia, transplant rejection and nephrotic syndrome, and may have therapeutic activity in polymyositis, dermatomyositis (see below) and severe glucocorticosteroid-dependent asthma (see Ch. 14).

The major adverse effect of ciclosporin is renal toxicity (primarily proximal renal tubular changes), which is usually dose-related and reversible. Other adverse effects include hypertension, hepatotoxicity, tremor, hirsutism and gingival hyperplasia. Bone marrow suppression is unusual. Lymphomas have been reported in some ciclosporin-treated renal transplant recipients. Ciclosporin interacts with a variety of drugs. Phenobarbital, phenytoin and rifampin decrease plasma ciclosporin levels through the induction of the hepatic P-450 system. On the other hand, macrolides, ketoconazole, itraconazole and grapefruit juice increase plasma levels of this drug. Therefore, monitoring of plasma ciclosporin levels is necessary in order to obtain adequate immunosuppressive effects and minimize adverse effects.

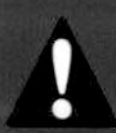

Immunosuppressive drugs

- **The major adverse effects of cytotoxic drugs are bone marrow suppression and opportunistic infections**
- **Cyclophosphamide causes hemorrhagic cystitis, amenorrhea and azoospermia, and an increased risk of malignancies**
- **Methotrexate causes hepatotoxicity and interstitial pneumonitis**
- **Ciclosporin causes renal toxicity**

Polymyositis and dermatomyositis

Polymyositis and dermatomyositis are immunologically mediated inflammatory muscle diseases characterized by lymphocyte infiltration in the skeletal muscle. Patients with polymyositis have symmetric proximal muscle weakness, elevated serum levels of muscle-associated enzymes such as creatine kinase (CK), electromyographic abnormalities characteristic of inflammatory myopathy, and histologic evidence of muscle damage and lymphocyte infiltration in a muscle biopsy. These features are also seen in patients with dermatomyositis in addition to a characteristic heliotrope skin rash and Gottron's erythema.

The underlying mechanisms of polymyositis and dermatomyositis may differ. Interstitial infiltration of CD8+ T cells surrounding and invading otherwise normal-appearing myocytes is a prominent feature in polymyositis. In contrast, perivascular infiltration of CD4+ T cells and B cells and perifascicular muscle fiber atrophy are prominent in dermatomyositis. The myositis-specific autoantibodies may also play a pathogenetic role: for example, anti-Jo-1 autoantibody is directed against histidyl-tRNA synthetase and is found in 20–30% of patients with myositis.

Glucocorticosteroids are the mainstay of therapy for polymyositis and dermatomyositis

Polymyositis and dermatomyositis are treated with high doses of glucocorticosteroids (prednisone or prednisolone 1–2 mg/kg/day). The glucocorticosteroid is continued in a high dose until the serum CK level returns to normal. The dose is then tapered very slowly. The condition may improve within 1–4 weeks, but in some patients treatment may be needed for 3 months before there is an improvement. Muscle strength may not improve for weeks to months after the serum concentrations of muscle-derived enzymes have normalized. Patients who have a poor prognosis (i.e. patients with acute severe myositis who are bedridden with muscle weakness, dysphagia or respiratory muscle weakness, and patients with interstitial pneumonitis) are treated with i.v. 'pulses' of 1000 mg methylprednisolone for 3 days, followed by maintenance with daily glucocorticosteroids. Sometimes it is difficult to distinguish glucocorticosteroid-induced myopathy (increasing muscle weakness during glucocorticosteroid therapy) from a relapse of the myositis.

Other immunosuppressive drugs are sometimes used

Immunosuppressive drugs are also used:

- For severe polymyositis or dermatomyositis.
- If the response to glucocorticosteroids is inadequate after 1–3 months of treatment.
- If there are frequent relapses.

Oral methotrexate is a major therapeutic option for glucocorticosteroid-resistant patients. Ciclosporin may be beneficial for conditions such as interstitial pneumonitis.

Systemic sclerosis

Systemic sclerosis (SSc) is a multisystem disorder of unknown etiology characterized by fibrosis of the skin, lungs and gastrointestinal tract, Raynaud's phenomenon, and microvascular abnormalities of the skin and visceral organs. Its characteristic immunologic and microvascular abnormalities include:

- Antinuclear antibodies, particularly anti-Scl-70 autoantibody found in 30–70% of patients and directed against the nuclear enzyme DNA topoisomerase I.
- Hypergammaglobulinemia.
- Perivascular infiltration of CD4+ T cells and macrophages in the dermis.
- Intimal thickening with narrowing of the vascular lumen in the skin and kidneys.

D-penicillamine has been used to reduce fibrosis and prevent the development of skin thickening and significant organ involvement. This drug interferes with

 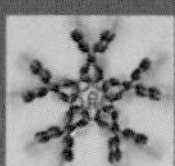

inter- and intramolecular cross-linking of collagen and is also immunosuppressive, including the inhibitory effect on TH-cell function. Its immunosuppressive activity may also lead to decreased collagen production.

Glucocorticosteroids are indicated for inflammatory myositis in SSc. They also reduce edema associated with the edematous phase of early skin involvement, but are not indicated in the long-term treatment of SSc. High doses of glucocorticosteroids may cause acute renal failure in such patients.

Polyarteritis nodosa

Polyarteritis nodosa (PN) is an immune complex-mediated necrotizing vasculitis that characteristically affects small and medium-sized muscular arteries, especially at their bifurcations. Most lesions occur in the kidney, heart, liver, gastrointestinal tract, musculoskeletal system, testes, peripheral nervous system and skin. The symptoms and signs depend on the severity and location of vessel involvement and the resulting ischemic changes. Non-specific features include fever, weight loss, malaise, neutrophilia, increased C-reactive protein and increased erythrocyte sedimentation rate. Circulating immune complexes have also been detected. The lesions contain immunoglobulins and complement components, and in some cases hepatitis B antigen is detected. The deposited immune complexes produce lesions by activating complement components and attracting and activating inflammatory cells.

Glucocorticosteroids are the mainstay of therapy, but the addition of cyclophosphamide nearly doubles the 5-year survival rate to 90%.

Transplantation rejection

Antilymphocyte globulin is used as an immunosuppressive drug for the treatment of transplantation rejection and certain types of aplastic anemia.

Many polyclonal antibodies have been prepared, but more recently a mouse anti-CD3 monoclonal antibody, muromonab, has been introduced for immunosuppression in an attempt to minimize the xenogeneic antibody response in the patient.

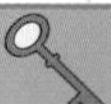

Characteristic features of autoimmune diseases

- **Autoimmune diseases are characterized by the presence of autoantibodies and autoreactive T cells against self-antigens**
- **Disease-specific autoantibodies are frequently detected: anti-DNA antibody in systemic lupus erythematosus; rheumatoid factor (autoantibody to IgG) in rheumatoid arthritis; anti-Jo-1 antibody in polymyositis; and anti-Scl-70 antibody in systemic sclerosis**
- **Glucocorticosteroids and immunosuppressive drugs are effective treatments**

Rejection of transplanted organs is another clinical setting where immunosuppressive drugs such as ciclosporin A are used because of their ability to inhibit T-lymphocyte function. Ciclosporin A is often used therapeutically for this purpose alongside glucocorticosteroids. Sirolimus is a newer immunosuppressant that also inhibits the activation and proliferation of T lymphocytes in response to antigens (such as presented on a foreign transplanted organ). Sirolimus is often used as an adjunct in combination with ciclosporin A and glucocorticosteroids for the prevention of acute renal allograft rejection. This combination of immunosuppressive drugs reduced the incidence of biopsy-proven acute rejection by about 40% during the first 6 months of therapy compared with placebo. Oral absorption of sirolimus is rapid (time to peak concentration in serum is 2 hours). The terminal elimination half-life (+ 1/2) is 72 hours in males and 61 hours in females. A loading dose of three times the maintenance dose will provide near steady-state concentrations within 1 day of treatment. The molecular mechanisms of action of this drug and its use in other diseases in discussed in Chapter 13.

FURTHER READING

Arshad S, Hassan. Allergy: an illustrated colour text. Edinburgh, Toronto: Churchill Livingstone, 2002.

Corrigan C, Rak S. Allergy. London: Mosby, c2004.

Frank MM, Austen KF, Calman HN, Unanue ER (eds). *Samter's Immunologic Diseases*, 6th edn. Boston: Little, Brown; 2001. [This book describes, in depth, the mechanism and therapy of immunologic diseases, including hypersensitivity and autoimmune diseases.]

Hele DJ, Belvisi MS. Novel therapies for the treatment of inflammatory airway disease. *Exp Opinion on Investigational Drugs* 2003; **12**: 5–18.

Levy BD, Serhan CN. Exploring new approaches to the treatment of asthma: potential roles for lipoxins and aspirin-triggered lipid mediators. *Drugs Today* 2003; **39**: 373–384.

Maddox L, Schwartz DA. The pathophysiology of asthma. *Ann Rev Med* 2002; **53**: 477–498.

Pelaia G, Vatrella A, Cuda G, Maselli R, Marsico SA. Molecular mechanisms of corticosteroid actions in chronic inflammatory airway diseases. *Life Sci* 2003; **72**: 1549–1561.

Roitt IM, Brostoff J, Male DK (eds). *Immunology*, 6th edn. London: Mosby; 2001. [This, and the above reference, are updated standard textbooks, with well-drawn illustrations, for understanding the basics of clinical allergy and immunology.]

Smith, Helen E, Frew AJ. Allergy: your questions answered. Edinburgh; New York: Churchill Livingstone, 2003.

Tobin MJ. Asthma, airway biology, and nasal disorders in AJRCCM 2001. *Am J Resp Critical Care Med* 2002; **165**: 598–618.

WEBSITE

http://www.allergyuk.org/

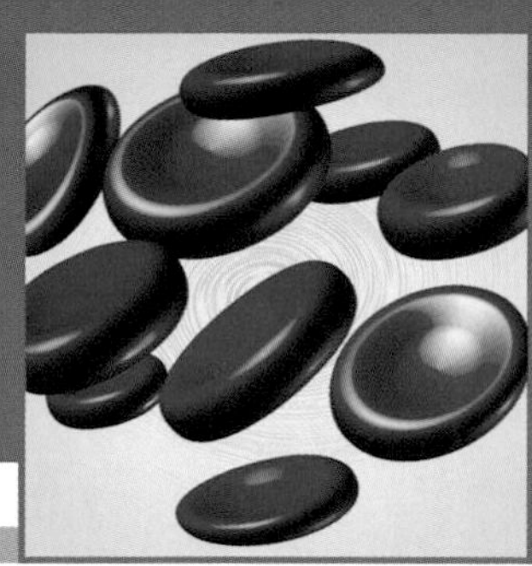

Chapter 10

Drugs and the Blood

PHYSIOLOGY OF THE HEMATOPOIETIC SYSTEM

Blood is a suspension of cells in plasma. The latter is a solution of proteins and salts. The cells are red blood cells (erythrocytes), white blood cells (leukocytes) and platelets (Fig. 10.1).

- Erythrocytes are anuclear, contain hemoglobin, and carry oxygen from the lungs to all tissues where it is exchanged for carbon dioxide.
- Leukocytes (neutrophils, monocytes, lymphocytes, eosinophils and others) defend the body against microorganisms.
- Platelets form plugs with coagulation proteins to stop leaks from blood vessels and have also been recently shown to act as inflammatory cells.

All blood cells are derived from hematopoietic stem cells

All blood cells originate in the bone marrow, except during early fetal life. The bone marrow provides a hematopoietic microenvironment to support the process of hematopoietic self-renewal and differentiation. Hematopoietic stem cells self-replicate and exist in very small numbers in the bone marrow and blood. Each stem cell has a great capacity for self-renewal. However, as a group, hematopoietic stem cells are relatively quiescent and only a minuscule fraction are proliferating and differentiating at any one time to replenish lost blood cells.

Hematopoietic growth factors and cytokines control hematopoiesis

Hematopoietic stem cells give rise to hematopoietic progenitor cells. Compared with stem cells, these cells have a decreased capacity for self-renewal and are more committed to differentiating into a particular cell type. With each generation, the descendants of the progenitor cells differentiate further into more mature cells with a more limited life span, becoming restricted to a particular blood cell lineage. Ultimately, the process ends with mature cells, which have no further capacity to divide and give rise to red cells, leukocytes and platelets (Fig. 10.2).

This maturation process is controlled by hematopoietic growth factors and cytokines that activate the appropriate growth factor, or cytokine, receptors leading to cell differentiation and proliferation. Many of these factors have been purified and cloned. Some have been

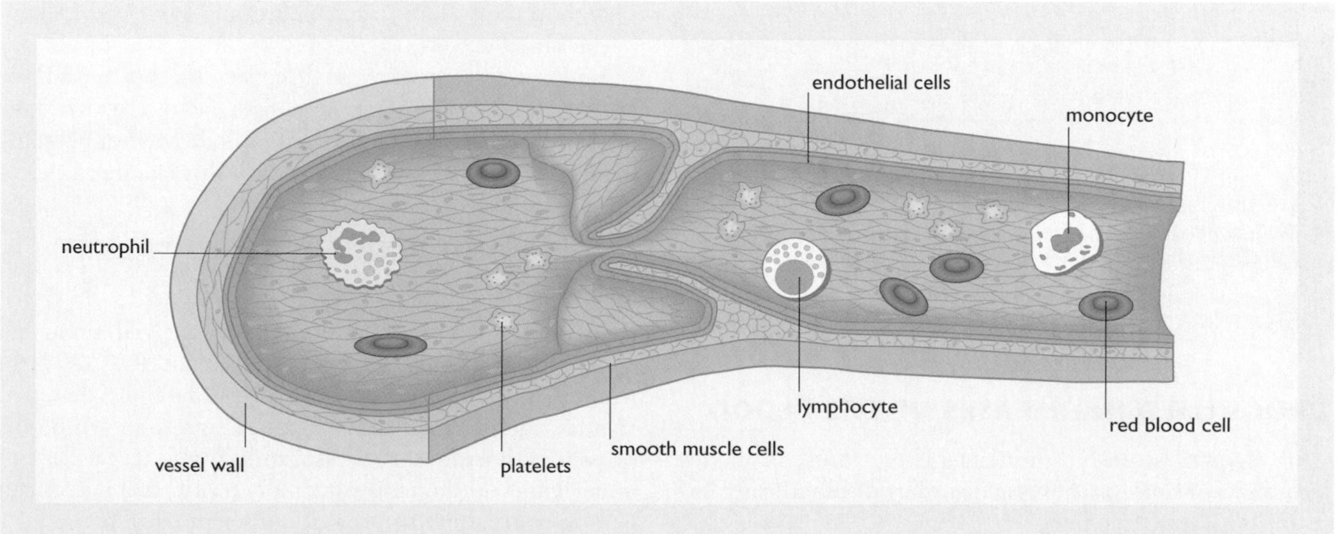

Fig. 10.1 Blood vessel (vein) and the blood cells. The blood vessel wall and its surrounding smooth muscle cells are lined by endothelial cells, which provide a nonthrombotic surface for smooth blood flow. White blood cells (neutrophils, monocytes and lymphocytes) interact with the blood vessel cells to defend the body against microbial invasion. Red blood cells carry oxygen to end organs. Platelets plug leaks in the blood vessels.

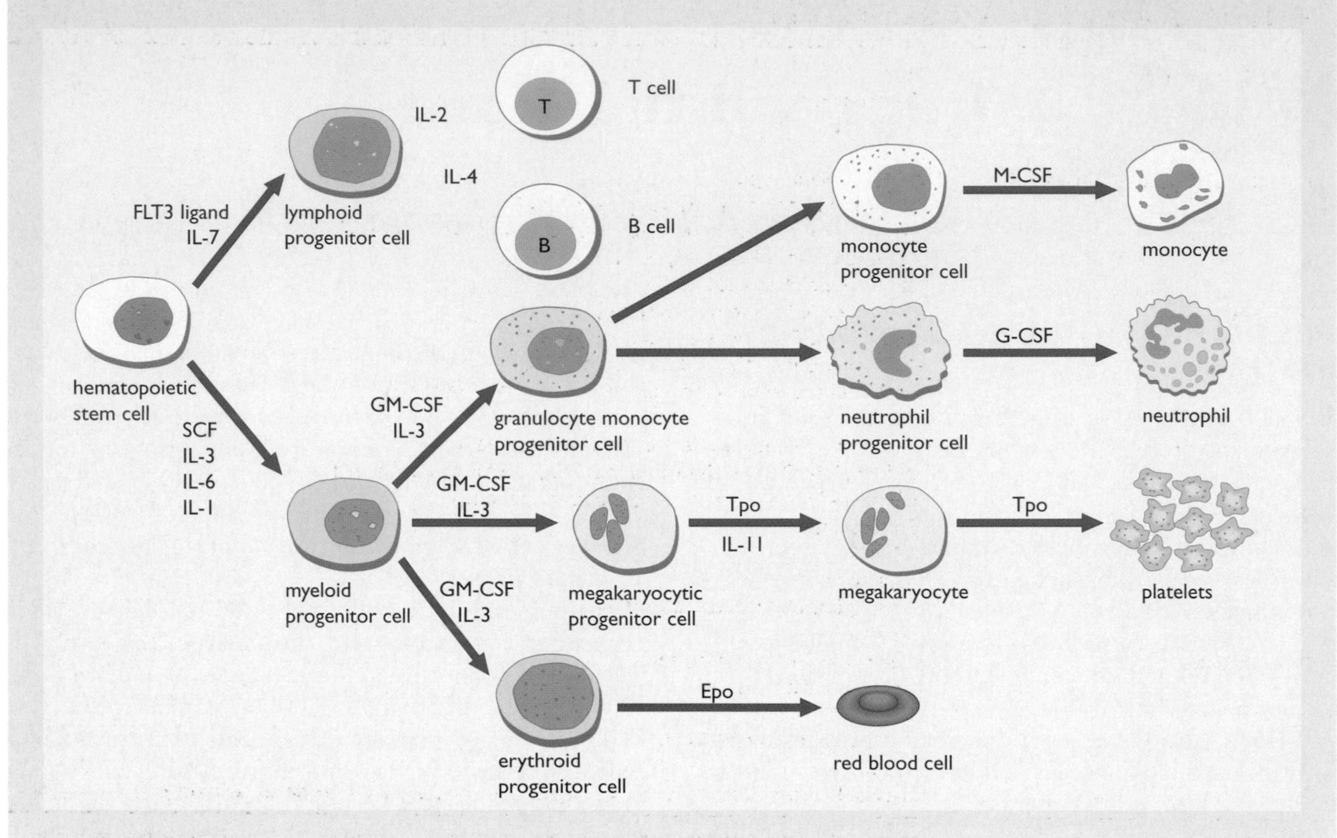

Fig. 10.2 Hematopoiesis and hematopoietic growth factors. Hematopoietic stem cells have a high regenerative potential, but with each generation the descendant cells acquire lineage-specific characteristics and decreased proliferative capacity. Growth factors including Epo, G-CSF, GM-CSF, IL, M-CSF, SCF and Tpo are needed for regulating each step of hemopoiesis (Epo, erythropoietin; FLT3, C-FMS-like tyrosine kinase; G-CSF, granulocyte colony-stimulating factor; GM-CSF, granulocyte–macrophage colony-stimulating factor; IL, interleukin; M-CSF, macrophage colony-stimulating factor; SCF, stem cell factor; Tpo, thrombopoietin).

produced by recombinant technology and are used as protein therapeutics for a variety of disorders, as discussed below.

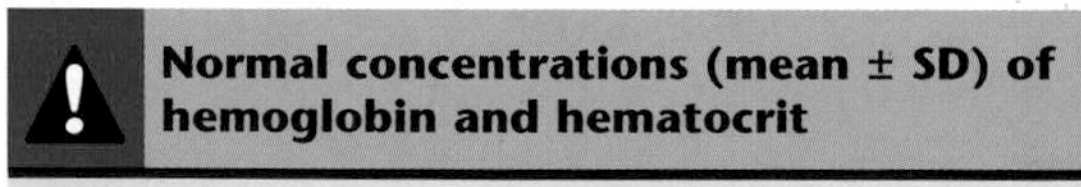

Normal concentrations (mean ± SD) of hemoglobin and hematocrit

	Hemoglobin g/dL	Hemoglobin (mmol/L)	Hematocrit %
Prepubertal child	12.5 ± 1.5	(7.37 ± 0.93)	38 ± 4
Male adult	15.4 ± 1.8	(9.56 ± 1.12)	44 ± 5
Female adult	13.5 ± 2.0	(8.38 ± 1.24)	38 ± 5

Hematocrit in third trimester for pregnant women may be as low as 30%

DRUGS USED IN DISEASES OF THE BLOOD

This chapter describes the drugs that are useful in the treatment of three pathologic disorders of blood: anemia, thrombosis and bleeding.

- Anemia is a subnormal circulating hemoglobin. Its symptoms result from the decreased oxygen-carrying capacity of red blood cells.
- Thrombosis is formation of unwanted clots in blood vessels, which can block delivery of blood to end organs or the return of blood to the heart.
- Bleeding disorders result from failure of the hemostatic system to form clots and to stop leaks in the blood vessels.

Drugs used to treat these disorders are shown in Table 10.1. Several hematopoietic growth factors, which have become standard drugs for hematologic or nonhematologic disorders, are also discussed in this chapter.

ANEMIA AND DRUGS USED TO TREAT ANEMIA

By definition, anemia is a reduction in the red blood cell mass with the hematocrit value less than 40% (37% in women), or hemoglobin below normal by more than two standard deviations. Anemia causes signs and symptoms of pallor, shortness of breath and fatigue (regardless of underlying etiologies) since all result from reduced hemoglobin failing to provide sufficient oxygen.

Based on the ability of bone marrow to produce red blood cells, and by measuring the number of young red blood cells (reticulocytes) in the blood, the causes of anemia can be placed into two categories:

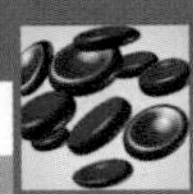

Table 10.1 Drugs used to treat blood disorders

Drugs for anemia	Iron Deseroxamine Vitamin B_{12} Folate
Hematopoietic growth factors	Erythropoietin (Epo) Granulocyte colony-stimulating factor (G-CSF) Granulocyte–macrophage colony-stimulating factor (GM-CSF) Oprelvekin (Interleukin-11, IL-11) Thrombopoietin (Tpo)
Antiplatelet agents	Irreversible COX inhibitor (aspirin) Reversible COX inhibitors (some NSAIDs) ADP antagonists (ticlopidine, clopidogrel) GPIIb/IIIa antagonists (abciximab, eptifibatide, tirofiban) Dipyridamole
Anticoagulants	Inhibitors of coagulant factor formation (warfarin) Indirect inhibitors of thrombin (heparin, LMWH [enoxaparin]) Direct inhibitors of thrombin (hirudin [lepirudin])
Thrombolytics	Streptokinase APSAC Urokinase Tissue plasminogen activator (tPA) Reteplase
Procoagulants	Coagulant factor concentrates Desmopressin (DDAVP) Vitamin K ε Aminocaproic acid (EACA) Aprotinin Topical hemostatics (thrombin, collagen, absorbable gelatin, oxidized cellulose)

COX, cyclooxygenase; ADP, adenosine diphosphate; APSAC, anisoylated plasminogen–streptokinase activator complex; NSAIDs, nonsteroidal antiinflammatory drugs; LMWH, low molecular weight heparin.

- A low reticulocyte count (hypoproliferative anemia), where the bone marrow is not making sufficient red blood cells.
- A high reticulocyte count due to a hemolytic anemia, consequent to increased peripheral destruction of red blood cells despite increased production.

Hypoproliferative anemias are further subdivided based on red blood cell size:

- Microcytic anemia (small red blood cells).
- Normocytic anemia (normal-sized red blood cells).
- Macrocytic anemia (large red blood cells).

Table 10.2 lists the etiologies of anemia according to these criteria.

Table 10.2 Causes of anemia

Hypoproliferative	
Microcytic	Iron deficiency Anemia due to chronic disease Sideroblastic anemia
Normocytic	Anemia due to chronic disease Endocrine anemia Bone marrow failure
Macrocytic	Vitamin B_{12} deficiency Folic acid deficiency Myelodysplastic syndrome
Hyperproliferative	
Hemolytic	Hemoglobinopathies Autoimmune Membrane disorder Drug-induced Metabolic abnormalities Glucose-6-phosphate dehydrogenase deficiency Infections

Iron and iron-deficiency anemia

Iron deficiency remains the most common cause of anemia worldwide

Although dietary iron deficiency may occur in infants and adolescence during their rapid growth phase, iron deficiency generally occurs only as a result of chronic bleeding. In women, it is usually due to blood loss from menstruation and pregnancy; in men and postmenopausal women, iron-deficiency anemia is often a clue to pathologic blood loss and thus warrants a search to discover the source of bleeding in these patients.

Two-thirds of the body's iron is in hemoglobin

Iron is needed to form the complex molecule heme, which is the oxygen-carrying component of hemoglobin. When aging red cells are destroyed, almost all their iron is salvaged for new red blood cells. However, a small but

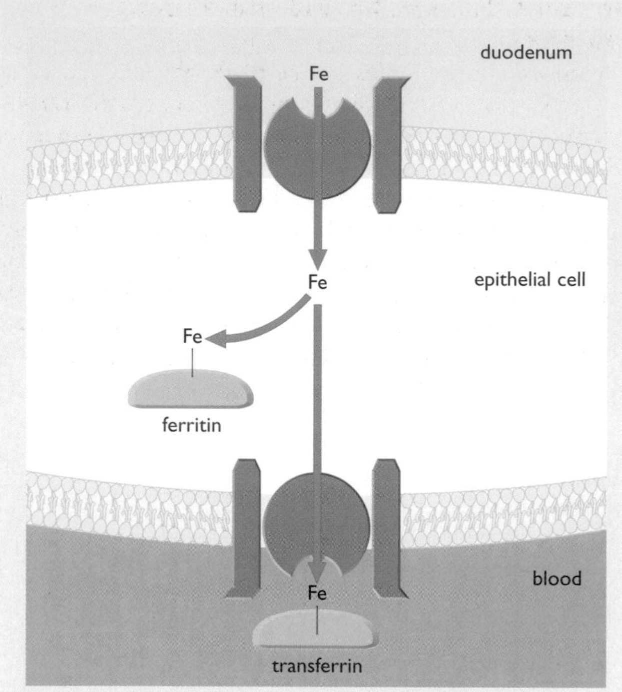

Fig. 10.3 Iron absorption by the gastrointestinal epithelial cell. Iron is absorbed via a cell surface receptor on the epithelial cell. Some of the iron passes through the cell and is carried in the blood by transferrin. Excess iron is stored as ferritin.

critical fraction of iron for red blood cells is obtained from the diet. Dietary iron is absorbed mostly in the duodenum and proximal jejunum in part as heme and in its elemental form via intestinal epithelial cell surface receptors. Heme iron is readily absorbed and released from the porphyrin ring by heme oxygenase in cells. Non-heme iron absorption is highly variable and many types of food, such as tea, egg yolk and bran, interfere with iron absorption. Excess iron is stored in cells as a ferritin complex.

Iron is transported in the plasma bound with transferrin. Iron-transferrin complexes bind to transferrin receptors, which are membrane glycoproteins expressed on maturing erythroid cells. This leads to the internalization with subsequent release of iron intracellularly. The free transferrin and transferrin receptors are recycled to the cell membrane (Fig. 10.3).

The physiologic daily loss of iron is approximately:

- 1 mg/day in men, and nonmenstruating women.
- 2–3 mg/day in menstruating women.
- 500–1000 mg with each pregnancy.

A patient's history and physical examination yields information suggesting iron-deficiency anemia, but the definite diagnosis of iron deficiency depends on one or more specific laboratory tests. Serum ferritin levels are helpful in the assessment of body iron stores since they are associated with iron-deficiency anemia unless there is a concurrent process that abnormally raises the level, such as infection or liver disease. Iron deficiency also results in a low serum iron level and a high total iron binding capacity (TIBC), i.e., a low iron:total iron binding capacity ratio. Microcytosis is a late finding. The most sensitive and specific test in diagnosing iron deficiency is a bone marrow examination of iron stores, the bone marrow iron stain, but this procedure is not usually needed in most clinical situations.

Treatment of iron-deficiency anemia consists of correction of the underlying causes and iron replacement therapy. Oral administration of ferrous sulfate is the standard treatment. Iron is best absorbed when taken on an empty stomach with ascorbic acid, which binds to iron and facilitates transport into intestinal cells. At the acidic pH of the stomach, mucin binds to inorganic iron and enhances its absorption, which may otherwise be impaired by antacids or medications that reduce stomach acid production. Commercial preparations of ferrous sulfate usually contain 60 mg of elemental iron. Only 10–20% of the ingested iron is absorbed by iron-deficient patients since bioavailability is relatively low. The usual dose is 150–200 mg elemental iron per day, divided into three or four doses. A prompt rise in reticulocyte count confirms iron deficiency. The hemoglobin concentration of patients optimally treated with 180 mg/day of elemental iron increases by about 1 g/dL/week (mass concentration 10 g/L/week; substance concentration 0.62 mmol/L/week). Iron supplementation should continue for another 6 months after the hemoglobin level has been normalized in order to replenish the body's iron stores.

The most common side effect of treatment with iron is gastrointestinal irritation and sometimes this is bothersome. Thus, physicians need to counsel patients in order to foster compliance. Lowering the daily doses of iron or taking iron with meals significantly reduces iron-induced adverse effects. A polysaccharide–iron complex preparation may cause less gastrointestinal irritation, but is more expensive. Parenteral iron preparations are also available but are only indicated for patients with iron-deficiency anemia unable to tolerate or absorb iron pills, or who have chronic bleeding disorders, or whose needs cannot be met by oral iron therapy alone. The intramuscular route is painful and may cause skin discoloration at the injection site. Alternatively, iron dextran can be slowly infused intravenously, but this requires close monitoring, because of a high incidence of anaphylactoid-like reactions.

Warning about oral iron preparations

- **Taking oral iron leads to black stools that may obscure the clinical diagnosis of gastrointestinal bleeding!**

Desferoxamine and iron overload

Excessive iron may result in acute or chronic iron toxicity (iron overload). Acute iron toxicity is usually seen in

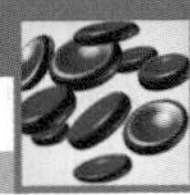

young children who ingest iron tablets that are used either as a pediatric or prenatal vitamin supplement, or for treatment of anemia in a family member or themselves. Iron pills are particularly tempting to young children, since they look like candies. Acute iron toxicity is the leading cause of poisoning death in children under 6 years. A chronic iron overload, on the other hand, is common with inherited hemochromatosis. This disorder is caused by excess iron absorption and blood transfusions over a long period of time in the absence of bleeding. For example, iron overload is a leading cause of death in thalassemia patients in industrialized nations due to the fact that the body cannot substantially increase elimination of iron.

Iron toxicity can be corrosive and/or cellular. Iron is an extremely corrosive substance to the mucosal tissues in the gastrointestinal system. Such corrosive effects can be manifest as hematemesis or diarrhea. Patients may become hypovolemic due to fluid and blood loss. The absorption of excessive quantities of ingested iron results in systemic iron toxicity with impaired oxidative phosphorylation, mitochondrial dysfunction, resulting in cell death. The organ most affected is the liver, although other organs, heart, kidneys, lungs and the hematologic systems, may also be damaged. With acute ingestion of elemental iron (>20 mg/kg body weight) patients typically show signs of gastrointestinal toxicity. When ingestion exceeds 40 mg/kg, patients generally have moderate to severe intoxication. Ingestion of >60 mg/kg may lead to death.

Iron overload can be prevented and treated with a chelating agent to complex iron and promote its excretion. The only iron chelating agent currently in clinical use is deferoxamine B, a trihydroxamic acid isolated from the bacterium *Streptomyces pilosus* with selectivity for ferric iron. It is given subcutaneously or intravenously to chelate iron in acute and chronic iron overload.

Deferoxamine subcutaneously is given at 20–50 mg/kg over 8–10 hours, three to five nights per week. Administration of deferoxamine should be continued until the ferritin level is consistently less than 1000 ng/mL. Ascorbic acid (vitamin C), 100 mg, increases excretion of iron and is given in combination with deferoxamine. If there is severe hemosiderosis, deferoxamine is given intravenously, 100 mg/kg over 12 hours. It is desired to keep the ferritin level below 2000 ng/mL; if the ferritin is above 4000 ng/mL hospital admission should be considered for high-dose deferoxamine therapy.

The most common adverse effects of deferoxamine include tinnitus and reversible transient hearing loss unrelated to dose. Decreased night vision is less common. Intravenous (i.v.) infusions exceeding 15 mg/kg/h may induce hypotension and even shock. Allergic reactions including anaphylaxis are not uncommon. Hydrocortisone can be mixed with deferoxamine to decrease this reaction. Diluting deferoxamine can reduce the irritation at the site of administration. Excessive iron chelation will cause growth disturbance in children and mineral deficiency.

Vitamin B_{12}, folate and macrocytic anemias

The macrocytic anemias can be megaloblastic, caused by a biochemical defect in deoxyribonucleic acid (DNA) synthesis, or nonmegaloblastic anemia, usually associated with a pathologic alteration in membrane lipids of red blood cells. The most common conditions causing megaloblastic anemia include vitamin B_{12} (cobalamin) deficiency, folate deficiency, myelodysplasia and medications that inhibit DNA synthesis. Both cobalamin and folate are critical cofactors in enzymatic reactions required for DNA synthesis (Fig. 10.4). The interdependency of

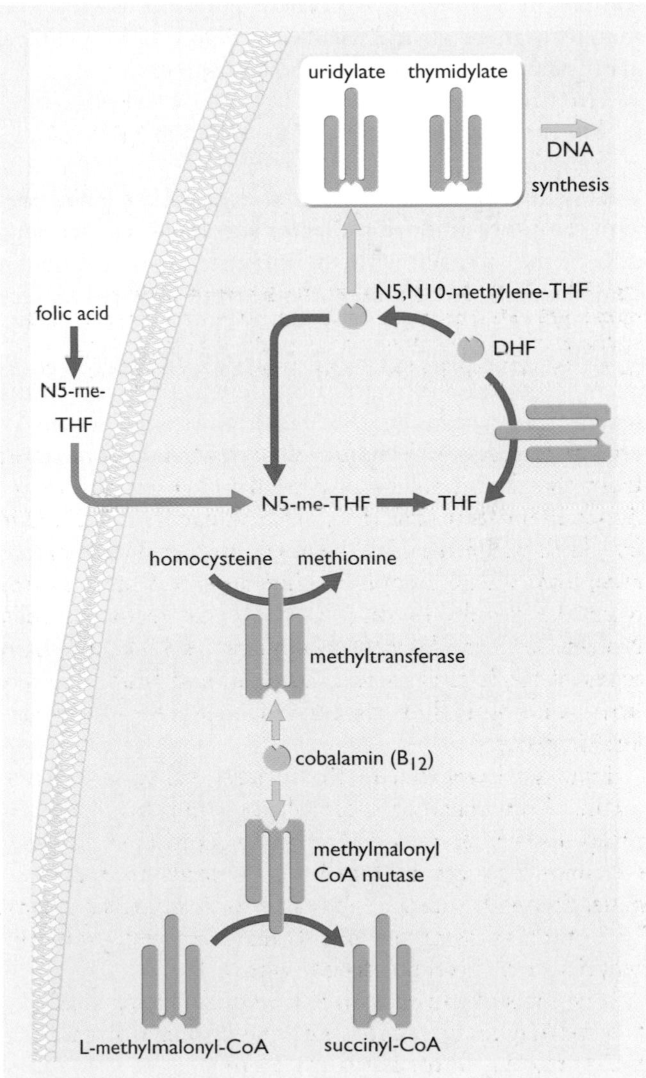

Fig. 10.4 Role of folate and vitamin B_{12} in DNA synthesis. Folate compounds are carbon donors in the conversion of deoxyuridine to deoxythymidine. Cobalamin is a cofactor for homocysteine–methionine methyltransferase, which transfers a methyl group from methyltetrahydrofolate to homocysteine to make methionine. Cobalamin is also required for methylmalonyl coenzyme A (CoA) mutase, which converts methylmalonyl coenzyme A to succinyl coenzyme A. Methotrexate inhibits DNA synthesis by inhibiting DHF reductase which converts DHF to THF (DHF, dihydrofolate; N5-me-THF, N5-methyl-tetrahydrofolate; THF, tetrahydrofolate).

cobalamin and methylfolate may explain why similar morphologic changes occur when either cobalamin or folate is deficient. Unlike folate deficiency, however, vitamin B_{12} deficiency also causes neurologic deficits. Paresthesia is the earliest symptom followed by loss of vibratory sense, ataxia, dementia and coma.

Vitamin B_{12} deficiency

Vitamin B_{12} (cobalamin) is a complex molecule consisting of a central cobalt atom linked to four pyrrole rings and attached to a nucleotide. Humans obtain vitamin B_{12} from dietary animal proteins. The daily requirement is 0.6–1.2 μg, and the biologic half-life of vitamin B_{12} (stored in the liver) is about 1 year with a total body content of 3–5 mg. The normal daily loss is very low; therefore, more than 2 years can elapse before clinical manifestations of deficiency become apparent.

The most common cause of B_{12} deficiency is pernicious anemia

Vitamin B_{12} is absorbed from the gastrointestinal tract with the aid of an intrinsic factor secreted by the parietal cells of the stomach with the intrinsic factor–cobalamin complex absorbed via receptors on the ileal cell surface (Fig. 10.5) (see also Ch. 22). Since vitamin B_{12} is widely available in animal products, dietary deficiency is an uncommon cause of vitamin B_{12} deficiency except in the strictest vegetarians (e.g. vegans). Breast-fed infants of vegans can develop vitamin B_{12} deficiency. The most common cause of vitamin B_{12} deficiency is pernicious anemia, a form of gastric secretory failure with atrophy of gastric parietal cells and failure to secrete the intrinsic factor. It is suspected that pernicious anemia is autoimmune in that antiparietal cell and anti-intrinsic factor antibodies are detected in many patients. In addition, vitamin B_{12} deficiency is seen in patients with partial or total gastrectomy, malabsorption syndrome, inflammatory bowel disease or small bowel resection.

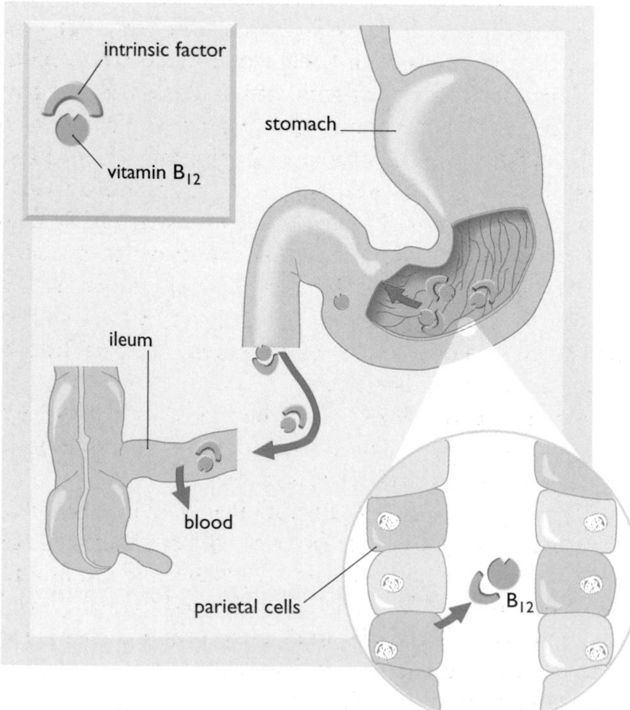

Fig. 10.5 Absorption of vitamin B_{12}. Intestinal absorption of vitamin B_{12} requires intrinsic factor, which is secreted by parietal cells in the stomach, and occurs in the distal ileum via cell surface receptors.

Diagnosis of vitamin B_{12} deficiency requires measuring serum vitamin B_{12} levels, although a minority of deficient patients have levels in the normal range. Vitamin B_{12} deficiency leads to increased serum and urine concentrations of methylmalonic acid, sensitive indices of vitamin B_{12} deficiency. A two-stage (Schilling) test, first with radiolabeled vitamin B_{12} alone and then with radiolabeled B_{12} plus intrinsic factor, can be performed to determine whether a vitamin B_{12} deficiency is due to pernicious anemia.

Treatment of vitamin B_{12} deficiency should start with parenteral B_{12}. There are two preparations of vitamin B_{12}, cyanocobalamin and hydroxycobalamin, for clinical use. The recommended initial dose is 0.1–1 mg of vitamin B_{12} intramuscularly daily for 1–2 weeks. The maintenance dose is monthly injections of 1 mg cyanocobalamin for life. However, oral therapy with 1 mg vitamin B_{12} five times a week is equally effective. Despite the lack of intrinsic factor, absorption in a passive diffusion can fulfil the 2–5 μg/day requirement. The application of a vitamin B gel intranasally (ENER-B gel) has been approved for dietary supplementation, but not for the treatment of pernicious anemia, although it does consistently raise serum vitamin B_{12} levels. Serum K^+ concentration may fall after treatment with vitamin B_{12} due to an increased need for intracellular K^+ to support new cell synthesis.

Megaloblastic anemia due to vitamin B_{12} deficiency can respond to large doses of folic acid administration. Conversely, supraphysiologic doses of vitamin B_{12} therapy can reverse megaloblastic anemia due to folate deficiency. Importantly, however, the neurologic damage due to vitamin B_{12} deficiency is not reversed by folate. Consequently, accurate diagnosis of the type of deficiency is essential.

Folic acid deficiency

Folates belong to the vitamin B family and are found in a wide variety of fresh foods, but are rapidly destroyed by heating food (see Ch. 22). Folic acid is widely distributed in nature as a conjugate with one or more molecules of glutamic acid. Naturally occurring folates must be reduced to mono- and diglutamates by conjugases present in the stomach before they can be efficiently absorbed from the proximal small intestine. Folates are transported to the liver where they are stored and transformed into 5-methyltetrahydrofolate, the form that enters tissue cells. In the cell, 5-methyltetrahydrofolate is converted into the metabolically active tetrahydrofolate

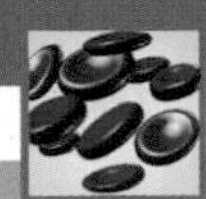

by vitamin B_{12}-dependent methyltransferase. The normal daily requirement of folate is about 100 µg, with tissue storage estimated at 10 mg. Inadequate dietary folate intake, therefore, leads to megaloblastic anemia much sooner than does vitamin B_{12} deficiency.

Warning about using folic acid

- Large doses of folic acid can reverse the megaloblastic anemia caused by vitamin B_{12} deficiency, but **do not** reverse the neurologic damage of vitamin B_{12} deficiency

Inadequate intake is the most common cause of folate deficiency

During pregnancy, the need for folates is markedly increased. Folate deficiency very early in pregnancy is associated with congenital neural tube defects. Folate supplementation is recommended for all pregnant women, or those who are likely to become pregnant, since there is increased requirement for folate even before a woman may realize that she is pregnant. Alcohol abuse is a common cause of folate-deficiency anemia as a result of reduced folate intake and diminished folate absorption. Since the concentration of folate in bile is several times higher than in plasma, bile deficiency will reduce the plasma concentration of folate. Patients with prolonged biliary drainage should therefore be given folate. People taking phenytoin and related anticonvulsants tend to have lower serum folate absorption, but they rarely have megaloblastic anemia. Antifolate drugs such as methotrexate are widely used to treat hematologic and inflammatory diseases. Methotrexate competes with dihydrofolate for the enzyme dihydrofolate reductase and, even at the relatively low doses of methotrexate used in the treatment of rheumatoid arthritis, there is evidence of red blood cell macrocytosis (see Fig. 10.4).

A patient's history, physical examination and finding of macrocytosis alert clinicians to possibile folate deficiency. Although folate deficiency and vitamin B_{12} deficiency cause similar morphologic changes in red blood cells, characteristic neurologic changes are only seen in megaloblastic anemia caused by vitamin B_{12} deficiency. Diagnosis of folate deficiency requires measuring serum or red blood cell folate levels; the latter is of greater diagnostic value.

Folate deficiency responds promptly to 1–5 mg/day oral folate. An injectable form is also available. Since vitamin B_{12} deficiency may cause concomitant folate deficiency, it is important to ascertain that the patient is not vitamin B_{12} deficient before starting folate treatment. Folate may correct the megaloblastic anemia of vitamin B_{12} deficiency, but will not correct neurologic damage. Indiscriminate use of folate may therefore mask the symptoms of vitamin B_{12} deficiency and lead to irreversible neurologic deficits.

Folic acid may help prevent atherosclerosis

Serum homocysteine concentrations are inversely correlated with serum folate levels. There is increasing evidence that an elevated serum homocysteine level is an independent risk factor for atherosclerosis. As a result, the effect of homocysteine-lowering treatment with folic acid in the prevention of atherothrombotic disease is being evaluated.

Hydroxyurea and sickle cell anemia

Sickle cell anemia is a common hemoglobinopathy, mainly in the black populations. Fifty years ago, Dr. Linus Pauling and colleagues discovered that sickle cell anemia was caused by the change in a protein molecule due to a single gene. The precise mechanism was later revealed as a point mutation in the β-chain gene of hemoglobin S resulting in substitution of valine for glutamate at the sixth amino acid position. This alteration markedly reduces the solubility of deoxygenated hemoglobin S, leading to polymerization of the deoxygenated hemoglobin S, and deformity of the red blood cell (sickling) and hemolysis. Patients with sickle cell anemia are homozygous for the sickle gene and have hemoglobin S but no hemoglobin A. In contrast, people with sickle cell trait are heterozygous for the sickle gene and have both kinds of hemoglobin. People with sickle cell trait (occurring in about one of 10 black people) are usually not symptomatic, but vigorous physical activity at high altitude, air travel and anesthesia are potentially dangerous.

Clinical manifestations result from episodic sickling leading to microvascular occlusion. Painful crises occur when rigid and deformed sickled cells interact with platelets, endothelium and coagulation factors to occlude the microcirculation. Patients with sickle cell disease have a severe hemolytic anemia that begins within weeks of birth, as hemoglobin S replaces hemoglobin F, and lasts throughout life. The average red blood cell life span in these patients is only 17 days versus the norm of 120 days, and thus patients are particularly sensitive to transient bone marrow suppression, caused by a variety of infections, that may lead to the development of aplastic crisis. Repeated episodes of ischemic necrosis lead to progressive organ damage.

Treatment of sickle cell anemia in the past was primarily supportive, with i.v. fluids, oxygen, analgesics for pain relief and blood transfusion.

Hydroxyurea (HU) is an inhibitor of the ribonucleotide reductase system that catalyzes the rate-limiting step in the de novo biosynthesis of purine and pyrimidine deoxyribonucleotides. It is currently used to treat chronic myelogenous leukemia and polycythemia vera (see Ch. 6). Recent clinical trials demonstrated that HU raises the population of reticulocytes containing hemoglobin F and stimulates a small rise in the hemoglobin F level. HU decreased painful crises in severely affected adults, and in children with sickle cell anemia. However, not all patients benefited from treatment, and crises were not eliminated in most patients. More clinical trials are needed to determine whether HU prevents chronic organ damage. Although HU has been widely used in the treatment of a variety of hematologic disorders, and is relatively well tolerated, the use of a cytotoxic drug in a nonmalignant condition raises questions about long-term safety. A clinical trial has recently shown that HU treatment at the maximum tolerated dose for 1 year results in a significant improvement in hematologic changes, including increased hemoglobin concentrations, with mild, transient and reversible toxicities in pediatric patients with sickle cell anemia. The dose of HU should be escalated slowly, a dose just below that which would produce significant cytopenia. The recommended final dose is 10–20 mg/kg body weight per day.

Hematopoietic growth factors

Hematopoietic growth factor receptors are members of the type I cytokine receptor family

More than 30 hematopoietic growth factors and cytokines that are involved in regulation of differentiation and proliferation of blood cells have been well characterized. These include factors regulating a specific cell lineage, factors regulating multiple cell lineages and factors indirectly regulating hematopoiesis by inducing gene expression of hematopoietic growth factors or cytokines. The structure of hematopoietic growth factors and cytokines is variable but the receptors for most of these factors are members of the type I cytokine receptor family. As a group, type I cytokine receptors usually consist of a receptor subunit and an associated transducer subunit. Three transducer subunits shared by the multiple members of this receptor family are glycoprotein 130 (GP 130), common β (βc) and common γ (γc). Unlike the tyrosine kinase receptor family, none of these type I cytokine receptors has an intrinsic tyrosine kinase domain. Instead, the receptors usually form homo- or heterodimers upon binding of their cognate growth factor or cytokines. The ligand-stimulated dimerization of the receptors triggers the activation of JAK/STAT tyrosine kinase signal pathways that mediate differentiation and proliferation of the growth factors or cytokines (Fig. 10.6; also see Ch. 3). Additionally, the Ras/MAP kinase and phosphatidylinositol 3 kinase signal pathways may also be utilized by these receptors to mediate stimulation of hematopoietic growth factors.

These factors have been rapidly introduced into the clinic for routine and experimental use. Currently, erythropoietin, G-CSF, GM-CSF and interleukin-11 have been approved for human use by the USA FDA, and many others, including thrombopoietin, are in the final phases of introduction.

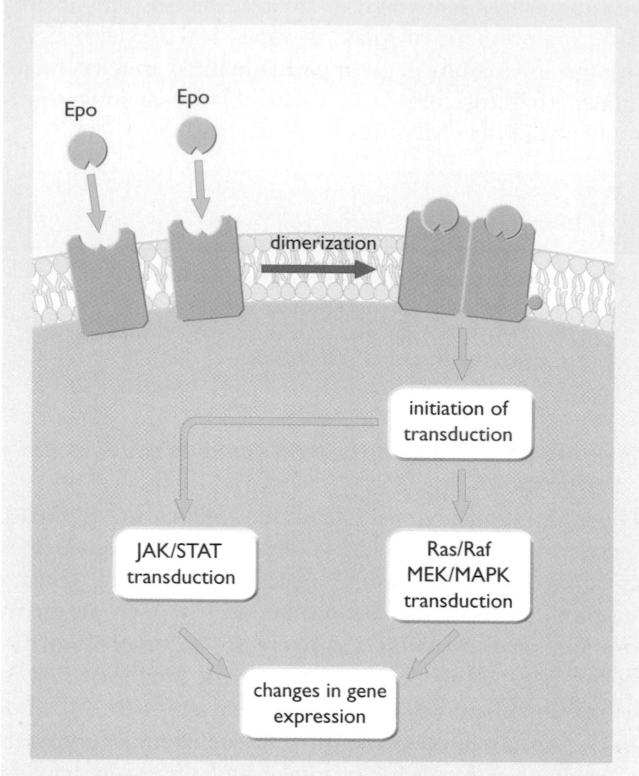

Fig. 10.6 Type I cytokine receptor signal transduction. Stimulation of type I cytokine receptors, in this case erythropoietin receptors (Epo), on hematopoietic progenitor cells induces dimerization of the receptors that trigger activation of JAK/STAT tyrosine kinase signal pathways and the Ras/MAP K signal pathway leading to the transcription of genes related to growth and differentiation.

Erythropoietin

Erythropoietin (Epo), a physiologic hormone, is the critical hematopoietic growth factor regulating red blood cell proliferation and differentiation in bone marrow. Natural erythropoietin was originally isolated and purified from the urine of patients with anemia. A recombinant form of human erythropoietin is a 165-amino acid glycoprotein with a 34–39 kDa molecular weight. The plasma half-life of intravenously administered erythropoietin is approximately 8 hours. The liver is a major site of erythropoietin degradation.

Erythropoietin is produced in response to tissue hypoxia in fetal liver and in adult kidney. Hemoprotein receptors (sensors in the peritubular cells of the kidneys that are responsive to tissue oxygen) regulate synthesis and subsequent release of erythropoietin (Fig. 10.7). Erythropoietin is rapidly released into the blood. In the bone marrow, erythropoietin binds to erythropoietin receptors on erythroid progenitor cells, activates the JAK/STAT and other tyrosine protein kinase signal pathways, and thereby stimulates cell proliferation and differentiation into red blood cells. (See discussion above, and Fig. 10.6.)

Erythropoietin is used for anemia due to renal failure, malignancies and chronic inflammation. The anemia of chronic renal failure results from a loss of erythropoietin. Recombinant human erythropoietin is now a standard

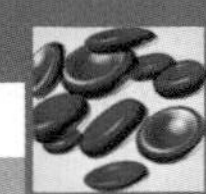

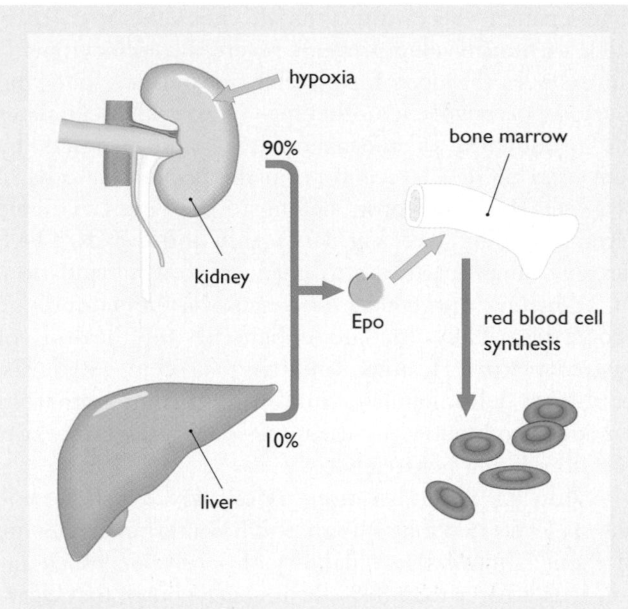

Fig. 10.7 Stimulation of erythropoietin (Epo) synthesis by hypoxia. Low oxygen tension is 'sensed' by renal peritubular cells inducing these cells to produce Epo. Epo stimulates the bone marrow to produce red blood cells. The liver also produces a small amount of Epo, which can be detected in anephric patients.

treatment for the anemia of chronic renal failure, and subcutaneous or i.v. erythropoietin 150 units/kg three times a week will correct anemia in 80% of such patients. The reticulocyte response to erythropoietin starts after 3 days of treatment and a significant rise in hematocrit occurs by 1 week. Maximum effects are achieved after 4–8 weeks. Erythropoietin has also been used to treat anemia due to primary bone marrow disorders and secondary anemia associated with inflammation, AIDS and cancer. Erythropoietin is also an effective treatment of zidovudine-induced anemia in patients with HIV and in cancer patients receiving chemotherapy.

Complications of erythropoietin treatment include hypertension and thrombosis, which can occur if hematocrit levels rise too rapidly. Seizures have been reported in patients with a pre-existing history of seizures. The iron stores in patients with anemia of renal failure are often rapidly depleted during erythropoietin treatment, due to erythropoiesis. Since it may be difficult to supplement with oral iron alone in these patients, because of continuing iron loss associated with blood loss, treatment with parenteral iron may be required.

The International Olympic Committee prohibits the use of erythropoietin in athletes because of the ability of this substance to increase red blood cell counts, oxygen delivery to tissues, and thus performance. In addition, this practice may be dangerous.

Drobepoetin α is a hyperglycosylated analog of erythropoietin which stimulates erythropoiesis by the same mechanism as endogenous erythropoietin.

Table 10.3 Drugs and disorders that can cause neutropenia

Myelosuppressive chemotherapy
Analgesics and antiinflammatory drugs
Antibiotics: sulfonamides, semisynthetic penicillins, chloramphenicol, cephalosporins
Antipsychotics
Anticonvulsants
H_2 antagonists
Autoimmune disorders: systemic lupus erythematosus, rheumatoid arthritis
Malignancy
Viruses: human immunodeficiency virus, Epstein–Barr virus
Tuberculosis

Myeloid growth factors and neutropenia

Neutrophils are the principal defense cells against bacterial and fungal infections. Their continuous turnover and replenishment in the tissues are critical for maintaining an uninfected state. Unlike other blood cells, neutrophils and neutrophil precursor cells spend most of their brief life span (15 days) in the bone marrow. Normal granulopoiesis supports cells in blood and tissue compartments that turn over rapidly. Neutrophils in blood and tissue are therefore susceptible to rapid depletion if the marrow storage pool is compromised.

Drugs are the most common cause of neutropenia

The most common cause of neutropenia is myelosuppression induced by cancer chemotherapy, but many commonly prescribed drugs can also cause neutropenia. Other causes include congenital, autoimmune and infectious disorders (Table 10.3). The proliferation and maturation of myeloid progenitor cells are regulated in part by specific hematopoietic growth factors called colony-stimulating factors.

Granulocyte colony-stimulating factor (G-CSF) and granulocyte–macrophage colony-stimulating factor (GM-CSF)

Granulocyte colony-stimulating factor (G-CSF) and granulocyte–macrophage colony-stimulating factor (GM-CSF) represent some of the most widely utilized therapeutic proteins. They were originally purified from human cell lines and are now made by recombinant technology. G-CSF and GM-CSF stimulate differentiation and proliferation of various myeloid progenitor cells by activating their specific receptors in the cell membrane of such cells. As with erythropoietin receptors, G-CSF and GM-CSF receptors are members of the type I cytokine receptor family that utilize JAK/STAT and other tyrosine protein kinase signal pathways to transduce cellular responses.

Although the specific physiologic roles of G-CSF and GM-CSF in the normal regulation of myelopoiesis are not clearly defined, both dramatically stimulate neutrophil production when administered exogenously. G-CSF and GM-CSF also enhance the functional responsiveness of mature neutrophils to inflammatory signals and may increase neutrophil-dependent host defenses by enhancing the functioning of neutrophils. G-CSF acts only on hematopoietic cells that are committed to become neutrophils, so it is relatively more lineage-specific than GM-CSF. The latter also stimulates macrophage development. When G-CSF or GM-CSF are given intravenously or subcutaneously, the neutrophil count usually rises within 24 hours. When the drug is stopped, the neutrophil count decreases by half within 24 hours and returns to baseline in 1–7 days. The response is decreased in patients extensively treated with radiation or chemotherapy due to their reduced number of progenitor cells.

Treatment with G-CSF is better tolerated than treatment with GM-CSF. Although administration of both may cause bone pain, GM-CSF therapy can also cause a pulmonary capillary leak syndrome with pulmonary edema and heart failure. Treatment with GM-CSF, unlike G-CSF, may also cause constitutional symptoms including fever, headache and malaise.

Pegfilgrastim is a covalent conjugate of recombinant methionyl human G-CSF and monomethoxy polyethylene glycol. It acts like other colony-stimulating factors to bring about the proliferation, differentiation and commitment of a variety of hematopoietic cells, but has the advantage of a very long plasma half-life (15–80 hours). It is used in the treatment of chemotherapy-induced suppression of bone marrow, particularly to correct neutropenia. The major adverse effects of this therapy are nausea, fatigue, neutropenia fever and generalized weakness.

Megakaryocyte growth factors and thrombocytopenia

Thrombocytopenia is a condition characterized by a decrease in the number of platelets circulating in the blood to less than 150 000/mm^3. Platelets have a pivotal role in several mechanisms of homeostasis, including blood coagulation, wound healing and the storage and release of cytokines. Patients with severe thrombocytopenia have a bleeding tendency. The etiologies of thrombocytopenia are complex. It may be due to any of the following mechanisms:

- Decreased bone marrow production (e.g. in patients with aplastic anemia).
- Increased splenic sequestration of platelets (e.g. in patients with portal hypertension or Gaucher's disease).
- Accelerated destruction of platelets in the peripheral circulation.
- Simple dilution in patients undergoing massive red blood cell replacement or exchange transfusions.
- As an adverse effect of many commonly used drugs.

Oprelvekin (interleukin-11)

Oprelvekin, a recombinant form of interleukin-11 (rIL-11), is the first growth factor approved by the FDA for use as secondary prevention of thrombocytopenia in cancer patients receiving cytotoxic chemotherapy. Treatment with oprelvekin prevents severe thrombocytopenia and reduces the need for platelet transfusions following myelosuppressive chemotherapy. Oprelvekin stimulates the production of megakaryocytes and platelets by activation of IL-11 receptors on the progenitor cells of platelets. IL-11 receptors belong to the type I cytokine receptor family (see Fig. 10.6) and utilize JAK/STAT tyrosine kinase pathways to produce growth regulation. In addition, oprelvekin possesses nonhematopoietic properties. They include enhancing the healing of gastrointestinal lesions, inducing protein synthesis, inhibiting adipogenesis, inhibiting proinflammatory cytokine production, increasing production of osteoclasts and stimulating neurogenesis.

Following administration, oprelvekin reaches peak plasma levels in about 3 hours and has a terminal half-life of about 7 hours. Bioavailability of oprelvekin subcutaneously is greater than 80%. It has been shown that clearance of oprelvekin decreases with age. The clearance of oprelvekin in infants and children is 20–60% higher than in adults and adolescents. In animal models, oprelvekin is eliminated via the kidney. However, only a very small amount of intact oprelvekin is recovered in urine, suggesting that the drug is metabolized before it is excreted.

The most common adverse effects associated with oprelvekin relate to sodium retention in the kidneys. The resulting changes in blood volume can lead to cardiovascular consequences (e.g. changes in blood pressure, arrhythmias, edema) and may explain the association between use of this drug and mild decreases in hemoglobin concentrations. These adverse effects may be prevented by the concomitant use of diuretics such as furosemide, which has proved successful in eliminating the fall in hematocrit associated with the administration of oprelvekin.

Thrombopoietin

Platelets are formed in the bone marrow by budding from large multinucleated cells termed megakaryocytes, which, like other hematopoietic cells, are derived from hematopoietic stem cells. Thrombopoietin (Tpo) is a primary growth factor regulating platelet production. It is a 65–85 kDa glycoprotein expressed in a variety of cells, particularly hepatocytes. Thrombopoietin stimulates platelet production in bone marrow by activating c-mpl receptors on the progenitor cells or platelets and Tpo has a platelet priming effect (it potentiates collagen-induced platelet aggregation). The c-mpl utilizes JAK/STAT, Ras/MAP kinase and phosphatidylinositol 3 kinase signal pathways to promote both the proliferation of megakaryocyte progenitor cells and their maturation into platelet-producing megakaryoctyes. Thrombopoietin was originally isolated from human urine and its recombinant form (PEG-rHuMGDF) is produced by expression in human cells. Thrombopoietin is being tested for treatment of patients with either primary or secondary thrombocytopenia.

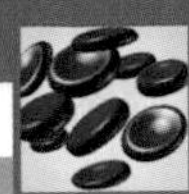

HEMOSTATIC DISORDERS AND ANTITHROMBOTIC THERAPY

Hemostasis

Normal hemostasis is a delicate balance between procoagulant, anticoagulant and fibrinolytic processes in blood vessels. Damage to vessel walls initiates a complex series of events involving platelets, endothelial cells and coagulation proteins that results in the formation of a platelet–fibrin clot. At the same time, physiologic anticoagulants and the fibrinolytic systems are activated by the products of the coagulation cascade to prevent excessive clotting (i.e. thrombosis).

Platelets play a critical role in hemostasis

Platelets do not normally interact with vascular endothelium. However, when endothelial cells are damaged, platelets bind to the site of damage through the interaction of platelet glycoprotein receptors with subendothelial collagen. The adhesive platelets undergo activation and degranulation, releasing a number of substances including thromboxane A_2 (TXA_2), adenosine diphosphate (ADP), epinephrine and serotonin. These in turn activate and recruit additional platelets into the growing platelet-rich thrombus. Activated platelets provide the phospholipid binding surfaces for supporting the assembly of coagulant factor Xase-activating complex (including factor IXa, platelet-bound factor VIIIa and calcium) and prothrombinase complex (including factor Xa, platelet-bound factor Va and calcium) thereby markedly increasing thrombin generation. Increased thrombin activates additional platelets and triggers the coagulation cascade (see below).

Activation of platelets by agonists such as ADP and TXA_2, particularly thrombin, leads to conformational activation of glycoprotein receptors IIb/IIIa on their surface. The activated IIb/IIIa receptors provide functional binding sites for fibrinogen and other adhesive molecules such as von Willebrand factor (VWF) and fibronectin. Binding of bivalent fibrinogen molecules to IIb/IIIa on adjacent platelets forms platelet aggregates. Thus, activation of the platelet glycoprotein receptor IIb/IIIa is the final pathway of platelet aggregation regardless of agonist type.

The platelet plug is reinforced by fibrin formed from activation of the coagulation cascade: a key role of thrombin

In addition to thrombin generated from platelet activation and aggregation, the tissue factor–factor VIIa complex plays a key role in initiating the coagulation cascade and generating thrombin. Tissue factor (TF) is an intrinsic membrane glycoprotein expressed in many cells in contact with blood. It becomes accessible only when proteases are formed, or cell injury occurs in vivo. After vascular injury, TF functions as a cofactor or receptor, in the presence of Ca^{2+}, binding to factor VII and activating factor VII to VIIa. TF/VIIa/Ca^{2+} complex then converts factor X to Xa, which in turn activates prothrombin (factor II) to thrombin (factor IIa). Thrombin then cleaves fibrinogen to fibrin, which stabilizes the primary platelet plug into a permanent plug (Fig. 10.8).

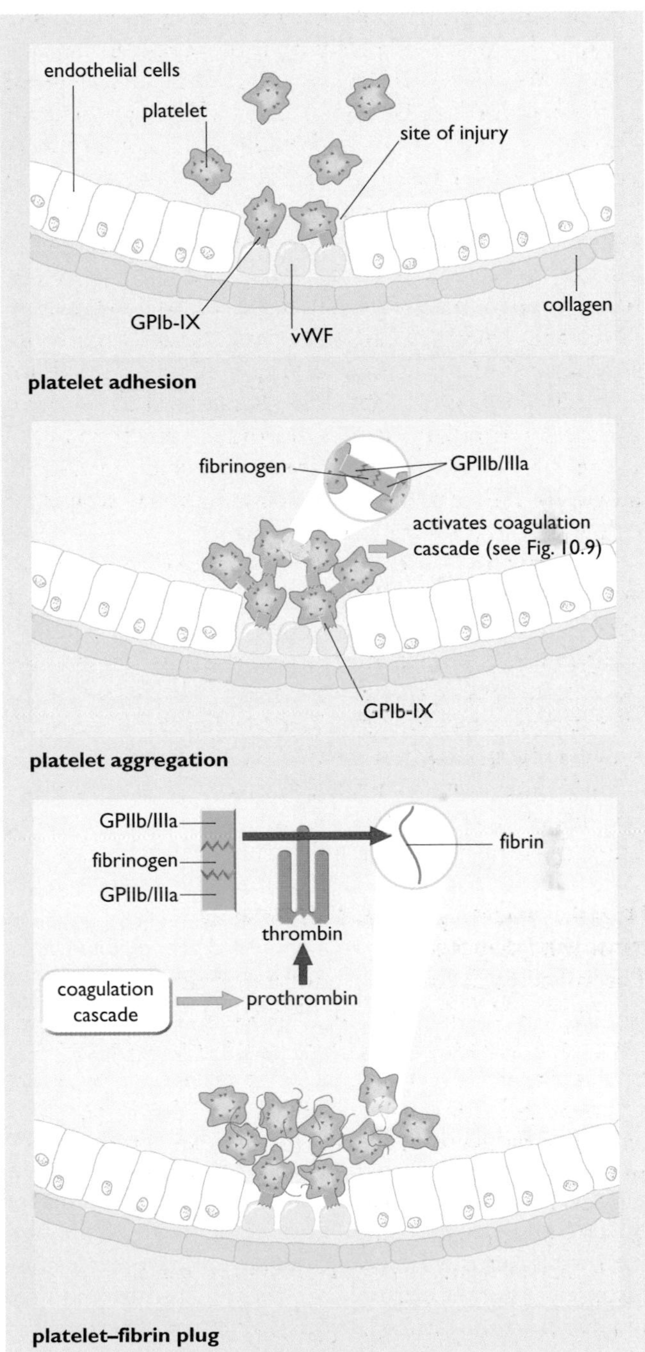

Fig. 10.8 Platelet function in hemostasis. There are three steps in the formation of the platelet–fibrin plug. The first is platelet adhesion: vascular injury damages the endothelial cells and exposes the underlying collagen matrix. Platelets adhere to the exposed collagen after von Willebrand factor (VWF) on collagen binds to platelet receptors, GPIb-IX. The second step, platelet aggregation, is activation of platelets by local factors such as thromboxane A_2, thrombin and collagen. It attracts other platelets, which aggregate through platelet receptors GPIIb/IIIa. The third step is the formation of a platelet–fibrin plug with platelets providing a phospholipid surface for the activated coagulation cascade to activate thrombin, which cleaves fibrinogen to produce fibrin to consolidate the initial platelet plug.

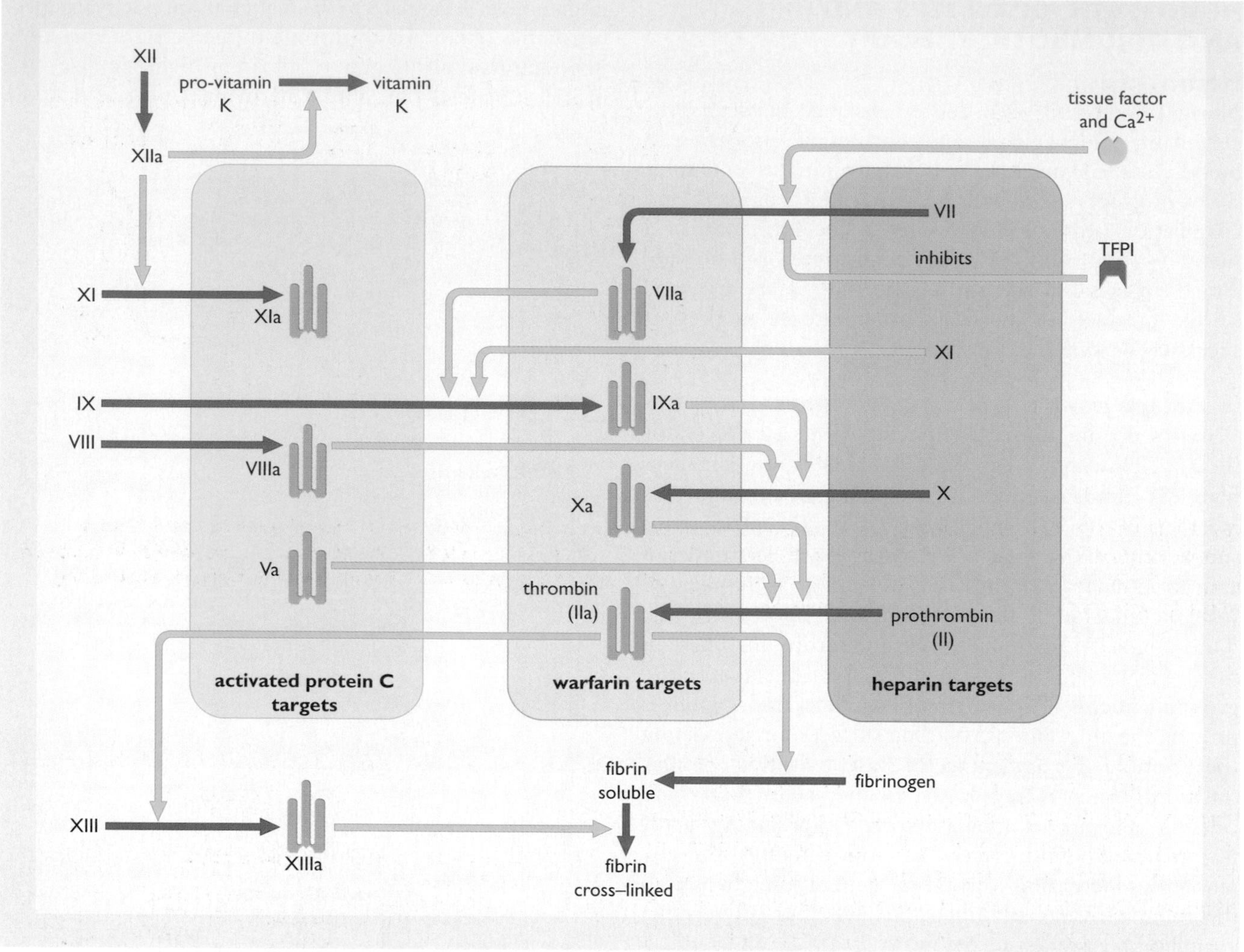

Fig. 10.9 The coagulation cascade. Initiation of coagulation by tissue factors activates factor VII, which activates factors IX and X. Factor IX activates factor X to Xa. Factor Xa cleaves prothrombin to thrombin, which cleaves fibrinogen to fibrin. By interacting with negatively charged surfaces, factor XII is autoactivated into XIIa that activates its substrates prekallikrein (PK) to kallikrein (K) and factor XI results in activation of the intrinsic coagulation pathway. TFPI, tissue factor pathway inhibitor. Factors in the gray rectangle are vitamin K dependent warfarin (heparin target). Factors in the yellow rectangle are vitamin K dependent (warfarin target). Factors in the green rectangle are negatively regulated by the activated protein C.

The tissue factor–factor VIIa complex also activates factor X indirectly by activating factor IX to IXa. Continued activation of factor X requires a factor IXa–factor VIIIa complex (Fig. 10.9). This explains why hemophiliacs with factor VIII or IX deficiency have a bleeding disorder. Another pathway to activate prothrombin to thrombin is the so-called intrinsic system that is triggered by the activation of factor XII, following its contact with highly charged surfaces (see Fig. 10.9).

In addition to fibrin conversion, thrombin activates coagulation factor XIII, which stabilizes and cross-links the soluble fibrin molecules into an insoluble fibrin clot (see Fig. 10.9). Thrombin activates other coagulation factors and cofactors to amplify its own generation, which recruit more platelets and promotes platelet aggregation. Thrombin also causes migration of white cells and regulates vascular tone. Finally, thrombin is a potent activator of vascular smooth muscle cell migration and proliferation. Given thrombin's central role in hemostasis and in thrombogenesis, the goal of many current antithrombotics is to block thrombin activity or prevent its generation (see below).

Hemostasis is tightly regulated by specific inhibitors of the activated coagulation factors

There are three groups of physiologic inhibitors of hemostasis in plasma. They are classified according to their mechanism of inhibition, and comprise kinins (pancreatic trypsin inhibitors), serpins (serine protease inhibitors), and α_2-macroglobulins. They limit the extent of hemostasis and protect against thrombus formation.

Tissue factor pathway inhibitor (TFPI) is a member of the kinin family. TFPI first binds to factor Xa and then inactivates tissue factor–factor VIIa complex by forming a quaternary complex. Administration of heparin releases endothelium-associated TFPI into the circulation.

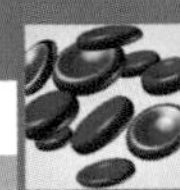

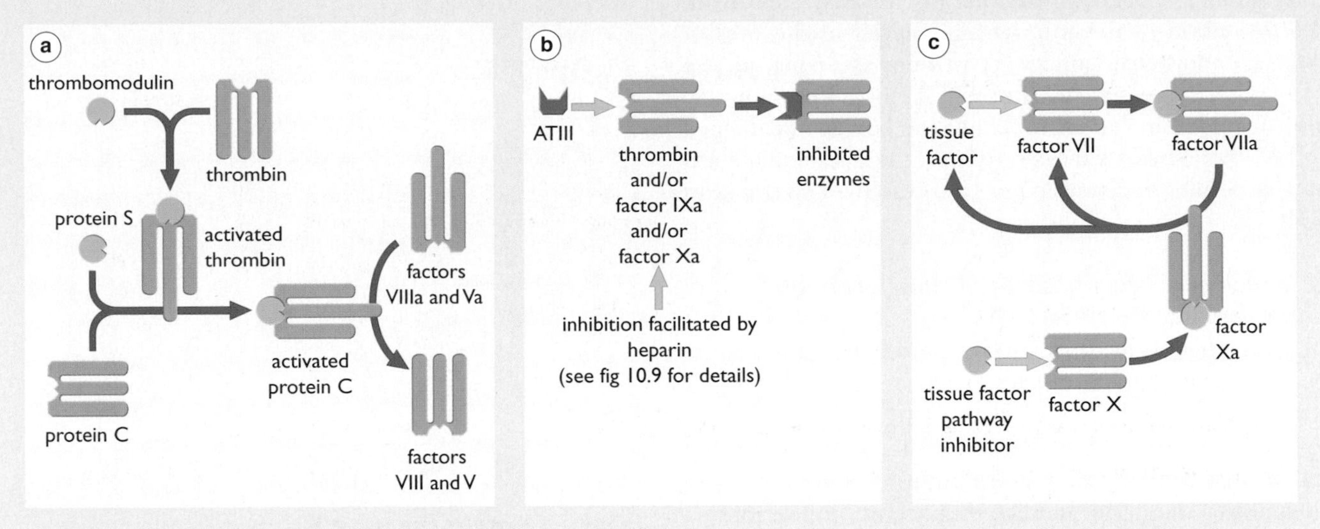

Fig. 10.10 Natural anticoagulants. There are three physiologic anticoagulation systems. (a) (1) Thrombomodulin stimulated by thrombin activates protein C, which with its cofactor protein S, inhibits cofactors Va and VIIIa in the coagulation cascade. (2) Antithrombin III (ATIII) stimulated by heparin inhibits thrombin, factor Xa and factor IXa (b). (3) Tissue factor pathway inhibitor inhibits tissue factor, which is a key activator of the coagulation cascade (c).

The important members of the serpin family include antithrombin III (ATIII), protein C and protein S. ATIII is a major inhibitor of thrombin, factor Xa and factor IXa. Heparin, as a cofactor for ATIII, greatly increases the ATIII inactivation of thrombin and factor Xa. Anticoagulant-activated protein C with its cofactor protein S is the major inhibitor of factors Va and VIIIa. Thrombin activates the protein C pathway by first binding to thrombomodulin, which activates protein C on endothelial cell surfaces. The physiologic relevance of ATIII, protein C and protein S is underscored by the greatly increased risk of venous thrombosis in people who have deficiencies of these natural anticoagulants (Fig. 10.10).

α_2-macroglobulin functions as a scavenger inhibitor of proteases such as plasmin.

The activity of the fibrinolytic system regulates hemostasis

In addition to physiologic anticoagulants, the plasma fibrinolytic system is the major endogenous mechanism that protects against thrombus formation by lysing established fibrin clots. This system consists of plasminogen, plasmin, plasminogen activators and their respective inhibitors. Fibrinolysis is mainly regulated by the enzyme tissue-type plasminogen activator (t-PA). Circulating t-PA is relatively inactive. Once incorporated into a fibrin clot, it converts fibrin-bound plasminogen to plasmin, which degrades the fibrin clot. The plasminogen and plasmin are subject to regulation by various inhibitors, including plasminogen activator inhibitors 1, 2 and 3 (PAI-1, -2 and -3) and α_2 antiplasmin (Fig. 10.11 and see below for more details).

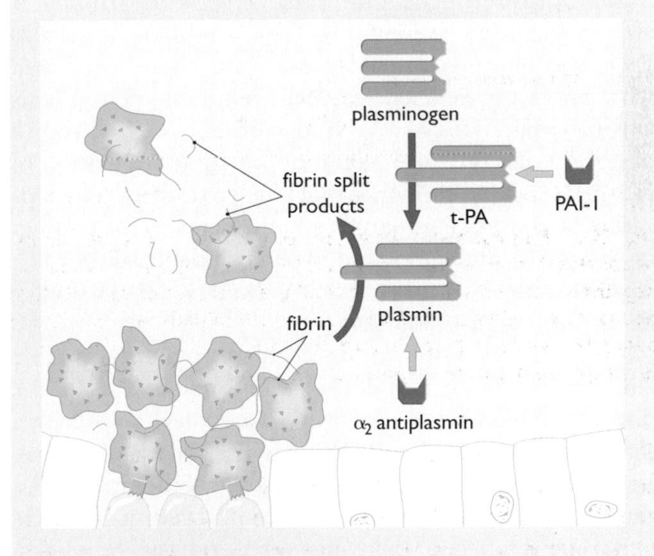

Fig. 10.11 The fibrinolytic system. Fibrin-bound tissue plasminogen activator (t-PA) changes fibrin-bound plasminogen to plasmin, which cleaves fibrin. Physiologic inhibitors are plasminogen activator inhibitor (PAI-1) and α_2 antiplasmin.

Thrombosis

Thrombosis is a major cause of death and disability as a result of:

- Arterial occlusion leading to myocardial infarction, stroke and peripheral ischemia.
- Venous occlusion causing deep venous thrombosis and pulmonary embolism.

Disabling or fatal thrombotic disease may stem from the formation of thrombi within arteries at the sites of arterial endothelial damage, or in veins as a consequence of stasis or increased system coagulability. Thrombi may also form within the chambers of the heart, on damaged or prosthetic heart valves, or within the microcirculation as the result of disseminated intravascular coagulation (DIC).

Endothelial injury is the main cause of arterial thrombosis

In the high-flow arterial system, endothelial injury is the dominant influence in thrombogenesis. Arterial thrombi form only at sites with underlying arterial wall pathology (e.g. damage caused by atherosclerosis, trauma following balloon angioplasty, or autoimmune vasculitis). Arterial thrombosis due to an increased concentration of plasma homocysteine probably results from its toxic effect on endothelial cells and damage to the arterial wall.

Stasis and hypercoagulability are the main causes of venous thrombosis

In contrast to arteries, in venous thrombosis the vessel wall is frequently intact. Stasis plays a dominant role and permits the build-up of platelet aggregates and nascent fibrin in areas of sluggish flow. Hypercoagulability is also an important contributor. The best-understood and prototypic hypercoagulable states are those associated with hereditary deficiencies of the natural anticoagulants antithrombin III, protein C or protein S. The recent discovery of a relatively common hereditary mutation of factor Va (Leiden), which is much more resistant to inactivation by activated protein C, greatly increases the number of patients with diagnosable hypercoagulable states.

Lifelong anticoagulation

Many patients with an underlying hypercoagulable abnormality require lifelong anticoagulation (see the discussion below for warfarin) once they have had a thrombotic event. In addition, hypercoagulability may also be an important mechanism in the pathogenesis of a thrombotic diathesis in common clinical settings, such as nephrotic syndrome, following severe trauma, or a burn, and in disseminated cancer.

Antithrombotic therapy

There are three easily identified classes of antithrombotic drugs for arterial and venous thrombotic disorders. Since platelets play a critical role in the pathogenesis of arterial thrombotic disorders, these cells are logical targets for antithrombotic drugs. Attenuation of platelet functions can be achieved by inhibition of prostaglandin synthases (to reduce TXA_2 production), inhibition of platelet membrane G protein-coupled receptors (e.g. ADP receptor, TXA_2 receptor and thrombin receptors), and antagonism of platelet adhesion receptor Ib-IX or platelet aggregation receptor GPIIb/IIIa (Fig. 10.12).

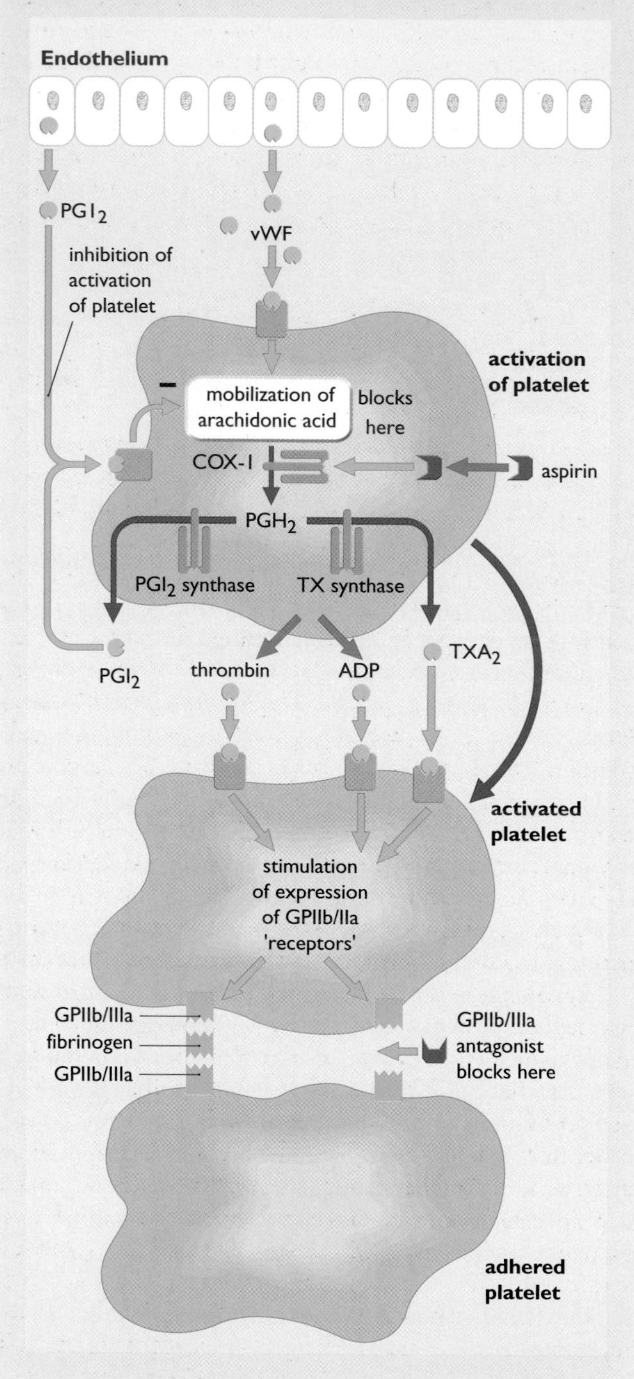

Fig. 10.12 Effects of antiplatelet agents on platelet activation and aggregation. After vascular injury, platelets bind to the vessel wall and undergo activation and degranulation, releasing a number of platelet activators that activate and recruit other platelets. The platelet activators cause the conformation change of platelet GPIIb/IIIa receptors that finally stimulate platelet aggregation. Aspirin, ADP receptor antagonists and GPIIb/IIIa antagonists block the process at different levels (PGI_2, prostaglandin I_2; PGH_2, prostaglandin H_2; TXA_2, thromboxane A_2; vWF, von Willebrand factor).

Given that thrombin-activated fibrin is a major component of thrombi, and that thrombin is the most potent activator of platelets, anticoagulant strategies have focused on inhibiting thrombin activity, or preventing

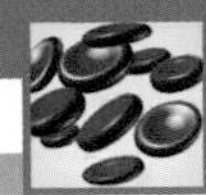

thrombin generation. These include the use of indirect inhibitors of thrombin such as oral coumarin derivatives, heparin or low molecular weight heparin (LMWH), and direct inhibitors of thrombin, such as argatroban, hirudin and its derivatives. The third class of antithrombotic therapeutics are thrombolytic agents that actively dissolve thrombi rather than interrupting progression of the thrombotic process by antiplatelet agents or thrombin inhibitors.

Inhibition of TXA_2 production: aspirin

In the hope of helping his father who was suffering from arthritis and the severe adverse effects of the sodium salicylate he used as treatment, Felix Hoffman, a German chemist at Farbenfabriken Friedrich Bayer, began synthesizing salicylic acid derivatives in hopes of preserving its anti inflammatory properties while reducing adverse effects on the stomach. The acetic acid ester of salicylic acid, acetylsalicylic acid, was synthesized in 1897 and Bayer began marketing it in 1899 as Aspirin. In the century since, Aspirin has become the most widely consumed drug in the world, mainly for its ability to act as an antiinflammatory and analgesic drug (see Ch. 12). However, in recent years it has also become the 'gold standard' for antiplatelet drugs used in the prevention and treatment of arterial thrombotic disorders such as angina pectoris, myocardial infarction (MI) and ischemic stroke. Aspirin has the best benefit:risk and cost:benefit ratio of any drug for acute coronary syndromes.

Aspirin prevents conversion of arachidonic acid to prostaglandin H_2 and subsequently reduces production of TXA_2 by acetylation of a serine residue of enzyme prostaglandin H_2 synthase (PGHS, usually referred to as cyclooxygenase, COX) and irreversibly inactivating it (see Fig. 10.12). There are two COX isoforms, COX-1 and COX-2, in mammalian cells. COX 1 is constitutively expressed in most cell types and COX-2 is an inducible enzyme that has increased expression in many clinical settings, such as inflammation and infection. Human platelets express only COX-1. Aspirin is a relatively selective COX-1 inhibitor, with an approximate 200-fold greater inhibition of COX-1 than COX-2. This is the rationale for the smaller dosage requirements for aspirin as an antithrombotic (involving COX-1) compared with its use as an antiinflammatory drug (involving COX-2). Inhibition of COX-1 and reduction of TXA_2 results in suppression of platelet aggregation for the whole 7–10-day life span of the platelet since COX-1 is irreversibly acetylated by aspirin and not resynthesized by platelets since they lack nuclei. However, ADP, epinephrine and thrombin can still activate platelets. Aspirin also blocks the synthesis of the platelet inhibitor PGI_2 in endothelial cells. However, this effect is limited with low doses of aspirin and short-lived (as endothelial cells possess a nucleus and can therefore synthesize new COX protein) compared with TXA_2 synthesis in platelets. The effect of aspirin on platelet function is demonstrated by prolonged bleeding times in patients taking aspirin.

Aspirin is rapidly absorbed from the gastrointestinal tract, partially hydrolyzed to salicylate on its first pass through the liver, and widely distributed to most body tissues. Following oral administration, salicylate can be present in the serum within 5–30 minutes and peak serum concentrations are attained within 1 hour. These properties of aspirin are discussed more fully in Chapter 15. However, in order to achieve therapeutic blood levels rapidly in patients who might be having an MI, chewed aspirin tablets are recommended, to promote buccal rather than gastric mucosal absorption. Hemostasis returns to normal approximately 36 hours after the last dose of the drug, presumably due to the release of new platelets from the bone marrow.

Aspirin is a cornerstone of therapy for unstable angina or non-Q-wave MI. It can reduce the incidence of death or MI in these conditions. Also, aspirin serves as the linchpin of therapy for acute MI and the foundation to which other therapies are added, both in the short and long term. It reduces the incidence of reinfarction by one-third and the composite end-point of MI, stroke or vascular death by one-quarter. Overall, aspirin has been found to be nearly as effective as streptokinase in reducing mortality in acute myocardial infarction. Combining the two agents has an additive effect on mortality. In addition, doses of aspirin as low as 80 mg/day are effective in the secondary prevention of MI, and in reducing mortality in postmyocardial infarction. Aspirin is also useful in preventing recurring transient ischemic attacks (TIAs) and reducing the risk of stroke in patients with TIAs. It is also used where there is an increased risk of arterial thrombosis, e.g. coronary catherization, balloon angioplasty and following vascular surgery. Aspirin is also used in conjunction with the other antiplatelet agents such as ADP antagonists or with anticoagulants such as heparin, or warfarin (see discussion below). A poor response to aspirin is found in 10–15% of patients, while others develop progressive resistance to aspirin. Patients with aspirin resistance may be more vulnerable to adverse vascular events.

A loading dose of 325 mg chewable aspirin for acute coronary syndromes is given to achieve therapeutic blood levels rapidly, followed by 160–325 mg/day during hospitalization. Virtually complete inhibition of COX-1 in platelets can be maintained with a low dose (80 mg/day).

Gastrointestinal irritation is the most common adverse effect of aspirin. Tinnitus and central nervous system toxicity do not occur with the low dose used in antithrombotic therapy. Aspirin, as with other nonsteroidal antiinflammatory drugs (NSAIDs), increases the risk of gastric bleeding in a dose-related manner (see Ch. 15). Aspirin may increase the risk of intracerebral hemorrhage; in prophylactic therapy, it is important to consider the risk/benefit of using aspirin, especially in patients at low risk for cardiovascular events. Some patients may develop severe bronchoconstriction with aspirin (see

ANAGRELIDE High platelet counts due to myeloproliferative diseases such as essential thrombocytosis, unlike the relatively benign reactive thrombocytosis, may have thrombotic consequences. The conventional treatment of these disorders has been with non-specific chemotherapeutic agents such as hydroxyurea. Anagrelide, an orally active quinazolin, is highly selective against megakaryocytes and therefore selectively lowers platelet counts. If long-term trials confirm that anagrelide does not have a leukemogenic potential, this drug may become the treatment of choice for thrombocythemia.

Inhibition of coagulant factor formation: warfarin

The discovery of the anticoagulant effects of coumarin in the 1940s led to the development of synthetic derivatives such as warfarin. A widely used oral anticoagulant, it acts on vitamin K-dependent synthesis of the coagulation factors II, VII, IX and X and cofactors (protein C and S) in the liver. The post-translational enzymatic carboxylation of the glutamic acid residues of these coagulation factors to γ-carboxyglutamic acid requires vitamin K as a cofactor. In the presence of calcium ions, the γ-carboxyglutamyl residues allow coagulation factors to undergo a conformational change, necessary for their biologic activity. Warfarin inhibits vitamin K epoxide reductase, leading to depletion of reduced vitamin K (KH) and decreased γ-carboxylation (Fig. 10.13), thereby indirectly impairing the function of coagulation factors. The anticoagulant effects of warfarin show only after disappearance of the existing γ-carboxylated coagulation factors. Prothrombin (factor II) has the longest half-life of 60 hours; therefore, 5 days of treatment are required if warfarin is to be fully antithrombotic. This is the rationale for overlapping heparin with warfarin for at least 5 days in the treatment of thrombotic diseases, even if the INR (see below) reaches therapeutic levels before 5 days.

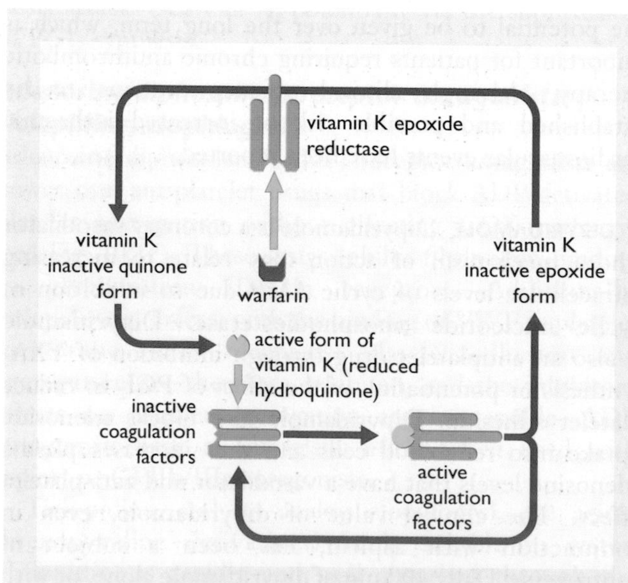

Fig. 10.13 Vitamin K-dependent synthesis of coagulation factors. Warfarin inhibits production of the reduced form of vitamin K, which is required for γ-carboxylation of the glutamic acids in factors II, VII, IX and X, protein C and protein S.

Table 10.4 Indications for oral anticoagulation with warfarin

Mechanical prosthetic heart valves
Atrial fibrillation
Treatment of venous thromboembolism
Previous myocardial infarction
Prevention of venous thromboembolism
Episodic systemic embolism

Warfarin is effective for:

- The prevention and treatment of venous thromboembolism and pulmonary embolism (see Ch. 13).
- The prevention of thrombotic and embolic strokes as well as recurrence of infarction in patients with acute myocardial infarction.

Patients with mechanical prosthetic heart valves should be treated with anticoagulants. A combined regimen of warfarin and low-dose aspirin seems to be superior to warfarin alone. Most patients with atrial fibrillation should be on lifelong anticoagulation treatment with warfarin (Table 10.4).

Treatment with warfarin begins with small daily doses (5–10 mg) for 1 week, to allow adjustment of the prothrombin times, followed by a maintenance dose. The prothrombin time should be maintained at 20–25% normal activity in long-term warfarin therapy. A standard coagulation assay method for the prothrombin time, the international normalized ratio (INR) (test/control), is used. Currently, one of two levels of warfarin therapy are usual: a medium response with an INR of 2.0–3.0, and a high response with an INR of 2.5–3.5. Higher INR values greatly increase the risk of bleeding. However, a lower INR (2.0–2.5) is effective in the prevention and treatment of most venous and arterial thrombotic disorders.

Warfarin is well absorbed orally and has excellent bioavailability. It is highly bound to plasma proteins (99% albumin) resulting in a small volume of distribution and a long half-life in plasma (30–40 hours), and no urinary excretion of unchanged drug. The drug is metabolized by hepatic microsomes CYP Cs and As to inactivate metabolites found in urine and feces.

Many clinical conditions and drug interactions can potentiate or attenuate the anticoagulant effects of warfarin (Table 10.5). Fluctuating levels of dietary vitamin K can be an important factor in patients on long-term warfarin therapy.

The major adverse effect of warfarin is bleeding, and this risk is correlated with the intensity of the treatment and the concomitant use of antiplatelet agents such as aspirin. The risk of bleeding is reduced by lowering the INR therapeutic range from 3.0–4.5 to 2.0–3.0. The

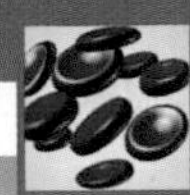

Table 10.5 Drugs and conditions interacting with warfarin

	Activity of warfarin
Antibiotics	+
Amiodarone	+
Cimetidine	+
Clofibrate	+
Fluconazole	+
Metronidazole	+
Phenytoin	+
Barbiturates	–
Carbamazepine	–
Griseofulvin	–
Nafcillin	–
Rifampin	–
Sucralfate	–
Age	+
Biliary disease	+
Congestive heart failure	+
Hyperthyroidism	+
Hypothyroidism	–
Nephrotic syndrome	–

+, increased activity; –, decreased activity.

most important nonhemorrhagic adverse effect is skin necrosis caused by extensive thrombosis of the microvasculature in subcutaneous fat. This phenomenon seems to be associated with protein C and S deficiency. (Proteins C and S are vitamin K-dependent anticoagulants as discussed above.) The thrombotic tendency may be mostly a transient procoagulant state during the initial treatment period with warfarin, due to proteins C and S having shorter half-lifes than prothrombin. The fall in protein C and S levels, therefore, occurs before a reduction in the prothrombin level. Skin necrosis can be avoided by using concurrent therapeutic doses of heparin when starting warfarin therapy.

Warfarin crosses the placenta and is teratogenic, so it must not be given to pregnant women. Women receiving warfarin should be informed of its teratogenic effect. Treatment with heparin and low molecular weight heparins (LMWHs) appears to be safe during pregnancy.

The anticoagulant effects of warfarin can be partially reversed by low doses of vitamin K acting through a warfarin-resistant pathway. Patients also become warfarin-resistant if large doses of vitamin K are given. Fresh frozen plasma or prothrombin complex concentrate can be infused if a rapid reversal of the warfarin effect is needed, as in severe bleeding.

Warfarin

- **Treatment with warfarin requires at least 4–5 days for full effect, even if the INR of prothrombin activity assay reaches the therapeutic level in 1–2 days**

Warning about using warfarin

- **Warfarin is a teratogen and can produce fetal central nervous system abnormalities or bleeding. Pregnant women with thrombosis should be treated with standard or low molecular weight heparin**

Indirect inhibition of thrombin activity: heparin and low molecular weight heparin

Heparin is a glycosaminoglycan of chains of alternating residues of D-glucosamine and uronic acid. Standard unfractionated heparin is a heterogeneous preparation with molecular weights ranging from 5000 to 30 000 kDa. The anticoagulant activity of heparin is variable because the chain length of the molecules affects activity and clearance. The higher molecular weight molecules are cleared from the circulation more rapidly. Furthermore, there are differential activities with lower molecular weight species being more active against factor Xa than against thrombin.

Heparin primarily exerts anticoagulant effects through binding to ATIII, thereby altering the conformation of ATIII and accelerating its inhibition of thrombin, factor Xa and factor IXa. ATIII is an α-globulin that inhibits serine proteases, including several of the clotting factors, by binding serine residue in the reaction center of coagulant factors, leading to this inactivation. Heparin participates as a catalytic agent, catalyzing the inactivation of thrombin by ATIII by acting as a template to which both ATIII and thrombin bind to form a ternary complex. In contrast, ATIII inactivation of factor Xa does not require the formation of a ternary complex. Low molecular weight species of heparin containing fewer than 18 polysaccharide chains are unable to serve as a template for ATIII inactivation of thrombin, but retain the ability to inactivate factor Xa (Fig. 10.14). However, heparin inhibition of thrombogenesis is incomplete because it is unable to inactivate platelet-bound Xa and fibrin-bound thrombin that remain enzymatically active. This contributes at least partially to the resistance of arterial thrombosis to heparin therapy.

Heparin is poorly absorbed orally and is given either subcutaneously or intravenously. It is often given intravenously as a bolus to achieve rapid anticoagulation and then maintained with continuous infusion. Subcutaneous boluses two or three times a day are equally effective. If immediate anticoagulation is needed, however, the i.v. route is preferred because there is a 1–2 hour delay with subcutaneous heparin. Treatment with heparin requires close laboratory monitoring. Heparin needs to be titrated to achieve an activated partial thromboplastin time (aPTT) of 1.5–2.5 times normal.

Heparin is highly negatively charged and binds to endothelial cells and a variety of plasma proteins such as lipoprotein, fibronectin, platelet factor 4 and von Willebrand factor. This binding contributes to reduced

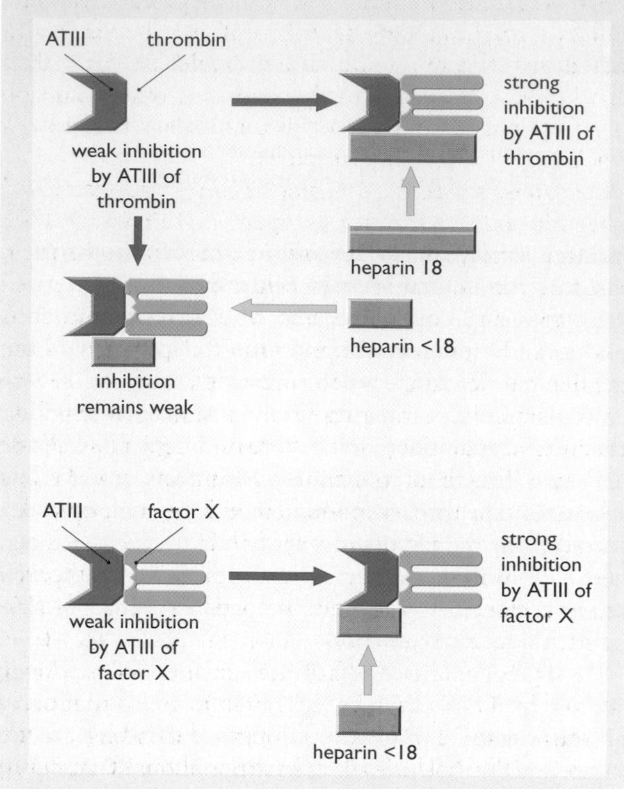

Fig. 10.14 Anticoagulation mechanism of heparin. Binding of heparin with antithrombin III (ATIII) greatly facilitates its inhibition of thrombin (IIa). However, this requires heparin molecules longer than 18 polysaccharide residues. Inhibition of factor Xa is not dependent on the size of the heparin molecule.

bioavailability at low concentrations and limits the amount of heparin available to interact with ATIII. Moreover, changes in plasma levels of heparin-binding proteins in patients with thrombotic disorders leads to unpredictable anticoagulant responses and a need for very high doses of heparin in some (heparin resistance).

The pharmacokinetic properties of heparin are complex. It binds to receptors on macrophages and the reticuloendothelial system, where it is rapidly internalized and degraded. Heparin thus has a longer half-life in patients with severe hepatic disease. However, this is a saturable mechanism giving zero-order kinetics. Heparin is also cleared more slowly with first-order kinetics by the kidney. As a result, the biologic half-life of heparin depends on dose. With an i.v. bolus of heparin at 25 units/kg, the biologic half-life is 30 minutes, but this increases to 60 minutes with 100 units/kg and 150 minutes after 400 units/kg.

Heparin is effective in:

- Preventing venous thrombosis.
- Treating deep venous thromboembolism and pulmonary embolism (see Ch. 14).
- The early treatment of patients with unstable angina and acute myocardial infarction.
- Preventing clotting in catheters used to cannulate blood vessels.
- Anticoagulating extracorporeal devices, as in cardiac bypass surgery and hemodialysis.
- Treating arterial thrombosis, as in acute myocardial infarction, in conjunction with antiplatelet and thrombolytic agents.

The therapeutic window of heparin is relatively narrow, and bleeding is a major complication. Not surprisingly, bleeding occurs much more frequently when a high dose of heparin is given. Since heparin is obtained from animals (pigs and cattle) it can be antigenic and cause hypersensitivity reactions, including chills, fever, urticaria and even anaphylactic shock. An uncommon but serious complication is heparin-induced thrombocytopenia. The platelet counts of patients receiving heparin should therefore be monitored, and heparin stopped if heparin-induced thrombocytopenia is suspected. Paradoxically, thrombocytopenia due to heparin can be a highly pro-thrombotic disorder. Long-term heparin therapy (usually longer than 3 months) is also associated with bone loss and elevation of liver enzymes may occur.

Heparin is contraindicated in patients who (1) are hypersensitive to it, (2) have bleeding disorders, (3) have severe hypertension or severe hepatic/renal disease, and are alcoholics, and (4) are undergoing surgery of the brain, spinal cord or eye.

Heparin-induced bleeding is rapidly reversed by administration of 100 units heparin/1 mg protamine, a basic peptide and specific antagonist of heparin, which combines with heparin to form a stable complex with loss of anticoagulant activity. Overdose of protamine should be avoided because it is also an anticoagulant agent. Neutralization of low molecular weight heparin by protamine is incomplete.

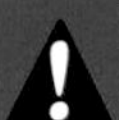

Adverse effects of heparin

- **Bleeding**
- **Thrombocytopenia and paradoxical thrombosis**
- **Osteoporosis**
- **Hypersensitivity**

Low molecular weight heparin: enoxaparin

Unfractionated heparin is commonly extracted from porcine intestinal mucosa or bovine lung. As a result of the extraction process, the polysaccharides are degraded into a heterogeneous mixture of fragments with molecular weights ranging from 300 to 30 000 kDa. All unfractionated heparin preparations have to be standardized.

LMWHs are obtained either by fractionation, chemical hydrolysis, or depolymerization of unfractionated heparin. Commercial preparations have a mean molecular weight of 5000 kDa, ranging from 1000 to 10 000 kDa. It should be noted, however, that LMWHs produced by

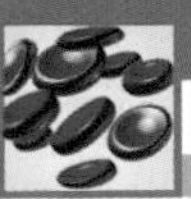

different methods should be considered as individual drug agents with different pharmacokinetic and pharmacodynamic properties, rather than being viewed as simply being interchangeable. Mechanistically, the anticoagulant effects of LMWHs differ from those of standard heparin because:

- The antithrombin:anti-factor Xa ratio is reduced from 1:1 to 1:4.
- The pharmacokinetic properties have diminished intersubject variability, at least in part due to decreased protein binding.
- There is decreased interaction with platelets compared to heparin.

LMWHs have a number of advantages over heparin. Maximum plasma levels after subcutaneous injections of LMWHs are reached within 2–3 hours. In comparison, the half-life of LMWHs is about 4 hours (i.e. twice as long as standard heparin). In addition, the bioavailability of LMWHs is about 90%, versus 20% after subcutaneous injection for heparin. LMWHs have a more predictable anticoagulant response, which means that they can be given subcutaneously once or twice a day without laboratory monitoring. LMWHs are as effective as standard heparin in the prevention and treatment of venous thrombosis and may be associated with fewer bleeding complications.

Enoxaparin sodium was the first LMWH approved in the USA for prevention of deep vein thrombosis following hip replacement surgery. Moreover, enoxaparin has been approved for use either in the hospital or at home with once a day dosage. Enoxaparin has been intensively compared for treatment of acute coronary syndromes, including unstable angina or acute myocardial infarction, with standard heparin. The data suggest that enoxaparin can be effectively substituted for standard heparin in acute myocardial infarctions. The dose of enoxaparin for treatment of deep vein thrombosis or pulmonary embolism is 30 mg subcutaneous injection twice a day for 6 days or longer depending on clinical requirements. Adverse effects of enoxaparin include bleeding, thrombocytopenia and local irritation.

Another low molecular weight heparin is reviparin, which has a half-life in serum of 3.3 hours.

Direct inhibition of thrombin activity: hirudin (lepirudin)

While multiple other factors may contribute to the pathogenesis of thrombotic disorders, the thrombogenic effects of thrombin play a central role. Inactivation of this enzyme, or prevention of thrombin generation, can inhibit thrombin-induced thrombosis.

Hirudin, a 65-amino acid (7 kDa) protein originally purified from the salivary glands of the leech *Hirudo medicinalis*, is a highly specific antagonist of thrombin. Its recombinant protein, lepirudin, derived from yeast cells, is also available. Lepirudin and similar analogs are potent direct inhibitors of thrombin. Unlike heparin, which needs ATIII to inhibit thrombin, lepirudin directly inhibits thrombin independently of ATIII. Theoretically, such direct thrombin inhibitors should be safer than heparin since they selectively inhibit thrombin and do not affect platelet function. Furthermore, they are not associated with thrombocytopenia.

Lepirudin is used for thrombosis complications related to heparin-induced thrombocytopenia (HIT) type II. HIT type II is a rare, allergy-like adverse reaction to heparin, caused by a complex immune mechanism and characterized by a rapid and serious decline in platelet count. It is presumed to be due to sequestration of platelets in the vasculature, leading to an increased risk of severe thromboembolic complications and resulting in crippling disability, amputation, or even death. Lepirudin allows HIT type II patients to maintain antithrombotic therapy and prevents thromboembolic complications. Lepirudin also reduces mortality, myocardial infarction and the need for invasive cardiac procedures, when compared with the standard treatment in patients with unstable angina. The recommended dose in HIT type II is 0.4 mg/kg/h (up to 110 kg) for an i.v. bolus slowly followed by 0.15 mg/kg/h (up 110 kg) as a continuously i.v. infusion for 2–10 days or longer depending on the situations. The half-life of lepirudin is about 60 minutes; it undergoes rapid hydrolysis. The parent drug and its fragments are eliminated in urine but can accumulate in renal insufficiency.

The major adverse effect of lepirudin is bleeding that can be exacerbated by concomitant antithrombotic therapy. Other adverse effects occurring with lepirudin treatment include abnormal liver function and allergic skin reactions. Chronic treatment with lepirudin may lead to development of antibodies against the lepirudin–thrombin complex that may enhance the lepirudin antithrombotic effect.

Bivalirudin is a synthetic 20-amino acid peptide that directly inhibits thrombin by specifically binding to both the catalytic site and the anion binding exosite of circulating and clot-bound thrombin. It has a very short serum half-life and has a number of side effects including back pain nausea, hypotension and headache.

Ximelagatran is another direct-acting thrombin inhibitor that is the pro-drug of melagatran. Ximelagatran is readily converted to biologically active melagatran by hydolysis of the ethyl–ester bond and reduction of the hydroxyamidine constituent. Melagatran then binds to thrombin on the arginine side pocket causing reversible inhibitory activity, which occurs very rapidly after treatment. The serum half-life is 3–5 hours and bleeding has been a major unwanted side effect, along with elevation of liver enzymes that occurs in up to 7% of treated patients.

Argatroban is a direct thrombin inhibitor that reversibly binds to the thrombin active site. Argatroban does not require the cofactor antithrombin III for antithrombotic activity. Argatroban exerts its anticoagulant effects by inhibiting thrombin-catalyzed or -induced reactions, including fibrin formation; activation of coagulation factors V, VIII and XIII; protein C; and platelet aggregation.

Agatroban is highly selective for thrombin with an inhibitory constant (Ki) of 0.04 μg/mL. At therapeutic concentrations, argatroban has little or no effect on related serine proteases (trypsin, factor Xa, plasmin and kallikrein).

Argatroban can inhibit the action of both free and clot-associated thrombin. In patients receiving continuous i.v. argatroban (100 μg/kg bolus) at 3 μg/kg/min in acute ischemic stroke it provided safe anticoagulation in acute ischemic stroke without major bleeding. Argatroban is 54% bound to human serum proteins. Metabolism is hepatic, mainly by CYP3A4/5. The only approved use for argatroban in the USA is for treating HIT, a potentially serious, immune-mediated complication of heparin therapy that is strongly associated with subsequent venous and arterial thrombosis during percutaneous coronary interventions. Whereas initial treatment of HIT is to discontinue administration of all heparin, patients may require anticoagulation for prevention and treatment of thromboembolic events. The recommended initial dose of argatroban for adult patients without hepatic impairment is 2 μg/kg/min, administered as a continuous i.v. infusion. The worst adverse effect is major bleeding, which may occur in about 5% of patients.

Thrombolytic agents

Unlike anticoagulant therapy, thrombolytic agents actively dissolve blood clots by promoting the conversion of plasminogen to plasmin, a serine protease that in turn hydrolyzes fibrin and fibrinogen, which leads to the dissolution of clots (Fig. 10.15). Consequently, selected acute thromboembolic disorders are treated with thrombolytic agents. However, thrombolytic agents can increase local thrombin concentrations as the clot dissolves, leading to enhanced platelet aggregation and thrombosis. Co-therapy with antiplatelet agents such as aspirin, or anticoagulant heparin, may prevent this.

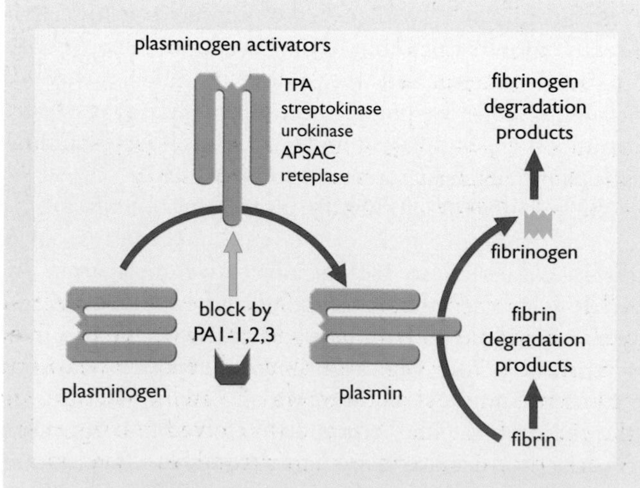

Fig. 10.15 The fibrinolytic system and mechanisms of thrombolytic agents. The plasminogen activators currently used as thrombolytic agents stimulate conversion of plasminogen to plasmin that degradates fibrin. The action sites of physiologic inhibitors are also illustrated (PAI-1, 2, 3, plasminogen activator inhibitor 1, 2, 3).

The use of thrombolytic agents to dissolve thrombi is standard therapy in acute myocardial infarction. Thrombolytics are also beneficial in the initial treatment of acute peripheral vascular occlusion, deep venous thrombosis and massive pulmonary embolism. Selected patients with acute ischemic stroke can receive recombinant tissue plasminogen activator (rtPA) within 3 hours of the onset of symptoms.

Hemorrhage is a major adverse effect of thrombolytics, since they do not distinguish between fibrin in unwanted thrombi and that in hemostatic plugs. Thrombolytics are contraindicated in patients with acute pericarditis, active internal bleeding, recent cerebrovascular accident, healing major wounds, or metastatic cancer. One complication of thrombolytic therapy in acute myocardial infarction is coronary artery re-occlusion following treatment.

Currently, five thrombolytic agents are commercially available in the USA. Their thrombolytic activities are either directly or indirectly based on the ability to enhance the generation of plasmin from precursor plasminogen. The pharmacologic and pharmacokinetic properties of these thrombolytics are summarized in Table 10.6.

- Streptokinase (SK) is derived from group A β-hemolytic streptococci and is highly antigenic. It has no intrinsic enzymatic activity. Following i.v. infusion, it combines with plasminogen to form a 1:1 complex that activates plasminogen to plasmin. The complex hydrolyzes fibrin plugs, fibrinogen and coagulation factors V and VII.
- Anisoylated plasminogen–streptokinase activator complex (APSAC) is modified so that it is pre-bound to a plasminogen molecule. It is also without enzymatic activity until its active site is deacylated following administration. It has a fourfold longer half-life than SK and can therefore be given as an i.v. bolus. Like SK, it is also highly antigenic.
- Urokinase (UK) is purified from human fetal kidney cells. UK directly converts plasminogen to plasmin by cleaving the arginine–valine bond in plasminogen. UK directly degrades both fibrin and fibrinogen. UK does not induce an antigenic response.
- Alteplase is a recombinant tissue plasminogen activator (rtPA) whose enzymatic activity depends on the presence of fibrin. Alteplase rapidly activates plasminogen bound to fibrin rather than free plasminogen in the circulation. Theoretically, it should cause less systemic fibrinolytic activation and reduce risk of bleeding. However, at clinical doses, rtPA also induces a system lytic state, and an increased bleeding tendency.

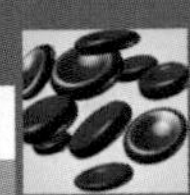

Table 10.6 Pharmacologic and pharmacokinetic properties of thrombolytics

	Streptokinase	APSAC	Urokinase	rtPA	Reteplase
Source of drug	Streptococcal culture	Mammalian cell	Streptococcal culture	Mammalian cell	Mammalian cell
Molecular weight (kDa)	47	131	32–54	70	55
Circulating half-life (min)	12–18	40–60	15–20	2–6	2–4
Fibrin specificity	1+	1+	2+	3+	3+
Dose (i.v. bolus in minutes)	1.5 MU (30–60)	30 mg (5)	3 MU (45–90)	15 mg bolus, then 50 mg/ 30 min, then 35 mg/ 30 min	10 mg bolus, then 10 mg bolus (30)
Duration of infusion (min)	60 or less	2–5	5–15	180 or less	30 or less
Patency at 90 min (%)	53–65	55–65	66	81–88	86–90
Lives saved per 100 treated	2.5	2.5	2.5	3.5	N/A
Early heparin required	No	No	No	Yes	No
Antigenic reactions	Yes	Yes	No	No	No
Intracerebral hemorrhage (%)	0.4	0.6	0.4	0.6	N/A
Hypotension	Yes	Yes	No	No	No
Relative cost per dose (US$)	300	1200	2200	2300	2500

APSAC, anisoylated plasminogen–streptokinase activator complex; rtPA, recombinant tissue plasminogen activator; MU, million units; N/A, not available.

Table 10.7 Novel antithrombotic strategies and agents

Strategy mechanism	Agents
Inhibit platelet functions	
Inhibit platelet adhesion	GPIa/IIa and GPIb/IX antagonists
Inhibit platelet recruitment	Thromboxane synthase inhibitors
	TXA_2 receptor antagonists
	Thrombin receptor antagonists
Inhibit platelet aggregation	Synthetic GPIIb/IIIa antagonists
Inhibit coagulation	
Prevent thrombin generation	Factor VII, tissue factor and VIIa/TF complex inhibitors
	Factor IXa inhibitors
	Factor Xa inhibitors
Inhibit thrombin activity	Active site inhibitors
Enhance natural anticoagulant activity	
Modulate protein C pathway	Protein C or activated protein C
	Soluble thrombomodulin
	Thrombin variants
	Allosteric modulators of thrombin
Enhance endogenous fibrinolysis	
Block type-I plasminogen activator inhibitor	Inhibitors of type-I plasminogen activator inhibitor synthesis
	Inhibitors of type-I plasminogen activator inhibitor activity
Inhibit procarboxypeptidase B	Inhibitors of procarboxypeptidase B

- Reteplase is a modified human tPA designed to improve the therapeutic properties of tPA without increasing its bleeding potential. Such modifications lead to faster reperfusion rates than with alteplase. Several additional second-generation thrombolytic agents produced by recombinant techniques are being developed.

Novel antithrombotic strategies and agents

The limitations of aspirin and heparin have led to new antithrombotic agents, including inhibitors of TXA_2-independent pathways (e.g. ADP antagonist), platelet adhesive receptor antagonists (e.g. GPIb/TX antagonist) and inhibitors of thrombin generation or activity. New antithrombotic strategies are focusing on the development of potent and specific inhibitors of platelet function, and the chain of enzymatic reactions involved in coagulation. Many promising novel antithrombotic agents are currently being assessed in the management of thrombotic diseases (Table 10.7). These include drugs to inhibit platelet adhesion, platelet recruitment and platelet aggregation; drugs to block thrombin generation or activity; and drugs to enhance natural anticoagulant activity or endogenous fibrinolysis.

STROKE

Stroke is a major cause of death in the Western world and may be the most important disease causing long-term disability. The management of strokes is changing since it is now possible to intervene and ameliorate neurologic deficits in many patients if treatment is initiated quickly after onset of symptoms. In this respect, stroke needs to be viewed in the same context as acute myocardial infarction so as to encourage prompt attendance at emergency medical departments.

The initial diagnosis of stroke is primarily clinical. The distinction between an ischemic and a hemorrhagic stroke must be made quickly since treatment for secondary prevention is quite different for these two. Computed tomography (CT), or possibly magnetic resonance imaging (MRI), may be the best way to make a differential diagnosis, even if the clinical presentation seems straightforward. Ischemic stroke is usually due to an occlusion of a cerebral artery. Clinical deficits found early in ischemic stroke are due to cessation of neuronal function, although at this stage function may recover if cerebral blood flow is restored. The time window for this is not clear. Once the window is exceeded, damage will be irreversible as a result of neuronal cell death. Thrombolytic therapy is appropriate in many patients with ischemic stroke, but contraindicated in patients with hemorrhages.

Thrombolytic therapy for acute strokes

Multiple controlled clinical trials have demonstrated that thrombolytic therapy decreases neurologic deficits and incapacity 3–6 months later. Although thrombolytic therapy with tPA, streptokinase or urokinase can cause intracranial bleeding, its benefits outweighs this risk. Moreover, in patients treated within 3 hours of onset, the risk of intracranial bleeding is less, and benefits are greater. These trials highlighted the importance of the emergency treatment of ischemic stroke. While further information is necessary in order to characterize the use of tPA in patients with concomitant diseases such as diabetes and hypertension, current evidence favors tPA therapy. This therapy is generally contraindicated in patients taking anticoagulants or those with clotting disorders, or low platelet counts.

There may be a small benefit in using aspirin in the early phases of acute stroke. The potential benefits of anticoagulants during acute stroke are not established; unfortunately, experimental neuroprotective agents have not been shown to be effective in clinical trials.

Stroke prophylaxis

Aspirin has a well-established benefit in preventing stroke, especially in patients who have had a TIA or have carotid atherosclerosis. Anticoagulation with warfarin has established benefit in preventing stroke in patients with atrial fibrillation.

BLEEDING DISORDERS

Defects in each of the components of the normal hemostatic mechanisms may cause abnormal bleeding. These defects can be acquired or hereditary, and are usually divided into four categories: namely, vascular, platelet, blood coagulation factors, or fibrinolytic defects, according to their actions (Table 10.8).

- Vascular defects include acquired or hereditary structural abnormalities of blood vessel walls.
- Platelet defects include acquired or hereditary abnormalities in platelet quantity (thrombocytopenia) or in platelet quality (thrombocytopathy).
- Von Willebrand's disease (vWD) is the most common inherited coagulopathy. Patients typically present with abnormal bruising and mucosal bleeding such as epistaxis and melena. In contrast, soft tissue bleeding and spontaneous hemarthroses are more characteristic of hemophilias (factor VIII or IX deficiency).
- Acquired defects of coagulant factors include severe liver disease, deficiency of vitamin K, increased fibrinolysis in DIC and platelet disorders.

Coagulation factor concentrates

Factor VIII concentrates with varying degrees of purity are commercially available for prophylactic and therapeutic use in patients with hemophilia A. Since 1985, all factor VIII concentrates have been treated with virus attenuation procedures, and the risk of HIV or hepatitis C transmission has essentially been eliminated. Recombinant factor VIII generated from genetically engineered mammalian cells is also now available (Table 10.9). The introduction of highly purified factor IX concentrate treated with viral attenuation procedures since 1991 has greatly improved the treatment of hemophilia A and B patients. Examples include the human recombinant factor VIII, moroctocog α for the treatment of hemophilia A and recombinant factor IX, nonacog α to treat hemophilia B. Headache, chills, fever and allergic reactions can occur with these treatments.

The development of alloantibodies that inhibit factor VIII or factor IX can be a severe problem in the treatment of hemophilias. Patients with high levels of factor

Table 10.8 Bleeding disorders
Hereditary
Hemophilia A (factor VIII deficiency)
Hemophilia B (factor IX deficiency)
Von Willebrand's disease
Platelet disorders (e.g. Glanzmann's thrombasthenia)
Acquired
Vitamin K deficiency
Liver disease
Disseminated intravascular coagulation
Thrombocytopenia (immune, infection, splenic sequestration)
Platelet disorder (uremia)

Table 10.9 Factor VIII concentrates

Product name	Purity
Recombinate	Recombinant
Monoclate-P	High
Koate-HP	Intermediate
Humate-P	Intermediate
Hyate-C	Porcine

VIII inhibitor can be treated with porcine factor VIII if the antibodies do not strongly cross-react with the porcine protein. Other options include using factor IX complex concentrates or recombinant factor VIIa concentrates. Recombinant activated factor VII is also used as a potent hemostatic agent.

Desmopressin

An infusion of desmopressin, 1-deamino-(8-D-arginine)-vasopressin (DDAVP), a synthetic analog of vasopressin, causes the release of von Willebrand factor (vWF) and factor VIII from body storage sites such as Weibel–Palade bodies in endothelial cells.

DDAVP is used in patients with mild factor VIII deficiency (>5%) prophylactically before minor surgical procedures. DDAVP cannot be used in patients with severe hemophilia A because they do not have any stored factor VIII. DDAVP is also used for the prevention and treatment of bleeding in patients with vWD. vWF is needed to mediate the formation of the platelet plug and also for factor VIII activity by forming a factor VIII–vWF complex. Patients with vWD subtypes that are deficient in vWF may respond to DDAVP treatment. Patients with defective vWF, or a severe deficiency of vWF, should be transfused with intermediate-purity factor VIII concentrates containing vWF. Recombinant factor VIII is not appropriate for these patients. DDAVP has been used for treatment of bleeding in patients with renal failure. Uremia causes complex abnormalities of hemostasis, reflected in part by a prolonged bleeding time. Intravenous infusion of DDAVP can normalize the prolonged bleeding time and ameliorate the tendency toward excessive bleeding.

DDAVP can be given as intranasal spray, intravenously or subcutaneously. Responses to DDAVP treatment vary, and diminish after several doses as a result of depletion of the factor VIII storage pools. The adverse effects of DDAVP include flushing, headache, hypertension and fluid retention.

Vitamin K

Vitamin K is an essential cofactor for the synthesis of prothrombin in the liver, as well as of factors II, VII, IX, X, protein C and protein S. These coagulation factors are synthesized, requiring an adequate dietary intake of vitamin K. Lack of vitamin K, or the presence of inhibitors such as warfarin, causes the production of non γ-carboxylated prothrombin, which is activated by factor Xa at only 1–2% of normal (see Fig. 10.13).

Vitamin K is used to reverse coagulation and bleeding caused by the vitamin K inhibitor warfarin. Vitamin K deficiency can also occur in patients with biliary obstruction and liver diseases, and after prolonged treatment with oral antibiotics, as a result of suppression of intestinal bacteria that synthesize vitamin K.

Natural vitamin K, derived from green, leafy vegetables, is vitamin K_1 (phytonadione). Vitamin K_2 (menaquinone) is synthesized by intestinal bacteria. Vitamins K_1 and K_2 are fat-soluble vitamins; therefore, bile salts are required for their gastrointestinal absorption. Synthesized vitamin K_3 (menadione sodium bisulfite) and vitamin K_4 (menadione diacetate) are water-soluble and can be injected. However, vitamin K_3 and K_4 are rarely used in the clinic because they are therapeutically ineffective (Fig. 10.16).

A major use of vitamin K is to prevent hypoprothrombinemia in the newborn. Vitamin K levels in the newborn may be marginal and exacerbated by inadequate nutritional intake in the first few days of life. The concentrations of factors II, VII, IX and X in newborn infants are approximately 20–50% of adult plasma levels; premature infants have even lower concentrations. Trace amounts of vitamin K will prevent hypoprothrombinemia by attenuating the decline in concentrations of vitamin K-dependent coagulation factors, although this treatment will not raise concentrations of these coagulation factors to adult levels. Prophylactic administration of small doses of vitamin K to newborn infants is routinely recommended and considered safe. Excess doses can provoke hemolytic anemia, hyperbilirubinemia and kernicterus in the newborn. Premature infants and newborn infants with a congenital deficiency in erythrocyte glucose-6-phosphate dehydrogenase are particularly sensitive to administration of vitamin K, including phytonadione, menadione, and menadiol. Phytonadione is the drug of choice for prophylactic treatment in newborn infants since it can be safely administered, orally or parenterally. Although menadione and menadiol do not require the presence of bile for gastrointestinal absorption, they can provoke toxic effects in newborns and are contraindicated in newborn infants and during later pregnancy. An alternative way to give prophylactic phytonadione to newborn infants is to administer it to mothers prior to delivery.

ε aminocaproic acid

ε aminocaproic acid (EACA) acts as a hemostatic agent by inhibiting the fibrinolytic system. It interferes with lysine-binding sites on plasminogen, blocking plasminogen association with fibrin, and thereby inhibiting the activation of plasminogen to plasmin. It is available in both oral and parenteral formulations, and has been used in the treatment of many bleeding conditions, but most commonly urinary tract bleeding.

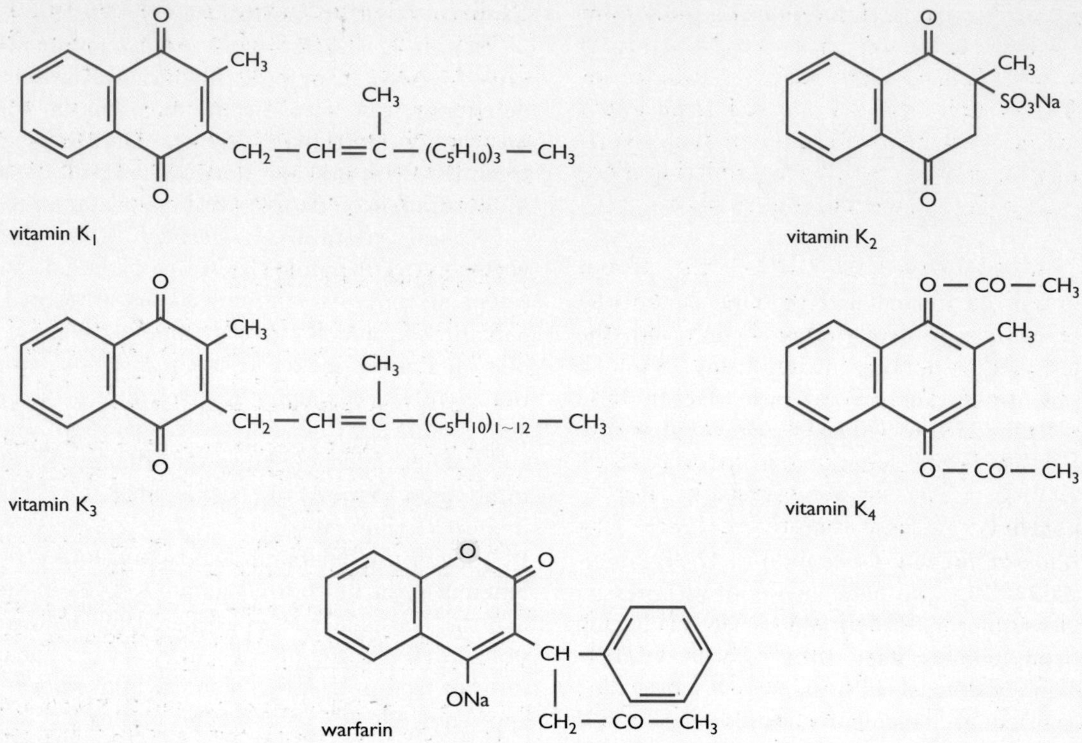

Fig. 10.16 Chemical structures of vitamin K and the antagonist warfarin.

The recommended dose of EACA is 6 g four times per day, or a loading dose of 5 g administered by i.v. injection over 30–60 minutes. It is rapidly absorbed orally and eliminated from the body by the kidney. The elimination half-life of EACA is approximately 2 hours.

Adverse effects of EACA include intravascular thrombosis due to inhibition of plasminogen activator, hypotension, myopathy, diarrhea and nasal stuffiness. Antifibrinolytic agents may exacerbate the thrombotic component of DIC and should be avoided in this condition.

Aprotinin

Aprotinin is a 6.5-kDa protein purified from bovine lung. It functions as an inhibitor of several serine proteases including tissue and plasma kallikrein by forming reversible enzyme–inhibitor complexes. Aprotinin inhibition of kallikrein results directly in a decreased formation of activated coagulation factor XII (see Fig. 10.9). Consequently, aprotinin inhibits the initiation of both coagulation and fibrinolysis due to contact of blood with a foreign surface. Aprotinin is administered intravenously. The enzymatic activity of the compound is expressed in kallikrein inactivation units (KIU). Plasma concentrations of 125 KIU/mL are necessary to inhibit plasmin, and 300–500 KIU/mL are needed to inhibit kallikrein.

Aprotinin is used for blood loss during cardiac surgery, particularly coronary artery bypass grafting, when the exposure of blood to artificial surfaces in the extracorporeal oxygenator and enzymatic and mechanical injury to platelets and coagulation factors leads to a hyperproteolytic and hyperfibrinolytic state. The use of aprotinin can reduce blood loss by as much as 50% in these surgical procedures.

The major adverse effect of aprotinin is hypersensitivity reactions. Therefore, a small test dose is necessary before a full therapeutic dose is given. In addition, aprotinin treatment may cause venous or arterial thrombosis. A lower prevalence of stroke among patients treated with aprotinin has been observed in a recent clinical trial.

Topical absorbable hemostatics

The purpose of chemical local hemostatics is to prevent and stop blood flow from blood vessels or from oozing wound sites. An ideal local hemostatic would be rapidly absorbed, cause no irritation and have a hemostatic action independent of the thrombotic mechanisms. Most absorbable hemostatics meet most of these requirements and can be placed on the wound. The most widely used local absorbable hemostatics include thrombin, micronized collagen, absorbable gelatin sponge and oxidized cellulose.

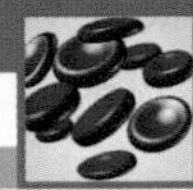

THROMBIN purified from bovine serum is applied topically to control capillary oozing in surgical procedures and to shorten the duration of bleeding from puncture sites in heparinized patients. One unit of thrombin causes 1 mL of standard fibrin solution to clot in 15 seconds. Thrombin may also be used for localized bleeding in the nose or mouth for patients with vWD. However, thrombin is never used by systemic injection, because of the high risk of generalized thrombosis.

MICROFIBRILLAR COLLAGEN HEMOSTAT is purified from bovine corium collagen. It acts by attracting and activating platelets to initiate clot formation. It is absorbable and is prepared as a dry, sterile, fibrous, water-insoluble product. Microfibrillar collagen has been found to be as effective as a topical hemostatic agent for large oozing surfaces. It is used during surgery to control capillary bleeding, and as an adjunctive hemostatic. It causes a mild, chronic cellular inflammatory response and may interfere with wound healing.

ABSORBABLE GELATIN is a simple protein complex made from animal gelatin. It is not antigenic. There are three preparations of gelatin for different clinical purposes, comprising absorbable gelatin sponge, absorbable gelatin film and absorbable gelatin powder. Gelatin sponge is produced as a sterile, absorbable, water-insoluble, gelatin-based sponge. It is used for the control of capillary vessel leakage and frank hemorrhage. When implanted in tissue it is absorbed completely in 3–5 weeks without inducing excessive scar formation. When applied to bleeding skin or nasal, rectal or vaginal mucosa, it completely liquefies within 2–5 days. Oral ingestion of 1–10 mg of gelatin powder has been employed to treat gastrointestinal bleeding.

OXIDIZED CELLULOSE is a specifically treated form of surgical gauze or cotton that promotes clotting by a physical effect, rather than by any alteration of the normal clotting mechanisms. It is used to control capillary, venous and small arterial hemorrhage when ligation or other methods are impractical or ineffective. It is also employed in oral surgery and exodontia. Oxidized cellulose should not be used with thrombin because its low pH interferes with the activity of the thrombin. Oxidized cellulose is nontoxic and relatively nonirritating but somewhat detrimental to wound healing. Phagocytosis is the route of removal. Moreover, it is not employed for permanent packing or implantation in fractures because of interference with bone regeneration and possible cyst formation. It is available as sterile cotton pledgets, gauze pads and gauze strips.

FURTHER READING

Colman RW, Hirsh J, Marder VJ, Salzman EW (eds). *Hemostasis and Thrombosis: Basic Principles and Clinical Practice*, 4th edn. Philadelphia: JB Lippincott; 2000. [An excellent textbook covering all aspects of hemostasis from molecular mechanism to clinical application.]

Gresle P, Fuster V, Page CP, Vermylen J (eds). *The platelet in Health and Disease*. Cambridge: Cambridge University Press; 2002. [A comprehensive overview of platelet biology and antiplatelet drugs.]

Handin RJ, Lux SE, Stossel TP. Blood: principles and practice of haematology. Philadelphia, Pa.: Lippincott Williams & Wilkins 2003.

Hirsh J, Dalen J, Anderson DR, Poller L, Bussey H, Ansell J, Deykin D. Oral anticoagulants: mechanisms of action, clinical effectiveness, and optimal therapeutic range. *Chest* 2001; **119**: 8S–21S.

Hirsh J, Warkentin TE, Shaughnessy SG, Anand SS, Halperin JL, Raschke R, Granger C, Ohman EM, Dalen JE. Heparin and low-molecular-weight heparin: mechanisms of action, pharmacokinetics, dosing, monitoring, efficacy, and safety. *Chest* 2001; **119**: 64S–94S. [The full pharmacology of heparin and heparin-like drugs in the treatment of coagulant pathologies.]

Patrono C, Coller B, Dalen JE, FitzGerald GA, Fuster V, Gent M, Hirsh J, Roth G. Platelet-active drugs: the relationships among dose, effectiveness, and side effects. *Chest* 2001; **119**: 39S–63S. [The pharmacology of antiplatelet drugs.]

Provan A, and Gribben J. Molecular haematology. Malden, Mass: Blackwell Pub., 2005. [The molecular biology of drugs used for their effects on coagulation.]

Provan A. Oxford handbook of clinical haematology. Oxford; New York: Oxford University Press, 2004. [One of the standard textbooks on haematology and the use of drugs for treating haematological conditions.]

WEBSITES

http://pathy.med.nagoya-u.ac.jp/atlas/doc/ [Atlas of Hematology.]

http://www.merck.com/mrkshared/mmanual/sections.jsp [Merck Manual.]

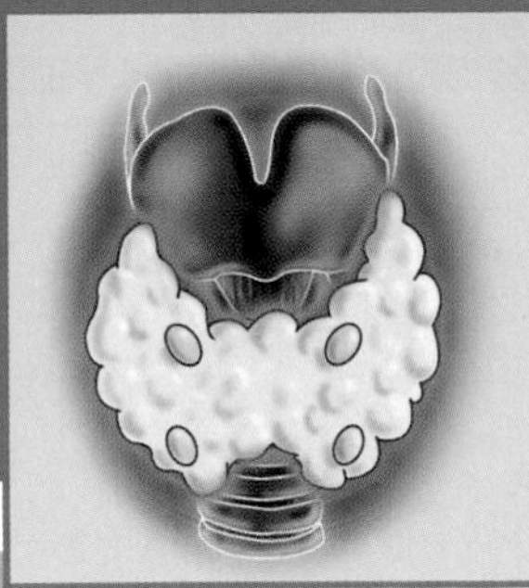

Chapter 11

Drugs and the Endocrine and Metabolic Systems

GENERAL PHYSIOLOGY OF THE ENDOCRINE AND METABOLIC SYSTEMS

The endocrine and metabolic system consists of a variety of organs (glands) that secrete substances (hormones) into the blood which affect the function of target tissues elsewhere in the body. Such glands include the hypothalamus, pituitary, thyroid, adrenals, gonads, pancreatic islets of Langerhans and the parathyroids. The endocrine system regulates seven major physiologic functions (Table 11.1). A cardinal feature of the drug therapy of endocrine diseases is the interaction between exogenously administered drugs and the 'endogenous pharmacology' of hormones.

The endocrine regulation of Ca^{2+} homeostasis is discussed in Chapter 15 and disorders of circulatory volume in Chapter 13. Additional information on disorders of the genitourinary function is presented in Chapter 17.

The hypothalamic–pituitary axis

- ***The hypothalamus and pituitary glands integrate physiologic signals and release hormones that regulate the function of other glands***

With the exception of energy metabolism and electrolyte homeostasis, pituitary hormones regulate most endocrine systems. The pituitary regulates thyroid, glucocorticosteroid, sex steroids and growth factor secretion by synthesizing and secreting specific hormones which regulate the appropriate glands. The pituitary, which secretes two hormones (prolactin and vasopressin) that act directly on target tissues, consists of anterior and

Table 11.1 Functional anatomy of the endocrine and metabolic systems

Endocrine function	Regulatory factors	Endocrine organ/hormone	Target tissues
Availability of metabolic energy (fuel)	Serum glucose, amino acids, enteric hormones (somatostatin, cholecystokinin, gastrin, secretin), vagal reflex, sympathetic nervous system	Pancreatic islets of Langerhans/insulin, glucagon	All tissues, especially liver, skeletal muscle, adipose tissue, indirect effects on brain and red blood cells
Metabolic rate	Hypothalamic thyrotropin-releasing hormone (TRH), pituitary thyrotropin (TSH)	Thyroid gland/ triiodothyronine (T_3)	All tissues
Circulatory volume	Renin, angiotensin II, hypothalamic osmoreceptor	Adrenals/aldosterone Pituitary/vasopressin	Kidney, blood vessels, CNS
Somatic growth	Hypothalamic growth hormone-releasing hormone (GHRH), somatostatin, sleep, exercise, stress, hypoglycemia	Pituitary/growth hormone Liver/insulin-like growth factors (IGFs)	All tissues
Calcium homeostasis	Serum Ca^{2+} and Mg^{2+} concentration	Parathyroid glands/parathyroid hormone, calcitonin, vitamin D	Kidney, intestines, bone
Reproductive function	Hypothalamic gonadotropin-releasing hormone (GnRH), pituitary follicle-stimulating hormone (FSH) and luteinizing hormone (LH), inhibins	Gonads/sex steroids Adrenals/androgens	Reproductive organs, CNS, various tissues
Adaptation to stress	Hypothalamic corticotropin-releasing hormone (CRH), pituitary adrenocorticotropic hormone (ACTH), hypoglycemia, stress	Adrenals/glucocorticosteroids, epinephrine	Many tissues: CNS, liver, skeletal muscle, adipose tissue, lymphocytes, fibroblasts, cardiovascular system

Endocrine and metabolic systems regulate seven major bodily functions. For each target tissue effect, endocrine glands release hormones in response to regulating factors, which include physiologic (e.g. sleep and stress), biochemical (e.g. glucose and Ca^{2+}) and hormonal (e.g. hypothalamic and enteric hormones) stimuli.

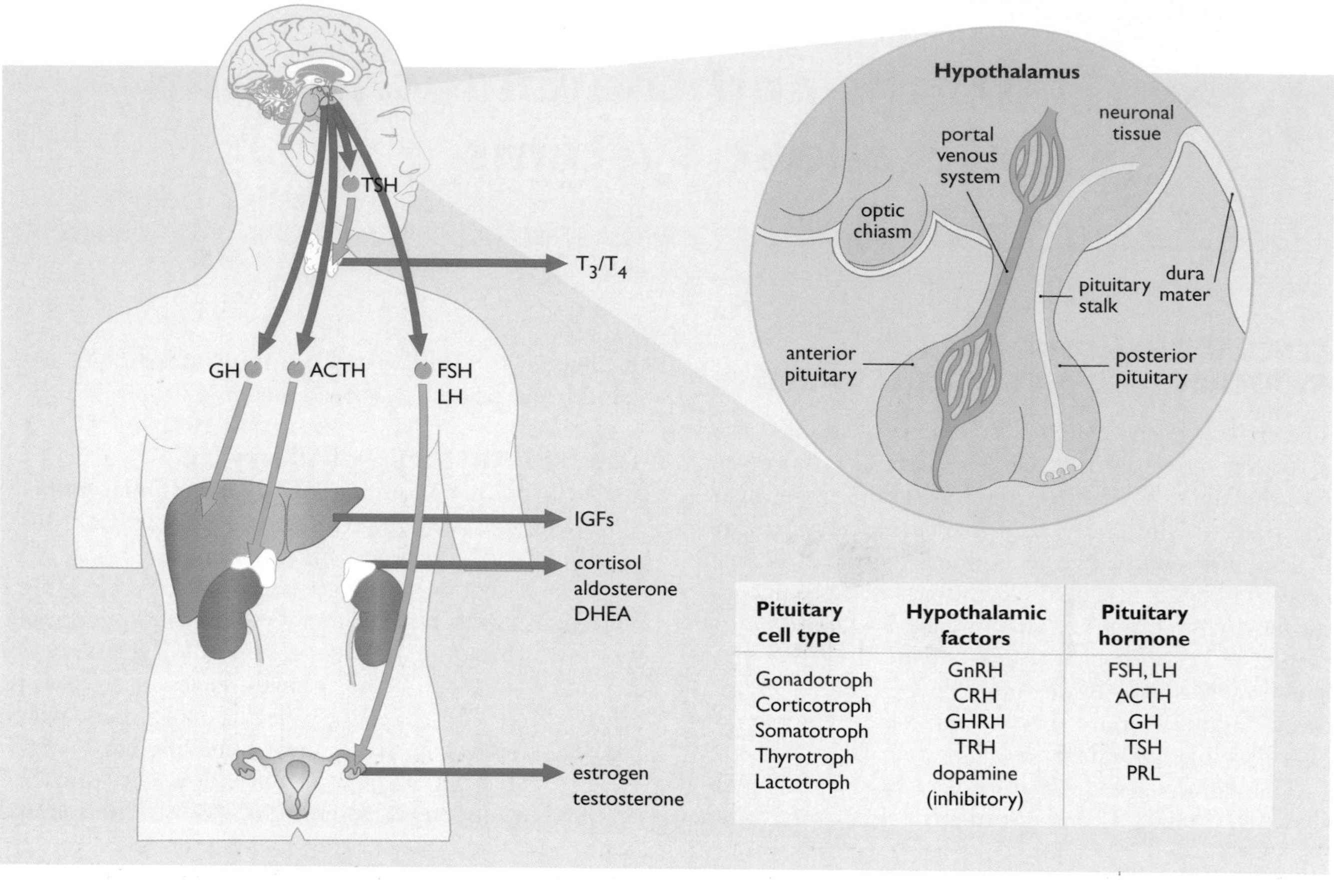

Pituitary cell type	Hypothalamic factors	Pituitary hormone
Gonadotroph	GnRH	FSH, LH
Corticotroph	CRH	ACTH
Somatotroph	GHRH	GH
Thyrotroph	TRH	TSH
Lactotroph	dopamine (inhibitory)	PRL

Fig. 11.1 The hypothalamic–pituitary axis. The cells of the anterior pituitary are regulated by hypothalamic hormones, which are released into portal veins leading from the hypothalamus to the anterior pituitary via the pituitary stalk. Anterior pituitary hormones are released into the inferior petrosal veins for delivery to endocrine organs elsewhere in the body. The posterior pituitary consists of specialized neurons that synthesize the peptide hormones, vasopressin and oxytocin, for release into the systemic circulation (ACTH, adrenocorticotropic hormone; CRH, corticotropin-releasing hormone; DHEA, dehydroepiandrosterone; FSH, follicle-stimulating hormone; GH, growth hormone; GHRH, growth hormone-releasing hormone; GnRH, gonadotropin-releasing hormone; IGFs, insulin-like growth factors; LH, luteinizing hormone; PRL, prolactin; T_3, triiodothyronine; T_4, tetraiodothyronine; TRH, thyrotropin-releasing hormone; TSH, thyroid-stimulating hormone).

posterior divisions (Fig. 11.1). The anterior pituitary (adenohypophysis) develops from Rathke's pouch in the embryonic oropharynx whereas the posterior pituitary (neurohypophysis) is an extracranial neuronal tissue derived from the diencephalon. The blood supply to the anterior pituitary flows to a capillary bed in the hypothalamus, then by conduit veins to the capillary bed of the pituitary. This portal venous system provides a pathway for delivery of hypothalamic hormones which regulate anterior pituitary function. As a result of low perfusion pressures in the portal venous system the anterior pituitary is vulnerable to ischemic damage, particularly during postpartum hemorrhage (Sheehan's syndrome). The cells of the anterior pituitary are a mixed population of cell types that secrete different peptide hormones.

Regulation of a thyroid hormone secretion is a typical example of a hypothalamic–pituitary–endocrine axis control loop (Fig. 11.2). If a low concentration of circulating thyroid hormone is detected by hypothalamic receptors sensitive to thyroid hormones, there is a resulting release of thyrotropin-releasing hormone (TRH) from the hypothalamus (tertiary level of regulation) into portal veins supplying the anterior pituitary. Stimulation of TRH receptors on pituitary thyrotroph cells leads to the release of thyroid-stimulating hormone (TSH, thyrotropin) into the systemic venous system (secondary level of regulation). TSH stimulates thyroid hormone release from the thyroid gland (primary level of hormone production). Thyroid hormone acts directly on target tissues and also has negative feedback effects on the hypothalamus and pituitary. The endocrine systems regulating the sex steroids and the adrenal response to physiologic stress share this four-tiered pattern of hypothalamic, pituitary, primary endocrine gland and target tissue response.

Many endocrine systems share a common pattern of diseases

Endocrine systems regulating metabolic rate (thyroid hormone), reproductive function (sex steroids), adaptation to physiologic stress (glucocorticosteroids) and somatic growth (growth hormone–IGF axis) share common disease patterns affecting each level of endocrine regulation. While disease at any level in the regulatory system may produce a similar effect (i.e. hypo-

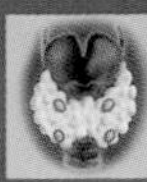

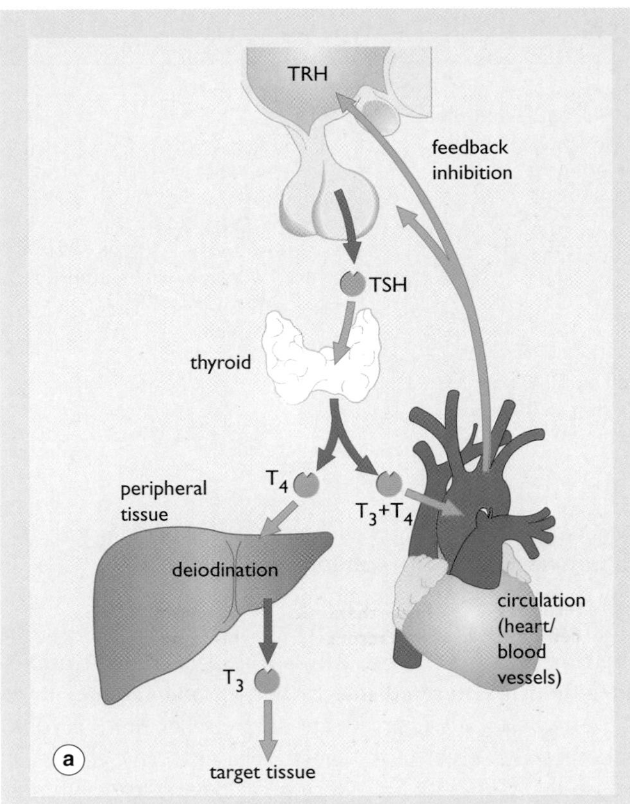

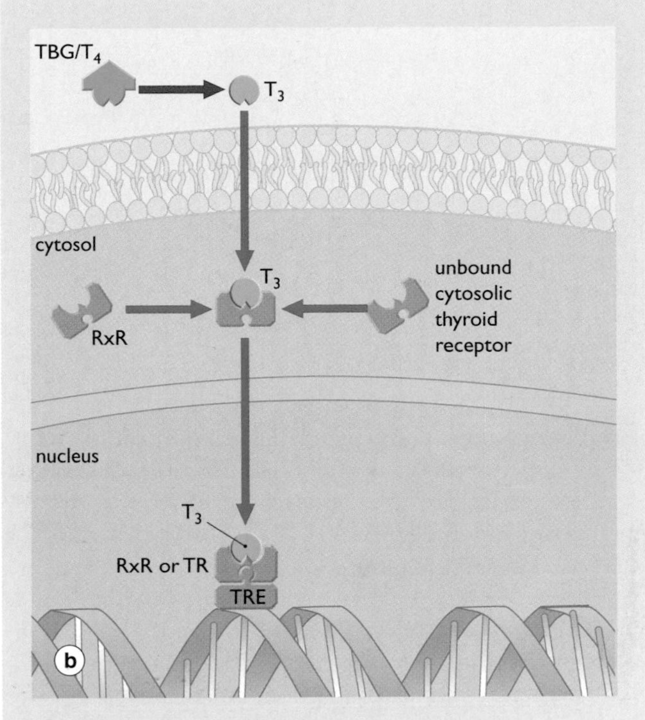

Fig. 11.2 The hypothalamic–pituitary–thyroid axis. (a) Thyroid hormone regulation illustrates the major features of endocrine systems regulated by the hypothalamus and pituitary. Hypothalamic thyrotropin-releasing hormone (TRH), released into the portal circulation, stimulates pituitary thyroid-stimulating hormone (TSH) release. Circulating TSH stimulates the thyroid to release thyroxine (tetraiodothyronine or T_4) and triiodothyronine (T_3) from stores in thyroid follicles. (b) The ligand-bound thyroid receptor may dimerize with itself or with the retinoic acid receptor (RxR) before translocation to the nucleus. Bound thyroid hormone receptors (TR) interact with specific thyroid response elements (TREs) of thyroid hormone-responsive genes. The hypothalamus and pituitary also contain thyroid hormone receptors, which mediate feedback inhibition by circulating thyroid hormone. Thyroid hormone is stored in the follicles of the thyroid gland. TSH stimulates endocytosis of thyroglobulin stores and release of thyroid hormone into the circulation. The scalloped margins of the thyroglobulin stores result from resorption by the cells lining the thyroid follicle.

or hyperstimulation of end-organ effects), different approaches to drug therapy may be preferred depending on the site of pathology. For example, hypogonadism due to failure of pituitary gonadotrophs may respond to therapy with exogenous gonadotropins, but gonadal failure will not. Diagnostic strategies in endocrine disease attempt to identify the site of pathology by identifying the pattern of hormonal responses, which is characteristic for different diseases. The primary alterations and compensatory responses of regulatory hormones accompanying the different patterns of endocrine disease must be understood to allow both diagnosis and treatment.

PATHOPHYSIOLOGY AND DISEASES OF THE ENDOCRINE AND METABOLIC SYSTEMS

Pharmacologic principles

Drugs affecting the endocrine and metabolic systems can act at any of a variety of steps in the process of hormonal signaling where they promote or inhibit target tissue responses. This provides different pharmacotherapeutic approaches to achieve the same pharmacologic effect, either by modifying hormone action or altering hormone production. Pharmacologic intervention can be in two forms: hormone replacement therapy drugs or hormone antagonists, or other drugs, that affect an endocrine system. Hormone replacement therapy sometimes utilizes a synthetic analog of an endogenous hormone.

In endocrine systems that are regulated by hormonal feedback on the hypothalamus and pituitary, drugs which reduce hormonal stimulation of target tissues can lead to increased hormone secretion. For example, the cortisol synthesis inhibitor metyrapone reduces glucocorticosteroid inhibition of adrenocorticotropic hormone (ACTH) release. Its use leads to increased ACTH stimulation of the adrenal gland, which may overcome the effect of metyrapone therapy.

Diseases of the pituitary

Hypothalamic and pituitary diseases affect either single or multiple hormonal systems and lead to symptoms which resemble those of diseases of the primary

Table 11.2 Causes of hypopituitarism

Neoplasms	Pituitary tumors Craniopharyngioma Meningioma
Infarction	Postpartum pituitary necrosis (Sheehan's syndrome)
Inflammatory/infiltrative diseases	Sarcoidosis Histiocytosis X Hemochromatosis Lymphocytic hypophysitis
Infectious diseases	Tuberculosis Syphilis
Physical insults	Trauma Surgery Radiation

Table 11.3 Causes of hyperprolactemia

Compression of pituitary stalk by neoplasms	
Pituitary lactotroph adenoma	
Physiologic stimuli	Breast-feeding
Hormonal status	Pregnancy Estrogen therapy Hypothyroidism
Drugs	Antipsychotic drugs (dopamine antagonists) Cimetidine Verapamil Opiates
Renal failure and hepatic cirrhosis	
Chest wall trauma	

endocrine glands. Thus, the critical role of the pituitary in the regulation of many endocrine functions means that pituitary disease can affect many body functions.

Diseases of the pituitary can lead to hypo- or hyperfunction of the pituitary gland.

Pituitary hypofunction (hypopituitarism)

Pituitary hypofunction is caused by destructive neoplasms, trauma, vascular infarction, inflammatory diseases or granulomatous infection of the pituitary (Table 11.2). In addition to the above, there are specific deficiencies in hypothalamic–pituitary axis with respect to a single hormone system that can lead to hypopituitarism. The cardinal features of hypopituitarism are: (1) hypofunction of several endocrine-responsive target tissues; (2) low concentrations of the primary hormones affecting these tissues; and (3) concentrations of pituitary hormones that are below the level that would normally elicit a compensatory response during hormone deficiency. In some cases, pituitary hormone concentrations may be increased, but not sufficient to fully correct the hormonal deficit. Pituitary hypofunction is treated by hormone replacement of thyroid hormone, sex steroids, glucocorticosteroids and vasopressin, and in some cases growth hormone.

Pituitary hyperfunction

PROLACTIN EXCESS (HYPERPROLACTINEMIA) Excess prolactin secretion by the pituitary is common and has multiple causes. Prolactin secretion is tonically inhibited by dopamine released by the hypothalamus which activates D_2 receptors located in the lactotrophs of the anterior pituitary to reduce cAMP. Excess prolactin usually results from either a secretory lactotroph adenoma or a variety of hypothalamic–pituitary conditions that reduce the tonic inhibition by dopamine (Table 11.3). Excess prolactin is a common cause of infertility and galactorrhea, and if the cause is associated with size of a pituitary tumor, other symptoms and signs such as headaches or disturbed vision due to compression of the optic nerves may appear.

■ *Prolactin secretion, even from pituitary adenomas, is suppressible by D_2 receptor agonists*

The D_2 agonists suppress prolactin secretion (Table 11.4). The drug is an ergot-derivative bromocriptine prototype which is effective in lowering prolactin concentrations but is poorly tolerated due to nausea and fatigue. Rare but dangerous adverse effects such as seizures, cardiac arrhythmias and cerebrovascular accidents have also been reported. The newer long-acting D_2 agonist, cabergoline, has fewer side effects than bromocriptine. In addition to reducing prolactin, D_2 agonists also shrink pituitary lactotroph adenomas by suppressing DNA synthesis and cell division. In many cases, shrinkage occurs within several days of initiating therapy. Normalization of prolactin is achieved in 70–80% of patients treated with D_2 agonists, whereas surgical cure is achieved in approximately 50–60% of microadenomas of the pituitary. For this reason, D_2 agonists have replaced surgery as the primary treatment for this type of pituitary tumor. Therapeutic effects also include reversal of amenorrhea and infertility, and prevention of hypogonadism-related bone loss.

Prolactin-lowering dopaminergic agents

- Nausea and vomiting
- Orthostatic hypertension
- Nasal congestion
- Exacerbation of psychosis
- Digital vasospasm

Abnormalities of the growth hormone–insulin-like growth factor axis

Growth hormone excess (acromegaly)

The growth hormone–insulin-like growth factor (IGF) axis is an endocrine system for which the pathology lies largely within the pituitary and hypothalamus. Growth

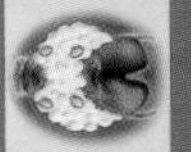

Table 11.4 Dopamine agonists used in the treatment of hyperprolactinemia

Drug	Pharmacology	Dose	Effectiveness	Pharmacokinetics	Adverse effects
Bromocriptine	D_2-selective agonist Ergot alkaloid derivative	1.25–5 mg b.i.d.	70–80% patients achieve normal prolactin levels	Limited absorption (30%) Extensive first-pass metabolism Rapid initial plasma clearance ($t_{1/2}$ = 2 hours) Distributes to tissues Slow terminal elimination	Nausea Fatigue Postural hypotension Nasal congestion Exacerbation of psychosis Seizures Cerebrovascular accident
Pergolide	D_1 and D_2 receptor agonist Ergot alkaloid derivative	0.025–0.5 mg q.d.	As for bromocriptine	Extensive hepatic metabolism $t_{1/2}$ = 27 hours after steady-state dosing	Nausea Postural hypotension Syncope Palpitation Arrhythmias Edema
Cabergoline	D_2-selective agonist Ergot alkaloid derivative	0.25–1 mg twice weekly	77% of patients achieve normal prolactin levels ~70% experience shrinkage (>25%) of prolactinoma 0.05 mg is more effective than 2.5 mg b.i.d. of bromocriptine	$t_{1/2}$ = 60 hours Biliary excretion No CYP metabolism	Nausea but less than bromocriptine
Quinagolide	D_2-selective agonist Nonergot derivative	0.025–0.3 mg q.d.	60–80% of patients achieve normal prolactin concentrations	$t_{1/2}$ = 17 hours Renal and hepatic excretion	Nausea Fatigue Postural hypotension

Iodide (I^-) found in dietary supplements, radiocontrast agents and some cough syrups can reduce thyroid hormone release. In addition, I^- reduces conversion of T_4 to T_3. In acute thyrotoxicosis due to Graves' disease, I^- administration (e.g. supersaturated potassium iodide solution (SSKI), Lugol's solution, or oral radiographic contrast agents) is the most rapidly acting suppressive treatment available.

β_1 adrenoceptor antagonists (e.g. propranolol and esmolol) are commonly used to counteract the effects of excess thyroid hormone. This form of 'functional' (physiologic) antagonism (see Ch. 3) occurs because many of the actions of thyroid hormone and β adrenoceptor agonism are the same (e.g. tachycardia, increased metabolic rate, nervousness and tremor). Thus the actions of thyroid hormone and epinephrine/norepinephrine can be additive or even synergistic. Thyroid hormone also up-regulates the number of adrenoceptors in many tissues, thereby exaggerating the interaction.

Antithyroid drug therapy

- **Propylthiouracil and methimazole inhibit thyroid hormone synthesis**
- **I^- blocks the release of stored thyroid hormone**
- **I^- and propylthiouracil inhibit conversion of thyroxine (tetraiodothyronine or T_4) to triiodothyronine (T_3)**
- **β adrenoceptor antagonists functionally antagonize the target organ effects of thyroid hormone**

Disorders of carbohydrate metabolism

Although thyroid hormone regulates basal metabolic rate, its effect on the delivery of fuel precursors to cells is minor. Instead, this critical endocrine function is performed mainly by the endocrine pancreas. Unlike most other endocrine systems, regulation of the endocrine pancreas does not occur through the hypothalamic–pituitary axis. Instead, carbohydrate and lipid metabolism is regulated by:

- Signals from the gut (gastric distention and food content).
- Signals from the blood stream (circulating glucose levels).
- Intracellular signals (intracellular energy stores).

The overall homeostatic function of carbohydrate (and lipid) metabolism is to deliver energy substrates for use and storage after eating, and to mobilize energy stores during the fasting (postabsorptive) state.

The regulation of carbohydrate and fatty acid metabolism is the key function of insulin and the associated counter-regulatory hormones. The maintenance of adequate levels of circulating glucose is essential for brain tissue and red blood cell intermediary metabolism since these lack insulin-dependent glucose transporters and depend on circulating glucose concentration for energy.

Insulin receptor stimulation activates glucose transporters on the plasma membranes of insulin-sensitive tissues

The intracellular mechanisms of action of insulin are not completely understood. The insulin receptor is a membrane-bound receptor linked to tyrosine kinase (Fig. 11.7). As with other intracellular kinases, phosphorylation of intracellular proteins alters their enzymatic activity, resulting in sequential phosphorylating and

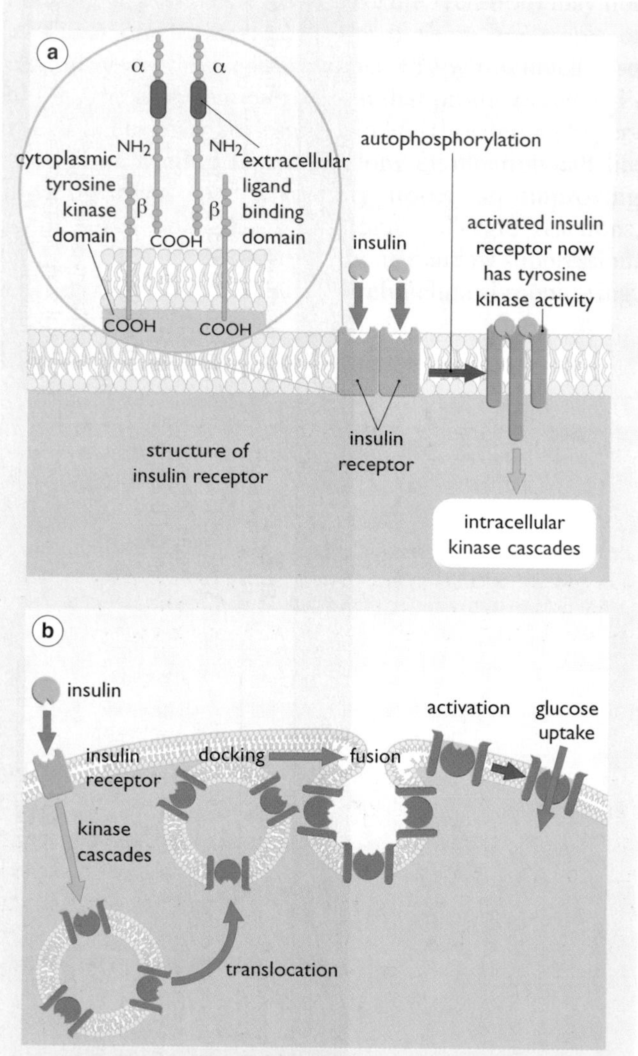

Fig. 11.7 Insulin action. (a) The insulin receptor is a heterodimeric transmembrane receptor consisting of two α and two β subunits. The intracellular portions of the β subunits contain tyrosine kinase activity (see Ch. 3). Insulin receptor stimulation leads to phosphorylation of multiple intracellular signaling molecules. Phosphorylation of tyrosine kinase residues on intracellular kinases leads to activation of serine/threonine kinase cascades. (b) Intracellular kinase cascades cause translocation of glucose transporters from an endosomal compartment to the plasma membrane where they increase glucose uptake.

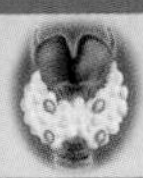

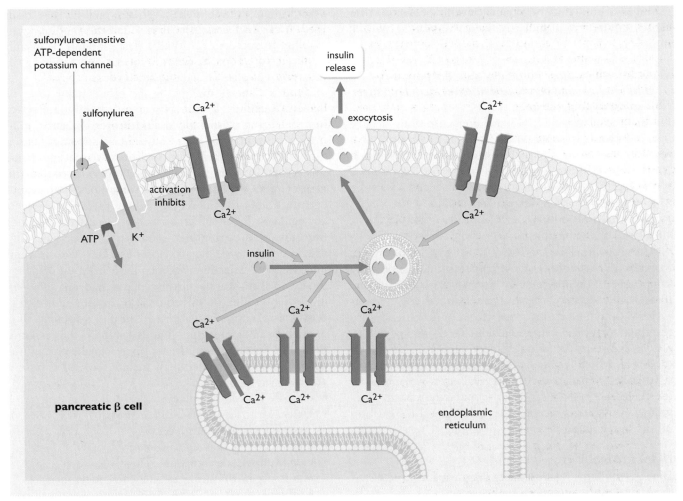

Fig. 11.8 Insulin secretion. Insulin release from pancreatic β cells is stimulated by the release of Ca^{2+} from the endoplasmic compartment by voltage-sensitive channels, and by influx of extracellular Ca^{2+}. The ATP-dependent K^+ channel on the plasma membrane maintains the intracellular resting potential. Inhibition of this K^+ channel by sulfonylurea or meglitinide drugs results in depolarization and activation of Ca^{2+} channels, resulting in enhanced insulin secretion.

dephosphorylating steps in an intracellular signaling cascade. Insulin receptor stimulation leads to translocation of glucose transporters from endosomal storage sites at the plasma membrane, leading to increased glucose uptake. The regulation of glucose transporters on peripheral tissues is essential to fuel delivery, while on pancreatic β cells it is essential to the glucose-sensing mechanisms that regulate insulin release.

Insulin release occurs in response to stimuli such as glucose, amino acids and gut-derived hormones, which reflect increasing fuel availability. These signals lead to depolarization of β cells in the pancreatic islets of Langerhans and Ca^{2+}-mediated exocytosis of insulin into the portal vein (Fig. 11.8). The resting membrane potential of β cells is regulated by ATP-sensitive potassium channels (iK_{ATP}), a target for sulfonylurea drugs. Insulin concentrations are high in the portal circulation, leading to greater effects on the liver, before being diluted in the general circulation. Although insulin has numerous effects on fuel metabolism (Table 11.11), the overall effect is coordinated glucose disposal, glycogen storage, fatty acid storage and protein synthesis. These different metabolic effects of insulin can occur at different concentrations. Inhibition of ketone body formation in

Table 11.11 Effects of insulin on fuel homeostasis

Carbohydrates	Increases glucose transport Increases glycogen synthesis Increases glycolysis Inhibits gluconeogenesis
Fats	Increases lipoprotein lipase activity Increases fat storage in adipocytes Inhibits lipolysis (hormone-sensitive lipase) Increases hepatic lipoprotein synthesis Inhibits fatty acid oxidation
Proteins	Increases protein synthesis Increases amino acid transport

the liver occurs at lower concentrations of insulin than those required to stimulate glucose uptake in skeletal muscle.

Counter-regulatory hormones from the pancreas, pituitary, adrenal cortex and adrenal medulla protect against hypoglycemia

In the fasting stage, as glucose concentrations decline insulin release is suppressed. Multiple neurohormonal responses occur if the plasma glucose falls below a critical concentration. These include:

- Pancreatic glucagon release.
- Sympathetic nervous system activation.
- Hypothalamic–pituitary–adrenal release of GH, cortisol and epinephrine.

These counter-regulatory processes and hormones increase glycogenolysis and inhibit insulin release. The symptoms of hypoglycemia, nervousness, tachycardia, tremor and sweating result from sympathetic nervous system activity. Failure of the counter-regulatory response, as seen in extreme insulin excess and panhypopituitarism, leads to an insufficient supply of glucose to the brain, which results in coma. Somatostatin, which is synthesized in pancreatic δ cells (and elsewhere), inhibits the release of both insulin and counter-regulatory hormones, providing a mechanism to dampen the escalating insulin and counter-regulatory hormone release.

Diabetus mellitus

Diabetes mellitus was originally diagnosed if urine tasted sweet due to the presence of glucose.

Two types of diabetes mellitus share the same features of hyperglycemia and vascular sequelae. They differ in their pathogenesis, and in the ability of residual insulin to suppress ketone formation from fatty acids (Table 11.12).

Type 1 diabetes mellitus (insulin-requiring, ketosis-prone diabetes mellitus) results from autoimmune destruction of pancreatic β cells. The autoimmune attack begins years before insulin secretion falls, and by the time diabetes mellitus is diagnosed the β cells are irreversibly damaged. Since this usually occurs before age 30, the description 'juvenile-onset' diabetes mellitus has been used. A cardinal finding in type 1 diabetes mellitus is an inability to secrete even the modest amounts of insulin required to suppress ketone formation, resulting in recurrent episodes of diabetic ketoacidosis.

Type 2 diabetes mellitus is the other major form of diabetes mellitus. Insulin is secreted, but is ineffective in normalizing plasma glucose. However, the circulating insulin concentrations are sufficient to suppress ketone formation under most circumstances, so patients with this condition do not have repeated episodes of diabetic ketoacidosis. Although insulin is sometimes used, type 2 patients do not usually require insulin therapy to prevent ketoacidosis. β-cell function in type 2 patients declines over time, to the extent that some type 2 patients develop insulin deficiency and may be prone to ketoacidosis when infection or serious illness occurs. Early in type 2 diabetes, the cardinal feature of this disorder is inadequate lowering of blood glucose in response to insulin administration. This phenomenon is termed 'insulin resistance.' It is not due to a receptor mutation that impairs the response to insulin. Insulin resistance and type 2 diabetes mellitus define a syndrome that may include several different processes including:

- Glucose transporter defects.
- Densensitization of insulin receptors.
- Toxic effects of hyperglycemia.
- The metabolic demands of obesity.
- Conditions associated with excessive counter-regulatory hormones (e.g. pheochromocytoma, Cushing's syndrome and acromegaly).
- Conditions associated with a loss of pancreatic function (e.g. surgical removal of pancreatic cancers and pancreatitis).

Type 1 and type 2 diabetes both exhibit hyperglycemia

Insufficient insulin action, whether due to insulin deficiency (type 1) or insulin resistance (type 2), results in hyperglycemia. Although impaired glucose intake by target tissues following food ingestion results in post-

Table 11.12 The main features of insulin-dependent and noninsulin-dependent diabetes mellitus

	IDDM (type 1)	NIDDM (type 2)
Age at onset	<30 years	>30 years
Family history of diabetes mellitus	Uncommon	Common
Body weight	Not obese	Obese
Ketoacidosis	Common	Rare
Insulin treatment requirement	All patients	Some patients
Presence of other autoimmune endocrine deficiencies	Yes (rare)	No
Prevalence in adult population	0.5%	5%
HLA association	Yes	No

IDDM, insulin-dependent diabetes mellitus; NIDDM,noninsulin-dependent diabetes mellitus.

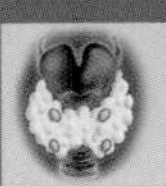

prandial hyperglycemia, deficient insulin-mediated suppression of hepatic gluconeogenesis is the primary cause of diabetic hyperglycemia. Dietary sugar accounts for a small fraction of the hyperglycemic state in most diabetics. Fasting plasma glucose concentrations >7 mmol/L (125 mg/dL) are associated with increased risk of long-term diabetic complications (see below). Symptomatic hyperglycemia (polyuria, polydipsia, unexplained weight loss) usually occurs at higher levels of hyperglycemia. Glucosuria only occurs when the concentration of glucose in the renal tubules exceeds the threshold for maximum absorption (Tm), which occurs at approximately 9 mmol/L (160 mg/dL). For this reason monitoring of urinary glucose is not a sensitive method for monitoring diabetic therapy. Elevated plasma glucose concentrations increase the rate of glycation (nonenzymatic covalent bonding of glucose) of many proteins in the body. Elevated glycated hemoglobin (HbA_{1c}) reflects prolonged hyperglycemia and is a useful test for monitoring glycemic control in diabetes.

Insulin resistance (an inability to respond appropriately to insulin) can occur in the absence of hyperglycemia

Severe insulin resistance leads to impaired glucose regulation and the development of clinical diabetes mellitus, but many patients with hypertension and hypercholesterolemia demonstrate insulin resistance without abnormal glucose regulation. The term 'syndrome X' describes patients with hypertension, hypercholesterolemia and insulin resistance. Such patients are a large fraction of the population at risk of premature arteriosclerosis. The pathogenesis of this syndrome is unknown, but impaired insulin action is associated with increased hepatic very low-density lipoprotein (VLDL) production and lower circulating high-density lipoprotein (HDL) concentrations (see below), which increase the risk of arteriosclerosis.

Both types of diabetes mellitus lead to microvascular and neuronal dysfunction, which result in 'end-organ complications'

Although type 1 and type 2 diabetes mellitus differ in disease etiology, the occurrence and prevalence of ketoacidosis and the role of insulin resistance, they both produce the same pathologic sequelae. So-called 'end-organ complications' include retinal disease, renal failure, peripheral nerve dysfunction, peripheral vascular disease and arteriosclerosis. Relating to the prevalence of obesity in affluent societies, type 2 diabetes mellitus is nine times more common in adults from such societies than type 1. Diabetes is a leading cause of blindness and renal failure, and a major cause of morbidity and mortality, due to arteriosclerosis resulting in cerebrovascular thrombosis, myocardial infarction and amputations of the extremities.

Insulin in the treatment of diabetes mellitus

Different insulin preparations (with different patterns of absorption) are used to match insulin delivery with caloric intake

Before the discovery and use of insulin in the 1930s, type 1 diabetes was lethal in childhood. A variety of insulin preparations provide a 'physiologic' pattern of insulin replacement (Table 11.13). An insulin pump attached to a small subcutaneous needle, delivering a basal rate of insulin and small boluses on demand at mealtimes, is the most successful way of mimicking physiologic insulin release. However, this method does not achieve better glucose control than that in compliant patients using multiple insulin injections. The success of such multiple injection regimens depends upon the availability of insulins with different pharmacokinetic absorption characteristics. The duration of action of different insulins (see below) vary since the hypoglycemic response to each type of insulin varies widely between patients, and requires careful monitoring.

Short-acting insulins (regular, semilente) are used for prompt, meal-related insulin delivery. Most 'regular' insulin is human insulin produced by recombinant DNA technology, although semisynthetic 'regular' insulin, produced from porcine insulin, is also available. 'Regular' insulin consists of an insulin/Zn^{2+} suspension, but has no additives or formulations to delay absorption. Short-acting insulins spontaneously form dimeric or hexameric aggregates to slow absorption. Absorption from the subcutaneous site is slower than pancreatic release and such preparations are injected 30–45 minutes before a meal and exert their action for approximately 6 hours afterwards.

Intermediate- and long-acting insulins are more gradual in the onset and offset of their actions. This is achieved by using a buffer which alters solubility (Lente), or by addition of the cationic protein protamine (neutral

Table 11.13 Different insulin preparations

Insulin preparation	Onset of action	Peak action (h)	Duration of action (h)
'Regular'	Rapid	1–3	5–7
Semilente	Rapid	3–4	10–16
Neutral protamine Hagedorn (NPH)	Intermediate	6–14	18–28
Lente	Intermediate	6–14	18–28
Ultralente	Prolonged	18–24	30–40

protamine Hagedorn or NPH), to 'regular' insulin Zn^{2+} suspensions. Depending on formulation, and species origin (human, pig or beef) of the insulin, intermediate insulins have an onset of action within 2 hours, a peak effect at 10 hours, and are usually inactive after 20 hours. Long-acting insulin (Ultralente) contains Zn^{2+} and an acetate buffer to delay absorption further. It begins to act within 4 hours and lasts up to 36 hours. Insulin glargine is a recently introduced insulin analog which is absorbed over 24 hours without a discernible absorption peak versus time profile. Insulin glargine differs from recombinant human insulin by the replacement of arginine by glycine at amino acid 21, and addition of two arginine residues to the C terminus of the B chain. Unlike Ultralente, insulin glargine starts to act within 1 hour of injection. It may provide adequate basal insulin concentrations in a single daily injection.

Insulin lispro and insulin aspart are genetically engineered recombinant insulin analogs which do not undergo spontaneous dimerization. These monomeric insulins are absorbed more rapidly than 'regular' insulin and have an onset and duration of action shorter than 'regular' insulin. They are therefore given immediately before meals. Due to their short time course of action, monomeric insulin analogs produce less hypoglycemia than 'regular' insulin.

Insulin regimens usually include combinations of short- or rapid-acting insulin with intermediate- or long-acting insulin to provide a maximal effect during hepatic neogenesis in the morning and during daytime meal ingestion, but minimal effects during fasting. Treatment of type 1 diabetes requires a close matching of insulin administration with caloric intake and therefore a combination of regular and intermediate insulin is usually necessary. Some type 2 patients, who have only residual β cell function, need intermediate- or long-acting insulin to improve glycemic control. Insulin administration is governed by the timing and pattern of food intake, but the early morning increase in activity of the hypothalamic–pituitary–adrenal (HPA) hormones such as cortisol and epinephrine may increase blood sugar even without food intake. This 'dawn phenomenon' of the HPA axis and the slow rate of absorption of intermediate insulin allows intermediate insulin to be taken at bedtime with minimal nocturnal hypoglycemia.

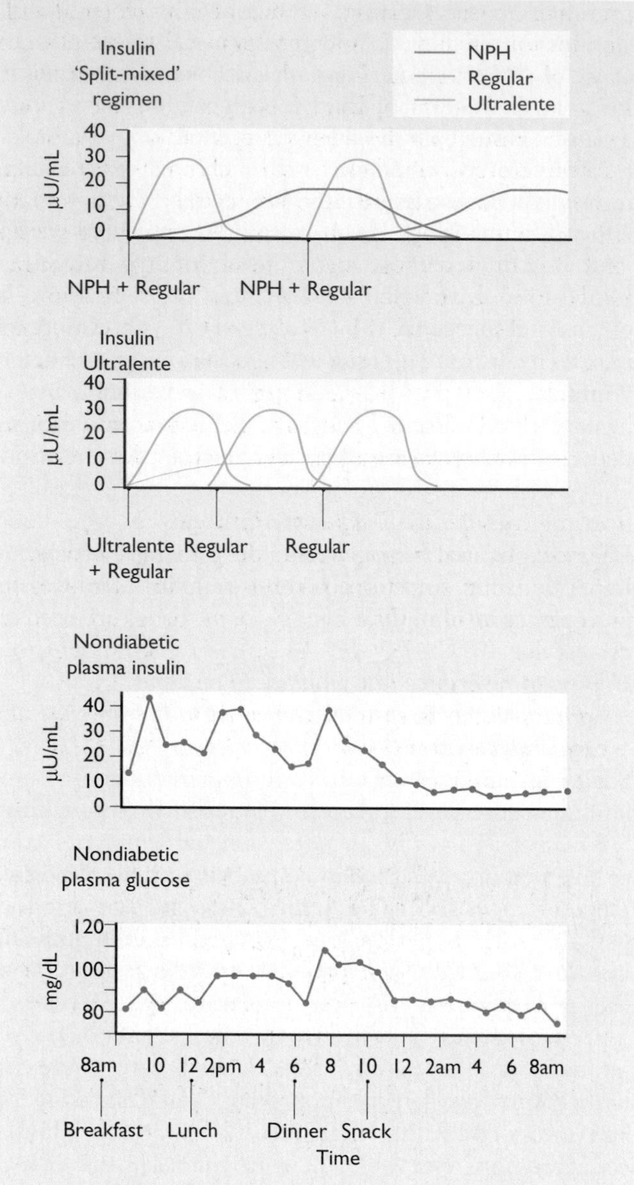

Fig. 11.9 Insulin therapy. Comparison of blood insulin levels following administration of different insulin preparations compared with insulin and glucose levels in nondiabetic controls. Exogenously administered insulin does not mirror the rapid meal-related increases of pancreatic insulin secretion because of delayed absorption from the site of injection. The goal of insulin dosing regimens is to coordinate peaks in insulin delivery with food intake. Systemic insulin levels are higher during insulin therapy of type 1 diabetes mellitus than with endogenous pancreatic regulation. Pancreatic insulin release into the portal venous system may suppress hepatic gluconeogenesis at lower doses than those needed with systemic insulin administration.

The goal of insulin therapy in type 1 diabetes is to mimic physiology

To reproduce the pattern of normal pancreatic function, type 1 diabetics require low levels of insulin from bedtime until early morning, higher levels of insulin from early morning until bedtime, and significant increases in short-acting insulin at the time of meal ingestion (Fig. 11.9). The first two objectives can be achieved by administration of intermediate (NPH, Lente) or long-acting insulin (Ultralente) twice per day, ideally at bedtime and in the morning. The evening dose of long-acting insulin is adjusted to achieve euglycemia before breakfast, without nocturnal hypoglycemia. When fasting morning euglycemia is achieved, then the morning dose of long-acting insulin is adjusted to achieve euglycemia before the evening meal. Insulin glargine permits basal insulin requirements to be met with a single dose of this long-acting insulin analog. Short-acting (regular or

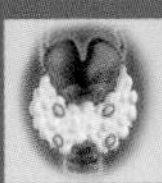

monomeric insulin analogs) should be administered with each meal to achieve 2-hour postprandial blood glucose levels of <160 mg/dL (9 mmol/L). Due to variation in physical activity and caloric intake, the dose of short-acting insulin should be adjusted according to the blood glucose before meals. Difficulty in administering insulin around midday may be accommodated by the use of intermediate-acting insulin (instead of long-acting insulin) in the morning, and adjustment of the size of the midday meal. Blood glucose at bedtime should be between 100 and 140 mg/dL (5.5–7.7 mmol/L) and subjects should check blood glucose at 2 a.m. on several occasions after any change in the insulin regimen.

As this book went to print, inhaled insulin preparations were nearing approval for the treatment of diabetes.

Oral hypoglycemic drugs for diabetes

The goals of oral hypoglycemic drug therapy can be to increase insulin secretion or the sensitivity of tissues to endogenous insulin. Oral hypoglycemic drugs are used to treat patients with diabetes mellitus who do not require insulin to prevent ketoacidosis. These drugs can be categorized according to whether they increase insulin release, increase sensitivity to insulin or block glucose uptake (Table 11.14).

Sulfonylureas and meglitinides enhance β-cell function by blocking ATP-dependent K^+ currents (iK_{ATP}) in pancreatic cells. As a result, they cause depolarization which activates voltage-sensitive Ca^{2+} channels, increasing intracellular Ca^{2+} concentrations, which in turn increases insulin exocytosis.

The antidiabetic actions of sulfonylurea were discovered serendipitously via the observation that sulfonamide antibiotics occasionally produced hypoglycemia. The second-generation sulfonylureas share similar effectiveness and safety profiles, although they differ slightly in dose and frequency of administration (see Table 11.14). The first-generation sulfonylureas (tolbutamide, chlorpropamide, acetohexamide and tolazamide) have lower molar potency but have the same efficacy as the more commonly used second-generation drugs. Second-generation drugs are metabolized in the liver to inactive forms; hence, they have less risk of hypoglycemia in patients with reduced renal function than renally excreted drugs such as chlorpropamide. Although glipizide and glyburide differ in their plasma elimination half-lifes (3 hours versus 10 hours, respectively) both are effective in single daily doses. Plasma drug concentrations do not closely correlate with glucose-lowering. Repaglinide is a recently introduced non-sulfonylurea

Table 11.14 Oral hypoglycemic drugs

	Principal mechanism of action	Typical doses	Effectiveness	Adverse effects
Biguanides	Inhibit hepatic gluconeogenesis		1.5–2% reduction in HbA1c Limited triglyceride lowering Limited LDL lowering No weight gain Reduced cardiac mortality In obese type 2 diabetes mellitus patients	Abdominal bloating, diarrhea Potential metabolic acidosis Contraindicated in renal insufficiency
Metformin	Increases glucose transporters Increases tissue insulin sensitivity	0.5–0.85 g t.i.d. 1 g b.i.d.		
Sulfonylureas	Stimulate insulin release from pancreas		1.5%–2% reduction in HbA1c Limited triglyceride lowering	Hypoglycemia Weight gain
Glyburide		5–10 mg q.d.–b.i.d.		
Glipizide		5–10 mg q.d.–b.i.d.		
Glipizide (extended-release)		5–20 mg q.d.		
Glimepiride		1–8 mg q.d.–b.i.d.		
Repaglinide	Stimulates insulin release from pancreas	0.5–4 mg ac (t.i.d. –q.i.d.)	1.7% reduction in HbA1c	Hypoglycemia
Thiazolidinediones	Increase tissue insulin sensitivity Inhibit hepatic gluconeogenesis		1–1.5% reduction in HbA1c 10–15% HDL increase 10–20% triglyceride reduction	Limited LDL increases Weight gain Worsens congestive heart failure Possible hepatotoxicity
Rosiglitazone		4–8 mg q.d. (or 2–4 mg b.i.d.)		
Pioglitazone		15–30 mg q.d.		
α-glucosidase inhibitors	Inhibit hydrolysis of disaccharides		0.7–1% reduction in HbA1c Limited triglyceride lowering	Abdominal bloating, diarrhea, flatulence Titration of dose q. 2 weeks recommended Hepatotoxicity (rare)
Acarbose	Reduce glucose absorption	25–100 mg b.i.d.–t.i.d. with meals		
Miglitol		25–100 mg t.i.d. with meals		

triglycerides (type IIb and type IV hyperlipidemias), and are particularly effective for familial dysbetalipoproteinemia (type III hyperlipidemia), which results from impaired remnant clearance due to Apo E abnormalities. A genetic deficiency of lipoprotein lipase (type I hyperlipidemia) is characterized by markedly elevated triglycerides, but is not responsive to fibrates. Gemfibrozil reduces the risk of a first myocardial infarction in middle aged men with non-HDL cholesterol concentrations >200 mg/dL (Helsinki Heart Study), and reduces the risk of recurrent myocardial infarction in men with HDL cholesterol concentrations <40 mg/dL (VA-HIT Study). Fibrates are well suited for the treatment of dyslipidemia in diabetic patients because they often demonstrate hypertriglyceridemia and low levels of HDL.

Niacin (nicotinic acid)

Niacin is a vitamin precursor of the nicotine adenine dinucleotides (NAD and NADP). Niacin's effects on lipoprotein metabolism are independent of its role as a precursor for nicotinamide, although niacin has been used to treat hyperlipidemia for many years. Its mechanism of action is poorly understood, but its major effect is to decrease production of VLDLs by reducing the flux of fatty acids from adipose tissue to the liver. Lower VLDL concentrations lead to a reduced exchange of cholesterol with HDL (and therefore higher HDL cholesterol concentrations) as well as reduced delivery of IDL to the liver for LDL formation. Due to these compensatory changes in lipoprotein metabolism, niacin optimizes the therapeutic effect of increasing HDL, while lowering LDL cholesterol and triglycerides. For these reasons, it is useful in the treatment of combined hyperlipidemias.

The adverse effects of niacin include dose-related acute effects such as flushing and pruritus. These are prostaglandin mediated as they are prevented by concurrent aspirin administration. Patients become tolerant to these effects, but not to the therapeutic effect on lipoproteins. Other adverse effects include aggravation of peptic ulcer disease, hyperuricemia, glucose intolerance, and hepatic and skeletal muscle toxicities. These can limit the use of niacin. Niacin is also given as a sustained-release preparation, which is well tolerated. Sustained-release niacin produces a greater LDL reduction compared with immediate-release niacin, although maximal efficacy is similar for the two formulations.

Other hypolipidemic agents

Probucol is a hypolipidemic agent with minimal cholesterol-lowering effects, but may reduce the oxidation of LDL. Oxidized LDL is taken up more avidly by macrophages to produce foam cells and atherosclerotic plaques. However, probucol is not commonly used because it reduces HDL to a greater degree than LDL cholesterol, while its use has been associated with ventricular arrhythmias.

Fish oils contain ω3 fatty acids such as eicosapentaenoic acid, which is an essential fatty acid constituent of cell membranes. Ingestion of fish oils results in decreased VLDL synthesis and improved clearance of remnant particles. These ω3 fatty acids reduce the production of arachidonic acid metabolites, and may thereby reduce platelet aggregation. The usual dose for reduction of hypertriglyceridemia is 5 g b.i.d. Nausea and malodorous eructation are the most common adverse effects. The hypolipidemic effect of this dietary constituent is thought to contribute to the low prevalence of coronary artery disease in some maritime cultures.

Dietary reduction of cholesterol as part of the treatment of hyperlipidemias

Dietary reduction of cholesterol intake and treatment of cholesterol-elevating conditions such as diabetes mellitus, renal disease, cholestatic disorders, hypothyroidism and hypogonadism are recommended before starting drug therapy for hyperlipidemia. Weight loss is associated with the combined health benefits of improved lipoprotein metabolism, reduced blood pressure and improved insulin sensitivity. If lifestyle modification is inadequate, and complicating medical conditions have been appropriately managed, cholesterol-lowering therapy can then be initiated according to the predominantly elevated component, for example:

- Nicotinic acid or fibric acid derivatives for triglycerides.
- Bile acid sequestrants or HMG CoA reductase inhibitors for LDL cholesterol.

Combined therapy with bile acid sequestrants and other agents is safe and usually produces additive cholesterol-lowering effects. Combinations of nicotinic acid, HMG CoA reductase inhibitors and fibric acid derivatives are effective, but may cause either hepatic or skeletal muscle toxicity.

Disorders of glucocorticosteroids and other stress response hormones

The hypothalamic–pituitary–adrenal (HPA) axis releases adrenal hormones such as glucocorticosteroids and epinephrine. These mediate a complex set of physiologic effects best characterized by the term 'general adaptation syndrome.' In the 1940s, Hans Selye coined this term to describe the adrenal response to 'fight or flight' situations. This concept of hormonally regulated adaptation to conditions of acute physiologic stress such as trauma, hypovolemia, systemic infection or environmental exposure provides a general framework for understanding the various actions of glucocorticosteroids and catecholamines (Fig. 11.13).

Under conditions of stress, the hypothalamic hormone, corticotropin-releasing hormone (CRH), causes pituitary ACTH release, resulting in increased production of cortisol in the zona fasciculata of the adrenals. The sympathetic nervous system, activated under similar conditions, releases neuronal norepinephrine and secretes epineph-

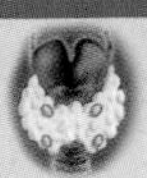

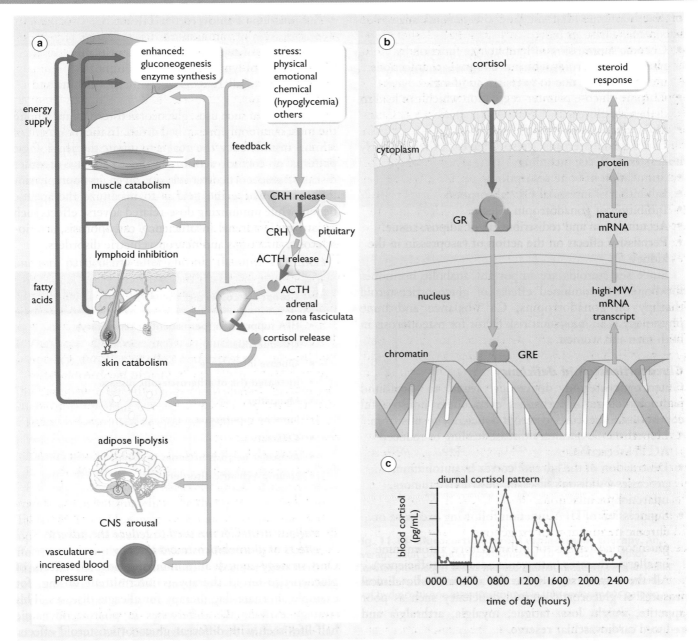

Fig. 11.13 Glucocorticosteroids and adaptation to stress. (a) A variety of sensorineural inputs regulate the pattern of corticotropin-releasing hormone (CRH) release in the hypothalamus. CRH releases adrenocorticotropic hormone (ACTH). ACTH leads to cortisol production in the adrenal zona fasciculata. Cortisol circulates to peripheral tissues where it binds cytosolic glucocorticosteroid receptors (GR) (b). After hormone binding, these receptors are translocated to the nucleus where they lead to transcription of glucocorticosteroid-responsive genes. The products of these genes lead to diverse target tissue effects such as enhanced gluconeogenesis, lipolysis, tissue catabolism, inhibition of lymphocyte function, pressor effects in the vasculature and CNS behavioral effects. (c) The diurnal cortisol pattern reflects peak activity of the hypothalamic–pituitary–adrenal axis in the early morning.

rine from the adrenal medulla. Among its various effects, cortisol enhances epinephrine synthesis and sensitizes the peripheral tissues to the effects of catecholamines. The overall effect of glucocorticosteroid and catecholamine action is to prepare the body for short periods of high physical or stressful activity. Thus, the various effects of glucocorticosteroids, i.e. increasing gluconeogenesis and lipolysis, mobilizing fuel substrates from muscle, increasing CNS arousal, increasing blood pressure, suppressing inflammation and delaying wound healing, seem to serve a common purpose. The sympathetic nervous system reinforces these effects by increasing blood pressure, cardiac output, blood glucose, lipolysis, CNS arousal, skeletal muscle blood flow and platelet coagulability.

The sustained increase of 'stress' hormones can lead to widespread physiologic disturbances (glucocorticoid excess)

While short-term activation of 'stress' hormones can be useful, major disorders can result from prolonged excess

In cases of refractory or malignant pheochromocytoma, the catecholamine biosynthesis inhibitor α-methyltyrosine may be used. Methyltyrosine is a competitive inhibitor of tyrosine hydroxylase, the rate-limiting step in catecholamine synthesis. Methyltyrosine has a relatively short plasma elimination half-life (4–7 hours) and is titrated from a starting dose of 250 mg to 1 g p.o. q.i.d. Adverse effects such as sedation, fatigue and extrapyramidal effects (rigidity, tremor) are frequent.

Mineralocorticosteroids, vasopressin and disorders of circulatory volume

The hypothalamus, pituitary and the adrenal glands are also involved in the hormonal regulation of extracellular fluid volume (Fig. 11.17). The pituitary and adrenal glands regulate circulatory volume by two interdependent mechanisms which regulate: (1) Na^+ balance (adrenal mineralocorticosteroids), and (2) free water balance (pituitary vasopressin).

Since Na^+ and its accompanying anions (Cl^- and HCO_3^-) are the main osmotic constituents of extracellular fluid, regulation of Na^+ loss through the kidney, gut and skin (sweat glands) is critical in determining extracellular fluid volume. Extracellular fluid is partitioned between the vascular and interstitial compartments, and therefore extracellular volume is a major determinant of circulatory blood volume and blood pressure homeostasis. The osmotic content of extracellular water drives free water from the large intracellular reservoir to the extracellular fluid compartments.

Sodium retention in the distal renal tubule is modulated by aldosterone acting on the genes responsible for the synthesis of Na^+/K^+ ATPase and the Na^+/H^+ exchanger

Na^+ levels are regulated in the kidney through the mineralocorticosteroid hormone aldosterone, angiotensin II, the sympathetic nervous system, atrial natriuretic peptides and intrinsic renal mechanisms.

The renal sensing mechanism for circulatory volume as well as its effector limb, the renin–angiotensin–aldosterone (RAA) axis, is also discussed in other chapters. Afferent inputs such as renal afferent arteriole baroreceptors, the renal tubular Na^+ sensor and volume

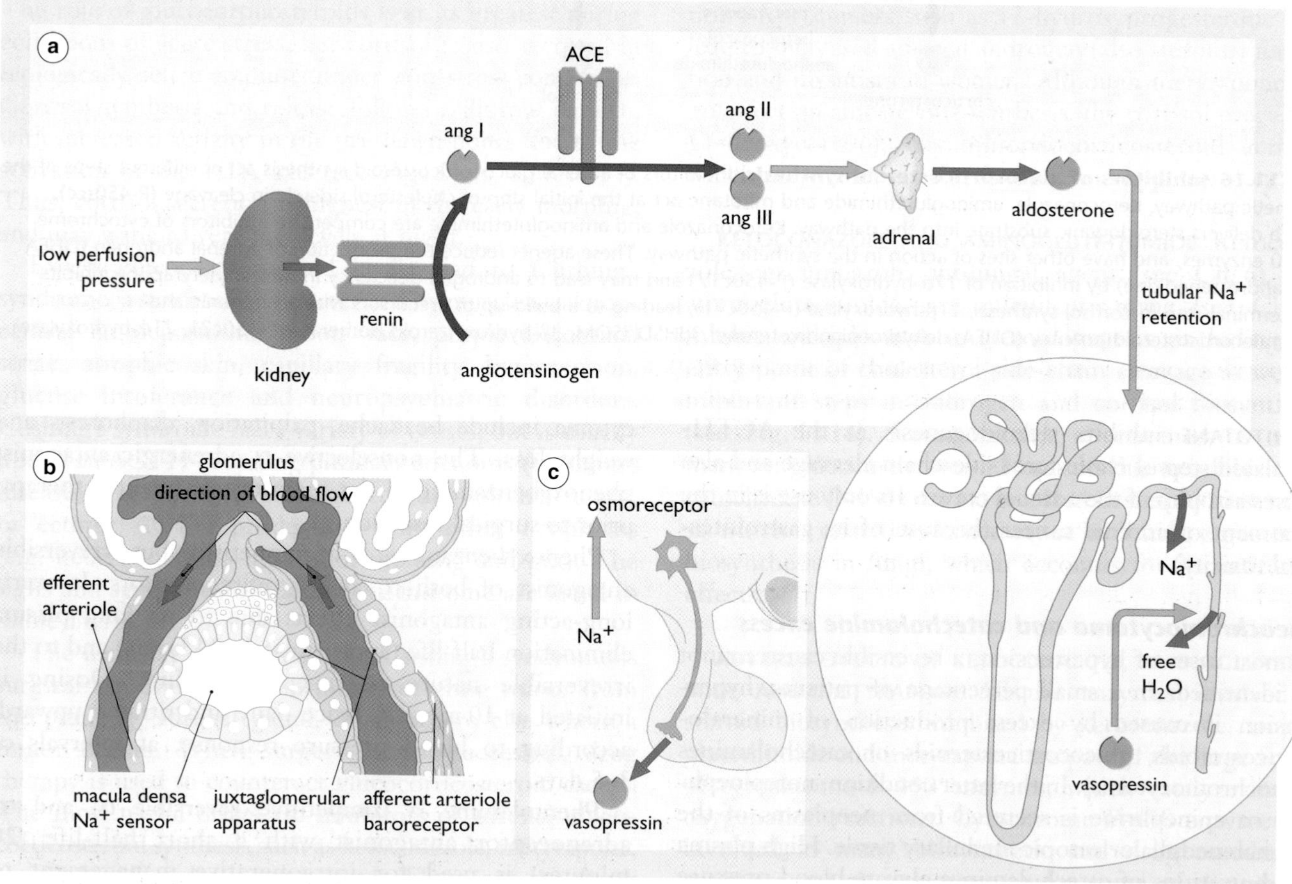

Fig. 11.17 Hormonal regulation of circulatory volume. Central cardiovascular reflexes, renal baroreceptors and the distal tubular Na^+ sensor provide physiologic input about circulatory volume (a, b). In response to decreased renal perfusion, the juxtaglomerular cells of the afferent glomerular arteriole release renin. Renin converts circulating angiotensinogen and angiotensin (ang) I, which is then converted to ang II by the converting enzyme (ACE) in the vascular endothelium (a). Ang II and ang III stimulate aldosterone production, which leads to Na^+ reabsorption in the distal convoluted tubule. Na^+ reabsorption increases the osmolality of extracellular fluids. This stimulates the hypothalamic osmoreceptor to release vasopressin from the posterior pituitary. Vasopressin leads to enhanced free water reabsorption in the collecting duct, which expands extracellular volume and reduces plasma osmolality (c).

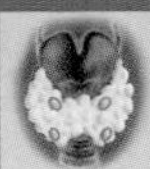

receptors in the central veins stimulate renin release in response to decreased blood volume or reduced renal perfusion. The actions of renin on precursors in the blood (angiotensinogen) leads to the synthesis of the peptide angiotensin I, which is converted to angiotensin II and angiotensin III in peripheral tissues, principally the lung. Angiotensin II and III act on the adrenal zona glomerulosa to increase the synthesis of aldosterone (Fig. 11.18). The synthetic pathways for aldosterone are similar to those for cortisol synthesis except for the two-step formation of the 18-aldehyde group by the angiotensin II-sensitive corticosterone methyloxidase I and II enzymes present only in the zona glomerulosa of the adrenal glands (see Fig. 11.18).

Like other steroid hormones, aldosterone induces genes in tissues expressing the mineralocorticosteroid receptor (i.e. kidney, brain, vasculature). Although the mineralocorticosteroid receptor can bind both aldosterone and cortisol, it is protected from glucocorticosteroid stimulation as a result of a unique enzyme, 11β-hydroxysteroid dehydrogenase. This enzyme, which is expressed in mineralocorticosteroid target tissues, selectively inactivates any cortisol in the proximity of mineralocorticosteroid receptors.

The classic target tissue for mineralocorticosteroids is the renal distal convoluted tubule epithelial cell where mineralocorticosteroid stimulation activates genes for Na^+/K^+ ATPase, ion channels and mitochondrial enzymes critical to Na^+ recovery and K^+ or H^+ excretion. Outside the kidney, mineralocorticosteroids conserve Na^+ in the gastrointestinal tract and sweat glands, and increase blood pressure by effects on the brain and the vasculature. Mineralocorticoid receptors also influence collagen synthesis by fibroblasts, and may thereby play an important role in remodeling of vascular tissues damaged by ischemia or hemodynamic stress. Aldosterone secretion is stimulated by high serum K^+. This stimulation is the major mechanism in the body for protection against life-threatening hyperkalemia. Excess mineralocorticosteroid action leads to a renal loss of K^+ and H^+ (i.e. hypokalemia and alkalosis) and increased extracellular fluid volume, while a lack of mineralocorticosteroid leads to hyperkalemia and volume depletion.

Free water balance is coupled to Na^+ balance via hypothalamic osmoreceptor stimulation and release of vasopressin from the posterior pituitary

While the RAA system and the sympathetic nervous system regulate the Na^+ content of extracellular water, such control extends to extracellular volume only if the free water balance is also regulated so as to maintain osmotic equilibrium. Marked Na^+ retention by aldosterone leads to both an increased Na^+ content and increased osmolality in extracellular water. As a result, water shifts from the intracellular to the extracellular space, and a hyperosmotic stimulus acts on osmoreceptor cells in the hypothalamus. The osmotic sensing mechanism in the

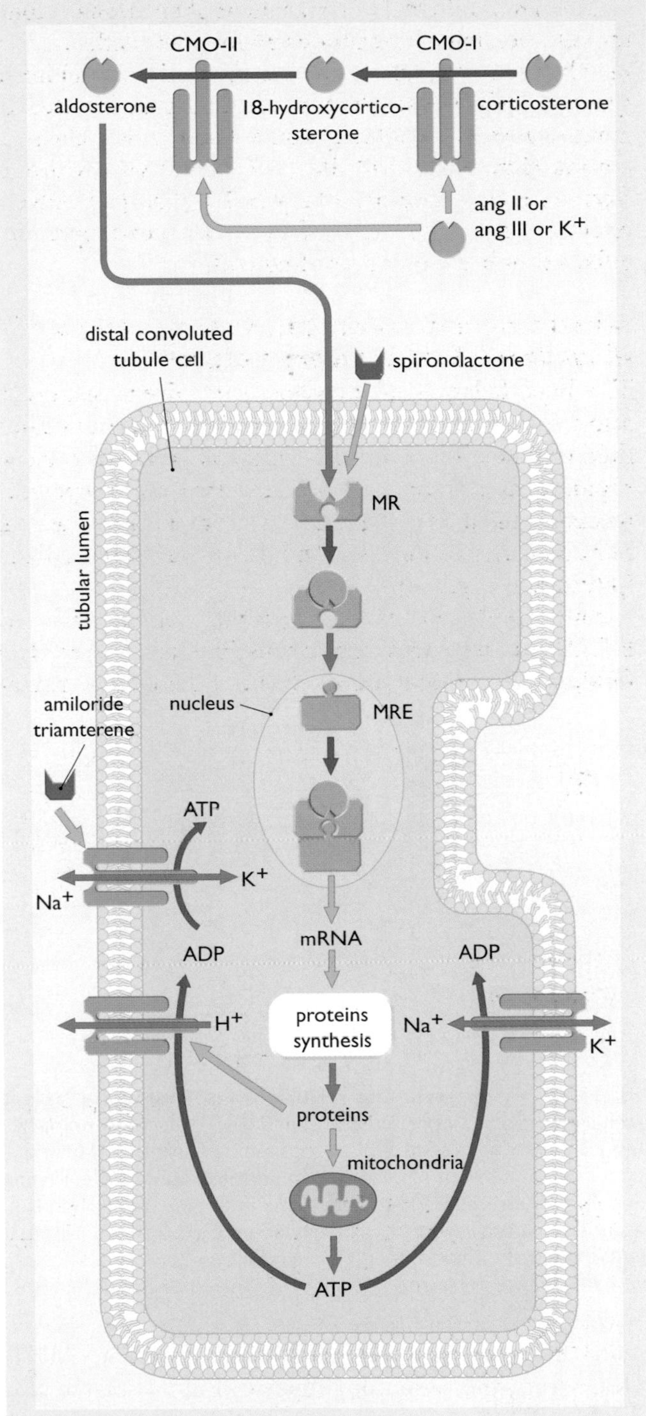

Fig. 11.18 Mineralocorticosteroids and regulation of Na^+ balance. Angiotensins (ang II and III) regulate the corticosterone methyloxidase (CMO) I and II enzymes, which catalyze the hydroxylation and aldehyde formation at the 18-C of corticosterone. Circulating aldosterone binds to cytosolic mineralocorticosteroid receptors (MR), which then translocate to the nucleus to regulate the expression of genes containing a mineralocorticosteroid response element (MRE). Renal tubular epithelial cells express Na^+/K^+ ATPase, the luminal Na^+ permease, luminal proton pumps and mitochondrial enzymes necessary for the production of ATP. The net effect of aldosterone stimulation in the distal convoluted tubule is to reabsorb Na^+ while excreting K^+ and H^+. Spironolactone is a competitive antagonist at mineralocorticosteroid receptors, while diuretics such as amiloride and triamterene functionally antagonize Na^+/K^+ ATPase.

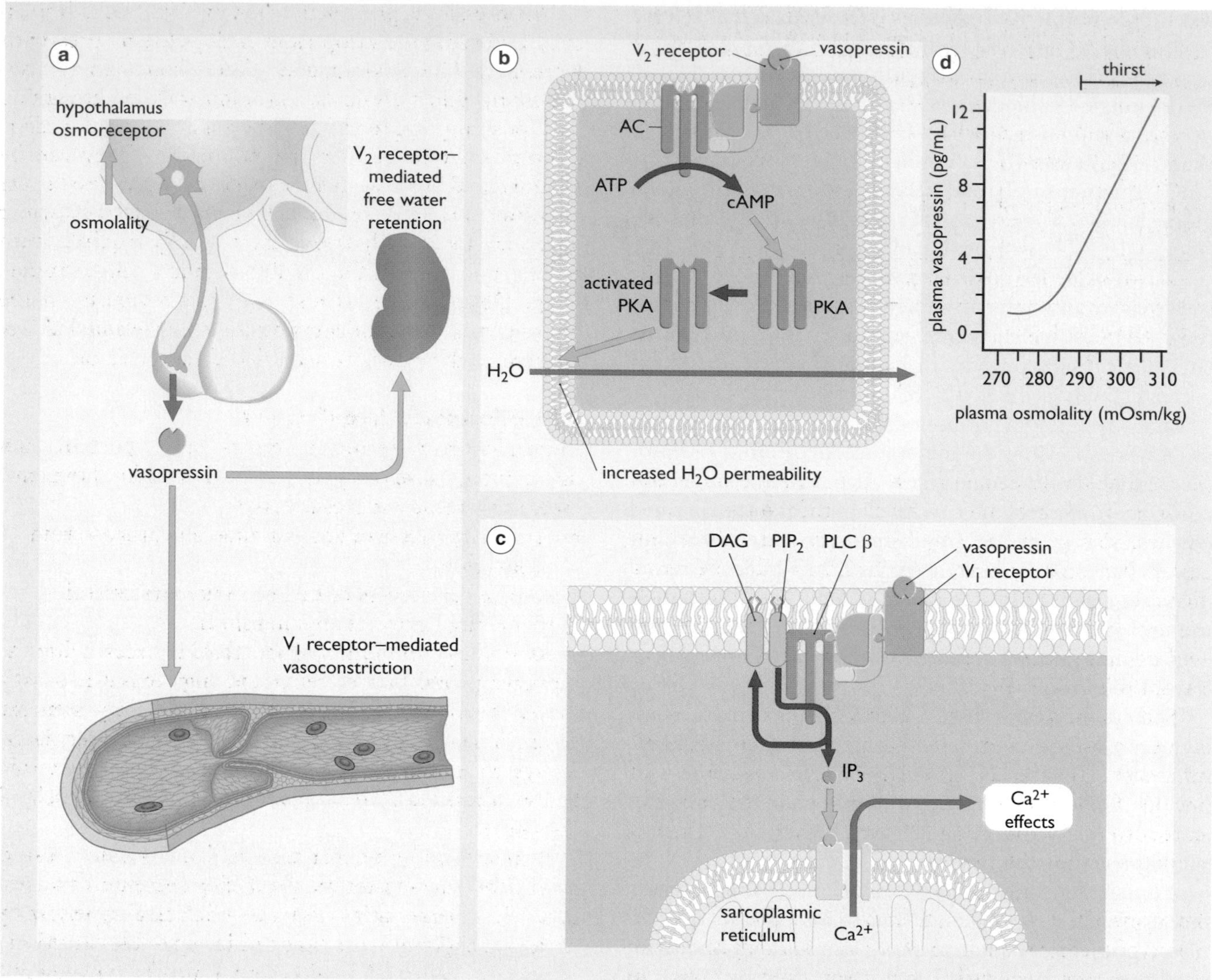

Fig. 11.19 Vasopressin and regulation of free water balance. Osmotic stimulation leads to vasopressin release from the posterior pituitary (a), and vasopressin then stimulates V_2 receptors on distal tubular epithelial cells. V_2 receptors are G protein-coupled receptors that stimulate adenylyl cyclase (AC) to increase intracellular cAMP and activate protein kinase A (PKA). This leads to enhanced permeability of the tubular epithelium (b). Increase in permeability of the collecting duct results in free water movement into the hypertonic renal medullary interstitium. PKA control of a water pore is shown in Fig. 12.11. Vasopressin also acts on other tissues: in the vasculature, via V_1 receptors that are linked to a phospholipase C (PLC β) signaling pathway. Release of inositol-1,4,5-triphosphate (IP_3) and diacylglycerol (DAG) from phosphoinositol (PIP_2) increases intracellular Ca^{2+} and potentiates vasopressor responses (c). As plasma osmolality increases with an increase in plasma vasopressin levels, so thirst mechanisms are activated (d).

brain causes vasopressin (antidiuretic hormone, ADH) release from the posterior pituitary (Fig. 11.19, see also Fig. 11.17C).

Vasopressin is a 9-amino acid peptide hormone. Circulating vasopressin stimulates V_2 GPCR receptors, which increase the permeability of the renal collecting tubules by a cAMP-mediated mechanism. This allows water in the tubule to move into the extracellular space of the renal interstitium. As a result, free water returns to the circulatory compartment, and then provides negative feedback to the osmoreceptors in the brain. Thirst is also activated and suppressed by similar circumstances. In addition to free water regulation, vasopressin stimulates V_1 receptors on the vasculature to cause vasoconstriction via a Ca^{2+}-dependent intracellular signaling pathway.

Vasopressin release is suppressed by reduced osmolality, resulting in increased free water losses in response to excess fluid intake. If there is a severe reduction in blood pressure (for example, in shock), vasopressin is released regardless of osmolality, and circulatory blood volume is maintained at the expense of osmolality.

Mineralocorticosteroid deficiency

Mineralocorticosteroid deficiency is usually due to destruction of the adrenal cortices (Addison's disease), associated with the expected symptoms of mineralocorticosteroid deficiency (hyperkalemia, acidosis, hypovolemia), as well as symptoms of glucocorticosteroid deficiency (anorexia, weakness, weight loss). The characteristics of mineralocorticosteroid deficiency are reduced

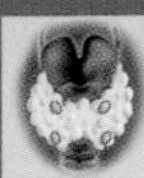

Table 11.19 Causes of diabetes insipidus

Neurogenic (vasopressin deficiency)
Hypothalamic and pituitary tumors
Lymphocytic hypophysitis
Sarcoidosis
Infections (tuberculosis, syphilis)
Histiocytosis X
Nephrogenic (renal vasopressin resistance)
Chronic renal disease
Hypokalemia
Drugs (lithium, demeclocycline, anesthetics)

extracellular volume and resulting postural hypotension, poor skin turgor and reduced urine output. Since intracellular water passively follows its osmotic gradient, serum Na^+ concentrations may be normal despite reductions in total body Na^+. Mineralocorticosteroid deficiency may also result from secondary deficiency of renin and/or angiotensin release in chronic renal disease (hyporeninemic hypoaldosteronism).

Sodium supplements and mineralocorticosteroid replacement are used to treat mineralocorticosteroid deficiency whatever the cause. Synthetic mineralocorticosteroids include 9α-fludrocortisone, which is a potent mineralocorticosteroid agonist with minimal glucocorticosteroid activity (see Fig. 11.18b).

Vasopressin deficiency (diabetes insipidus)

Some of the consequences of vasopressin deficiency, and the receptors responsible for vasopressin actions, are described in Chapter 12.

A deficiency of action of vasopressin results from either impaired release or impaired action on the kidney:

- Impaired vasopressin release is usually due to destructive lesions (neoplasms, granulomatous inflammation or trauma) of the posterior pituitary.
- An impaired renal response to vasopressin is caused by renal disease and certain drugs (Table 11.19).

Vasopressin deficiency is diagnosed by an inability to concentrate urine when the extracellular fluid osmolality increases (hypernatremia). In contrast to the normal serum Na^+ concentration found with mineralocorticosteroid deficiency, serum Na^+ concentration is increased in free-water deficiency states.

Treatment of diabetes insipidus requires differentiation between pituitary and renal causes

Nephrogenic diabetes insipidus is treated by removal of any causative drugs and treatment of the intrinsic renal disease.

Pituitary disease leading to vasopressin deficiency is not usually reversed by treatment of the underlying tumor or inflammation.

Vasopressin replacement therapy involves administration of synthetic vasopressin analogs (desmopressin or lypressin). These compounds differ from native vasopressin by either a lysine substitution at the eighth amino acid position (lypressin) or deamination of the first-position cysteine residue (desmopressin). They can be administered by nasal spray (currently the preferred route of administration) or subcutaneous or intramuscular injection. Twice-daily treatment is usually required, with at least one dose in the evening to allow uninterrupted sleep. Desmopressin is also used intravenously in the treatment of hemophilia owing to its unexplained ability to increase the activity of von Willebrand's factor.

Mineralocorticosteroid excess

Mineralocorticosteroid excess is an important, but uncommon, cause of hypertension. Like other hormonal excess syndromes, it is caused by:

- A primary excess of adrenal mineralocorticosteroid production.
- A secondary excess of the mineralocorticosteroid-regulating hormone angiotensin II.

Secondary mineralocorticosteroid excess due to excessive production of renin and angiotensin is usually caused by renal diseases such as renal artery stenosis, which impair the kidney's ability to respond appropriately to systemic arterial pressure. Mineralocorticosteroid excess is mild and the pressor effects of angiotensin II dominate.

Primary mineralocorticosteroidism usually results from either an aldosterone-producing adenoma or angiotensin II hypersensitivity leading to bilateral hypertrophy of the zona glomerulosa (idiopathic hyperaldosteronism). Surgical resection of an aldosterone-producing adenoma often reverses the hypertension, but bilateral adrenalectomy will not correct the hypertension in idiopathic hyperaldosteronism.

Mineralocorticosteroid excess increases extracellular Na^+

As a result of the increased extracellular Na^+ and indirect stimulation of vasopressin release produced by mineralocorticosteroid excess, water moves from the intracellular space and extracellular fluid volume increases. As circulatory volume and renal perfusion increase a pressure–natriuresis response occurs in the kidney and Na^+ excretion increases. The effects of mineralocorticosteroid-related Na^+ retention and pressure–natriuresis reach equilibrium at a modest level of volume expansion, but do not progress to overt volume excess (edema). Serum Na^+ concentrations remain normal, but K^+ is progressively lost, leading to hypokalemia.

Diseases that reduce renal perfusion by reducing circulatory volume as a result of hypoalbuminemia or reduced cardiac output lead to progressive Na^+ and volume retention, which is not corrected by the pressure–natriuresis response. This accounts for the edema seen in conditions such as congestive heart failure, cirrhosis and the nephrotic syndrome. Although mineralocorticosteroid levels are high in such conditions, they are elevated by an appropriate physiologic response to reduced renal perfusion.

The major therapy for an aldosterone-producing adenoma is surgery, but many cases of mineralocorticosteroid excess require medical therapy.

Spironolactone (see Ch. 12 for full details) is a steroidal mineralocorticosteroid and androgen receptor antagonist. As an antagonist of mineralocorticoid receptors in the distal tubule and collecting duct, its potassium-sparing diuretic effect is useful in states of secondary mineralocorticoid excess such as congestive heart failure and hepatic cirrhosis. Low doses of spironolactone in patients with congestive heart failure demonstrate greater mortality reduction than would be expected on the basis of its diuretic effect. This observation suggests mineralocorticoid effects on tissues other than the kidney in the regulation of the cardiovascular system. Spironolactone is metabolized to at least two active metabolites that have long plasma half-lifes. As an androgen receptor antagonist, spironolactone can cause gynecomastia and hypogonadism in some males. It is also used for the treatment of hirsutism in women. In contrast to other androgen receptor antagonists that interrupt pituitary feedback and result in compensatory increases of testosterone, spironolactone also reduces androgen synthesis, which may also contribute to the androgen-reducing effect of spironolactone.

Diuretics (see Ch. 12) are a drug class that functionally antagonize the effects of mineralocorticosteroid on renal tubules and are commonly used to treat mineralocorticosteroidism. The potassium-sparing diuretics amiloride and triamterene reduce tubular Na^+ reabsorption but do not interact with androgen receptors to cause hypogonadal symptoms in male patients. However, they may cause hyperkalemia and their use requires close monitoring.

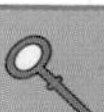

Clinical and laboratory diagnosis of volume disorders

- Clinical findings of hypervolemia (edema) reflect Na^+ excess, while signs of hypovolemia (orthostatic hypotensions, dehydration, oliguria) reflect Na^+ deficiency
- The laboratory finding of hypernatremia reflects free water deficiency, while hyponatremia usually reflects free water excess

Vasopressin excess

Vasopressin excess is a common cause of hyponatremia. Vasopressin excess has numerous causes, including vasopressin-secreting tumors, adverse effect of drugs, pulmonary disease and neurologic disease. Through poorly understood mechanisms, these conditions can lead to release of vasopressin which is not inhibited by low serum osmolality, a condition termed 'syndrome of inappropriate ADH secretion.' Excess vasopressin secretion leads to renal free water retention. Since Na^+ regulation is not similarly affected, the excess water retention leads to a dilutional hyponatremia. Most of the excess free water diffuses into the intracellular space, and therefore increases in circulatory volume (hypertension) and extracellular water (edema) do not occur. However, the mild expansion of extracellular water is sufficient to increase renal perfusion and lead to increased tubular Na^+ excretion. Increased Na^+ excretion is an inappropriate response to hyponatremia, but is an appropriate physiologic response to increased circulatory volume.

Treatment of elevated vasopressin release is usually directed toward correcting its underlying cause. In some cases, vasopressin secretion by tumors or neurologic disease requires medical therapy, including restriction of free water intake. Antibiotic tetracyclines such as demeclocycline antagonize the action of vasopressin on the kidney, but can cause renal toxicity. Paradoxically, diuretics improve the hyponatremia, probably by reducing the renal medullary osmotic gradient for free water reabsorption.

DRUGS AFFECTING THE ENDOCRINE CONTROL OF THE REPRODUCTIVE SYSTEM

The following section concentrates on the endocrine control of the reproductive tract. The genitourinary aspects of this system are covered in greater detail in Chapter 17. Unlike other endocrine systems, which regulate important physiologic functions on a short-term basis, the hypothalamic–pituitary–gonadal (HPG) axis regulates the differential expression of secondary sexual characteristics that take place over a lifetime. Functions such as sustaining spermatogenesis, follicular development and the menstrual cycle require short-term regulation, while others such as puberty and menopause take place over long periods. Hypothalamic gonadotropin hormone-releasing hormone (GnRH) and pituitary gonadotropin release are coordinated by complex neuroendocrine mechanisms. The major regulator of sex steroid production is luteinizing hormone (LH), while that for gamete development is follicle-stimulating hormone (FSH). These hormones are secreted in an episodic or 'spiking' pattern with lower basal levels during much of the day. Androgens and estrogens exert feedback inhibition on gonadotropin secretion, but these effects vary during the menstrual cycle.

Androgens are produced in the gonads and adrenals, while estrogens are produced from androgen precursors in the gonads and adipose tissue

LH and FSH stimulate gonadal steroidogenesis and conversion of adrenal androgens to testosterone and estrogens, as shown in Figure 11.20. The syntheses of

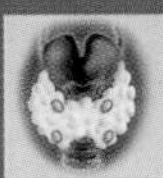

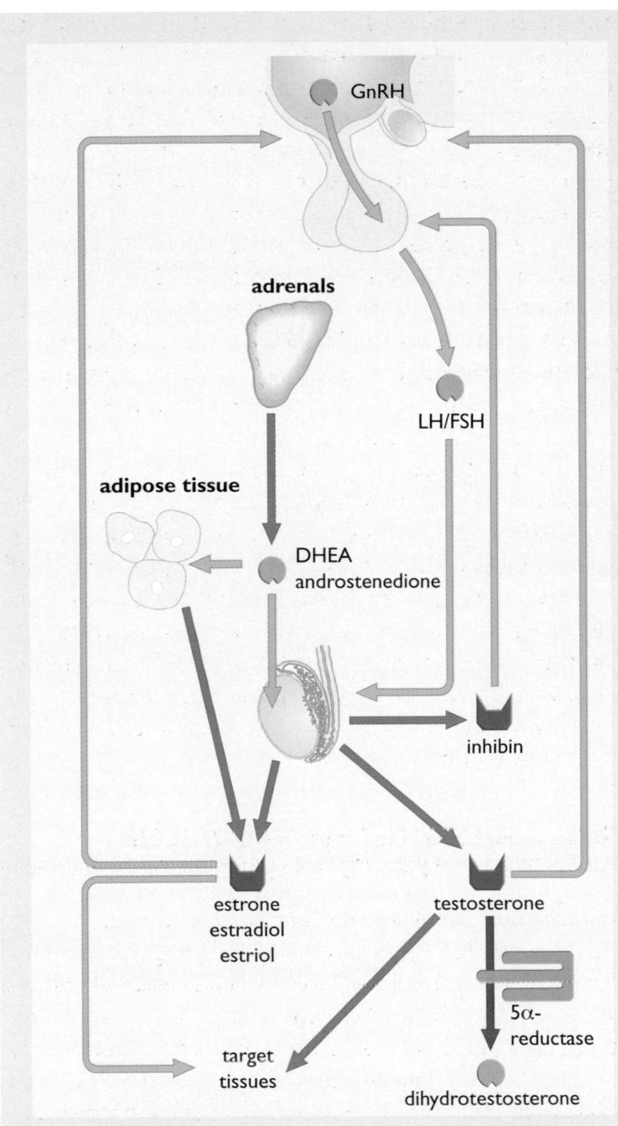

Fig. 11.20 Regulation of sex steroids. Hypothalamic gonadotropin-releasing hormone (GnRH) stimulates the release of luteinizing hormone (LH) and follicle-stimulating hormone (FSH) from the gonadotrophs of the anterior pituitary. LH and FSH stimulate sex steroid production in the gonads. Adrenal androgens are further metabolized to more potent androgens in the gonads. The aromatase enzyme in both the gonads and adipose tissue converts androgens to estrogens. In certain target tissues, the enzyme 5α-reductase converts testosterone to the more potent androgen dihydrotestosterone. In postpubertal males, sex steroid production is constant. In females, gonadotropins and sex steroids are released in a complex pattern during the menstrual cycle (see Fig. 11.24) (ACTH, adrenocorticotropic hormone; DHEA, dehydroepiandrosterone).

estrogens and androgens share biosynthetic steps with other adrenocortical steroids, but glucocorticosteroids and mineralocorticosteroids are not synthesized in gonadal tissues as such tissues lack the appropriate enzymes. Under normal conditions, most sex steroids are produced in the gonads. With adrenal disease, however, production of large quantities of the steroid dehydroepiandrosterone in the zona reticularis can lead to the production of substantial amounts of sex steroids. Dehydroepiandrosterone (DHEA) has only slight androgenic activity but is readily converted to other sex steroids in the gonads, leading to the production of potent androgens. DHEA, when administered orally, is extensively conjugated by the liver, and produces small increases in concentrations of active androgens. Estrogens are also produced as a result of aromatase activity in the gonads and adipocytes. The aromatase enzyme converts androgens to estrogens and is expressed in adipose tissue where it is responsible for most postmenopausal estrogen production and higher estrogen levels in obese men and women.

Physiology of the female reproductive tract

The ovary provides the gametes for fertilization and synthesizes hormones for reproductive tissues and to maintain the secondary female sex characteristics

The ovary consists of spherical follicles embedded in a stroma, surrounded by a membrane, the tunica albuginea (Fig. 11.21). Each follicle contains a gamete (oocyte, ovum, egg). There are originally about 7 million ova, but a large proportion die before birth and during childhood, leaving some 400 000 at puberty, of these about 0.1% (i.e. 400) will ovulate. The most important hormones from the ovary are the sex steroids estrogen (mainly estradiol, but also estrone and estriol) and progesterone. Their production is controlled by the HPA (Fig. 11.22).

The menstrual cycle, the period between two ovulations, lasts 24–32 days

Day 1 of menstruation begins with shedding of the uterine endometrium, which takes 3–5 days. This is followed by the follicular or proliferative phase of the cycle until day 14 (or midcycle) when ovulation occurs (Fig. 11.23). In the follicular phase, the developing follicles produce estradiol, which causes the uterine endometrium to proliferate. If the ovum is not fertilized, there is a luteal or secretory phase lasting 14 days until the endometrium is shed at menstruation. During the luteal phase, the ruptured follicle becomes a corpus luteum, which produces progesterone and causes the endometrium to become secretory.

Luteinizing hormone (LH) increases androgen and progesterone production, while follicle-stimulating hormone (FSH) increases estrogen production from androgens

The production of estrogen and progesterone is controlled by the HPA (see Fig. 11.22):

- LH increases production of androstenedione and testosterone via receptors on the follicular thecal wall.
- FSH induces aromatization of the androgens to estrogens via receptors on granulosa cells.

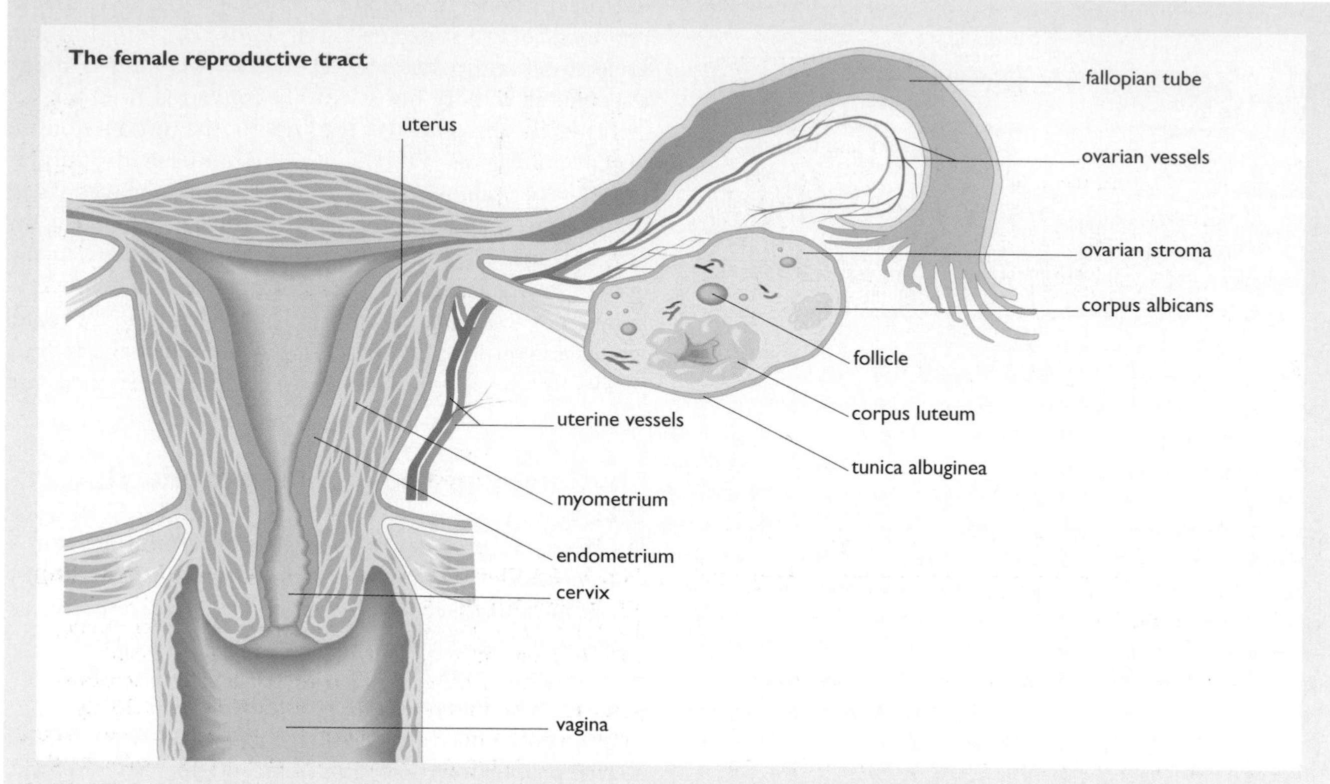

Fig. 11.21 Structure of the female reproductive tract. This consists of two ovaries, each surrounded by a fallopian tube that is approximately 10 cm long and joins a short muscular organ, the uterus. The lower end of the uterus narrows to form the cervix, which is a muscular structure containing many secretory glands and protruding into the vagina. The cervix produces mucus to act as a barrier to infection between the vagina and uterus. The vagina is a thick-walled muscular tube lined by stratified nonkeratinized squamous epithelium. The outer layers of epithelium are constantly shed and these cells form the bulk of the cells seen in vaginal smears, which are taken to determine whether the vaginal mucosa is atrophic or being stimulated by estrogen, and to reveal the presence of infection or cancers.

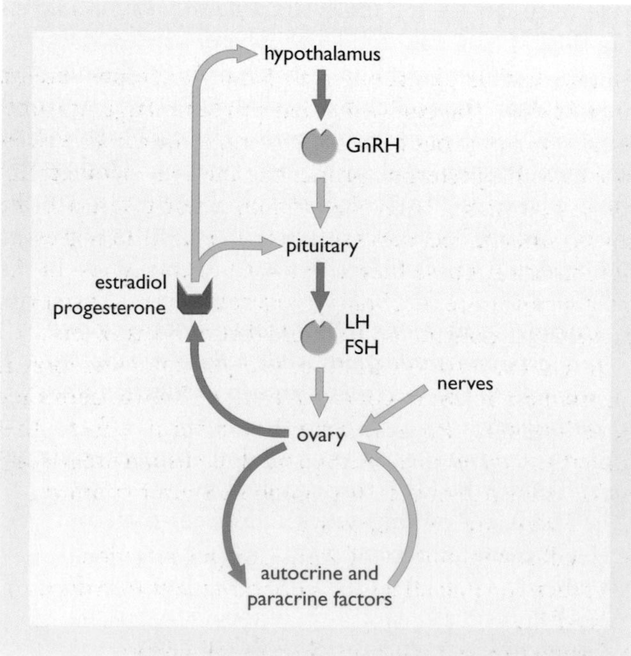

Fig. 11.22 The hypothalamic–pituitary–ovarian (HPA) axis. Endocrine control of ovarian function is exerted by hormones, the most important being estrogen and progesterone. Their production is controlled by the HPA. Neurons within the preoptic area of the hypothalamus secrete pulses of a decapeptide called gonadotropin-releasing hormone (GnRH), which enters the hypophysial portal system and reaches the pituitary. It acts on specific receptors on the gonadotropin-secreting pituitary cells, and stimulates the pulsatile release of both follicle-stimulating hormone (FSH) and luteinizing hormone (LH). These two gonadotropins then act on specific receptors in the ovary and stimulate the production of steroid and peptide hormones and ovulation.

- In the late follicular phase, some granulosa cells differentiate so that they express LH receptors and respond to LH by secreting progesterone. This is the first step in the conversion of the granulosa cells to luteal cells. Only the follicle possessing this second set of receptors will respond to the LH surge and ovulate.

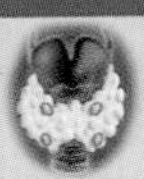

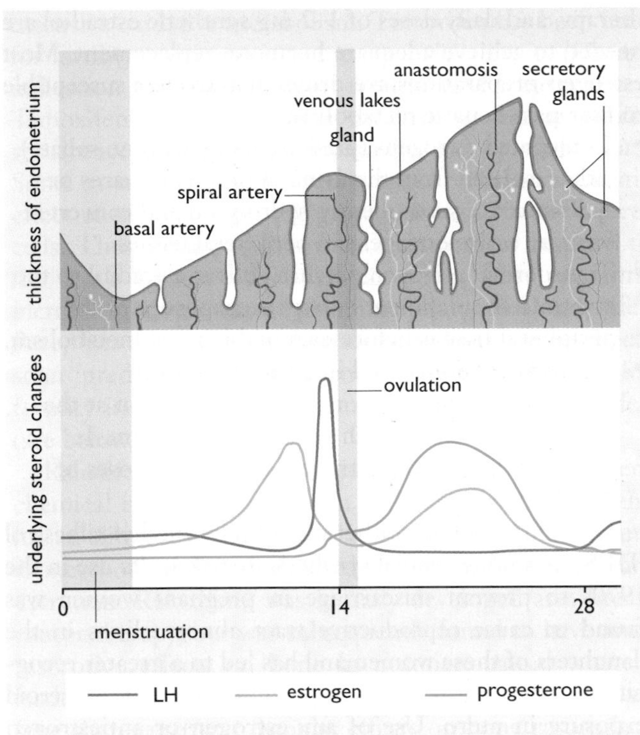

Fig. 11.23 Changes in human endometrium during the human menstrual cycle. Underlying steroid changes are indicated (LH, luteinizing hormone).

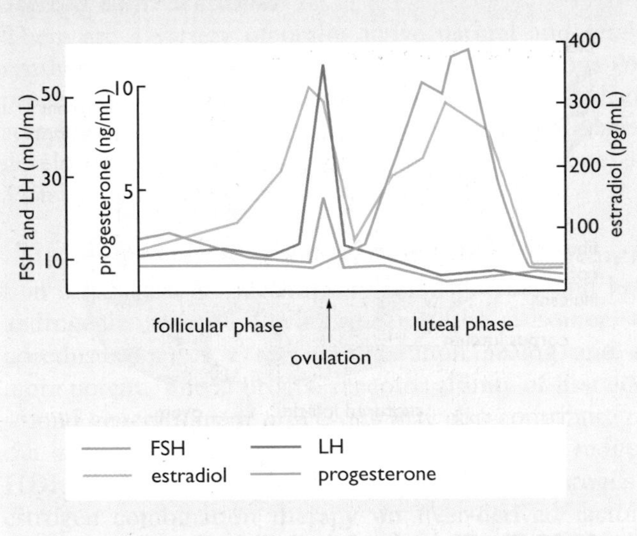

Fig. 11.24 Changes in the concentrations of circulating hormones during the menstrual cycle. Note that the hormone concentrations are drawn to different scales. During menstruation and in the early follicular phase, the steroid concentrations are low, and, as there is little steroid negative feedback, gonadotropin secretion (especially FSH) is slightly elevated. FSH stimulates the follicles in the ovary to grow, mature and secrete estrogen. The increasing estrogen concentration then exerts negative feedback, reducing gonadotropin concentrations. However, when the estrogen concentration reaches a critical concentration (>200 pg/mL) for a critical length of time (2 days), the negative feedback switches to a positive feedback, stimulating a dramatic transient release of LH (the LH surge) and to a lesser extent FSH from the pituitary. The increased concentration of LH appears to desensitize the LH receptors on the theca, thereby terminating androgen and therefore estrogen synthesis, resulting in a rapid decline of the circulating estrogen concentration. However, LH receptors on the differentiated granulosa cells continue to respond to LH and start to secrete progesterone.

An LH surge induces ovulation, reduces androgen and estrogen synthesis, and increases progesterone production

Estrogen concentrations rise as the follicles mature. Normally the sex steroids control the rate of their own secretion by negative feedback on the hypothalamus and pituitary to reduce LH and FSH secretion. Through a poorly understood mechanism, this feedback effect is reversed at midcycle when high estradiol concentrations (>200 pg/mL) promote LH secretion for a 2-day period. The LH surge (Fig. 11.24):

- Appears to desensitize the LH receptors on the theca, thereby terminating androgen/estrogen synthesis.
- Stimulates LH receptors on the differentiated granulosa cells to start secretion of progesterone.
- Stimulates resumption of meiosis in the ovum. The second meiotic division then starts, but is arrested in the metaphase and is completed only at fertilization.
- Induces the release of ovarian cytokines, plasminogen activators, prostaglandins and histamine, causing the first dissolution of the thecal wall and then contraction of the weakening structure resulting in its rupture (ovulation). This occurs approximately 36 hours after the surge.

The corpus luteum forms after ovulation and produces large quantities of progesterone, which maintains the uterine endometrium

Under LH stimulation the granulosa cells of the ruptured ovarian follicle differentiate to form the corpus luteum (Fig. 11.25). The corpus luteum produces large amounts of 17-hydroxyprogesterone and progesterone as well as estrogen. Progesterone primes the uterine endometrium for implantation. If fertilization does not take place the corpus luteum becomes senescent and starts to regress in the midluteal phase (day 21 onward of the cycle). In the later luteal phase, declining progesterone concentrations cause the endometrium to be shed at menstruation.

In response to fertilization, progesterone secretion is maintained by rising concentrations of human chorionic gonadotropin. Progesterone has several effects that inhibit the menstrual cycling and thus sustain pregnancy:

- Maintenance of secretory endometrium for embryo and placental development.
- Feedback inhibition of gonadotropin secretion.
- Antiestrogenic effects on cervical mucus to reduce fertility.
- Promotion of mammary duct development.

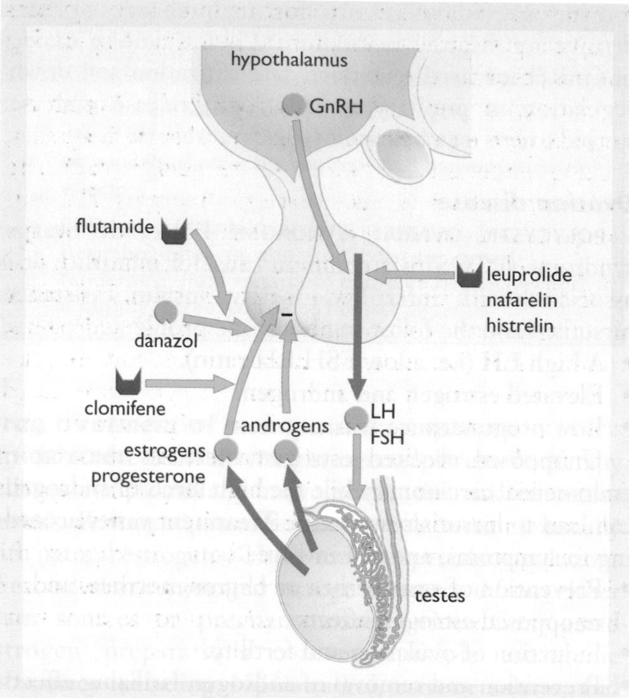

Fig. 11.28 Modulation of the gonadotropin axis. Several drugs alter the function of the hypothalamic–pituitary–gonadal axis. Agonists of the gonadotropin receptor (leuprolide, nafarelin, histrelin) produce desensitization of gonadotroph responses, leading to reduced concentrations of luteinizing hormone (LH) and follicle-stimulating hormone (FSH). Danazol mimics the feedback inhibition of endogenous androgens and reduces gonadotropin secretion without marked peripheral androgenic adverse effects. Androgen and estrogen receptor antagonists interrupt the feedback inhibition of gonadotropin secretion by sex steroids. The resultant rise in gonadotropins that occurs with the estrogen antagonist clomifene promotes ovarian folliculogenesis in the treatment of infertility, whereas the reflex LH increase that occurs with the androgen receptor antagonist flutamide may stimulate testosterone synthesis and lead to failure of the antiandrogen effect. Flutamide may therefore be combined with a gonadotropin-releasing hormone (GnRH) agonist in the treatment of prostatic cancer.

synthesis. More recently, leuprolide, nafarelin and histrelin (all GnRH agonists) have proven useful. These drugs have greater potency for the GnRH receptor on the pituitary than the endogenous agonist GnRH. After a brief stimulation, they desensitize the GnRH receptor and so reduce gonadotropin secretion. However, these drugs require parenteral administration and lead to menopausal-type adverse effects such as vasomotor symptoms, bone loss and genitourinary atrophy.

Androgen excess in women

Hirsutism and acne are common in women, and are only occasionally related to androgen excess. Hirsutism is a common symptom of PCOS. Androgenic action on the pilosebaceous unit (sebaceous gland and hair follicle) induce conversion of vellus to terminal hair and increasing growth rate. Removal of androgenic stimulation does not reverse the process, but prevents further growth.

Steroidal antiandrogens include:

- Spironolactone, an aldosterone antagonist which has a higher potency on androgen receptors than cyproterone. It inhibits cytochrome P-450 mono-oxygenases and alters steroidogenesis, reducing testosterone synthesis and increasing its metabolism. The potassium retention it produces requires monitoring.
- Cyproterone, which also has progestogen actions which require periodic interruption of therapy to allow breakthrough menstrual bleeding. Alternatively, it can be given with ethinyl estradiol and so provide contraceptive protection. It is not used in the US.

Combined oral contraception is used for PCOS-related androgen excess when infertility is not an immediate issue

Nonsteroidal antiandrogens include flutamide and nilutamide, and the 5α-reductase inhibitor, finasteride, and have no greater efficacy than steroidal antiandrogens in the treatment of female androgen excess.

Small-scale clinical trials using thiazolidenedione or biguanide (metformin) insulin-sensitizing agents have demonstrated reduction in androgen excess in PCOS. GnRH agonists reduce ovarian steroidogenesis, but are poorly tolerated due to menopausal symptoms.

Androgen excess and deficiency in males

The adrenals and the testes produce various compounds that stimulate androgen receptors. Dihydrotestosterone and testosterone are the most potent, but precursors such as dehydroepiandrosterone and androstenedione also have androgenic effects. 17-carbon androgenic precursors from either the adrenals or the gonads can be converted to testosterone by 17-hydroxysteroid dehydrogenase in the testis or ovary. The enzyme 5α-reductase produces the potent androgen dihydrotestosterone in the prostate, skin, sebaceous glands and brain. Due to this tissue-specific expression of 5α-reductase, androgenic effects on prostate growth and male pattern baldness are largely mediated by dihydrotestosterone. The androgen receptor is a DNA-linked ligand-activated transcription factor with homology to mineralocorticoid and progesterone steroid receptors.

Androgens are important in the treatment of disorders of puberty, prostatic disease and hirsutism

Androgen excess in prepubertal boys due to unregulated testicular testosterone production ('testotoxicosis') leads to premature puberty, short adult stature and behavioral problems. Conversely, pubertal delay can be treated with short courses of androgen therapy to stimulate the HPG axis in adolescent boys. After puberty, androgen excess produces no effects in males, but leads to androgenic responses ranging from hirsutism to virilization in women. Androgen deficiency in adult males is an important cause of male osteoporosis.

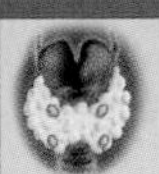

Androgen replacement therapy

- **Intramuscular preparations (testosterone enanthate, cypionate) are inexpensive and can be given at 2–4-week intervals**
- **Transdermal testosterone delivery systems are effective, but expensive**
- **Oral androgens are associated with a high risk of hepatic disease**

ANDROGEN REPLACEMENT As with the estrogens, testosterone has poor bioavailability owing to hepatic metabolism. As a result, synthetic analogs, transdermal delivery patches and intramuscular formulations are used clinically (Table 11.21). Intramuscular testosterone preparations (testosterone enanthate, testosterone cypionate, testosterone propionate) use an oil-based vehicle to slow absorption from the injection site with dosing intervals of 2–4 weeks, in contrast to the 3-day interval for aqueous testosterone. Transdermal testosterone delivery systems or topical gels provide another mechanism of bypassing first-pass hepatic metabolism.

Testosterone replacement therapy is for hypogonal men who demonstrate clinical (reduced shaving frequency, exercise endurance, libido and testicular size) and laboratory findings (reduced free or free plus albumin-bound testosterone). Testosterone replacement therapy improves physical performance, sexual function, mood and lipid profiles within 4 weeks in most cases. In healthy men, high-dose testosterone, or synthetic androgens, produce small increases in muscle mass and exercise performance, while posing the risks of aggressive mood disorder, priapism, erythrocytosis, oligospermia and worsened lipid profile. Adverse hepatic effects such as blood-filled hepatic cysts (peliosis hepatis), hepatic adenomas and cholestatic hepatic injury have been reported primarily with oral synthetic androgens. In elderly men, androgen supplementation increases serum concentrations of prostate-specific antigen and may

Table 11.21 Androgen agonists

	Use	Typical dose	Pharmacokinetics	Adverse effects
Testosterone	Male hypogonadism		Elimination half-life 0.3–1.5 hours Hepatic metabolism	Testosterone class effects: erythrocytosis, priapism, HDL lowering
Transdermal		Truncal 4–6 mg q.d. Scrotal 5 mg q.d. Topical gel (1%) 5–10 g q.d.		Testosterone class effects
Intramuscular (enanthate, cypionate or propionate esters)		200–400 mg i.m. q. 2–4 weeks		Testosterone class effects
Nandrolone decanoate		Anemia of bone marrow failure (50–200 mg i.m. q. week)	Prolonged absorption, elimination half-life 4 hours, hepatic metabolism	Testosterone class effects
Oral synthetic androgens				
Methyltestosterone	Male hypogonadism Delayed puberty Cryptorchidism Breast cancer palliation Breast engorgement	10–50 mg q.d. p.o. 75 mg q.d. × 5 days for postpartum breast engorgement	45% Hepatic first-pass metabolism, $t_{1/2}$ = 0.2–2 hours 90% renally excreted as testosterone sulfates and glucuronides Extensive protein binding	Oral androgen class effects: fluid retention, erythrocytosis, priapism, acne, reduced HDL cholesterol, prostate hypertrophy, oligospermia, gynecomastia, peliosis hepatis, hepatic adenoma (rare)
Fluoxymesterone	Delayed puberty Breast cancer palliation	50–200 mg q.d. p.o.	$t_{1/2}$ = 9 hours	Class effects
Oxymetholone	Aplastic anemia	50–150 mg p.o. q.d.		Class effects
Oxandrolone	Delayed puberty Cachexia	5–10 mg q.d.–b.i.d. p.o.	$t_{1/2}$ = 5–13 hours Less hepatic first-pass metabolism 30% renal excretion High protein binding (95%)	Class effects

worsen prostate hypertrophy.

The orally active androgens methyltestosterone and fluoxymesterone are not commonly used for androgen replacement, but are commonly abused by body builders. Other orally active androgenic steroids (testolactone, oxandrolone, stanozolol, oxymetholone) and intramuscular preparations (nandrolone) have androgenic effects and are used clinically for their anabolic actions in cancer and refractory anemia. Close monitoring for hepatic dysfunction is needed during oral androgen therapy as well as for a variety of androgen-related adverse effects (Table 11.22).

Antiandrogenic therapies (Fig. 11.29) are used to treat prostatic disease in men:

- Nonsteroidal androgen antagonists (flutamide, nilutamide) are selective for testosterone receptors and are devoid of effects on other steroid receptors. Their use leads to increased LH secretion and testosterone synthesis, possibly resulting in therapeutic failure.
- A gonadotropin-suppressing progestogen, megestrol acetate, is used to reduce androgen in metastatic prostate cancer, but has no direct androgen receptor antagonist actions. Orchiectomy is also used to reduce endogenous androgens.
- Spironolactone, the mineralocorticosteroid antagonist, is also an androgen agonist and is commonly used for female hirsutism, but is not efficacious in prostate cancer treatment.

Table 11.22 The effects of androgen therapy

Central nervous system	Gonadotropin suppression
	Behavioral effects
Body habitus	Hirsutism
	Virilization
	Acne
	Baldness
	Gynecomastia
Hematologic	Erythrocytosis
Metabolic	Dyslipidemia
Hepatic	Cholestatic jaundice
	Peliosis hepatis
	Hepatocellular carcinoma
Genitourinary	Priapism
	Prostatic hypertrophy
	Prostatic cancer

In men, the observation that androgen effects such as prostatic growth and male pattern baldness depend on androgen receptor stimulation by dihydrotestosterone has led to the therapeutic use of the 5α-reductase inhibitor finasteride. Testosterone is converted to the more potent dihydrotestosterone by the enzyme 5α-reductase, which is expressed in the skin, liver and genital tissues. Finasteride is moderately effective in improving the symptoms of prostatic hypertrophy, but less so than α adrenoceptor antagonists.

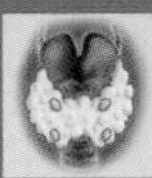

testosterone

testes

5α–reductase

inhibits

finasteride

dihydro-
testosterone

testosterone

receptor
dimerization

receptor
dimerization

GRE

GRE

androgen
antagonists:
spironolactone
cyproterone
flutamide
nilutamide
bicalutamide

occurs in:
prostate
seminal vesicles
hair follicles
brain

occurs in:
genitalia
muscle
sebaceous glands
vocal cords

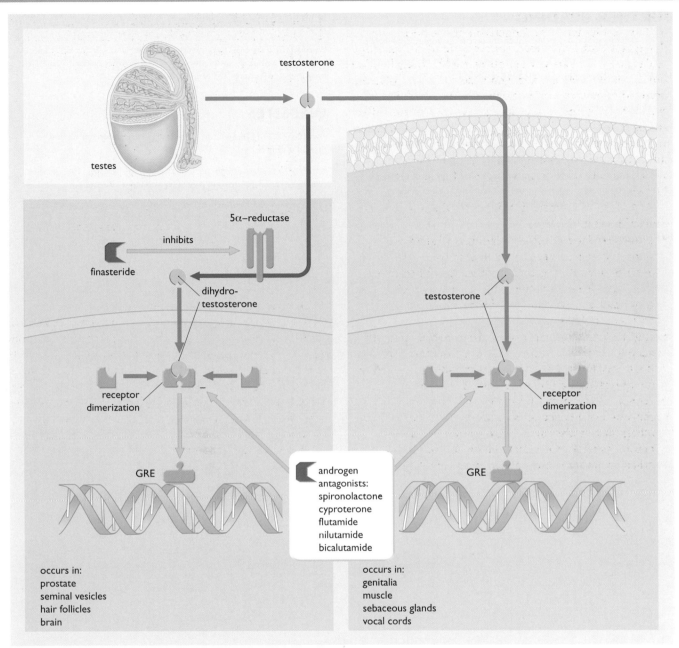

Fig. 11.29 Antiandrogen therapy. The endogenous androgens testosterone and dihydrotestosterone bind and dimerize cytosolic androgen receptors (AR), translocate to the nucleus and regulate gene transcription through the glucocorticoid response element (GRE). Dihydrotestosterone is produced from testosterone in selective target tissues that express the enzyme 5α-reductase. Androgen antagonists competitively inhibit androgen binding to the AR. The steroidal antiandrogen spironolactone may also inhibit testosterone synthesis. 5α-reductase inhibitors selectively reduce dihydrotestosterone synthesis in target tissues such as the prostate gland.

FURTHER READING

Bar RS. Early diagnosis and treatment of endocrine disorders. Totowa, N.J.: Humana Press, c2003.

DeGroot LJ. Endocrinology. Oxford Elsevier 2005.

Melmed S, Conn PM. Endocrinology: basic and clinical principles. Totowa, N.J.: Humana Press, c2005.

Mino-Leon D, Figueras A, Amato D, Laporte JR. Treatment of type 2 diabetes in primary health care: a drug utilization study. *Annals Pharmacother* 2005; **39**: 441–445.

Padwal R, Majumdar SR, Johnson JA, Varney J, McAllister FA. A systematic review of drug therapy to delay or prevent type 2 diabetes. *Diabetes Care* 2005; **28**: 736–744. [Drug treatment of type 2 diabetes.]

Racine Ms, Barkan AL. Medical management of growth hormone-secreting pituitary adenomas. *Pituitary* 2002; **5**: 67–76.

Sanders S. Endocrine and reproductive systems. London; New York; Mosby, 2003.

Woelfle J, Chia DJ, Massart-Schlesinger MB, Moyano P, Rotwein P. Molecular physiology, pathology, and regulation of the growth hormone/insulin-like growth factor-I system. *Ped Nephrol* 2005; **20**: 295–302.

WEBSITES

www.thyroid.org [This website provides updated treatment options to thyroid disorders.]

http://www.healthinsite.gov.au/topics/Endocrine_Diseases [This website provides general information regarding endocrine diseases.]

http://www.merck.com/mrkshared/mmanual/sections.jsp [Merck Manual.]

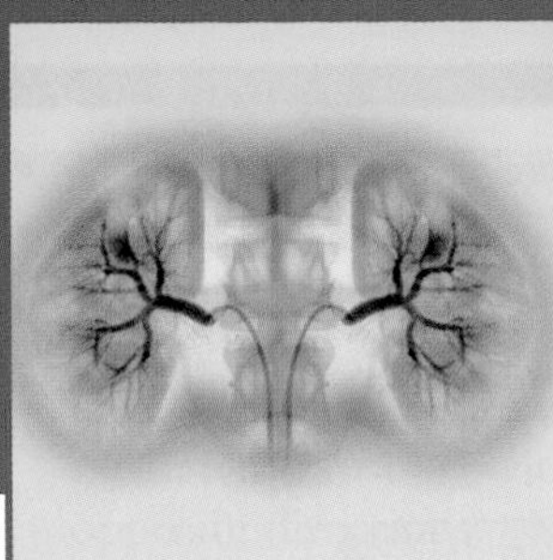

Chapter 12

Drugs and the Renal System

PHYSIOLOGY OF THE KIDNEY

Essential functions of the kidney include:

- Excretion of nitrogenous waste products of metabolism such as urea and creatinine.
- Regulation of extracellular fluid.
- Regulation of the concentration of various ions.
- Regulation of the pH of body fluids.

The renal system includes the bladder, where urine is stored before excretion through the urethra (see Ch. 17).

The kidney has two distinct regions: cortex and medulla

Two distinct regions can be macroscopically identified in the kidney: a dark outer region, the cortex, and a paler inner region, the medulla. The medulla is further divided into a number of conical areas, the renal pyramids (Fig. 12.1).

The individual functional unit of the kidney is the nephron, with each kidney containing approximately one million nephrons. The nephron is a blind-ended tube with the blind end forming a capsule, the Bowman's capsule, which surrounds a knot of capillaries, the glomerulus. Glomerular capillaries receive their blood from the afferent arteriole, a resistance blood vessel. Blood leaves the glomerulus not in a vein (capacitance vessel) but in a second resistance vessel, the efferent arteriole. This arrangement of afferent and efferent vessels permits generation of a hydrostatic force that drives ultrafiltration (see below). The other parts of the nephron are the proximal tubule, loop of Henle, distal tubule and the collecting duct (see Fig. 12.6 below). Many distal tubules join a collecting duct which merges into larger ducts before draining into a renal calyx and, finally, into the renal pelvis.

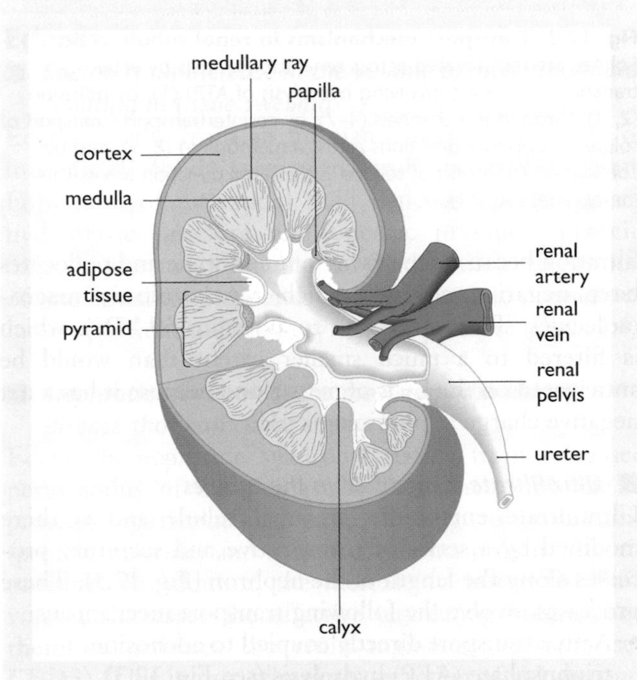

Fig. 12.1 Structure of the kidney. The kidney consists of two visible regions, the cortex and medulla, with the latter being divided into the renal pyramids.

There are two distinct populations of nephrons: cortical and juxtamedullary nephrons

- Cortical nephrons have glomeruli in the outer two-thirds of the cortex with short loops of Henle, which either extend a short distance into the medulla, or do not reach the medulla. These nephrons account for 85% of all nephrons. The efferent arteriole of cortical nephrons forms a network of peritubular capillaries that encircle all parts of the nephron.
- Juxtamedullary nephrons (15% of all nephrons) have glomeruli in the inner third of the cortex with long loops of Henle extending deep into the medulla (see Fig. 12.6 below) and are responsible for generating hypertonic fluid within the medullar interstitium. The efferent arteriole of juxtamedullary nephrons gives rise to peritubular capillaries, but also forms a series of vascular loops (the vasa recta) which descend into the medulla and surround the loop of Henle.

Urine is a modified ultrafiltrate of plasma produced through three filtration barriers

The force that drives ultrafiltration (i.e. filtration of small molecules) is glomerular capillary hydrostatic pressure. This pressure is dependent on the ratio of the resistance in the afferent arteriole to that in the efferent arteriole. In contrast to other vascular beds, the presence of a second arteriole, the efferent arteriole, ensures that the hydrostatic pressure in glomerular capillaries declines very little along their length.

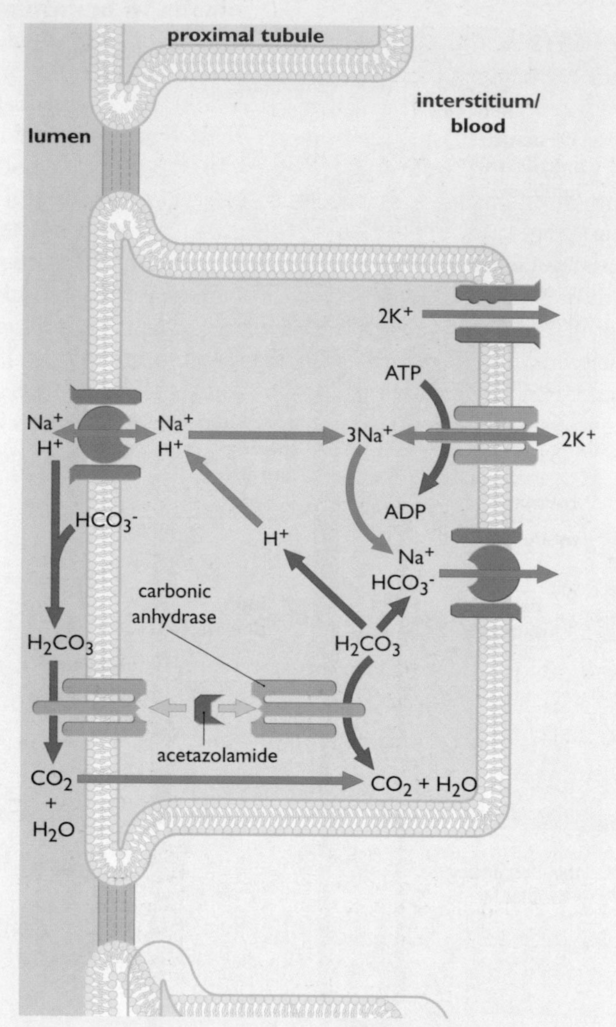

Fig. 12.7 Sodium bicarbonate reabsorption in the proximal tubule and site of action of the carbonic anhydrase inhibitor acetazolamide. Countertransport of Na^+ and H^+ across the apical membrane moves Na^+ into the cell and H^+ into the lumen. The latter reacts with tubule fluid bicarbonate (HCO_3^-), producing carbonic acid (H_2CO_3) that dissociates to form CO_2 and H_2O, a reaction catalyzed by carbonic anhydrase bound to the apical membrane. Both CO_2 and H_2O readily enter the cell, where carbonic acid is formed by the action of cytoplasmic carbonic anhydrase. Carbonic acid dissociates into HCO_3^-, which is transported across the basolateral membrane with Na^+, and H^+. The latter moves into the lumen via the Na^+/H^+ countertransporter to begin the cycle again. Inhibition of both membrane-bound and cytoplasmic forms of the enzyme by acetazolamide inhibits Na^+ and HCO_3^- reabsorption.

(bumetanide-sensitive cotransporter-1, BSC-1) (Fig. 12.8). Loop diuretics have the greatest efficacy of all diuretics and cause a maximum excretion of 15–25% of the Na^+ filtered at the glomerulus.

The thick ascending limb of the loop of Henle is impermeable to water and therefore movement of Na^+ and Cl^- ions into the medullary interstitium (see Fig. 12.6), without accompanying water, increases the osmotic pressure in this region. High osmotic pressures in the medullary interstitium causes reabsorption of water from the collecting duct but only in the presence of antidiuretic hormone (such as vasopressin) (see below). Loop diuretics inhibit water reabsorption from the collecting duct by reducing ion concentrations in the medullary interstitium.

Reabsorption of Ca^{2+} and Mg^{2+} is also inhibited by loop diuretics since absorption of these ions is driven by a lumen-positive potential produced by recycling of K^+ across the apical membrane via a K^+-selective channel (see Fig. 12.8). Loop diuretics increase the delivery of Na^+ to the collecting duct, which increases K^+ and H^+ secretion, leading to a hypokalemic alkalosis (see below).

Loop diuretics are water-soluble weak acids, highly bound to plasma albumin (>90%) at therapeutic concentrations. Most furosemide is excreted by the kidneys as a result of secretion in the proximal tubule (see Table 12.3). Bumetanide and torsemide are largely cleared by metabolism in the liver and, as a result, accumulate less in renal failure than furosemide, meaning the risk of adverse drug effects in renal failure is less with bumetanide and torsemide.

In addition to their diuretic properties, loop diuretics have indirect venodilator activity as a result of the release of a substance from the kidney (most probably a prostaglandin). This action leads to a fall in left ventricular filling pressure and helps relieve pulmonary edema before diuresis occurs.

Furosemide (20–80 mg orally) acts within an hour and its effect is short-lived (complete within 6 hours). Thus, furosemide can be given twice daily without diuresis interfering with sleep. Once-daily dosing leaves an 18– hour gap when the kidney can reabsorb Na^+, resulting in 'rebound Na^+ retention.' This may be of sufficient magnitude to negate any prior diuresis. This is avoided if furosemide is given by continuous intravenous (i.v.) infusion.

Clinical indications for loop diuretics include:

- Acute pulmonary edema where they are administered intravenously to ensure a rapid onset of action. In congestive heart failure, with or without pulmonary edema, furosemide is orally used routinely to reduce the signs and symptoms of heart failure as well as to increase longevity (see Ch. 13).
- Other edematous states such as the nephrotic syndrome, ascites of liver cirrhosis and chronic renal failure (oral administration).
- Hypertension in patients who have not responded to other diuretics or antihypertensive drugs, especially in patients with renal insufficiency (see Ch. 13).
- Acute renal failure, when they are given to increase urine production (see below).
- Hyponatremia: this can produce swelling of brain cells that results in neurologic dysfunction characterized by lethargy, confusion and even coma. Loop diuretics dissipate the high solute concentration in the medullary interstitium. This promotes

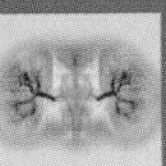

Table 12.1 Adverse effects of diuretic drugs

	Carbonic anhydrase inhibitors	Loop diuretics	Thiazide and thiazide-like diuretics	Potassium-sparing diuretics
Effects that are a consequence of diuretic action	Metabolic acidosis Hypokalemia Abnormal taste, lethargy, decreased libido (reduced by administration of $NaHCO_3$)	Hypokalemia (corrected by K^+ supplements or combination with potassium-sparing diuretics) Metabolic alkalosis Hypovolemia and hypotension Hypocalcemia Hypercalcemia	Hypokalemia (corrected as for loop diuretics) Metabolic alkalosis Hyponatremia Hypovolemia and hypotension Hypomagnesemia Hypomagnesemia	Hyperkalemia Metabolic acidosis
Effects unrelated to diuretic actions	Occasionally hepatitis and blood dyscrasias as a result of immunologic hypersensitivity reactions	Hyperuricemia which may precipitate gout (enhanced uric acid absorption in proximal tubule as a result of volume depletion or decreased secretion due to competition at organic acid secretion sites) Ototoxicity (hearing loss, tinnitus; most likely to occur with ethacrynic acid)	Hyperuricemia(mechanism as for loop diuretics) Hyperglycemia which may reveal latent diabetes mellitus (due to reduced insulin secretion and alterations in glucose metabolism) An increase in plasma levels of low-density lipoproteins (LDL) and cholesterol Male sexual dysfunction	Nausea and vomiting (amiloride and triamterene) Diarrhea and peptic ulcer (spironolactone) Spironolactone binds to other steroid receptors. This can result in: Gynecomastia Menstrual disorders Impotence Hirsutism Loss of libido

Table 12.2 Notable interactions between diuretics and other drugs

Diuretic drug(s)	Drug(s) interactions	Consequence	Comment
Acetazolamide	Phenytoin Phenobarbital Primidone	Osteomalacia and rickets	Uncertain mechanism
Acetazolamide	Aspirin or salicylates	Lethargy, confusion and coma	Acetazolamide-induced acidosis results in more salicylate entering the central nervous system and salicylate intoxication
Thiazide, thiazide-like and loop diuretics	Cardiac glycosides	Increased cardiac glycoside-induced arrhythmias	Hypokalemia potentiates action of cardiac glycosides
Thiazide, thiazide-like and loop diuretics	Sulfonylureas (oral hypoglycemic drugs) and insulin	Hyperglycemia	Thiazides and to a lesser extent loop diuretics decrease insulin secretion
Thiazide, thiazide-like and loop diuretics	Lithium	Increased plasma levels of lithium with risk of toxic effects	Increased tubular reabsorption of lithium
Thiazide, thiazide-like and loop diuretics	Uricosuric agents	Reduced effect of uricosuric agents	Decreased tubular secretion of uricosuric agents
Thiazide, thiazide-like and loop diuretics	Nonsteroidal antiinflammatory drugs	Reduced diuretic response	Interaction a result of inhibition of prostaglandin synthesis
Loop diuretics	Aminoglycosides Cisplatin	Increased risk of ototoxicity	Synergism of ototoxicity
Potassium-sparing diuretics	ACE inhibitors and K supplements	Increased risk of hyperkalemia	Additive hyperkalemic effects

Table 12.3 Pharmacokinetic parameters of some diuretic drugs

Drug	Routes of administration	Oral absorption (%)	Half-life (h)	Volume of distribution (L/kg)	Elimination	Comments
Acetazolamide	p.o., i.v., i.m.	100	8 (6–9)	0.2	Unchanged in urine	Decrease dose in elderly and other patients with diminished renal function Alkalinization of urine may decrease urinary excretion of weak bases (e.g. quinidine) and increase their pharmacologic effect
Furosemide	p.o., i.v., i.m.	52 (27–80)	1.5 (0.5–2.0)	0.2–0.3	About 75% of dose is excreted unchanged in urine	Food intake reduces absorption
Chlorothiazide	p.o., i.v.	7–33	15–27	0.3	Unchanged in urine	Oral absorption decreases with dose
Indapamide	p.o.	High	17 (10–22)	60 L	Extensive metabolism	
Triamterene	p.o.	30–83	1.5–2.5	2.2–3.7	Rapid metabolism	
Spironolactone	p.o.	60–70	1.3 ± 0.3 (SD)	Not known	Extensive metabolism	Absorption is variable because of poor solubility in water but is improved after food Canrenone is an active metabolite

p.o., oral administration; i.v., intravenous; i.m., intramuscular.

additional water loss in relation to Na^+ excretion and accounts for the use of loop diuretics, combined with hypertonic saline, in the treatment of hyponatremia.

The main adverse effects and principal drug interactions that occur with loop diuretics, compared with other diuretics, are shown in Tables 12.1 and 12.2.

Thiazide and thiazide-like diuretics

Thiazide diuretics include bendroflumethiazide, chlorothiazide, polythiazide and hydrochlorothiazide. More recently discovered thiazide-like diuretics have a similar mode of action, but not a thiazide structure. These include indapamide, chlortalidone and metolazone. Thiazides and thiazide-like diuretics all possess a sulfonamide moiety (see Fig. 12.5).

The molecular mechanism of action of thiazide diuretics is inhibition of the Na^+/Cl^- cotransporter (TSC; thiazide-sensitive cotransporter) in the distal convoluted tubule (Fig. 12.9). Compared with loop diuretics, thiazides have moderate efficacy. One reason for this is physiologic in that by the time the filtrate has reached the distal tubule, 90% of the filtered Na^+ has already been reabsorbed. The action of thiazides results in the urinary excretion of up to half the Na^+ that passes to the distal nephron; that is 5% of Na^+ filtered at the glomerulus. However, in contrast with loop diuretics, which are used to treat hyponatremia, thiazides are prone to produce this potentially fatal problem. Thiazides can precipitate hyponatremia since they increase Na^+ excretion without affecting the kidney's ability to concentrate urine.

Differences among thiazide and thiazide-like diuretics

Thiazide and thiazide-like drugs given orally are well absorbed. They are eliminated by the kidney via secretion in the proximal tubule (see Table 12.3). However, a significant fraction of doses of bendroflumethiazide, polythiazide and indapamide is also eliminated by metabolism. Chlortalidone has a particularly prolonged action, such that it can be given on alternate days for the control of edema. Indapamide differs from other drugs in this class in that it lowers blood pressure (see treatment of hypertension in Ch. 13) at doses below those required to elicit a diuresis, an effect attributed to L-type calcium channel blockade. In addition, indapamide has less effect on uric acid secretion and glucose metabolism than other members of the group (see Table 12.1).

In contrast with loop diuretics, thiazides decrease excretion of Ca^{2+}. The exact mechanism underlying this effect is uncertain. In the distal tubule, Ca^{2+} is reabsorbed from the lumen via an epithelial calcium channel (ECaC) that is distinct in structure and function from other types of calcium channel. Entry of Ca^{2+} is followed by exchange across the basolateral membrane via a Na^+/Ca^{2+} exchange countertransporter (see Fig. 12.9). Since the intracellular concentration of Na^+ is reduced as a consequence of the primary molecular action of thiazide, the increase in the Na^+ concentration gradient across the basolateral membrane may be sufficient to enhance the removal of Ca^{2+} across the basolateral membrane via the Na^+/Ca^{2+} exchanger. There is a parallel here with the cellular mechanism by which digitalis affects intracellular Ca^{2+} in

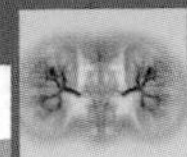

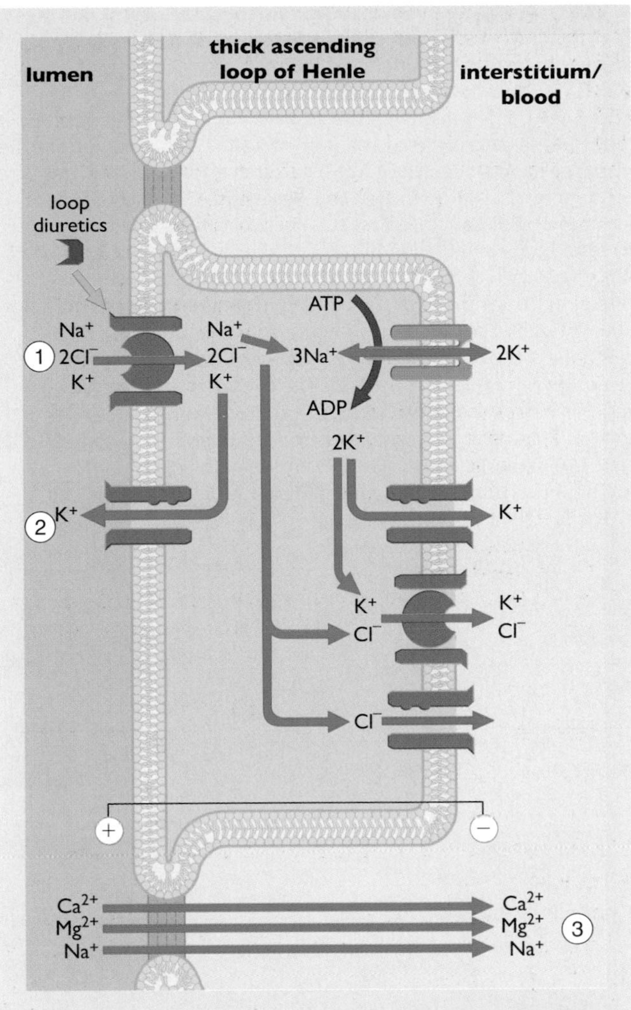

Fig. 12.8 Transport mechanism in the thick ascending loop of Henle. Loop diuretics block the $Na^+/K^+/2Cl^-$ cotransporter (1), thereby preventing the absorption, and hence increasing tubular excretion, of Na^+ and Cl^-. These drugs also decrease the potential difference across the tubule cell which is generated by the recycling of K^+ (2). As a result, increased excretion of Ca^{2+} and Mg^{2+} occurs because of inhibition of paracellular diffusion (3). + and – indicate a voltage difference.

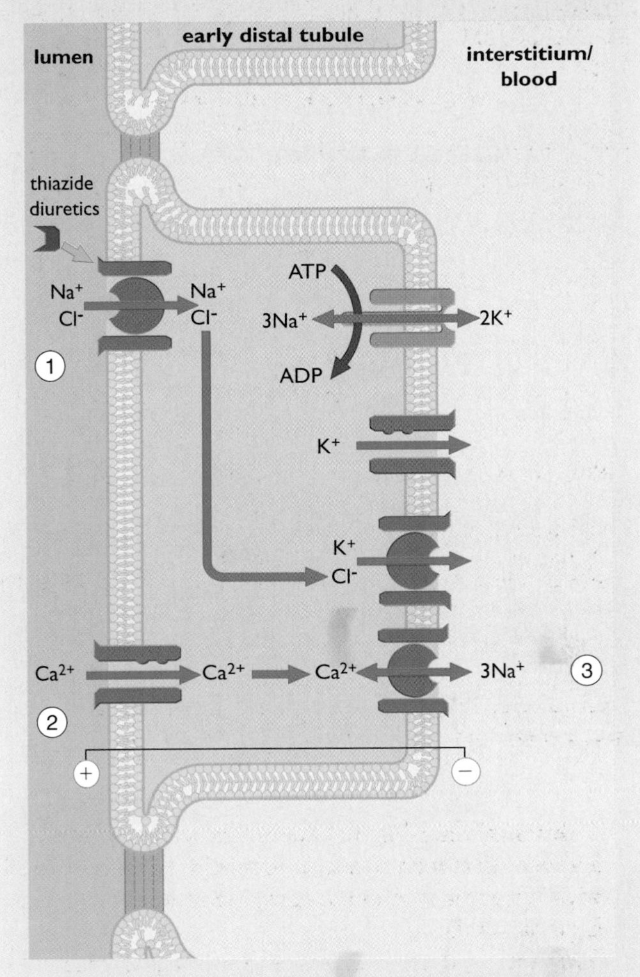

Fig. 12.9 Transport mechanisms in the early distal tubule. Thiazide diuretics increase the excretion of Na^+ and Cl^- by inhibiting the Na^+/Cl^- cotransporter (1). The reabsorption of Ca^{2+} (2) is increased by these drugs through a mechanism that may involve stimulation of Na^+/Ca^{2+} countertransport (3) due to an increase in the concentration gradient for Na^+ across the basolateral membrane. + and – indicate a voltage difference.

the heart in the treatment of heart failure (see Ch.13), which also involves an indirect effect on the Na^+/Ca^{2+} exchanger secondary to a change in Na^+ homeostasis.

Pharmacotherapeutic indications for thiazide diuretics include:

- Edema associated with congestive heart failure, hepatic cirrhosis and nephrotic syndrome.
- Hypertension (see Ch. 13), where they are used either alone or in combination with other antihypertensive drugs. Clinical studies have shown that, when used alone to treat hypertension, a daily dose of thiazide not exceeding 25 mg of hydrochlorothiazide, or its equivalent, produces a maximal benefit. Higher doses produce a greater diuresis with no proportional decrease in blood pressure, but a greater risk of hypokalemia, which predisposes to cardiac arrhythmias such as ventricular fibrillation and torsades de pointes (see Ch. 13).
- Renal stone disease (nephrolithiasis) (see below).

Common adverse effects of thiazide and loop diuretics

These drugs can cause metabolic alkalosis and hypokalemia. These effects are due to increased K^+ and H^+ secretion in the late distal tubule (connecting tubule) and collecting duct. There are two types of cells in the late distal tubule and collecting duct:

- Principal cells, which are sites for Na^+, K^+ and water transport.
- Intercalated cells, which are sites for H^+ secretion into the lumen (Figs 12.10, 12.11).

Na^+ reabsorption across the apical membrane of principal cells occurs mostly via Na^+ channels as opposed

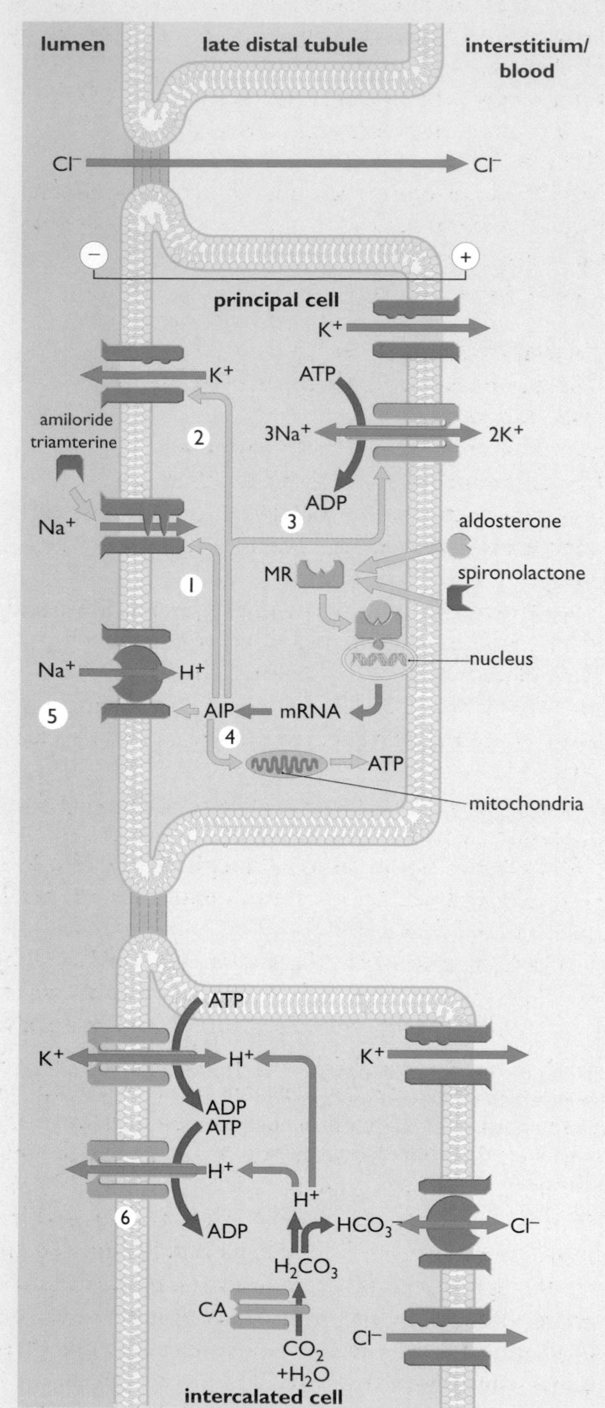

Fig. 12.10 Transport mechanisms in the late distal tubule and collecting duct, and mode of action of potassium-sparing diuretics. Amiloride and triamterene block apical Na^+ channels resulting in a diminished potential difference across the principal cell (lumen negative with respect to interstitium). The loss of potential results in a decreased driving force for K^+ secretion from the principal cell and H^+ secretion from the intercalated cell. The net effect is increased Na^+ excretion and decreased K^+ and H^+ excretion. Aldosterone binds to a cytoplasmic mineralocorticosteroid receptor (MR) resulting in stimulation of the synthesis of aldosterone-induced proteins (AIP), which (1) activate silent (nonfunctional) Na^+ channels; (2) increase the synthesis of K^+ channels; (3) increase the synthesis of Na^+/K^+ ATPase; (4) increase mitochondrial production of ATP; (5) increase the synthesis of the Na^+/H^+ countertransporter; and (6) increase the synthesis of H^+ ATPase. The overall effect of these changes is a decrease in Na^+ excretion and an increase in K^+ and H^+ excretion. Spironolactone, an aldosterone antagonist, has opposite effects. CA, carbonic anhydrase; this enzyme also catalyzes the formation of carbonic acid in principal cells which provide H^+ for Na^+/H^+ countertransport.

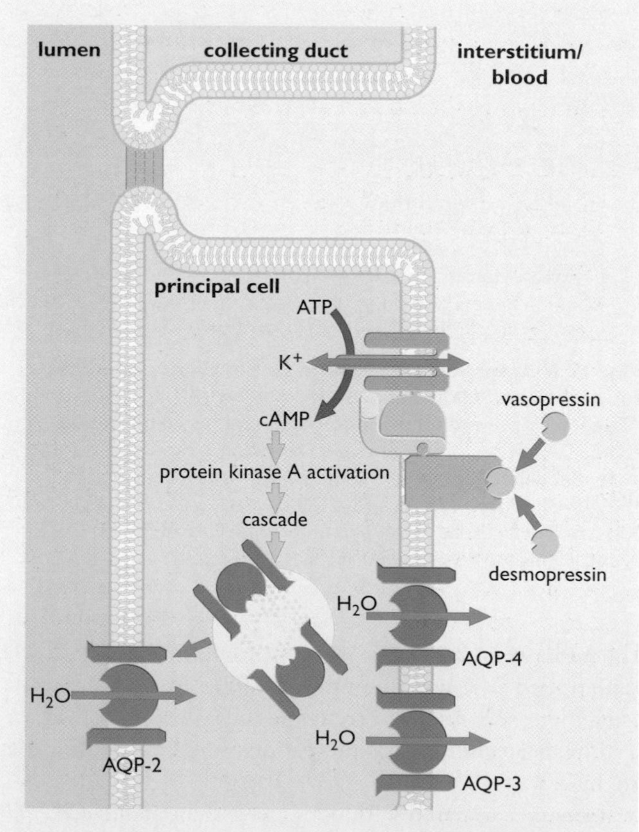

Fig. 12.11 The mechanism for controlling water permeability of the collecting duct. Vasopressin or its analog (e.g. desmopressin) bind to G protein-coupled V_2 receptors on the basolateral membrane of principal cells in the collecting duct. This, via activation of adenylyl cyclase and protein kinase A, leads to the migration of vesicles containing preformed water channels (aquaporin-2; AQP-2) to the apical membrane. AQP-2 channels are released from the vesicle and inserted into the membrane, thereby increasing water permeability. Water channels of the aquaporin -3 and -4 types (AQP-3, AQP-4) are present in the basolateral membrane to allow passage of water into the interstitium.

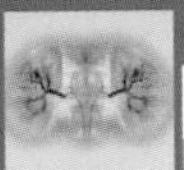

to transporters. This amiloride-sensitive epithelial Na^+ channel (ENaC) differs in structure and function from the voltage-regulated Na^+ channel in nerves and cardiac muscle. The epithelial Na^+ channels provide a high-conductance pathway for Na^+ to move across the apical membrane and down the electrochemical gradient generated by Na^+/K^+ ATPase in the basolateral membrane (see Fig. 12.10). The high permeability of the apical membrane to Na^+ results in depolarization of this membrane but not the basolateral membrane. This creates a potential difference across the cell with the lumen negative with respect to the interstitium. This potential difference provides a driving force for the secretion of K^+ into the tubular lumen. K^+ is transported into the cell by Na^+/K^+ ATPase and moves across the apical membrane via ROMK-1, an inwardly rectifying channel of the ROMK (rat outer medullary K^+ channel) family of K^+ channels. A proportion of K^+ that enters via Na^+/K^+ ATPase moves back across the basolateral membrane via K^+ channels.

The action of thiazides and loop diuretics result in an increase in apical Na^+ concentration in the late distal tubule and collecting duct. This increases K^+ secretion because:

- Increased Na^+ delivery results in enhanced Na^+ reabsorption that increases the lumen-negative potential, which is the driving force for K^+ secretion.
- Increased intracellular Na^+ concentration in the principal cell increases the activity of Na^+/K^+ ATPase; this increases uptake of K^+, which is then available for secretion.
- Increased flow in the distal parts of the nephron generated by the diuretics flushes away secreted K^+, thus maintaining the concentration gradient for further secretion.

In addition, thiazides and loop diuretics can cause contraction of extracellular fluid and a fall in blood pressure which activate the renin–angiotensin system (see Ch.13). This system is the primary stimulus for the secretion of aldosterone, a hormone that promotes the secretion of K^+ (see below).

Intercalated cells are the site of H^+ secretion either via H^+ ATPase or a H^+/K^+ ATPase. The H^+ ions for these transport enzymes are generated by carbonic anhydrase (see Fig. 12.10). In addition, there is an Na^+/H^+ countertransporter in principal cells that reabsorbs Na^+ in exchange for H^+. With regard to overall Na^+ reabsorption, Na^+/H^+ transport in the late distal tubule and collecting ducts is of minor importance compared with this transport system in the proximal tubule (see above). Secreted H^+ is buffered in the lumen by HCO_3^- and other ions such as HPO_4^{2-}.

Thiazide and loop diuretics produce a metabolic acidosis because of increased urinary loss of H^+ with a corresponding greater reabsorption of HCO_3^-. This occurs because:

- Increased Na^+ delivery to the distal tubule stimulates Na^+/H^+ exchange.
- The increased lumen-negative potential produced by increased Na^+ reabsorption enhances H^+ secretion by H^+ ATPase.
- Enhanced secretion of K^+, due to increased Na^+ reabsorption, increases the activity of H^+/K^+ ATPase.
- Elevated aldosterone secretion, due to extracellular volume reduction, produces increased expression of the transporters and enzymes involved in H^+ secretion (see Fig. 12.10).

Potassium-sparing diuretics

These drugs act on the late distal tubule and collecting duct

These drugs are divided into two groups:

- ENaC channel blockers, of which there are two, triamterene and amiloride. (These compounds are organic bases that do not contain the sulfonamide group; see Fig. 12.5.)
- The aldosterone antagonists (e.g. spironolactone and its metabolite, potassium canrenoate) that block mineralocorticosteroid receptors, which are DNA-linked receptors (see Ch. 3). Spironolactone has a 4-ring structure that is characteristic of steroids (see Fig. 12.5).

Both types of potassium-sparing diuretic drug have limited diuretic actions, resulting in the loss of 2–3% of Na^+ filtered at the glomerulus, although the magnitude of the diuresis produced by aldosterone antagonists depends on the levels of aldosterone.

Blockade of apical Na^+ channels in principal cells by amiloride or triamterene reduces Na^+ movement across the apical membrane (see Fig. 12.10). Amiloride also inhibits Na^+/H^+ exchange, although this occurs at concentrations much higher than are likely to be achieved during therapeutic use. The resultant lowering of intracellular Na^+ concentration by amiloride and triamterene reduces activity of basolateral Na^+/K^+ ATPase activity such that less Na^+ is pumped out and less K^+ moves into the cells. The reduction in Na^+ movement across the apical membrane reduces the lumen-negative potential difference and consequently decreases the driving force for K^+ secretion. The net effect of these drugs is therefore to reduce Na^+ reabsorption and decrease K^+ secretion; hence the term potassium-sparing diuretics. The latter effect can, however, result in the development of hyperkalemia.

Amiloride and triamterene can cause metabolic acidosis

The diuretic action of amiloride and triamterene indirectly decreases H^+ secretion, which can cause metabolic acidosis. The reduction in the lumen-negative potential difference produced by these ENaC blockers decreases H^+ secretion via H^+ ATPase whilst the reduction in K^+ secretion decreases H^+ secretion via K^+/H^+ ATPase.

Aldosterone antagonism affects renal Na^+, K^+ and H^+ metabolism

The cells of the late distal tubule and collecting duct contain cytoplasmic receptors for mineralocorticosteroids which, when bound to aldosterone, migrate to the nucleus and initiate DNA transcription, translation and production of specific proteins (aldosterone-induced proteins). These proteins:

- Activate silent Na^+ channels (cause inactive channels present in the membrane to become functional conducting channels, although the exact mechanism for this effect is unclear).
- Increase the synthesis of K^+ channels.
- Increase the synthesis of Na^+/K^+ ATPase.
- Increase mitochondrial production of ATP.
- Increase the synthesis of the Na^+/H^+ antiporter (exchanger).
- Increase the synthesis of H^+ ATPase (see Fig. 12.10).

As a result of these actions, the net effect of aldosterone is to increase Na^+ reabsorption, and K^+ and H^+ secretion.

Spironolactone indirectly reduces Na^+ reabsorption and K^+ and H^+ secretion

Spironolactone competitively inhibits the binding of aldosterone to its receptor (see Fig. 12.10), thus blocking stimulation of the synthesis of proteins that modify the transport functions of the late distal tubule and collecting duct. The effects of spironolactone are therefore to reduce Na^+ reabsorption and K^+ and H^+ secretion. The latter actions can lead to hyperkalemia and metabolic acidosis.

Mineralocorticoid receptors are expressed not only in epithelial cells but also in tissues such as brain, heart and blood vessels. Chronic stimulation of these receptors in heart and blood vessels by aldosterone has been shown to induce harmful effects such as fibrosis and hypertrophy. Spironolactone improves survival of patients with severe heart failure when added to conventional treatment, such as angiotensin-converting enzyme inhibitors. Such beneficial effects may owe more to blockade of nonepithelial receptors than blockade of epithelial receptors in the kidney.

Both amiloride and triamterene are effective when given orally and, whilst amiloride is eliminated predominately unchanged in the urine, triamterene is extensively metabolized to the active metabolite 4-hydroxytriamterene. Spironolactone is well absorbed following oral administration and is extensively metabolized in the liver (see Table 12.3). It has a short half-life of 1.3 hours but is metabolized to the longer-acting active metabolite canrenone (half-life 17 hours), which prolongs the diuretic effect.

CLINICAL INDICATIONS Triamterene, amiloride and spironolactone are used in combination with potassium-losing diuretics (thiazides and loop diuretics) to preserve K^+ balance. The inclusion of potassium-sparing diuretics in diuretic treatment is an alternative to the use of K^+ supplements with potassium-losing diuretics. Amiloride and triamterene are used in combination with thiazide and loop diuretics to treat edema associated with congestive heart failure and liver disease. One example of such a diuretic combination is 50 mg of triamterene plus 40 mg furosemide contained in one tablet with 0.5 to 2 tablets taken once daily. These drugs are also used in combination with thiazides for the treatment of hypertension (see Ch. 13) but only when hypokalaemia develops.

Eplerenone

Eplerenone is a new, more selective aldosterone antagonist. Its actions in treatment of hypertension in patients with heart failure is described in Chapter 13. Its advantage over spironolactone is that it is more selective for the aldosterone receptor than spironolactone, so produces less sex hormone-related adverse effects (e.g. gynecomastia).

Aldosterone antagonists

These are additionally useful in the treatment of:

- Primary aldosteronism (Conn's syndrome): a tumor of the adrenal gland that secretes large amounts of aldosterone which results in hypertension, hypokalemia and an increase in extracellular fluid. This condition can be managed by dietary Na^+ restriction and spironolactone (100–200 mg daily) although adverse effects limit long-term use of spironolactone (see Table 12.1). Surgical excision of the tumor is the usual treatment.
- Secondary aldosteronism: increased production of aldosterone in response to activation of the renin–angiotensin system that occurs in an accelerated phase of hypertension due to overproduction of renin or as a consequence of edema (see above).
- Chronic heart failure: primarily for extrarenal effects as discussed above and in Chapter 13.

Osmotic diuretics

Osmotic diuretics such as mannitol (given intravenously) and isosorbide (given orally) are freely filtered at the glomerulus and undergo little, if any, reabsorption. These are rare examples of drugs whose action does not involve a particular molecular target but is a general function of their physicochemical properties. Osmotic diuretics increase the osmotic pressure of tubular fluid, thereby reducing the reabsorption of water and lowering luminal Na^+ concentration, with a subsequent decrease in Na^+ reabsorption in the proximal tubule and descending loop of Henle. Osmotic diuretics increase the extracellular fluid volume by increasing water loss from intracellular compartments, and this increase inhibits renin release and decreases blood viscosity, which in turn increase

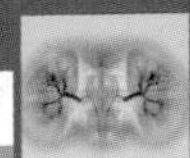

renal blood flow. In addition, renal vasodilation and the subsequent increase in medullary blood flow produced by osmotic diuretics may involve the release of prostaglandins. The increase in medullary blood flow contributes to the overall diuretic effect by reducing medullary hypertonicity. When administered parenterally, mannitol is confined to the extracellular space, only slightly metabolized, and rapidly excreted by the kidney. Approximately 80% of a typical dose appears in the urine within 3 hours. Mannitol is freely filtered by the glomeruli with less than 10% tubular reabsorption; it is not secreted by tubular cells.

CLINICAL INDICATIONS Osmotic diuretics are rarely used because of the greater therapeutic effectiveness of other diuretics. However, they are sometimes used in the treatment of oliguria (see below), but not in the treatment of edema. If given to patients with heart failure, they may cause pulmonary edema as a result of extracting water from intracellular compartments and expanding the extracellular fluid volume. As a result of increasing the osmotic pressure of plasma, osmotic diuretics induce the movement of water out of the eye and brain. Such effects are used in the treatment of acute attacks of glaucoma and in the reduction of a raised intracranial pressure due to cerebral edema. These uses are unrelated to the renal actions of osmotic diuretics, with their useful effects disappearing following filtration in the kidney.

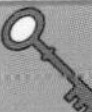

Mechanisms of action of diuretic drugs

- Loop diuretics block the $Na^+/K^+/2Cl^-$ cotransporter in the thick ascending loop of Henle, resulting in the excretion of 15–25% of filtered Na^+
- Thiazide diuretics block the Na^+/Cl^- cotransporter in the distal convoluted tubule, resulting in the excretion of 5% of filtered Na^+
- Potassium-sparing diuretics increase the Na^+ excretion by 2–3% and decrease K^+ excretion by acting on the late distal tubule and collecting duct
- Potassium-sparing diuresis is produced by blockade of luminal Na^+ channels (e.g. with amiloride or triamterene) or by blockade of cytoplasmic mineralocorticosteroid receptors (e.g. with spironolactone)
- Osmotic diuretics reduce water reabsorption, resulting in a subsequent decrease of Na^+ reabsorption in the proximal tubule and descending limb of the loop of Henle
- Carbonic anhydrase inhibitors indirectly block Na^+/H^+ exchange in the proximal tubule, which results in the excretion of up to 5% of Na^+ filtered at the glomerulus

Polyuria

Polyuria is excessive production of a dilute urine and is usually accompanied by polydipsia (increased drinking). The main causes of polyuria are:

- Diabetes mellitus (see Ch. 11).
- Diabetes insipidus, which is caused either by a failure to produce sufficient vasopressin (central diabetes insipidus) or because the collecting ducts fail to respond to vasopressin (nephrogenic diabetes insipidus).

Therapeutic targeting of vasopressin (ADH) receptors in polyuria

Antidiuretic hormone (ADH), also known as 8-arginine vasopressin, is a nonapeptide released from the posterior pituitary in response to increases in plasma osmolality, or reductions in blood volume and/or arterial blood pressure (see Ch. 11). There are two subtypes of receptor for ADH, V_1 and V_2, and both are G protein linked. Stimulation of V_1 receptors produces smooth muscle contraction, particularly of vascular smooth muscle. V_2 receptors mediate the effects of vasopressin on water permeability in the collecting duct. The affinity of V_2 receptors for ADH is greater than that of V_1 receptors and therefore blood pressure responses are seen only at higher doses than those having renal actions.

In addition to ADH itself, other ADH agonists used to treat diabetes insipidus include:

- Lypressin (8 lysine vasopressin): a nonselective agonist with similar potency and duration of action to vasopressin, but administered as a nasal spray.
- Desmopressin (dDVAP, 1-deamino-8-D-arginine-vasopressin) which is approximately 3000 times more selective for V_2 receptors and has a longer duration of action (half-life 75 minutes) than vasopressin (half-life 10 minutes).

ADH acts to increase the number of water channels (aquaporins) in the apical membrane of collecting ducts. This increases the permeability of collecting ducts to water, whereas in its absence the collecting ducts are impermeable to water. Vasopressin binds to V_2 receptors on the basolateral membrane of principal cells of the collecting ducts (see Fig. 12.11). These receptors are positively coupled to adenylyl cyclase and the resultant increase in cAMP activates protein kinase A. By ill-defined mechanisms, protein kinase A-induced protein phosphorylation triggers a shuttling of vesicles, that contain preformed water channels to the apical membrane where there is exocytosis of the vesicles and insertion of the channels into the membrane. A further effect of activation of protein kinase A is to decrease the rate of removal of water channels from the membrane. The overall effect of V_2 receptor activation is an increased number of water channels and increased water permeability. As mentioned above, water channel proteins are called aquaporins and the protein inserted in the apical membrane of the collecting duct is a particular type designated aquaporin-2 (AQP-2). The basolateral membrane also contains water channels to allow movement of water into the interstitium; these channels are of the aquaporin-3 and -4 types (AQP-3 and AQP-4) (see Fig. 12.11).

Desmopressin is the drug of choice for central diabetes insipidus. Administration of desmopressin distinguishes between central and nephrogenic diabetes insipidus. The drug will increase urine osmolality in a patient with central diabetes insipidus but has little or no effect in patients with the nephrogenic form. Desmopressin via nasal spray is the drug of choice for treating central diabetes insipidus and, in most patients, therapy is life-long. A single nasal dose (10–40 μg) lasts 6–20 hours and has no vasoconstrictor effects, unlike arginine vasopressin and lypressin, due to low affinity for V_1 receptors. If nasal administration is not possible, desmopressin can be given by oral or subcutaneous routes.

Lypressin is also administered as a nasal spray but has a short duration of action of 4–6 hours. Since it is a nonselective agonist, lypressin can produce V_1 receptor effects, such as cutaneous vasoconstriction and increased intestinal activity (belching and abdominal cramps). For patients who do not respond to desmopressin, lypressin is a viable alternative.

Arginine vasopressin is not used in long-term treatment due to its short duration of action and V_1 receptor-mediated effects. It is an alternative to desmopressin in the evaluation of patients with suspected diabetes insipidus and for treatment of transient polyuria, when it is administered by i.v. infusion, or subcutaneous or intramuscular injection.

Some patients with polyuria release vasopressin, but in insufficient amounts. Such patients have partial central diabetes insipidus, and are treated with nonhormonal drugs such as chlorpropamide or carbamazepine. Both drugs potentiate the antidiuretic effect of residual vasopressin, but the mechanisms responsible for this action are unclear.

Desmopressin is also effective in treating nocturia, especially in the elderly. The main adverse effect in this situation is hyponatremia.

Nephrogenic (renal) diabetes insipidus is treated with long-acting thiazides and indometacin. In some patients, nephrogenic diabetes insipidus is attributed to mutations of the V_2 receptor or aquaporin-2 and in such cases polyuria of nephrogenic diabetes insipidus can be controlled by long-acting thiazides (e.g. chlorothiazide) alone or in combination with amiloride. Amiloride prevents the development of hypokalemia and is particularly useful in the treatment of lithium-induced nephrogenic diabetes insipidus (see below). The cyclooxygenase inhibitor indomethacin also reduces the polyuria of diabetes insipidus and is used together with thiazide diuretics.

The paradoxical antidiuretic action of thiazides and of indometacin in nephrogenic diabetes insipidus are poorly understood:

- The response to thiazides begins with a reduction in circulating fluid volume. This may increase the oncotic pressure of plasma proteins and reduce the hydrostatic pressure in the peritubular capillaries of the proximal tubule. This would favor Na^+ and water reabsorption in this region of the nephron, with decreased fluid delivery to collecting ducts, and thereby a reduction in polyuria.
- Indometacin can decrease glomerular filtration rate and enhance fluid reabsorption from the proximal and distal tubules. In addition, it potentiates the effect of vasopressin on the collecting duct. Prostaglandins attenuate the effect of vasopressin in the presence of an effective V_2 receptor. Thus, the effects of indometacin are a consequence of inhibition of cyclooxygenase-1 (COX-1).

Diabetes insipidus

- **Is characterized by polyuria**
- **Is due to either decreased production of vasopressin (central diabetes insipidus) or insensitivity to the renal effects of vasopressin (nephrogenic diabetes insipidus)**
- **Central diabetes insipidus is treated with desmopressin (desamino vasopressin)**
- **Nephrogenic diabetes insipidus can be treated with thiazide diuretics**

Syndrome of inappropriate vasopressin secretion

The syndrome due to inappropriate (excess) vasopressin secretion is water retention, hyponatremia and reduced plasma osmolality. Urine osmolality often exceeds that of the plasma. Although plasma Na^+ concentrations are diminished, Na^+ excretion in urine may be normal, and the patient is neither edematous nor dehydrated. The causes of inappropriate (excess) vasopressin secretion include:

- Tumors such as carcinomas of bladder, prostate or pancreas.
- Pulmonary infections such as tuberculosis.
- Head injury.

Treatment of inappropriate vasopressin secretion is with demeclocycline

The tetracycline demeclocycline reduces the action of vasopressin on collecting ducts, an action attributed to inhibition of adenylyl cyclase. The resulting fall in cAMP reduces aquaporin-2 insertion, resulting in decreased water permeability.

Renal stones (nephrolithiasis)

Renal stones develop when poorly soluble substances form crystals in the urine and these aggregate to form stones large enough to lodge within the urinary system. Large stones in the upper urinary tract (renal pelvis and

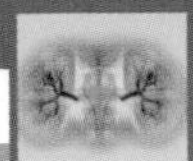

ureter) increase resistance to urine flow, resulting in back pressure that opposes glomerular filtration. Accordingly, prolonged or severe obstruction results in functional impairment of the affected kidney.

Thiazide diuretics prevent renal Ca^{2+} stone formation

Most renal stones are composed of calcium oxalate and/or calcium phosphate. Management consists of removing the stones (by means of surgery or ultrasound) and preventing further stone formation. Thiazide diuretics prevent stone formation because in the long term they diminish urinary excretion of Ca^{2+} (see above) in patients whose stones are caused primarily by impaired renal absorption of Ca^{2+}. A variety of other measures, such as in adjusting diet according to the mechanism of stone formation, may be of great value.

Allopurinol prevents uric acid stone formation

Renal stone disease also results from precipitation of uric acid. Treatment with allopurinol, a xanthine oxidase inhibitor, is beneficial because it reduces urinary uric acid levels and stone formation (see treatment of gout in Ch. 15). Oxalic acid stones can be caused by excess dietary oxalate, pyridoxine (vitamin B_6) deficiency, polyethylene glycol (antifreeze) intoxication, or may arise secondarily to gastrointestinal diseases such as inflammatory bowel disease.

D-penicillamine prevents cystine stone formation

Some rare inherited disorders are associated with stone formation. Cystinuria is an autosomal recessive condition that impairs cystine, ornithine, arginine and lysine transport in the proximal renal tubules. Cystine is less soluble than the other dibasic amino acids and renal stones develop in homozygous individuals. Stone formation can be prevented by D-penicillamine, which, by thiol exchange, reacts with cystine to form a soluble penicillamine–cysteine product. (See Ch. 15 for details on penicillamine.)

Hyperuricemia

One cause of gout is hyperuricemia with sodium urate crystal formation in tissues (see Ch. 15). It can be treated by drugs that facilitate urinary excretion of uric acid (uricosuric drugs). Uric acid excretion is mainly by glomerular filtration with secretion into the proximal tubule. However, the bulk of uric acid in tubular fluid is reabsorbed by countertransport systems in both the apical and basolateral membranes of tubular cells. These exchange urate for either organic or inorganic anions. Uricosuric drugs inhibit the transport of urate across the apical membrane.

The principal uricosuric drugs probenecid and sulfinpyrazone are useful in patients who have a low urine clearance of uric acid. To prevent urate crystallization in the early stage of uricosuric therapy, a high fluid intake (2 L/day) is needed, plus sodium bicarbonate or potassium citrate to produce an alkaline urine (pH ≥6.0). Interestingly, losartan may enhance clearance of uric acid independently of its capacity to block angiotensin II receptors.

ADVERSE EFFECTS Uricosuric drugs are avoided in patients who overproduce uric acid. Paradoxically, uricosuric drugs can cause gout in some patients and hence they are not given during an acute attack.

Probenecid and sulfinpyrazone cause gastrointestinal disturbances and are contraindicated in patients with peptic ulceration. Probenecid blocks renal tubule secretion of organic acid drugs, such as benzylpenicillin, which may prolong their effects and increase the risk of toxicity.

Oliguria

Oliguria is reduced urine volume. In adults, urine output is about 1.5 L/24 h, but in oliguric patients urine volume is inappropriately low, generally less than 400 mL/24 h. When urine production is less than 50 mL/24 h, the patient is said to be anuric.

Oliguria is a clinical feature of acute renal failure

Severe hypoperfusion of the kidneys, acute tubular damage to the tubules, or blockade of the urinary tract can cause acute renal failure. Hypoperfusion of the kidney can be corrected by restoring the effective circulating volume, while obstruction of the urinary tract is rectified by surgery. In both situations, renal function usually returns to normal. If the tubular cells are damaged, oliguria persists for 2–4 weeks before there is recovery and a gradual return to normal renal function in most patients.

No drugs prevent or treat acute renal failure, but mannitol or furosemide can be useful

There are no satisfactory drugs for prevention or treatment of acute renal failure. However, diuretic therapy with either mannitol or furosemide may be of value if intratubular obstruction plays a role in the pathogenesis of renal dysfunction. These drugs increase renal blood flow. The diuresis they evoke helps maintain tubule patency by eliminating debris from the tubule lumen. In order to produce diuresis in acute renal failure, the doses of furosemide may need to be 250 mg daily compared with 20–80 mg used to relieve edema.

Many organs or body systems are adversely affected by acute renal failure and various drugs are used in the management of such secondary effects. For example:

- Antihypertensive drugs for hypertension (see Ch. 13).
- Anticonvulsant drugs for seizures (see Ch. 8).
- H_2 antagonists in preventing gastric ulceration (see Ch. 16).
- Antibacterial drugs, since infections develop in many cases and are a major cause of morbidity and mortality.

Chronic renal failure

Chronic renal failure is deteriorating renal function due to a loss of functioning nephrons and is common to the later stages of all chronic renal disease. Common causes include:

- Severe hypertension.
- Diabetes mellitus.
- Glomerulonephritis.
- Obstruction of the urinary tract.

Drugs are used to treat the symptoms of chronic renal failure

The only effective treatments for chronic renal failure are chronic dialysis or renal transplants. However, some drugs are used to aid management; these include:

- Loop diuretics, to increase urine volume and Na^+ excretion.
- Acetazolamide, to correct metabolic alkalosis associated with the vomiting of renal failure.
- Antihypertensive drugs (see Ch. 13) to control the hypertension associated with chronic renal failure. They reduce the rate of decline in renal function. Angiotensin-converting enzyme (ACE) inhibitors are particularly effective. Most patients with chronic renal failure have hypertension. This can damage the kidneys, leading to proteinuria and hyperfiltration with subsequent loss of glomeruli.
- Antiemetics (see Ch. 8) to control the nausea and vomiting experienced by many patients in late renal failure.
- Recombinant human erythropoietin to treat the anemia that develops following the loss of a major source of erythropoietin from peritubular cells in the renal cortex. Erythropoietin stimulates production of red blood cell precursors in the bone marrow (see Ch. 10).
- Hydroxylated derivatives of vitamin D (1α-hydroxycholecalciferol and 1,25-dihydroxycholecalciferol) to maintain plasma Ca^{2+} and prevent hyperparathyroidism. In chronic renal failure, vitamin D metabolism (see Ch. 11) is abnormal because there is impaired hydroxylation of 25-hydroxycholecalciferol to 1,25-dihydroxycholecalciferol within the kidney. As a result, absorption of dietary Ca^{2+} is reduced and plasma Ca^{2+} is low. Secondary hyperparathyroidism (see Ch. 11) then develops, which can lead to bone disease.

Many drugs should be prescribed with care in those with impaired renal function because of:

- Diminished excretion of drugs primarily excreted via the kidney, may cause drug concentrations to increase dangerously.
- Some drugs are ineffective when renal function deteriorates.
- Impaired health resulting from renal failure lowers the threshold for adverse effects to some drugs.

Examples of such drugs are given in Table 12.4. Nephrotoxic drugs should not be used in patients with renal disease, if possible, because the consequences of nephrotoxicity are likely to be more severe if the functional capacity of the kidney is already limited.

Glomerulonephritis

The term 'glomerulonephritis' describes a range of kidney diseases characterized by inflammatory changes to the glomerulus. Typically, patients with glomerulonephritis exhibit both hematuria and proteinuria, as well as diminished renal function often associated with fluid retention, hypertension and edema. Glomerulonephritis can occur as primary renal disease or result from a systemic disease such as systemic lupus

Table 12.4 Key classes of drugs to be avoided or used with caution in renal failure

Adverse response	Drug	Comment
Increased effects of drug	Opioid analgesics	Morphine and its analogs may produce prolonged central nervous system (CNS) depression and unusual neurologic effects
	Anxiolytics/sedatives	Dosage should be reduced because of increased CNS sensitivity in severe renal failure
Reduced response to drugs	Uricosuric agents	Probenecid and sulfinpyrazone become ineffective
	Antibacterial drugs	Nitrofurantoin and nalidixic acid fail to achieve effective urinary concentrations
Increased risk of toxicity	Cardiac glycosides	Reduced renal excretion of digoxin and increased risk of arrhythmias
	Potassium-sparing diuretics	Aggravation of the hyperkalemia of acute renal failure Potassium supplements are also contraindicated
	Antibacterial drugs	Increased risk of peripheral neuropathy with isoniazid and nitrofurantoin
Adverse effects poorly tolerated	Biguanide antihypoglycemics	Metformin increases the risk of lactic acidosis
	Tetracyclines	Tetracyclines (except doxycycline and minocycline) inhibit protein synthesis and induce a catabolic effect that results from increased metabolism of amino acids. This may aggravate renal failure

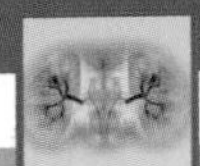

erythematosus (Ch. 15). Causes of primary glomerulonephritis can be unclear but may occur subsequent to bacterial or viral infections.

Drugs are used to slow the progression of glomerulonephritis

Drug treatment of glomerulonephritis is similar to that in nephrotic syndrome (see above). There are no drug therapies effective in every form of glomerulonephritis, but in some patients preservation or an improvement in renal function can be achieved with:

- Antihypertensive drugs to control blood pressure. ACE inhibitors such as captopril are the drugs of choice because they decrease intraglomerular pressure and proteinuria.
- Thiazides or loop diuretics to reduce fluid retention.
- Immunosuppression with either glucocorticosteroids alone, or in combination with cytotoxic drugs such as cyclophosphamide.

Dialysis and drug therapy

Dialysis may complicate drug therapy

Dialysis separates diffusible solutes from less diffusible ones by the semipermeable membranes in dialysis equipment. The technique is used for end-stage renal disease to remove waste products and excess water from the body. Furthermore, dialysis is a useful adjunct in the management of overdose and poisoning.

There are two types of dialysis:

- Hemodialysis, where blood is passed through a system containing dialysis solution separated from blood by a semipermeable membrane.
- In peritoneal dialysis, the dialysis solution is given into the peritoneal cavity. In this case, peritoneal tissues act as the semipermeable membrane.

In both techniques, solutes diffuse from blood into the dialysis fluid.

Dialysis complicates drug therapy because drug is cleared from blood not only by the body's own elimination mechanisms but also by the dialysis. If clearance by dialysis significantly contributes to drug elimination, it may be necessary to give supplementary doses of drug.

The clearance of drugs by dialysis depends upon the nature of the dialysis technique, the fraction of drug unbound in blood and its molecular size. Hemodialysis clears drugs more efficiently than peritoneal dialysis. Accordingly, it is the method of choice in drug overdose or poisoning. Only unbound drug contributes to the concentration gradient that drives diffusion from blood into the dialysis fluid. With a high degree of plasma protein binding, clearance by dialysis is limited. Most drugs are small enough to diffuse readily across either artificial or endogenous tissue membranes.

Nephrotoxic drugs

The kidney's central role in removal of drugs (plus metabolites) makes it susceptible to adverse drug effects. Renal tissue is exposed to drug in both blood and the renal tubule. Concentrations in tubules can be much higher than in the blood and consequently more toxic. Many nephrotoxic drugs have their primary effects on discrete parts of the nephron. This results from factors such as regional differences in transport characteristics, cellular energetics, repair mechanisms and capacity to bioactivate or detoxify potential toxins. The reasons for the selective renal toxicity of some drugs are still to be elucidated. The sites of action of some nephrotoxic drugs are shown in Figure 12.12.

Certain antimicrobial drugs may have nephrotoxicity

The aminoglycosides, amphotericin B and some first-generation cephalosporins are nephrotoxic. The order of such drugs, in terms of toxicity, is gentamicin, tobramycin, amikacin and netilmicin.

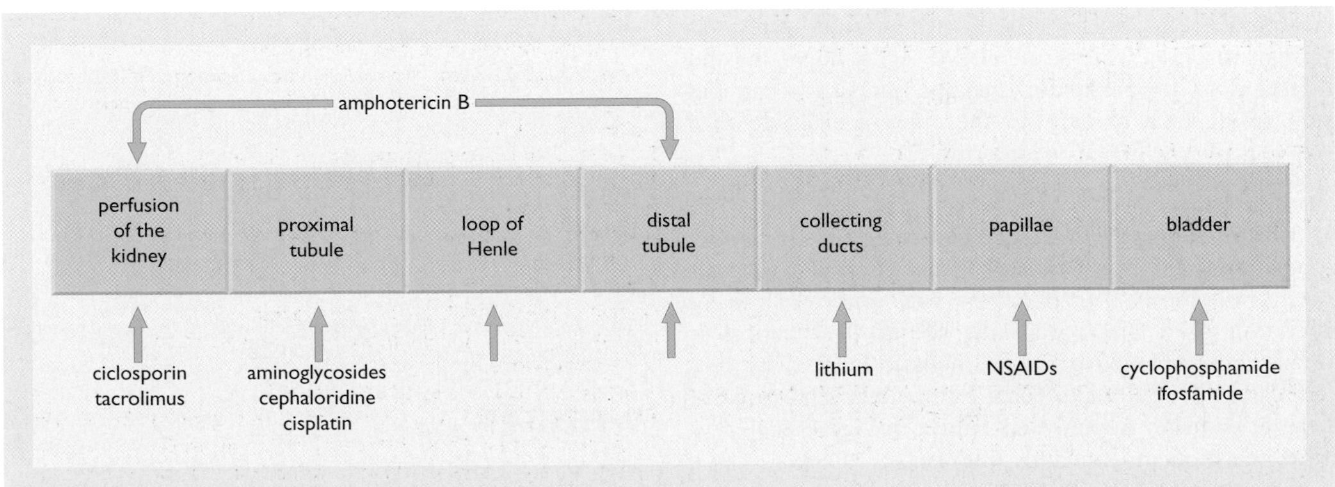

Fig. 12.12 Primary renal sites of action of some nephrotoxic drugs.

Aminoglycosides are important in the treatment of severe Gram-negative infections, but 10–15% of patients develop acute renal failure. The primary site of injury is the proximal tubule.

The systemic antifungal drug amphotericin B is nephrotoxic and up to 80% of patients given amphotericin B develop impaired renal function. This drug causes renal vasoconstriction, and although several regions of the nephron are damaged, the primary site of toxicity is the distal tubule.

Some first-generation cephalosporins (cephaloridine and cephalothin) are potentially nephrotoxic, but are not so toxic as aminoglycosides and amphotericin B.

Antineoplastic drugs

Anticancer alkylating agents and platinum derivatives can cause renal damage

Nephrotoxicity is prominent with alkylating agents. Cyclophosphamide and ifosfamide cause release of acrolein, a nephrotoxic compound that induces hemorrhagic cystitis. This can be prevented by the simultaneous administration of mesna (2-mercaptoethane sulfonate), which reacts with acrolein, rendering it nontoxic in the urinary tract.

Cisplatin, and to a lesser degree carboplatin, are also nephrotoxic. Cisplatin-induced injury mainly affects the straight portion of the proximal tubule. To minimize renal damage due to these drugs, it is routine to hydrate the patient with an infusion of 1–2 L of saline before drug administration.

Cell destruction with antineoplastic drugs releases large amounts of purines. Catabolism of purines leads to excessive urate formation and excretion and an increased risk of renal stone formation and hyperuricemic gout.

Immunosuppressant drugs

Ciclosporin and tacrolimus can cause renal damage

The nephropathy due to ciclosporin and tacrolimus is unique since both drugs adversely affect renal vasculature. Ciclosporin usually causes acute reversible impairment of renal function early after beginning treatment. This is associated with afferent arteriolar vasoconstriction, which can be reversed by dopamine and nifedipine. Chronic nephrotoxicity can also occur and may result from damage to the afferent arteriole with sclerosis of downstream glomeruli.

Analgesics

Acetaminophen and NSAIDs can cause renal damage

Acute renal failure as a result of acute tubular necrosis occurs in about 2% of cases with an overdose of acetaminophen (paracetamol). Renal dysfunction is usually accompanied by severe hepatic failure, but in a few cases there is acute renal failure in the absence of hepatic damage. Acute renal failure occurs several days after ingestion and is mainly oliguric.

Chronic NSAID-induced nephropathy is characterized by interstitial nephritis and renal papillary necrosis. Renal damage results from long-term ingestion of NSAIDs and is unusual in patients under 30 years of age. It occurs mainly in women aged 40–60 years. The loss of papillary tissue may lead to secondary nephron damage and eventually to impaired renal function.

Lithium can cause renal damage

A minority of patients treated with lithium for affective disorders develop nephrogenic diabetes insipidus, which usually reverses on stopping the drug. The mechanism is a reduction in V_2 receptor-mediated stimulation of adenylyl cyclase by vasopressin. Amiloride can be used to reverse lithium-induced diabetes insipidus by inhibiting reabsorption of lithium through Na^+ channels in the collecting ducts.

Some drugs cause acute interstitial nephritis

Many drugs can lead to an acute deterioration of renal function by causing inflammation of the renal interstitium (acute interstitial nephritis), possibly due to a hypersensitivity reaction. Such drugs include:

- Penicillins.
- Sulfonamides (including co-trimoxazole).
- NSAIDs.
- Diuretics (thiazides and furosemide).
- Allopurinol.
- Cimetidine.

Patients often have an accompanying fever, skin rash and hematuria.

FURTHER READING

Carter BL, Ernst ME, Cohen JD. Hydrochlorothiazide versus chlorthalidone: evidence supporting their interchangeability. *Hypertension* 2004; **43**: 4–9. [Nuanced discussion of the clinical pharmacology and therapeutics of two important diuretics.]

Casas JP, Chua W, Loukogeorgakis S, Vallance P, Smeeth L, Hingorani AD, MacAllister RJ. Effect of inhibitors of the renin-angiotensin system and other antihypertensive drugs on renal outcomes: systematic review and meta-analysis. *Lancet* 2005; **366**: 2026–2033. [An attempt to provide a clear view of the interactions of antihypertensive drugs on kidney functioning.]

Cretkovic RS, Plasker GL. Desmopressin. *Drugs* 2005; **65**: 99–107. [Pharmacokinetics and dynamics of desmopressin.]

Kote CJ. *Principles of Renal Physiology*, 4th edn. Dordrecht, The Netherlands: Kluwer Academic; 2000. [A clear and concise introduction to renal physiology.]

Pattison JM. A colour handbook of renal medicine. London: Manson Pub., 2004.

Subramanian S, Ziedalski TM. Oliguria, volume overload, Na+ balance, and diuretics. *Crit Care Clin* 2005; **21**: 291–303. [A basic primer for understanding sodium and water balance and its adjustment.]

Wilson WC, Aronson S. Oliguria. A sign of renal success or impending renal failure? *Anesthesiol Clin N Am* 2001; **19**: 841–883.

WEBSITES

http://www.healthinsite.gov.topics/Kidney_and_Urinary_Tract_Diseases [This website provides general information regarding renal disorders.]

http://www.merck.com/mrkshared/mmanual/sections.jsp [Merck Manual.]

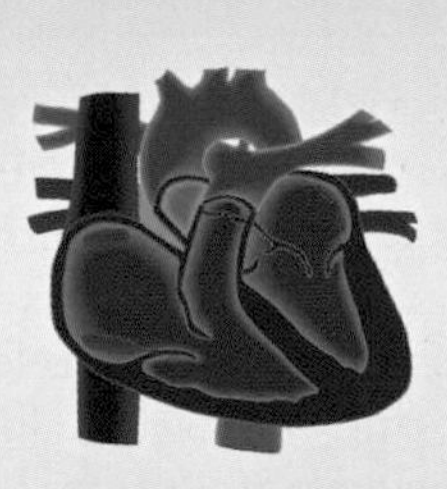

Chapter 13

Drugs and the Cardiovascular System

PHYSIOLOGY OF THE CARDIOVASCULAR SYSTEM

The cardiovascular system consists of the heart and blood vessels

The cardiovascular system ensures a blood supply that maintains optimal environments for body tissues by supplying oxygen and nutrients, and removing waste products. The normal partial pressures of oxygen and carbon dioxide in oxygenated arterial blood are:

- pO_2 100 mmHg.
- pCO_2 40 mmHg.

The resting human heart rate is approximately 70 beats/min, pumping approximately 5 L/min of blood. The adult heart weighs approximately 300 g. It has four chambers: two smaller ones, located towards the base called the atria, and two larger ones, located towards the apex, called ventricles (Fig. 13.1). The wall of the heart chambers has three layers: the epicardium (outer layer), the mid-myocardium (the middle layer) and the endocardium (the inner layer).

Cardiac valves ensure that blood flows in one direction. The right atrium and ventricle receive deoxygenated blood from the body, and pump it via the pulmonary artery to the lungs. The left atrium and ventricle receive the re-oxygenated blood via the pulmonary veins and pump it out through the aorta to the rest of the body. The location and names of the valves are shown in Figure 13.1.

> **Heart valves**
>
> - **Valves prevent backward flow of blood through the heart**
> - **Atrioventricular valves are between atria and ventricles**
> - **Backflow into arteries is prevented by semilunar valves**
> - **Artificial valves can replace valves damaged by diseases such as rheumatic fever**

Vascular tree

The body's vascular system (vascular tree) has two main types of blood vessels, namely arteries and veins. Both are lined with endothelial cells which are in contact with the blood. The endothelium is more than a simple barrier between the blood and the surrounding vessel, as it releases many important vasoactive substances such as nitric oxide (NO) that affect vessel diameter and blood clotting, thereby locally regulating blood flow (Fig. 13.2).

Typical resting systolic/diastolic blood pressure is 120/80 mmHg, although there are differences among subpopulations (e.g. values are often lower in females). Blood pressure is proportional to the output of the heart (cardiac output) and resistance to flow in arterioles. Resistance depends on vessel caliber, elasticity and

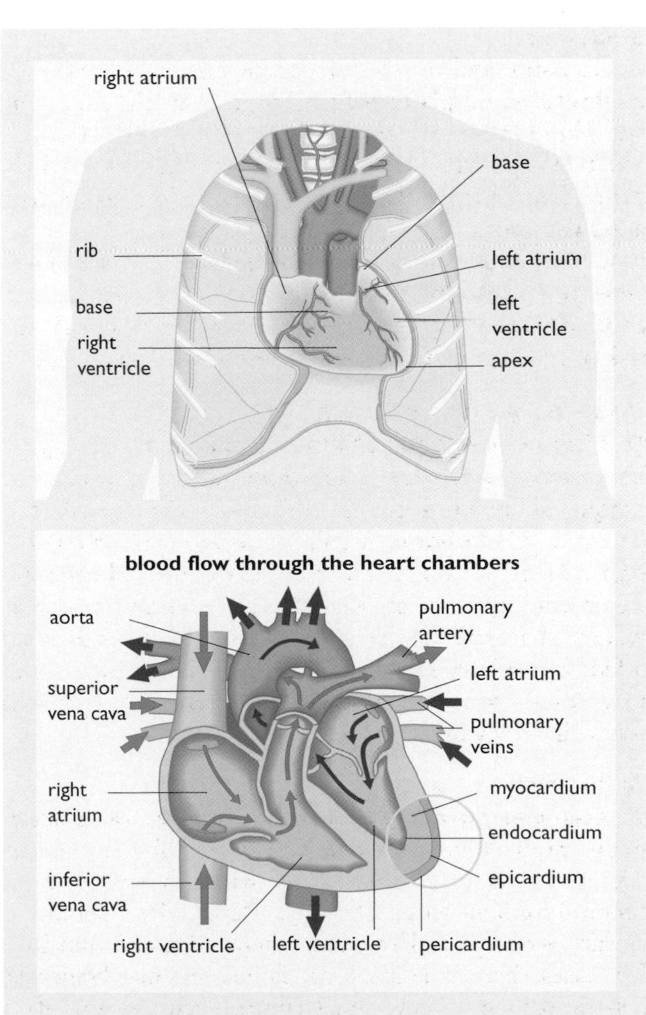

Fig. 13.1 The heart consists of four chambers and is located in the chest cavity. The circulation of blood flow through the heart is shown.

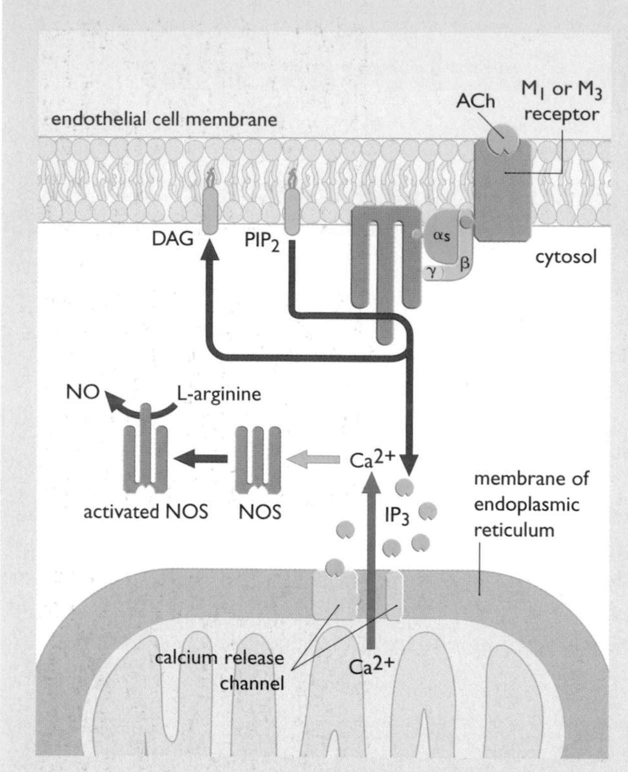

Fig. 13.2 Example of release of vasoactive substance (here, nitric oxide) from endothelium. Acetylcholine (ACh), bradykinin, thrombin, serotonin, shear stress, and other substances can release nitric oxide (NO). ACh utilizes numerous intermediates in the cellular response that ultimately facilitates nitric oxide release (DAG, diacylglycerol; NOS, nitric oxide synthase; IP_3, inositol-1,4,5-triphosphate; PIP_2, phosphatidylinositol).

geometry, and blood viscosity. Arterial blood pressure is expressed as systolic pressure/diastolic pressure. Peak blood pressure occurs during systole as the left ventricle contracts and pumps blood into the aorta. The trough occurs during diastole when the left ventricle relaxes and fills with blood returning to the heart (Fig. 13.3). Mean pressures range from approximately 90 mmHg in arteries, to about 5 mmHg in major central veins. Blood pressure is intermediate in the capillaries that connect arterioles and venules.

Nutrients and metabolites leave and enter the vasculature through capillary membranes. Regulation of blood flow by alteration of blood vessel diameter is complex. Each vascular bed has its own properties. Some are regulated by autonomic nerves (e.g. skin) while others are autoregulated (e.g. heart and skeletal muscle). Autoregulation involves the local release of vasoactive substances such as NO from the endothelium. Cardiac muscle and vascular smooth muscle share common features but in addition have differences that are vital to their function, as will be explained.

Cardiac electrophysiology

- ***Normal beating starts as a result of spontaneous depolarization (pacemaker activity) in specialized cells in the sinoatrial node***

The sinoatrial (SA) node in humans at rest (Fig. 13.4) rhythmically generates impulses at a rate of approximately 70 beats/min, a rate that is faster than in any other region of the heart. The node is innervated by autonomic nerves; release of acetylcholine from the vagus

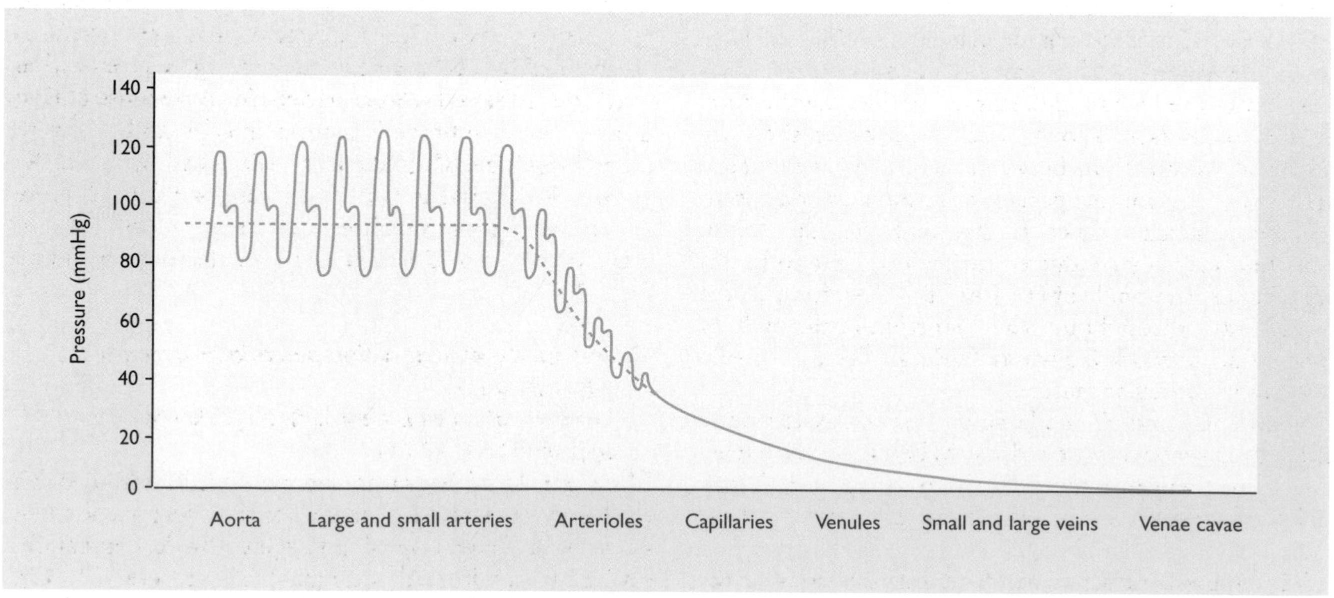

Fig. 13.3 Blood pressure in various blood vessel types. Systolic and diastolic blood pressures are shown, as well as mean arterial pressure. (Adapted from *Principles of Anatomy and Physiology*, 8th edn. by Tortora and Grabowski.)

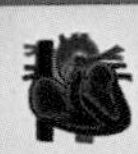

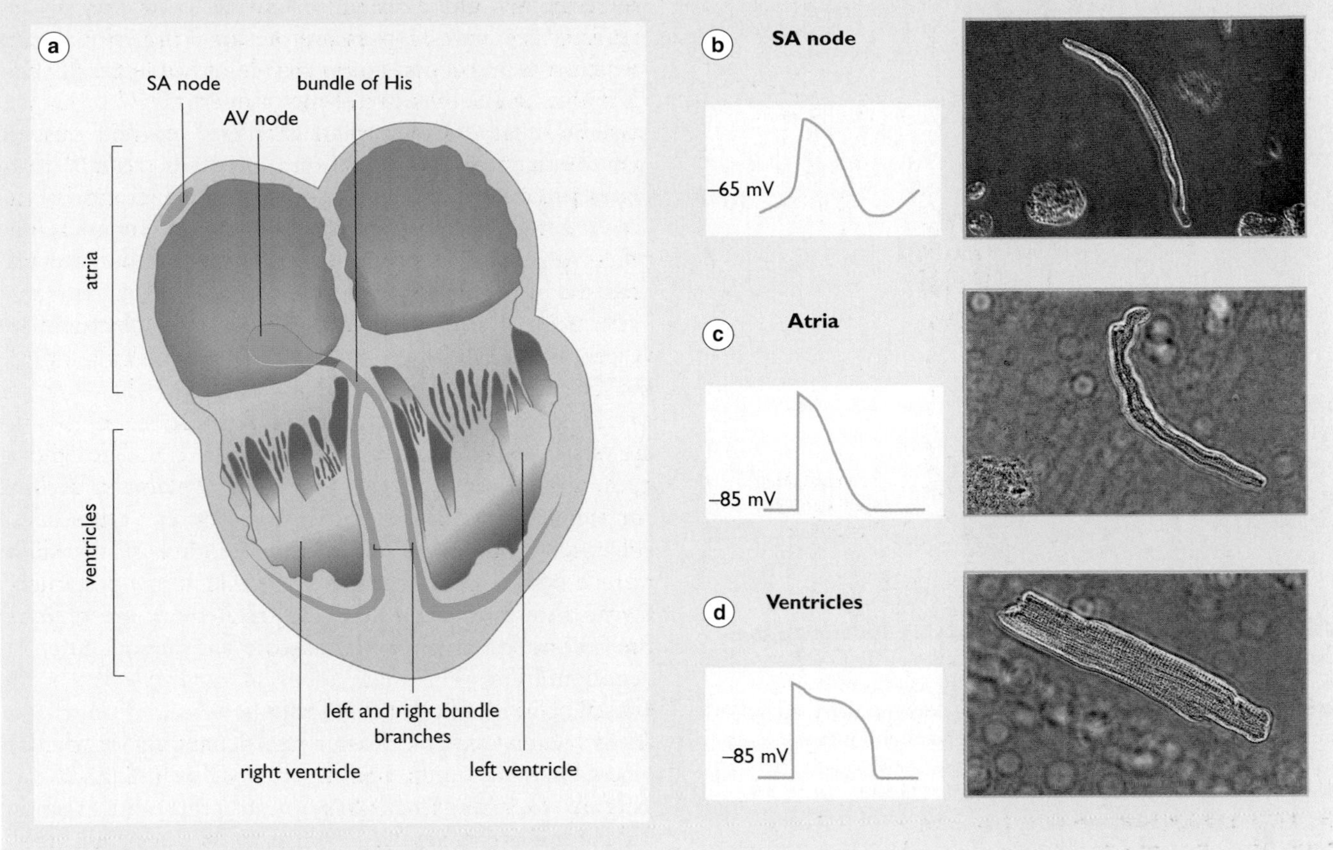

Fig. 13.4 Regional variation in cell structure and action potential configuration throughout the heart. Action potential from different heart regions are quite different due to differences in the ion channels that underlie action potentials in these regions. (a) Location of the sinoatrial (SA) node, the atrioventricular (AV) node and the bundle of His. (b) An action potential from the SA node and an SA node cell. (Courtesy of Dr. Hilary F. Brown.) (c) An action potential from the atria and an atrial cell. (d) An action potential from the ventricles and a ventricular cell.

nerve decreases the rate while norepinephrine increases it. The SA node action potential activates atrial cells, which then conduct the impulse to the atrioventricular (AV) node. Conduction is delayed at the AV node for about 70 milliseconds (msec) because of the small diameter of the fibers and the nature of the ionic currents in these cells (see below). The AV node is the only electrical connection between atria and ventricles; therefore it controls the passage of action potentials from atria to ventricles. Once in the ventricle, the action potential is rapidly conducted through the left and right branches of the bundle of His (see Fig. 13.4), from where it spreads throughout the ventricles through a conduction network known as Purkinje fibers to finally reach the ventricular muscle.

Ventricular and SA node action potentials are quite different in shape (height and width) because the currents that cause them (produced by the opening and closing of ion channels) are not exactly the same (Figs 13.4–, 13.6).

The unequal distribution of K^+ and Na^+ ions across ventricular and atrial cell membranes results in resting (diastolic) membrane potentials ranging from –65 in SA node cells to –90 mV in ventricles. In SA and AV nodal cells, diastolic membrane potential is unstable and the value it attains is more positive than that in atrial or ventricular cells. Resting membrane potential is determined by a K^+ gradient due to a high concentration of K^+ inside the cell relative to outside and because during diastole the membrane is more permeable to K^+ than to other ions. The K^+ gradient is maintained by a Na^+/K^+ pump (also known as Na^+/K^+ ATPase, see Ch. 12). The Na^+/K^+ pump moves three Na^+ ions out of cells in exchange for two K^+ ions (i.e. it is an electrogenic pump, Fig. 13.7).

Sodium-dependent action potential is generated when an atrial or ventricular cell is depolarized quickly to approximately –70 mV

The upstroke of the action potential (see Fig. 13.6) is due to the opening of Na^+ channels with voltage-dependent gates, with channel opening triggered by depolarization, giving rise to inward movement of Na^+ (see Ch. 12). Opening of Na^+ channels is transient and, if the membrane remains depolarized for more than a few

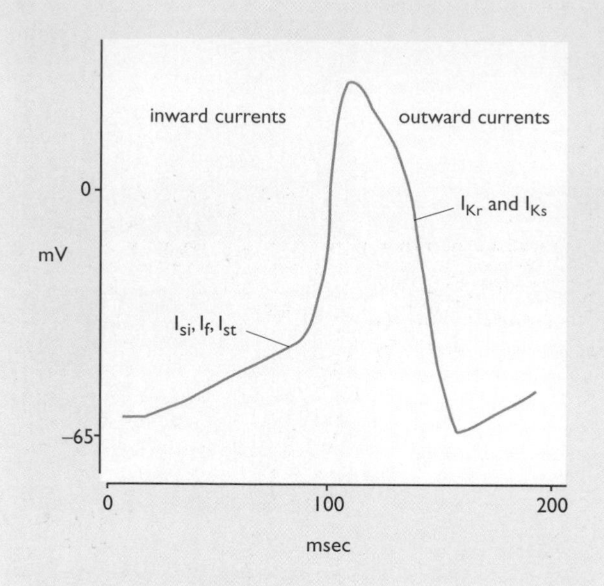

Fig. 13.5 Ion channels and currents (I) underlying the sinoatrial node action potential (I_{si}, an inward current carried by Ca^{2+} ions; I_f, 'funny' or hyperpolarization-activated cation current that may have a role in pacemaking and is carried by Na^+ and Ca^{2+} ions; I_{st}, the sustained inward Na^+ current that may be important in pacemaker activity; I_{Kr} and I_{Ks} rapid kinetics delayed rectifier K^+ current and slow which is an outward current; note that there is no I_{Na} (inward Na^+ current) or I_{K1} (inward rectifier K^+ current).

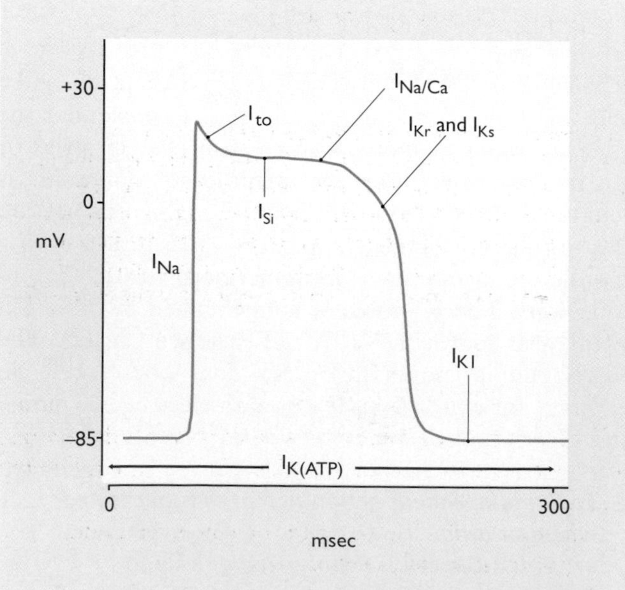

Fig. 13.6 Configuration of a typical ventricular action potential showing the activation of the most important ionic currents (I_{Na}, fast inward Na^+ current; I_{si}, slow inward Ca^{2+} current; I_{to}, transient outward K^+ current; I_{Kr} and I_{Ks}, rapid and slow kinetics delayed rectifier K^+ currents; I_{K1}, inward rectifier K^+ current; $I_{K(ATP)}$, ATP-sensitive K^+ current; note, the last of these is activated only during ischemia or hypoxia).

milliseconds, the channel inactivates and the inward current terminates. Inactivation results in a period during which a second action potential cannot be triggered. This is known as the effective refractory period.

The characteristic plateau phase of the cardiac ventricular and atrial action potentials results from opening of L-type Ca^{2+} channels and the operation of the Na^+/Ca^{2+} exchanger (see later). L-type Ca^+ channels, like the Na^+ channels, are voltage dependent, but the Ca^+ current has a much slower time course. The currents that arise from the opening of Na^+ and Ca^{2+} channels are therefore specifically referred to as:

- The fast inward Na^+ current (I_{Na}).
- The slow inward Ca^{2+} current (I_{Ca} or I_{si}).

During the depolarization phase of the action potential, other voltage-dependent channels become activated, particularly a variety of different types of K^+ channel. These carry K^+ ions in the outward direction, which causes repolarization of the membrane potential.

As shown partially in Figure 13.4 there are regional variations in cardiac cell structure and action potential configuration. The main types of cardiac cell are the nodal cells, atrial cells, His/Purkinje cells and ventricular cells (which vary in characteristics depending on whether located in the mid-, endo-, or epicardium). As shown Figure 13.4, these cells vary in structure and function. Some cells (e.g. ventricular) are rod-shaped and highly striated, whereas others (e.g. SA node cells) are plate-like and poorly striated. Only certain cells (SA and AV node and His/Purkinje) depolarize spontaneously.

Cardiac K^+ currents

- **Delayed rectifier current (I_K), which is activated by depolarization and has two components (r and s)**
- **Transient outward current (I_{to}) which causes the initial repolarization phase, referred to as the 'notch' of the action potential, which is important in some, but not all, regions of the heart**
- **Inward rectifier current (I_{K1}), with a main role of stabilizing the resting membrane potential**
- **ATP-sensitive current ($I_{K(ATP)}$), which is blocked by basal levels of ATP, and is therefore important when ATP is reduced (e.g. in disease conditions such as ischemia)**

Excitation is coupled to contraction in atria and ventricles

One of the most important events in the cardiac action potential is the voltage-dependent opening of L-type Ca^{2+} channels (see Ch. 3 and Fig. 13.6). This leads to a relatively small inward movement of Ca^{2+} ions across the sarcolemmal membrane, which in turn activates a process known as Ca^{2+}-induced Ca^{2+} release, whereby a much larger amount of Ca^{2+} is released from intracellular stores (especially the sarcoplasmic reticulum). As a result, intracellular Ca^{2+} rises from 100 nM in diastole to 10 μM

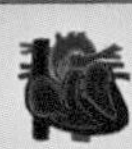

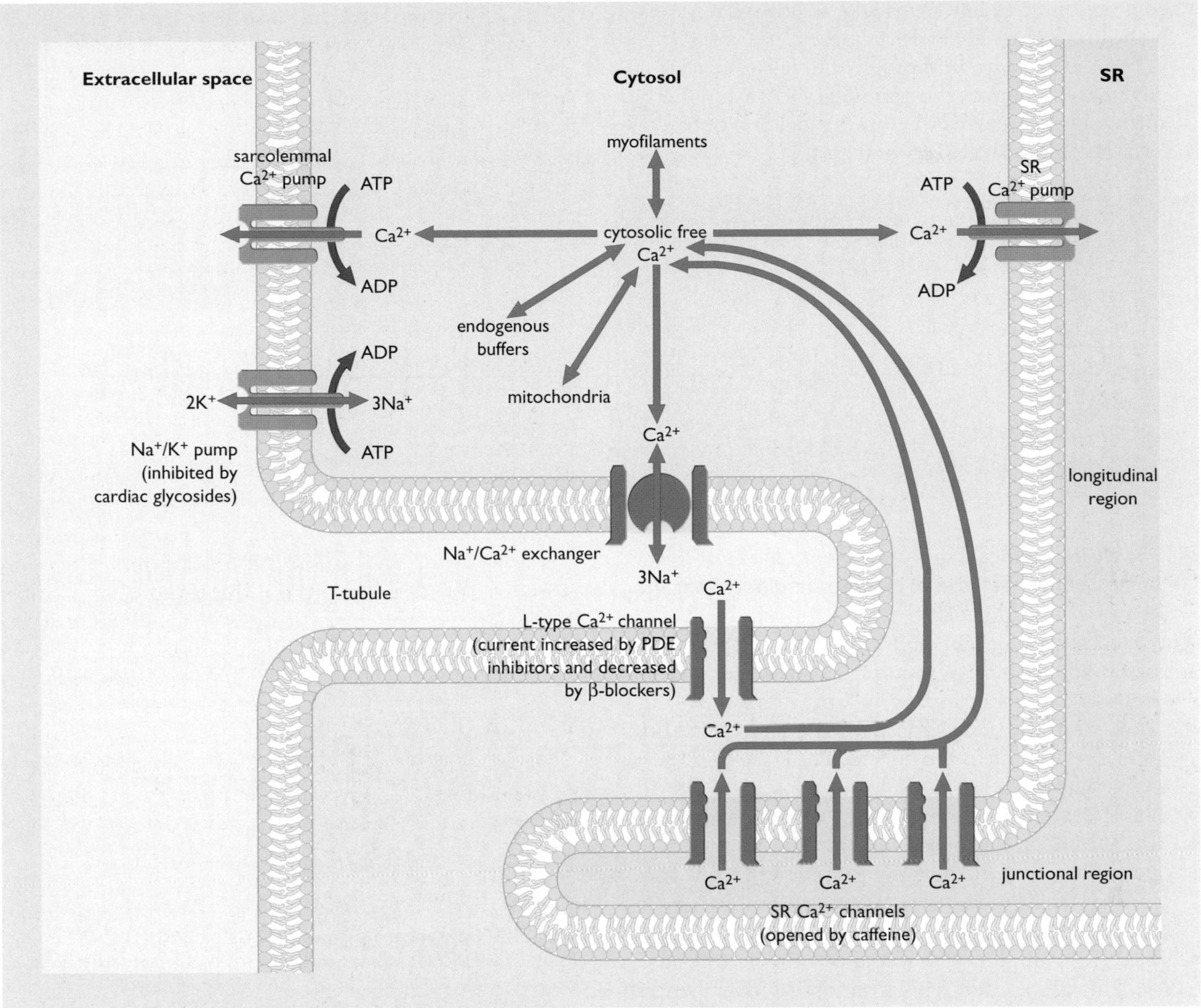

Fig. 13.7 Ion transport pathways in the heart, focusing on Ca^{2+} movements during the cardiac cycle. Membrane depolarization at the start of the action potential is the trigger for the opening of Ca^{2+} channels which span the cells surface membrane (the sarcolemma). The local increase in Ca^{2+} concentration in the interior of the cell (cytosol) causes further release of Ca^{2+} from the intracellular stores (sarcoplasmic reticulum; SR). Some Ca^{2+} may also enter the cell via the Na^+/Ca^{2+} exchanger. Once inside the cytosol, Ca^{2+} is bound to buffers, which include the inner surface of the sarcolemma and the contractile machinery (myofilaments; not shown functioning in this mode), which are activated by the presence of Ca^{2+}, leading to contraction. At the end of the action potential, Ca^{2+} leaves the cell by the Na^+/Ca^{2+} exchanger and the ATP-dependent sarcolemmal Ca^{2+} pump, and is also taken up again into the SR by ATP-dependent Ca^{2+} pumps (PDE, phosphodiesterase).

during systole. As the cytosolic Ca^{2+} concentration rises, Ca^{2+} binds to troponin C, which regulates the position of actin and myosin filaments, causing them to ratchet past one another, leading to contraction.

After contraction, Ca^{2+} is re-sequestered into the stores by an adenosine triphosphate (ATP)-dependent Ca^{2+} pump, whereupon it is ready to take part in the next cycle. In addition, Ca^{2+} is extruded from the cell during diastole via the electrogenic Na^+/Ca^{2+} exchanger. Figure 13.7 shows schematically how cellullar Ca^{2+} is controlled, as well as how drugs may modulate the processes involved.

The sequence of electro-mechanical events during one heart beat, the cardiac cycle, takes place in the following order:

- Generation of an impulse in the sinoatrial node.
- Depolarization of the atria.
- Right atrial contraction and generation of pressure which ejects blood through the open tricuspid valve into the right ventricle.
- Left atrial contraction and generation of pressure which ejects blood through the open mitral valve into the left ventricle.
- After a short interval, ventricular depolarization and

contraction, with left ventricular contraction preceding right ventricular contraction.
- When the pressure in the right and left ventricles increases, this opens the pulmonary valve and the aortic valve, respectively, allowing ejection of blood into the pulmonary artery and aorta.

Pharmacologic tools used to block ion currents experimentally

- Tetrodotoxin to block I_{Na}
- Nicardipine to block I_{si}
- 4-Aminopyridine to block I_{to}
- Dofetilide to block I_{Kr}
- Barium to block I_{K1}
- Glyburide to block $I_{K(ATP)}$

The electrocardiogram is a recording made at the body surface of electrical changes resulting from the heart's electrical activity

The electrocardiogram (ECG or EKG) records the average body potential resulting from depolarizations and repolarizations occurring in cardiac myocytes. It is recorded from the body surface using contact electrodes.

An understanding of the normal EKG (see Fig. 13.8) is essential. The sequence of events in the normal EKG is:
- The P wave, which results from atrial depolarization.
- The PR interval, which is timed from the beginning of the P wave to the beginning of the QRS complex. It is equivalent to the time taken for the wave of depolarization to pass through the AV node.
- The QRS complex, which results from ventricular depolarization; atrial repolarization is hidden beneath this large complex.
- The T wave, which results from ventricular repolarization.
- The ST segment is the interval between the QRS complex and the T wave. Its position above or below the baseline is characteristically changed during ischemic heart disease (so-called elevation or depression of the ST segment).
- The QT interval is the time from the start of the QRS complex to the end of the T wave and is equivalent to the time taken for the wave of depolarization and repolarization to pass through the ventricles

PATHOPHYSIOLOGY AND DISEASES OF THE HEART

Arrhythmias

Arrhythmia literally means no rhythm, whereas dysrhythmia means abnormal rhythm. In practice, both terms are used interchangeably to mean an abnormal or irregular heart beat, with 'arrhythmia' favored in the USA. There are many pathologic causes of arrhythmias,

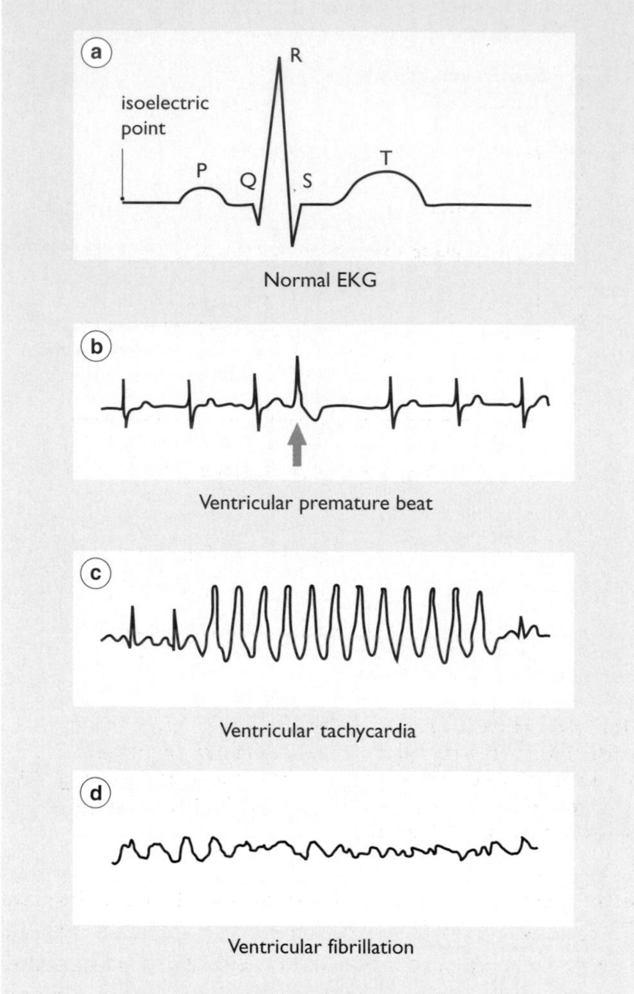

Fig. 13.8 Electrocardiograms (EKGs or ECGs). (a) The normal EKG. (b) Ventricular premature beats. (c) Ventricular tachycardia. (d) Ventricular fibrillation. In (a), the P wave represents depolarization of atria, the QRS is depolarization of the ventricles and the T wave, is repolarization of the ventricles. Arrhythmias are manifest as abnormalities in the configuration of the EKG.

Causes of cardiac arrhythmias

- AMI (acute ischemia and subsequent necrosis/apoptosis).
- Heart failure (hypertrophy, high preload and diastolic myocardial stretch).
- Hyperthyroidism (fully reversible when euthyroid).
- Hypokalemia (especially in anorexia nervosa).
- Autonomic dysfunction (including pheochromocytoma).
- Drugs (including many antiarrhythmic drugs).
- Inherited mutations of cardiac ion channels (e.g. inherited long QT syndromes).
- Fever.

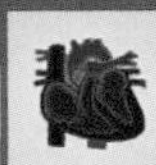

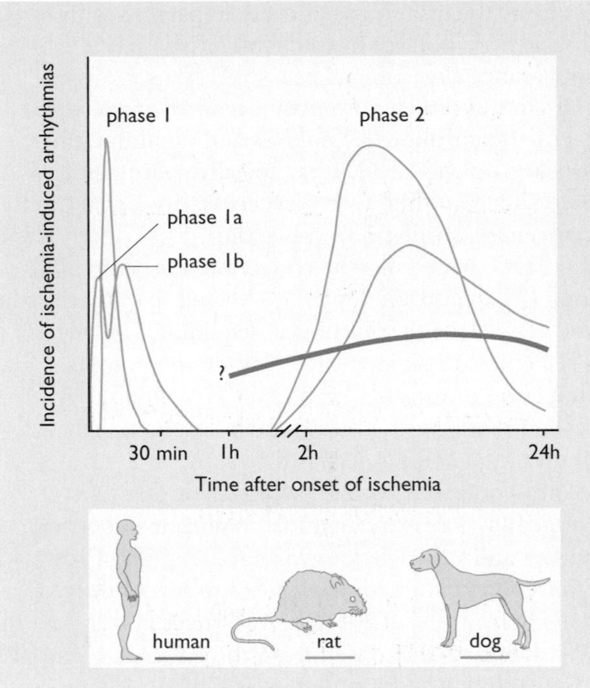

Fig. 13.9 Time course of arrhythmias during AMI. The characteristics of arrhythmias in AMI in the human are clear. Time course of lethal ventricular arrhythmias in the hours following AMI. Although there are data from animal models, there is very little accurate data for the human.

such as acute myocardial infarction (AMI; see p. 396 and Ch. 11). Additionally, arrhythmias may occur as adverse effects of therapeutic drugs, paradoxically including many antiarrhythmic drugs. During cardiac ischemia/infarction arrhythmias occur with a characteristic time course (Fig. 13.9).

Arrhythmias may be classified according to their anatomic origin:

- Supraventricular (originating in the SA node, atria or AV node).
- Ventricular (originating in the ventricles).

Arrhythmias vary in their importance. Arrhythmias range from the innocuous (some supraventricular arrhythmias) to the life-threatening (i.e. asystole and some fast ventricular arrhythmias). Lethal ventricular arrhythmias are the most common cause of death in the USA and in other economically developed countries, with around 350 000 such deaths every year in the USA alone. Sudden cardiac death (death without prior symptoms, or symptoms of less than 30 minutes duration) is primarily due to lethal ventricular arrhythmias: ventricular fibrillation (most commonly) or asystole (in a minority of cases). Sudden cardiac death often occurs without warning, and almost always out of hospital.

Acute myocardial infarction is an important cause of serious ventricular arrhythmias

Acute myocardial infarction (AMI) is a clinical syndrome comprising myocardial ischemia (lack of blood flow in part of the heart) leading to myocyte necrosis (infarction) or apoptosis. It occurs when, for example, a coronary artery becomes obstructed by a clot (thrombus) or a dissecting aneurysm. As a result of the obstruction, insufficient blood reaches the myocardium to meet the tissues' needs for oxygen and nutrients, and removal of metabolic waste. The causes of arrhythmias in AMI are not clear. Possibilities include accumulation of extracellular K^+ (which causes diastolic depolarization and abnormal repolarization) and cyclic adenosine monophosphate (cAMP) which may trigger spontaneous action potentials.

Reperfusion, which means readmission of blood supply to the previously ischemic region, is essential if the tissue is to recover and infarction is to be avoided. Early reperfusion, especially after a brief period of ischemia, can itself cause arrhythmias, and this is sometimes used as an indication of successful therapeutic reperfusion.

Ischemia

- **Ischemia resulting from a reduced blood flow is associated with contractile failure, EKG abnormalities and chest pain**
- **Silent ischemia is characterized by contractile failure and EKG abnormalities without chest pain**
- **Myocardial infarction occurs if sustained ischemia results in myocardial cell death**
- **Stunning is a reversible impairment of cardiac or vascular function that is detectable during the first few hours or days after the start of reperfusion**
- **Hibernating myocardium occurs if the myocardial function is depressed during relative ischemia. It preserves energy substrates, thereby aiding recovery when reperfusion occurs**
- **Preconditioning is caused by a short period of ischemia and describes the resulting protection (from arrhythmias, infarction and contractile dysfunction) afforded to the heart against the effects of a longer period of ischemia**

Arrhythmis are diagnosed according to their EKG characteristics

Diagnosis of arrhythmias (see Fig. 13.8) depends on the appearance of the EKG:

- A flat-line EKG indicates asystole.
- SA nodal arrhythmias are associated with a normal EKG configuration, but an abnormal heart rate (fast or slow), and are often asymptomatic.
- Atrial premature beats appear on the EKG as abnormally timed P waves and are often asymptomatic.
- In atrial flutter, the atria beat rapidly (>300 beats/min) and partial AV block occurs (resulting from the inability of the normal AV node to conduct each atrial beat). Thus not every atrial beat is conducted to the ventricles. In the EKG, the P waves are

repetitive. Atrial flutter is relatively common in the elderly.

- In atrial fibrillation, the atria beat asynchronously so that the active pumping function is impaired. In the EKG, the P waves are generally not identifiable. Atrial fibrillation is common in the elderly and in people with mitral valve disease.
- Paroxysmal supraventricular tachycardia is an arrhythmia originating in the AV node. It can result from retrograde conduction through the node and can cause tachycardia in the atria. In itself this is not life-threatening but it can become so if it sustains a dangerously rapid ventricular rate.
- Ventricular premature beats (VPBs; Fig. 13.8b) are sometimes referred to as ventricular ectopic beats, and are defined as discrete and identifiable premature QRS complexes (usually of an abnormal shape). They are common in AMI.
- Ventricular tachycardia (Fig. 13.8c) is defined as consecutive VPBs (a minimum of at least two). Sustained ventricular tachycardia may cause marked hemodynamic effects such as hypotension in some patients and yet have relatively little effect in others. It occurs in many conditions.
- Ventricular fibrillation (Fig. 13.8d) is usually lethal since the heart cannot pump any blood. In ventricular fibrillation individual EKG deflections vary in size and frequency from moment to moment. This arrhythmia is probably the main cause of death in patients with AMI.
- Torsades de pointes has a characteristic EKG appearance ('twisting of peaks'). It is a serious arrhythmia similar to ventricular fibrillation, with rapid asynchronous complexes and an undulating baseline on the EKG. It is typically spontaneously reversible and therefore not necessarily lethal (unlike ventricular fibrillation). A prolonged QT interval in the EKG, which may be congenital (in congenital long QT syndrome) or drug induced (e.g. by class Ia and class III antiarrhythmics, see Table 13.3 below) is a recognized risk factor for torsades de pointes. Induction of torsades de pointes is facilitated by several predisposing factors including hypokalemia, bradycardia and numerous drugs.
- Wolff–Parkinson–White syndrome is due to a congenital accessory anatomic connection between atrium and ventricle known as the bundle of Kent. This connection allows impulses to be conducted quickly from the atria to the ventricles and bypass the AV node. It is diagnosed from the EKG as a short PR interval followed by a 'delta wave' on a wide QRS complex. It may give rise to atrial fibrillation.

Mechanisms of arrhythmia initiation and maintenance

Arrhythmias are initiated and maintained by a combination of abnormal impulse (action potential) generation

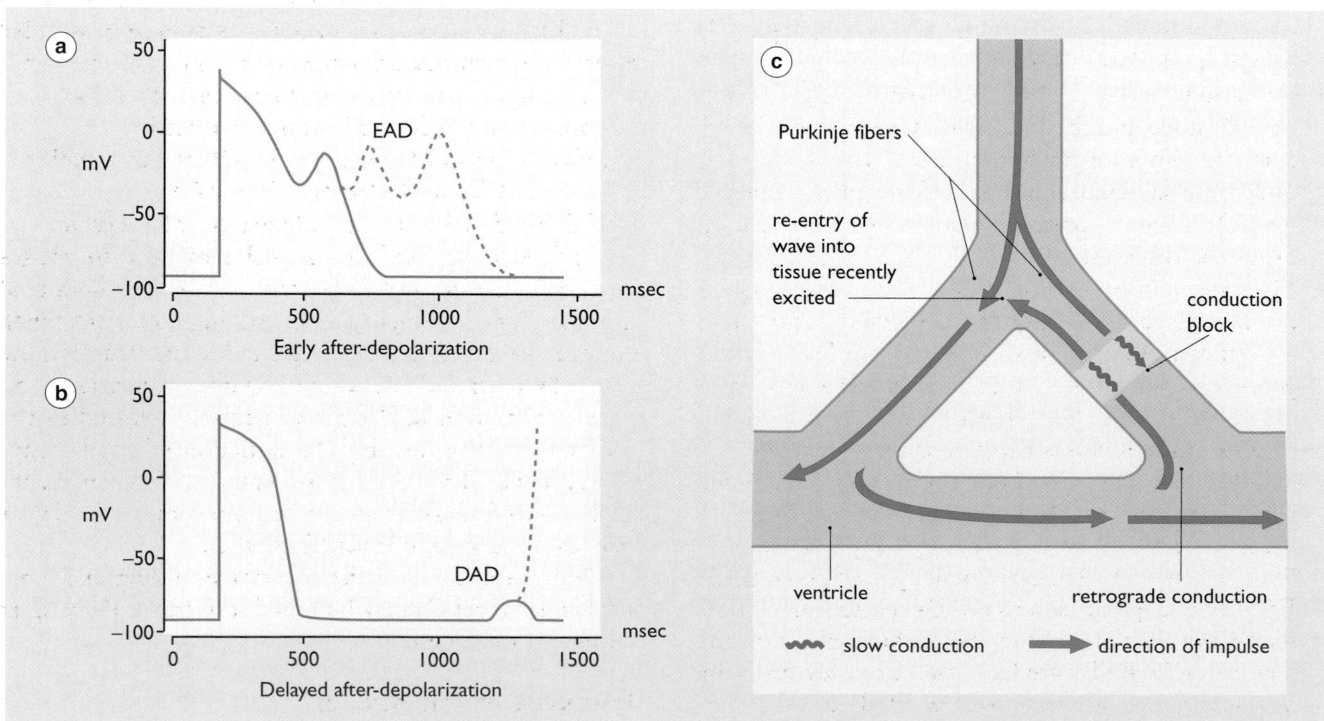

Fig. 13.10 Main mechanisms of arrhythmogenesis. (a) Early after-depolarizations (EADs) occur during the repolarization phase of the action potential. The dotted line indicates repetitive EADs. (b) Delayed after-depolarizations (DADs) occur after repolarization of the action potential, during diastole. The dotted line shows an action potential generated from a DAD. (c) Unidirectional block. Excitation moves into the Purkinje fibers, from where it should pass into ventricular tissue. However, conduction is blocked in one area in a unidirectional fashion; this allows retrograde conduction of an impulse from the ventricle back into the Purkinje fibers, hence re-exciting tissue that is no longer refractory and is excitable once more.

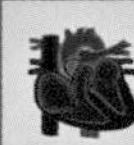

Table 13.1 Mechanisms of arrhythmogenesis

Abnormal impulse generation
- Automaticity
  - Enhanced normal automaticity
  - Abnormal automaticity
- Triggered automaticity
  - Early after-depolarizations
  - Delayed after-depolarizations

Abnormal impulse conduction
- Conduction block
  - First-, second- or third-degree block
- Re-entry
  - Circus movement
  - Reflection

and abnormal impulse conduction. Normal and abnormal impulse generation is known as automaticity. Normal and abnormal impulse conduction is described by its pathway, which is either normal (orthograde), blocked or abnormal (re-entrant) (Fig. 13.10). Automaticity can initiate an arrhythmia if it occurs ectopically (out of place, i.e. not in the SA node).

Examples of arrhythmias likely caused by automaticity are:

- Nodal tachycardias.
- VPBs associated with developing myocardial infarction.

There are three types or automaticity that can give rise to arrhythmias (Table 13.1):

- Enhanced normal automaticity occurs in tissues (the AV node and the His bundles) capable of slow automatic impulse generation that is overdriven under normal conditions by the faster rate of the SA node. Normal automaticity can become enhanced by drugs and diseases.
- Abnormal automaticity occurs in tissue that is not normally capable of automatic impulse generation (i.e. atrial and ventricular). During pathologic processes (such as myocardial infarction) abnormal automaticity often arises in the Purkinje fibers. Catecholamines may enhance this automaticity.
- Triggered automaticity (known as triggered activity), is similar to abnormal automaticity, but here the aberrant impulses are triggered by the previous 'normal' impulse. Triggered activity is of two types. Early after-depolarizations (EADs) occur during the repolarization phase of the action potential (i.e. during phase 2 or 3). EADs are facilitated by bradycardia and drugs that prolong the action potential duration (e.g. class III antiarrhythmics). The mechanism underlying EADs is not known. Delayed after-depolarizations (DADs; see Fig. 13.10) occur after the action potential has ended (i.e. during phase 4). DADs typically occur as a result of cellular Ca^{2+} overload, as may occur during AMI, reperfusion or digitalis intoxication. Ca^{2+} overload leads to oscillatory release of Ca^{2+} from the sarcoplasmic reticulum (SR) and the production of an inward current (resulting in the DAD) carried by the Na^+/Ca^{2+} exchanger.

Re-entry and conduction block (heart block) are examples of arrhythmogenic conduction

The most common site of heart block is the AV node:

- In first-degree AV block conduction through the AV node is slowed, manifest in the EKG as a prolonged PR interval.
- In second-degree AV block some of the impulses are not conducted to the ventricles (i.e. beats are missed) and, in the EKG, QRS complex does not always follow the P wave.
- In third-degree AV block, clinically the most serious, there is a complete block of conduction through the AV node. This generally leads to a slow ventricular escape rhythm that may not maintain adequate cardiac output. Abnormal conduction of this type can unmask VPBs.

Re-entry maintains (and may initiate) ventricular tachycardia and ventricular fibrillation

Re-entry is defined as a circuit of conduction that re-excites tissue with no diastolic interval. In 1914, Mines established the conditions necessary for re-entry to occur as an area of unidirectional block of the impulse that can allow reverse (retrograde) conduction to re-excite the tissue beyond the block. The following criteria must be fulfilled to provide definitive evidence of a re-entry mechanism:

- The length of the path must be greater than its wavelength (ω) determined by the effective refractoriness of the pathway (ERP) and conduction velocity (CV), such that ω = ERP × CV.
- Unidirectional conduction block must be present.

Unidirectional conduction block may be anatomic (as in Wolff–Parkinson–White syndrome), or functional (e.g. prolonged refractoriness resulting from ischemia), or both. Re-entry can be terminated by interrupting the circuit by premature activation, by overdrive pacing and by administration of drugs. Re-entry is involved in the maintenance and possibly the initiation of atrial tachycardia, atrial fibrillation, atrial flutter, AV nodal tachycardia, Wolff–Parkinson–White syndrome, ventricular tachycardia and ventricular fibrillation.

There are many other putative arrhythmogenic mechanisms; details may be found in Further Reading at the end of the Chapter.

Treatment of arrhythmias

Automaticity and conduction are targets for antiarrhythmic drugs

There are several different objectives when treating arrhythmias:

- To restore cardiac rhythm to normal – the first objective.

- To prevent arrhythmia recurrence.
- To ameliorate hemodynamic consequences of arrhythmias.
- To reduce the risk of a more severe arrhythmia such as ventricular fibrillation.

Although it is most desirable to restore normal sinus rhythm, this is not always necessary. It has been shown, for instance, that in atrial fibrillation the control of ventricular rate is as useful a goal of drug therapy as restoring normal sinus rhythm. Cardiac arrhythmias are treated by drugs, and also by nonpharmacologic methods such as electrical defibrillation, surgery and implantation of artificial pacemakers. The nonpharmacologic methods are growing in importance. The first objective of drug treatment, to restore sinus rhythm without producing adverse effects, is not well achieved with many available drugs. Typical antiarrhythmic drugs used in the USA are shown in Table 13.2. Monitoring of plasma drug concentrations is required for many of these drugs and target values are given in the table.

Table 13.2 Mean plasma concentration and route of administration of antiarrhythmic drugs used in the USA

Drug	Mean effective plasma concentration (μg/mL)	Route of administration
Disopyramide	3	i.v./p.o.
Lidocaine	3	i.v.
Procainamide	7	i.v./p.o.
Quinidine	4	i.v./p.o.
Mexiletine	1	i.v./p.o.
Tocainide	7	i.v./p.o.
Phenytoin	15	i.v./p.o.
Flecainide	0.7	i.v./p.o.
Encainide	0.75	i.v./p.o.
Propafenone	1.5	i.v./p.o.
Bretylium	1	i.v./p.o.
Amiodarone	1.5	i.v./p.o.
Verapamil	0.1	i.v./p.o.

i.v., intravenous; p.o., oral.

The Vaughan Williams classification of antiarrhythmic drugs

Antiarrhythmic drugs may, in theory, be classified according to their mechanism of action at molecular, cellular or tissue levels. Since the first antiarrhythmic drug, quinidine, was discovered in 1914 by Wenckebach, the list of antiarrhythmic drugs has grown, but a fully coherent system of classification has not grown with it. The first classification system devised by Vaughan Williams in 1970 (Table 13.3) describes distinguishing properties of drugs used as antiarrhythmics, although these properties do not necessarily correspond with mechanisms of action.

Classification of antiarrhythmic drugs might be expected to assist selection of appropriate treatments. However, there are few arrhythmias for which a single class of drug is the only available choice. This is partly because the available drugs are not necessarily effective in a majority of patients. For supraventricular arrhythmias this is not necessarily a major problem since if one drug is ineffective, another can be administered. However, the need to select a drug that is likely to work is more critical in the case of ventricular arrhythmias as these may be debilitating or lethal. Because ventricular arrhythmias are particularly unresponsive to antiarrhythmic drugs, drug selection is often based on sequential testing of drugs' abilities to suppress arrhythmias induced by 'programmed' electrical stimulation of a ventricle in individual patients in the hospital. However, evidence-based studies demonstrate that this method does not very well predict improvement in survival in the long term. Nevertheless, it continues to be used as a guide to

Table 13.3 Vaughan Williams approach to classification of antiarrhythmic drugs

Class	Type of drug	Eletrophysiologic actions	Examples
Ia	Na^+ channel blocker that also blocks K^+ channels.	Blocks conduction, increases ERP	Quinidine Disopyramide
Ib	Na^+ channel blocker; more effective at high rates.	Blocks conduction, decreases ERP	Lidocaine Mexiletine
Ic	Na^+ channel blocker; not rate dependent	Blocks conduction, no effect on ERP, or an increase	Flecainide Encainide
II	β adrenoceptor antagonist	Decreases sinus node automaticity, sympatholytic activity	Propranolol Sotalol
III	A drug that prolongs the action potential duration	No effects on conduction, delays repolarization	Bretylium Amiodarone Sotalol
IV	Ca^{2+} antagonist	Slows conduction velocity in the atrioventricular node	Verapamil Diltiazem

ERP, effective refractory period.

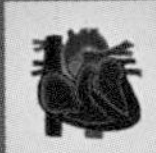

selecting therapy targeted to the individual. Drugs of a different antiarrhythmic class are often used in combination in prophylaxis against ventricular arrhythmias. In view of these considerations, the most important treatment for life-threatening ventricular arrhythmias is nonpharmacologic: the automatic implantable cardiac defibrillator (AICD).

The Vaughan Williams classification does not help drug selection on the basis of mechanism of the arrhythmia. EADs and re-entry, for example, may represent targets for drugs yet they may also represent targets for arrhythmia facilitation (pro-arrhythmia) by drugs (including some antiarrhythmics). The prevalent effect (pro- or antiarrhythmic) of a drug will depend on the underlying condition and drug dose. In animal experiments it is possible to evoke EADs with class III antiarrhythmic drugs, yet prevent re-entry with the same drugs. Class I drugs can facilitate re-entry by slowing conduction velocity, and block re-entry by converting unidirectional block of conduction to bidirectional block. Thus, it is not easy to predict whether the overall effect of an antiarrhythmic drug will be beneficial or detrimental.

The characteristic molecular action of class I antiarrhythmic drugs is blockade of cardiac Na^+ channels

The overriding molecular mechanism of action of class I drugs is block of Na^+ channels. This results in blockade of the inward (depolarizing) Na^+ current (cellular action). The resultant tissue mechanism of antiarrhythmic action is less clear, but animal experiments suggest that conversion of unidirectional block to bidirectional block may prevent the occurrence of re-entry. Some class I drugs also have additional molecular actions, i.e. block of K^+ channels, and therefore block of repolarizing K^+ currents. This prolongs the effective refractory period and may contribute to the drug's effects on re-entry (see class III drugs for explanation; p. 384). Quinidine, identified by Frey in 1918, was the first antiarrhythmic drug to be used. Since then, many other class I drugs have been synthesized.

Class I antiarrhythmics were subclassified in the late 1970s by Harrison because, although all class I drugs share the property of slowing ventricular conduction (manifested as a widening of the QRS complex), they fall into three groups depending on their effect on ventricular effective refractory period (see Table 13.3). Quinidine is a class Ia drug, meaning that it widens QT interval (because it blocks K^+ currents), as well as slowing conduction at therapeutic doses. Quinidine (and other class Ia drugs) lack selectivity for Na^+ versus K^+ channels. As a result, some investigators now attribute quinidine's antiarrhythmic effects not to Na^+ channel blockade but to its ability to widen QT interval via block of cardiac K^+ channels. This serves to illustrate that classifying a drug according to the Vaughan Williams system does not necessarily provide a precise description of the molecular action let alone define the tissue mechanism of action.

The typical oral dose of quinidine varies from 200 to 300 mg every 3 to 4 hours because of interindividual variations in pharmacokinetics. Quinidine is used to treat atrial fibrillation and flutter (restoring sinus rhythm), Wolff–Parkinson–White syndrome and ventricular tachycardia, but it is not a first-choice drug. Like other class Ia drugs, quinidine does not reduce the incidence of sudden cardiac death (i.e. ventricular fibrillation) following AMI. Its atropine-like effects may elicit adverse sinus tachycardia. Another less common adverse effect, 'quinidine syncope,' is now thought to result from quinidine-induced torsades de pointes, especially in hypokalemic patients, and may relate to the QT widening effect of the drug. Meta-analyses (see p. 57 for explanation) suggest that quinidine when used to treat atrial arrhythmias may increase the chance of sudden cardiac death. With quinidine, gastrointestinal irritation is common (30% of cases), and the rarer 'cinchonism' syndrome (deafness, tinnitus, blurred vision, flushing and tremor) may also occur. Quinidine elevates blood concentrations of digoxin, potentially leading to an adverse drug interaction. Quinidine, along with other class Ia drugs, is contraindicated in patients with AV block or a history of long QT/torsades de pointes.

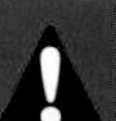

Adverse effects of quinidine

- Nausea
- Fever
- Syncope
- Blood dyscrasia
- Torsades de pointes

Procainamide has similar electrophysiologic and pharmacologic properties to quinidine. Its differences include a more rapid absorption by mouth, and the availability of intravenous (i.v.) and intramuscular formulations. It has an active metabolite, *N*-acetylprocainamide (NAPA), which possesses relatively selective class III antiarrhythmic properties. Unlike quinidine, procainamide has approval in the USA only for treatment of ventricular arrhythmias (not supraventricular). It is a first-line drug for suppression and prophylaxis of ventricular tachycardia, especially when given intravenously in emergency settings. There is no evidence that procainamide reduces the prevalence of mortality from ventricular fibrillation following AMI. A requirement for frequent dosing, resulting from rapid metabolism, limits patient compliance and hence may jeopardize therapeutic effectiveness. Gastrointestinal side effects are common (as for quinidine). Procainamide can cause leukopenia and (sometimes lethal) agranulocytosis, and blood counts are recommended during the first

12 weeks of therapy. Thrombocytopenia and positive Coomb's tests are rare. Long-term use (>6 months) is associated with a 'lupus-like-syndrome,' which differs from systemic lupus erythematosus only in terms of its lack of renal involvement, lesser severity and greater reversibility.

Disopyramide, another class Ia drug, has similar indications and properties to quinidine. It has particularly pronounced atropinic effects. The anticholinergic adverse profile includes blurred vision, dry mouth and urinary retention in elderly males. It has an advantage over quinidine in that there is no adverse drug interaction with digoxin.

Ethmozine (also known as moricizine) is a class Ia antiarrhythmic that, at daily oral doses of 600–900 mg, produces a dose-related reduction in the occurrence of frequent VPBs and reduces the incidence of nonsustained and sustained ventricular tachycardia in patients with and without organic heart disease. In clinical trials, moricizine has antiarrhythmic activity that is similar to that of disopyramide, propranolol (see later) and quinidine at the doses studied. Activity is maintained during long-term use. Moricizine may be effective in patients in whom other antiarrhythmic agents are ineffective, not tolerated and/or contraindicated. It is not greatly used, however.

Lidocaine is the prototypical class Ib antiarrhythmic but is distinct from other Ib agents in that it is administered exclusively by the i.v. route. This results in a high concentration of drug reaching the heart. Lidocaine's rapid metabolism in the liver makes oral administration unfeasible. Characteristically for class Ib drugs, lidocaine has few effects on the normal EKG. Its electrophysiologic actions occur selectively in the ischemic myocardium and during ventricular tachycardia. It was used for many years in the early phase of AMI (see p. 398) to reduce the incidence of ventricular fibrillation. However, despite its ability to reduce the frequency of VPBs and even VF in this setting, lidocaine has no beneficial influence on long-term survival. Overdose results in actions on nervous tissue, leading to paresthesias and convulsions. This is particularly a risk in patients with hypotension, who may have diminished liver blood flow, decreasing elimination of lidocaine. Therapy monitoring is important in the safe use of this drug. Its mode of administration means that it is used only in emergency settings, and not for maintenance therapy. Lidocaine's other use as a local anesthetic is discussed in Chapter 21.

Mexiletine is an orally active class Ib antiarrhythmic, originally but no longer used as an anticonvulsant. It is now exclusively used for suppression of VPBs and ventricular tachycardia. Following AMI, mexiletine has little or no effect on survival as is typical of class Ib drugs. Neurologic adverse effects, which are not closely dose-related, are the most common (dizziness, paresthesias, ataxia and tremor). Pharmacokinetic-based drug interactions occur with antacids (which increase mexiletine's gastric absorption), but low plasma protein binding means that displacement of highly plasma protein-bound drugs is not a concern. The combination of mexiletine with a β_1 adrenoceptor antagonist is more effective than either drug alone, and allows dose reduction of each in the suppression of ventricular arrhythmias.

Tocainide is an orally active class Ib agent, used less often than mexiletine.

Phenytoin is an orally active anticonvulsant with class Ib antiarrhythmic properties similar to those of lidocaine. Its general and anticonvulsant properties are discussed in detail in Chapter 8. As an antiarrhythmic, phenytoin has been used to treat ventricular arrhythmias, digitalis overdose-induced arrhythmias and torsades de pointes.

Flecainide is the prototypical class Ic antiarrhythmic. The characteristics of class Ic agents are high potency and selectivity for cardiac Na^+ channels, with slow dissociation of the drug from the Na^+ channels. This causes detectable EKG effects (QRS widening) associated with slowed ventricular conduction in healthy cardiac tissue at normal heart rates (this is potentially hazardous; see below). Flecainide is used exclusively to treat supraventricular arrhythmias (paroxysmal supraventricular tachycardia, atrial flutter and fibrillation), and is contraindicated in patients with structural heart disease. This is because it was shown in the Cardiac Arrhythmia Suppression Trial (CAST study) that flecainide may double the likelihood of death in patients with myocardial infarction (Fig. 13.11). This adverse effect is assumed to result primarily from a seemingly paradoxical pro-arrhythmic effect: nonlethal VPBs are suppressed but lethal arrhythmias (especially ventricular fibrillation) are

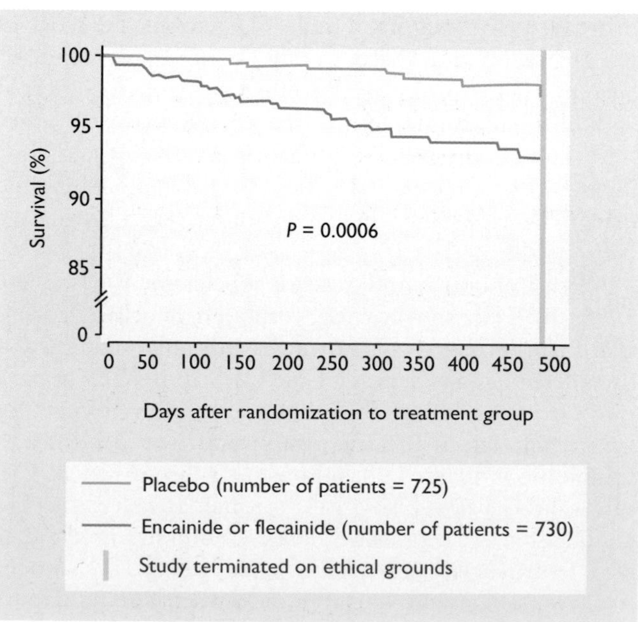

Fig. 13.11 Survival of patients in the Cardiac Arrhythmia Suppression Trial. Note that patients were allocated to their groups in a randomized blinded fashion and that the cause of death in each case was cardiac-related.

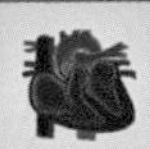

facilitated. This is now presumed to be due to slowed conduction in healthy parts of the ventricle. Aside from this, the adverse effects of flecainide are minor.

Encainide is a class Ic drug with similar properties to flecainide, and a similar risk of pro-arrhythmia.

Propafenone is another class Ic agent that is little used. Although it appears to share a qualitatively similar pharmacologic and pro-arrhythmic profile with flecainide and encainide, it was not evaluated in the CAST study and therefore there is less of a perception that it is strongly contraindicated in patients with structural heart disease and myocardial infarction. Furthermore, propafenone possesses weak β_1 adrenoceptor antagonist activity which may offset pro-arrhythmic effects.

Overall, class I drugs were once widely used but owing to emerging evidence of limited effectiveness, they are now used much less frequently. It is generally regarded that mexiletine, quinidine, disopyramide and procainamide are equally effective in suppressing ventricular arrhythmias. No class I drug reduces the likelihood of death following AMI, and many are pro-arrhythmic.

Class II antiarrhythmics act by reducing sympathetic activity

β adrenoceptor antagonists (β blockers) are one of the most commonly used classes of drug for cardiovascular diseases. Their use as antiarrhythmics is very limited as compared with their use in the treatment of hypertension, angina pectoris and congestive heart failure (see later). Norepinephrine and epinephrine may precipitate or aggravate arrhythmias in animal models by stimulating myocardial β_1, β_2 and α_1 adrenoceptors. Inappropriate cardiac adrenoceptor activation (especially β_1) may contribute to arrhythmogenesis in humans, although this is probably the case only during exercise or mental stress (where sympathetic tone is high) or in diseased hearts. The prototype class II drug is propranolol, a nonselective β_1 and β_2 antagonist. Conventionally, β_1 antagonism has been regarded as the molecular mechanism of action of class II antiarrhythmics, although β_2 antagonism (and even α_1) may also contribute. Metoprolol and esmolol are 'cardioselective' class II agents, meaning that they are relatively

Table 13.4 The main Ca^{2+} antagonists used in cardiovascular disease

Drug	Main uses	Usual doses (mg/day)	Plasma half-life (h)	Metabolism and elimination	Adverse effects (all may cause pedal edema)
Verapamil	Hypertension Angina pectoris Supraventricular tachycardias	160–480 p.o. 2.5 i.v. repeated	2–7	Hepatic metabolism by CYP3A/CYP1A2 Urinary excretion	Constipation Hypotension Bradycardia
Diltiazem	Angina pectoris Hypertension Supraventricular tachycardia Raynaud phenomenon	180 p.o. 180–360 p.o. 20 i.v. over 2 min	2–6, prolonged in elderly	Hepatic metabolism High first-pass + urinary excretion of metabolites	Hypotension Bradycardia
Nifedipine	Hypertension Angina pectoris Raynaud phenomenon	15–30 or 40 sublingual 30–90 mg long-acting p.o.	5	Hepatic metabolism by CYP3A4 High first-pass + urinary excretion of metabolites	Hypotension
Amlodipine	Hypertension	5–10 p.o. in single daily dose	30–60	Hepatic metabolism (slow, no first pass)	Hypotension
Nicardipine	Angina pectoris Hypertension	30–120 p.o. 60–120 p.o. (30–60 sustained release)	1–2	Similar to nifedipine	Hypotension
Felodipine	Hypertension	10–20 p.o.	24	Similar to nifedipine (but slower)	Hypotension
Barnidipine	Essential hypertension	20 p.o. in single daily dose	30–60	Similar to amlodipine	Hypotension
Lacidipine	Essential hypertension	4 mg p.o. in single daily dose	30–60	Like amlodipine	Hypotension Edema (less so than amlodipine)
Lercanidipine	Essential hypertension	10 or 20 p.o. in single daily dose	<24, but effect lasts >24 h	Hepatic metabolism, 10% first pass metabolism	Tachydardia, Edema (less so than amlodipine)
Manidipine	Essential hypertension	10 to 40 mg p.o. in single daily dose	<24, but effect lasts >24 h	Hepatic metabolism, 10% first-pass metabolism)	Tachydardia, Edema (less so than amlodipine)

p.o., orally; i.v., intravenously.

selective β_1 antagonists (selectivity is not 100% and it diminishes if dosage is increased).

Class II agents, especially propranolol, are particularly useful in suppressing atrial fibrillation and flutter associated with exercise or mental stress. Several β blockers have been shown to reduce mortality in patients with myocardial infarction, a benefit that has not been reproducibly demonstrated for any other antiarrhythmic drug class. This favorable action of β blockers may be due to therapeutic actions unrelated to arrhythmia suppression. The dosages, uses and adverse effects of β_1 adrenoceptor antagonists are described in detail in the section on treatment of angina.

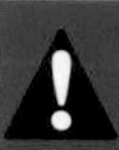

β blockers should be avoided in patients with:

- Asthma
- Diabetes mellitus with hypoglycemic reactions
- Severe intermittent claudication

Adverse effects of propranolol

- Bradycardia
- Depression
- Fatigue
- Cold extremities

Class III antiarrhythmics act by prolonging the action potential duration

Prolongation of the cardiac action potential duration by class III antiarrhythmics is seen on the EKG as an increase in QT interval. This leads to suppression of re-entry although, as noted earlier, it may exacerbate EADs. Thus anti- and pro-arrhythmic effects are possible, depending on the underlying mechanism of the arrhythmia (EAD versus re-entry). Bretylium, amiodarone, sotalol (which is also a β blocker) d-sotalol (not a β blocker) and dofetilide are all class III drugs.

Bretylium is the oldest, but least effective class III agent, and its adrenergic neuron-blocking effects (see Ch. 8) represent a lack of molecular selectivity and account for adverse effects such as hypotension.

Amiodarone was developed as a coronary vasodilator, and its antiarrhythmic effects were found by chance. Although amiodarone is generally referred to as a class III antiarrhythmic, it also blocks Na^+ and Ca^{2+} channels and to some extent α adrenoceptors. Amiodarone may also decrease expression of β_1 adrenoceptors in cardiac myocytes but does not interact directly with these receptors. This nonselectivity means that its molecular mechanism of action is unclear, and its classification as a class III agent questionable. Its onset of action is quite fast (within 60 minutes) when given intravenously, but by the oral route the drug must be administered for up to 3 weeks before a pharmacotherapeutic effect is achieved. Amiodarone has a very long half-life of >50 days, which means that it is not possible to achieve rapid modification of effects (beneficial or adverse) by altering dose. Amiodarone has been shown to be effective against atrial and ventricular arrhythmias. It is much more effective than quinidine, class II agents, verapamil and digitalis in suppressing paroxysmal supraventricular tachycardia related to Wolff–Parkinson–White syndrome. Its effectiveness against supraventricular tachycardia is enhanced when used in combination with digoxin, although care must be taken as serum digoxin concentrations are commonly increased via a drug–drug interaction. Combination with class IV antiarrhythmics (see below) may provide benefit against severe supraventricular tachycardia, although care must be taken to avoid AV block. Prevention of sudden cardiac death may occur with amiodarone, but serious side effects jeopardize long-term therapy (see adverse effects box). One advantage over β blockers, however, is that amiodarone is not contraindicated in patients with common disorders such as asthma, diabetes, coronary artery disease or renal failure. Amiodarone is now the most commonly used antiarrhythmic for life-threatening ventricular arrhythmias. Early clinical data in patients resuscitated and surviving ventricular fibrillation showed amiodarone to be inferior to AICD in terms of 3-year survival. More recently in patients with dilated cardiomyopathy, a study of 400 mg amiodarone twice a day for 1 week followed by 400 mg amiodarone once a day for 51 weeks, then 300 mg once a day was stopped early because the endpoint was not going to be reached. Arrhythmia-free survival was better in amiodarone patients than in ICD patients (arrhythmias are stopped with an ICD, not prevented), and overall mortality at 4 years was the same whether the patient was treated with amiodarone or AICD. In another trial (MADIT-II), the AICD improved survival versus conventional therapy post MI, which included amiodarone. The widespread use of amiodarone in comparison with use of the AICD relates in part to the perceived similarity of effectiveness versus the relative simplicity of taking a drug (versus AICD implant surgery) and the lower levels of patient anxiety associated with drug versus AICD use.

The effects of amiodarone on the thyroid activity are complex and therapeutically important, with 14–18% of patients experiencing either hyper- or hypothyroidism. In the liver, amiodarone inhibits the activity of type I 5′-deiodinase activity, an enzyme that deiodinates thyroid hormone T_4 to generate T_3. Inhibition of 5′-deiodinase activity may persist for months after amiodarone withdrawal. Amiodarone also inhibits T_4 entry into peripheral tissues. These actions give rise to increased serum T_4 concentration and decreased serum T_3 concentration in euthyroid subjects. Amiodarone can also alter serum thyroid stimulating hormone (TSH) levels. Doses higher than 400 mg/day may initially increase serum TSH concentra-

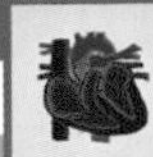

tion followed by a return to normal. Amiodarone may also directly affect TSH synthesis and secretion in the pituitary. During long-term amiodarone therapy, clinically euthyroid patients may show modest increases or decreases in serum TSH concentration, possibly reflecting hypo- or hyperthyroidism, respectively. Amiodarone also reduces the number of β adrenoceptors and the effect of T_3 on β adrenoceptors. Furthermore, amiodarone causes a decreased hepatic transcription of the T_3-responsive gene encoding for the low-density lipoprotein receptor, and down-regulates thyroid hormone receptors. Amiodarone-induced thyrotoxicosis occurs more frequently in geographical areas with low iodine intake (e.g. Tuscany) whereas hypothyroidism is more common in areas with normal iodine intake (e.g. Massachusetts). Type II amiodarone-induced thyrotoxicosis is a destructive thyroiditis leading to release of preformed thyroid hormones from the damaged thyroid follicular cells. This appears to be the more common form of amiodarone-induced thyrotoxicosis in regions with normal dietary iodine intake. It is generally regarded that because the indication for amiodarone is life-threatening (arrhythmias), then discontinuation is to be avoided. An alternative approach is to treat type II thyrotoxicosis with 30–40 mg prednisone (or equivalent) for 3 months, and treat type I thyrotoxicosis with methimazole and potassium perchlorate for up to 30–40 days. Often, the two types cannot be distinguished, in which case thionamide, potassium perchlorate and glucocorticoids may be used. If withdrawal of amiodarone is not feasible and medical therapy has failed, thyroidectomy may be required. Amiodarone-induced hypothyroidism has an autoimmune component in some patients and is associated with Hashimoto's thyroiditis (an established risk factor). It is more common than thyrotoxicosis, and is easier to treat (with T_4).

Until recently, all the class III drugs used clinically were believed to share a common molecular action, i.e. block of cardiac K^+ channels. However, other molecular actions can lead to action potential prolongation. These include α_1 adrenoceptor agonism and inhibition of Na^+ channel inactivation. The latter may contribute to the molecular mechanism of action of ibutilide, a class III agent approved in the USA for the treatment of supraventricular tachycardia.

Adverse effects of amiodarone

- **Thyroid abnormalities**
- **Corneal deposits**
- **Pulmonary disorders**
- **Skin pigmentation**

DL-sotalol (commonly referred to simply as sotalol) is a mixed class II/class III agent. It combines β adrenoceptor and K^+ channel blockade. This drug led a shift of focus onto more selective ('pure') class III agents that began in the 1980s. The premise was that greater selectivity would lead to greater efficacy.

A second generation of class III agents began with the introduction of D-sotalol, the sotalol enantiomer that possesses class III effects on K^+ channels without effects on β_1 adrenergic receptors. It was the first 'pure' and potent class III agent with actions on K^+ channels at submicromolar concentrations. Despite this, it is less effective than DL-sotalol for supraventricular arrhythmias, and is contraindicated in patients with a myocardial infarct. In the Survival With Oral D Sotalol (SWORD) clinical trial, D-sotalol, was found to increase mortality following myocardial infarction. Most currently used class III agents (including dofetilide and clofilium) selectively block the rapid kinetics isoform of the delayed repolarizing potassium current, I_{Kr} (an important repolarizing K^+ current in atria and ventricles). This includes amiodarone (although amiodarone blocks other non-K^+ channels and receptors as noted earlier). Other class III drugs act on I_{Kr} plus other K^+ currents, targeting the channels responsible for the transient outward K^+ current, I_{to} (tedisamil), the inward rectifying K^+ current, I_{K1} (terikalant) or the ATP-dependent K^+ current $I_{K(ATP)}$ (glyburide). None of these drugs are used clinically as an antiarrhythmic owing to adverse effects. A fear that torsades de pointes may be a class effect has meant that most of the second generation of I_{Kr}-selective class III agents (as well as most of the nonselective K^+ channel blockers) have been withdrawn. One exception is dofetilide, which remains in widespread clinical use, exclusively for atrial arrhythmias.

Class IV antiarrhythmics are Ca^{2+} antagonists

Ca^{2+} channel blockers (Ca^{2+} antagonists) are drugs that block L-type Ca^{2+} channels. There are three classes of this type of drug characterized by verapamil (a phenethylalkylamine derivative of papaverine), diltiazem (a benzothiazepine derivative) and nifedipine (a 1,4-dihydropyridine derivative). They are used to treat a variety of cardiovascular conditions including hypertension, angina pectoris (all three types, see p. 392) and arrhythmias (verapamil and diltiazem only).

Verapamil is the prototype of class IV antiarrhythmics (Table 13.4). It:

- Decreases AV nodal conduction velocity.
- Decreases SA nodal rate.
- Causes negative inotropy.
- Causes coronary and peripheral vasodilation.

Adverse effects of verapamil

- **Bradycardia**
- **Nausea and vomiting**
- **Constipation**

Diltiazem has a similar pharmacologic profile to verapamil. The antiarrhythmic application of these drugs is in the treatment of supraventricular arrhythmias. Clinical trials of Ca^{2+} antagonists in patients with coronary artery disease have failed to identify effective suppression of ventricular arrhythmias or reduced mortality. One reason for this may be that, as a result of the vasoselective nature of these drugs, the maximum safe doses used are insufficient to act in the ventricles to inhibit arrhythmias. Although verapamil and diltiazem have sufficient actions in the AV node to confer antiarrhythmic activity against supraventricular tachycardia despite their overall vascular selectivity, in contrast the dihydropyridines are so very vascular selective that they have no antiarrhythmic action even on the AV node. The basis for Ca^{2+} antagonist selectivity for blood vessels is explained in the section on treatment of angina (p. 392).

Adenosine as an antiarrhythmic falls outside the Vaughan Williams classification

Adenosine is not orally active but can be very effective when used intravenously for paroxysmal supraventricular nodal tachycardia. It has an ultra short half-life (seconds), and its effects are blocked by commonly used drugs (theophylline) and by caffeine. It is an agonist at A_1 adenosine receptors in the SA node, AV node and atria. Following receptor stimulation, a cascade begins with activation of an inhibitory G protein (Gi), which leads to inhibition of adenylyl cyclase activity and other actions mediated by Gi including reduction in L-type Ca^{2+} currents. Activation of A_1 receptors leads to opening of the same K^+ channels as those affected via this transduction cascade by acetylcholine. Because these channels are absent in the ventricles, adenosine has no effect on ventricular arrhythmias by this mechanism. The tissue action is hyperpolarization and a decrease in action potential duration leading to termination of re-entry. These actions account for a range of possible effects that include slowing of ventricular rate during atrial fibrillation, termination of sinoatrial re-entrant tachycardia (a rare condition of re-entry within the SA node), termination of paroxysmal supraventricular tachycardia involving re-entry through the AV node and termination of Wolff–Parkinson–White syndrome involving retrograde conduction through the AV node (however, in the latter, class Ia and Ic agents are preferred since adenosine may accelerate the tachycardia as a result of its ability to shorten the atrial refractory period.) In addition, through mechanisms that are less well established, A_1 activation by adenosine activates K_{ATP} channels, and this may account for the anti-ischemic effects of adenosine in ventricles reported in preclinical studies. Adenosine's ability to evoke bronchospasm in subjects with asthma means that its use is contraindicated in such patients.

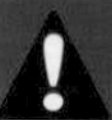

Adverse effects of adenosine

- Acceleration of tachycardia in Wolff–Parkinson–White syndrome
- Atrial fibrillation in Wolff–Parkinson–White syndrome
- Bronchospasm and hypotension

CVT-510 (tecadenoson) is a selective A_1 agonist currently in clinical development as a treatment for supraventricular tachycardia. It has greater selectivity for the AV node than adenosine.

There are four types of adenosine receptor (A_1, A_{2A}, A_{2B} and A_3). Coronary vascular A_{2A} receptor activation leads to coronary vasodilation, although this has not been exploited clinically (in angina, for example).

Digitalis cardiac glycosides are used primarily to treat heart failure, with additional antiarrhythmic actions

Digitalis can be used to treat atrial arrhythmias. Its mechanism of action is unusual. Atrial arrhythmias can result in ventricular rates that are too fast for effective diastolic filling so cardiac output falls. Digitalis converts atrial flutter to fibrillation by shortening the atrial refractory period, but its effects on the AV node mean that ventricular rate actually slows (Fig. 13.12).

Once the ventricular rate has stabilized, atrial fibrillation can be terminated by electroshock. However, it may be necessary to pretreat patients with heparin or warfarin depending on the suspected duration of the

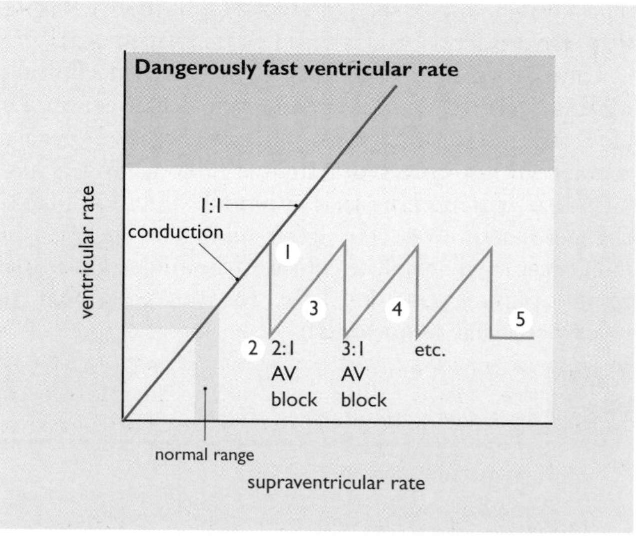

Fig. 13.12 The unusual mechanism by which digitalis ameliorates supraventricular tachycardia. (1) Digitalis prolongs AV refractory period by releasing acetylcholine from vagus. **(2)** This causes 2:1 AV block. **(3)** However, digitalis also shortens atrial refractory period increasing supraventricular tachycardia rate. **(4)** This exacerbates the AV block (since the AV recovery time is reduced). **(5)** Eventually AV dissociation occurs leading to a safer ventricular rate.

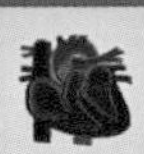

atrial fibrillation. This is because in atrial fibrillation (especially chronic fibrillation) a stasis thrombus may form in the atrial cavity, and restoration of sinus rhythm may dislodge the thrombus into the circulation, causing stroke. Digitalis must not be used for supraventricular tachycardia caused by Wolff–Parkinson–White syndrome, as the accessory pathway would allow the ventricles to 'follow' the atria and fibrillate. Digoxin is the antiarrhythmic cardiac glycoside of choice.

The 'Sicilian Gambit' Classification of antiarrhythmic drugs is based upon the deliberations of the Task Force of the Working Group on Arrhythmias of the European Society of Cardiology, and is an alternative approach to the Vaughan Williams classification of antiarrhythmic drugs (Fig. 13.13). It is not clear whether or to what extent the Sicilian Gambit provides a more precise or accurate description of antiarrhythmic drug mechanisms of action, and so the Vaughan Williams classification system is still pre-eminent.

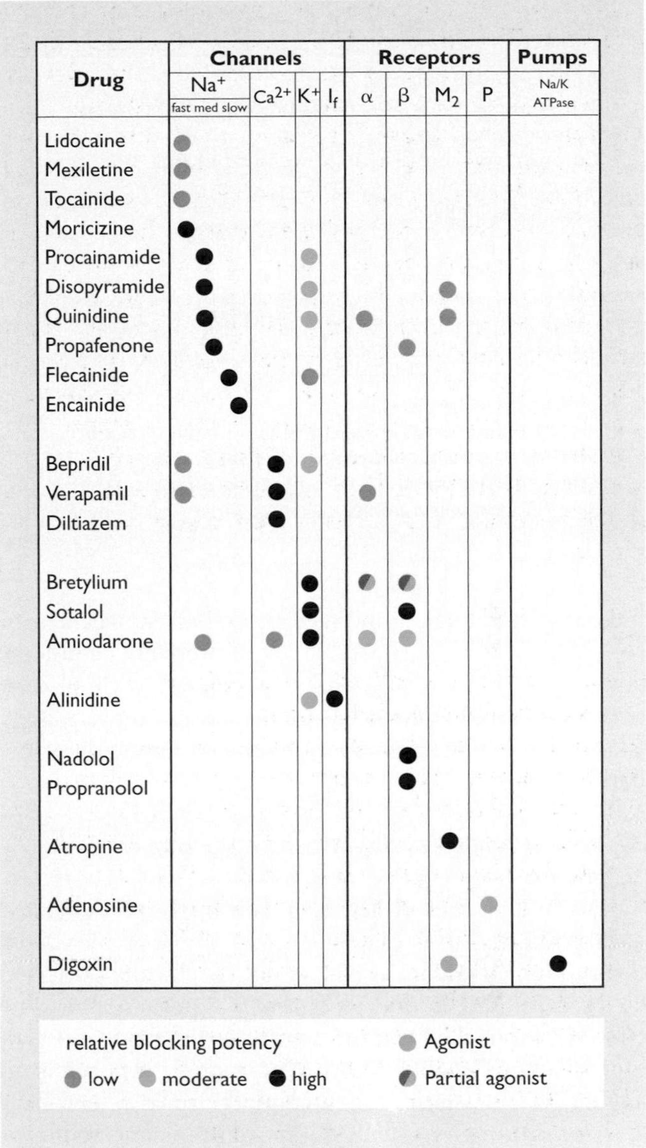

Angina pectoris

There are a number of disease conditions in which insufficient blood flow occurs in one or more coronary arteries. The resultant regional (localized) myocardial ischaemia can produce characteristic pain in the chest (angina pectoris, see below) although pain may not necessarily occur (silent ischemia). In medicine, there are different types of angina. The most important, in terms of prevalence, angina pectoris (which is a symptom, not a disease) is the paroxysmal pain in the chest (especially in the pectoral region) that is generated by episodes of ischemia in the ventricular myocardium. Myocardial ischemia results from coronary artery obstruction which can be partial or complete; it can be temporary, lasting for a few minutes, or permanent leading to the death of tissue by necrosis or apoptosis.

Myocardial ischemia can result from:

- Fixed partial obstruction of an artery or arteries due to atheroma or other pathologic processes.
- Inappropriate arterial vasospasm.
- A thrombus.

If myocardial ischemia is sufficiently severe, and maintained for a sufficient period of time, death of tissue (infarction or apoptosis) occurs. For this reason, despite the apparent advantage of the lack of chest pain, the silent form of ischemia is potentially more dangerous than the other form, because there is no pain to warn that intervention is required.

Drug	Channels: Na^+ fast	Na^+ med	Na^+ slow	Ca^{2+}	K^+	I_f	Receptors: α	β	M_2	P	Pumps: Na/K ATPase
Lidocaine	low										
Mexiletine	low										
Tocainide	low										
Moricizine	high										
Procainamide		high			moderate						
Disopyramide		high			moderate				low		
Quinidine		high			moderate		low		low		
Propafenone		high						low			
Flecainide			high		low						
Encainide			high								
Bepridil	low			high	moderate						
Verapamil	low			high			low				
Diltiazem				high							
Bretylium					high		partial agonist	partial agonist			
Sotalol					high			high			
Amiodarone	low			low	high		moderate	moderate			
Alinidine					moderate	high					
Nadolol								high			
Propranolol								high			
Atropine									high		
Adenosine										Agonist	
Digoxin									Agonist		high

relative blocking potency: low, moderate, high; Agonist; Partial agonist

Fig. 13.13 The Sicilian Gambit approach to antiarrhythmic drug classification. This is an alternative approach to antiarrhythmic drug classification introduced by the Task Force of the Working Group on Antiarrhythmias of the European Society of Cardiology. This scheme summarizes the actions of a variety of antiarrhythmic drugs on ion channels, drug receptors and ion pumps. I_f, hyperpolarization activated current; M_2, muscarinic subtype 2 receptors; P, purinergic receptors; Na/K ATPase, Na^+/K^+ pump. (Reproduced from *Circulation* 1991; **84**: 1831. Copyright 1994 American Heart Association.

Angina pectoris results from an imbalance between coronary blood supply and myocardial oxygen demand

Angina pectoris is often precipitated, or worsened, by exercise, emotion, meals and cold, and is characteristically alleviated by rest. Triggering stimuli result in an increase demand for cardiac work and hence coronary flow. If the coronary flow cannot increase enough to meet demand, ischemia is the result. Thus, angina pectoris may be regarded as an expression of a coronary blood supply–demand mismatch. Various possible reasons for this are given in Table 13.5.

Unstable angina is commonly associated with pathologic changes in atherosclerotic plaques lining coronary arteries

Unstable (also known as crescendo) angina occurs suddenly at rest, or with minimal physical activity, and

Table 13.5 Conditions that cause angina

- Coronary arteriosclerosis
- Transient platelet aggregation and coronary thrombosis
- Coronary artery spasm
- Coronary vasoconstriction following adrenergic stimulation
- Accumulation of potent vasoconstrictors at sites of endothelial injury

Table 13.6 Clinical features of variant angina pectoris

- Chest pain at rest
- Pain at the same time of day (early morning)
- ST segment elevation during chest pain
- Chest pain accompanied by ventricular arrhythmias
- Nitroglycerin relieves chest pain and ST segment elevation

increases in frequency and severity and often occurs prior to AMI. Very often, unstable angina reflects pathologic changes in a coronary artery associated with platelet aggregation and atherosclerotic plaque anatomy; therapy is aimed at relieving pain and halting progression of the coronary lesion.

Variant angina and syndrome X are rare forms of angina

Variant angina pectoris (Prinzmetal's angina) is associated with coronary arteries that are usually free of a fixed obstruction. It occurs at rest, is not specifically provoked by exercise and is due to coronary artery spasm. The clinical features of variant angina differ from those of typical angina (Table 13.6). Syndrome X also refers to angina in the setting of apparently normal coronary arteries, although its clinical importance is uncertain.

Types of angina

- **Angina pectoris presents as a radiating (to the arm and jaw) chest pain, is due to insufficient oxygen supply to the myocardium and can occur during exercise and stress**
- **Chronic stable angina is caused by fixed coronary stenosis (narrowing)**
- **Unstable angina occurs at rest or with physical activity and has a crescendo pattern**
- **Variant angina or Prinzmetal's angina occurs at rest and is caused by coronary vasospasm**

Treatment of angina

The mechanisms of action of the drugs used in each type of angina are described in detail later. General guidelines are as follows.

- For acute attacks of angina, sublingual nitrates provide rapid relief by reducing preload and afterload (defined in the heart failure section, p. 402) or relaxing coronary artery spasm. Nitrates can be used for preventing an attack if given just before the precipitating activity.
- For stable angina, in which anginal attacks occur in a predictable manner during exercise, several different classes of drug may be used on a prophylactic basis to prevent attacks, including long-acting nitrates, nonselective or β_1-selective adrenoceptor antagonists and Ca^{2+} antagonists. Each of these differ in their molecular, cellular and tissue mechanisms of action, but all affect one or more of preload, afterload, myocardial oxygen consumption and heart rate. The general pharmacology of β blockers is shown in Table 13.7.
- For unstable angina, therapy is aimed at relieving pain and preventing progression to an AMI. Because unstable angina is unpredictable by definition, the nature of its treatment varies greatly according to clinical presentation. The American College of Cardiology and the American Heart Association jointly publish and update guidelines for unstable angina and non-ST segment elevation type AMI (unstable angina) which is also known as non-ST segment elevation acute myocardial infarction (UA/NSTEMI), most recently in 2002.
- Maintained acute anginal pain, especially when caused by coronary thrombosis (heart attack), may be treated with morphine.
- There are no specific therapies for syndrome X.

The American College of Cardiology (ACC)/American Heart Association (AHA) guidelines for the management of unstable angina and non-ST segment elevation myocardial infarction (UA/NSTEMI), last revised in 2002, uses the following classifications

- **Class I: conditions for which there is evidence and/or general agreement that a given procedure or treatment is useful and effective.**
- **Class II: conditions for which there is conflicting evidence and/or a divergence of opinion about the usefulness/efficacy of a procedure or treatment.**
- **Class III: conditions for which there is evidence and/or general agreement that the procedure/treatment is not useful/effective and in some cases may be harmful.**
- **Levels of evidence for the above:**

  A: Weight of evidence/opinion is in favor of usefulness/efficacy
  B: Usefulness/efficacy is less well established by evidence/opinion

Class I

- **Aspirin 162–325 mg should be administered as soon as possible and 75–160 mg daily continued indefinitely (level of evidence: A)**

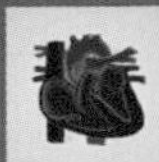

- Clopidogrel 75 mg daily should be administered to patients who are unable to take aspirin (level of evidence: A)
- When a noninterventional approach is planned, clopidogrel added to aspirin as soon as possible and administered for at least 1 month (level of evidence: A), and for up to 9 months (level of evidence: B)
- A platelet GP IIb/IIIa antagonist should be administered, in addition to aspirin and heparin, to patients in whom catheterization and percutaneous coronary interventions (PCI) are planned. The GP IIb/IIIa antagonist may also be administered just prior to PCI (level of evidence: A)
- When PCI is planned and the risk for bleeding is not as high, clopidogrel should be started and continued for at least 1 month (level of evidence: A) and for up to 9 months (level of evidence: B)
- In patients taking clopidogrel in whom elective coronary artery bypass graft surgery (CABG) is planned, the drug should be withheld for 5–7 days (level of evidence: B)
- LMWH (specifically enoxaparin) should be the preferred anticoagulant in patients managed with an early conservative strategy
- ACE inhibitors should remain an important therapy in those at higher risk

Class II

- Eptifibatide or tirofiban should be administered, in addition to aspirin and low molecular weight heparin (LMWH) or unfractionated heparin (UFH), to patients with continuing ischemia, elevated plasma troponin C, or with other high-risk features in whom invasive management is not planned (level of evidence: A)
- A platelet GP IIb/IIIa antagonist should be administered to patients already receiving heparin, aspirin and clopidogrel in whom catheterization and PCI are planned. The GP IIb/IIIa antagonist may also be administered just prior to PCI (level of evidence: B)
- Eptifibatide or tirofiban, in addition to aspirin and LMWH or UFH, is given to patients without continuing ischemia who have no other high-risk features and in whom PCI is not planned (level of evidence: A)

Class III

- Intravenous fibrinolytic therapy in patients without acute ST-segment elevation, posterior MI, or a presumed new left bundle-branch block (level of evidence: A)

Abciximab administration in patients in whom PCI is not planned (level of evidence: A)

Organic nitrates and nitrates are effective in all forms of angina

Several preparations of nitrates are available:

- Nitroglycerin.
- Erythrityl tetranitrate.
- Isosorbide dinitrate.
- Pentaerythritol tetranitrate.

They vary in whether they are used orally, sublingually or dermally. Sublingual nitroglycerin is used to treat an acute attack, although the other nitrates are used to prevent attacks. The major pharmacologic action of nitrates is relaxation of contracted smooth muscle of all types, in particular vascular smooth muscle. Nitrates, when administered sublingually (to achieve rapid absorption), may relieve angina within a few minutes. The main beneficial action in angina is dilation of systemic veins. This reduces preload, which in turn reduces myocardial wall tension and cardiac oxygen demand. The molecular mechanism of action for this effect is activation of vascular guanylyl cyclase activity, which increases cyclic guanosine monophosphate (cGMP) levels (Fig. 13.14). cGMP is an important transduction component (see Ch. 3). Most nitrates are pro-drugs, and decompose to form NO, which activates guanylyl cyclase (see Fig. 13.14). By the same mechanism, nitrates also cause vasodilation of large and medium-sized coronary arteries, thereby increasing coronary blood flow and oxygen delivery to the subendocardial region of the myocardium. However, this is clinically relevant only if vasospasm is present. Indeed, if there is a fixed partial coronary artery obstruction (arteriosclerosis) dilation of adjacent healthy coronary arteries can shunt blood away from the ischemic region (coronary 'steal'). Peripheral arteriolar dilation also occurs, but this is short-lived and its clinical significance is unclear. Sympathetic reflexes usually overcome the short-lived ability of nitrates to reduce afterload.

Long-acting nitrates such as isosorbide dinitrate are usually given at 6–8-hour intervals during the day, whereas the shorter-acting drug, nitroglycerin, may be applied as a patch preparation on the chest at any time, although it is generally not applied overnight. These treatment regimens minimize the effect of nitrate tolerance, which can occur over time with repeated nitrate administration. As a general principle, tolerance is avoided by careful planning of dosing in relation to the drug's pharmacokinetics to ensure that a steady-state plasma concentration is not sustained over a 24-hour period. The patient must be free of nitrate for at least 8 hours of the day to prevent development of tolerance.

Nitrates are used primarily to treat angina pectoris of all types. However, they also have minor uses such as relaxation of smooth muscle sphincters, as in the radiographic examination of the bile duct. Nitrates are also used as specific therapy in cyanide poisoning.

β adrenoceptor antagonists (β blockers) reduce myocardial oxygen demand

β blockers were mentioned briefly in the section on treatment of arrhythmias (p. 383), The first clinically useful β blocker was created by Nobel prizewinner James Black in the 1960s. He argued that since an increase in heart rate often precipitated angina, a drug that blunted the effects of the sympathetic nerves on the heart would

Table 13.7 β Adrenoceptor antagonists used in cardiovascular disease

Drug	Relative selectivity	Main uses	Usual dose (mg/day)	Plasma half-life (h)	Elimination route	Adverse effects
Propranolol	$\beta_1=\beta_2$	Essential and renal hypertension Angina pectoris AMI Atrial arrhythmias Hypertrophic obstructive cardiomyopathy	40–320 p.o. 120–240 p.o. 160 p.o. 30–160 p.o. 30–160 p.o.	3–6	Hepatic metabolism and renal excretion	Bronchospasm Bradycardia Fatigue Lassitude Headache Asthenia Dyspepsia Sweating Impotence
Metoprolol	$\beta_1>\beta_2$	Hypertension AMI Congestive heart failure Angina pectoris	100–200 p.o.	3–4	Hepatic metabolism	Similar to propranolol
Atenolol	$\beta_1>\beta_2$	Hypertension Angina Atrial arrhythmias AMI	50 p.o. 100 p.o. 50–100 p.o. Up to 10 i.v.	3–6	Mainly renal excretion	Similar to propranolol
Acebutolol	β_1 partial agonist $>\beta_2$	Hypertension Angina pectoris Atrial arrhythmias	400 p.o. 400–1200 p.o. 400–1200 p.o.	3–6	Mainly renal	Similar to propranolol
Carvedilol	$\beta_1=\beta_2$	Hypertension Angina Congestive heart failure	12.5–50 p.o.	7	Hepatic metabolism and renal excretion	Similar to propranolol + postural hypotension
Betaxolol	$\beta_1>\beta_2$	Hypertension (Glaucoma)	20–40 p.o. (Eyedrops)	3–6	Mainly renal	Similar to propranolol
Bisoprolol	$\beta_1>\beta_2$	Hypertension Angina	5–20 p.o. 5–20 p.o.	10–12	Hepatic metabolism (50%) and renal (50%)	Similar to propranolol
Timolol	$\beta_1=\beta_2$	Hypertension AMI (Migraine prophylaxis) (Glaucoma)	10–60 p.o. 20 p.o. (Eyedrops)	4	Hepatic metabolism and renal excretion	Similar to propranolol
Nadolol	$\beta_1=\beta_2$	Hypertension Angina Arrhythmias	80–240 p.o. 40–160 p.o. 40–160 p.o.	14–17	Mainly fecal + hepatic metabolism and renal excretion	Similar to propranolol
Pindolol	$\beta_1>\beta_2$ (partial agonist)	Hypertension Angina	5–45 p.o. 5–15 p.o.	2.5–4	Hepatic (50%) and renal (50%)	Similar to propranolol
Labetalol	β_1/α_1 $\beta_1=\beta_2>\alpha$	Hypertension	100–2400 p.o.	6	Hepatic metabolism and renal excretion (60%) + fecal (40%)	GI disturbance Male sexual dysfunction Liver damage (rare)
Sotalol	$\beta_1=\beta_2=I_{Kr}$	Ventricular and supraventricular arrhythmias	80–320 p.o.	12	Mainly renal	Similar to propranolol plus torsades de pointes
Celiprolol	β_1 (with weak β_2 agonism)	Hypertension	200–600 p.o.	5–6 (but pharmaco-dynamic $T_{1/2}$ is 24)	Renal	Similar to propranolol but little risk of bronchospasm
Penbutolol	$\beta_1>\beta_2$ (partial agonist)	Hypertension	20 p.o.	5	Hepatic metabolism and renal excretion	Similar to propranolol but less asthenia and bradycardia

p.o., orally; i.v., intravenously.

be antianginal. Subsequently, β blockers were found to have many other useful therapeutic actions, as discussed in this chapter and elsewhere.

β blockers block activation of the β adrenoceptors by the peripheral autonomic nervous system, and by epinephrine released from the adrenal medulla. Most of their beneficial effects in cardiovascular disease are presumed to result from β_1 rather than β_2 antagonism. β_1 antagonism will:

- Decrease exertionally induced increases in heart rate.

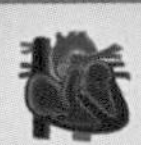

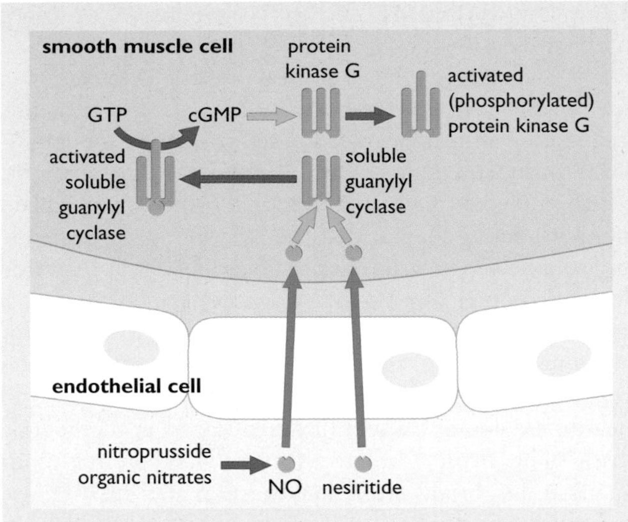

Fig. 13.14 Molecular and cellular mechanisms of action of nitrate and nitrite vasodilators, nitric oxide (NO) and nesiritide. The primary molecular target, soluble guanylyl cyclase, is accessed by drug or NO diffusion between cells. The product, phosphorylated protein kinase, causes vascular smooth muscle relaxation by phosphorylating (and inactivating) myosin light chain kinase.

- Decrease systolic blood pressure, particularly if hypertension is present.
- Decrease cardiac contractile activity.

As a result, β blockers reduce myocardial oxygen demand by blunting the heart's response to sympathetic tachycardic stimuli. The details of their molecular mechanisms of action are shown in Figure 13.15. Drugs in this class include those listed in Table 13.8.

At relatively low doses, β_1-selective antagonists such as metoprolol, atenolol and acebutolol tend to reduce heart rate responses and myocardial contractile activity with lesser effects on bronchial smooth muscle (in which circulating epinephrine may effect a physiologically important bronchodilation due to β_2 agonism). However, at higher doses, selectivity is lost and the effects resemble those of nonselective β blockers (β_1 and β_2), such as propranolol, which may exacerbate bronchospasm in some asthmatics as a result of β_2 antagonism. β_1 partial agonists are also useful in angina. Although partial agonists can elevate heart rate when the rate is low, they prevent tachycardia mediated via the sympathetic system.

In unstable angina, β blockers are useful through their sympatholytic effects in reducing cardiac workload and myocardial oxygen demand. They achieve a 13% relative risk reduction in the rate of progression to an acute MI and a 29% relative risk reduction in death among high-risk individuals with a threatened or evolving MI. Thus, i.v. β_1 blockers are recommended on appearance of chest pain, followed by long-term oral use for low- to intermediate-risk patients with angina and for all high-risk patients unless contraindicated.

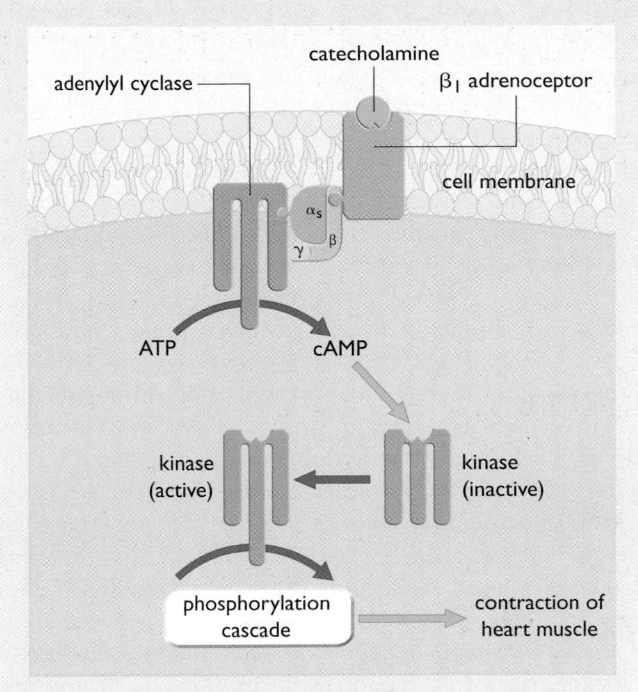

Fig. 13.15 Molecular mechanism of action of β_1 adrenoceptor antagonists. Stimulation of β_1 adrenoceptors by catecholamines leads to activation of adenylyl cyclase and an elevation of cAMP. This process is inhibited by β_1 adrenoceptor antagonists.

Table 13.8 β Adrenoceptor antagonists used in patients with angina

Drug	Selectivity	Classification
Acebutolol	β_1 selective	Partial agonist
Atenolol	β_1 selective	Antagonist
Metoprolol (low doses)	β_1	Antagonist
Pindolol	β_1	Partial agonist
Propranolol	β_1, β_2 nonselective	Antagonist
Sotalol	β_1, β_2 nonselective	Antagonist
Timolol	β_1, β_2 nonselective	Antagonist

β blockers are associated with a variety of adverse effects including fatigue, insomnia, dizziness, male sexual dysfunction, bronchospasm, bradycardia and heart block

β blockers should be used cautiously, or may be contraindicated, in patients with bradycardia (heart rate less than 55 beats/min), bronchospasm, hypotension (systolic pressure less than 90 mmHg) or any degree of heart block. β blockers can promote acute pulmonary edema in patients with compensated heart failure or severe congestive heart failure (although, apparently paradoxically, these drugs are now used to treat heart failure).

Ca^{2+} antagonists block L-type Ca^{2+} channels to alleviate angina pectoris

Ca^{2+} antagonists including nifedipine, nicardipine, felodipine and amlodipine (the 1,4-dihydropyridines), verapamil, bepridil and diltiazem possess slightly different tissue and system actions when used to treat angina, despite having similar molecular actions on L-type Ca^{2+} channels and identical cellular actions (inhibition of I_{si}).

Verapamil, bepridil and diltiazem act directly on cardiac tissue (reducing cardiac contractility and in high doses slowing atrioventricular conduction) as well as the blood vessels (causing vasodilation). They reduce myocardial oxygen consumption at rest and during exercise by reducing heart rate and cardiac contractile activity, increasing coronary blood flow, and reducing preload and afterload. Verapamil and diltiazem may adversely slow conduction through the AV node, leading to AV block (see antiarrhythmic drugs, p. 385).

The 1,4-dihydropyridines are very vascular selective, causing vasodilation without slowing AV conduction or heart rate or reducing cardiac contractility. As they are always used as a slow-release formulation, reflex tachycardia is avoided. The basis for vascular selectivity is a marked voltage dependence such that the ability to block L-type Ca^{2+} channels is minimal at membrane potentials encountered in (the relatively hyperpolarized) working myocardium and cardiac nodal tissue during diastole, compared with effects in the relatively depolarized blood vessels. Verapamil and diltiazem also show voltage dependence, but this is not as marked as with dihydropyridines, so AV conduction slowing is possible with therapeutic doses (see section on antiarrhythmic effects of Ca^{2+} antagonists, p. 385). The beneficial actions of 1,4-dihydropyridines in angina are attributed to increases in coronary blood flow to the epicardial regions of the myocardium, and peripheral vasodilation (a reduction in afterload).

Ca^{2+} antagonists are effective in preventing chest pain in patients with stable angina following exercise or stress, either alone or in combination with nitrates and/or β_1 adrenoceptor antagonists. If nifedipine, nicardipine, felodipine or amlodipine is combined with a β_1 adrenoceptor antagonist there is only a low risk of AV block, and of impairing cardiac output as a result of reduced ventricular contractility (effects that would be particularly hazardous if the patient has congestive heart failure or AV conduction abnormalities). Nifedipine, nicardipine, felodipine and amlodipine can therefore be used in patients with these conditions. However, there is a greater risk for this type of adverse drug interaction if verapamil, diltiazem or bepridil is combined with a β_1 adrenoceptor antagonist. Since verapamil, diltiazem and bepridil have negative inotropic effects they should not be given to patients with severe heart failure. Bepridil is less selective for L-type Ca^{2+} channels than verapamil or diltiazem, because it blocks cardiac Na^+ and K^+ channels at high doses, possibly sufficiently to slow cardiac conduction and delay repolarization. This has been associated with the adverse effect of torsades de pointes. Because of this, bepridil is recommended only for severe stable angina that is not fully responsive to other interventions.

Ca^{2+} antagonists have several adverse effects, with nifedipine being the least well tolerated. The systemic vasodilating effects of nifedipine (primarily the rapid-onset formulations) may cause dizziness and palpitations. Nifedipine also causes venodilation, which may explain the peripheral edema that occurs in some patients. Amlodipine and nicardipine are generally better tolerated than nifedipine, causing little or no peripheral edema, and have no adverse interactions with β_1 adrenoceptor antagonists (owing to their lack of direct effect on myocardial L channels). Moreover, amlodipine and nicardipine do not cause reflex tachycardia at therapeutic doses. The main adverse effect of verapamil is constipation, but bradycardia, hypotension and heart failure may also occur. Verapamil in combination with a β_1 adrenoceptor antagonist is contraindicated owing to precipitation of hypotension and AV block. Diltiazem use is associated with bradycardia.

Reducing the risk of AMI in angina patients

■ ***Aspirin is used in the treatment of angina patients to decrease the risk of AMI***

Although aspirin is considered primarily as a treatment for unstable angina (see below) it is also recommended in stable angina at moderate doses (80–325 mg/day). The therapeutic aim is to reduce the chance of coronary thrombosis, rather than specifically to treat the stable angina. Aspirin inhibits cyclooxygenase enzymes (COX-1 and COX-2), which play a pivotal role in the biosynthesis of thromboxanes in platelets and prostacyclin in vascular endothelium (Fig. 13.16 and see Chs 9 and 10):

- Platelet-derived thromboxane is a potent vasoconstrictor, and aspirin inhibits its synthesis.
- Endothelium-derived prostacyclin is a potent vasodilator and inhibits platelet aggregation, so inhibition of its synthesis is potentially hazardous.

By irreversibly blocking cyclooxygenase in platelets, which are unable to synthesize proteins, the thromboxane synthesizing ability of platelets is lost. On the other hand, small doses of aspirin have lesser effects in endothelial cells where new cyclooxygenase is being constantly synthesized allowing for the generation of prostacyclin. Thus, the thromboxane to prostacyclin ratio is shifted in the direction of prostacyclin thereby preventing platelet adhesion.

Variant angina and its treatment with drugs that dilate coronary arteries

Variant angina caused by coronary vasospasm is also known as Prinzmetal's angina. Variant angina is the only form of angina in which dilation of coronary arteries is the principal action of the drugs used to treat it. It is initially treated with nitrates, either alone, or with a Ca^{2+} antagonist:

- Nifedipine (40–160 mg/day) alone may be sufficient

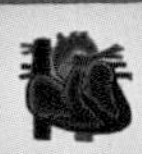

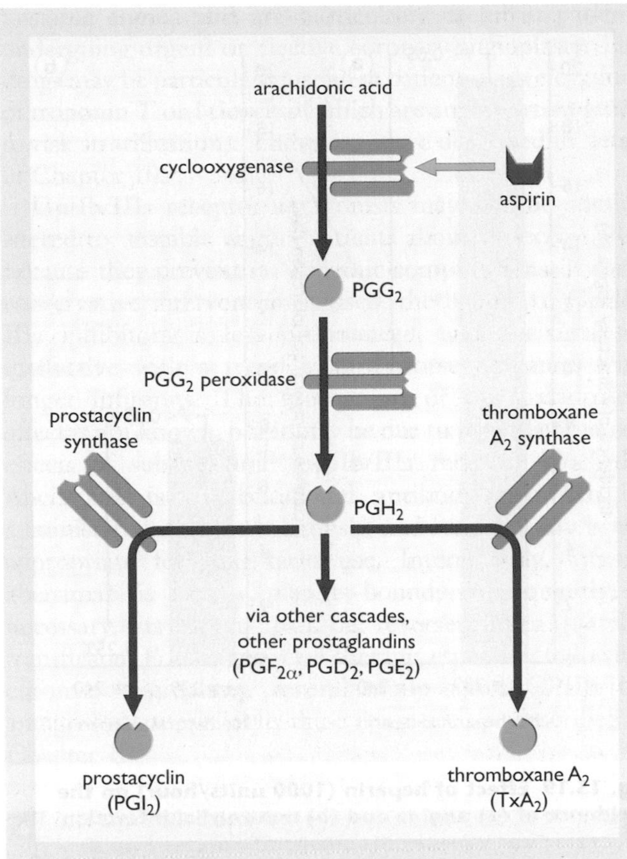

Fig. 13.16 Mechanism of action of aspirin. Aspirin blocks the activity of cyclooxygenase and reduces the formation of prostacyclin and thromboxane A_2. PGG_2 and PGH_2 are both prostaglandin cyclic endoperoxides and are unstable intermediates.

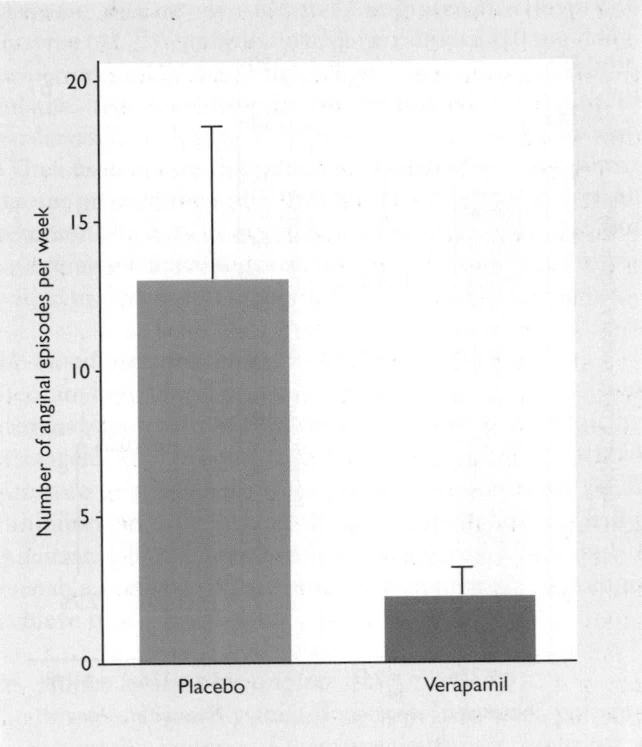

Fig. 13.17 Effect of verapamil in patients with variant angina.

to prevent variant angina in up to 75% of patients. Its effectiveness is not modified by the presence of concurrent partially obstructive coronary arteriosclerosis.

- Verapamil (Fig. 13.17) and diltiazem may also be used, as well as nicardipine, israpidine and amlodipine.

Despite differences in tissue selectivity (vasculature versus AV node), all these Ca^{2+} antagonists appear to be equally effective in variant angina, although individual patients may respond better to one drug than to another. For unknown reasons, the combination of diltiazem and nifedipine may be beneficial if the agents are less than completely effective when used alone. β blockers are not recommended in these patients because they are often ineffective and may increase the frequency and severity of spasm.

Treatment of unstable angina and non-ST segment elevation myocardial infarction

Unstable angina is particularly life-threatening and careful treatment strategies are employed. The main concern in unstable angina is the possibility of progression to AMI, a condition discussed later.

The main use of aspirin in unstable angina is to prevent thrombosis and AMI

Aspirin may reduce the platelet aggregation that is initiated by coronary endothelial injury and can participate in the etiology of unstable angina. If platelets aggregate they can occlude severely narrowed coronary arteries and release potent vasoconstrictors, which worsens the angina. These vasoconstrictors include thromboxane A_2, serotonin (5-HT), adenosine diphosphate (ADP), thrombin and platelet-activating factor.

The optimal aspirin regimen for patients with unstable angina remains to be defined. Low-dose aspirin (typically 100 mg/day) is insufficient to block the activity of cyclooxygenase completely, so its use can achieve a maintained suppression of thromboxane synthesis, with only a transient inhibition of prostacyclin synthesis, and an overall effect of reduced platelet aggregation. These actions contribute to the benefit achieved by prophylactic use of aspirin against AMI (see below and Fig. 13.18). By inhibiting platelet activation and aggregation, aspirin reduces the incidence of death and nonfatal AMI in patients with unstable angina with only a small increased risk of major bleeding (0.2%). Higher doses of aspirin (>100 mg) do not provide greater benefit and may increase bleeding, especially when combined with the antithrombotic ADP receptor blocker clopidogrel. Current guidelines, therefore, recommend that all patients with unstable angina receive 162–325 mg of aspirin initially, followed by 75–160 mg daily thereafter.

- β blockers and aspirin may have little immediate effect, but can improve long-term survival.
- Once the patient has stabilized, continued administration of aspirin and β blockers is strongly recommended.

Sympathomimetic drugs are used for cardiogenic shock in AMI

Cardiogenic shock can complicate AMI. This occurs if cardiac output is severely impaired, typically due to a large loss in cardiac muscle. Prognosis is very poor, with a high death rate. Emergency treatment (prior to surgical intervention; see below) has been with i.v. adrenoceptor agonists which activate β_1 receptors in the heart (norepinephrine, dopamine or dobutamine). The aim is to use the lowest dose sufficient to achieve improvement of CNS and coronary blood flow, without increasing afterload or preload. The therapeutic window is narrow, and pulmonary edema and exacerbation of heart failure are common. Supportive surgical intervention by intra-aortic balloon (which is inflated and deflated in time with the cardiac cycle so as to direct more of the cardiac output to the coronary and carotid arteries) is instigated as soon as possible.

Antiarrhythmics are used for suppressing arrhythmias in the acute phase of AMI

If non-life-threatening ventricular arrhythmias occur, these may be suppressed by i.v. lidocaine. Procainamide (i.v.) may be used if ventricular tachycardia is present on hospital admission. If ventricular fibrillation occurs, electrical cardioversion is necessary. Amiodarone (i.v.) may be used for treatment and prophylaxis of frequently recurring ventricular fibrillation and hemodynamically unstable ventricular tachycardia in patients refractory to other therapy. The use of these drugs varies greatly among different countries and hospitals. Accelerated idioventricular rhythm resulting from abnormal automaticity in infarcting Purkinje fibers (2 hours or more after the acute event) can be overdrive-suppressed by administering atropine which, by blocking M_2 muscarinic receptors in the sinoatrial node, allows sinus rate to increase, recapturing cardiac rhythm.

The use of antiarrhythmics post-AMI for improving survival once the patient has stabilized is controversial

Intravenous lidocaine has been shown by meta-analysis to have no effect on death rate in 1-year follow-ups, but is still administered immediately following AMI (even if ventricular arrhythmias are minimal or absent) in some parts of the world. Although lidocaine may immediately suppress non-life-threatening arrhythmias, it has no beneficial effect on long-term survival, and may disturb the patient by eliciting adverse effects in the CNS (particularly paresthesias) and cardiovascular system (asystole). The maintained use of class I antiarrhythmics (procainamide, quinidine) or class III antiarrhythmics (sotalol, amiodarone) in the days and weeks after the acute events is questionable owing to lack of effectiveness against ventricular fibrillation and possible adverse effects (including proarrhythmia), as discussed earlier in this chapter. Other class I and III antiarrhythmics have been, and may continue to be used, but their effects on survival are dubious at best (see the CAST and SWORD studies mentioned earlier). Class II agents are the only antiarrhythmics proven to reduce death rate in the year following hospital discharge after AMI, although the mechanism of action is unclear (it may not even be the result of suppression of arrhythmias).

Restenosis and drug-eluting stents post-AMI (and in unstable angina)

Coronary artery surgery is considered during the immediate post-AMI period and also in the general unstable angina setting. Stents are artificial blood vessels used to repair severely atherosclerotic arteries, particularly coronary, that are not amenable to reperfusion by other means. Drug-eluting stents release a drug from their matrix. The stent provides a high local release of drug. This means that effective drugs that may have serious adverse effects when equilibrated systemically may be used by this manner of administration. Currently, there are numerous and varied drug-eluting stents with antithrombotic, antiproliferative and antiinflammatory actions, including sirolimus, tacrolimus, everolimus, ABT-578, biolimus, paclitaxel, QP2, dexamethasone, 17/3-estradiol, batimastat, actinomycin-D, methotrexate, angiopeptin, tyrosine kinase inhibitors, vincristine, mitomycin, ciclosporin, and C-myc antisense technology (Resten-NG, AVI-4126). Only three of drugs have proven their efficacy in randomized studies: paclitaxel, sirolimus and everolimus. A significant effect on an angiographic primary end-point does not necessarily translate into a significant clinical effect. The safety and efficacy of PCI in unprotected left main coronary arteries are still a matter of debate. In the USA, the use of drug-eluting stents remains under investigation.

Sirolimus (previously known as rapamycin) and tacrolimus inhibit T-lymphocyte activation, although the exact mechanisms of action is not known, and appear to differ. Experimental evidence suggests that tacrolimus binds to an intracellular protein, FKBP-12. A complex of tacrolimus-FKBP-12, Ca^{2+}, calmodulin and calcineurin is then formed and the phosphatase activity of calcineurin inhibited. This effect may prevent the dephosphorylation and translocation of nuclear factor of activated T cells (NF-AT), a nuclear component thought to initiate gene transcription for the formation of lymphokines (such as interleukin-2, γ interferon). The net result is the inhibition of T-lymphocyte activation (i.e. immunosuppression). Although sirolimus resembles tacrolimus and binds to FKBP-12, tacrolimus blocks lymphokine (e.g. IL-2) gene transcription, whereas sirolimus acts later to blocks IL-2-dependent T-lymphocyte proliferation and the stimulation caused by cross-linkage of CD28, possibly by blocking activation of a kinase referred to as mammalian target of rapamycin or 'mTOR,' a serine-threonine kinase that is important for cell cycle progression. Therefore, sirolimus is believed to act in synergy with tacrolimus in suppressing the immune system. Tacrolimus is also used in atopic dermatitis and sirolimus is approved for prevention of renal allograft rejection. Cilostazol (see section on deep vein thrombosis) is being evaluated for prevention of restenosis in patients undergoing coronary angioplasty and stent implantation, and in patients with a history of prior stroke for secondary prevention of cerebral infarction.

Treatment of syndromes related to AMI (acute coronary syndromes)

Although treatments for the various aspects of AMI exist, overall success (in terms of survival) is poor. The reduction in 1-year mortality with optimal use of all available interventions is 20–30%. Unfortunately, in many AMI patients, the first symptom is ventricular fibrillation, so 35–50% die outside of hospital from their first AMI before medical attention can be received. Thus, those patients most at risk of death are not included in most statistics on effectiveness of interventions. In the long term, prevention of coronary artery disease by diet and avoidance of risk factors such as cigarette smoking, combined with AICDs for those identified as being at risk of acute coronary obstruction, will probably be more effective than pharmacologic intervention after the acute event.

Congestive heart failure

Congestive heart failure (CHF) is the most common reason for hospitalization of people over 65 years of age in the USA, with over 400 000 new cases each year. Diagnosis is made on the basis of impaired cardiac function and reduced tolerance to exercise. The major causes of congestive heart failure are ischemic heart disease, hypertension, valvular heart disease and cardiomyopathy. The identity of the cause influences the choice of drug treatment.

Heart failure refers to the inability of the heart to provide a sufficient cardiac output for the body's needs

Congestive describes the engorgement of the venous system and the associated tissue edema. The central venous pressure that determines edema is known as preload. The heart can fail to provide sufficient cardiac output for various underlying reasons including:

- Loss of viable myocytes (cardiomyopathy) due to infarction, infection or exposure to chemicals/drugs (e.g. cobalt/Adriamycin).
- Excessive resistance to cardiac output (known as afterload) owing to arterial hypertension or aortic stenosis.

Table 13.9 Symptoms associated with congestive heart failure

Acute	Chronic
Tachycardia	Various arrhythmias
Shortness of breath	Hypertension
Edema (peripheral and/or pulmonary)	Cardiomegaly
Decreased exercise tolerance	Edema (peripheral/ pulmonary)

The severity of the symptoms depends upon the degree of heart failure.

- Valvular defects (e.g. mitral regurgitation) and tachycardia (e.g. in thyrotoxicosis) that reduce cardiac stroke volume.

In each case, acute impairment of cardiac output is commonly followed by a progressive worsening of hemodynamics. This is because the reflex responses to impaired cardiac output forces the viable myocardium to work harder. This can lead to hypertrophy and thickening of the ventricular wall (known as adverse remodeling). The adversely remodeled heart is intrinsically less efficient as a pump. CHF becomes symptomatic if insufficient oxygenated blood is supplied to the organs of the body, or if central venous pressure rises sufficiently to cause edema (Table 13.9):

- Acute CHF can result from exposure of cardiac muscle to toxic levels of drugs or as a result of coronary artery occlusion, usually due to thrombosis.
- Chronic CHF occurs when the heart is damaged by conditions such as primary hypertension or myocardial ischemia and infarction, Adriamycin or cobalt exposure, and surviving myocytes often become hypertrophic.
- Cardiomyopathic CHF may be acute or chronic and usually involves both ventricles. Classification of cardiomyopathies is based upon physiologic and anatomic considerations (Figs 13.20 and 13.21). Cardiomyopathic myocarditis resulting from bacterial infection may involve loss of myocytes, and a failure of cardiac excitation–contraction coupling in surviving myocytes.

Common diseases that contribute to the development of congestive heart failure

- Cardiomyopathy
- Myocardial ischemia and infarction
- Hypertension
- Cardiac valve disease
- Congenital heart disease
- Coronary artery disease

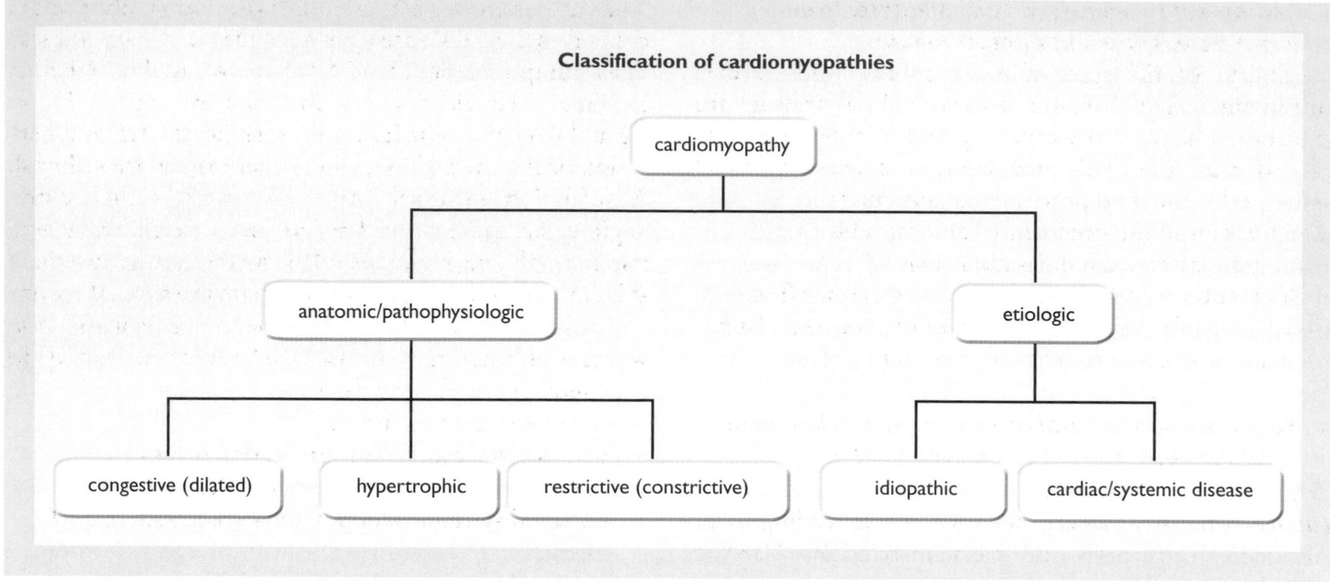

Fig. 13.20 Classification of cardiomyopathies based upon anatomic, pathophysiologic and etiologic considerations.

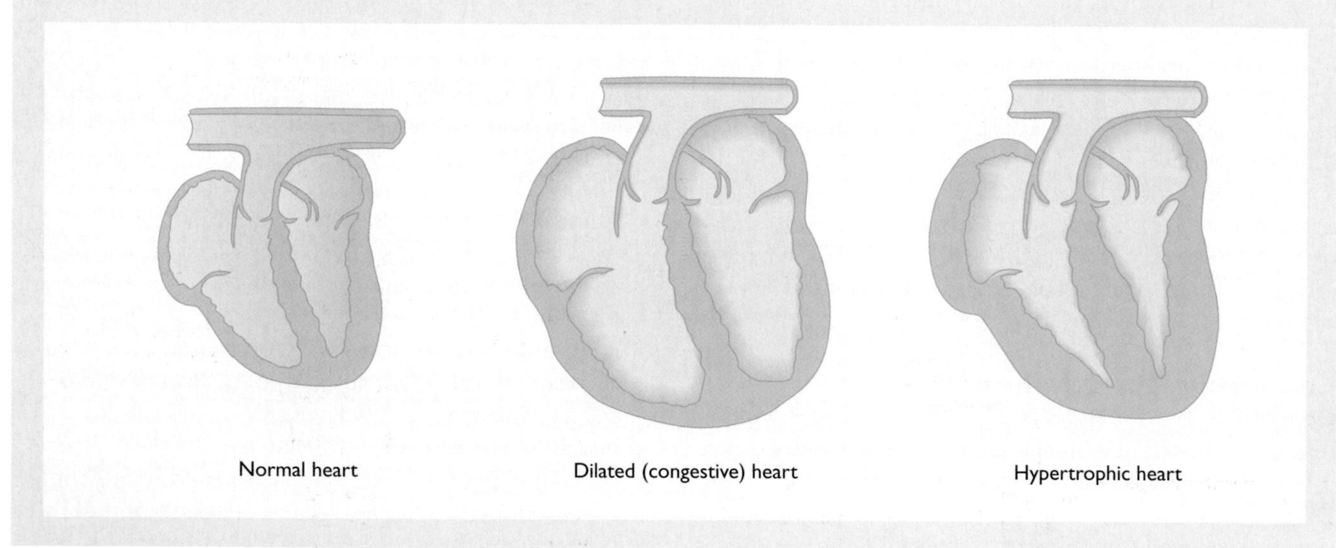

Fig. 13.21 Types of cardiomyopathies involving both the right and left ventricle.

Clinical features of congestive heart failure

- **Reduced force of cardiac contraction**
- **Reduced cardiac output**
- **Reduced tissue perfusion**
- **Increased peripheral vascular resistance**
- **Edema**

Left ventricular heart failure (the most common form) is characterized by reduced cardiac output and blood pressure, as well as pulmonary congestion

Left ventricular heart failure produces 'forward failure' of reduced cardiac output and blood pressure, and 'backward failure' of pulmonary venous congestion. Blood pressure may not necessarily fall as fluid retention may compensate for the impaired cardiac output but, if so, edema is a likely occurrence.

Right ventricular heart failure is characterized by dyspnea, edema and fatigue

The characteristics of right ventricular heart failure (dyspnea, edema and fatigue) result from backward failure. In this condition central venous and right atrial pressures are both high, producing general venous congestion. Any obstruction to right ventricular inflow or excessive load imposed on the right ventricle can precipitate this condition. It ultimately leads to left ventricular failure since the left ventricle's demand for oxygenated pulmonary venous blood cannot be met.

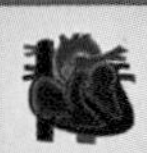

Compensatory reflexes initially alleviate, then exacerbate, symptoms of heart failure

Regardless of the type of heart failure, both cardiac output and (often, though not always) blood pressure are reduced. The cardiovascular system compensates for these decreases, initially maintaining adequate organ and tissue perfusion. Two processes usually occur:

- Activation of extrinsic neurohumoral reflexes.
- Intrinsic cardiac compensation (Fig. 13.22).

Both work in conjunction, improving cardiac function. However, in the long term the symptoms of heart failure are made worse as a result of adverse remodeling.

Extrinsic neurohumoral reflexes initially help maintain cardiac output and blood pressure in CHF

Hypotension activates baroreceptors, which increase the activity of the sympathetic nervous system, leading to an increased heart rate and vasoconstriction. Cardiac contractility and arteriolar resistance therefore increase. The latter increases cardiac afterload. Cardiac afterload is defined as the resistance against which the cardiac muscle must pump to expel blood from the ventricles. When it increases, the ejection fraction (the amount of blood ejected from the ventricles with each heart beat) and perfusion of the liver, kidneys and other organs are reduced. A reduction in renal perfusion activates the renin–angiotensin system, leading to renin secretion which increases plasma angiotensin II formation. Angiotensin II subsequently releases aldosterone from the adrenal cortex.

Angiotensin II causes peripheral vasoconstriction whereas aldosterone increases Na^+ retention leading to the following sequence of events:

- Increased water retention.
- Increased venous and arterial blood pressures.
- Increased vascular and interstitial fluid volume.
- Increased systemic and pulmonary congestion and edema.
- Increased cardiac preload (Fig. 13.22).

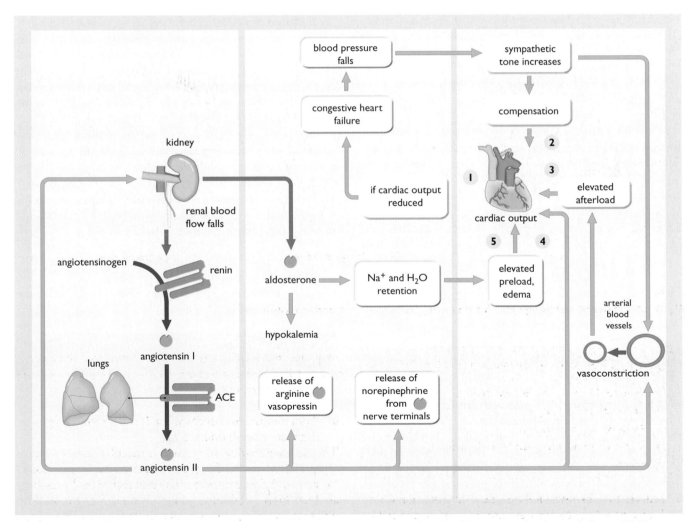

Fig. 13.22 The major extrinsic neurohumoral compensatory mechanisms involved in congestive heart failure. (1) The initial event is a reduction in cardiac output. **(2)** Reflex sympathetic compensation can increase cardiac output, but **(3)** an associated increase in afterload can reduce cardiac output. The cascade of other events can lead to hypertrophy **(4)** owing to actions of angiotensin II on the heart, which increases cardiac output and Na^+ retention. This may increase cardiac output **(5)** by raising preload and left ventricular end-diastolic pressure, but this may cause death by initiating pulmonary edema.

Intrinsic cardiac compensatory mechanisms are activated by an increase in cardiac preload

The cardiac changes that occur include:

- Ventricular dilation. Ventricular chamber volume increases as a consequence of stretch- and neurohumorally-driven hypertrophy and remodeling. Initially this increases the volume of blood ejectable per heart beat.
- An increase in the pressure generated by the ventricles.

As preload increases, there is increased filling of the ventricles and a resultant increase in end-diastolic pressure which, initially, maintains cardiac output by increasing the force of muscle contraction (inotropy). In cardiac muscle, chamber pressure generation depends on the degree of resting stretch of the muscle fiber (i.e. preload at the onset of contraction). This relationship is described by the cardiac muscle length–tension curves, the equivalent of which in the intact heart is known as the Frank–Starling ventricular function curve (see Fig. 13.26).

The hypertrophy and dilation that develop as a consequence of CHF increase cardiac muscle mass, which facilitates ventricular systole and increases the efficiency of blood ejection from the ventricles. It is also an adaptive mechanism which reduces ventricular wall tension.

The relationship between heart wall tension (also known as wall 'stress') and ventricular chamber pressure is known as Laplace's law: $T = (P \times r)/w$ (where T is the tension developed in the heart muscle wall, P is the transmural pressure, r is the radius of the ventricle and w is wall thickness). If ventricular wall tension is not relieved, severe damage results. From Laplace's law, however, ventricular wall tension varies inversely with wall thickness, and the ventricular hypertrophy may reduce the developing wall tension as preload increases. However, this adaptive process cannot compensate for CHF indefinitely and, with time, the ventricles usually become much less compliant than normal, and cardiac output falls.

Compensatory mechanisms activated during CHF result in positive inotropism

An increase in the rate of contractility ($[+dP/dt]_{max}$) is defined as positive inotropism. This is achieved as a consequence of increased sympathetic drive to the heart, and activation of ventricular β_1 adrenergic receptors. This leads to increased efficiency in systolic emptying. However, the benefit of this compensatory mechanism is not well maintained. Failure results from ventricular overload due to increased ventricular filling pressures, systolic wall stress and increased myocardial energy requirements.

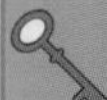

Positive inotropes that improve cardiac contractility

- Cardiac glycosides (e.g. digoxin)
- Phosphodiesterase inhibitors (e.g. inamrinone)
- β_1 agonists (e.g. dobutamine)

Treatment of congestive heart failure

There are two phases of treatment of CHF: acute and chronic. Drug treatment should not only provide relief from symptoms but also reduce mortality. CHF is most amenable to drug treatment if it is the result of cardiomyopathy or arterial hypertension. The immediate objectives are to:

- Reduce congestion (edema).
- Improve cardiac systolic and diastolic function (ventricular emptying and filling, Table 13.10). Many drugs can be used to achieve this purpose (Fig. 13.23).

Cardiac glycosides have been used for heart failure for more than 200 years

Digoxin is the prototype cardiac glycoside extracted from the leaves of the purple (*Digitalis purpurea*) and white (*D. lanata*) foxglove, a common flower. These naturally occurring compounds are known collectively as cardiac glycosides. Although there are many cardiac glycosides, digoxin has the most widespread clinical use in the US.

All cardiac glycosides share a similar chemical structure. Digoxin, digitalis and ouabain all possess an aglycone steroid nucleus that is essential for pharmacological activity. An unsaturated (C17-linked) lactone ring is present, which confers the cardiotonic actions, and C3-linked sugar moieties which influence potency and pharmacokinetic characteristics.

Cardiac glycosides inhibit membrane-bound Na^+/K^+ ATPase to improve symptoms in CHF

Cardiac glycosides achieve their effects at the molecular level by inhibiting membrane-bound Na^+/K^+ ATPase

Table 13.10 Pharmacotherapeutic approach to congestive heart failure

Problem	Approach
Fatigue	Rest, positive inotropes
Edema	Diet (salt restriction), diuretics, digitalis
Poor cardiac contractility	Positive inotropes
Dyspnea	Diuretics (thiazides/loop)
Congestion	Nitrovasodilators
Increased cardiac preload and afterload	Angiotensin-converting enzyme inhibitors, venodilators, vasodilators
Irreversible heart failure	Heart transplantation

The most important approach is to reduce congestion (edema) and improve cardiac contractility.

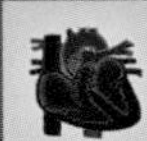

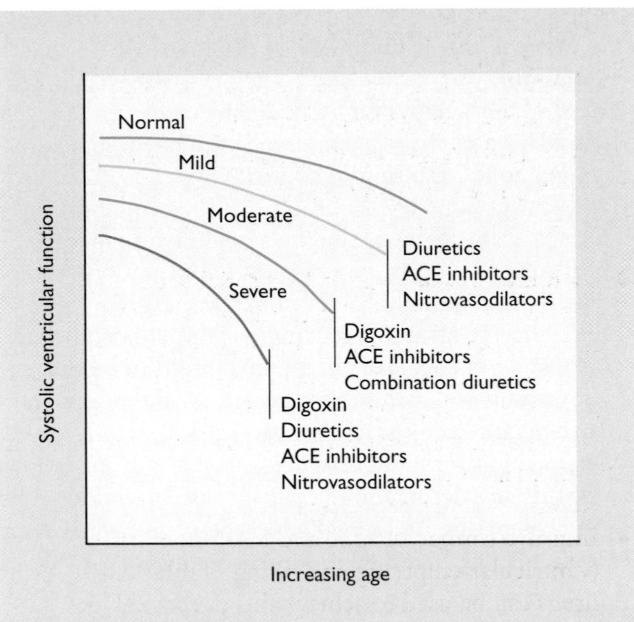

Fig. 13.23 Drugs used in the treatment of the various stages of congestive heart failure. The slow decline in ventricular function with age is exacerbated by disease (ACE, angiotensin-converting enzyme).

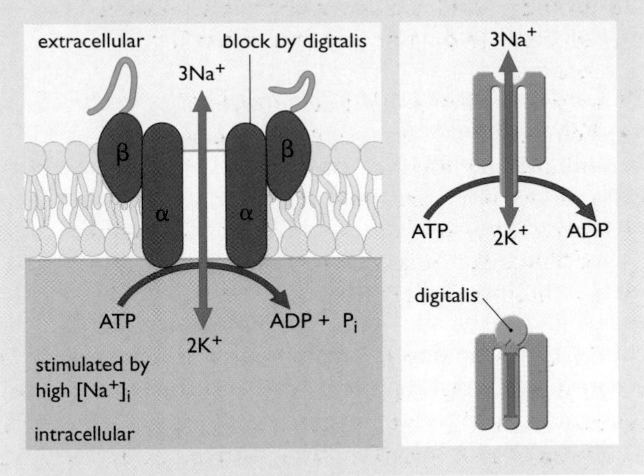

Fig. 13.24 Mechanism of action of digitalis glycosides. The binding site for digitalis is on the extracellular aspect of the α–β heterodimer structure of the Na^+/K^+ ATPase enzyme. Inhibition of this enzyme raises intracellular Na^+ concentration, which raises intracellular Ca^{2+}, and mediates the positive inotropic actions of cardiac glycosides.

(Fig. 13.24). This enzyme is involved in establishing the resting membrane potential of most excitable cells by virtue of its ability to pump three Na^+ ions out of the cell in exchange for two K^+ ions into the cell against their concentration gradients, thereby establishing intracellular concentrations which are high (140 mM) for K^+ and low (25 mM) for Na^+. The pump's energy is derived from the hydrolysis of ATP. Inhibition of the pump results in an increased intracellular cytoplasmic Na^+ concentration.

The increase in Na^+ concentration leads to inhibition of a membrane-bound ion exchanger (Na^+/Ca^{2+} exchanger), and as a consequence, to an increase in cytoplasmic Ca^{2+} concentration. The exchanger is an ATP-independent antiporter (see Ch. 3) that normally causes a net extrusion of Ca^{2+} from cells. The increased cytoplasmic Na^+ concentration passively reduces the exchange function so that less Ca^{2+} is extruded. The raised cytoplasmic Ca^{2+} concentration is then actively pumped into the SR and becomes available for release during subsequent cellular depolarizations, thereby enhancing excitation–contraction coupling. The result is a greater contractility, known as positive inotropism (Fig. 13.25).

In the failing heart, the positive inotropic actions of the cardiac glycosides change the Frank–Starling ventricular function curve. Figure 13.26 outlines the actions of positive inotropic agents on cardiac output.

Despite widespread use, there is no convincing evidence that digitalis, the most commonly used cardiac glycoside, has a beneficial effect on the long-term prognosis of patients with CHF. The symptoms are

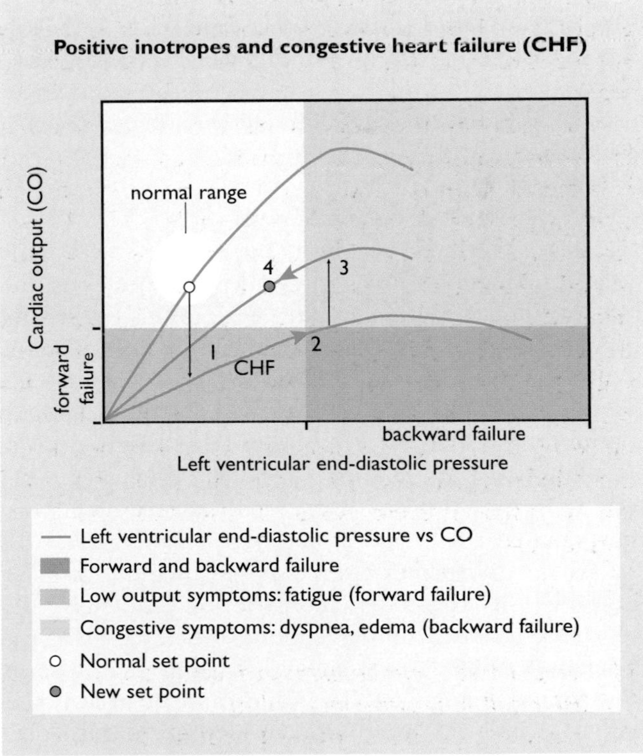

Fig. 13.25 The Frank–Starling curve, positive inotropes and congestive heart failure (CHF). Normal cardiac output is determined by the pressure in the left ventricle at end-diastole. In CHF, the set point for cardiac output is reduced and cardiac output falls **(1)**. Compensatory neurohumoral responses become activated which increase end-diastolic pressure and improve cardiac output; however, this can give rise to backward failure **(2)**. Positive inotropic agents increase cardiac output **(3)**. The improved cardiac output reduces the drive for a high end-diastolic pressure, and decompensation occurs to a new set point **(4)**.

improved in many patients but digitalis does not reduce mortality due to CHF.

Cardiac glycosides additionally alter the electrical activity in the heart

In addition to improving the force of contraction, cardiac glycosides alter the electrical activity in the heart, both directly and indirectly.

Cardiac glycosides indirectly alter heart rate by increasing the activity of the vagus nerve (cranial nerve X) as a result of the stimulation of afferent elements in the paravertebral (nodose) ganglion and a reflex increase in activity of the vagus nerve arcs. Increased vagal firing activity predominates in the supraventricular regions and causes:

- Slowing of the SA node firing rate.
- Slowing of the AV node conduction velocity (widening the PR interval of the EKG).
- Shortening of the atrial action potential.

At toxic doses, cardiac glycosides increase efferent cardiac sympathetic tone. However, the rate of neural discharge is not uniform for all sympathetic nerves and this can result in nonuniform myocardial excitability and arrhythmias, including AV node block, AV junctional tachycardia and ventricular premature beats.

The direct effects of cardiac glycosides on cardiac tissue are most marked at high doses and relate to the loss of cytoplasmic K^+ due to inhibition of Na^+/K^+ ATPase. The continued loss of cytoplasmic K^+ to the extracellular space reduces the resting membrane potential of the cell, resulting in:

- Enhanced automaticity.
- Decreased cardiac conduction velocity.
- Increased AV node refractory period.

With increasing cardiac glycoside concentrations, the free Ca^{2+} concentration reaches toxic levels, saturating the SR sequestration mechanism, resulting in oscillations in free cellular Ca^{2+} due to Ca^{2+}-induced Ca^{2+} release from the SR and resultant oscillations in membrane potential (oscillatory afterpotentials). Arrhythmias, including single and multiple ventricular premature beats and tachyarrhythmias, may result from oscillatory afterpotentials.

Cardiac glycosides increase peripheral vascular resistance by direct vasoconstriction and centrally mediated increases in sympathetic tone. In CHF, the elevated peripheral resistance that is present falls as treatment is maintained. The improvement in hemodynamics occurring as a result of the increased cardiac output results in diuresis (due to increased renal blood flow).

All cardiac glycosides have a low therapeutic ratio because their pharmacotherapeutic and their toxic actions each result from increased cytoplasmic Ca^{2+} concentrations. The most important adverse effects are cardiac arrhythmias.

In addition to the heart, other organ and system toxicities are common with cardiac glycosides, but usually only during prolonged therapy. The most frequent noncardiac adverse effects of cardiac glycosides involve:

- Actions on the gastrointestinal tract (gastric irritation).
- Central nervous system (CNS) effects due to stimulation of the vagal afferents and chemoreceptor trigger zone, resulting in nausea, vomiting, diarrhea and anorexia.
- Other CNS effects, including visual disturbances, headaches, dizziness, fatigue and hallucinations. These are especially common in the elderly.
- Rare adverse effects, including eosinophilia and skin rash, and gynecomastia in men (thought to be due either to hypothalamic stimulation, or the peripheral estrogenic actions of cardiac glycosides).

Plasma monitoring of cardiac glycoside concentrations is useful in determining causes of toxicity. The pharmacokinetics of individual cardiac glycosides vary according to the lipophilicity of the compound.

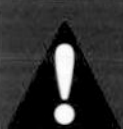

Adverse effects of cardiac glycosides

- **Toxicity, because the therapeutic dose ratios are narrow**
- **May promote cardiac K^+ loss and hypokalemia which precipitate life-threatening arrhythmias when used with diuretics**
- **Abdominal discomfort, emesis and anorexia**
- **Arrhythmias with cardioversion, which should therefore be used with extreme caution**

Cardiac glycoside toxicity is affected by blood K^+

Cardiac glycoside toxicity may be worsened by hypokalemia (which may be associated with the use of diuretics or secondary aldosteronism). Cardiac glycosides and K^+ ions compete for a common binding site on Na^+/K^+ ATPase. Hypokalemia facilitates cardiac glycoside binding to the enzyme, thereby enhancing pharmacologic activity, and toxic effects, in equal measure.

Treatment of cardiac glycosides toxicity is achieved by:

- Oral administration of K^+ supplements to raise serum K^+ concentration.
- Antiarrhythmic drugs such as procainamide and phenytoin to reverse cardiac glycoside-induced arrhythmias.
- Monoclonal antibodies to bind cardiac glycosides.
- Intravenous digoxin-immune fragment for antigen binding (Fab), derived from specific antibodies to digoxin, for patients with life-threatening intoxication. The high affinity of cardiac glycosides for the antibody prevents binding to Na^+/K^+ ATPase and the drug can be cleared from the circulatory system.

Although cardiac glycoside toxicity may be reversed by these treatments, it can be minimized or prevented by monitoring of serum electrolytes and cardiac glycoside

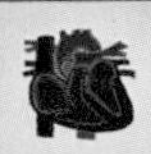

blood concentrations. A very important factor in the risk of developing digoxin toxicity is renal function. Since digoxin is primarily excreted unchanged by the kidneys, maintenance doses of digoxin must be adjusted in patients with renal insufficiency.

Phosphodiesterase inhibitors in CHF

Phosphodiesterase (PDE) inhibitors have been used in patients with CHF unresponsive to other treatment. The isoform PDE3 is found in myocardial and vascular smooth muscle. The inhibition of cAMP degradation results in an elevation of cytosolic Ca^{2+} content.

There are many tissue-specific PDE isoforms. Inhibitors such as inamrinone (known as amrinone in the UK), milrinone and vesnarinone are bipyridines that increase cAMP levels by inhibiting PDE3. Inhibition results in a more prolonged influx of Ca^{2+} during the cardiac action potential and increases contractility. cAMP breakdown is also inhibited in arterial and venous smooth muscle, resulting in marked vasodilation.

PDE inhibitors increase cardiac output, decrease pulmonary capillary wedge pressure (an indirect measure of left atrial pressure and the likelihood of pulmonary edema) and reduce total peripheral resistance, without producing any significant changes in heart rate or arterial blood pressure.

Inamrinone is a PDE inhibitor useful for short-term (acute) treatment of CHF

Inamrinone is used clinically for the short-term treatment of patients with CHF that is unresponsive to digitalis and diuretic therapy. It can be used alone or in conjunction with β_1 agonists to:

- Improve cardiac output.
- Increase stroke volume.
- Reduce right atrial and pulmonary capillary wedge pressure.

Prolonged i.v. use does not result in a loss of response, i.e. tachyphylaxis does not occur, but such use can cause adverse effects. There is a high incidence of nausea and vomiting in patients treated with inamrinone, but liver function abnormalities and thrombocytopenia are the adverse effects that cause most concern. These adverse effects disappear on discontinuation of treatment. Inamrinone can also cause supraventricular and ventricular arrhythmias and can therefore only be used clinically if the EKG is frequently monitored.

Milrinone is a potent PDE3 inhibitor not used in long-term therapy of CHF

Milrinone is an inamrinone analog, but is more potent. It has a similar spectrum of dose-limiting adverse effects to that of inamrinone, and may also cause thrombocytopenia in a minority (0.4%) of patients. There is less gastrointestinal irritation if it is used orally. Its use is limited, however, because it can precipitate lethal arrhythmias; therefore, it is not used for chronic therapy. Similar findings have limited the use of a similar agent, enoximone. Neither are approved for use in the USA.

Vesnarinone is a PDE inhibitor with additional potentially useful actions, but is not approved for CHF treatment in the USA

Studies suggest that vesnarinone may increase cardiac contractility by additional mechanisms such as activation of the Na^+/Ca^{2+} exchange antiporter, which will lead to an increase in cytosolic Ca^{2+} during systole. This may be a direct effect or indirect (secondary to the drug's ability to widen the cardiac action potential duration by a mechanism that appears to involve I_{Kr} blockade). In addition, vesnarinone may stimulate I_{si}. The major limiting adverse effect is agranulocytosis, which occurs in 1–3% of patients. However, this is reversible when the drug is stopped. Like milrinone, in the long-term therapy of heart-failure vesnarinone is not recommended owing to a dose-dependent increase in the likelihood of death, and the drug is not approved for use in the USA.

β_1 adrenoceptor antagonists have a surprising benefit in CHF

These agents may seem a surprising addition to the range of drugs for CHF, given that β adrenoceptor agonists have long been used in emergency treatment of acute CHF (discussed below). Although difficult to prove, it is suspected that their system mechanism of action is antagonism of the adverse remodeling effects of a raised sympathetic tone (commonly seen in heart failure). At the cellular level, it is suspected that β_1 adrenoceptor antagonists such as carvedilol reduce down-regulation of β_1 adrenoceptor expression that occurs in response to the high level of sympathetic tone. Consequently, there may be a resetting of β_1 adrenoceptor expression which is more consistent with a healthy cardiovascular status. The G protein-coupled receptor kinase (GRK)–arrestin system is involved in the transduction of desensitization and down-regulation of the myocardial β_1 adrenoceptor. GRK2 is predominantly located in vascular endothelial cells, whereas another isoform, GRK3 is located in cardiac myocyte. However, the myocardial GRK2 isoform (also known as β adrenergic receptor kinase 1; βARK1) is up-regulated in patients with CHF. Inhibition of GRK2 activity may impair adverse cardiac remodeling in dilated cardiomyopathy and CHF. Even though the mechanisms of action are not clear, two β_1-selective antagonists, metoprolol and bisoprolol, have been shown to reduce death rate during long-term treatment, suggesting that at the molecular level, β_1 antagonism is the mechanism of action. Therapeutically, both cardiac output failure and sudden cardiac death (exact cause of death uncertain) are reduced. Another β_1 antagonist, carvedilol, has also been shown to reduce death rate in CHF patients. However, this drug, in addition to blocking β_1 adrenoceptors, also blocks β_2 adrenoceptors and α_1 adrenoceptors and possesses antioxidant actions,

Aldosterone receptor blockade reduces mortality in CHF

Eplerenone was the first aldosterone receptor blocker to receive approval for improving the survival in patients with clinical evidence of stable CHF after an AMI and left ventricular systolic dysfunction (ejection fraction < 40%). In the EPHESUS (Eplerenone Post-AMI Heart Failure Efficacy and Survival Study) trial, compared with post-MI heart failure patients on placebo and standard therapy (ACE inhibitors and β blockers), eplerenone plus standard therapy reduced mortality by 15%. Treatment should be initiated at 25 mg once daily and titrated to the target dose of 50 mg orally, once daily, preferably within 4 weeks as tolerated by the patient.

The mechanism of action of eplerenone is unclear. It may achieve its affects in heart failure by acting on unique fast-response receptors (as opposed to slow-response nuclear receptors) located in cardiac cell membranes, resulting in inhibition of aldosterone-mediated apoptotic cell death. Activation of the plasma membrane receptor by aldosterone in cardiomyocytes results in the following cascade of intracellular events:

- Activation of phospholipase C.
- Rapid elevation of intracellular Ca^{2+}.
- Activation of protein kinase C and calcineurin (a Ca^{2+}-dependent phosphatase).
- Dephosphorylation of the pro-apoptotic protein BAD.
- Mitochondrial depolarization and release of cytochrome C.
- Activation of the apoptotic enzyme caspase-3.

BAD, when dephosphorylated in the aldosterone-induced cascade, heterodimerizes with two other proteins, bcl-2 and bcl-xL, suppressing their actions (they signal the continued survival of the cell) which include stabilization (closure) of the mitochondrial porin channel (a voltage-operated anion channel). With porin channels open, cytochrome C escapes into the cytosol where it activates caspase-3 (Fig 13.27).

Eplerenone has also been in use for treatment of hypertension for some years, and its characteristics are described further in the treatment of hypertension section.

Nitrovasodilators achieve benefit in CHF without directly acting on the heart

Nitrovasodilators are chemically diverse agents that mediate a potent vasodilating action on both arterial and venous smooth muscle. The molecular mechanism of action remains poorly characterized. However, these agents:

- Are thought to produce vascular relaxation at the cellular level by nitrosothiol intermediate enhancement of cGMP activity.
- May regulate intracellular Ca^{2+} release from the sarcoplasmic reticulum, alter sympathetic tone, and produce smooth muscle-relaxing autacoids such as PGI_2 and PGE_2.
- Reduce diastolic pressure and improve diastolic function in the heart (see Fig. 13.26).

Nitroprusside is a standard first-choice nitrovasodilator in the treatment of acute CHF, especially in patients with elevated arterial blood pressure, because it reduces both cardiac preload and afterload. It reduces left ventricular filling pressures by reducing venous tone, and by doing so increases venous capacitance and produces a shift in blood volume distribution.

Since nitroprusside has no important direct effect on ventricular contractility, the increase in cardiac output and stroke volume occur as a result of a reduction in cardiac afterload. The increase in cardiac output is not accompanied by a reflex increase in blood pressure or heart rate, and nitroprusside lowers myocardial oxygen consumption.

Nitroprusside must be given intravenously at 0.10–0.20 mg/kg/min with dose titration, and is used as an acute short-term treatment of CHF.

Liver metabolism of nitroprusside produces cyanide, which is then cleared by the kidney. Cyanide can accumulate in patients with renal insufficiency, resulting in nausea, confusion and convulsions. Nitroprusside can also be metabolized to prussic acid, which avidly binds hemoglobin.

The major adverse effect of nitroprusside is hypotension, which may be severe.

Nitroglycerin (glyceryl trinitrate) and isosorbide dinitrate predominantly decrease cardiac preload, but produce a slight reduction in cardiac afterload. Tolerance develops rapidly and thus administration has to be intermittent. A high first-pass metabolism can be avoided by sublingual administration or topical application. Hypotension is the most common adverse effect.

Hydralazine used in combination with nitrates has been shown to increase the life expectancy of patients with CHF. This combination is therefore an alternative first-line therapy to ACE inhibitors, especially for patients who are unable to tolerate the latter.

In addition to reducing cardiac afterload, hydralazine has an indirect positive inotropic effect, resulting from enhanced sympathetic nervous system activity due to arterial vasodilation. It is therefore useful when withdrawing dobutamine or β_1 agonist treatment. Hydralazine also increases renal blood flow. Hydralazine alone is insufficient to reduce vascular congestion adequately, and is therefore used with topical nitroglycerin or oral isosorbide dinitrate to induce venodilation.

The adverse effects of hydralazine include:

- Reflex activation of the sympathetic nervous system.
- Drug-induced systemic lupus erythematosus, which is rare with doses of hydralazine less than 200 mg/day.

Hydralazine is contraindicated in patients with CHF who have ischemic coronary artery disease, unless nitrates are used at the same time, since myocardial oxygen consumption increases with hydralazine owing to increased sympathetic drive to the heart.

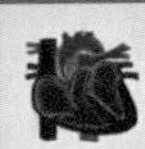

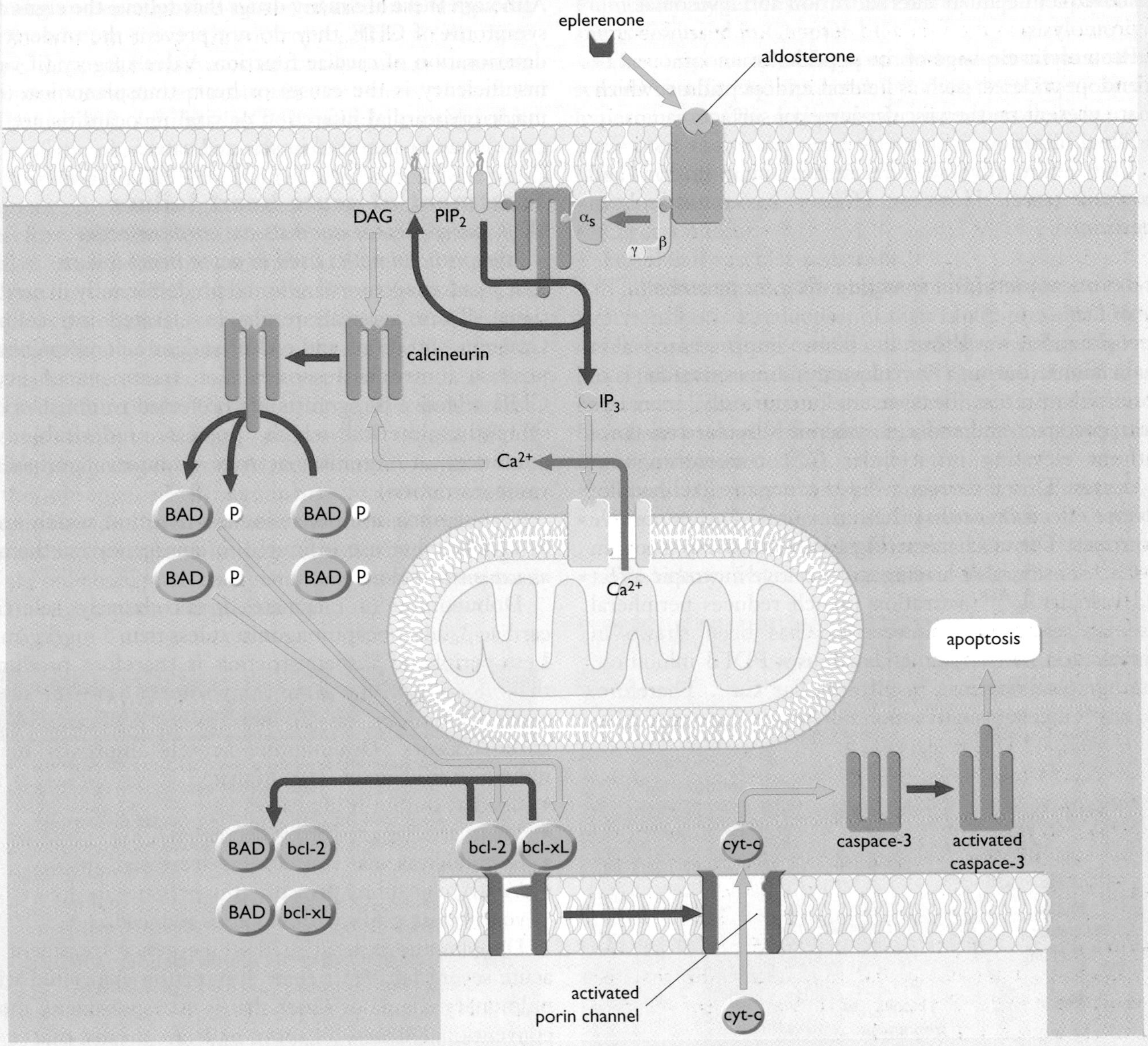

Fig. 13.27 Postulated mechanism by which aldosterone causes apoptotic cell death and by which eplerenone inhibits this in the treatment of heart failure. Aldosterone receptor activation leads to activation of calcineurin, which dephosphorylates the protein BAD, which heterodimerizes with bcl-2 and bcl-xL. The heterodimers can no longer block the mitochondrial porin channel, allowing cytochrome c (cyt-c) to escape and activate the pro-apoptotic enzyme caspase-3. DAG, diacycloglycerol; PIP_2 phosphotidylinositol; IP_3 inositol-1,4,5-triphosphate.

Nesiritide has a unique mechanism of action in CHF

Nesiritide is a purified recombinant preparation of a new drug class, human B-type (brain) natriuretic peptide (BNP). Nesiritide is indicated for the i.v. treatment of patients with acutely decompensated CHF who have dyspnea at rest or with minimal activity. In this population, nesiritide reduces pulmonary capillary wedge pressure and improves dyspnea. Nesiritide binds to particulate guanylate cyclase in vascular smooth muscle and endothelial cells, leading to increased intracellular concentrations of cGMP and smooth muscle cell relaxation (mimicking endogenous NO; see Fig 13.14). Nesiritide is administered intravenously. The recommended dosing regimen is a 2 μg/kg bolus followed by an infusion of 0.01 μg/kg/min. The pharmacodynamic half-life (3 hours) is longer than the pharmacokinetic half-life (18 minutes). At steady state, plasma BNP levels increase from baseline endogenous levels by approximately three- to sixfold with nesiritide infusion doses of 0.01–0.03 μg/kg/min.

BNP is cleared from the circulation via the following three mechanisms, in order of decreasing importance:

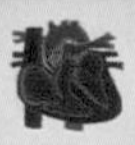

- The heart, which generates cardiac output.
- The arterioles, which determine peripheral vascular resistance.
- Endothelial cells, which regulate the synthesis or degradation of endogenous hypertensive and hypotensive agents such as angiotensin II and NO.
- The CNS, which senses the blood pressure and controls it by regulating the systems involved in blood pressure control.

Hypertension

- **Hypertension is commonly diagnosed when the diastolic pressure is consistently found to be higher than 90 mmHg**
- **Blood pressure can be raised by increased cardiac output, increased peripheral resistance, or increased blood volume**
- **Primary hypertension has no apparent cause**
- **Secondary hypertension results from disease, e.g. pheochromocytoma and venovascular stenosis**

Hypertension is classified into essential (or primary) and secondary

Primary hypertension is an elevation of blood pressure with no apparent cause. It accounts for 90–95% of all cases and usually occurs in adulthood, typically at ages above 40 years. Several risk factors are associated with primary hypertension, including a genetic predisposition, obesity, high alcohol consumption and physical inactivity. Some of these may represent additional systems targets for antihypertensive drugs.

Secondary hypertension accounts for 5–10% of all cases and, by definition, is due to an identifiable cause, for example renovascular disease, which elevates blood pressure by activating the renin–angiotensin–aldosterone system (Fig. 13.30). A variety of endocrine diseases (e.g. pheochromocytoma, an adrenal medulla tumor that secretes excessive epinephrine) may also cause secondary hypertension.

Both primary and secondary hypertension can be classified by the degree of increased cardiovascular risk and the extent to which blood pressure is elevated

In most patients, treatment of hypertension is a lifetime project designed to reduce cardiovascular risk over many years. In some patients, typically with markedly elevated blood pressure, it may also be necessary to decrease blood pressure over the course of hours or days. These relatively uncommon situations are often called hypertensive emergencies or urgencies, respectively.

In most patients with hypertension the blood pressure increases progressively over months to years. As a result, an increased risk of cardiovascular disease develops slowly

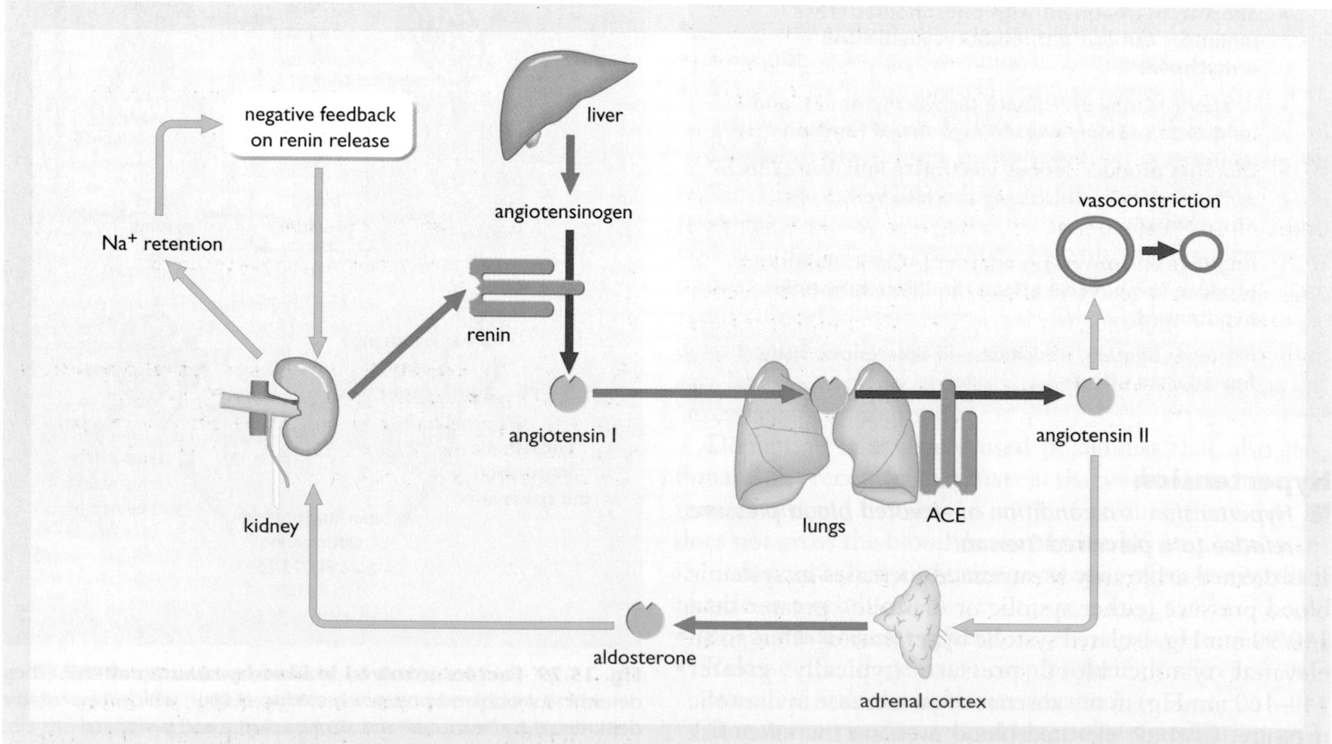

Fig. 13.30 Renin–angiotensin–aldosterone system. Release of renin stimulates conversion of angiotensinogen (from the liver) to angiotensin I, which in turn is converted to angiotensin II under the influence of angiotensin-converting enzyme. Angiotensin II leads to vasoconstriction, release of aldosterone (adrenal cortex) and Na^+ retention. The latter increases blood pressure but reduces renin release, so the system is a homeostatic process.

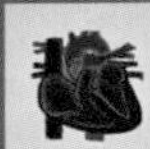

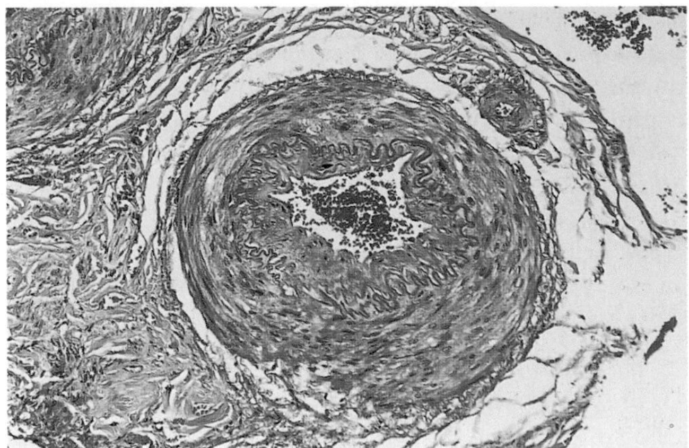

Fig. 13.31 Changes of chronic hypertension in the blood vessel wall. These occur slowly over time. Medial smooth muscle cells migrate into the intima so that the intima becomes thicker. (Courtesy of Dr. Alan Stevens and Professor Jim Lowe.)

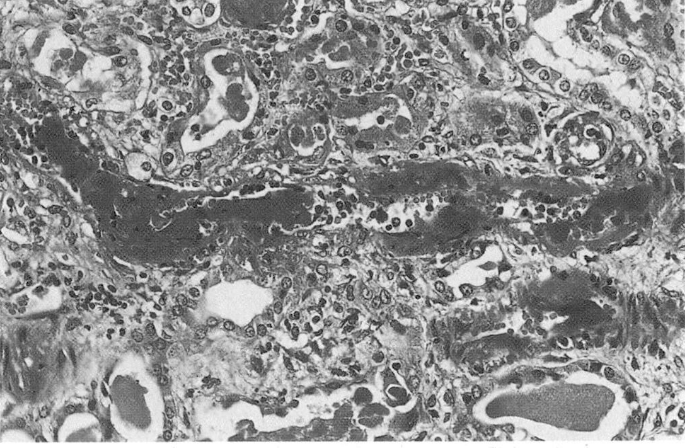

Fig. 13.32 Changes of accelerated hypertension in the blood vessel wall. Accelerated hypertension damages the blood vessel wall. Damage to the endothelial lining leads to adhesion and activation of platelets and release of various mediators (platelet-activating factor, thromboxane A_2, serotonin, ADP, thrombin). (Courtesy of Dr. Alan Stevens and Professor Jim Lowe.)

over a period of years (Fig. 13.31). The loss of vascular elasticity and compliance in blood vessels then contributes to the establishment of chronic hypertension. Consequently, therapy involves long-term control of blood pressure.

In hypertensive emergencies, acutely elevated blood pressure, typically over a short period, may lead to immediately life-threatening organ damage in the heart, aorta, brain or kidneys (Fig. 13.32). In this situation the objective is to lower blood pressure within minutes or hours. Hypertensive emergencies are becoming increasingly rare as antihypertensive therapy improves, but emergencies may occur if the therapy is inadequate, if the patient stops taking their medication because they falsely think they are 'well,' or if the patient is undiagnosed and has never been treated. Presentation involves high, and rising, blood pressure and signs of end-organ damage, e.g. encephalopathy. If an emergency occurs it is important to reduce the blood pressure quickly by i.v. drug administration, but carefully and in stages (usually chosen arbitrarily) to avoid low cerebrovascular pressure and thereby inducing cerebral ischemia (Fig. 13.33).

Cerebral blood flow
Mean arterial pressure
Normal relationship
Relationship in severe hypertension

Fig. 13.33 The relationship between cerebral blood flow (CBF) and mean arterial pressure (MAP). In severe hypertension, particularly in emergency hypertension, a rapid reduction of MAP may cause an excessive reduction in CBF, cerebral ischemia and possibly stroke.

Treatment of hypertension

Nondrug treatment is the first-choice therapy

Patients with hypertension are advised to avoid activities that may predispose to cardiovascular disease. The major recommendations are:

- To exercise.
- To reduce body weight, if overweight.
- In some cases, to restrict dietary salt intake.
- To stop smoking.
- To restrict ethanol intake.
- To treat lipoprotein disorders.

Drug treatment of a hypertensive emergency is different from treatment of chronic hypertension

The Seventh Report of the Joint National Committee on Prevention, Detection, Evaluation, and Treatment of High Blood Pressure (2003) provides a guideline for hypertension prevention and management of chronic hypertension (see Key Facts on p. 414 ; Fig. 13.34).

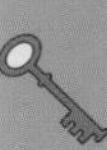

Key components of The Seventh Report of the Joint National Committee on Prevention, Detection, Evaluation, and Treatment of High Blood Pressure (2003)

- In persons older than 50 years, systolic blood pressure (blood pressure) of more than 140 mmHg is a much more important cardiovascular disease risk factor than diastolic blood pressure
- The risk of cardiovascular disease, beginning at 115/75 mmHg, doubles with each increment of 20/10 mmHg; individuals who are normotensive at 55 years of age have a 90% lifetime risk for developing hypertension
- Individuals with a systolic blood pressure of 120 to 139 mmHg or a diastolic blood pressure of 80 to 89 mmHg should be considered as prehypertensive and require health-promoting lifestyle modifications to prevent cardiovascular disease
- Thiazide diuretics should be used in drug treatment for most patients with uncomplicated hypertension, either alone or combined with drugs from other classes. Certain high-risk conditions are compelling indications for the initial use of other antihypertensive drug classes (ACE inhibitors, angiotensin-receptor blockers, β-blockers, Ca^{2+} antagonists)
- Most patients with hypertension will require two or more antihypertensive medications to achieve goal blood pressure (<140/90 mmHg, or <130/80 mmHg for patients with diabetes or chronic kidney disease)
- If blood pressure is more than 20/10 mmHg above goal blood pressure, consideration should be given to initiating therapy with two agents, one of which usually should be a thiazide diuretic
- The most effective therapy will control hypertension only if patients are motivated

Classes of drugs used for treating hypertension

- Diuretics
- β_1 adrenoceptor antagonists (β blockers)
- α_1 adrenoceptor antagonists
- β_2 adrenoceptor agonists
- Direct-acting vasodilators
- Ca^{2+} antagonists
- ACE inhibitors
- Angiotensin II antagonists
- Aldosterone antagonists
- Adrenergic neuron blockers and reserpine
- Imidazoline I_1 antagonists
- Dopamine D_1 antagonists

All antihypertensive drugs have adverse effects which can affect compliance

Although true for all disease treatments, to a greater or lesser extent, adverse effects are particularly important in the treatment of hypertension since most hypertensive patients are free of symptoms for most of the time (except during an emergency). It is only when secondary complications such as a stroke ensue that the disease becomes symptomatic. Therefore, any adverse drug effect, no matter how trivial, will make the patient feel worse. This explains why compliance is poor in long-term treatment of hypertension.

The pharmacotherapeutic goal in treating hypertension can be achieved by diverse mechanisms of drug action using a wide range of drugs

Choice of drugs is influenced by demonstration of beneficial effects on clinically important end-points, by cost, by tolerability in individual patients, and by concomitant disorders (such as congestive heart failure or diabetes which mandate use of an angiotensin-converting enzyme inhibitor as the primary drug).

Several classes of drug are currently used to treat hypertension, but their classification is heterogeneous

The choice of drug therapy may be influenced by the type of hypertension and any other clinical conditions.

Generally, there is little difference between patient populations in terms of the ability of the different classes of drug to reduce blood pressure acutely. However, certain groups of people may be more responsive in the long term to certain classes of drugs than others. For example, the Caucasian population responds better than people of African origin to adrenoceptor antagonists and ACE inhibitors, whereas the elderly population responds better than the young to Ca^{2+} antagonists and diuretics. However, variation in drug responses is greater from individual to individual than between populations. The ultimate aim of therapy is to reduce the increased mortality found in the hypertensive population. The few drugs that have been shown to achieve this include thiazide diuretics and ACE inhibitors. There are suggestions that some classes of drugs may increase, rather than decrease, mortality.

Diuretics are useful antihypertensives, but benefit may be unrelated to diuresis

The pharmacology of diuretics is discussed in detail in Chapter 12. Three types of diuretic are used in hypertension:

- Thiazides.
- Loop diuretics.
- Potassium-sparing agents.

Diuretics were once thought to lower blood pressure via increased water excretion in the kidney, leading to a reduction of plasma volume, extracellular fluid volume and cardiac output. However, there are several reasons for questioning this, the most important of which is that, for a range of diuretic drugs, antihypertensive activity is not directly proportional to diuretic activity:

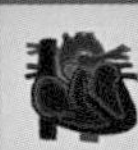

lifestyle modifications

not at goal BP
(<140/90mmHg or <130/80 mmHg for those with diabetes or chronic kidney disease)

initial drug choice

hypertension without compelling indications		hypertension with compelling indications
Stage 1 hypertension (systolic BP 140-159 mmHg) thiazide diuretics for most may consider ACE inhibitor, ARB, β-blocker, CA or combination	Stage 2 hypertension (systolic BP 160 mmHg or diastolic BP 100 mmHg) 2 drug combination for most (usually thiazide diuretic and ACE inhibitor or ARB or β-blocker or CA)	drug(s) for the compelling indications (see text) other antihypertensive drugs (diuretics, ACE inhibitor, ARB, β-blocker, CA as needed)

not at goal BP

optimize dosages or add additional drugs until goal BP is achieved
consider consultation with hypertension specialist

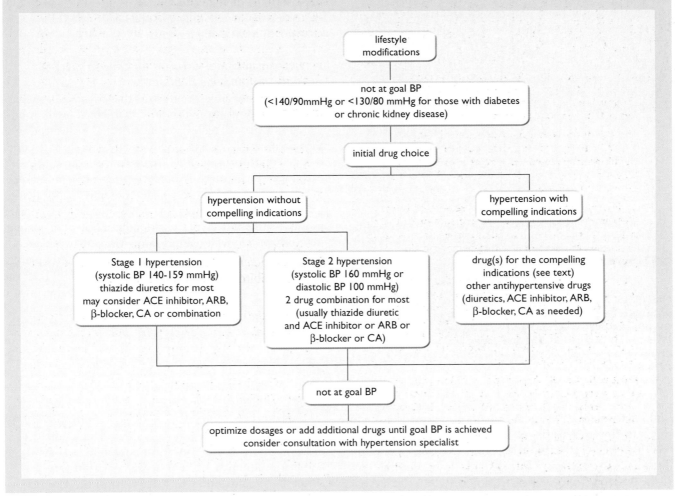

Fig. 13.34 Algorithm for treatment of hypertension. BP, blood pressure; ARB, angiotenisin AT-1 receptor blocker; CA, Ca^{2+} antagonist. (Adapted from Chobanian AV et al. *JAMA* 2003; **289**: 2560–2571.)

- Thiazides are relatively effective antihypertensive agents, but are only moderately effective diuretics.
- Loop diuretics are relatively ineffective antihypertensive agents (in patients with normal renal function) but are powerful diuretics.

If the diuretic effect of thiazides were responsible for their antihypertensive effect, the dose–response relationship for the two effects would be superimposable. This is not the case (Fig. 13.35). Triamterene is not an antihypertensive drug despite having a diuretic effect similar to the antihypertensive agent amiloride. On the other hand, thiazides lose effectiveness in patients with moderate renal insufficiency.

Thus, although diuresis has been the conventional explanation for the beneficial effect provided by diuretics in hypertension, there is increasing awareness that their mechanisms of action in hypertension are not well understood.

It has been suggested that diuretics (especially the thiazides) may produce their effects in hypertension by modulating the activity of K^+ channels. ATP-regulated K^+ channels in resistance arterioles may be activated by thiazides. This molecular action leads to membrane hyperpolarization, which opposes smooth muscle Ca^{2+} entry and contraction and, at the system level, reduces peripheral vascular resistance.

Thiazides are the most commonly used antihypertensive diuretics

Thiazide diuretics (e.g. bendroflumethiazide, hydrochlorothiazide) and thiazide-like drugs which are sulfonamide derivatives, such as chlortalidone, are actively transported by a probenecid-sensitive secretory mechanism into the proximal renal tubule. As diuretics, this group of drugs acts on the luminal membrane of the cortical diluting segment of the distal convoluted tubule (see Ch. 12).

Thiazides may cause male sexual dysfunction. Since hypertension (in the elderly male) is commonly associated with impotence, the prevalence and impact of this adverse effect are difficult to determine. Relatively high doses of thiazide diuretics may induce hyperuricemia, and have adverse effects on serum concentrations of

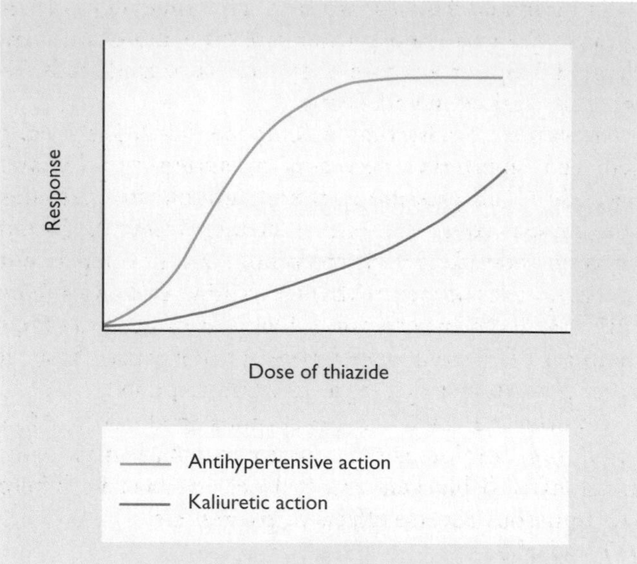

Fig. 13.35 Dose–response relationship for thiazide antihypertensive agents and blood pressure (antihypertensive action) and as a diuretic (shown here as effect on K^+ excretion, the kaliuretic action). The lack of overlap of the curves suggests that the two effects may not be related.

lipids and glucose. In addition to the more well-know thiazide diuretics discussed elsewhere, there are others.

Quinethazone has a profile similar to other thiazide diuretics. It may be used to treat hypertension (and reduce edema following heart failure) after one or two 50 mg tablets, orally, once a day. Because of its relatively prolonged duration of activity, a single daily dose is generally sufficient. A total daily dose of 150–200 mg may be necessary in some patients. When quinethazone is used in combination with other antihypertensive agents, the dosage of each drug may often be reduced.

Metolazone was described above in connection with treatment of edema associated with heart failure. In mild to moderate essential hypertension, 2.5–5 mg orally is taken once daily. A rapid-availability tablet may be used, 0.5 mg once daily, usually in the morning. If hypertension is inadequately controlled, the dose may be increased to 1 mg once a day. Increasing the dose higher than 1 mg does not increase the effect.

Benzthiazide was discussed earlier for its role as a treatment for edema in heart failure. In hypertension, benzthiazide may be used either as the sole therapeutic agent or to enhance the effectiveness of other antihypertensive drugs in the more severe forms of hypertension. Initiation of therapy requires 50–100 mg orally daily in two doses. This dosage may be continued until a therapeutic drop in blood pressure occurs. In maintenance of antihypertensive therapy the dosage should be adjusted according to the patient response, either upward to as much as 50 mg q.i.d. or downward to the minimal effective dosage level. Other thiazides used in treating hypertension include methylclothiazide 5 mg and polythiazide 2 mg, both orally and once daily, used alone or in combination with other agents.

Hypokalemia may occur as an adverse effect of long-term thiazide treatment

A characteristic adverse effect of thiazides is an increase in Na^+ concentration in the distal convoluted tubule which impairs K^+ reabsorption, since K^+ reabsorption is mediated here by Na^+/K^+ ATPase and therefore depends on an appropriate Na^+ gradient to allow Na^+/K^+ exchange. Thus, thiazide diuretics may cause an increase in K^+ excretion (kaliuresis) and possibly hypokalemia. However, if appropriately low doses of thiazides are used in the treatment of hypertension, these potential changes may not be clinically significant. Marked hyperkalemia induced by low doses of a thiazide diuretic in a patient with hypertension may prompt the suspicion that the patient has underlying primary hyperaldosteronism. Fortunately, the maximum antihypertensive effect of thiazides occurs with very low doses of 25–50 mg/day. Hypokalemia, should it occur, may give rise to, or exacerbate pre-existent, cardiac arrhythmias. Potassium supplements (oral potassium chloride) may be used to avoid hypokalemia. Alternatively, potassium-sparing drugs may be given in combination with thiazides.

Thiazides may increase plasma renin (owing to increased removal of blood Na^+ as a consequence of diuresis) and therefore increase angiotensin II synthesis and, consequently, the release of aldosterone. As aldosterone contributes to K^+ loss from the kidney, this action therefore contributes to the hypokalemic effect of thiazides. Concomitant use of a β adrenoceptor antagonist or an ACE inhibitor reduces plasma renin activity or plasma angiotensin II activity, respectively. This can ameliorate the aldosterone-dependent component of the hypokalemic effect of thiazides. In addition, ACE inhibitors potentiate the hypotensive effects of thiazides.

Diuretic-induced hypokalemia may be avoided by using potassium-sparing diuretics

Avoidance of hypokalemia may be achieved by using so-called potassium-sparing diuretics. These act at the cortical collecting duct, where exchange of Na^+ for K^+ and H^+ ions occurs via an exchanger that is regulated by endogenous aldosterone (see Ch. 12):

- Drugs such as amiloride and triamterene act at the luminal membrane. Their molecular mechanism is blockade of Na^+ channels and noncompetitive antagonism of aldosterone.
- Spironolactone is a reversible competitive antagonist of aldosterone at its intracellular receptor in the luminal membrane of the cortical collecting duct. It acts by antagonizing the mineralocorticoid effects of aldosterone (Fig 13.36). In addition to its fast time-course cell membrane effects, aldosterone binds to

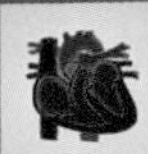

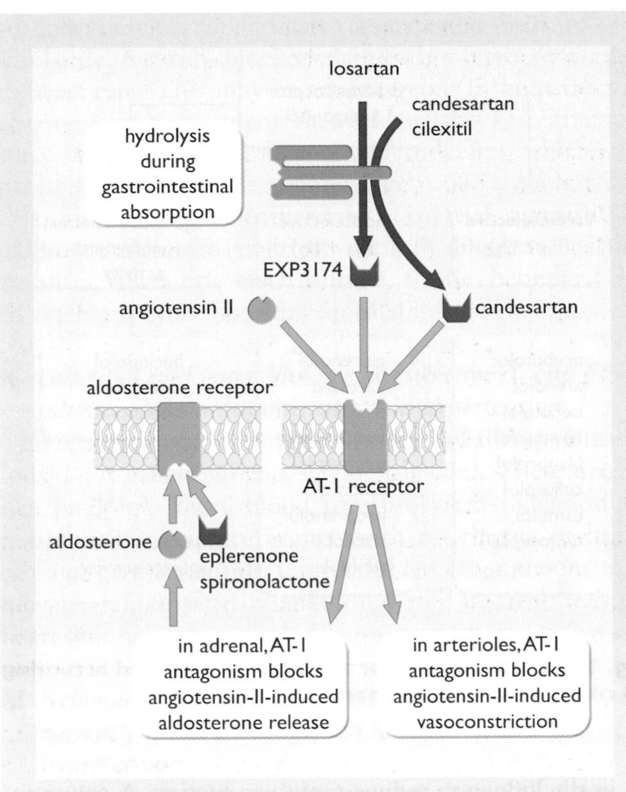

Fig. 13.36 Losartan and candesartan are used to treat hypertension primarily as a consequence of angiotensin AT-1 receptor antagonist activity, by reducing blood levels of aldosterone and by dilating arterioles. Eplerenone treats hypertension by blocking aldosterone receptors.

intracellular mineralocorticoid receptors in both epithelial (e.g. kidney) and nonepithelial (e.g. heart, blood vessels and brain) tissues and increases blood pressure through induction of sodium reabsorption and possibly other mechanisms. It is generally not used in the treatment of primary hypertension due to potentially severe adverse effects, especially in male patients where it interferes with testosterone synthesis and action.

Eplerenone is the first of a new class of aldosterone antagonist antihypertensive agent

Eplerenone was described earlier in connection with treatment of heart failure. It is described in more detail here (see Fig. 13.36). Very importantly, the substitution of a carboxymethyl group on carbon-17 markedly decreases eplerenone's affinity at other steroid receptors compared to spironolactone. Diminished interactions with sex hormone receptors may explain the low likelihood of adverse effects such as gynecomastia with eplerenone. The recommended starting dose of eplerenone is 50 mg orally, administered once daily. The full therapeutic effect is apparent within 4 weeks. For patients with an inadequate blood pressure response to 50 mg once daily, the dosage should be increased to 50 mg twice daily. Higher dosages are not recommended either because they have no greater effect on blood pressure than 100 mg or because they are associated with an increased risk of hyperkalemia.

In clinical trials, oral eplerenone 50–200 mg daily achieved significant decreases in sitting systolic and diastolic blood pressure at trough and effectiveness was maintained over the entire dosing interval. Blood pressure reductions with eplerenone are not dependent on age, gender or race, with the exception that, in patients with low renin hypertension, blood pressure reductions in those of African origin were smaller than those in other patients during the initial titration period.

Eplerenone may be co-administered with ACE inhibitors, angiotensin II receptor antagonists, Ca^{2+} antagonists, β blockers and hydrochlorothiazide. There are numerous adverse effects of eplerenone:

- Headache.
- Dizziness.
- Diarrhea.
- Stomach pain.
- Cough.
- Excessive tiredness.
- Flu-like symptoms.
- Breast enlargement or tenderness.
- Abnormal vaginal bleeding.

Some more uncommon adverse effects can be serious:

- Chest pain.
- Tingling in arms and legs.
- Loss of muscle tone.
- Weakness or heaviness in legs.
- Confusion.
- Lack of energy.
- Cold, gray skin.
- Irregular heartbeat.

Eplerenone is contraindicated in the following situations:

- Hyperkalemia.
- Type II diabetes (noninsulin dependent) with microalbuminuria (protein in the urine).
- Kidney disease.
- With concurrent potassium supplements or a potassium-sparing diuretic such as amiloride, triamterene or spironolactone.

Plasma protein binding is about 50%. Eplerenone is metabolized by the liver primarily mediated via CYP4503A4 with an elimination half-life of 4–6 hours. For these reasons, there is scope for drug–drug interactions at the level of plasma protein binding and metabolism (especially with ketoconazole).

Other diuretics used in hypertension include indapamide and torsemide. Indapamide 1.5 mg orally (single daily dosage) has been reported to be the most effective drug for a significant reduction in systolic blood pressure within 2–3 months of beginning therapy, which is an essential element in optimizing secondary cardiovascular risk prevention (e.g. stroke) among hypertensive

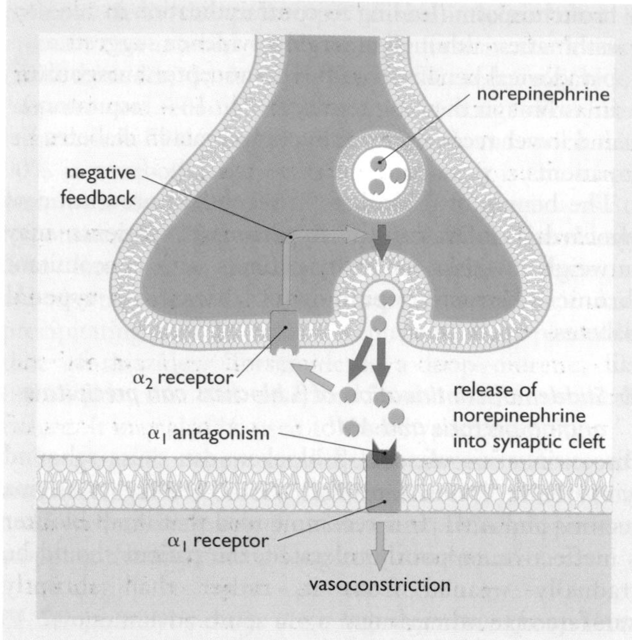

Fig. 13.38 Antagonism at postsynaptic α_1 adrenoceptors. Praosin (α_1 antagonist) prevents vasoconstriction by norepinephrine. The effects of norepinephrine are further reduced by negative feedback since presynaptic α_2 adrenoceptors are not blocked by prazosin and can be occupied by norepinephrine to activate a negative feedback pathway.

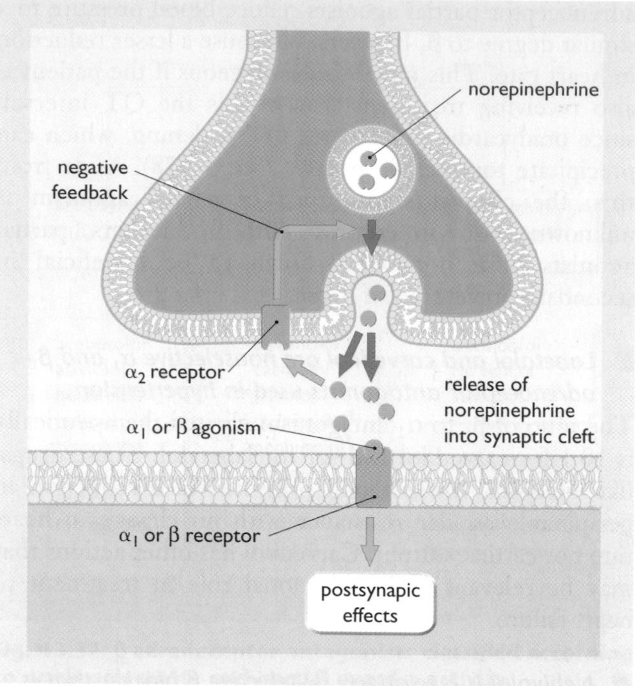

Fig. 13.39 Presynaptic α_2 agonism. This prevents the release of norepinephrine and subsequent postsynaptic α_1 agonism. Clonidine is an α_2 selective agonist. The postsynaptic receptor is β_1, in the heart and mediates tachycardia. In blood vessels it is a mediating vasoconstriction.

of postsynaptic β_1 adrenoceptors and tachycardia. Consequently, nonselective α antagonists are not useful antihypertensives. Because prazosin has selectivity for α_1 receptors, the negative feedback mechanism remains intact, meaning that the drug's therapeutic effectiveness is not compromised by tachycardia (Fig. 13.38).

α_1 adrenoceptor antagonists modify plasma levels of LDL cholesterol, and apoprotein B, so that overall LDL cholesterol levels are reduced as well as very low density lipoprotein (VLDL) levels and total triglyceride levels. These drugs also increase high-density lipoprotein (HDL) cholesterol levels and therefore reduce one of the risk factors associated with coronary artery disease (see Ch. 11). The clinical relevance of this is unknown.

Prazosin is given twice a day, whereas doxazosin and terazosin are given once daily because of their long plasma half-life, affording better patient compliance. Other uses of prazosin are described in Chapter 17.

Urapidil is an α_1 adrenoceptor antagonist with additional 5-HT_{1A} agonist activity. The latter action in the CNS (medulla) causes a reduction in sympathetic tone. Consequently, urapidil can lower blood pressure without eliciting the reflex tachycardia typically seen with other α_1 adrenoceptor antagonists. Oral urapidil has demonstrated efficacy comparable to most other antihypertensive agents in all grades of hypertension; i.v. urapidil is effective in hypertensive crises and for controlling hypertension during surgery. The primary use of the drug, where approved (it has been available since the 1980s in Europe, South America and Asia, but is not approved for use in the USA), is as an alternative in hypertensive patients with relative contraindications to other agents, and in patients unresponsive to or intolerant of other regimens.

Adverse effects of α_1 antagonists include postural hypotension, dizziness, weakness, fatigue, reflex tachycardia (except urapidil) and headaches, but little sedation, dry mouth or ejaculation failure.

α_2 adrenoceptor agonists are not a generally the preferred choice for treating hypertension

Centrally acting α_2 adrenoceptor agonists such as clonidine, guanfacine, guanabenz and α methyldopa mimic the autoinhibitory effects of norepinephrine on sympathetic activity without producing other sympathomimetic effects (Fig. 13.39). The reason for this is their relative selectivity for α_2 receptors. The mechanisms of action are as follows:

- The molecular mechanism of action is α_2 adrenoceptor agonism which reduces the activity of the vasomotor center in the brain, leading to falls in sympathetic nervous activity.
- This leads to a reduction in peripheral resistance as a result of arteriolar relaxation. However, with maintained therapy, a reduction in heart rate and cardiac output appear to be the predominant effects, especially with clonidine.

 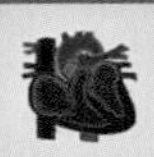

OH, OH, CH_2—C(CH_3)(COOH)—NH_2

DOPA-decarboxylase

α methyldopamine

OH, OH, CH_2—CH(CH_3)—NH_2

dopamine β hydroxylase

α methylnorepinephrine

OH, OH, CH(OH)—CH(CH_3)—NH_2

Fig. 13.40 Metabolism of a methyldopa to α methylnorepinephrine. Note that a CH_3 group is absent in DOPA, the endogenous precursor to dopamine, which is metabolized, by the same enzymes, to norepinephrine.

Clonidine is a widely used α_2 agonist, whereas α methyldopa is a pro-drug metabolized via a two-step enzymatic process to α methylnorepinephrine (Fig. 13.40), an α_2 agonist. Because renal blood flow is well maintained with α methyldopa, it has been widely used in hypertensive patients with renal insufficiency or cerebrovascular disease. α methyldopa is also used in hypertensive pregnant women because it has no adverse effects on the fetus, despite crossing the blood–placenta barrier.

Adverse effects of α_2 agonists are sedation (more so with clonidine and guanabenz than guanfacine and guanadrel), dry mouth, orthostatic hypotension (particularly in the elderly), male sexual dysfunction (impotence) and galactorrhea. α methyldopa is now used very infrequently owing to more serious adverse effects (including diffuse parenchymal injury in the liver resembling the effects of viral hepatitis and, rarely, fever and hemolytic anemia) with the exception that it is still used extensively in treating hypertension during pregnancy on account of its long safety record.

The use of clonidine in hypertensive patients has been associated with a rapid rebound of blood pressure to pretreatment levels when the treatment is stopped abruptly. The withdrawal syndrome includes tachycardia, restlessness and sweating. The rebound of blood pressure may be treated by reintroducing the drug or using a peripherally acting α_1 adrenoceptor antagonist to prevent sympathetic nervous system-mediated peripheral vasoconstriction. These adverse effects can be avoided by gradually decreasing the dose of clonidine over time.

Clonidine is available as a transdermal preparation for control of blood pressure for up to 7 days with the potential for fewer adverse effects. However, adverse effects of the patch on the skin may be troublesome.

Rauwolfia alkaloids such as reserpine have adrenergic neuron blocking actions resulting in arteriolar vasodilation and a reduced cardiac output in patients with hypertension

Reserpine is transported into peripheral sympathetic nerve terminals by uptake-1 (a mechanism for norepinephrine re-uptake into nerves) and its mechanisms of action are as follows:

- Its molecular mechanism is inhibition of the norepinephrine pump (an ATP-and Mg^{2+}-dependent uptake) located on the storage vesicles for norepinephrine in the neuronal cytoplasm. This reduces the norepinephrine content of neuronal storage vesicles and nerve action potential-mediated release of norepinephrine from sympathetic nerve terminals.
- Its resulting tissue and system actions are arteriolar vasodilation and reduced cardiac output. Reserpine effectively reduces blood pressure.

Like other rauwolfia compounds, this action is characterized by slow onset of action and sustained effects. In the average patient not receiving other antihypertensive agents, the usual initial dosage is 0.5 mg daily, orally, for 1 or 2 weeks. For maintenance, the dose is reduced to 0.1–0.25 mg daily. Higher dosages should be used cautiously, because serious psychologic depression and other side effects may increase considerably. This may be lessened by careful dose titration. Both cardiovascular and central nervous system effects may persist for a period of time following discontinuation of the drug.

Adverse effects of rauwolfia alkaloids as a class include dryness of mouth, stuffy nose and (more rarely) psychologic depression. They are contraindicated with monoamine oxidase inhibitors. In view of these factors, the use of reserpine and related compounds has declined.

Other rauwolfia alkaloids used in the treatment of hypertension include deserpidine, rauwolfia serpentina, and rescinnamine. Deserpidine is given orally, 250–500 μg/day as a single dose or divided into two doses. Rauwolfia serpentina is given orally, 250–500 mg/day as a single dose or divided into two doses. Rescinnamine's initial dose is 0.5 mg orally, twice daily. Maintenance doses may vary from 0.25 mg to 0.5 mg daily. Higher doses should be used cautiously because serious psychologic depression and other side effects may be increased considerably.

Guanethidine has two molecular and cellular mechanisms acting in parallel to achieve adrenergic neuron block

Guanethidine and related guanidine compounds including guanadrel (and others no longer used therapeutically in the USA, such as bethanidine, and those never approved for use in the USA such as debrisoquine) are, like reserpine, transported into peripheral sympathetic nerve terminals by uptake-1. However, their mechanisms of action differ from those of reserpine:

- One molecular mechanism is competition with norepinephrine for the intracellular norepinephrine pump. The drugs are actually taken up and stored in the adrenergic vesicles in preference to norepinephrine, thereby reducing the content of norepinephrine in the storage vesicles.
- A second molecular mechanism is binding to the inner surface of the neurolemma and this reduces fusion between storage vesicles and the neurolemma – an 'adrenergic neuron blocking' action. This reduces release of norepinephrine from sympathetic nerve terminals.

Reserpine and the guanidine analogs share two common adverse effects. These are:

- Postural hypotension.
- A generalized block of sympathetic neurotransmission.

Postural hypotension (a fall in blood pressure on standing up) results from a loss of the sympathetic-mediated reflex arterial and venous constriction in the lower body that normally occurs on standing. There is venous pooling of blood in the lower limbs, reducing venous return and cardiac output. Because of this, and the availability of newer, safer drugs, guanethidine is now used only for patients with severe hypertension who are unresponsive to other drugs.

Ca^{2+} antagonists are used in the treatment of hypertension

As discussed, these drugs fall into three main groups, based on their chemical structure (see above):

- The 1,4-dihydropyridines, nifedipine, nicardipine and amlodipine, are the most vascular-selective group and the most effective antihypertensive Ca^{2+} antagonists.
- The phenethylalkylamine, verapamil, and the benzothiazepine, diltiazem, are less vascular-selective and may also affect the AV node, causing AV block. Verapamil and diltiazem are therefore associated with cardiac conduction problems, especially in patients receiving β_1 adrenoceptor antagonists.

Elderly hypertensive patients respond well to Ca^{2+} antagonists. However, people of African descent are less responsive. In general, Ca^{2+} antagonists have a rapid onset of action and reduce blood pressure within half an hour of administration. Occasional adverse effects include a throbbing headache, palpitations, sweating, tremor and flushing (due to vasodilation), which occur with rapid-onset formulations, but are almost absent with slow-onset, long-acting formulations, which are preferred. The main adverse effect with verapamil is constipation, but more importantly both verapamil and diltiazem can have negative inotropic effects in patients with pre-existing cardiac failure, and are therefore contraindicated in such patients. Nifedipine and amlodipine do not do this (their adverse effects are discussed in the section on treatment of stable angina).

Newer Ca^{2+} antagonists approved in the US for treatment of hypertension include barnidipine (also known as mepirodipine), lacidipine, lercanidipine and manidipine. Their characteristics are included in Table 13.4. Generally these are longer-acting agents similar to amlodipine, with low adverse effect risk, including a lower risk of edema.

Barnidipine 20 mg once a day orally provides 24-hour blood pressure lowering equivalent to that with amlodipine and nitrendipine, but produces fewer class-specific side effects, and its effectiveness and safety profile are maintained in long-term therapy. Lacidipine has a similar profile, although grapefruit juice adversely affects its metabolism. Lercanidipine, another similar drug, appears to reduce the risk of atherosclerosis by a mechanism unrelated to its antihypertensive effect. Manidipine has similar pharmacology to lercanidipine.

Importantly, despite their ability to control hypertension, there is a growing awareness that Ca^{2+} antagonists may actually increase mortality in patients with hypertension, with a possible association with an increased risk of AMI, gastrointestinal hemorrhage and cancer. For individual drugs, as opposed to the class as a whole, a small but significant increase in total mortality has been reported only for nifedipine, and some drugs (amlodipine, felodipine, verapamil and diltiazem) have been reported to not increase mortality by the same study criteria. Nifedipine should not to be used to treat hypertension within 2 weeks of AMI.

Direct-acting vasodilators

Drugs that dilate arterioles by a molecular mechanism that is not α_1 adrenergic receptor antagonism or L-type Ca^{2+} channel blockade have traditionally been called 'direct-acting vasodilators.' These drugs are used for the treatment of hypertensive emergencies.

Hydralazine is a third-line drug for mild to moderate hypertension. Hydralazine is the only direct-acting vasodilator drug used in treating mild to moderate hypertension, usually as a second- or third-line drug. It is also still used as a parenteral treatment in hypertensive emergencies and in hypertensive pregnant patients, because of a long safety record in this setting.

The molecular and cellular mechanisms of action of hydralazine are to increase cGMP following activation of guanylyl cyclase, resulting in relaxation of smooth muscle in the precapillary resistance vessels and thereby reducing blood pressure by a reduction in peripheral resistance (see Fig. 13.2).

Hydralazine, in doses in excess of 200 mg/day, is associated with a lupus-like syndrome in some patients. Its other use in treatment of CHF was described above.

Minoxidil is useful for severe hypertension with renal failure. Minoxidil is highly effective in reducing blood pressure, especially in severe hypertension, and if there is renal failure. Diazoxide is similar to minoxidil, but is rarely used except in emergencies because of its adverse effects.

Minoxidil is a more effective vasodilator than hydralazine and produces dilation of resistance vessels. It acts at the molecular level by activating ATP-sensitive K^+ channels leading to hyperpolarization of the smooth muscle sarcolemma, and subsequently a reduced Ca^{2+} influx via L-type Ca^{2+} channels. Minoxidil is given once or twice a day, and is very effective in patients with severe hypertension and renal insufficiency. Like hydralazine, it should also be given in combination with diuretics and adrenergic receptor antagonists, to prevent reflex increases in cardiac output and fluid retention, which may be profound in some patients.

A common adverse effect of minoxidil is facial hair growth, which limits the use of this drug in women but has resulted in its use to treat male-pattern baldness.

ACE inhibitors

ACE inhibitors and angiotensin receptor blockers were discussed in the section on treatment of heart failure but are dealt with in greater depth here. The inactive decapeptide angiotensin I is converted to the active octapeptide angiotensin II by ACE (see Fig. 13.31). Angiotensin II has a variety of effects that contribute to elevating blood pressure (Fig. 13.41). It constricts arterioles and stimulates aldosterone release from the adrenal cortex. In turn, aldosterone stimulates Na^+ reabsorption in the kidney (see use of spironolactone and eplerenone, above). As a result of reducing the synthesis of angiotensin II, captopril causes vasodilation and reduces Na^+ retention. A reduction in blood pressure may be achieved either by blocking ACE or angiotensin II receptors. ACE inhibitors are widely used in all types and severities of hypertension. They reduce mortality. They are classified chemically on the basis of whether they contain sulfhydryl, carboxyl or phosphinyl moieties. ACE inhibitors have the following mechanisms of action:

- Their molecular mechanism is inhibition of ACE activity.
- This results in reduced angiotensin II synthesis and reduced metabolism of some vasodilating kinins (such as bradykinin).

Captopril interacts with ACE via its sulfhydryl moiety, and was the prototype ACE inhibitor. Other commonly

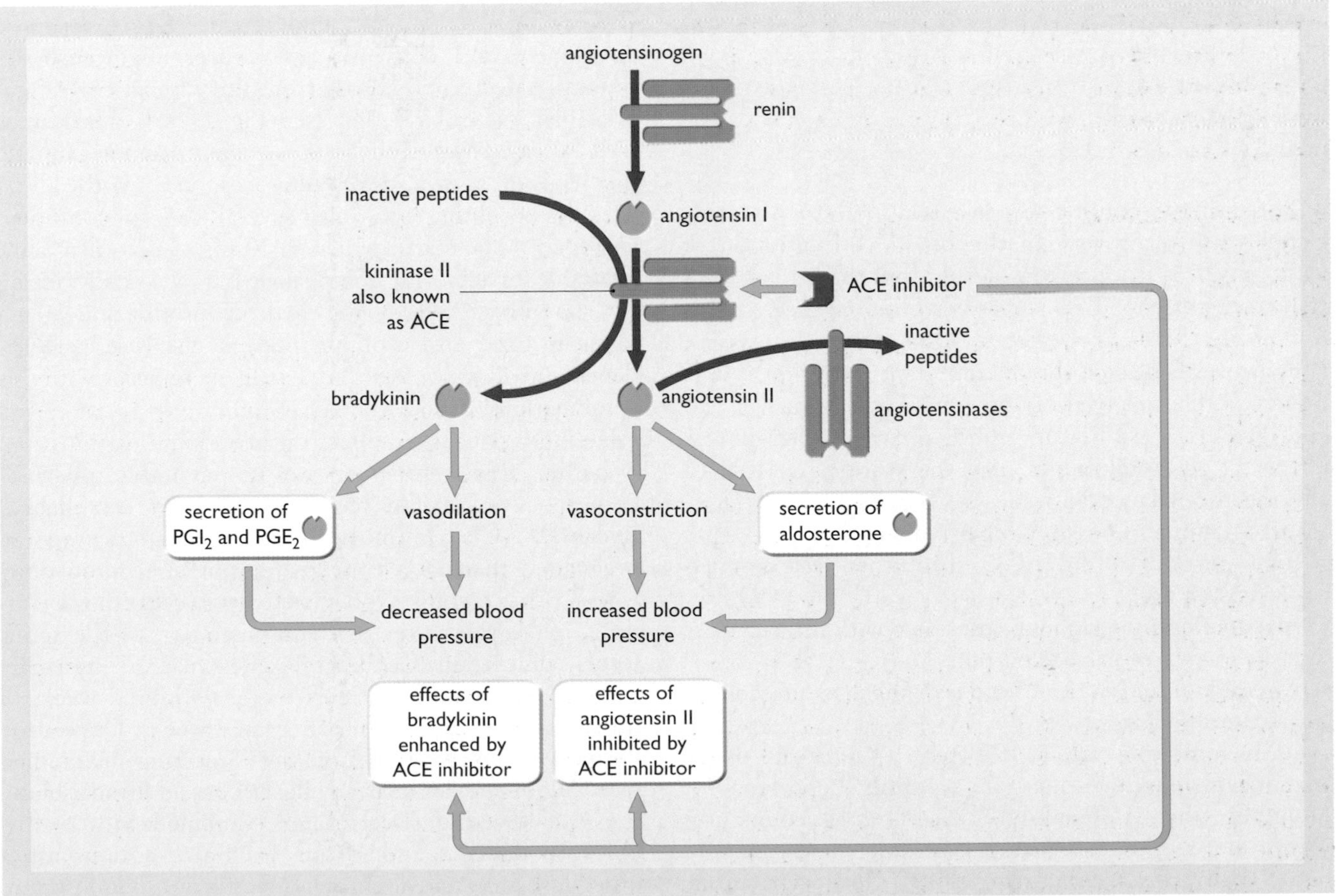

Fig. 13.41 Effects of angiotensin-converting enzyme (ACE) inhibitors. ACE inhibitors reduce angiotensin II (vasoconstrictor) concentrations and elevate bradykinin (vasodilator) concentrations. The accumulation of bradykinin shown in the lower part of the figure results from the action of the ACE inhibitors on kininase II. Note, kininase II and ACE are actually the same enzyme (peptidyl-dipeptidase).

used ACE inhibitors are lisinopril (the most commonly used in the USA), enalapril, benazepril, cilazapril, ramipril and quinapril (all of which interact with ACE via carboxyl moieties) and fosinopril (via its phosphinyl moiety) (see Table 13.11). The carboxyl-containing ACE inhibitors (enalapril, lisinopril, etc.) have a slower onset and longer duration of action than captopril. Many ACE inhibitors are pro-drugs and the suffix '-at' is used to denote active metabolite of ACE inhibitors. For example, enalapril and ramipril are metabolized to active metabolites, enalaprilat and ramiprilat. Perindopril and zofenopril, two newer ACE inhibitors, are both pro-drugs (of perindoprilat and SQ26333, respectively).

ACE inhibitors

- Captopril
- Enalapril
- Benazepril
- Cilazapril
- Fosinopril
- Perindopril
- Quinapril
- Ramipril
- Zofenopril
- Moexipril
- Trandolapril

Surprisingly, chronic use of ACE inhibitors is associated with a recovery in the blood concentration of angiotensin II to previous levels, but blood pressure reduction persists. This suggests additional mechanisms for antihypertensive effects. One possibility is an alteration of plasma bradykinin concentration. ACE catalyzes the inactivation of bradykinin, which is an endogenous vasodilator. The pharmacotherapeutic effects of ACE inhibitors may therefore be related to altering the balance between the actions of angiotensin II, bradykinin and possibly other kinins (see Fig. 13.41).

The responses to ACE inhibitors relevant to hypertension are:

- A reduction in peripheral resistance with little change in heart rate or cardiac output.
- A reduction in Na^+ retention secondary to altered aldosterone levels.

ACE inhibitors are as effective as diuretics or β_1 adrenoceptor antagonists in treating hypertension. However, when ACE inhibitors are used concomitantly with a diuretic, overall therapeutic effectiveness may be better than that for either drug alone. This may result in part because the ability of diuretics to adversely activate the renin–angiotensin system is ameliorated by ACE inhibitors.

Both experimental and clinical evidence suggest that the reduction in efferent arteriolar resistance resulting from a reduction in angiotensin II following treatment with ACE inhibitors may be useful in patients with renal dysfunction, particularly those with diabetic nephropathy or a reduced renal functional mass. This is because inhibition of angiotensin II activity may cause a substantial reduction in perfusion pressure. As a result, renal failure may develop in these patients.

ACE inhibitors are associated with few adverse effects (which increases patient compliance). One unusual adverse effect is a characteristic cough that is believed to be a consequence of the actions of bradykinin, the metabolism of which is inhibited by ACE inhibitors (see Ch. 14). This adverse effect appears to be least marked with fosinopril, which is structurally distinct from other ACE inhibitors.

Angiotensin II receptor antagonists

The prototype drug, saralasin, was unsuitable for therapeutic use since it is a peptide that is immunogenic and not orally active. Therefore, nonpeptide, orally active compounds were developed. These include losartan, candarsatan, irbesartan and olmesartan. Losartan was the first angiotensin-II antagonist introduced to treat hypertension. It is a pro-drug with an active metabolite (EXP3174). It is an angiotensin AT-1 receptor antagonist, and consequently reduces angiotensin-II-induced aldosterone release from the adrenal cortex and arteriolar vasoconstriction (see Fig 13.36). Losartan is well tolerated and as effective as enalapril and nifedipine. There is a slowly developing response, with blood pressure becoming lower over several weeks of continued treatment. The starting dose is 50 mg orally once daily, favorable for achieving compliance, but twice-daily dosing can be used. A 12.5 mg hydrochlorothiazide–50 mg losartan fixed-dose combination is also used. Dose-dependent adverse effects are less likely to occur with this combination. Unlike the ACE inhibitors, losartan and related drugs have no effect on bradykinin degradation. Whether this contributes to its favorable pharmacotherapeutic profile has not yet been established. Because ACE inhibitors are contraindicated in pregnancy, there is a concern for potential fetotoxicity with AT-1 antagonists too. Candesartan cilexetil is a pro-drug, hydrolyzed after oral administration to the active form, candesartan. Candesartan cilexetil 2–32 mg orally can achieve an antihypertensive effect within 2 weeks of initial dosing, with the full effect in 4 weeks. Once-daily dosing can achieve blood pressure lowering maintained over 24 hours. Candesartan cilexetil has additional blood pressure lowering effects when combined with hydrochlorothiazide. Candesartan is more potent on a dose–dose basis and slightly more effective than losartan. Reflex tachycardia does not occur. In long-term studies the antihypertensive effectiveness of candesartan cilexetil was maintained. Candesartan is >10 000-fold selective

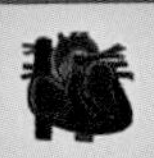

for the AT-1 versus AT-2 receptor. Oral bioavailability iscandesartan cilexetil is 15%, with C_{max} reached after 3–4 hours. The volume of distribution is 0.13 L/kg with candesartan highly bound to plasma proteins (>99%). It undergoes minor hepatic metabolism by O-deethylation to an inactive metabolite. Total plasma clearance is 0.37 mL/min/kg, and about 26% of the dose is excreted unchanged in urine and approximately 67% in feces. The elimination half-life is approximately 9 hours. Adverse effects of candesartan are few and minor. The most common reasons for discontinuation of therapy with candesartan cilexetil are headache (0.6%) and dizziness (0.3%).

Irbesartan is another AT-1 antagonist. It has a higher bioavailability (60–80%), lower plasma protein binding (90%) and less selectivity for AT-1 versus AT-2 receptors (8500-fold) than candesartan. Once-daily oral doses of 150 and 300 mg produce statistically and clinically significant decreases in systolic and diastolic blood pressure.

Olmesartan medoxomil is used to treat hypertension at doses of up to 40 mg once daily. Like candesartan cilexitil and losartan it is a pro-drug. Other AT-1 antagonists used to treat hypertension include eprosartan, telmesartan and valsartan. The usual recommended starting dose of eprosartan mesylate tablets is 600 mg orally once daily when used as monotherapy in patients who are not volume depleted. Eprosartan mesylate tablets can be administered once or twice daily with total daily doses ranging from 400 mg to 800 mg.

Mechanisms of action of major classes of antihypertensive drugs

- **Thiazide diuretics increase Na^+ excretion and transiently reduce blood volume, but the mechanism by which they reduce blood pressure is uncertain**
- **Sympatholytics reduce the ability of the sympathetic nervous system to raise blood pressure**
- **Vasodilators relax vascular smooth muscle and reduce peripheral resistance**
- **ACE inhibitors reduce peripheral resistance and blood volume with no effect on heart rate**

Imidazoline I_1 antagonists

Moxonidine 200 or 400 μg orally achieves a blood pressure lowering action by two mechanisms. It is an imidazoline I_1 receptor agonist in the rostroventrolateral medulla, thereby reducing the activity of the sympathetic nervous system. Moxonidine is also thought to have an agonist effect on α_2 receptors in the brain, achieving an action similar to that produced by clonidine (see Fig. 13.39). However it is more selective for I_1 than α_2 receptors, and it lacks the respiratory depressant effect attributed to central α_2 activation. This may be the reason why moxonidine has fewer adverse effects than clonidine. Blood pressure reduction with moxonidine is usually accompanied by a reduction in heart rate, which is of shorter duration and lesser magnitude than the fall in blood pressure. The terminal half-life of elimination is 2 hours. The major route of elimination is renal. Adverse effects are minor and mild and include dry mouth, headache, dizziness and tiredness.

Dopamine D_1 antagonists

Fenoldopam is a selective dopamine D_1 agonist, which produces vasodilation, increases renal perfusion and enhance natriuresis in hypertensive patients. Fenoldopam has a short duration of action due to an elimination half-life of less than 10 minutes. Fenoldopam is used as a parenteral therapy for high-risk hypertensive surgical patients, in the perioperative management of patients undergoing renal and other organ transplantation, and following radiocontrast medium injection in high-risk patients. It is a prototype drug and is approved in the USA for in-hospital, short-term (up to 48 hours) management of severe hypertension, when rapid but quickly reversible reduction of blood pressure is required, including malignant hypertension with deteriorating end-organ function. Its short duration of action facilitates avoidance of sustained excessive blood pressure lowering in the emergency setting.

Combination treatment

A useful pharmacotherapeutic approach in hypertension is to use two or more drugs in combination. By combining drugs with different mechanisms of action, doses may be reduced, thereby reducing adverse effects. There is a large range of fixed-dose ratio combinations approved in the USA (Table 13.13), a few of which come in single-dosing (tablet or capsule) form. The combinations achieve lower individual doses of each drug, and consequently fewer side effects, and are also intended to improve compliance. All of the combination use drugs are discussed elsewhere in this chapter, except for piretanide, which is a loop diuretic that inhibits the renal $Na^+/K^+/Cl^-$ cotransporter.

β adrenoceptor antagonists and Ca^{2+} antagonists (dihydropyridine Ca^{2+} antagonists only) are usually well tolerated when used in combination, provided that care is taken with dose. The combination of nifedipine with β adrenoceptor antagonists has been associated with bradycardia and heart failure owing to synergism of their effects (one mediated via cardiac β_1 adrenoceptor antagonism, the other via ventricular L-type Ca^{2+} antagonism).

Diuretics plus ACE inhibitor (e.g. hydrochlorothiazide and perindopril) provide an effective combination for treating hypertension that is well tolerated in many patients with mild to moderate hypertension. The advantage of combining diuretics and ACE inhibitors is an additive effect in reducing blood pressure. The combination of ACE inhibitors and Ca^{2+} antagonists is

Table 13.13 Fixed-dose ratio combination antihypertensive therapy

Amiloride hydrochloride; hydrochlorothiazide
Amlodipine besylate; benazepril hydrochloride
Atenolol; chlortalidone
Benazepril hydrochloride; hydrochlorothiazide
Bendroflumethiazide; nadolol
Bisoprolol fumarate; hydrochlorothiazide
Candesartan cilexetil; hydrochlorothiazide
Captopril; hydrochlorothiazide
Chlorothiazide; methyldopa
Chlorothiazide; reserpine
Chlortalidone; clonidine
Chlortalidone; reserpine
Deserpidine; methyclothiazide
Diltiazem; enalapril
Enalapril; felodipine
Enalapril; hydrochlorothiazide
Eprosartan mesylate; hydrochlorothiazide
Fosinopril; hydrochlorothiazide
Guanethidine; hydrochlorothiazide
Hydralazine; hydrochlorothiazide
Hydralazine; hydrochlorothiazide; reserpine
Hydrochlorothiazide; irbesartan
Hydrochlorothiazide; lisinopril
Hydrochlorothiazide; losartan
Hydrochlorothiazide; methyldopa
Hydrochlorothiazide; metoprolol
Hydrochlorothiazide; moexipril
Hydrochlorothiazide; olmesartan medoxomil
Hydrochlorothiazide; propranolol
Hydrochlorothiazide; quinapril
Hydrochlorothiazide; reserpine
Hydrochlorothiazide; spironolactone
Hydrochlorothiazide; telmisartan
Hydrochlorothiazide; timolol maleate
Hydrochlorothiazide; triamterene
Hydrochlorothiazide; valsartan
Hydroflumethiazide; reserpine
Perindopril; indapamide*
Piretanide (acenocoumarol); ramipril*
Polythiazide; prazosin
Polythiazide; reserpine
Reserpine; trichlormethiazide
Trandolapril; verapamil*

* Indicates available in a single tablet or capsule form.

also effective at lowering blood pressure and is usually well tolerated. Ca^{2+} antagonist and diuretics in combination do not usually have additive effects.

Using β_1 adrenoceptor antagonists with Ca^{2+} antagonists, other than the dihydropyridines, is dangerous

Using β_1 adrenoceptor antagonists in combination with non-dihydropyridine Ca^{2+} antagonists (e.g. verapamil) is dangerous since such combinations have been reported to cause asystole, severe bradycardia and hypotension, because of the combination of the mechanisms described above. Each, by lowering cardiac intracellular Ca^{2+}, reduces myocardial contractility. Dihydropyridines such as nifedipine do not do this because they are highly vascular selective and do not affect cardiac tissue to any great extent.

Emerging therapy for the treatment of hypertension

Renin inhibitors are a new class of drugs that reduce angiotensin II levels. Several renin inhibitors with high potency and long duration of action have been developed. However, the oral bioavailability of currently available agents is too low to achieve effective plasma concentrations in humans. Endopeptidase 24.11 (neutral endopeptidase) is an enzyme that hydrolyzes the polypeptide atrial natriuretic peptide (ANP). ANP has diuretic, natriuretic and vasodilator properties; it is released following changes in atrial volume or pressure, and plays a role in regulating blood pressure. Theoretically, inhibition of neutral endopeptidase should reduce ANP degradation and thereby increase circulating levels of ANP. This form of drug treatment may prove beneficial in patients with hypertension. However, the prototype agent, omapatrilat, has yet to gain approval for use in the USA owing to concerns over its safety (possible angioedema). Omapatrilat is not selective, blocking neutral endopeptidase and ACE.

Treatment of hypertensive emergencies

Hypertensive emergencies are situations in which the target organ damage is so extensive and acute that the patient's life is in immediate jeopardy. There is no particular level of blood pressure that provides the diagnosis since the latter depends on clinical presentation. Conditions associated with hypertensive emergencies include hypertensive encephalopathy, dissecting aortic aneurysm, pulmonary edema, myocardial ischemia and accelerated renal failure due to hypertensive nephropathy. Treatment is summarized in Table 13.14.

Sodium nitroprusside is a direct-acting vasodilator used in hypertensive emergencies

Sodium nitroprusside is given intravenously to produce a controlled rapid reduction in blood pressure during a hypertensive emergency. It has a short half-life of 30–40 seconds. Sodium nitroprusside is a profound arterial and venous dilator (see Table 13.14). The molecular mechanism of action for its effect is brought about by NO (see Fig. 13.2). It is a pro-drug that spontaneously degrades to NO inside smooth muscle cells. NO increases cGMP in vascular smooth muscle cells by stimulating cytosolic guanylyl cyclase activity (see Fig. 13.14).

Sodium nitroprusside achieves a rapid onset of action and efficacy. An infusion can be used to reduce blood pressure rapidly, but it is important to monitor the blood pressure constantly. This is because nitroprusside can cause an abrupt fall in blood pressure, resulting in hypoperfusion of vital organs; dose must be titrated carefully, depending on the blood pressure response.

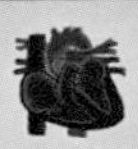

Table 13.14 Drugs used in hypertensive crises

Vasodilators	Onset of action (min)
Nitroprusside	Immediate
Diazoxide	2–4
Hydralazine	10–20
Enalaprilat	15
Nicardipine	10
Sympatholytics	
Trimethaphan	1–5
Esmolol	1–2
Labetalol	5–10

The drugs are shown in order of preference based on their rapidity of action.

Ganglion-blocking drugs are used only for emergency hypertension

Trimethaphan is a nicotinic receptor antagonist with relative selectivity for the nicotinic receptors found in autonomic ganglia. It is used only for emergency hypertension associated with a dissecting aortic aneurysm. When given intravenously it produces generalized antagonism of both parasympathetic and sympathetic ganglia (i.e. gastric motility ceases, the bladder fails to empty, etc.) and is therefore unsuitable for maintenance therapy of hypertension.

Hypertensive emergency

- **Occurs when elevated arterial pressure is an immediate threat to life**
- **Intravenous nitroprusside is an efficacious drug in this setting**

Other treatments of acutely high blood pressure

A very high blood pressure on its own, in the absence of acute illness, does not usually require parenteral therapy, which can be dangerous. Patients with a less severe emergency can be given oral drug treatment. Any class of drug may be used, but the four classes most commonly used are:

- Diuretics.
- β adrenoceptor antagonists.
- Ca^{2+} antagonists.
- ACE inhibitors.

Adverse effects of drugs on the heart

Some examples are listed in Table 13.15.

PATHOPHYSIOLOGY AND DISEASES OF BLOOD VESSELS

A variety of diseases involve a generalized or localized impairment of blood flow to specific tissues or organs and are grouped together here as peripheral vascular disease.

Table 13.15 Adverse effects of drugs on the heart

Drug	Adverse effects	Comments
Doxorubicin	Cardiopathy	Total dose must be limited
Ibuprofen and related drugs	Elevation of blood pressure	Not a major concern
Cocaine/ amphetamines	Elevation of blood pressure	Dangerous effect of abuse

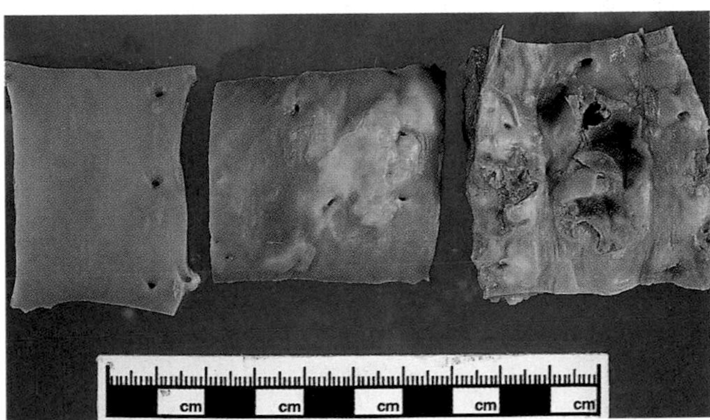

Fig. 13.42 Arteriosclerosis is characterized by thickening and hardening of walls of arteries and arterioles. The earliest changes are small fatty streaks, which are visible as pale areas beneath the endothelium in the aortic segment on the left. The central segment shows pearly white fibrolipid plaques, and the segment on the right shows advanced ulcerated plaques with adherent fibrin-platelet thrombus. (Courtesy of Dr. Alan Stevens and Professor James Lowe.)

In most cases the mechanisms of action of the drugs used to treat peripheral vascular diseases are described elsewhere in this book. Specifically, the pharmacology of drugs that dilate arterioles (e.g. Ca^{2+} antagonists) is described in the section on hypertension, and antithrombotic drugs are described in the section on unstable angina and Chapter 10. Blood vessel diseases for which drug therapy is not used have not been discussed.

Peripheral vascular disease

This affects arteries and can be caused by a number of pathologic processes. These include:

- Arteriosclerosis is one of the pathologic processes that leads to peripheral vascular disease (Fig. 13.42).
- Dystrophic calcification of the arterial media is observed in Mönckeberg's sclerosis, which is common in the major lower limb arteries of the elderly and is most common in people with chronic diabetes mellitus.
- Cystic medial necrosis or degeneration describes mucoid degeneration of the collagen and elastic tissue of the media, often with cystic changes, and occurs predominantly in elderly patients with hypertension. Indeed, peripheral vascular disease is a

feature commonly associated with longstanding hypertension.

In patients with pre-existing peripheral vascular disease, aspirin and dipyridamole are effective in delaying or preventing thrombosis formation and so are used as prophylaxis. It is presumed that:

- Aspirin prevents thrombosis in peripheral vascular disease.
- Dipyridamole prevents thrombosis and dilates arterioles.

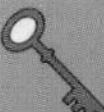

Principles of treatment of peripheral vascular disease

- Drugs are targeted at the perfusion deficit and at the underlying cause (e.g. vasospasm) if known
- Thrombolytics are used if thrombosis has impaired perfusion
- Arteriodilators are used if vasospasm has impaired perfusion

Local treatment is needed for peripheral vascular disease

- Drugs that prevent, or disperse thrombosis or relieve vasospasm are used to treat peripheral vascular disease and act locally. In contrast, in the treatment of coronary artery disease (angina), vasodilation at distant sites is effective by reducing preload or afterload on the heart.

Chronic ischemia of the legs and intermittent claudication

These conditions arise as a consequence of atheromatous disease involving the aorta, iliac arteries and/or any other peripheral vessels. Treatment is directed towards prophylaxis against thrombosis and comprises low-dose aspirin therapy (325 mg/day) and surgery.

Vasculitis

Vasculitis is inflammation in blood vessels, caused by immune complex deposition. Arteries, venules or capillaries affected by such inflammation show necrosis and infiltration with lymphocytes and eosinophils, resulting in ischemia of the related tissue. The different forms of vasculitis include systemic necrotizing vasculitis (e.g. polyarteritis nodosa, allergic angiitis), hypersensitivity vasculitis (e.g. serum sickness, Henoch–Schönlein purpura), and vasculitides associated with cardiac transplant rejection as discussed in Chapter 15. Takayasu's syndrome, a rare condition, except in Japan, is characterized by a vasculitis involving the aortic arch as well as other major arteries. Glucocorticosteroids are used to treat this disease, but heart failure and cerebrovascular accidents may eventually supervene.

Raynaud's disease

This is a condition in which episodes of intense arteriolar vasoconstriction occur in the arteries supplying the fingers or toes. It is usually precipitated by cold or vibration.

Initially, treatment includes avoidance of exposure to cold and smoking. More severe symptoms may require vasodilator treatment. Drugs are used to cause arteriolar vasodilation, although their effectiveness may be modest in this disease.

α_1 adrenoceptor antagonists such as prazosin are used to reduce the vasospasm, but they are not selective for the spasm and can adversely lower blood pressure. Direct-acting vasodilators (e.g. nitroglycerin and nitrates; see Fig. 13.14) and Ca^{+} antagonists such as diltiazem and nifedipine are also used

The molecular mechanism of action of diltiazem and nifedipine is blockade of L-type Ca^{2+} channels, and the cellular response is a reduction in Ca^{2+} entry and the cascade of events that leads to vasoconstriction (see section on treatment of hypertension, above).

In four separate clinical trials investigating the use of nifedipine in Raynaud's disease, the majority of patients improved symptomatically. Nifedipine is more effective than prazosin and can be given by mouth before cold exposure to avoid attacks. ACE inhibitors and prostacyclin may also be beneficial treatments of Raynaud's disease because they cause vasodilation.

Varicose veins

The two main peripheral vascular diseases affecting veins are varicose veins and venous thrombosis (including thrombophlebitis). Varicose veins develop when veins lose their elasticity and become engorged with blood They are treated by injection of sclerosing agents or surgery. Sodium tetradecyl sulfate is injected into the vein as sclerotherapy. It causes inflammation of the intima and thrombus formation, which usually occludes the vein. The subsequent formation of fibrous tissue results in complete occlusion and subsequent loss of that vein.

Venous thrombosis ('red clots')

Venous thrombosis consists predominantly of coagulated blood with a lesser component of platelet aggregation. Superficial thrombophlebitis is a local superficial inflammation of the vein wall with secondary venous thrombosis. Superficial thrombophlebitis is treated with NSAIDs, including aspirin, because the inflammatory process, rather than the tendency for thrombosis, is the primary target.

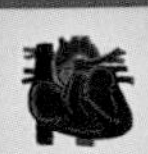

Venous thrombosis and its treatment

- Venous peripheral vascular disease is characterized by vascular inflammation and venous thrombosis
- Treatment of superficial thrombophlebitis is targeted towards inflammation, using nonsteroidal antiinflammatory drugs (NSAIDs)
- Treatment and prophylaxis of deep vein disease is directed towards preventing thrombosis
- Heparin and warfarin are used prophylactically against thrombosis
- Streptokinase is used to disperse established thrombi

Hyaluronidase is used to improve the circulation in superficial thrombophlebitis

It is a 'spreading' or 'diffusing' enzyme that modifies the permeability of connective tissue by hydrolyzing hyaluronic acid. This temporarily decreases the viscosity of the cellular cement and promotes the diffusion of injected fluids, or of localized transudates and exudates.

In deep vein thrombosis a thrombus forms in a vein, commonly deep in the leg. Any inflammation is secondary. It is necessary to inhibit formation of the thrombus rather than direct therapy towards the secondary inflammation. The important secondary aim of treatment is to prevent pulmonary embolism due to a venous thrombus becoming lodged in the pulmonary circulation.

Large doses of the anticoagulant heparin (or LMWH such as enoxaparin) can be given as prophylaxis in the event of venous thrombosis for 1 week to 3 months.

Heparin initiates anticoagulation but has a short duration of action

It inhibits the reactions that lead to the clotting of blood and formation of fibrin clots and, in combination with antithrombin III, inhibits thrombosis by inactivating activated factor X and inhibiting the conversion of prothrombin to thrombin (a mechanism described in more detail in Ch. 10). Heparin does not disperse established thrombi.

Oral anticoagulants such as warfarin are given if a venous thrombus remains localized. Warfarin, another prophylactic agent, antagonizes the ability of vitamin K to facilitate the synthesis of clotting factor II, VII, IX and X (see Ch. 10). However, it takes at least 49–72 hours for these anticoagulant effects to develop. Heparin and warfarin can cause inappropriate bleeding, so careful titration between effective and adverse doses is required.

Streptokinase (or the various forms of tPA) is used in the treatment of established thrombi, and is followed by anticoagulant prophylaxis to prevent recurrence

It acts with plasminogen to produce an 'activator complex,' which converts plasminogen to plasmin. Plasmin degrades fibrin clots as well as fibrinogen and other plasma proteins (see Ch. 10).

Ximelagatran is under investigation for treatment of venous thromboembolism

Ximelagatran is administered orally as a pro-drug for melagatran. Melagatran binds reversibly to fibrin-bound thrombin and freely circulating thrombin. Oral ximelagatran inhibits thrombin activity rapidly, and also delays and suppresses thrombin generation. It has anticoagulant, antiplatelet and profibrinolytic effects, with only minor prolongation of the capillary bleeding time. Oral ximelagatran exhibits a stable and predictable pharmacokinetic profile and a low potential for interaction with other medications. It is excreted primarily as melagatran via the kidney. Clinical trials have evaluated oral ximelagatran in the prevention of venous thromboembolism (comprising deep venous thrombosis with or without pulmonary embolism) after elective hip or knee replacement surgery, treatment and long-term secondary prevention of venous thromboembolism, the prevention of stroke and other systemic embolic events associated with nonvalvular atrial fibrillation and the prevention of cardiovascular events after an AMI. The results of these trials suggest that the benefit–risk profile of a fixed dose, without coagulation monitoring, compares favorably with that of currently approved standard therapy such as enoxaparin/warfarin for treatment of deep vein thrombosis with or without pulmonary embolism. However, increased levels of liver enzymes have been reported in 9.6% of ximelagatran-treated patients require regular monitoring.

Reviparin is an LMWH useful in venous thromboembolism

At 1750 IU anti-XA subcutaneously, reviparin is as effective as unfractionated heparin in preventing deep vein thrombosis in moderate-risk surgery (general and abdominal) and significantly reduces deep vein thrombosis in patients with brace immobilization of the legs. At a daily dose of 4200 IU anti-Xa reviparin is as effective as unfractionated heparin or enoxaparin in preventing deep vein thrombosis in high-risk orthopedic surgery and as effective as unfractionated heparin in prevention of deep vein thrombosis and/or pulmonary embolism and/or mortality in high-risk orthopedic surgery. In patients with acute venous thromboembolism, reviparin is more effective than unfractionated heparin in thrombus reduction and at least as effective as unfractionated heparin in the prevention of clinical recurrence of deep vein thrombosis and/or pulmonary embolism. The use of reviparin is associated with a similar or lower incidence of bleeding complications than unfractionated heparin. Tinzaparin is another thrombin inhibitor. Anti-Xa subcutaneously, 4500 IU, has a half-life of 3.4 hours. The mean anti-Xa to anti-IIa activity ratio is 2.8 and is higher than that of unfractionated heparin (approximately

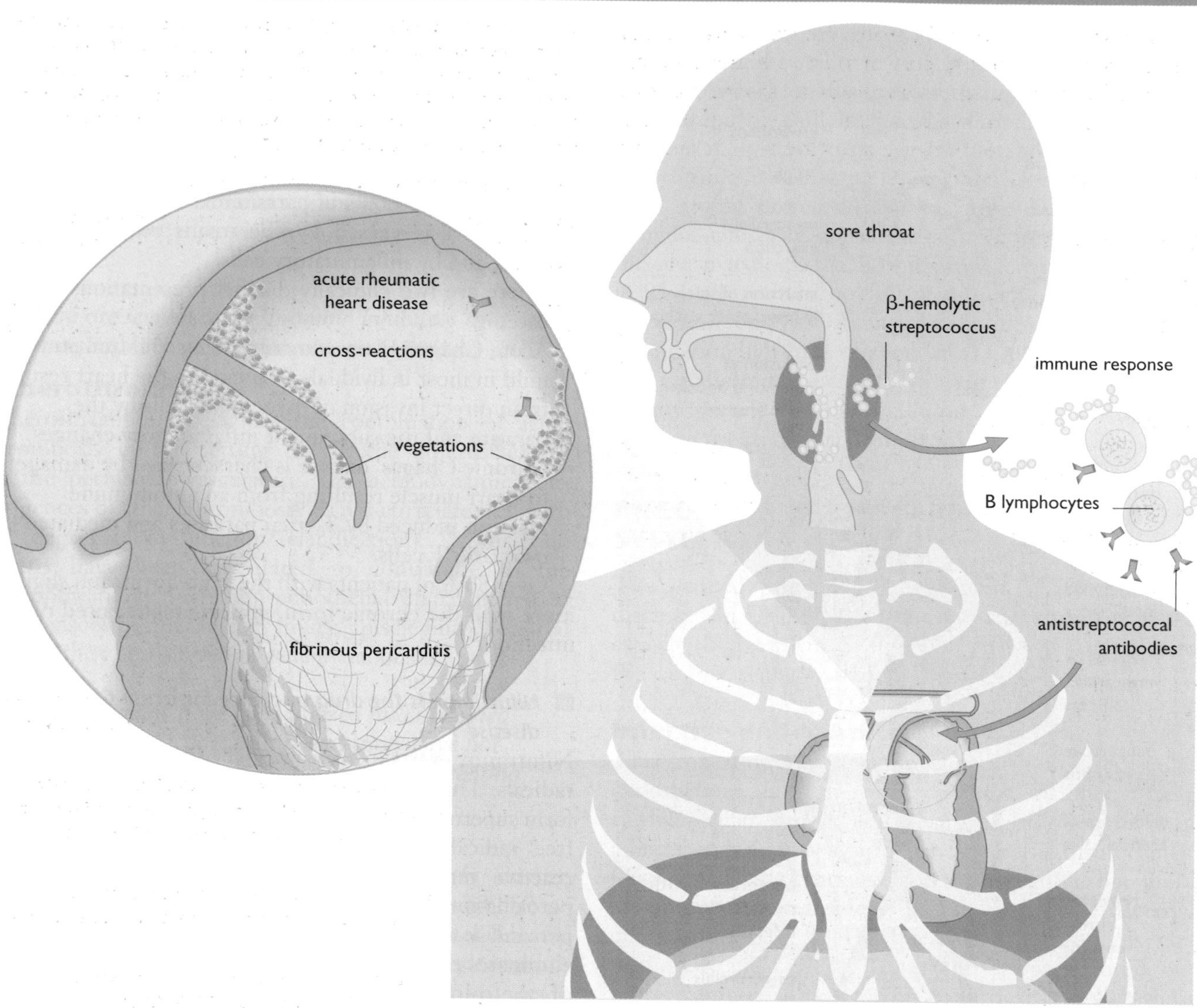

Fig. 13.44 Pathogenetic sequence and main morphologic features of acute rheumatic heart disease. Acute rheumatic fever often causes mitral valvulitis characterized by a linear arrangement of vegetations along the line of closure of the leaflets.

Kawasaki's disease

This is a generalized vasculitis causing extensive damage to the vessels of the heart, and can be fatal. Although the etiology is unknown, current evidence suggests that is probably not an autoimmune disease and instead may be triggered by a virus. During the acute phase, Kawasaki's disease may be characterized by medium and large vessel arteritis, arterial aneurysms, valvulitis and myocarditis. Of particular concern are coronary artery aneurysms, which may precipitate thrombosis or rupture. Lymphocyte and macrophage activation is evident in this disease. Experimental studies have shown the presence of antibodies that can kill endothelial cells previously treated with interleukin-1 or tumor necrosis factor. The function of these antibodies in the disease process is unknown: they may simply be a marker of the disease, or have a pathogenic role.

Treatment of Kawasaki's disease

Patients with Kawasaki's disease can be classified according to their relative risk of myocardial ischemia, on a scale of 1 to 5. No therapy is recommended until level 3, at which small- to medium-sized solitary coronary artery aneurysms are observed. Aspirin is then prescribed. Level 4 is characterized by the presence of one or more large coronary artery aneurysms, or multiple small- to medium-sized aneurysms without obstruction. It is treated with aspirin, with or without the addition of warfarin. Patients at the highest risk of myocardial infarction have evidence of coronary artery obstruction and are classified as level 5. They are treated with aspirin with or without the addition of warfarin, as well as Ca^{2+} antagonists to reduce myocardial oxygen demand.

Recent studies have found that the use of i.v. gammaglobulin therapy before the tenth day of the

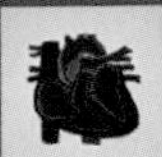

illness has reduced morbidity from Kawasaki's disease and the apparent incidence of coronary artery abnormalities. Gammaglobulin contains antibodies against various viruses. The antibodies are directed against the virus envelope and can 'neutralize' some viruses, and prevent their attachment to host cells.

Rheumatic fever

Rheumatic fever is an inflammatory disease with long-lasting outcomes that occurs in children and young adults. It is most common in the Middle East, Far East and Eastern Europe. It occurs in a small proportion of individuals (those who have significant streptococcal antibodies) weeks after a pharyngeal infection with group A streptococcus, at which stage autoantibodies against the heart can be detected (Fig. 13.44). Evidence suggests that carbohydrate antigens on streptococci cross-react with an antigen on the heart valves and myocardium. Rheumatic fever is therefore thought to develop as a result of an abnormal host–immune response, both cellular and humoral, triggered by streptococcus A. It is likely that the disease is due to a complex inter-relationship between the genetics of the host's immune system and the streptococcus bacillus.

Treatment of rheumatic fever

Treatment is aimed at the infection and its effects

This initially involves eradication of residual streptococcal infections with a single intramuscular injection of benzathine penicillin or oral phenoxymethylpenicillin four times daily for 1 week. High-dose salicylate therapy inhibits cyclooxygenase activity and is given to the limit of tolerance determined by the development of tinnitus. If there is carditis, systemic glucocorticosteroids can be given. Recurrences are common if there is persistent cardiac damage and are prevented by the continued use of oral phenoxymethylpenicillin daily or by monthly injections of benzathine penicillin, until the age of 20 years, or for 5 years after the last attack.

FURTHER READING

Cardiovascular therapeutics and experimental therapeutics are large and fast-moving fields. The best way to stay in touch is to scan the journal *Circulation* (American Heart Association) for review articles and publications on multicenter clinical trials.

Ashrafian H, Violaris AG. Beta-blocker therapy of cardiovascular diseases in patients with bronchial asthma or COPD: The pro viewpoint. *Pri Care Resp J* 2005; **14**: 236–241.

ASSENT-2 Investigators. Single-bolus tenecteplase compared with front-loaded alteplase in AMI: the ASSENT-2 double-blind randomised trial. *Lancet* 1999; **354**: 716–722.

Baguet J-P, Robitail S, Boyer L, Debensason D, Auquier P. A meta-analytical approach to the efficacy of antihypertensive drugs in reducing blood pressure. *Am J Cardiovasc Drugs* 2005; **5**: 131–140.

Blasi F, Tarsia P, Cosentini R, Valenti V. Newer antibiotics for the treatment of respiratory tract infections. *Curr Opin Pulm Med* 2004; **10**: 189–196.

Braunwald E, Antman EM, Beasley JW et al. ACC/AHA guideline update for the management of patients with unstable angina and non-ST-segment elevation myocardial infarction – 2002: summary article: a report of the American College of Cardiology/American Heart Association Task Force on Practice Guidelines (Committee on the Management of Patients With Unstable Angina). *Circulation* 2002; **106**:1893–1900.

Brown NJ. Eplerenone. *Circulation* 2003; **107**: 2512–2518.

Chieffo A, Stankovic G, Bonizzoni E et al. Early and mid-term results of drug-eluting stent implantation in unprotected left main. *Circulation* 2005; **111**: 791–795.

Cleophas TJ, Zwinderman AH. Beta-blockers and heart failure: meta-analysis of mortality trials. *Int J Clin Pharm Ther* 2001; **39**: 383–388. [An appraisal of the topic.]

Chobain AV, Bakris GL, Black HR et al. Joint National Committee on Prevention, Detection, Evaluation, and Treatment of High Blood Pressure. The Seventh Report of the Joint National Committee on Prevention, Detection, Evaluation, and Treatment of High Blood Pressure. *JAMA* 2003; **289**: 2560–2572.

Connolly SJ. Meta-analysis of antiarrhythmic drug trials. The American Journal of Cardiology 1999; **84**(Suppl 1): 90–93.

Domanski MJ et al. Effect of angiotensin converting enzyme inhibition on sudden cardiac death in patients following AMI. A meta-analysis of randomized clinical trials. *J Am Coll Cardiol* 1999; **33**: 598.

Eikelboom JW, Quinlan DJ, Mehta SR et al. Unfractionated and low-molecular-weight heparin as adjuncts to thrombolysis in aspirin-treated patients with ST-elevation acute myocardial Infarction: a meta-analysis of the randomized trials. *Circulation* 2005; **112**: 3855–3867.

Fiessinger JN, Huisman MV, Davidson BL et al. THRIVE Treatment Study Investigators. Ximelagatran vs low-molecular-weight heparin and warfarin for the treatment of deep vein thrombosis: a randomized trial. *JAMA* 2005; **293**: 736–739.

Freedman JE. Molecular regulation of platelet-dependent thrombosis. *Circulation* 2005; **112**: 2725–2734. [Biology of current and future putative drug targets.]

Gaziano TA. Cardiovascular disease in the developing world and its cost-effective management. *Circulation* 2005; **112**: 3547–3553.

Gluckman TJ, Sachdev M, Schulman SP, Blumenthal RS. A simplified approach to the management of non-ST-segment elevation acute coronary syndromes. *JAMA* 2005; **293**: 349–357.

Goldschmidt-Clermont PJ, Creager MA, Lorsordo DW, et al. Atherosclerosis 2005: Recent Discoveries and Novel Hypotheses. *Circulation* 2005 **112**: 3348–3353

Healey JS, Baranchuk A, Crystal E et al. Prevention of atrial fibrillation With angiotensin-converting enzyme inhibitors and angiotensin receptor blockers: a meta-analysis. *J Am Coll Cardiol* 2005; **45**: 1832–1839.

Heidenreich PA et al. Meta-analysis of trials comparing beta-blockers, Ca^{2+} antagonists, and nitrates for stable angina. *JAMA* 1999; **281**: 1927.

Hiatt WR. Treatment of disability in peripheral arterial disease: new drugs. Current drug Targets. *Cardiovasc Hematolog Disord* 2004; **4**: 227–231.

Jabbour S, Young-Xu Y, Graboys TB et al. Long-term outcomes of optimized medical management of outpatients with stable coronary artery disease. *Am J Cardiol* 2004; **93**: 294–299.

La Rosa JC et al. Effect of statins on risk of coronary disease: a meta-analysis of randomized controlled trials. *JAMA* 1999; **282**: 2340.

Lawes CMM, Bennett DA, Feigin VL, Rodgers A. Blood pressure and stroke: an overview of published reviews. *Stroke* 2004; **35**: 1024.

Loscalzo J. Clinical trials in cardiovascular medicine in an era of marginal benefit, bias, and hyperbole. *Circulation* 2005; **112**: 3026–3029. [An opinion on how to assimilate cardiovascular clinical trial data.]

Martino E, Bartalena L, Bogazzi F, Braverman LE. The effects of amiodarone on the thyroid. *Endocrine Rev* 2001; **22**: 240–254.

Mebazaa A, Barraud D, Welschbillig S. Randomized clinical trials with levosimendan. *Am J Cardiol* 2005; **96**(Suppl 1): 74–79 [Update on an emerging drug.]

Patrono C, García Rodríguez LA, Landolfi R, Baigent C. Drug therapy: low-dose aspirin for the prevention of atherothrombosis. *N Engl J Med* 2005; **353**: 2373–2383.

Peng H, Carretero OA, Vuljaj N et al. Angiotensin-converting enzyme inhibitors: a new mechanism of action. *Circulation* 2005; **112**: 2436–2445. [An animal study that reveals a possible new explanation for some of the long term benefit with this class of drug on the heart in hypertensive patients.]

Pitt B, White H, Nicolau J et al. Eplerenone reduces mortality 30 days after randomization following acute myocardial infarction in patients with left ventricular systolic dysfunction and heart failure. *J Am Coll Cardiol* 2005; **46**: 425–431.

Prandoni P. Emerging strategies for treatment of venous thromboembolism. *Expert Opin Emerg Drugs* 2005; **10**: 87–94.

Roccaforte R, Demers C, Baldassarre F, Teo KK, Yusuf S. Effectiveness of comprehensive disease management programmes in improving clinical outcomes in heart failure patients. A meta-analysis. *Eur J Heart Failure* 2005; **7**: 1133–1144.

Silber S. When are drug-eluting stents effective? A critical analysis of the presently available data. *Z Kardiol* 2004; **93**: 649–663.

Taylor AL, Wright JT Jr, Cooper RS, Psaty BM. Importance of race/ethnicity in clinical trials: lessons from the African-American Heart Failure Trial (A-HeFT), the African-American Study of Kidney Disease and Hypertension (AASK), and the Antihypertensive and Lipid-Lowering Treatment to Prevent Heart Attack Trial (ALLHAT). *Circulation* 2005; **112**: 3654–3666.

Teerlink JR. Overview of randomized clinical trials in acute heart failure syndromes. *Am J Cardiol* 2005; **96**(Suppl 1): 59–67.

Williams B. Recent hypertension trials: implications and controversies. *J Am Coll Cardiol* 2005; **45**: 813–827.

Yan AT, Yan RT, Liu PP. Narrative review: pharmacotherapy for chronic heart failure: evidence from recent clinical trials. *Ann Intern Med* 2005; **142**: 132–145.

Yusuf S, Mehta SR, Xie C et al; CREATE Trial Group Investigators. Effects of reviparin, a low-molecular-weight heparin, on mortality, reinfarction, and strokes in patients with AMI presenting with ST-segment elevation. *JAMA* 2005; **293**: 427–435.

WEBSITES

http://www.americanheart.org/presenter.jhtml?identifier=3034115 [Americal Heart Association Summaries of key research and free access to scientific journal content.]

http://www.healthinsite.gov.au/topics/Respiratory_Tract_Infections [This website provides general information regarding respiratory tract infections.]

http://www.merck.com/mrkshared/mmanual/sections.jsp [Merck Manual.]

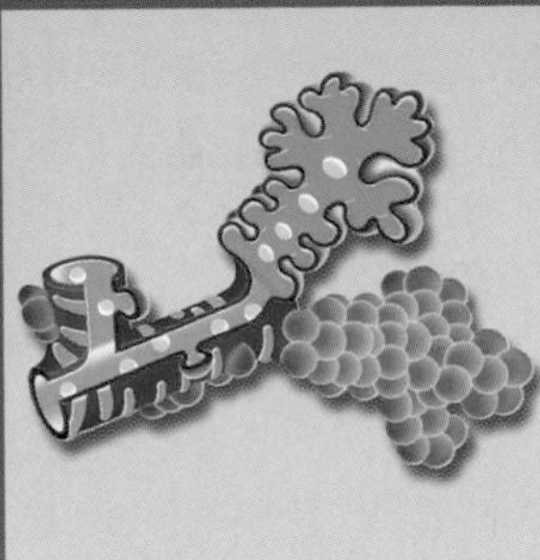

Chapter 14

Drugs and the Pulmonary System

PHYSIOLOGY OF THE PULMONARY SYSTEM

Blood is oxygenated and carbon dioxide removed by the pulmonary system

The body's metabolic processes use large quantities of oxygen and produce large amounts of carbon dioxide. The oxygen-absorbing surface of the lung (the gas-exchange surface) is therefore large (80 m^2). It can fit into the body because it is folded and shaped into a branching tree-like system of air-conducting tubes (bronchi and bronchioles), which end in millions of tiny sacs called alveoli (Fig. 14.1).

Respiration is controlled by spontaneous rhythmic discharges from the respiratory center in the medulla of the brain, which is regulated by higher centers in the brain and vagal afferents from the lungs (Fig. 14.2) and influenced by:

- Changes in blood pCO_2, which activate chemoreceptors in the medulla.
- Changes in blood pO_2, which activate chemoreceptors in the aortic arch and carotid bodies.

Respiration can be influenced by certain drugs. Doxapram is a respiratory stimulant used for patients in respiratory failure which is thought to work via stim-

Upper respiratory tract transport passages
nasal cavity
nasopharynx
epiglottis
larynx
esophagus
trachea
main bronchi
branch bronchi
small bronchi
bronchioles
distal respiratory tree
(gas exchange region)
terminal bronchiole
respiratory bronchioles
smooth muscle
alveolar duct
alveolar sacs
alveoli

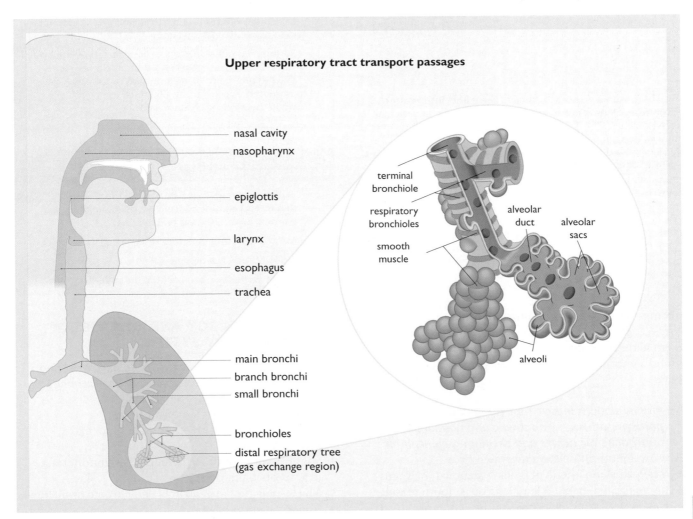

Fig. 14.1 Structure of the respiratory tract.

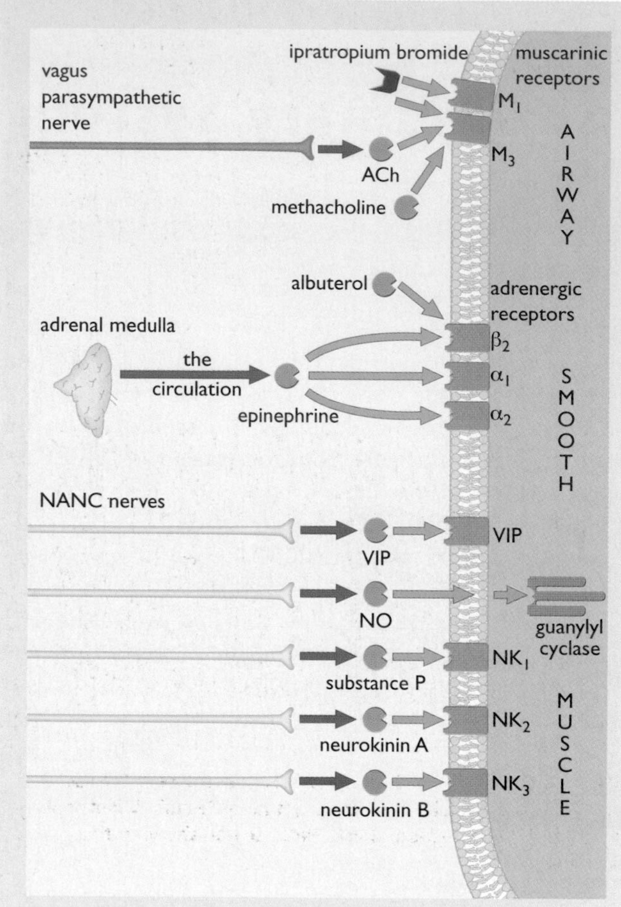

Fig. 14.2 Airway smooth muscle tone and innervation. A constrictor tone is provided by the vagus nerve and release of acetylcholine (ACh). This is blocked by the mixed M_1/M_3 muscarinic antagonist, tiotropium bromide. Methacholine challenge, used to assess airway irritability in subjects with asthma (see Fig. 14.4), activates these receptors. Circulating epinephrine relaxes airway smooth muscle by activating β_2 receptors. This is mimicked by β_2 agonist drugs such as albuterol. The major inhibitory influence on airway smooth muscle tone is via the release of nitric oxide (NO) from nonadrenergic noncholinergic (NANC) nerves, and to a lesser extent, vasoactive intestinal peptide (VIP). NANC nerves also carry fibers that can release sensory neuropeptides (such as substance P and neurokinins) which can cause airway smooth muscle constriction.

ulating carotid chemoreceptors and those in the respiratory center. Several drugs will also cause respiratory depression including narcotic analgesics, barbiturates, older centrally acting H_1 receptor antagonists and ethanol.

Airway smooth muscle tone is regulated by parasympathetic, sympathetic and nonadrenergic noncholinergic nerves and circulating epinephrine

Airway smooth muscle is innervated by:

- The parasympathetic nervous system via the vagus nerve (cranial nerve X), and airway smooth muscle tone is generated by acetylcholine acting on muscarinic receptors (see Fig. 14.2).
- The so-called 'third nervous pathway,' with the neurotransmitters (nitric oxide and vasoactive intestinal polypeptide [VIP]) used by the nonadrenergic noncholinergic (NANC) nerves of this system (see Fig. 14.2) producing smooth muscle relaxation (bronchodilation).

Bronchodilation is also produced by circulating epinephrine binding to β_2 adrenoceptors on the muscle (see Fig. 14.2). Although the bronchial smooth muscle has little or no direct sympathetic innervation, there is a sympathetic (inhibitory) supply to the parasympathetic ganglia.

Airway smooth muscle tone therefore depends on the balance between the:

- Parasympathetic input.
- Inhibitory influence of circulating epinephrine.
- NANC inhibitory nerves.
- Sympathetic innervation of the parasympathetic ganglia.

Drugs that alter respiration

- **Narcotic analgesics, barbiturates, certain H_1 receptor antagonists and ethanol cause respiratory depression**
- **Doxapram is a respiratory stimulant and is used for patients in ventilatory failure**
- **Respiratory stimulants are believed to stimulate both carotid chemoreceptors and the respiratory center. They should be used with caution as they may have unwanted effects on the CNS such as convulsions, while their efficacy is uncertain**

Noninfectious diseases of the respiratory tract

- **The most common diseases are asthma, allergic rhinitis and chronic obstructive pulmonary disease (chronic bronchitis and emphysema)**
- **Asthma is an inflammatory disease**
- **Cystic fibrosis is a genetic disease**
- **Cough is usually a symptom of an underlying disease**

PATHOPHYSIOLOGY AND DISEASES OF THE PULMONARY SYSTEM

Pulmonary disease can cause coughing, wheezing, shortness of breath and abnormal gas exchange

Coughing, wheezing, shortness of breath (dyspnea) and abnormal gas exchange can result from:

- Changes in airway smooth muscle tone (e.g. bronchial asthma).
- Vascular congestion of the upper respiratory tract (e.g. nasal congestion).
- Mucus plugging (e.g. asthma and chronic bronchitis).
- Abnormal gas exchange (e.g. emphysema).
- Hypersecretion (rhinitis, component of asthma)

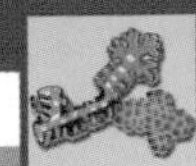

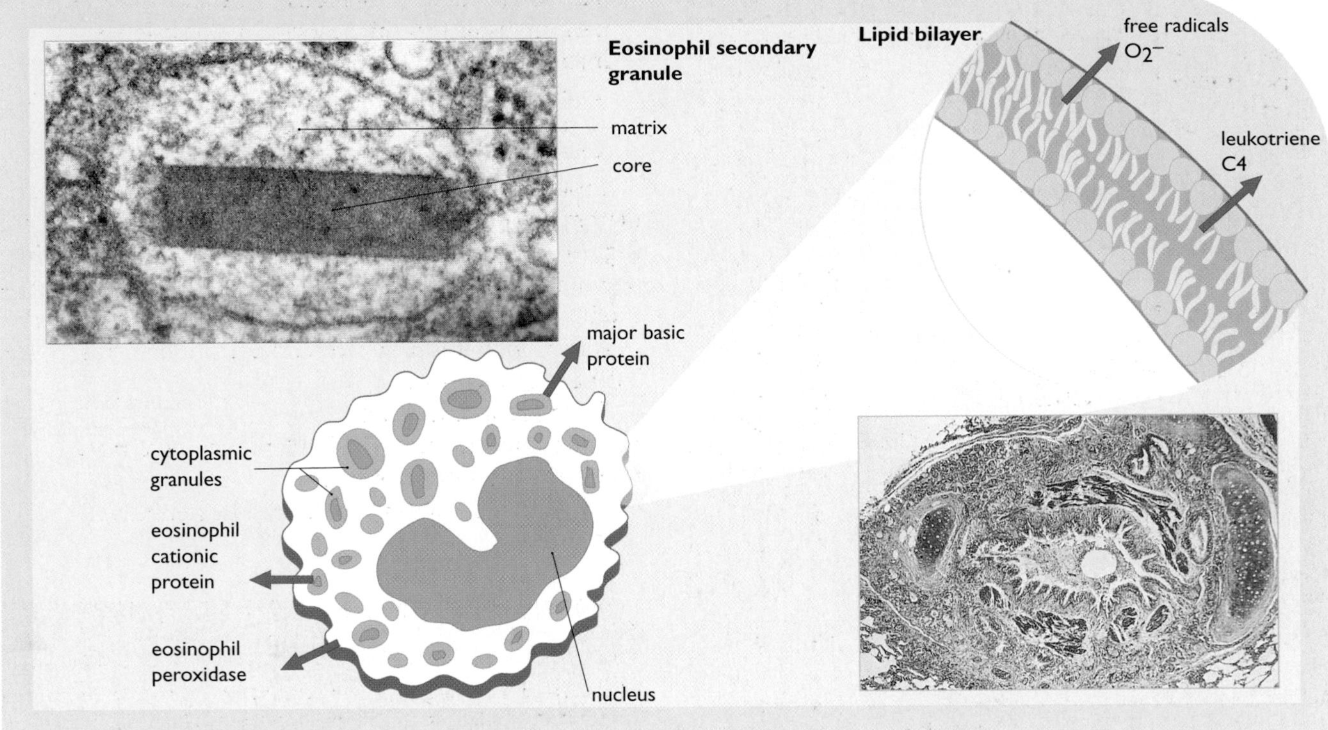

Fig. 14.3 Cytotoxic mediators released by eosinophils lead to epithelial damage. Infiltrating eosinophils release cytotoxic mediators, including major basic protein, eosinophil peroxidase and eosinophil cationic protein, from their granules. Certain inflammatory mediators can be released from the lipid bilayer upon eosinophil activation. Lower right, a section of asthmatic airway showing the pathophysiologic changes. (Courtesy of Dr. Alan Stevens and Professor James Lowe.)

Bronchial asthma

Bronchial asthma is a chronic inflammatory disease of the airways that causes acute bronchospasm and dyspnea

Bronchial asthma is a common disease, affecting up to 20% of the population in some countries. Its associated morbidity and mortality are rising in most countries despite increasing use of antiasthma drugs.

The characteristic clinical features of bronchial asthma are associated with a chronic inflammatory response in the airways involving local lymphocyte and eosinophil accumulation, which is evident following bronchoalveolar lavage (BAL) on biopsy and at autopsy (Fig. 14.3). It is thought that the granules of infiltrating eosinophils release cytotoxic mediators (see Fig. 14.3), which damage the respiratory ciliated epithelium. The tissue damage is associated with increased airway irritability (bronchial hyperresponsiveness), which causes coughing and wheezing in response to stimuli that do not normally provoke such responses in healthy people (Fig. 14.4).

Bronchial hyperresponsiveness may result from exposure of sensory nerves beneath the damaged epithelium (Fig. 14.5). Activation of these nerves on exertion or following exposure to environmental irritants results in local axon and vagal reflexes, which can produce bronchoconstriction, mucus secretion and airway vasodilation (see Fig. 14.5).

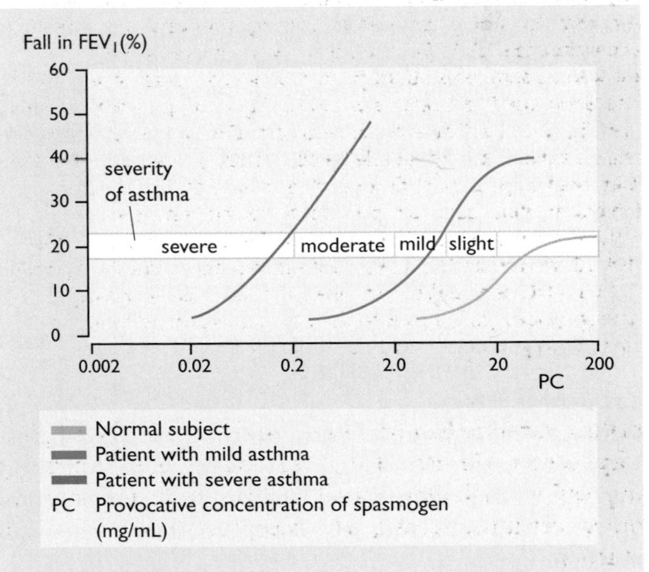

Fig. 14.4 Bronchial hyperresponsiveness. People with bronchial asthma have bronchial hyperresponsiveness, which causes them to cough and wheeze in response to stimuli that would not provoke such responses in normal subjects. Clinically, this hyperresponsiveness can be demonstrated by measuring the change in lung function, which is shown by a reduction in FEV_1 (forced expiratory volume in one second) in response to an inhaled spasmogen such as histamine or the muscarinic agonist methacholine. Increased irritability is observed with increasing disease severity.

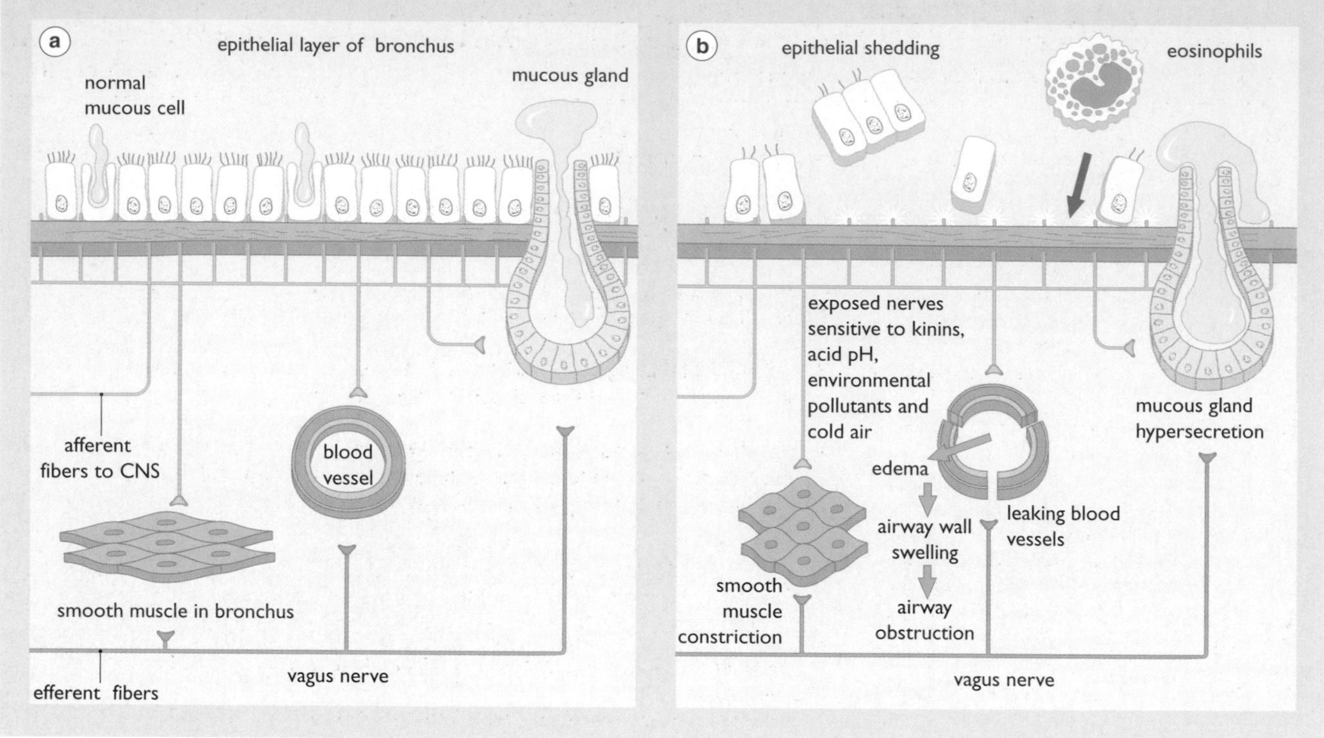

Fig. 14.5 Mechanism of bronchial hyperresponsiveness. This may result from exposure of sensory airway nerves following damage to the ciliated epithelial layer by cytotoxic mediators released by infiltrating eosinophils, which may then become hypersensitive as a result of exposure to inflammatory mediators such as prostaglandins and cytokines. (a) Normal lung; (b) asthmatic lung.

Clinical features of bronchial asthma

- **Acute attacks of dyspnea associated with acute airway obstruction due to contraction of airway smooth muscle**
- **Mucus hypersecretion, which may lead to mucus plugging**
- **Airway inflammation**
- **Bronchial hyperresponsiveness**

Bronchodilators and antiinflammatory drugs are used in the treatment of asthma

Bronchodilators

Acute reversible bronchospasm contributes to the characteristic wheezing of asthma. It is readily treated by three different classes of bronchodilator drugs: β_2 adrenoceptor agonists, anticholinergics (muscarinic receptor antagonists) and xanthines.

β_2 ADRENOCEPTOR AGONISTS are the most widely prescribed drugs for the treatment of bronchoconstriction in asthma and are available by inhalation from a metered-dose inhaler or nebulizer, systemically as well as orally (Table 14.1). Short-acting β_2 adrenoceptor agonists are widely used for the acute relief of bronchospasm and include albuterol, terbutaline and fenoterol. Epinephrine, isoproterenol, isoetharine and metaproterenol are sometimes used but are not selective for β_2 receptors, having various degrees of activity at α receptors and β_1 receptors, which are essentially unwanted effects. Most β_2 agonists are available as racemic mixtures, but recently the single enantiomer R-albuterol has been introduced into clinical practice.

β_2 adrenoceptor agonists relax airway smooth muscle through the activation of G protein-coupled receptors, leading to their activation and an increase in cAMP in airway smooth muscle. They are excellent functional (physiologic) antagonists of the bronchoconstriction caused by a wide range of stimuli. One of the drawbacks of albuterol, terbutaline and fenoterol, however, has been their short biologic half-life (2–3 hours), but a variety of long-acting β_2 adrenoceptor agonists have now been introduced that produce bronchodilation for up to 15 hours, including salmeterol, aformoterol and bambuterol. The prolonged action of salmeterol is believed to be due to the presence in the molecule of a long lipophilic tail, which binds to an 'exoreceptor' in the vicinity of the β_2 adrenoceptor on airway smooth muscle. These long-acting drugs are intended for long-term prevention of asthma attacks, but are not recommended for acute relief, particularly salmeterol, which has a delayed onset (>15 mins) of action. They are particularly useful for treating nocturnal asthma but are not recommended as monotherapy and are usually combined with inhaled glucocorticosteroids (see below). However, a number of

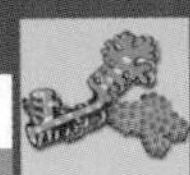

Table 14.1 Commonly used β_2 agonists for the treatment of respiratory diseases

β_2 agonists	Route of administration	Dose range	Half-life (hours)
Albuterol	Oral: Extended release	2 mg/12 hours pediatric 4–8 mg/12 hours adult	5–6
Terbutaline	Oral: Tablets	5 mg 3 times daily for adults and children over 12 years 2.5 mg 3 times daily for children 6–12 years	3–4
	Injection: Subcutaneous	0.255 mg (0.25 mL) for adults and children over 12 years 0.006–0.01 mg/kg for children 6–12 years	3–4
	Inhalation: Micronized metered dose	2 inhalations of 0.2 mg separated by a 60-second interval every 4–6 hours for adults and children over 12 years	3–4
Fenoterol	Inhalation: Aerosol	1–2 inhalations (0.1 mg) up to 3 times daily in adults 1 inhalation (0.1 mg) up to 3 times daily for children over 6 years 1–2 inhalations (0.2 mg) up to 3 times daily in adults	6–7
Aformoterol	Inhalation: Breath-activated inhaler	1–2 capsules (12 μg) twice daily 6–12 μg twice daily in adults	
	Breath-activated dry powder		
Salmeterol	Inhalation: Aerosol	2 inhalations of 21 μg twice a day for adults and children over 12 years	17
	Powder	1 inhalation of 50 μg twice daily for adults and children over 4 years	17
Isoproterenol	Inhalation: Aerosol	1–2 inhalations of 0.131 mg up to 5 times a day in adults and children	
	Solution	5–15 deep inhalations of a 1:200 dilution of a 0.5% solution administered via a nebulizer in adults and children	
Bambuterol	Oral	10–20 mg daily at night in adults	

regulatory agencies have recently put a 'black box' warning on all medicine containing salmeterol, as the use of such drugs may increase the risk of death in certain patients.

The adverse effects of β_2 adrenoceptor agonists include tremor and hypokalemia, and, when given in excessive amounts, tachycardia. The adverse effects of β_2 adrenoceptor agonists are reduced when they are inhaled and this is the preferred route of administration.

ANTICHOLINERGICS Muscarinic receptor antagonists cause bronchodilation by binding to muscarinic receptors on airway smooth muscle and thereby preventing the action of acetylcholine released from parasympathetic nerves in the vagus nerve. Anticholinergics do not therefore prevent all types of bronchospasm, but are particularly effective against irritant-induced changes in respiratory function. Muscarinic receptor antagonists also decrease mucus secretion.

Currently available muscarinic receptor antagonists do not discriminate between M_2 and M_3 receptors (Fig. 14.6), and it is likely that M_2 autoreceptor antagonism on cholinergic presynaptic terminals may reduce the effectiveness of the antagonism at M_3 receptors on smooth muscle. Selective M_3 receptor antagonists could therefore be a therapeutic advance.

Muscarinic antagonists include short-acting drugs such as atropine, ipratropium bromide and oxitropium bromide and the longer-acting drug tiotropium bromide (Table 14.2). These drugs are used clinically by the inhaled route to reduce the systemic adverse effects otherwise associated with muscarinic receptor antagonists. When inhaled, they are poorly absorbed into the circulation from the lung, do not cross the blood–brain barrier and have few adverse effects. Maximum bronchodilation is usually observed from 30 minutes after administration and lasts for up to 5 hours with the short-acting drugs and up to 15 hours with tiotropium bromide. However, their efficacy in asthma is usually modest compared with inhaled β_2 agonists and their use is primarily in the treatment of COPD (see below).

XANTHINES have been widely used in the treatment of asthma since the start of the twentieth century following observations that 'strong coffee' relieved the symptoms of asthma. Coffee, tea and chocolate-containing beverages contain naturally occurring xanthines such as caffeine and theobromine. The main xanthine used clinically is theophylline, which is sometimes used as theophylline ethylenediamine salt (aminophylline). Other xanthines that are used are bamifylline and elixophylline. Xanthines are usually given orally, but are rapidly metabolized, and

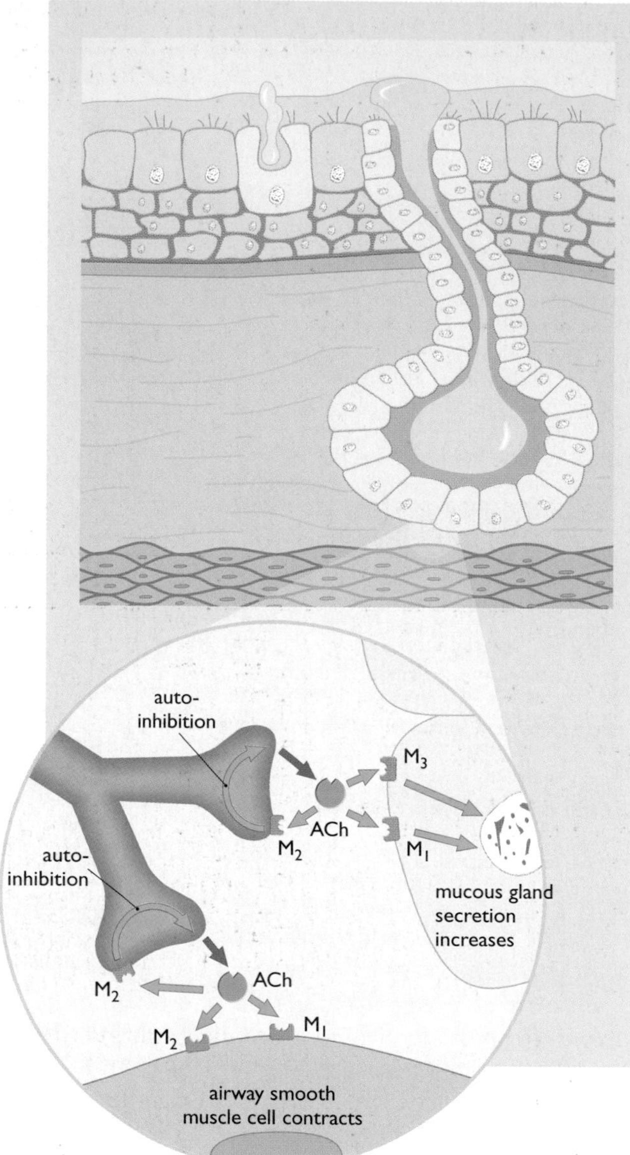

Fig. 14.6 Action of acetylcholine (ACh) on airway smooth muscle. ACh released from parasympathetic neurons acts on M_1 and M_3 muscarinic receptors on airway smooth muscle and submucosal glands to bring about muscle constriction and mucus secretion. In addition, some of the released ACh acts on presynaptic M_2 muscarinic receptors on the nerve terminal to reduce further release of ACh. These M_2 receptors are known as 'autoreceptors.'

have a short biologic half-life. However, this limitation is overcome by using 'slow-release' preparations, which will maintain effective plasma concentrations over 16–18 hours.

The major problem with using xanthines as bronchodilators is that they have a very narrow therapeutic window; consequentially, plasma concentrations over 10 μg/mL are required for effective bronchodilation, but plasma concentrations over 20 μg/mL are associated with an increased likelihood of adverse effects, including nausea, cardiac arrhythmias and convulsions. Plasma xanthine concentrations should therefore be measured routinely. Aminophylline can be given as a slow intravenous (i.v.) infusion with a loading dose for acute severe asthma.

For treatment of acute asthma in patients not receiving theophylline products, a loading dose of 5 mg/kg should be administered and maintained at 4 mg/kg every 6 hours in young children (1–9 years), 3 mg/kg every 6 hours in children (9–16 years) and smokers, 3 mg/kg every 8 hours in nonsmoking adults and 2 mg/kg in older patients.

Drug interactions are important as the serum theophylline concentration can be increased (barbiturates, benzodiazepines) or decreased (cimetidine, erythromycin, ciprofloxacin, allopurinol) by a variety of drugs. These interactions can cause variations in serum theophylline levels among patients, so that the dose of theophylline must be titrated to suit the individual. Initially, start at the lowest dose and, if tolerated and adequate control of symptoms is not achieved, the dose can be increased in stages up to the maximum dosage recommended. An interval of 3 days must be left between increases in dosage to allow for serum levels to stabilize. In the case of acutely ill patients the serum levels should be monitored every 24 hours. In all cases the dose should be adjusted to give serum concentrations of 5–15 μg/mL.

Sustained-release preparations are not suitable for the treatment of acute asthma, which should be treated with other medications or an immediate-release preparation.

For the treatment of nocturnal asthma the medication should be given at 8 pm and serum theophylline levels should be monitored. It is preferable to titrate the dose with small increments, allowing 3 days between increments, and increasing the dose only if it is tolerated and no adverse effects become apparent.

Drugs for asthma

- **All β adrenoceptor agonists promote bronchodilation**
- **The principal action of glucocorticosteroids is suppression of the inflammatory response**
- **Xanthines combine bronchodilator and antiinflammatory properties**
- **Muscarinic receptor antagonist-induced bronchodilation is occasionally useful**

Drugs that modify serum theophylline concentrations

Drugs that increase serum theophylline concentrations include:
- Oral contraceptives
- Erythromycin
- Ca^{2+} antagonists
- Cimetidine (but not ranitidine)

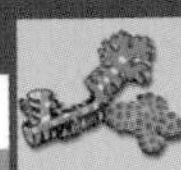

Table 14.2 Commonly used muscarinic receptor antagonists for the treatment of respiratory diseases

Muscarinic receptor antagonists	Route of administration	Dose range	Half-life (hours)
Ipratropium bromide	Oral inhalation:		
	Aerosol	20–80 μg 3 or 4 times daily in adults and children over 12 years	
		20–40 μg 3 times a day in children 6–12 years	
		20 μg 3 times daily	
	Dry powder	20–80 μg 3 or 4 times daily in adults	
	Nasal inhalation:		
	Nasal spray	42 μg in each nostril 2–3 times daily	
Oxitropium bromide	Oral inhalation:	200 μg 2–3 times daily in adults	2–4
	Aerosol		
Tiotropium bromide	Oral inhalation:		
	Aerosol		10

Table 14.3 Classification of phosphodiesterase isozymes

Family	Isozyme	Tissue	Inhibitors
1	Ca^{2+}/calmodulin dependent	Brain, airway smooth muscle	Vinpocetine Theophylline
2	cGMP stimulated	Heart, vascular smooth muscle, platelets, airway smooth muscle	Theophylline
3	cGMP inhibited	Lymphocyte, platelets, heart, vascular smooth muscle, airway smooth muscle	Milrinone Theophylline
4	cAMP selective	Inflammatory cells (neutrophil, macrophage, mast cell, eosinophil, lymphocyte) airway smooth muscle, heart, brain, striated muscle	Rolipram Theophylline Cilomilast Roflumilast
5	cGMP selective	Trachea, platelets, vascular smooth muscle	Zaprinast Theophylline Sildenafil

Drugs that decrease serum theophylline concentrations include:

- **Rifampin**
- **Phenobarbital**
- **Phenytoin**
- **Carbamazepine**

Xanthines are believed to produce bronchodilation by inhibiting a family of enzymes called phosphodiesterases (Table 14.3). These enzymes take part in the metabolism of the second messengers involved in relaxing airway smooth muscle (i.e. cAMP and cGMP). In particular, inhibition of phosphodiesterase 3 and 4 in airway smooth muscle leads to intracellular accumulation of cAMP and therefore smooth muscle relaxation (see Table 14.3 and Fig. 14.7).

Antiinflammatory and prophylactic drugs

Antiinflammatory drugs may resolve existing bronchial inflammation and/or prevent subsequent inflammation in patients with asthma. Most antiinflammatory drugs prevent subsequent inflammation and are therefore classed as prophylactic antiasthma drugs. Since antiinflammatory drugs do not cause bronchodilation, they are not recommended for acute asthma attacks.

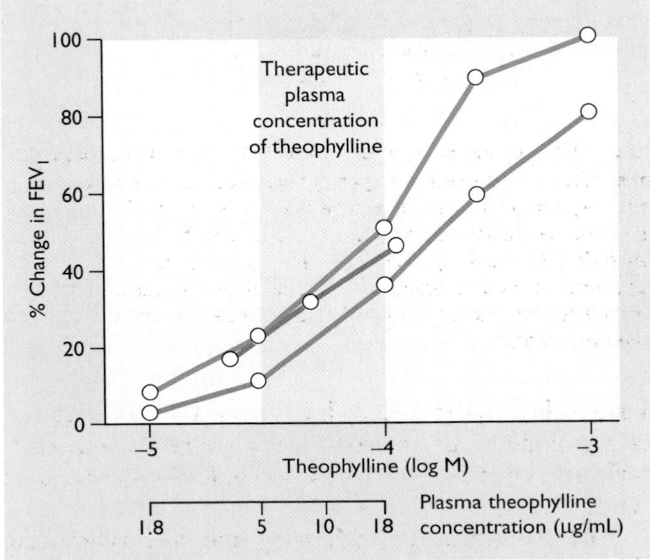

Fig. 14.7 Effects of theophylline at therapeutic concentrations. Percentage change in FEV_1 (red), percentage inhibition of airway smooth muscle relaxation (green), or percentage inhibition of phosphodiesterase activity in airway smooth muscle (purple) in relation to plasma concentrations of theophylline (μg/mL) or theophylline concentration (log M in an isolated tissue experiment). (Adapted from Rabe et al. *Eur Resp J* 1995; **289**: 600–603.)

GLUCOCORTICOSTEROIDS are the best established antiinflammatory drugs for the treatment of chronic inflammatory process underlying asthma. They inhibit inflammatory cell infiltration into the airways and reduce edema formation by acting on the vascular endothelium. Their mechanism of action is discussed in detail in Chapter 9.

Glucocorticosteroids can be given prophylactically by inhalation to achieve a local antiinflammatory effect without causing systemic adverse effects. Inhaled glucocorticosteroids used for bronchial asthma include beclometasone dipropionate, budesonide, fluticasone propionate, triamcinolone, mometasone and ciclesonide. Oral glucocorticosteroids may be required for severe asthma unresponsive to inhaled glucocorticosteroids, and usually prednisone, methylprednisolone, or prednisolone is prescribed (Table 14.4).

Both oral and i.v. glucocorticosteroids are useful in the treatment of acute severe asthma. However, oral glucocorticosteroids have major systemic adverse effects involving suppression of the hypothalamus–pituitary axis (see Ch. 11 and Table 14.4). Chronic use can lead to a variety of serious adverse effects, including stunting of growth in children (see Ch. 11 and Table 14.4).

Combination inhalers containing a glucocorticosteroid with a long-acting β_2 agonist are now widely used to optimally control the underlying inflammation as well as the symptoms of bronchospasm that characterize asthma. The most frequently prescribed combination inhalers are salmeterol/fluticasone propionate or budesonide/formoterol. One advantage of having both drugs combined in one inhaler is that both drugs can be administered at lower does than when administered individually, thereby reducing likely side effects; it is particularly important to minimize the side effects of the glucocorticosteroids.

XANTHINES not only produce bronchodilation, as described above, but also inhibit inflammatory cell activation and infiltration in the airways of asthmatics. Furthermore, xanthine withdrawal after chronic treatment in some asthmatics leads to a worsening of asthma, even in patients taking glucocorticosteroids. The antiinflammatory effects are associated with plasma concentrations lower than those required to produce bronchodilation (5–10 mg/mL). Such findings have led to a reappraisal of the place of xanthines in the treatment of asthma (see Fig. 14.7), particularly because:

- Xanthines are administered orally, which greatly enhances patient compliance compared with that for inhaled drugs.
- Low plasma concentrations of theophylline have fewer adverse effects.

The antiinflammatory action of xanthines may be mediated through inhibition of phosphodiesterase 4, the isozyme found predominately in inflammatory cells (see Table 14.3). Recent evidence suggests that theophylline, which is an established agent for the treatment of acute bronchospasm in asthmatics, may be effective when used at low doses for long-term maintenance treatment in asthmatics as a result of this antiinflammatory action.

PDE4 INHIBITORS PDE4 isoenzymes are the predominant enzymes found in most inflammatory cells. Recent Phase III clinical studies have shown that roflumilast *N*-oxide, an orally active PDE4 selective inhibitor, is effective in treating mild to moderate asthma.

Antiallergy drugs, including cromolyn sodium, ketotifen and nedocromil sodium, are used prophylactically in the treatment of bronchial asthma. Cromolyn and nedocromil sodium are active by inhalation. Ketotifen is orally active and is used worldwide except in the USA. Other antiallergy drugs include ebastine and mizolastine. The mechanisms of action of these prophylactic drugs are not clearly understood, but cromolyn sodium was originally thought to be a 'mast cell stabilizer,' so preventing the release of histamine and other inflammatory mediators (see Ch. 9). It is now clear that this action is not the only effect of these prophylactic drugs. They are capable of affecting many inflammatory cell types such as alveolar macrophages, thereby preventing inflammatory cell recruitment into the airway wall. In addition, cromolyn sodium and nedocromil sodium can depress the exaggerated neuronal reflexes triggered by irritant receptors in the airways, probably by suppressing the response of exposed irritant nerves (see Fig. 14.5). This action has also led to their use in the treatment of 'asthmatic cough.' Recently, an immunoglobulin G (omalizumab) exhibiting antihuman immunoglobulin EFc region activity has been introduced into clinical practice. Omalizumab is administered subcutaneously and has a very long half-life, allowing it to be administered monthly for the treatment of allergic asthma.

Drugs affecting leukotriene synthesis and actions

ZAFIRLUKAST AND MONTELUKAST are orally active cysteinyl-leukotriene receptor antagonists that antagonize the actions of LTC_4 and LTD_4 on airway smooth muscle and vascular endothelium. They are particularly effective in patients with aspirin-induced asthma. They are also very effective in treating exercise-induced asthma and are available as once-a-day formulation, which may improve compliance, which is a major clinical problem in the treatment of asthma, particularly in children. Zileuton is an orally active inhibitor of the synthesis of cysteinyl-leukotrienes and other 5-lipoxygenase metabolites derived from arachidonic acid metabolism (see Table 14.3) which has also been shown to have a modest clinical effect in the treatment of asthma.

Ciclosporin analogs

Ciclosporin has been successfully used in the treatment of immune disorders involving lymphocytes (see Ch. 9) and has recently been shown to have some clinical benefit in

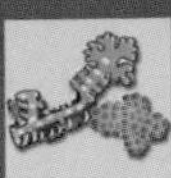

Table 14.4 Commonly used glucocorticosteroids for treatment of respiratory diseases

Glucocorticosteroids	Route of administration	Dose range	Drug interactions
Beclometasone dipropionate	Nasal inhalation:		
	Aerosol	1 inhalation (42 µg/inhalation) in each nostril 2–4 times a day in adults and children over 12 years	
		1 inhalation (42 µg/inhalation) in each nostril 3 times a day in children 6–12 years	
	Suspension	1–2 inhalations (42 µg/inhalation) in each nostril twice a day in adults and children over 12 years	
		1 inhalation (42 µg/inhalation) in each nostril twice a day in children 6–12 years	
	Oral inhalation:		
	Aerosol	2 inhalations (42 µg/inhalation) given 3 or 4 times a day in adults and children over 12 years	
		1–2 inhalations (42 µg/inhalation) 3 or 4 times a day in children 6–12 years	
	Aerosol	2 inhalations (84 µg/inhalation) twice daily in adults and children over 12 years	
		2 inhalations (84 µg/inhalation) twice daily in children 6–12 years	
	Dry powder	200 µg twice daily or 100 µg 4 times daily in adults and children over 12 years	
		50–100 µg 2–4 times daily in children	
Budesonide	Nasal inhalation:		
	Nasal inhaler	256 µg daily either 2 sprays per nostril twice daily or 4 sprays per nostril once daily in adults and children over 6 years	Cytochrome P-450 3A inhibitors
	Nasal spray	64 µg per day (one spray of 32 µg per nostril once daily) in adults and children over 6 years	Cytochrome P-450 3A inhibitors
	Oral inhalation:		
	Dry powder	200–400 µg twice daily in adults and 200 µg twice daily in children previously maintained with bronchodilators alone	Cytochrome P-450 3A inhibitors
		200–400 µg twice daily in adults with 200 µg twice daily in children previously maintained with inhaled corticosteroids	Ketoconazole
		400–800 µg twice daily in adults and 400 µg twice daily in children previously maintained with oral corticosteroids	
	Aerosol	200 µg twice daily in adults and children	Cytochrome P-450 3A inhibitors
Fluticasone propionate	Oral inhalation:		
	Dry powder	100 µg twice daily in adults and children over 12 years and 50 µg twice daily in children 4–7 years previously maintained with bronchodilators alone	Cytochrome P-450 3A inhibitors
		100–250 µg twice daily in adults and children over 12 years and 50 µg twice daily in children 4–7 years previously maintained with inhaled corticosteroids	
		1000 µg twice daily in adults and children over 12 years previously maintained with oral corticosteroids	
	Aerosol	88 µg twice daily in adults previously maintained with bronchodilators alone	Cytochrome P-450 3A inhibitors
		88–220 µg twice daily in adults previously maintained with inhaled corticosteroids	
		880 µg twice daily in adults previously maintained with oral corticosteroids	
	Intranasal:		
	Nasal spray	220 µg/day given once or twice a day in adults	Cytochrome P-450 3A inhibitors
		100–200 µg/day given once a day in children 4 years and older	
Mometasone furoate	Intranasal:		
	Nasal spray	200 µg/day given once a day in adults and children over 12 years	
		100 µg/day given once a day in children 6–12 years	
Triamcinolone	Oral inhalation:		
	Aerosol	200 µg 3–4 times a day in adults and children over 12 years	
		100–200 µg 3–4 times a day in children 6–12 years	

continued

Table 14.4—*cont'd*

Glucocorticosteroids	Route of administration	Dose range	Drug interactions	
	Nasal inhalation:			
	Nasal spray	220 μg once a day in adults and children over 6 years		
	Systemic:			
	Oral tablets	8–16 mg/day	Phenytoin Phenobarbital Primidone Rifampin Carbamazepine Aminoglutethimide Ephedrine Diuretics Antihypertensives Estrogens Anticholinesterases Cardiac glycosides	Hypoglycemics Oral anticoagulants NSAIDs Salicylates Live vaccines Amphotericin Acetazolamide Carbenoxolone Methotrexate Ciclosporin Erythromycin
	Intramuscular injection	2.5–60 mg/day		Azole antifungals As above
Dexamethasone	Systemic:			
	Oral	0.75–9 mg/day		See triamcinolone
Prednisone	Systemic:			
	Oral	5–60 mg/day		See triamcinolone
Methylprednisolone	Systemic:			
	Oral	4–48 mg/day		See triamcinolone
	Intramuscular injection	4–48 mg/day		As above
	Intravenous infusion	30 mg/kg over 30 minutes every 4–6 hours for 48 hours		As above
Cortisone	Systemic:			
	Oral	25–300 mg/day		See triamcinolone
	Intramuscular injection	25–300 mg/day		As above

asthmatics resistant to therapy with glucocorticosteroids. However, it has considerable adverse effects and so there is ongoing research to find safer analogs of this drug to use in the treatment of asthma.

Antiinflammatory treatment is now used much earlier in asthma than in the past

Since asthma is a chronic inflammatory disease of the airways, and not just a disease associated with bronchoconstriction, a number of organizations and societies around the world including the National Institutes of Health in the United States, the World Health Organization and the Canadian Thoracic Society have issued guidelines on the optimal treatment of bronchial asthma. These are based on a stepwise approach, but stress the need for antiinflammatory treatment much earlier in the disease than has been used in the past, since this has been demonstrated to have a good effect on disease progression.

! Adverse effects of antiasthma drugs

- **β_2 adrenoceptor agonists may cause tremor and their long-term use may worsen the underlying disease**
- **A 'black box' warning has recently been introduced on medicines containing the long acting β_2 against salmeterol**
- **Xanthines cause tremor, tachycardia and gastrointestinal irritation**
- **Oral glucocorticosteroids should be reserved for patients who do not adequately respond to other therapy, because they have a wide spectrum of adverse effects**
- **Aerosol glucocorticosteroids cause fewer adverse effects than oral glucocorticosteroids, and mainly overgrowth of *Candida* in the mouth and hoarseness**

Chronic obstructive pulmonary disease

Chronic bronchitis and emphysema often occur together in heavy smokers, a condition referred to as chronic

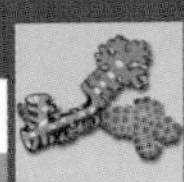

obstructive pulmonary disease (COPD). COPD mainly occurs in older smokers, although it can also occur in younger patients genetically deficient in the enzyme α_1 antitrypsin. Chronic bronchitis is defined in functional terms as a disorder associated with the excessive production of sputum and cough daily, or on most days. Airway obstruction is the result of luminal narrowing and mucus plugs, and may lead to secondary respiratory infection (Fig. 14.8). Typically, chronic bronchitis causes alveolar hypoventilation, hypercapnia and hypoxia, although some patients hyperventilate in order to avoid severe hypoxia. Secondary pulmonary hypertension may develop and lead to right heart failure (cor pulmonale). Patients typically have a productive cough, sputum production, breathlessness on exertion and airway obstruction. Respiratory infection is common and can exacerbate the disease. In long-term smokers, emphysema can occur with destructive loss of alveolar structures and subsequent chronic impairment of gas exchange. Patients with emphysema have very poor prognosis and have very poor respiratory performance. There are no drugs that prevent or reverse emphysema, although smoking cessation will reduce disease progression. Patients are treated symptomatically with various drugs (see below) and such patients also often require nebulized oxygen.

Bronchodilators, mucokinetic drugs and antibiotics are used to treat the symptoms associated with chronic bronchitis and emphysema

Bronchodilators

β ADRENOCEPTOR AGONISTS (short- and long-acting) are used to treat airway obstruction and breathlessness on exertion in patients with chronic bronchitis and emphysema, but they are generally less effective in such patients than in the treatment of bronchial asthma because less of the airway obstruction is due to abnormal airway smooth muscle contraction.

Long-acting β_2 agonists are also sometimes used in a combination inhaler with glucocorticosteroids, although the evidence for a clear clinical benefit of glucocorticosteroids in the treatments of COPD is wanting.

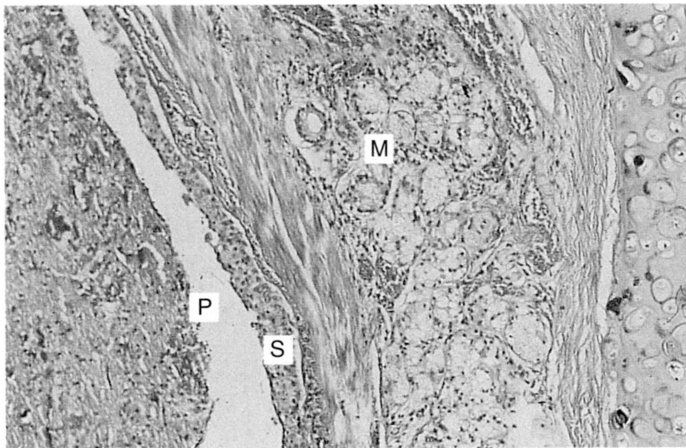

Fig. 14.8 Chronic bronchitis. The main abnormality is hypersecretion of mucus, which plugs the airway (P). Hypersecretion is associated with hypertrophy and hyperplasia of bronchial mucus-secreting glands (M). The Reid index, which is the ratio of gland:wall thickness in the bronchus, is increased in chronic bronchitis. Inflammation is typically absent, although excessive mucus production is frequently associated with the development of coincidental respiratory tract infections, leading to secondary inflammation. Squamous metaplasia (S) is common in patients who have persistent or recurrent superimposed infections. (Courtesy of Dr. Alan Stevens and Professor James Lowe.)

XANTHINES are used in the treatment of chronic bronchitis, particularly for their effects on airway smooth muscle. They also have central nervous system (CNS) effects, leading to increased alertness, which may be important in chronic bronchitis, and can increase diaphragm contractility.

Mucokinetic drugs

N-ACETYLCYSTEINE breaks the disulfide bonds that hold mucus glycoproteins together and thereby reduce the viscosity of mucus. *N*-acetylcysteine and a related drug ambroxol have been shown to produce some clinical benefit in the treatment of COPD. Other mucokinetic agents include guaifenesin, potassium iodide and even saline. Erdosteine is a mucolytic drug that is also an inhibitor of elastase that can be used in the treatment of COPD.

MUSCARINIC RECEPTOR ANTAGONISTS are the mainstay of therapy for chronic bronchitis because they can reduce much of the bronchospasm associated with smoking and the subsequent inhalation of irritants. Their ability to reduce mucus secretion in the airway by antagonizing acetylcholine acting on muscarinic receptors in mucous glands is also very beneficial (see Fig. 14.6). Increasingly the long-acting muscarinic receptor antagonist tiotropium bromide is used for the maintenance treatment of symptoms in patients with COPD.

Antibiotics

Patients with chronic bronchitis commonly get secondary bacterial infections colonizing the sputum. Antibiotics are therefore often prescribed for these patients and are discussed in more detail in Chapter 6 and below.

PDE4 inhibitors

Recent clinical studies have suggested that the orally active PDE4 selective inhibitors roflumilast and cilomilast show clinical benefit in the treatment of COPD. α_1 antitrypsin is also used to treat patients having a genetic deficiency of this enzyme that results in early onset of emphysema. It has also been tried in patients with emphysema.

Respiratory distress syndrome(s)

Adult respiratory distress syndrome (ARDS) is an acute life-threatening condition. It results from increased leakiness of the pulmonary capillary network leading to hypoxia, reduced lung compliance, alveolar infiltrates and noncardiogenic pulmonary edema. It is common in patients with sepsis, who account for 50% of ARDS cases. The mortality rate of ARDS is approximately 60–70%.

Current therapy for ARDS is inadequate

No drug specifically prevents the onset of ARDS or lessens its lethality. However, there are promising studies in animals as well as case reports of emerging therapies for the future including monoclonal antibodies directed against cytokines, PAF, TNF and IL-1 receptor antagonists.

There is also an infant respiratory distress syndrome that occurs in premature infants lacking surfactant. There are several surfactant preparations used clinically until infants start to manufacture their own lung surfactant. These include calfactant and poractant alfa.

Cystic fibrosis

Cystic fibrosis is caused by mutations in specific proteins essential for apical Cl^- clearance

Cystic fibrosis is an inherited disease that starts early in childhood and affects the airways and the ducts in various organs, principally lungs, pancreas and sweat glands. Patients with cystic fibrosis have mutations in specific proteins essential for apical Cl^- clearance (Fig. 14.9). This results in defective Cl^- clearance and excessive Na^+ reabsorption and, as a consequence of osmotic changes, excessive water reabsorption. The defect results in thick and viscous secretion in ducted organs, typically in the airways of the lung, and ducts of the pancreas and sweat glands in homozygotes. In the lungs this gives rise to areas in which inspired air is poorly circulated. The subsequent bacterial infection (involving *Staphylococcus aureus*, *Pseudomonas aeruginosa*, or other organisms) results in irreversible lung damage (bronchiectasis). Analogous processes involving retained secretions occur in other organs.

Mucokinetic drugs, antisecretory agents, antibiotics and physical therapy are used to treat cystic fibrosis

People with cystic fibrosis have a markedly reduced life expectancy, but it can be significantly extended by aggressive therapy with drugs and physical therapy (Table 14.5). Current therapy of the pulmonary effects centers on:

- Thinning secretions and thereby keeping airways and organ ducts patent.
- Combating opportunistic infections.

The purulent mucus secreted by people with cystic fibrosis is characteristically yellow and rich in DNA tangles (from killed cells), which has led to the use of DNAases to loosen secretions further (see below).

Mucokinetic drugs and antisecretory agents

Respiratory tract fluid secretion is reduced by muscarinic receptor antagonists. A variety of other drugs will increase the movement of fluid and reduce its viscosity.

- Expectorants increase the fluidity of the secretions and thereby improve the productivity of coughing.

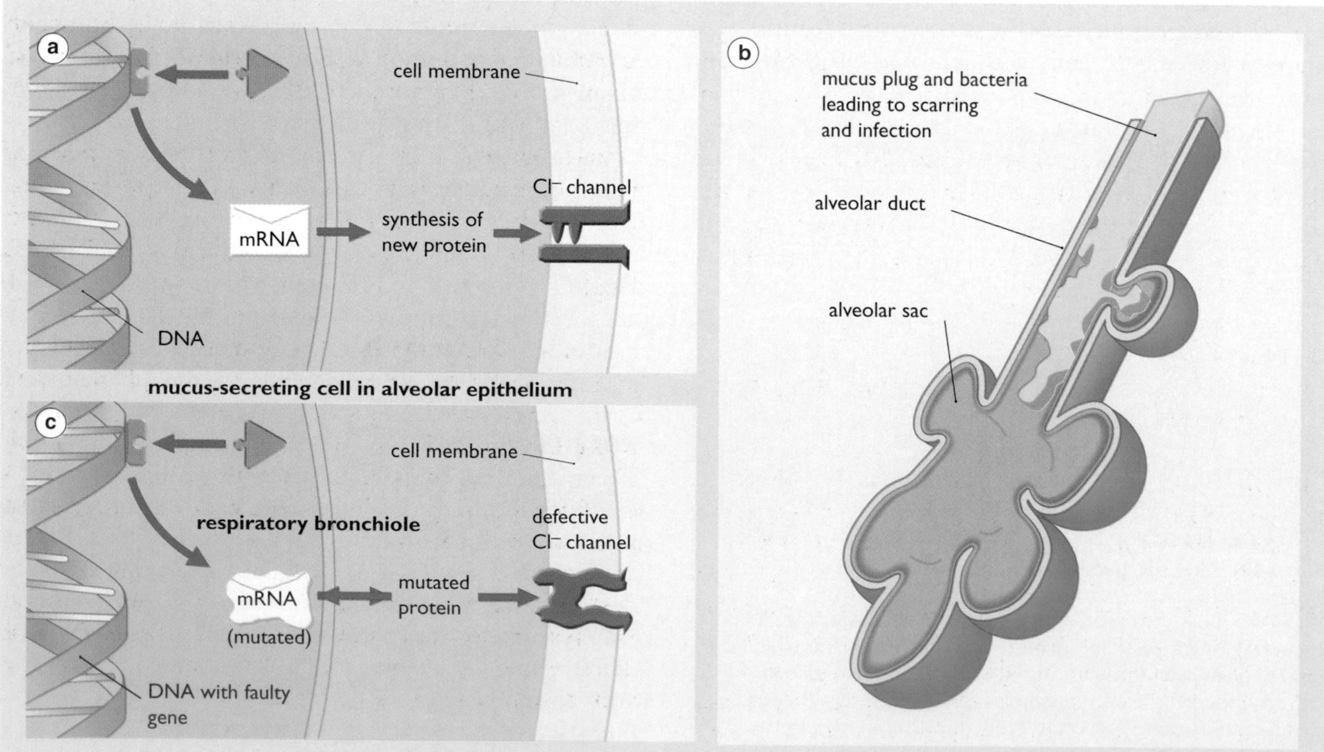

Fig. 14.9 Pathogenesis of cystic fibrosis. Mutations in a specific protein essential for the Cl^- channel in respiratory epithelial cells result in defective Cl^- clearance and water resorption. This results in thick and viscous secretions in ducted organs which harbor infections.

 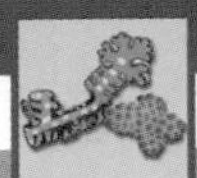

Table 14.5 Possible therapeutic approaches to cystic fibrosis

Problem	Approach
Defective gene	Replace
Defective gene product	Add
Increased Na^+ reabsorption	Increase Na^+ excretion (amiloride)
Thick stagnant mucus	Expectorants, mucolytics, DNAases, physical therapy
Bacterial infection (*Staphylococcus aureus, Pseudomonas aeruginosa*)	Antibiotics
Irreversible lung damage	Lung transplant

Typical expectorants include glyceryl guaiacolate, which can be given orally, and menthol and camphor, which are given as a vapor, but the effectiveness of these agents is limited. Potassium iodide may have better expectorant properties.

- Mucolytic agents decrease the viscosity of secretions. *N*-acetylcysteine breaks the disulfide bonds that help pack the mucin molecule and thereby make it more viscous. However, it has many adverse effects including nausea, vomiting, stomatitis and rhinorrhea.
- Agents that break down DNA tangles (e.g. recombinant DNAases given by aerosol) have recently been shown to be effective in the treatment of cystic fibrosis.

Antibiotics

The typical bacteria found in the lungs of patients with cystic fibrosis are *S. aureus* (early in the disease) and *P. aeruginosa*. Pneumonia is therefore particularly common. The first-line antibiotics used to treat this are gentamicin, tobramycin or amikacin together with one of the following: ciprofloxacin, ticarcillin, imipenen, ceftazidime and piperacillin. Tobramycin is often given as an aerosol. If there is excessive lung damage the patient may require a lung transplant.

Gene therapy

Early predictions of a genetic cure for cystic fibrosis have yet to be verified.

Cough

Coughing is a valuable reflex, but may require treatment if it becomes distressing and exhausting

Cough is a very common respiratory symptom, often associated with the presence of other respiratory conditions such as rhinitis or asthma. Sometimes it results from gastroesophageal reflux and coughing can be reduced with adequate treatment of the primary disease. However, sometimes cough occurs without a known cause or persists despite treatment of the primary condition which requires specific antitussive therapy. Cough is a reflex triggered by mechanical or chemical stimulation of the upper respiratory tract, or by central stimuli (Fig. 14.10). It is a protective mechanism that serves to expel foreign bodies and unwanted material from the airways (Table 14.1). However, coughing is sometimes both useless and distressing and can psychologically and physically exhaust the patient. Use of specific antitussive therapy is then indicated.

As a reflex mechanism, a cough involves a reflux arc (see Fig. 14.10) with sensor, central and efferent components. The exact nature of the sensory receptors for cough is unknown although a cough receptor has recently been identified. However, anatomically, cough-sensitive nerves extend from the larynx to the division of the segmental bronchi. The exact pathway of afferent fibers involved in cough and the exact location of the CNS relay (cough center) are also unknown but are thought to involve the nucleus tractus solitarius. The efferent pathway for cough involves the intercostal and phrenic nerves. Abrupt contraction of the respiratory muscles leads to an explosive rise in intrathoracic pressure, which forces air out of the alveoli and through the airways.

The sensor and central components of the reflex arc are targets for drugs used to suppress cough

Drugs to suppress cough reduce either:

- Receptor activation and therefore activity in afferent nerves.
- The sensitivity of the 'cough center.'

Peripherally acting antitussive drugs

A variety of agents act at peripheral sites. These drugs act directly in some way to reduce the sensitivity of 'cough receptors' to substances such as irritant chemicals and autacoids, which activate the receptors.

MENTHOL VAPOR inhalation reduces the sensitivity of peripheral cough receptors in animals. This probably also occurs in humans. Sucking lozenges impregnated with menthol or eucalyptus oil will also reduce the tendency to cough.

TOPICAL LOCAL ANESTHETICS such as benzocaine, bupivacaine or lidocaine applied to the pharynx and larynx can reduce the sensitivity of the 'cough receptors' in these areas to irritant chemical or physical stimuli. These are typically used to treat the cough associated with bronchoscopy and in patients who are refractory to other cough therapies.

BENZONATATE is taken orally and is thought to act on both peripheral and central receptors. It is probably less effective than codeine (see below) and is chemically related to the local anesthetic tetracaine.

Centrally acting antitussives

The opioids are drugs that reduce the sensitivity of the 'cough center.' Morphine and codeine possess central

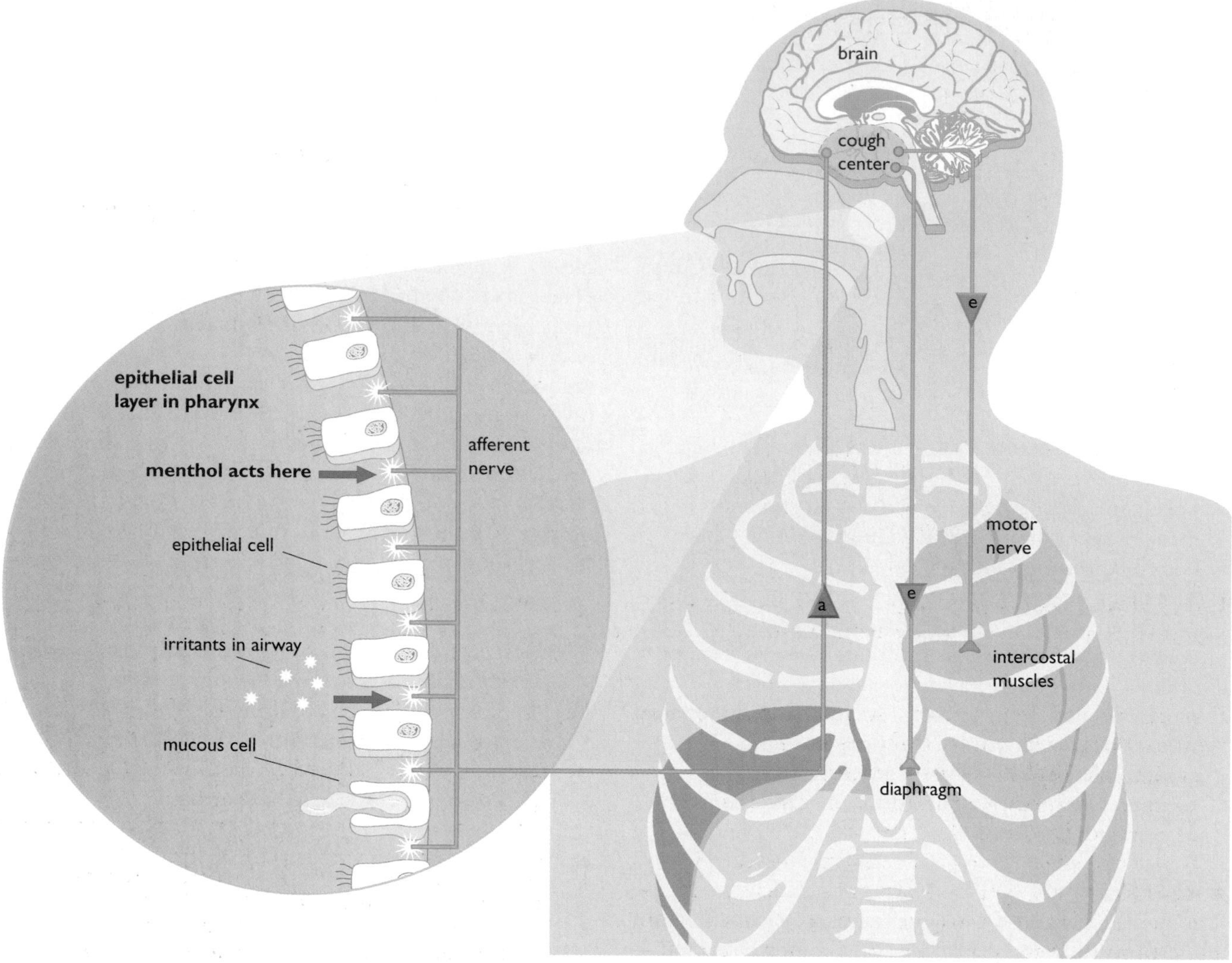

Fig. 14.10 Cough reflex arc. Coughing may be triggered by mechanical, chemical or central stimuli (a, afferent nerves; e, efferent nerves).

Table 14.6 Causes of cough.

Mechanical	Inflammatory	Extrathoracic	Abnormal cough reflex	Central
Bronchitis Pneumonia Cystic fibrosis and asthma Tumor, granuloma, blood, edema Foreign body	Asthma Viral infection Pollutants ACEI Interstitial disease	Postnasal drip Esophageal reflux Middle ear disease	Viral infection Asthma ACEI Idiopathic	Psychogenic

ACEI, angiotensin-converting enzyme inhibitor (Adapted from Fuller. Cough. In: Crystal and West. *The Lung*. New York: Raven Press; 1991.)

antitussive actions by virtue of their agonist actions on opiate receptors in the cough center. This action can be separated from other opioid effects. Codeine is usually used therapeutically in proprietary 'cough mixtures' in some countries but not the USA.

Dextromethorphan is the *d*-isomer of the methyl ether opiate, levorphanol, and is devoid of analgesic properties. It is as effective as codeine as a cough suppressant, but very high doses can cause CNS depression.

Chlophedianol is generally less effective than codeine. High doses can produce CNS effects such as excitation and nightmares.

Rhinitis and rhinorrhea

■ ***Rhinitis and rhinorrhea are manifestations of mucosal inflammation in the nose***

Rhinitis is acute or chronic inflammation of the nasal mucosa, while rhinorrhea is characterized by the produc-

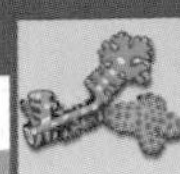

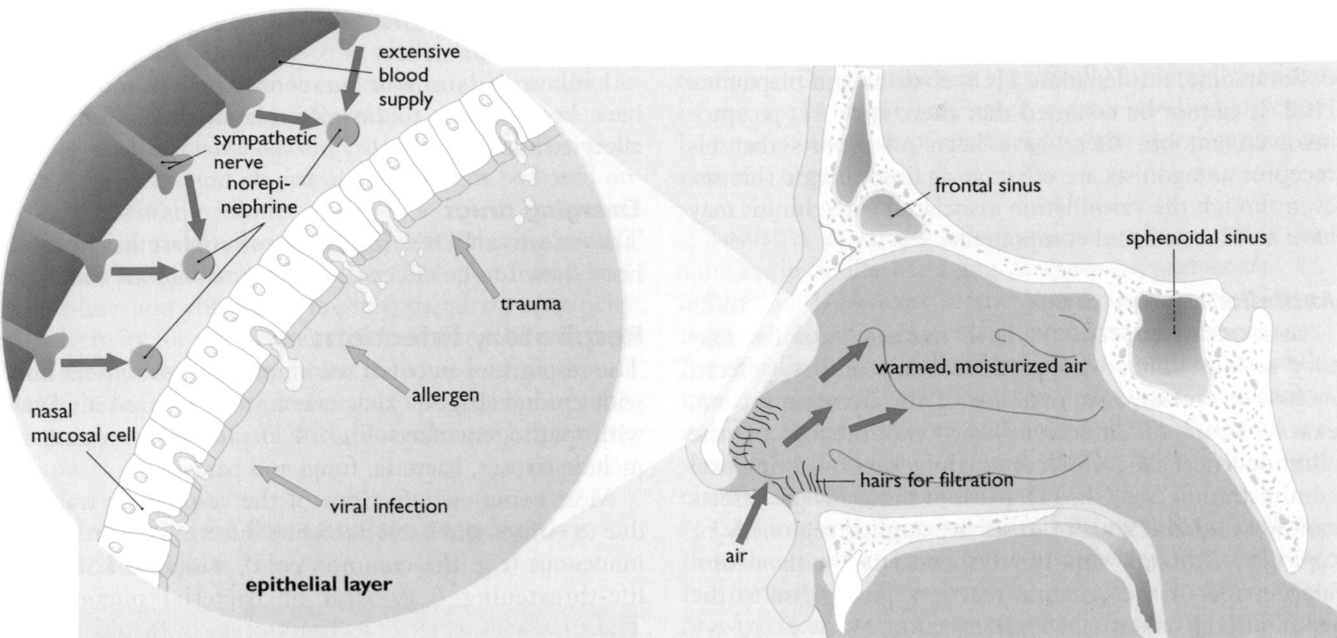

Fig. 14.11 Mechanisms of rhinitis and rhinorrhea. Sympathetic input is the most important physiologic controlling system regulating the extensive blood supply to the nasal mucosa. Fluid hypersecretion occurs in response to a variety of stimuli.

tion of excessive watery nasal secretions by the nasal mucosa. Both occur mainly as the result of either:

- A viral infection of the nasal mucosa.
- An interaction between antigens and tissue-bound IgE antibodies within the nasal mucosa.

These interactions lead to increased nasal mucosal blood flow, or blood vessel permeability, or both. As a result, the volume of the nasal mucosa increases and inspiration of air through the nasal passages becomes more difficult.

The blood supply to the nasal mucosa includes extensive collaterals and venous sinuses to provide sufficient blood flow to keep the nasal mucosa warm and moist. The most important physiologic controlling mechanism for nasal blood flow is sympathetic neural tone, though autacoids also play a role (Fig. 14.11). Sympathetic nerve activity reduces rhinitis and rhinorrhea, clears the nasal passages, and facilitates breathing. Sympatholytic drugs (adrenergic neuron blockers and α adrenoceptor antagonists) can cause nasal congestion. In contrast, α_1 agonists that elicit vasoconstriction can be used to treat the symptoms of rhinitis (see below).

H_1 receptor antagonists (antihistamines), antiinflammatory drugs and nasal vasoconstrictors are used to treat rhinitis and rhinorrhea

There are a variety of targets at which drugs can be aimed to suppress rhinitis and control rhinorrhea (Table 14.7). Ideally, rhinitis should be controlled by targeting its cause, but there is no treatment effective against the viruses causing the common cold and so treatment is symptomatic. Allergic reactions release autacoids such as histamine, cysteinyl leukotrienes that affect the nasal mucosa. Histamine can also induce sneezing and itching.

Table 14.7 Targets in the treatment of rhinitis and rhinorrhea

Target	Treatment
Nasal blood flow	Vasoconstrictors
Antiinflammatory	Glucocorticosteroids
Suppression of mediator release	Cromolyn sodium Omalizumab
Mediator receptor blockade	H_1 receptor antagonists Leukotriene antagonists

The control of the symptoms of rhinitis can be achieved in a number of ways:

- The inflammatory response can be reduced by a local application of glucocorticosteroids sprayed directly onto the nasal mucosa.
- The next level of control is to prevent the antibody interaction resulting in release of autacoids by using an anti-IgE preparation (omalizumab).
- Cromolyn sodium can be applied to the nasal mucosa to inhibit the release of histamine and other autacoids from mast cells and other inflammatory cells.

The hypersecretory phase of rhinitis can be prevented or reduced by using a drug to vasoconstrict the nasal mucosa, and α adrenoceptor agonists (sympathomimetics) are most commonly used for this purpose.

H_1 receptor antagonists

The major autacoid released during an allergic reaction in the nasal mucosa is histamine, which acts on the nasal mucosa, predominantly via H_1 receptors. H_1 receptor antagonists (see Ch. 9) are therefore useful in the

The second-line antibiotics are floxacillin and ciprofloxacin.

- If there is an acute infective exacerbation of chronic bronchitis in the presence of bronchiectasis and infection due to *H. influenzae*, *S. pneumoniae*, *M. catarrhalis* or *P. aeruginosa*, the first-line antibiotics are tetracycline and trimethoprim/sulfamethoxazole. The second-line antibiotics are floxacillin, ciprofloxacin, cefaclor, cefuroxime axetil, amoxicillin/clavulanate and any one of the above with erythromycin or clarithromycin.

PNEUMONIA is an infection of the alveoli and small bronchioles that can involve the pleura (pleurisy). It can occur in a variety of situations and treatment varies according to the situation (Table 14.10).

In bronchopneumonia the primary infection is centered on the bronchi and spreads to involve adjacent alveoli, which become filled with an acute inflammatory exudate. Affected areas of lung become consolidated, at first in a patchy distribution involving only the lobules but, if untreated, the consolidation becomes confluent and involves one or more lobes. This pattern of disease is most common in infancy and old age, and predisposing factors include debility and immobility. Immobility leads to retention of secretions, which gravitate to the dependent parts of the lungs and become infected; bronchopneumonia, therefore, most commonly involves the lower lobes. The causative organisms depend upon the circumstances predisposing to infection.

Macroscopically, affected areas of the lung are firm and airless, and have a dark red or gray appearance in

Table 14.10 Treatment of bacterial pneumonia

Type of infection	First-line antibiotics	Second-line antibiotics
Adults		
When community-acquired and mild to moderate disease. No comorbidity *S. pneumoniae, M. pneumoniae, C. pneumoniae, H. influenzae*	Tetracycline, erythromycin	Doxycycline, clarithromycin
With comorbidity. Mixed infections with *S. pneumoniae, H. influenzae,* oral anaerobes, Gram-negative bacilli, *S. aureus, Legionella* sp.	Cefaclor, cefuroxime axetil, amoxicillin/clavulanate or any of these plus erythromycin or clarithromycin	Trimethoprim/sulfamethoxazole plus erythromycin
When community-acquired severe disease in hospital, with or without comorbidity *S. pneumoniae, H. influenzae, Legionella* sp., *M. pneumoniae, S. aureus, C. pneumoniae.* Comorbidity pathogens: anaerobes, Gram-negative bacilli	Cefuroxime axetil, cefuroxime, cefotaxime, ceftriaxone, or any of these plus erythromycin or clarithromycin ± rifampin	
With severe disease in intensive care environment *S. pneumoniae, H. influenzae, Legionella* sp., Gram-negative bacilli, *P. aeruginosa, S. aureus, M. pneumoniae, C. pneumoniae*	Erythromycin ± rifampin plus one of ciprofloxacin, imipenem, or ceftazidime	
In institutionalized elderly patients with mild to moderate disease *S. pneumoniae, H. influenzae,* oral anaerobes, Gram-negative bacilli, *S. aureus, Legionella* sp.	Trimethoprim/sulfamethoxazole, cefaclor, cefuroxime axetil, amoxicillin/clavulanate, or any one of the above ± erythromycin or clarithromycin	
With severe disease *S. pneumoniae, H. influenzae,* oral anaerobes, Gram-negative bacilli, *S. aureus, Legionella* sp.	Cefaclor or cefuroxime axetil or amoxicillin/clavulanate or ceftriaxone or combinations, penicillin or amoxicillin plus ciprofloxacin	Ciprofloxacin plus clindamycin
Children		
With mild disease *S. pneumoniae, S. aureus,* streptococci Group A, *M. pneumoniae, H. influenzae*	Amoxicillin, pivampicillin, erythromycin estolate	Trimethoprim/sulfamethoxazole, clarithromycin, erythromycin/sulfisoxazole, amoxicillin/clavulanate, cefixime, cefaclor, cefuroxime axetil chloramphenicol ± erythromycin or clarithromycin
With severe disease *S. pneumoniae, S. aureus,* streptococci Group A, *M. pneumoniae, H. influenzae*	Cefuroxime ± erythromycin estolate or clarithromycin	Trimethoprim/sulfamethoxazole, clarithromycin, erythromycin/sulfisoxazole, amoxicillin/clavulanate, cefixime, cefaclor, cefuroxime axetil, chloramphenicol ± erythromycin or clarithromycin

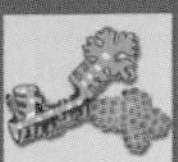

bronchopneumonia. There may be pus in peripheral bronchi. Histologically, there is acute inflammation of the bronchi and the alveoli contain an acute inflammatory exudate. The pleura is commonly involved, leading to pleurisy.

If the pneumonia is treated, recovery usually involves focal organization of the lung by fibrosis. Common complications include lung abscess, pleural infection and septicemia.

Antitubercular drugs

- Mycobacteria readily develop drug resistance
- The main antitubercular drugs are isoniazid, rifampin, streptomycin, ethambutol and pyrazinamide
- Drug combinations are always required in the treatment of tuberculosis

WHOOPING COUGH is a potentially debilitating condition resulting from infection with *Bordetella pertussis*, and children can be vaccinated against it. Erythromycin (the estolate is preferred for children) is the first-line antibiotic, while trimethoprim/sulfamethoxazole is second-line therapy and tetracycline, amoxicillin and ampicillin are third-line therapy.

Treatment of tuberculosis

- The first-line treatment of tuberculosis is a combination of rifampin, isoniazid and pyrazinamide
- Treatment is usually for 6 months and the pyrazinamide may be discontinued after 2 months

Tuberculosis

Tuberculosis is a bacterial infection with unique characteristics that make it difficult to treat. Infections with the mycobacteria (*Mycobacterium tuberculosis*) responsible for tuberculosis are more common where there is crowding and poverty. With the general improvement in world economies, housing and hygiene, the incidence of tuberculosis, particularly in the wealthier countries, decreased remarkably in the latter half of the twentieth century, but the disease has recently increased in incidence and importance. Much of the increase is associated with AIDS, and strains of tubercle bacillus resistant to previously effective therapy continue to emerge.

M. tuberculosis can infect tissue other than respiratory tissue (e.g. brain and intestine), and the mycobacteria can be found in both closed and caseous cavity lesions and in macrophages. Often the disease is self-limiting and the mycobacteria are sealed in a calcified lesion, where they remain dormant. This prevents spread of the infection, but also prevents drugs from readily penetrating to the bacterium. Therefore, there is a risk of subsequent rupture of the lesion and renewed infection. An additional complication of the dormant phase is that antimycobacterial drugs act on actively growing organisms. Such features mean therapy must be continued for 9–18 months and combinations of drugs are used. Prophylactic therapy is required for the contacts of people with active disease. The main therapeutic aim is to achieve the lowest relapse rate possible, which is ideally less than 5%.

For a detailed description of drugs used to treat tuberculosis see Chapter 6. Briefly, combinations of drugs are used for extended periods. The major drugs for non-resistant tuberculosis are isoniazid, rifampin, ethambutol, pyrazinamide and streptomycin. Other useful drugs include capreomycin, cycloserine, ethionamide and para-aminosalicylic acid.

Hypersensitivity pneumonitis

Hypersensitivity pneumonitis (allergic alveolitis) is a lymphocytic and granulomatous interstitial pneumonitis caused by type III and IV hypersensitivity reactions to repeated inhalation of a variety of antigens. Farmer's lung, caused by repeated inhalation of dusts in hay containing thermophilic actinomycetes, is the prototype of this disorder. The causative agents are most commonly thermophilic actinomycetes, fungi or animal proteins inhaled in large quantities.

Hypersensitivity pneumonitis is characterized by the development of a cough, fever, chills, malaise, and dyspnea in a previously sensitized person (6–8 hours after exposure to the antigen), bilateral inspiratory crackles on auscultation, and poorly defined patchy or diffuse infiltrates on the chest radiograph. Pulmonary function tests show a restrictive pattern with decreased lung volumes, decreased diffusion capacity and hypoxemia. Neutrophilia and an increase in C-reactive protein are common following exposure to the antigen.

Precipitating antibodies against the antigen are usually demonstrated in the serum of patients with hypersensitivity pneumonitis, and bronchoalveolar lavage consistently demonstrates an increase in T cells in lavage fluids (predominantly the CD8+ T_C cell subset). In patients with very recent exposure to antigen, however, the CD4+ T_H cells in lavage fluids may be increased.

MANAGEMENT The most effective treatment of hypersensitivity pneumonitis is avoidance of the offending antigen or environment. Dust control or use of protective masks to filter the offending dust particles in contaminated areas may also be effective. Glucocorticosteroids are the drug treatment of choice and markedly reduce the pulmonary inflammatory process.

FURTHER READING

Barnes PJ. Novel signal transduction modulators for the treatment of airway diseases. *Pharmacology & Therapeutics* 2006; **109**: 238–245. [A perspective on emerging treatment strategies].

Berti I, Longo G, Visintin S et al. Treatment of mild asthma. *N Engl J Med* 2005; **353**: 424–442.

Boushey HA, Sorkness CA, King TS et al. The national heart, lung, and blood institute's asthma clinical research network. Daily versus as-needed corticosteroids for mild persistent asthma. *N Engl J Med* 2005; **352**: 1519–1528.

Cazzola M, Matera MG, Page CP. Novel approaches for the treatment of pneumonia. *Trends Pharmacol Sci* 2003; **29**: 306–318.

Dinwiddie R. Anti-inflammatory therapy in cystic fibrosis. *Journal of Cystic Fibrosis* 2005, **4**(Suppl 2): 45–48.

Griffiths MJD, Evans TW. Drug therapy: inhaled nitric oxide therapy in adults. *N Engl J Med* 2005; **353**: 2683–2695.

Leath TM, Singla M, Peters SP. Novel and emerging therapies for asthma. *Drug Discovery Today* 2005; **10**: 1647–1655.

Minasian C, McCullagh M, Bush A. Cystic fibrosis in neonates and infants. *Early Human Development* 2005; **81**: 997–1004.

Page CP, O'Connor B, Spina D (eds) *Drugs for the Treatment of Respiratory Diseases*, Cambridge: Cambridge University Press; 2003. [An account of drugs used in the treatment of respiratory diseases.]

Reynolds SM, MacKenzie AJ, Spina D, Page CP. Pharmacology of cough. *Trends Pharmacol Sci* 2004; **25**: 569–576. [An overview of the pharmacology of cough.]

Sears MR, Greene JM, Willan AR et al. A longitudinal, population-based, cohort study of childhood asthma followed to adulthood. *N Engl J Med* 2003; **349**: 1414–1422.

Sutherland ER, Cherniack RM. Current concepts: management of chronic obstructive pulmonary disease. *N Engl J Med* 2004; **350**: 2689–2697.

Thomas CF Jr, Limper AH. Medical progress: pneumocystis pneumonia. *N Engl J Med* 2004; **350**: 2487–2498.

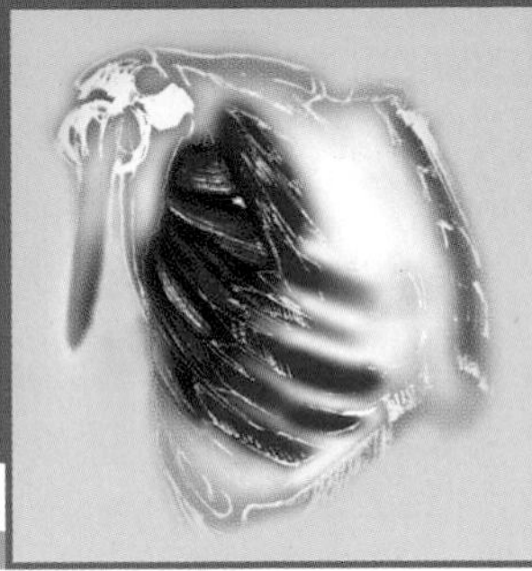

Chapter 15

Drugs and the Musculoskeletal System

PHYSIOLOGY OF THE MUSCULOSKELETAL SYSTEM

The musculoskeletal system protects vital organs and is responsible for body movements. The integrity of the musculoskeletal system depends on interactions between skeletal muscles, which usually cross joints and move the bones to which they are attached. Joints link two or more bones and provide a low-friction surface on which bones can move. Muscle function is controlled by voluntary and involuntary discharges from the motor cortex in the central nervous system (CNS). Muscle tone is modulated by spinal reflexes at the level of the spinal cord where the motor nerve exits.

The skeleton is made up of a series of bones and joints that maximize range of movement while maintaining stability. The two types of bone are:

- Cortical compact bone (80%), which provides strength when torsion is the dominant force, is dense, and is the main component of long bones.
- Trabecular bone (20%), which resists compressive forces, is found at the end of long bones, and makes up the major component of the vertebral body.

There are also two types of joint:

- A synovial (true) joint (e.g. the knee joint) allows extensive movement. Its stability is maintained by ligaments as well as muscles that pass across it.
- A fibrocartilaginous joint (e.g. the sacroiliac joint) maximizes joint stability, but limits movement of the skeleton.

PATHOPHYSIOLOGY AND DISEASES OF THE MUSCULOSKELETAL SYSTEM

Bone diseases

- Can cause fractures and pain
- Osteoporosis is characterized by a reduced quantity of bone
- Osteomalacia is characterized by a lack of mineralization
- Paget's disease is characterized by the production of abnormal bone

Osteoporosis

Osteoporosis is a thinning of normal bone with aging, but may be accelerated by a premature natural or surgical loss of ovarian function, drugs (e.g. glucocorticosteroids), or lifestyle factors (e.g. alcohol, smoking). It is a common disorder in women and may result in forearm, hip and spinal fractures. The increasing morbidity and mortality due to osteoporosis in Europe and North America reflects the increasingly aging population.

An assessment of bone density using imaging studies provides the best estimate of fracture risk

Bone quality is normal in osteoporosis, but its quantity is reduced (Fig. 15.1). The balance between formation (a function of osteoblasts) and bone resorption (a function of osteoclasts) determines whether the amount of bone increases or decreases over time. Bone mass is determined by the net effect of these two active ongoing processes. It increases from birth to about 30 years of age in both men and women (Fig. 15.2), and then slowly declines, with a more rapid decline in women in the early postmenopausal years.

Bone formation and resorption can be semiquantified by histomorphologic analysis on bone biopsy or indirectly assessed using markers of bone formation and resorption. Serum Ca^{2+} concentrations and Ca^{2+}-regulating hormones are normal.

Osteomalacia and rickets

Osteomalacia is a relatively uncommon condition of bone in which there is decreased mineralization of new bone matrix (Fig. 15.3). In children this lack of calcification may result in growth failure and deformity, and is called rickets. Adults may present with bone pain, proximal myopathy or fractures with minor trauma.

Osteomalacia is most commonly due to acquired vitamin D deficiency. Biochemical markers include hypocalcemia, a secondary elevation of parathyroid hormone (PTH) concentration and a low plasma 25-hydroxyvitamin D concentration. Other less common hereditary types of osteomalacia also occur.

The major source of vitamin D is the skin, where it is produced by a photochemical reaction. It is also contained in food, particularly fortified milk. Individuals who lack exposure to sunlight because of climate, type of clothing or institutionalization (such as long-term

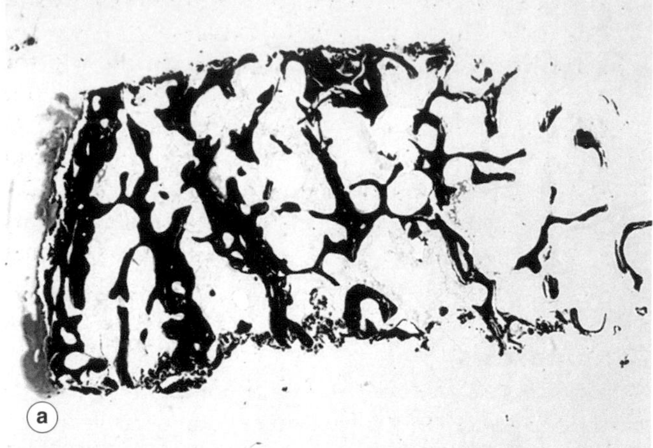

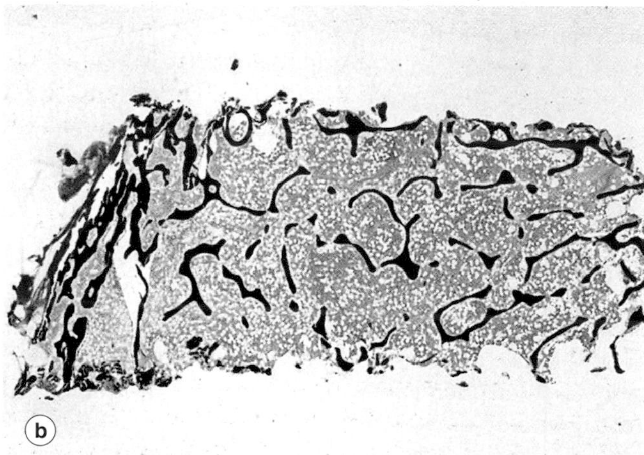

Fig. 15.1 Osteoporosis. (a) Micrograph of a resin section of a bone biopsy from the iliac crest showing normal cortical and trabecular bone stained with a silver method, which makes calcified bone show up as black. (b) Micrograph of bone from a patient with osteoporosis. When compared with (a), which shows the bone mass of a healthy patient of the same age, it is clear that the cortical zone is narrower and that the trabeculae are thinner and less numerous. (Courtesy of Dr. Alan Stevens and Professor Jim Lowe.)

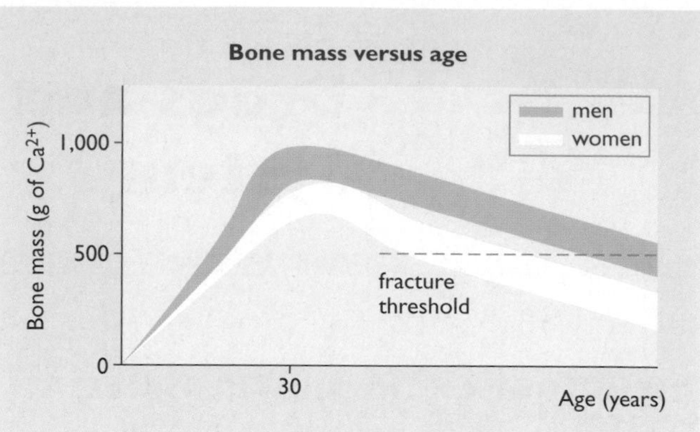

Fig. 15.2 How bone mass changes with age in men and women.

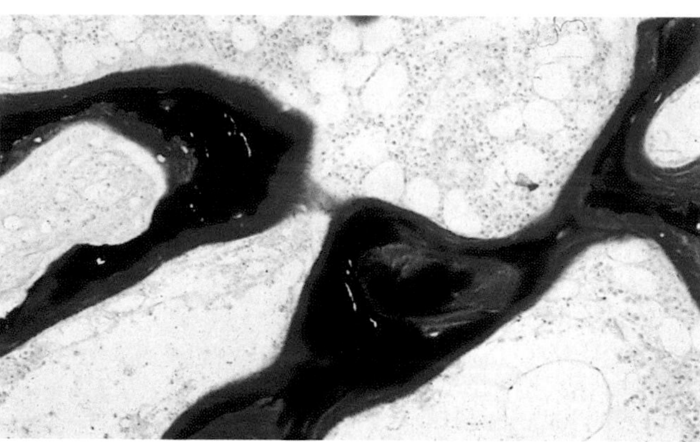

Fig. 15.3 Osteomalacia. Micrograph of iliac crest bone embedded in acrylic resin without previous decalcification from a patient with osteomalacia. There is a broad zone of unmineralized osteoid (red) and a central zone of mineralized bone (black) in this section stained by the von Kossa's silver technique. (Courtesy of Dr. Alan Stevens and Professor Jim Lowe.)

geriatric care) are at risk of vitamin D deficiency (see Ch. 22).

Paget's disease of bone

Paget's disease is a bone condition that presents with bone pain, skeletal deformity, neurologic complications or fractures. The incidence is highly variable: it is common in Central Europe, the UK, Australia, New Zealand and the USA, and rare in Africa, the Middle and Far East, and Scandinavia.

The pathology reveals excessive bone resorption and formation (Fig. 15.4). There are three phases: osteolytic, osteoblastic and quiescent. All three patterns may be present in one patient at the same time. The presence of inclusion bodies on histopathology has led to the suggestion that the disease may have a viral origin.

Osteoarthritis

Osteoarthritis is the most common joint disease. It is characterized pathologically by a loss of articular cartilage, bone remodeling and hypertrophy, subchondral bone sclerosis, and bone cysts. It may be the result of either:

- Excessive loads on the joint.
- The presence of abnormal cartilage or bone.

The most characteristic feature of osteoarthritis is gradual progressive cartilage loss. The early biochemical changes with osteoarthritis include: (1) a reduction of glycosaminoglycan content in cartilage (with lower chondroitin sulfate, keratan sulfate and hyaluronic acid); (2) increased enzymes that break down cartilage (matrix metalloproteinase); and (3) increased water content. The increased enzyme activity of matrix metalloproteinase is partly responsible for the breakdown of proteoglycan and collagen. The chondrocyte initially is stimulated to increase the number of chondrolytes and also produce cytokines such as interleukin-1 (IL-1) and tumor necrosis factor α (TNF-α). Naturally occurring small proteins are present to inhibit these catabolic enzymes. The

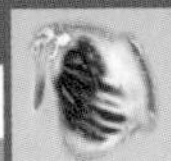

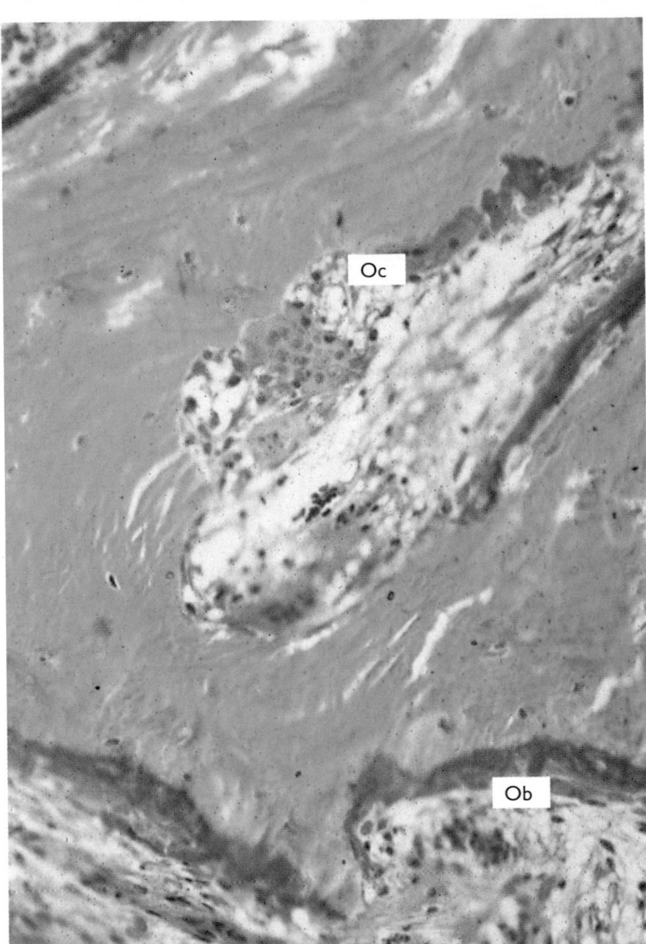

Fig. 15.4 Paget's disease. Micrograph of a resin-embedded, Gouldner-stained section from a patient with active Paget's disease. There is uncontrolled osteoclast (Oc) resorption of a bone, and osteoblasts (Ob) are attempting to fill in sites of recent osteoclast erosion in an adjacent site. (Courtesy of Dr. Alan Stevens and Professor Jim Lowe.)

pathophysiologic changes cause the localized pain that initially occurs with use and is relieved with rest, but which later occurs with minimal activity or movement. Joint stiffness, which is characteristic of inflammatory arthritis, is minimal or short lived.

Rheumatoid arthritis

Rheumatoid arthritis is a chronic inflammatory disease of joints that results in joint pain, swelling and destruction. It affects an estimated 1% of the adult population throughout the world. Progression of the disease results in joint destruction, deformity and significant disability.

Rheumatoid arthritis is characterized by chronic inflammation in the synovium, which lines the joint. The synovium is inflamed, with an accumulation of polymorphonuclear leukocytes in the superficial layers and mononuclear cells (CD4+ T lymphocytes and plasma cells) beneath the lining cell layer and deep in the synovial tissues. With disease progression there is massive synovial hypertrophy, with invasion by both inflammatory cells and fibroblast-like cells. Fibrovascular tissue known as 'pannus' invades and destroys both bone and cartilage. Mediators of inflammation contribute to the inflammatory synovitis, cartilage breakdown and bone erosions. Proinflammatory cytokines including TNF-α, IL-1, granulocyte-macrophage colony stimulating factor (GM-CSF), IL-6 and other chemokines are produced in the rheumatoid joint. In addition antiinflammatory cytokines such as IL-4 and IL-10 are present and may suppress the inflammatory state. TNF-α has direct effects on synovitis, osteoclasts and chondrocytes. Knowledge of such activities has led to specific biologic therapies being developed that counter the actions of these cytokines (see below).

Rheumatoid arthritis is associated with a variety of nonarticular clinical syndromes including vasculitis, subcutaneous nodules, interstitial pulmonary fibrosis, pericarditis, mononeuritis multiplex (vasculitis of peripheral nerves), Sjögren's syndrome (inflammation of the salivary and tear glands), Felty's syndrome (splenomegaly and leukopenia) and ocular inflammation.

Gout and other types of crystal arthritis

Gout is a common disease characterized by the precipitation of monosodium urate crystals in tissues

Gout predominantly affects men in their thirties and forties, but also occurs in postmenopausal women. The clinical manifestations include acute inflammatory arthritis (acute gout), chronic articular and periarticular inflammation, uric acid kidney stones (urolithiasis) and, rarely, gouty nephropathy. Hyperuricemia is common, but, unless associated with symptoms and signs, should not generally be treated.

Uric acid production and secretion is usually balanced to keep the tissue uric acid concentration below values at which urates precipitate and crystals form (Figs 15.5 and 15.6). Genetic and environmental factors may affect both the production and renal secretion of uric acid. Hyperuricemia is associated with obesity, diabetes mellitus, hypertension and renal insufficiency, and with thiazide diuretics and low-dose salicylates.

Uric acid overproduction, which is seen in 10% of individuals with gout, can be associated with inherited enzyme deficiencies or myeloproliferative disorders. A reduced renal clearance of uric acid is responsible for the remaining 90% of cases. Decreased renal excretion of urate is associated with chronic renal failure, lead nephrology, ketoacidosis, hypothyroidism and diabetes insipidus.

Calcium pyrophosphate dihydrate deposition disease and hydroxyapatite deposition

Calcium pyrophosphate dihydrate (CPPD) deposition disease has been reported in association with a variety of conditions and may result in acute inflammation (pseudogout) or joint degeneration. Pseudogout is a relatively common disease with clinical features indistinguishable

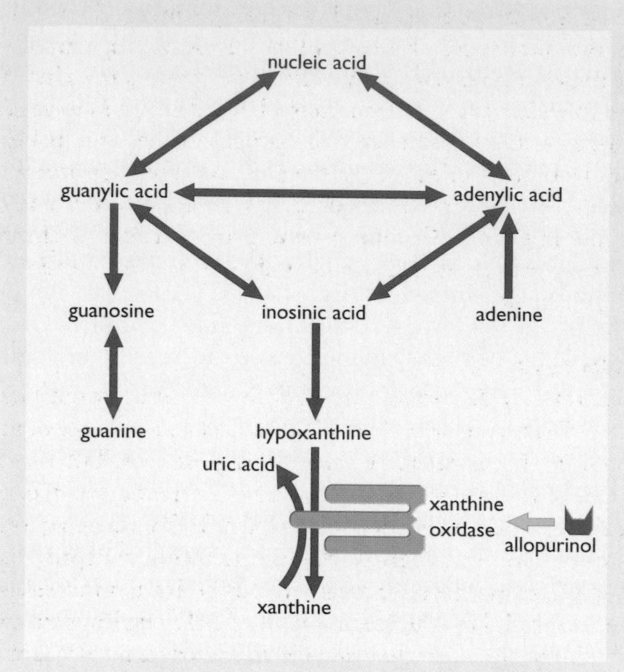

Fig. 15.5 Simplified outline of purine metabolism.

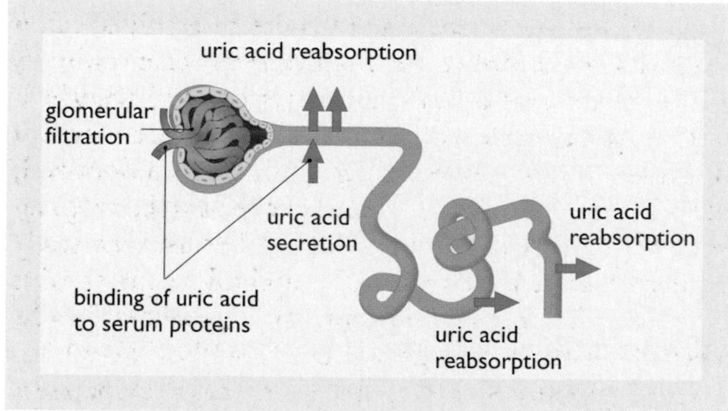

Fig. 15.6 Uric acid secretion and reabsorption in kidney. Uricosuric agents block uric acid reabsorption in the proximal tubules.

from those of acute gout. The characteristic acute inflammatory response involves neutrophils reacting to calcium pyrophosphate crystals. The tissue inflammation responds to the same medical treatment as gout. Hydroxyapatite deposition may result in acute joint inflammation, periarticular inflammation and subcutaneous tissue deposition. It is frequently associated with osteoarthritis, but the importance of apatite crystals in the pathogenesis of osteoarthritis is not clear.

Systemic lupus erythematosus

Systemic lupus erythematosus (SLE) is an autoimmune disease that affects approximately 1 in 1000 individuals. It is more prevalent in young females. Its morbidity and mortality are decreasing in most parts of the world as a result of early recognition and treatment. Associated complications are higher in poorer socioeconomic groups, and the incidence of SLE is higher in certain individuals of African, Hispanic or Asian descent. SLE is characterized by a variety of clinical features, which include skin and musculoskeletal manifestations. Renal, pulmonary, serosal, neuropsychiatric and reticuloendothelial involvement are less common, but potentially more serious. Pathologic findings include inflammation, blood vessel abnormalities and immune complex deposition.

The immunologic disturbance includes antibodies to a variety of 'self' tissues. Antinuclear antibodies (ANA) against components of the cell nucleus are most common. The contribution of ANA to the clinical events is unclear because of the presence of antibodies in nondisease states and because the target antigen in the nucleus would normally be protected from antibody binding. The immune disturbance promotes B-cell hyperactivity to both self and foreign antigens. Activation of an antibody response to a foreign antigen such as a virus may be a triggering mechanism.

Seronegative spondyloarthropathies

Seronegative spondyloarthropathies are a group of inflammatory types of arthritis characterized by common clinical features and associated to a varying degree with the HLA-B27 gene. Sacroiliitis is the characteristic feature of this disorder that includes ankylosing spondylitis, psoriatic arthritis, reactive arthritis and the arthritis associated with inflammatory bowel disease.

Pathologically, granulation tissue erodes the fibrocartilaginous joint, resulting eventually in ossification and possible bony fusion. An inflammatory process similar to that seen in rheumatoid arthritis may involve the peripheral synovial joints. Enthesitis (inflammation of tendinous insertions to bone) is another characteristic feature. Extra-articular features include ocular inflammation, cutaneous inflammation and occasionally cardiac involvement.

DRUGS USED TO TREAT MUSCULOSKELETAL DISEASES

Drugs for osteoporosis

Drugs used to treat osteoporosis in postmenopausal women include hormone replacement therapy, calcitonin, bisphosphonates, selective estrogen receptor modulators (SERMs), calcium and vitamin D.

Hormone replacement therapy

Estrogen replacement therapy (ERT) at the time of the menopause inhibits the effect of osteoclasts on bone resorption (see Ch. 11). It therefore slows bone loss and may actually increase bone quantity in the first few years following cessation of normal ovarian function. It can be provided orally, by injection or transdermally, as estrogens and their esters are easily absorbed through

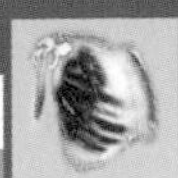

the skin, mucous membranes and gastrointestinal tract. The different routes of administration have different pharmacokinetics and other properties. Oral estrogens (e.g. conjugated equine estrogen, estrone sulfate and micronized estradiol-20β) are the most widely prescribed drugs to treat postmenopausal osteoporosis.

Estrogens circulate in the blood in association with sex hormone binding globulin and albumin. Like other steroid hormones, they act in the cell nucleus. They diffuse passively through cell membranes and bind to the nuclear estrogen receptor found in estrogen-responsive tissues. Following activation, the estrogen receptor binds to specific DNA sequences that result in transcription of adjacent genes. There are at least two types of estrogen receptors: α and β. Estrogen has been shown to bind to the α receptor and forms an estrogen-receptor complex which thus binds to the estrogen response element. The α receptor is located in reproductive tissues including breast and endometrium. The β receptor is predominant in nonreproductive tissues including bone, liver and the cardiovascular system. This partly explains why estrogen and estrogen-like substances have different effects in different tissues.

The decision to start estrogen replacement therapy and patient adherence to therapy depend not only on its effect on bone but also on its other clinical effects

Estrogen replacement therapy will relieve vasomotor symptoms if given in the first few years of the menopause. Usually, treatment can be tapered, but occasionally long-term treatment is required. ERT inhibits bone loss and may initially increase bone density. In addition, it influences lipoprotein metabolism (see Ch. 11), resulting in decreased low-density lipoprotein (LDL) cholesterol and increased high-density lipoprotein (HDL) concentrations, thereby potentially protecting against cardiovascular disease. Some clinical studies have shown a reduced rate of myocardial infarction, decreased mortality from cardiovascular disease and an overall reduction in total mortality in postmenopausal women who receive ERT. However, a 4-year prospective study in postmenopausal women with a history of heart disease has shown increased cardiovascular events with estrogen replacement at 1 year of study, although there is a trend towards reduced events in the last 3 years of this study. Transdermal estrogen usually controls postmenopausal symptoms and osteoporosis, but has less effect on lipoproteins.

Progesterone should be considered for all patients started on ERT who have not had a hysterectomy, because it will reduce the significantly increased risk of endometrial cancer associated with ERT to below the native risk. Unopposed estrogens should only be given to women who have had a hysterectomy and therefore have no risk of developing endometrial hyperplasia. The addition of cyclic progesterone therapy usually results in the continuation of monthly menstruation, but menstrual bleeding can be reduced by using lower doses or continuous progesterone. Continuous use of progesterone inhibits endometrial proliferation and reduces the risk of endometrial cancer, but can cause 'breakthrough bleeding.' There is some evidence that progesterone diminishes the favorable effect of estrogens on the lipoprotein profile. Progesterone can be given orally, transdermally or by injection. Common oral progesterones include medroxyprogesterone, norethindrone and micronized progesterone.

Calcitonin

Calcitonin, a 32-amino acid peptide that directly inhibits osteoclasts, can slow bone loss. It acts on a calcitonin receptor that is expressed in a variety of cells, but most importantly on osteoclasts. There is homology between this receptor on osteoclasts and the PTH receptor on osteoblasts. The cell surface calcitonin receptor is coupled to adenylyl cyclase so that its activation increases the intracellular concentration of cAMP, resulting in an inhibitory effect on the osteoclasts. Calcitonin may exert an effect on the osteoblasts, but this is less clear.

Oral calcitonins are ineffective because they are broken down by aminopeptidases and proteases in the gastrointestinal tract. Parenteral calcitonin is well absorbed, but this inconvenient route of administration limits its widespread use. Intranasal calcitonin is therefore used instead. Although it is not well absorbed, with low peak plasma concentrations, it is more practical and has wider patient acceptance. Randomized, controlled trials of nasal calcitonin have demonstrated an improved bone density of 1–2% over 2 years. One study has demonstrated reduction of vertebral fractures with intranasal calcitonin 200 IU daily, but not at 400 IU daily. Injected calcitonin at higher doses (50–100 IU/day) has analgesic properties and is frequently used in patients with severe pain due to recent vertebral compression fractures.

Intranasal or subcutaneous calcitonin can be given to produce beneficial effects on bone without causing serious systemic adverse effects. Marine (salmon or eel) calcitonins are usually used because they are more potent than human calcitonin. Minor adverse effects include flushing and gastrointestinal symptoms (nausea, vomiting or diarrhea). However, neutralizing antibodies may develop which inhibit calcitonin's actions.

Bisphosphonates

Bisphosphonates are analogs of pyrophosphate, but have a carbon rather than an oxygen atom. This P–C–P structure allows for many variations by changing the side chains on the carbon atom which can result in significant physicochemical, biologic and therapeutic differences. Thus every phosphonate needs to be considered individually.

Bisphosphonates have a strong affinity for calcium phosphate and act exclusively in calcified tissues where they inhibit bone resorption, although the mechanism of this effect is unclear. Unlike calcitonin, which has an immediate effect on resorption, bisphosphonates take about 48 hours to block resorption.

Different bisphosphonates have significantly different antiresorptive potency, the potencies of etidronate, clodronate, tiludronate, pamidronate, alendronate and risedronate being 1, 10, 10, 100, 1000 and 5000, respectively.

Oral absorption of most bisphosphonates is at best 1–10% of a given dose. They should never be given with milk products, food, or at the same time as Ca^{2+} supplements, as this further inhibits absorption by up to 90%.

Several large prospective studies in osteoporosis have shown that at least three bisphosphonates (etidronate, alendronate, risedronate) increase bone density by 4–9% over the first 3 years of treatment and reduce vertebral fractures by approximately 50%. If given continuously, etidronate can cause osteomalacia. This can be avoided by intermittent administration over 2 weeks with periods of several weeks to 3 months off the drug. Bone biopsy studies up to 7 years after cyclic etidronate have not shown mineralization defects. Bisphosphonates such as alendronate and risedronate do not have this effect and can be given continuously.

Alendronate 10 mg daily or risedronate 5 mg daily have shown significant improvement in bone density in 3-year prospective placebo-controlled trials. Fracture reduction is 50% for a single further vertebral fracture and up to 90% reduction in multiple vertebral fractures.

Other studies have supported taking bisphosphonates such as alendronate in larger doses (35–70 mg) orally once weekly, which has the advantage that patients are less inconvenienced than when taking bisphosphonates daily and then having to wait 30–120 minutes for a meal.

The most common clinical adverse effects of bisphosphonates are gastrointestinal (heartburn, nausea, abdominal pain). Short-term upper endoscopy studies show incidence of gastric ulcers to be 4–14%, with erosive esophagitis occurring much less frequently. It is recommended to take these medications with water and then to avoid lying supine for 30 minutes.

Bisphosphonates are slowly released from the skeleton and may have actions on bone tissue for years. There is some concern that this prolonged action may have an undetermined cumulative effect 10–20 years later. Most experts are reluctant to use bisphosphonates in very young people for this reason.

Selective estrogen receptor modulators

Selective estrogen receptor modulators (SERMs) are drugs that have tissue-specific effects in different areas. This is similar to estrogen in bone and cardiovascular system but not in other tissues such as breast and endometrium (Fig. 15.7). SERMs are believed to act competitively on the α estrogen receptor and may function as competitive inhibitors in tissues with α receptors. SERMs can also bind to β estrogen receptor complexes and have agonist effects in tissues where these β estrogen receptors predominate (see Fig. 15.7). The SERM tamoxifen has been shown to prevent the recurrence of breast cancer, and this is likely due to antiestrogen effects. It also shows benefit in protecting against osteoporosis and cardiovascular disease, but has been found to increase the incidence of endometrial cancer. Raloxifene is a benzothiophene derivative that is also a SERM. The raloxifene–estrogen receptor complex binds to a unique area of DNA, different from the estrogen-response element, to produce estrogen-antagonist effects in some tissues and agonistic action in others. Long-term clinical trials of 3 years with raloxifene 60 mg/day have shown improvement of bone density of the hip (2–3%) and lumbar spine (3–4%). Fracture studies have shown reduction of new vertebral fractures by approximately 50%. In these same studies there was no evidence of increased risk of endometrial cancer and an improvement in the lipoprotein profile. These studies also show a highly significant reduced risk of breast cancer in patients taking raloxifene compared with patients taking placebo.

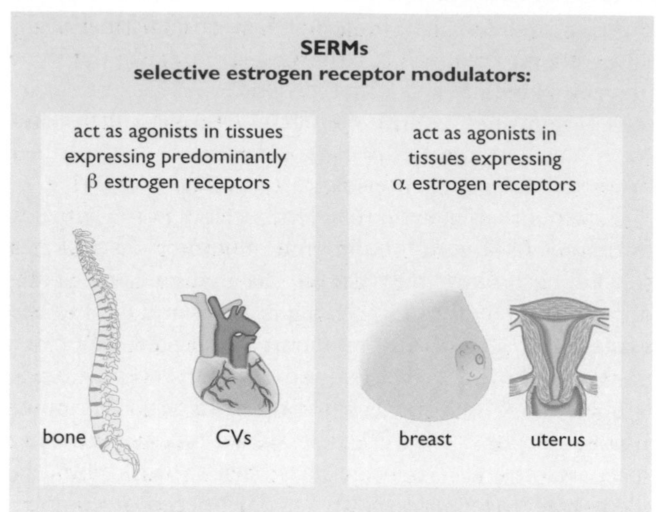

Fig. 15.7 Effect of SERMs on estrogen tissues.

Adverse effects of SERMs include an increased risk of venous thromboembolic events similar to estrogen. Also, women sometimes report a slight increase in hot flushes and leg cramps.

Other therapies

Calcium supplements have a small beneficial effect in preventing bone loss. Calcium, in the form of either dietary Ca^{2+} or oral Ca^{2+} supplements, is inexpensive and safe and should be recommended to all patients to slow bone loss. It is recommended that postmenopausal women have a Ca^{2+} intake of more than 1500 mg daily.

Vitamin D analogs facilitate Ca^{2+} absorption from the gastrointestinal tract and may have an effect on both

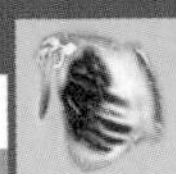

bone resorption and formation. However, their efficacy in reducing the risk of fractures remains to be determined.

Tibolone is a synthetic C-19 steroid with weak hormonal properties. In animal studies tibolone has 1/50th the potency of ethinyl estradiol, 1/8th that of norethisterone, and much less androgenic potency. Tibolone does not stimulate the endometrium and at a daily dose of 2.5 mg reduces vasomotor menopausal symptoms. Tibolone at 1.25 mg and 2.5 mg/day has had favorable effects on biochemical markers of bone resorption (urinary C telepeptides) and bone formation (serum osteocalcin). Short-term studies have shown increases in bone mass in the spine and prevention of bone loss in the forearm in postmenopausal women. However, long-term studies are needed to demonstrate fracture reduction.

PTH hormone analogs such as teriparatide (a parathyroid hormone agonist) used in cyclic doses are also effective when administered subcutaneously in the treatment of osteoporosis. They stimulate osteoblasts and thereby result in increased bone formation. Although they can only be given by injection, they may be a highly effective treatment for increasing bone in the first few years after menopause.

Drugs for osteomalacia

Vitamin D is used to treat and prevent osteomalacia. Vitamin D-deficient osteomalacia responds well to vitamin D, 25-hydroxyvitamin D, 1α-hydroxyvitamin D, or 1,25-dihydroxyvitamin D. Patients with osteomalacia may also respond to sun exposure. In the USA, where dairy products are fortified with vitamin D, osteomalacia is relatively rare.

Drugs for Paget's disease

Drugs used to treat Paget's disease of bone include analgesics, calcitonin and bisphosphonates.

SIMPLE ANALGESICS AND NSAIDs (aspirin, acetaminophen) are often used for pain due to Paget's disease, but do not reduce the long-term complications.

CALCITONIN inhibits resorption and can reduce pain by a variety of potential mechanisms. Marine (salmon and eel) calcitonins are more potent than human calcitonin, but can be associated with the development of antibodies, resulting in resistance to treatment. The treatment needs to be given subcutaneously in high doses (50–100 IU/day) to achieve adequate blood concentrations to be effective in reducing bone pain, but this is commonly associated with adverse effects including cutaneous flushing and gastrointestinal effects.

BISPHOSPHONATES are an effective treatment of Paget's disease and currently are the mainstay of treatment. They reduce the turnover of both 'pagetic' and normal bone. Large studies with alendronate and risedronate in Paget's disease have shown that they effectively reduce the activity of pagetic bone. The doses used are generally higher than the daily dose used for osteoporosis. Gastrointestinal intolerance is the main adverse effect seen with the higher doses used in Paget's disease.

In patients that are not able to tolerate alendronate or risedronate because of gastrointestinal adverse effects, intravenous (i.v.) pamidronate infusions over a few hours can be effective. Tiludronic acid is a hypocalcemic drug that can be used for the treatment of Paget's disease.

Drugs for osteoarthritis

Drug treatment of osteoarthritis includes analgesics and NSAIDs.

ANALGESICS, particularly acetaminophen, often relieve the pain of osteoarthritis and are the preferred drug. Data from large clinical studies show the effectiveness of analgesics in comparison to NSAIDs in osteoarthritis, showing they are as effective. Narcotic analgesics can also be used for short periods, intermittently, or for acute flares.

NSAIDs are frequently used to treat pain in patients with osteoarthritis. They are effective analgesics and can help reduce disease inflammation, but have no major effect on the underlying process. NSAIDs inhibit cyclooxygenase, the enzyme that converts arachidonic acid to prostaglandins (see Ch. 9, Figs 15.8–15.11).

NSAIDs are associated with a high incidence of gastrointestinal adverse effects. The most common GI adverse effects are nausea, vomiting, dyspepsia, abdominal pain and diarrhea. Less common but more clinically significant side effects are gastric ulcers and gastrointestinal bleeding. Traditional NSAIDs include ibuprofen, naproxen, ketoprofen, flurbiprofen, indometacin, ketorolac, nabumetone, oxaprozin, piroxicam, sulindac, and tolmetin (Table 15.1).

There are two different cyclooxygenase (COX) enzymes that convert arachidonic acid to prostaglandins. COX-1 produces a class of prostaglandins that are important in normal physiologic functions including gastrointestinal mucosal protection, and regulation of platelet function and renal cells. COX-2 enzymes are inducible in disease states and are responsible for pain and inflammation. The COX-2 isoform also has an important function in producing prostaglandins involved in normal renal function.

The structures of COX-1 and COX-2 have considerable homology, but because of a number of amino acid differences, drugs (coxibs) have been developed recently with selectivity for the COX-2 isoform (Figs 15.8–15.10).

Celecoxib and rofecoxib are two highly selective inhibitors of COX-2 (Fig. 15.11). Large clinical trials effectiveness with these two drugs have demonstrated similar efficacy in reducing pain as compared with

Table 15.1 Nonsteroidal antiinflammatory drugs

	Maximum recommended doses	Approximate half-life (hours)
NSAIDs		
Diclofenac	150 mg/day	1–2
Etodolac	1200 mg/day	5–10
Fenoprofen	2400 mg/day	2
Ibuprofen	3200 mg/day	2
Indometacin	150 mg/day	2
Ketoprofen	300 mg/day	5 (?)
Ketorolac	40 mg/day	5
Meloxicam	15 mg/day	1–3
Nabumetone	2000 mg/day	22
Naproxen	1500 mg/day	15
Oxaprozin	1800 mg/day	24–48
Piroxicam	20 mg/day	30–60
Sulindac	400 mg/day	7–15
Tolmetin	1800 mg/day	7
Coxibs		
Celecoxib	400 mg/day	10
Rofecoxib	50 mg/day	15–20

Adverse effects of traditional NSAIDs

- Gastrointestinal tract: gastric irritation, peptic ulcers, bleeding, perforation
- Kidney: decreased renal blood flow, decreased creatinine clearance, increased blood pressure, rarely interstitial nephritis or nephrotic syndrome
- CNS: headaches, confusion, tinnitus, aseptic meningitis (rare)
- Hematopoietic system: bleeding, inhibited platelet function (irreversible effect with aspirin persisting 10–12 days)

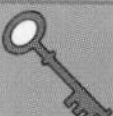

Treatments for osteoarthritis

- Mechanical devices to relieve stress in the joint
- Analgesics
- Antiinflammatory drugs
- Surgical intervention

traditional NSAIDs such as ibuprofen, naproxen and diclofenac, with an apparent reduction in gastrointestinal adverse effects such as gastric ulcers.

Adverse effects of coxibs include minor GI side effects, but more importantly coxibs are thought to increase the risk of cardiovascular events (myocardial infarctions) and this had led to rofecoxib being recently voluntarily withdrawn from clinical use by the manufacturer and other coxibs being used with caution.

Drugs for rheumatoid arthritis

Drugs used in the treatment of rheumatoid arthritis can be categorized on the basis of their therapeutic effects, primarily based on their symptomatic or antiinflammatory actions compared with their capacity to induce a remission or delay progress of the disease and associated joint destruction. The treatment of patients with rheumatoid arthritis is based on an understanding of the biology and natural history of the disease coupled with

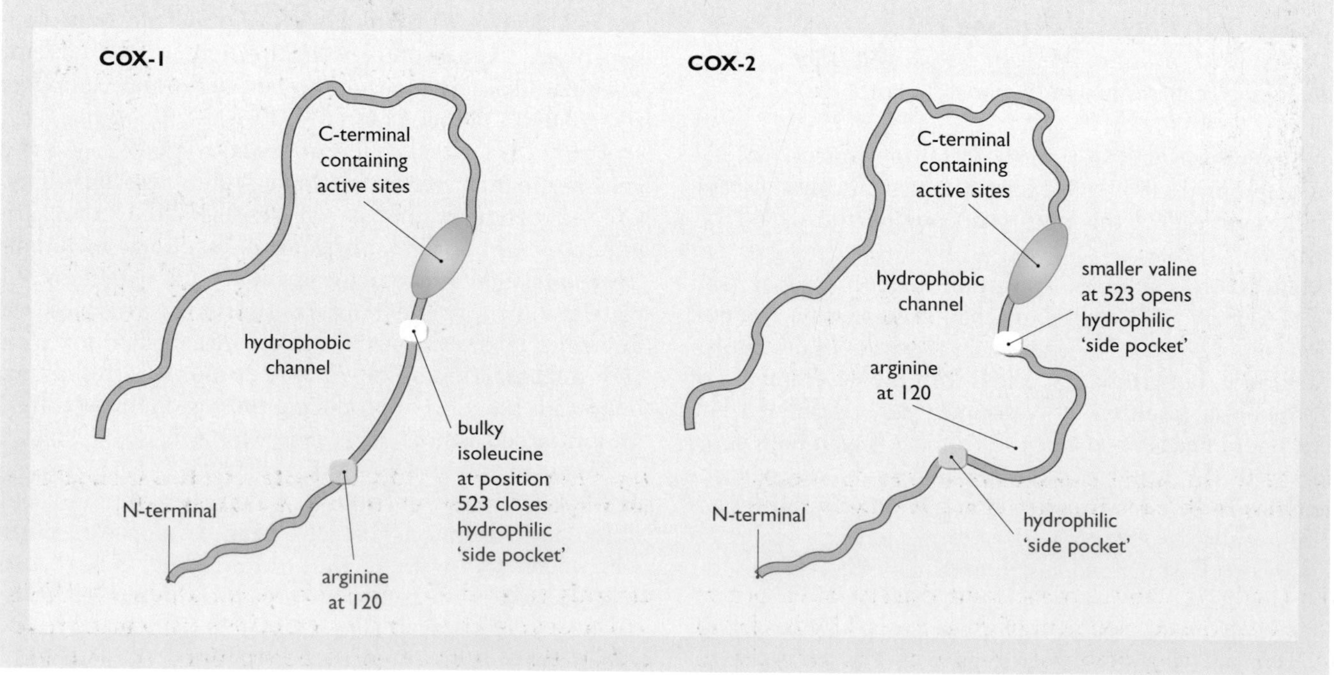

Fig. 15.8 Schematic structure of COX-1 and COX-2 enzyme. Arachidonic acid is converted to endoproxides equally well by COX-1 and COX-2.

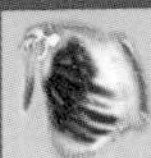

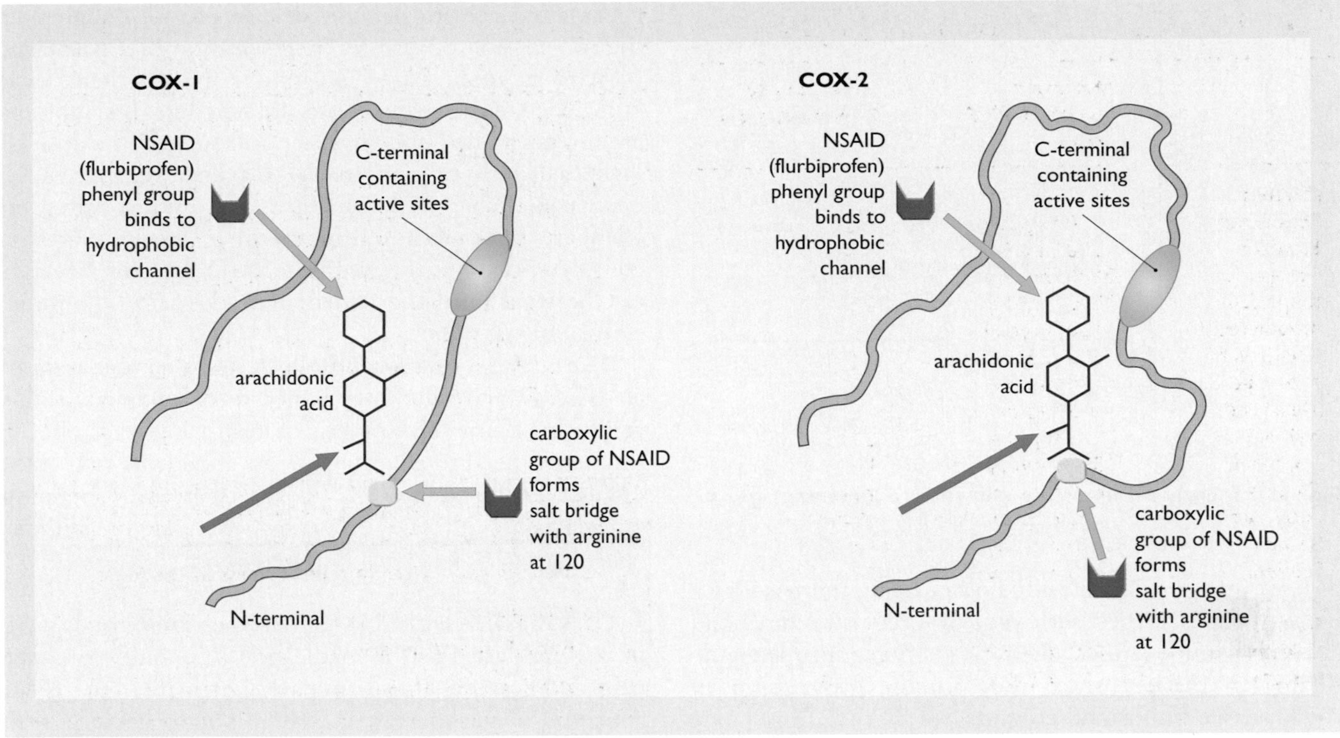

Fig. 15.9 Classical NSAIDs block both COX-1 and COX-2 enzyme by excluding arachidonic acid from its active site.

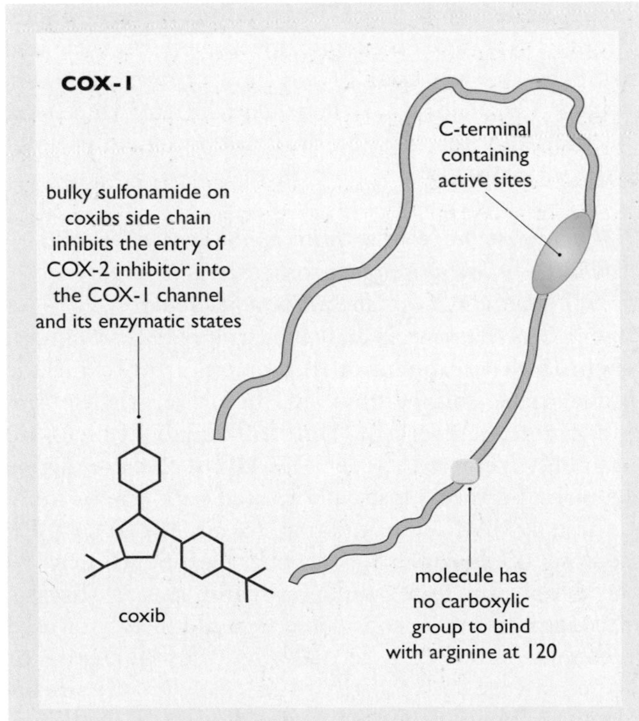

Fig. 15.10 Schematic demonstration of coxib or COX-2 selective inhibitor having less effect on COX-1 enzyme.

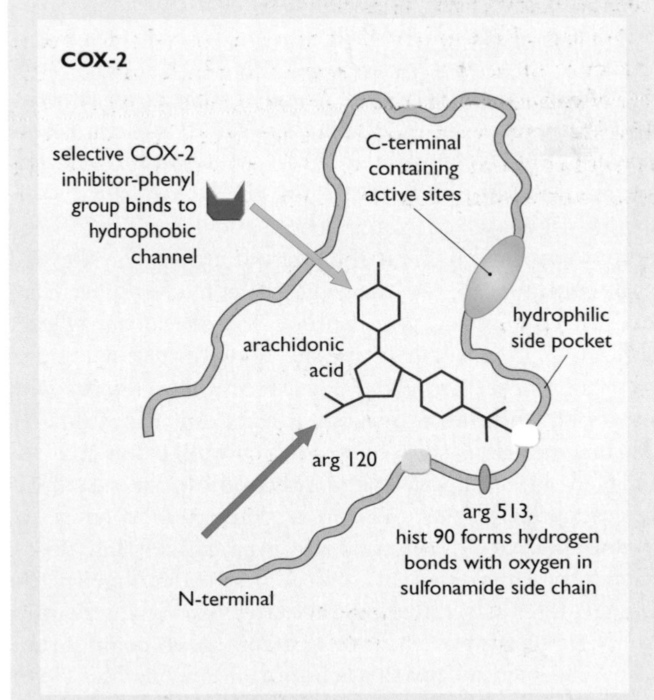

Fig. 15.11 Coxibs or COX-2 selective medications inhibit prostaglandin production from arachidonic acid.

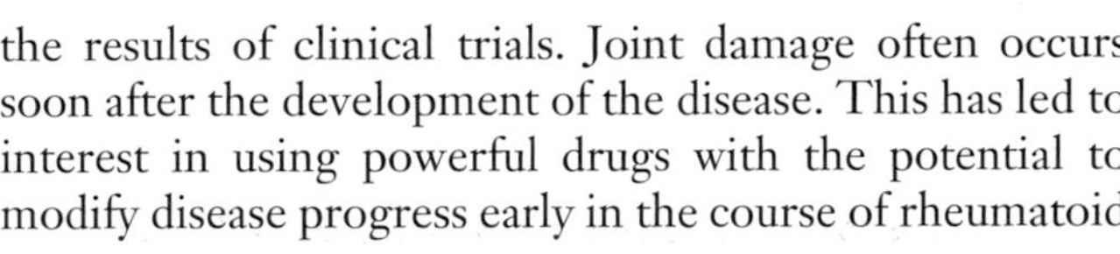

the results of clinical trials. Joint damage often occurs soon after the development of the disease. This has led to interest in using powerful drugs with the potential to modify disease progress early in the course of rheumatoid arthritis (Fig. 15.12). Acetaminophen, aspirin, NSAIDs and coxibs are used initially to provide symptomatic relief rather than prevent joint destruction. In addition, glucocorticoids have been used to suppress exacerbation

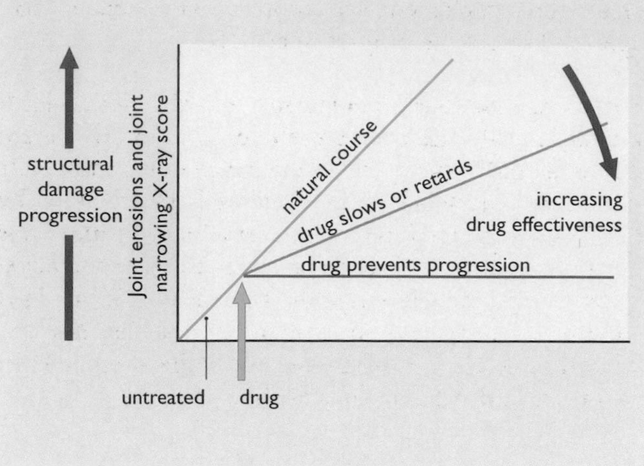

Fig. 15.12 Early intervention will reduce joint damage.

of joint inflammation. On the other hand, there is now a large group of drugs with very different structures and actions that are termed disease modifying antirheumatic drugs (DMARDs) since they inhibit progression of the disease. Important examples of DMARDs include antimalarials, methotrexate, gold, D-penicillamine, sulfasalazine, azathioprine, ciclosporin, leflunomide, etanercept and infliximab. In recent years there has been a growing trend to treat rheumatoid arthritis aggressively with early, potent DMARDs.

ASPIRIN is an acetylated salicylate that is an effective and inexpensive antiinflammatory drug. It is distinct from other NSAIDs because it is an irreversible cyclooxygenase inhibitor and acetylates the active site in the cyclooxygenase enzyme. The salicylates have been commonly used to treat rheumatoid arthritis in the past and continue to be used by patients and physicians because of their low cost. Enteric-coated aspirin is better tolerated than aspirin in the gastrointestinal tract. Typically, doses are given 3–4 times a day, usually with meals to minimize adverse effects on the stomach. Absorption is usually rapid and complete but may be delayed with enteric-coated preparations or sustained-release preparations. Aspirin is converted to an active metabolite with a long half-life. At relatively low doses, aspirin is eliminated by typical first-order kinetics. At higher doses salicylates exhibit zero-order kinetics with a constant amount of active drug metabolized per unit time (see Ch. 4). Clinically this is important in that high doses of aspirin can be given twice daily if desired. However, at high doses when toxicity appears, it may be of prolonged duration. The maximum concentration should be 200–300 mg/mL; it is not often necessary to measure serum concentrations as adverse effects (gastrointestinal disturbance, decreased hearing or tinnitus) usually limit doses.

NSAIDs have, in the last two decades, been the mainstay of treatment to reduce the symptoms of rheumatoid arthritis but, like salicylates, they do not alter the progression of disease. The selection of a particular NSAID is often based on physician experience and knowledge of the correct dose and schedule. If symptoms are not controlled, the physician will suggest the dose be increased with caution to the maximal recommended dose (see Table 15.1). Failure of response after an adequate trial of a minimum of 2 weeks warrants consideration of an alternative NSAID. Various NSAIDs can be tried until the patient has adequate or optimal control of symptoms.

The addition of a second NSAID or a combination of an NSAID and salicylates is not recommended as this results in additive risk of gastrointestinal adverse effects. Physicians need to educate patients about this risk, since often over-the-counter (OTC) medications containing salicylates or NSAIDs are used by patients without consultation.

COXIBS (selective COX-2 enzyme inhibitors) were increasingly used as the medication of choice to reduce pain and swelling in inflammatory arthritis, but recent concerns about increased cardiovascular liability with these drugs has meant they are now used more cautiously.

LOW-DOSE GLUCOCORTICOSTEROIDS Intra-articular glucocorticosteroids such as prednisone are highly effective, have fewer systemic adverse effects than oral treatment and are used if only one or two joints are affected. The major risk is the potential to introduce joint infection and the possible risk of accelerating joint cartilage destruction.

If active rheumatoid arthritis is not controlled with NSAIDs or low-dose glucocorticosteroids, other antirheumatic drugs should be considered

Other drugs that have been demonstrated to have clinical benefit in the treatment of rheumatoid arthritis include antimalarials, sulfasalazine, azathioprine, ciclosporin, leflunomide, etanercept and infliximab, which are commonly referred to as DMARDs. Severe active rheumatoid arthritis is usually treated with one or more of these DMARDs in addition to an NSAID and/or low-dose prednisone. Second-line treatments may be considered for mild, moderate and severe disease. Antimalarials may be considered for mild disease or used in conjunction with a second agent for moderate or severe disease. Methotrexate is usually the initial treatment for moderate or severe disease. Sulfasalazine may be considered instead of methotrexate based on adverse effect concerns with the latter drug. The recent introduction of leflunomide has decreased the use of gold, azathioprine, penicillamine and ciclosporin. The newer biologic agents that inhibit the actions of TNF-α include etanercept and infliximab (see below) are increasingly considered if there is not a good response to therapy with less expensive treatments, if adverse effects

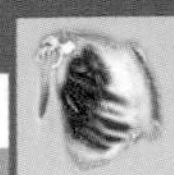

limit use of other treatments or if rapid disease remission is considered a priority.

ANTIMALARIALS Hydroxychloroquine and chloroquine are examples of antimalarials used to induce remission or help reduce inflammation in rheumatoid arthritis. However, although antimalarials are thought to be the least-effective DMARDs, they have the lowest toxicity. The dose should be maintained for a trial of 6 months to determine their effectiveness. Color vision and peripheral vision should be monitored for 6–12 months, depending on the dose.

The antiinflammatory mechanism of action of chloroquine and hydroxychloroquine is unclear. There is some evidence that they interfere with a wide variety of leukocyte functions. They may inhibit IL-1 production by macrophages, lymphoproliferative responses and cytotoxic responses of T lymphocytes. At high doses (now rarely used) they also have an inhibitory effect on DNA synthesis.

SULFASALAZINE Sulfasalazine is frequently used in the UK as the first-choice DMARD, but is used less commonly in the USA. It is thought to be as effective as gold, but probably has fewer adverse effects. Sulfasalazine is a combination of 5-aminosalicylic acid linked covalently to sulfapyridine. It is poorly absorbed orally, but is cleaved to its active components by colonic bacteria. It is believed that sulfapyridine is absorbed systemically and is possibly responsible for its therapeutic effect. Sufapyridine is eventually excreted in urine. The mechanism of action is unclear, but there is some evidence that it reduces natural killer cell activity and alters other lymphocyte functions.

The adverse effects are primarily caused by sulfapyridine. Severe reactions include acute hemolysis in individuals with glucose-6-phosphate dehydrogenase deficiency, and rarely agranulocytosis. Rashes occur in 20–40% of patients. Other adverse effects include nausea, fever and arthralgias.

GOLD Intramuscular gold salts have historically been the major DMARD used in the USA to treat rheumatoid arthritis. Adverse effects include dermatitis, proteinuria and bone marrow suppression. Monitoring should include a complete blood count and urinalysis before each injection. Oral gold preparations such as auranofin have been available for a number of years, but they appear to be less effective than injectable gold. There are two parenteral gold salts available, gold sodium thiomalate and aurothioglucose.

Gold salts are taken up by reticuloendothelial cells (i.e. in the bone marrow, lymph nodes, liver and spleen), and in these tissues they impair macrophage function and cytokine activity. Other possible mechanisms of action include inhibition of prostaglandin synthesis, interference with complement activation, cross-linking of collagen and inhibition of lysosomal activity.

PENICILLAMINE Oral penicillamine, which is a chelator of heavy metals, has been a useful drug in the treatment of rheumatoid arthritis and its effectiveness is comparable to that of injectable gold. It is well absorbed orally (40–70%), although food will decrease its absorption. It is metabolized in the liver and is excreted in urine and feces.

Penicillamine will suppress autoantibodies to IgM and has other effects on immune complexes, but the mechanism of action of this drug in the treatment of rheumatoid arthritis remains unclear.

Adverse effects of penicillamine

- Cutaneous: macular or papular rashes, urticaria, pemphigoid, lupus erythematosus, dermatomyositis
- Hematologic: fatal hematologic reactions are rare but include thrombocytopenia, leukopenia, agranulocytosis, aplastic anemia
- Renal: reversible proteinuria in the nephrotic range
- Unusual adverse effects: acute pneumonitis, myasthenia gravis (with long-term treatment)
- Less serious effects: nausea, other gastrointestinal effects, transient anosmia

METHOTREXATE Methotrexate (see Ch. 9) is a folic acid antagonist that is effective in the treatment of rheumatoid arthritis if given orally or parenterally in weekly doses of 5–25 mg/week. Methotrexate decreases inflammatory cells in the synovium which may prevent erosion and joint damage. There is concern that methotrexate is associated with liver damage with cumulative doses over 1.5 g. In patients with certain coexisting diseases, including alcoholic liver disease, obesity and diabetes mellitus, the increased risk of liver toxicity may warrant avoidance of the drug. Monthly complete blood counts and measurement of liver enzymes and serum albumin concentrations are recommended. If there are persistent elevations of liver enzyme concentrations, or hypoalbuminemia, methotrexate should be discontinued and appropriate investigations done to determine the cause of the liver disease. Investigations might include a liver biopsy to look for evidence of early fibrosis or cirrhosis, which warrants permanent discontinuation of methotrexate. Other common adverse effects of methotrexate include nausea, oral ulcers, hair loss, acute pneumonitis (1–2%) and bone marrow suppression.

AZATHIOPRINE Azathioprine is an orally active purine analog that is cytotoxic for inflammatory cells (see Chs. 7 and 9). Treatment may be necessary for 3–6 months to be clinically effective. As azathioprine can cause serious adverse effects, including bone marrow suppression and liver toxicity, close monitoring is necessary.

LEFLUNOMIDE Leflunomide is an isoxazole immunomodulatory agent which inhibits dihydro-orotate dehydrogenase, an enzyme important in the synthesis of pyrimidine. As a result of its action it has antiproliferative activity and an antiinflammatory effect. Leflunomide has been shown to inhibit the de novo synthesis of uridine. After oral administration, leflunomide is metabolized to its active metabolite, which is responsible for all of its activity. Leflunomide may be given orally in a loading dose of 100 mg/day for 3 days to attain rapid steady-state concentrations. Maintenance dosing would take an estimated 2 months to achieve this concentration. The active drug is extensively bound to albumin (>99%) in healthy subjects. The active metabolite is eliminated by further metabolism and excreted in the biliary system and urine.

Large clinical trials indicate that leflunomide is effective in decreasing joint swelling and tenderness over 12 months. Studies have compared leflunomide to placebo, methotrexate and sulfasalazine, and responses were evident by 1 month with stabilization of clinical response by 6 months. Leflunomide showed similar clinical improvement to both methotrexate and sulfasalazine.

The main toxicity with leflunomide is elevation of liver enzymes. Increases of transaminase (ALT + AST) are usually less than twofold, and revert rapidly to normal with discontinuation of the drug. If elevation is twofold, but less than threefold, dose reduction can be considered. In the presence of persistent elevations greater than threefold, a liver biopsy should be considered if treatment is continued. There is potential concern of increased hepatotoxicity when leflunomide is used concomitantly with methotrexate. Women of childbearing potential should use reliable contraception methods since animal studies suggest there could be a risk of fetal death or teratogenic effects. In situations where rapid drug elimination is warranted, a drug elimination schedule using colestyramine three times a day for several days can be employed. It is presumably efficacious on account of an enterohepatic circulation of leflunomide.

CICLOSPORIN Lymphocytes are important in rheumatoid arthritis and there is evidence suggesting that the immunosuppressive drug ciclosporin is effective in the treatment of rheumatoid arthritis and in selective patients it may control resistant synovitis. Ciclosporin acts at a number of levels on the immune response which are discussed in Chapters 7 and 9.

ETANERCEPT is a genetically engineered fusion protein of two identical chains of a recombinant human TNF-α receptor with the P 75 monomer fused to the Fc domain of human IgG1. This protein binds and inactivates TNF-α which has direct effects on synoviocytes, osteoclasts and chondrocytes (Fig. 15.13). It is many times more effective in binding TNF-than natural, soluble TNF-α receptors thus sequestration of TNF-α by etanercept inhibits cell lysis.

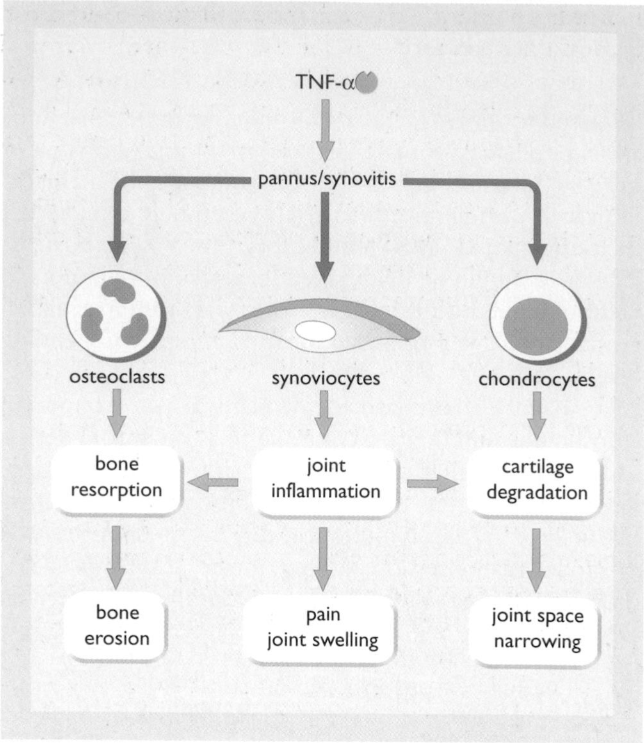

Fig. 15.13 Role of TNF-α in rheumatoid arthritis.

Etanercept is given by a subcutaneous injection twice a week. The median half-life is 115 hours (range 98–300).

Etanercept can be used safely with salicylates, NSAIDs, analgesics, glucocorticoids and methotrexate, but little is known about the effect of this drug on renal or hepatic function.

Etanercept has shown reduced joint pain and swelling in a number of clinical trials as measured in terms of the American College of Rheumatology (ACR) criteria of response over a 12-month period. Studies comparing it to methotrexate show a similar reduction in joint space narrowing but patients treated with etanercept show less progression of erosion over a 2-year period.

Serious allergic adverse reactions were reported in less than 2% of patients treated with etanercept. However, reactions at local injection sites were common (37%) and included erythema, itching, pain or swelling. These reactions were described as mild to moderate and generally did not lead to discontinuation of etanercept. In clinical trials that were placebo controlled, 4% of patients treated with etanercept had a serious adverse event compared with 5% of placebo-treated patients. However, patients developing an infection should be monitored carefully and, with a serious infection or sepsis, etanercept should be at least temporarily discontinued.

INFLIXIMAB Infliximab is a chimeric IgG1 anti-TNF-α monoclonal antibody which binds soluble cytokine TNF-α and also binds membrane-bound TNF-α, leading to

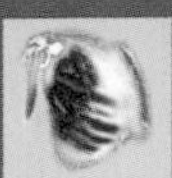

loss of functioning TNF-α. It is a synthetic product made from both human and as mouse components. Clinical studies have shown the half-life to be 8–12 days, and it can be detected in the circulation for approximately 50 days. Treatment consists of an i.v. induction dose and maintenance doses every few weeks (4–8 weeks). Efficacy studies have shown that infliximab, if used with low-dose methotrexate in rheumatoid arthritis, will significantly prevent disease progression in the first 2 years of treatment. Radiographic studies have shown little progression in joint erosion and joint space loss, and in higher doses have demonstrated reversal of joint erosion.

The safety profile of infliximab has been demonstrated in a number of clinical trials and in over 50 000 treated patients. In 5% of patients, early hypersensitivity reactions may be observed during or shortly after infusions. Reactions include hypotension, urticaria and shortness of breath. Mild reactions usually can be treated by slowing of infusion rates and premedication with an H_1 receptor antagonist. Serious infections have occasionally been observed in patients taking infliximab. Patients that have a new infection while taking infliximab should be monitored closely and treatment should be held or discontinued in a patient with a serious infection or sepsis. Recently, it has been recognized that patients may reactivate dormant TB infections. Some patients treated with infliximab develop antibodies against the drug, referred to as human anti-chimeric antibodies (HACA). The presence of HACA is associated with a higher rate of infusion reactions. Concomitant administration of methotrexate or azathioprine results in a lower incidence of these antibodies and therefore, in patients with rheumatoid arthritis, it is recommended that infliximab be used with concomitant oral weekly methotrexate. Adalimumab is an IgG1 (anti-TNF-α) monoclonal antibody, which can be administered subcutaneously (40 mg), and has a relatively long half-life.

ANAKINRA is a recombinant IL-1 receptor antagonist (IL-1ra). This protein results in a notable reduction of macrophages and lymphocytes in synovial tissue on biopsy. Anakinra is given by daily subcutaneous injections up to 150 mg/day. In large multinational clinical trials in patients with rheumatoid arthritis, anakinra has been shown to be effective as a monotherapy and in combination with methotrexate in reducing joint pain and swelling. Similarly to etanercept and infliximab, it also significantly reduces radiographic joint narrowing and erosions. Serious adverse effects are rare. Injection site reactions are common (over 40%) at higher daily doses (150 mg/day) but result in discontinuation in fewer than 5% of patients.

Drugs for crystal arthritis

Drugs used to treat acute crystal arthritis include NSAIDs, colchicine and glucocorticosteroids.

NSAIDs are usually started at the first sign of an acute attack of crystal arthritis and continued until the signs of inflammation resolve. Most commonly indometacin is started in a dose of 50 mg three times a day and then slowly tapered over 10–14 days. Other NSAIDs that may be effective include diclofenac, ketoprofen, tolmetin, naproxen, celecoxib and rofecoxib, although good clinical efficacy studies are lacking comparing different NSAIDs in acute crystal arthritis.

COLCHICINE is effective in the treatment of acute gout and other types of crystal arthritis. It penetrates inflammatory cells and enters into the microtubular system where it has a direct inhibitory action on the microtubules so that the inflammatory cells lose their ability to respond. Colchicine disrupts the structure of tubulin, which impairs the capacity of inflammatory cells to move to the site of inflammation (chemotaxis) and decreases phagocytosis. The maximal dose of 6 mg (10 tablets) over 24 hours should not be exceeded and then no further colchicine should be given for the next 7 days. Intravenous colchicine should be used rarely, if at all.

Adverse effects include gastrointestinal toxicity, with nausea, vomiting and diarrhea in up to 80% of individuals at higher doses. Colchicine has also been associated with bone marrow suppression, renal failure, disseminated intravascular coagulation, hypocalcemia, seizures and death. Rarely, chronic use is associated with a neuromuscular disorder resembling polymyositis. Colchicine toxicity is increased with renal impairment. An overdose of colchicine may be fatal, in part due to disruption of intestinal epithelial cells which ordinarily turn over rapidly.

GLUCOCORTICOSTEROIDS may be an effective treatment in acute crystal arthritis including gout when alternatives, including NSAIDs or colchicine, are not tolerated or are contraindicated. Options include oral prednisone or i.v. or intra-articular glucocorticosteroids (often useful when only one or two joints are involved). Intramuscular adrenocorticotropic hormone (ACTH, corticotropin) which also stimulates secretion of adrenal androgens in addition to glucocorticosteroids, is sometimes used but offers no known advantage over glucocorticosteroids alone.

Regulating serum uric acid concentrations provides an effective method of preventing recurrent episodes of gout

Initial preventive management of gout should include weight and blood pressure control, a low purine diet (i.e. reduced intake of red meats or seafood) and avoidance of medications that can contribute to hyperuricemia. Drugs such as low-dose aspirin, ethanol, thiazide diuretics, ciclosporin and ethambutol can decrease urate clearance.

Increasing uric acid excretion

Blood uric acid concentration can be decreased by

increasing clearance of uric acid (uricosuric agents) or by decreasing uric acid synthesis (xanthine oxidase inhibitors). Measurement of the amount of uric acid excreted in the urine should be done prior to using a uricosuric drug. Increasing uric acid clearance in patients overproducing uric acid could result in production of uric acid stones in the urine.

URICOSURIC AGENTS are the treatment of choice for individuals who:

- Have diminished renal clearance of uric acid (i.e. do not overproduce uric acid).
- Do not have renal stones or renal dysfunction, as increasing renal excretion of uric acid could transiently increase risk of worsening stone disease.
- Have had a previous reaction to a xanthine oxidase inhibitor.

Uricosuric agents such as probenecid and sulfinpyrazone block the reabsorption of filtered and secreted uric acid in the renal tubules, leading to increased clearance of uric acid and a subsequent decrease in its plasma concentration (see Fig. 15.6). Probenecid blocks tubular reabsorption of organic anions such as uric acid and decreases serum urate levels. The most common adverse effects are rash and gastrointestinal upset. Sulfinpyrazone is a congener of phenylbutazone, and similarly blocks urate reabsorption in the renal tubule. The most frequently reported adverse effects of sulfinpyrazone are gastrointestinal, including nausea and aggravation of peptic ulcer disease. Blood dyscrasias including aplastic anemia have been reported but are rare.

Inhibition of uric acid synthesis

ALLOPURINOL is a xanthine oxidase inhibitor; it competitively binds to the enzyme which controls the last two steps in purine metabolism, of both adenine and guanine, to uric acid.

Allopurinol is useful for lowering uric acid in patients with:

- Uric acid overproduction.
- Nephrolithiasis.

Allopurinol is commonly preferred to a uricosuric agent by patients because of the ease of administration. The typical dose is 300 mg/day orally, but may need to be increased to 600–800 mg/day. The dose must be decreased if glomerular filtration is decreased, and should be less than 200 mg/day when the creatinine clearance is 10–20 mL/min (0.20–0.33 mL/s).

The adverse effects of allopurinol are not dose related; the relatively minor problems include headaches, dyspepsia and diarrhea. A pruritic rash develops in 5% of patients and rarely a syndrome of hypersensitivity to allopurinol may occur with fever, renal failure and toxic epidermal necrolysis which can be life threatening and precludes the further use of this drug.

Allopurinol is readily absorbed, with 80% being bioavailable within 2–6 hours. It is oxidized by xanthine oxidase to oxypurinol. Both allopurinol and oxypurinol inhibit xanthine oxidase, thereby decreasing the conversion of hypoxanthine and xanthine to uric acid. The advantage is that these precursors of uric acid are readily soluble and excreted in urine (see Fig. 15.5).

Drug interactions with allopurinol are common. For example, allopurinol interferes with:

- The metabolism of other purine analogs such as azathioprine and 6-mercaptopurine and the doses of these drugs need to be reduced by 25–50% when allopurinol is given.
- Hepatic inactivation of other drugs, including that of oral anticoagulants. Prothrombin activity must be closely monitored if allopurinol is given, and the dose of oral anticoagulant may need adjusting.

Drugs for systemic lupus erythematosus

Treatment of systemic lupus erythematosus involves antiinflammatory and immunosuppressive drugs.

GLUCOCORTICOSTEROIDS The symptoms and signs of acute inflammation in the skin and joints in SLE are readily treated with glucocorticosteroids. Options include:

- Topical preparations for inflammatory rashes.
- Low-dose oral therapy for mild disease.
- Higher-dose oral or pulse i.v. infusions for severe and life-threatening disease.

The mechanism of action of glucocorticosteroids in the treatment of SLE is unclear. They have a direct effect on the bone marrow cells, resulting in demargination of circulating neutrophils (neutrophilia) and, at the same time, leukopenia, with fewer circulating eosinophils and monocytes. At high doses, glucocorticosteroids inhibit cytokine release and action, and high-dose glucocorticosteroids may also inhibit phospholipase A_2, which controls both prostaglandin and leukotriene production (see Ch. 9).

The dose of glucocorticosteroid is chosen to minimize the risk of adverse effects yet provide adequate levels to suppress the inflammatory response. Oral prednisone or prednisolone is used in preference to other longer-acting oral drugs, such as dexamethasone, and is usually given in a single morning dose. Prednisone is available in convenient doses (5 mg tablets) to facilitate dose increases or reductions. Adverse effects of glucocorticosteroids include skin thinning and bruising, central obesity, muscle wasting, hypertension, glucose intolerance and osteoporosis.

ANTIMALARIALS are a particularly effective treatment for cutaneous lesions and inflammatory arthritis in patients with SLE. Once they have been started and have produced clinical benefit, their discontinuation may result in a recurrence of disease manifestations. Antimalarial drugs include hydroxychloroquine, quinacrine

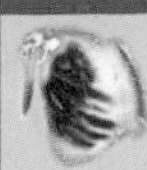

and chloroquine and their pharmacology is discussed in Chapter 6. The first two drugs are used extensively in many countries, while chloroquine is a less expensive but less well-tested alternative. The relative safety of antimalarials makes them attractive drugs for early intervention. Common adverse effects include non-specific symptoms, cutaneous rashes and gastrointestinal complaints. Less frequently, there are CNS reactions. Retinal toxicity is the major clinical concern, but is rarely seen at low doses of antimalarials. Visual field and color vision should be tested at baseline and then every 6 months in patients treated with antimalarials.

AZATHIOPRINE (see Ch. 9) is widely used for many of the manifestations of SLE including renal disease to reduce the requirement for glucocorticosteroids. Azathioprine reduces inflammation in lupus nephritis and improves renal function. However, it can have major adverse effects, including bone marrow suppression. Significant hepatic toxicity has also been observed, but is usually reversible if the drug is discontinued. It is not clear whether azathioprine increases the risk of malignancy, particularly hematopoietic and lymphoreticular malignancy.

ALKYLATING AGENTS are the most effective agents after glucocorticosteroids for treating life-threatening SLE (Table 15.2). They inhibit the activation and division of cells and act in SLE by inhibiting the division of inflammatory cells such as T lymphocytes. However, because of this mechanism of action, cyclophosphomide has significant adverse effects (see Ch. 9). Cyclophosphamide is usually added to high-dose glucocorticosteroids to treat severe SLE that is either life threatening or does not respond to glucocorticosteroids and azathioprine. The dose of glucocorticosteroid should be reduced slowly following clinical improvement. Cyclophosphamide is a more effective treatment of diffuse lupus nephritis than other treatments.

Table 15.2 Drugs affecting inflammation and the immune system in the treatment of diseases of the musculoskeletal system

	Disease indication	Adverse effects
Antimalarials	RA, SLE	Retinopathy
Gold salts	RA	Dermatits GI symptoms Proteinuria
Penicillamine	RA, scleroderma	Dermatitis GI symptoms Proteinuria
Methotrexate	RA, psoriasis Polymyositis Dermatomyositis SLE	Myelosuppression Pneumonitis Ulcerations Hepatotoxicity
Sulfasalazine	RA Inflammatory bowel disease	Dermatitis GI symptoms Hepatitis
Azathioprine	RA, SLE Polymyositis Transplantation	Myelosuppression GI symptoms Hepatotoxicity
Cyclophosphamide	Vasculitis SLE	Myelosuppression Alopecia GI symptoms Infertility Hemorrhagic cystitis Malignancy
Ciclosporin	RA Transplantation SLE Psoriasis Uveitis	Hypertension Renal toxicity Neurotoxicity Hepatotoxicity
Glucocorticosteroids	RA SLE Transplantation Vasculitis Connective tissue disease	Cushing's syndrome Osteoporosis Cataracts Ulcers
Leflunomide	RA	Myelosuppression GI symptoms Liver
Etanercept	RA	Rash Infection
Infliximab	RA	Rash Infection Hypersensitivity reaction
Anakinra	RA	Injection site reaction

GI, gastrointestinal; RA, rheumatoid arthritis; SLE, systemic lupus erythematosus.

Drugs for seronegative arthritis

NSAIDs are the most widely used drugs for treating the inflammation of seronegative spondyloarthropathies.

The most effective NSAIDs including indomethacin, diclofenac, naproxen, tolmetin, celecoxib and rofecoxib are often recommended first. Other NSAIDs may be effective and can be tried if the above are not effective or are associated with adverse effects. Although various clinical trials suggest that certain NSAIDs are more effective than others, clinical experience and familiarity with doses is probably more important for selecting any one NSAID.

GLUCOCORTICOSTEROIDS do not affect the long-term outcome of seronegative spondyloarthropathies, but might be beneficial in low doses to control symptoms. Sulfasalazine, which is frequently used to treat rheumatoid arthritis, may control the peripheral arthritis in this disease. All drugs used to treat rheumatoid arthritis can be used to treat psoriatic arthritis.

Some common drugs have adverse effects on the musculoskeletal system

Low-dose aspirin (less than 2 g/day) can raise serum uric acid levels by interfering with the excretion of uric acid in the renal tubule. These doses of aspirin are commonly used to prevent cardiovascular events including myocardial infarct and stroke. Considerations for treatment would include switching to sulfinpyrazone or adding allopurinol if acute attacks are severe or frequent.

Hydralazine has been commonly used to treat hypertension in the past and may be used to treat select patients with congestive heart failure. In up to 50% of patients antinuclear antibodies (ANA) may be found in the blood of patients taking hydralazine long term. Individuals who are slow acetylators (see Ch. 4) or who take relatively large doses are more likely to develop an SLE-like syndrome that includes rash, arthralgia and fever. With the development of this syndrome there should be rapid withdrawal of the drug. Usually, symptoms resolve but they may require treatment with glucocorticosteroids and sometimes the symptoms will be prolonged.

Glucocorticosteroids are commonly used to treat both musculoskeletal and nonmusculoskeletal immune disorders. Unfortunately, they can cause osteoporosis and steroid myopathy. The mechanism of glucocorticosteroid osteoporosis is multifactorial and includes direct inhibition of osteoblasts, increased calcium urinary excretion and decreased calcium absorption from the gastrointestinal tract. Preventive measures include minimizing the dose and duration of glucocorticoid use, encouraging appropriate calcium and vitamin D supplementation, weight-bearing exercises and consideration of drugs used in the treatment of osteoporosis. The best-studied drugs to prevent glucocorticosteroid-induced osteoporosis are alendronate and risedronate (see treatment of osteoporosis above).

Glucocorticosteroids may induce muscle atrophy and weakness. If this complication develops, an exercise program may improve general function but dose reduction is the only treatment that will provide long-term benefit.

The statins are synthetic lipid-lowering agents that may be associated with both myalgias and myositis. In clinical studies elevations of CPK have been reported in up to 5% of patients. Rarely, patients develop an acute myopathy with severe proximal muscle weakness and marked elevations of CPK. The risk of myopathy is increased with concomitant use of fibrate and other lipid-lowering treatments including niacin. Patients starting therapy with statins should be advised of this risk and should promptly report unexplained muscle pain, tenderness or weakness. Usually, symptoms remit with prompt withdrawal of the drug.

Musculoskeletal infections

Septic arthritis

Septic arthritis is characterized by fever, pain, swelling and a reduced joint range. In sexually active individuals there should be a high index of suspicion for infection with *Neisseria gonorrhoeae*. Otherwise, most cases are caused by Gram-positive organisms (*Staphylococcus aureus* and streptococci, Table 15.3). Important host factors include:

Table 15.3 Organisms causing septic arthritis

Nongonococcal	Gram-positive (65–85%) Gram-negative bacilli (10–15%) Mixed aerobic and anaerobic (5%) Mycobacteria and fungi (<5%)
Neisseria gonorrhoeae	

- Underlying joint disease (rheumatoid arthritis, osteoarthritis).
- Chronic illnesses (diabetes mellitus, chronic renal failure).
- Alcohol abuse.
- Drugs (glucocorticosteroids, cytotoxics, i.v. drug abuse).
- Extra-articular infections (urinary tract, skin).
- Most joint infections are single, but 20% are polyarticular.

Early effective management is important to prevent muscle contractures and, more importantly, joint destruction. If infection is suspected, the joint should be promptly aspirated and the fluid analyzed for manifestations of infection. Treatment involves the use of appropriate antibiotics and an effective method of drainage (e.g. arthroscopy, arthrotomy, repeated needle aspiration). Initial selection should be based on the patient's age and any associated diseases, and the Gram stain. The regimen can be adjusted at 24–48 hours when the culture results are available, and later modified when the sensitivities are known. Suggested initial antibiotic regimens include:

- Intravenous methicillin or cloxacillin with or without an i.v. aminoglycoside.
- Intravenous imipenen.
- Intravenous ceftriaxone.

Parenteral antibiotics produce excellent synovial and intra-articular antibiotic concentrations. Intra-articular antibiotics are not needed.

The duration of therapy is determined by the clinical response, the effectiveness of drainage and the organism present. Streptococcal infection can usually be effectively treated with 2 weeks of i.v. therapy followed by 2–4 weeks of oral high-dose treatment. Staphylococcal infections may require longer treatment. Convincing clinical studies comparing short versus long (i.e. 2–6 weeks) periods of i.v. antibiotic therapy are not available.

Osteomyelitis

Bacteria can invade bone in a variety of ways: as a result of direct trauma, surgery, or extension from a soft tissue infection, and in the blood. The resulting osteomyelitis may present acutely, subacutely or chronically with bone pain, fever and leukocytosis. Patients with sickle cell

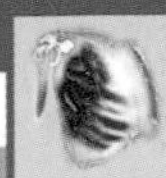

disease are 100 times more likely to present with osteomyelitis than the general population. Bone destruction with periosteal elevation may be seen radiographically. Abscess and sinus formation may occur. A bone scan is the most commonly used primary diagnostic tool for evaluating osteomyelitis in both adults and children. The diagnosis is often made late clinically so it is important to recognize early imaging findings.

Treatment includes:

- Splinting to prevent fractures.
- Consideration of surgical drainage.
- Intravenous antibiotics.

Prosthetic joint infections

Prosthetic joint infections are increasingly common, but are difficult to diagnose and treat. Over 100 000 total hip replacements are carried out each year in the USA and one of the main clinical concerns is the risk of bacterial infection of the prosthetic implant. Such an infection may occur early postoperatively (i.e. within a year) or be a late complication and result from a bacteremia. Skin contaminants are isolated from early postoperative infection (i.e. *Staphylococcus epidermidis*, *S. aureus*, anaerobes). Late infections are usually due to staphylococci, streptococci and Gram-negative bacilli. There is increasing concern about the emergence of methicillin-resistant *S. aureus* (MRSA).

■ ***All bacteriologically confirmed infections should be treated with high-dose i.v. antibiotics, appropriate surgical debridement and reimplantation***

Six weeks of high-dose i.v. antibiotics alone results in low rates of cure (i.e. less than 20%). Adding antibiotic to the cement at the time of revision surgery may be beneficial. Results are further improved by carrying out a two-stage revision procedure, with a temporary prosthesis for 6 weeks to several months and then permanent reimplantation.

Prophylactic perioperative antistaphylococcal antibiotics are believed to prevent infection if used in a short course starting immediately before surgery and continuing 24–72 hours after surgery. In addition, antibiotics are often used empirically in the first 3–6 months following joint replacement to prevent prosthetic joint infection with procedures such as dental surgery and genitourinary manipulation, but this topic needs further study.

FURTHER READING

Bermas BL. Oral contraceptives in systemic lupus erythematosus — a tough pill to swallow? *N Engl J Med* 2005; **353**:2602–2604.

Bone HG, Hosking D, Devogelaer J-P, et al. The alendronate phase III osteoporosis treatment study group. Ten years' experience with alendronate for osteoporosis in postmenopausal women. *N Engl J Med* 2004; **350**:1189–1199.

Drazen JM. COX-2 Inhibitors — a lesson in unexpected problems. *N Engl J Med* 2005; **352**:1131–1132

Geusens P, Reid D. Newer drug treatments: their effects on fracture prevention. *Best Practice & Research Clinical Rheumatology* 2005; **19**: 983–989

Heaney RP, Recker RR. Combination and sequential therapy for osteoporosis. *N Engl J Med* 2005; **353**: 624–625.

O'Dell JR. Drug therapy: therapeutic strategies for rheumatoid arthritis. *N Engl J Med* 2004; **350**: 2591–2602.

Olsen NJ. Tailoring arthritis therapy in the wake of the NSAID crisis. *N Engl J Med* 2005; **352**: 2578–2580.

Olsen NJ, Stein CM. Drug therapy: new drugs for rheumatoid arthritis. *N Engl J Med* 2004; **350**: 2167–2179.

Papapoulos SE. Who will benefit from antiresorptive treatment (bisphosphonates)? *Best Practice & Research Clinical Rheumatology* 2005, **19**: 965–973.

Rhen T, Cidlowski JA. Mechanisms of disease: antiinflammatory action of glucocorticoids — new mechanisms for old drugs. *N Engl J Med* 2005; **353**: 1711–1723.

Sambrook P. Who will benefit from treatment with selective estrogen receptor modulators (SERMs)? *Best Practice & Research Clinical Rheumatology* 2005; **19**: 975–981.

Thatayatikom A, White AJ. Rituximab: A promising therapy in systemic lupus erythematosus. *Autoimmunity Reviews* 2006; **5**: 18–24.

Tolar J, Teitelbaum SL, Orchard P. J. Mechanisms of Disease: Osteopetrosis. *N Engl J Med* 2004; **351**: 2839–2849.

Walsh JP, Ward LC, Stewart GO, et al. A randomized clinical trial comparing oral alendronate and intravenous pamidronate for the treatment of Paget's disease of bone. *Bone* 2004; **7**: 747–754.

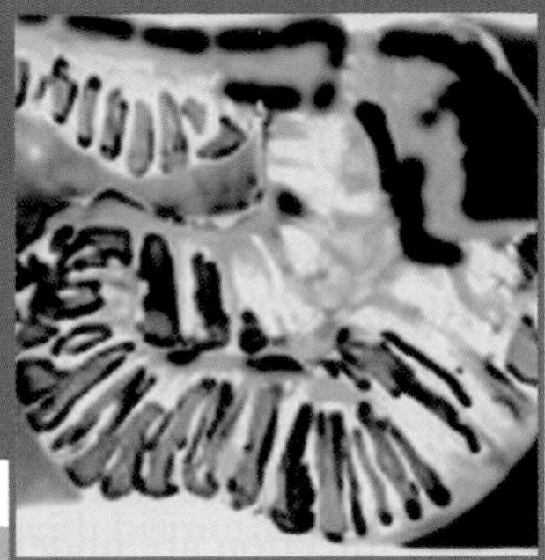

Chapter 16

Drugs and the Gastrointestinal System

PHYSIOLOGY OF THE GASTROINTESTINAL SYSTEM

The alimentary tract is a smooth muscle tube lined internally by an epithelium that varies in structure depending on its functions. Functions of the alimentary tract include:

- Food ingestion.
- Breaking food up into small portions.
- Converting large food molecules into smaller molecules (amino acids, small peptides, carbohydrates, sugars and lipids) by enzymes and other secretions so that they can be absorbed into the blood and lymph. Most of the small molecules are then transported to the liver where they are used as building blocks for essential proteins, carbohydrates and lipids.
- Excretion of undigested and previously digested matter as waste products.
- Water and electrolyte balance.
- Regulation of hormone secretion in various segments of the alimentary tract to enable controlled digestion and excretion.

The esophagus transports undigested fragmented food from the pharynx to the stomach where digestion begins

The esophagus is about 25 cm long and opens into the stomach at the esophagogastric junction. The stomach is a dilated portion of the digestive tract where the fragmented food is retained while it is macerated and partially digested.

The gastric epithelium secretes hydrochloric acid, digestive enzymes and mucus. It also contains hormone-secreting cells. The acid and digestive enzymes convert food into a thick semi-liquid paste (chyme), while mucus lubricates ingested food and protects the stomach from the corrosive effects of the acid and enzymes.

The liver is a metabolic, secretory and immunologic organ

The liver's metabolic role includes:

- Anabolism and catabolism of many endogenous substances, including glycogen and hemoglobin.
- Metabolism of many drugs and foods.

The metabolic and secretory systems metabolize, transport, or secrete endogenous and exogenous chemicals, and can be modified by chemicals, including drugs. The Kupffer cells of the liver play an important role in immune responses.

The liver is also part of the biliary tract. It manufactures and secretes bile, which is collected by the bile ducts and stored in the gallbladder, from where it is discharged into the duodenum to aid fat digestion.

The liver has two blood supplies (Fig. 16.1). Blood from these supplies then flows into the hepatic venous system and hepatic vein.

The liver is exposed to drugs that enter the circulation from any site of administration

All substances, including drugs, absorbed from the upper intestine are carried immediately to the liver by the portal vein, while substances in the systemic circulation can reach the liver through the hepatic artery. Drugs given orally can therefore have a double exposure to the liver via the portal vein and the systemic circulation. Drugs

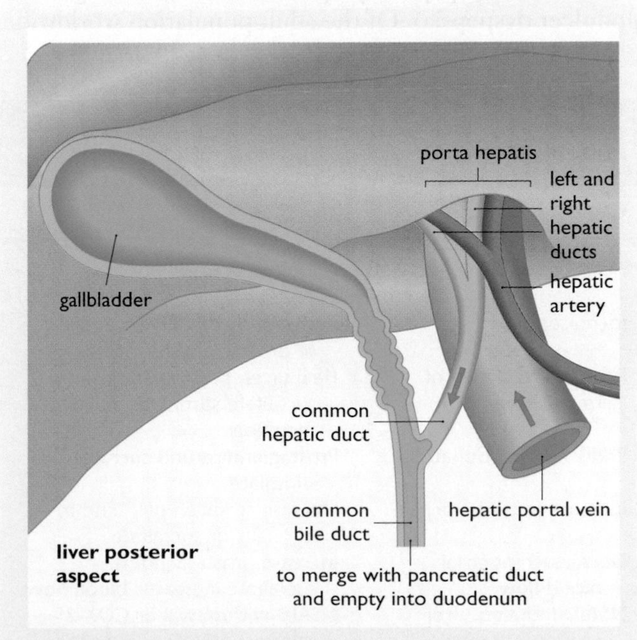

Fig. 16.1 The liver has two blood supplies. The liver is supplied by the systemic circulation via the hepatic artery to serve the nutritional needs of the hepatic cells. It is also supplied by the portal vein, which delivers blood that has already perfused the upper intestine.

used for treating nausea and vomiting, and further details are discussed below.

Constipation

Regulation of normal gastrointestinal motility involves the CNS, the enteric nervous system and gastrointestinal hormones. There are many causes of constipation, but ultimately it results from an absence of propagating contractions in the colon, which may be associated with either decreased or increased segmenting contractions. In some patients there may be abnormalities of propulsion in just the proximal or distal parts of the colon. Normal defecation of formed stools can vary from three times a day to only once every 3 days.

The incidence of severe chronic constipation, excluding that due to organic disease or an iatrogenic cause, is not known, but it is significantly greater in women than in men. The definition of constipation is also clouded; it is sometimes described as an altered frequency of defecation, and sometimes as difficult defecation.

- ***Constipation is managed by dietary improvement, eliminating any drugs that can cause constipation, excluding the presence of underlying pathology, and laxatives***

Laxatives

The mechanisms of action of laxatives are illustrated in Figure 16.4. Details commonly used laxatives are given in Table 16.5. Laxatives are widely misused in some societies for many reasons, including eating disorders where they are used to reduce caloric intake. Sometimes the use of laxatives may disguise the presence of underlying disease (e.g. obstruction).

BULK LAXATIVES Constipation and diarrhea can be treated with bulk provided in the form of dietary fiber. Unprocessed fiber (e.g. bran from unprocessed wheat or citrus sources) forms a readily available nondigestible source of bulk-forming laxative that can be used if sufficient fiber cannot be obtained from a normal, balanced diet. It may take several days for full effectiveness to be seen and may cause flatulence. Dietary fiber acts by absorbing water and promoting bacterial growth, since as it swells it distends the colon and increases peristaltic motility. Other bulk laxatives include preparations of ispaghula husk, sterculia gum and methylcellulose, which are available in more palatable forms than unprocessed fiber and are gluten-free; some preparations are also

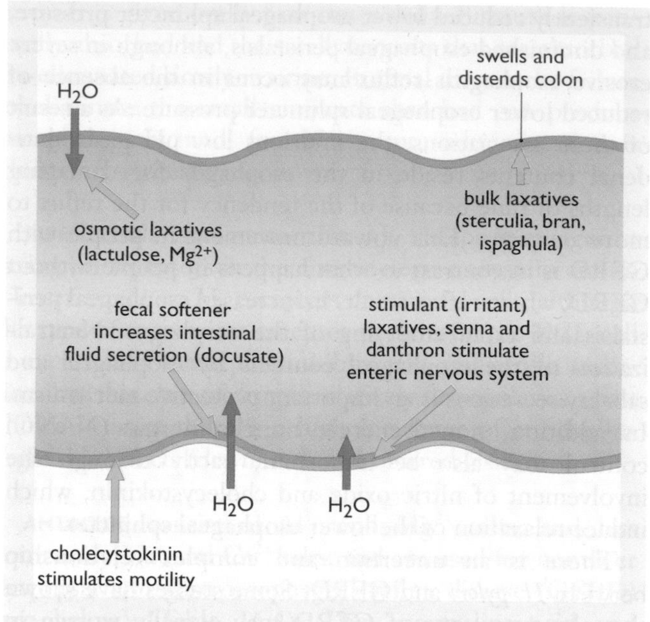

Fig. 16.4 Mechanism of action of laxatives. Bulk laxatives absorb water and on swelling slowly distend the colon and increase peristaltic motility; osmotic laxatives enhance peristalsis by osmotically increasing the bowel fluid volume; stimulant (irritant) laxatives stimulate the enteric nervous system; fecal softeners increase intestinal fluid secretion.

Table 16.5 Drugs used for the treatment of constipation*

A variety of bulk-forming laxatives including bran, ispaghula, sterculia, methylcellulose	*
Senna	Minimal absorption: action takes up to 12 hours given orally and less than 2 hours rectally
Bisacodyl	Administered orally or rectally Minimal absorption but relatively quick action after 6–8 hours orally but less than 60 minutes rectally
Lactulose	Poorly absorbed orally and broken down to active acids in the colon Takes 1–2 days to act
Docusate	Surfactant action. Minimally absorbed. Acts in up to 3 days
Magnesium sulfate	Acts within 6 hours. Up to 30% absorbed. Renal elimination
Danthron	An animal carcinogen restricted for use in the terminally ill Liver damage
Sodium picosulfate	Used only as a preoperative bowel preparation

* Because most drugs are minimally absorbed in most situations, plasma levels are insignificant. Side effects of all these preparations are flatulence, cramps and abdominal discomfort; individual unwanted effects are described in the text.

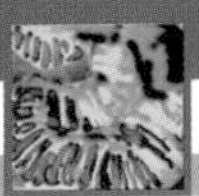

sugar-free. They have essentially the same action as bran, but sterculia contains polysaccharides, which are broken down by bacteria, and the resulting fatty acids can have an additional osmotic effect. Fiber is thought to normalize stool texture, and is also used to treat patients with loose stools (see below).

OSMOTIC LAXATIVES are widely prescribed. They are poorly absorbed and increase the small and large bowel fluid volume by osmosis and as a result increase peristaltic motility.

Lactulose is widely used and is a semisynthetic disaccharide of galactose and fructose. It passes unchanged to the colon and is then broken down by bacteria to lactic and acetic acids, which act osmotically to increase fluid volume and lower pH. It is effective within 2–3 days. Mg^{2+} salts and Na^{+} acid phosphate are used less often than lactulose. They are poorly absorbed and are osmotically active. Mg^{2+} also increases the synthesis of cholecystokinin, which increases colon motility and fluid secretion into the lumen.

STIMULANT CONTACT OR IRRITANT LAXATIVES should not be given over the long term. They have limited or restricted uses and can cause long-term pathologic problems. They act within hours and include:

- Senna, which is a plant alkaloid obtained from plantains. The constituent anthroquinones are hydrolyzed by gut bacteria to yield glycosides and subsequently anthracenes. These stimulate the enteric nervous system and alter fluid balance across the gut wall to promote propulsive motility.
- Bisacodyl, which is a diphenolic compound similar to phenolphthalein that can be given rectally for a rapid response.
- Danthron, which has similar properties to senna, but is carcinogenic in animal studies and is reserved for use only in the terminally ill.
- Sodium picosulfate, which is frequently used for bowel preparation before endoscopy or surgery.

The mechanisms of action of this group of drugs are poorly understood, but is has been suggested that they damage intestinal cells and weaken intercellular junctions. They also stimulate PG, cAMP, and possibly cholecystokinin, and vasoactive intestinal polypeptide (VIP) synthesis. These changes can all affect fluid balance and motility.

Chronic use of the anthroquinone laxatives can lead to melanosis coli, a black discoloration of the colonic mucosa, which can persist for years. Chronic administration of stimulant laxatives can also lead to the development of a 'cathartic colon,' which is a progressive deterioration of colon function that can exacerbate an existing bowel dysfunction.

FECAL SOFTENERS Docusate is dioctyl sodium sulfosuccinate. It has detergent properties, increases intestinal fluid secretion, and has weak stimulatory activity on intestinal motility. It relieves constipation within 1–2 days.

PROKINETIC DRUGS Bethanechol, metoclopramide and naloxone can stimulate colon motility, but descriptions of their use in the treatment of severe chronic constipation are insubstantial and require further clarification.

Chronic laxative use

- **Chronic use of stimulant (irritant) laxatives can lead to the development of a 'cathartic colon' with reduced propagative motility, dilation and exacerbation of any underlying disease**
- **Can damage the enteric nervous system**
- **Can lead to electrolyte imbalance**

Diarrhea

There are many causes of diarrhea including:

- An existing chronic disease (e.g. loss of functioning mucosa in inflammatory bowel diseases and gut reactions, motor abnormalities of irritable bowel syndrome, malabsorption diseases, endocrine abnormalities such as thyrotoxicosis).
- Infectious agents.
- Drugs.
- Psychologic factors.

Acute secretory diarrhea usually results from an infection.

Acute infectious diarrhea is extremely common and usually lasts just a few days. A common cause is acute viral gastroenteritis, and in children a rotavirus is usually the identified cause. In many cases, particularly adults, viral causes are often not identified, but bacterial pathogens such as *Campylobacter* are commonly cultured.

Worldwide, acute diarrhea (mainly of infectious origin) causes up to five million deaths every year as a result of dehydration. Approximately 85% of these deaths are in children less than 2 years of age and many could be prevented by simple measures. In Britain about 12 children younger than 1 year of age die each year from infectious diarrhea, while 20% of all health service consultations in the UK are for children less than 2 years of age with acute diarrhea.

The vigor of treatment for acute diarrhea depends upon the differential diagnosis and the patient's age. Young children are particularly prone to dehydration as 15% of the body weight turns over each day as water. Classifying enteropathogenic bacteria according to whether or not they invade the intestine is also important when deciding upon treatment (Table 16.6).

- Generally, invasive bacteria cause bloody, relatively small-volume diarrhea.

Table 16.11 Emetic potential of chemotherapeutic drugs

Severely emetogenic in almost all patients	Moderately emetogenic	Least emetogenic
Cisplatin Mustine Cyclophosphamide Dacarbazine Doxorubicin	Mitomycin C Procarbazine Nitrosoureas	5-Fluorouracil Cytarabine 6-Mercaptopurine Bleomycin Vinblastine Vincristine

- Cancer chemotherapy and radiation.
- Apomorphine, levodopa and ergot derivatives (e.g. bromocriptine, lergotrile) with dopamine agonist properties, used in the treatment of Parkinson's disease.
- Morphine and related opioid analgesics.
- Cardiac glycosides such as digoxin.
- Drugs enhancing 5-HT function.
- Miscellaneous agents (e.g. heavy metals, ipecacuanha alkaloids, *Veratrum* alkaloids).

Many cytotoxic treatments cause dose- and regimen-related severe nausea and vomiting (Table 16.11). Nausea and vomiting induced by radiation is also related to the dose used and to the area and extent of the body irradiated. In addition, cytotoxic or radiation treatment frequently causes severe disruption to the gastrointestinal tract where products of tissue destruction may be released and a local inflammatory response influence vagal afferent nerve endings within the gut to trigger the emetic reflex. The release of 5-HT from the enterochromaffin cells provides an important example. Such substances may be transported in the blood and, with the cytotoxic agents themselves, directly stimulate the central components mediating the emetic reflex.

Apomorphine, levodopa and ergot derivatives with dopamine agonist properties, used in the treatment of Parkinson's disease, directly stimulate the central chemoreceptor mechanisms. They also induce gastric stasis.

Morphine and related opioid analgesics have probably the most complex mechanisms of action of any drugs that cause nausea and vomiting. Acute administration of such agents to opioid-naive patients frequently induces nausea and sometimes vomiting. However, tolerance develops rapidly to such effects and the first treatment antagonizes the emetic effects to a second opioid injection or other emetogens. The emetic potential may be mediated in the chemoreceptor trigger zone (CTZ), whereas the 'broad-spectrum' antiemetic effect may be mediated 'downstream' from the CTZ and close to the 'vomiting center.' The antiemetic effect may relate to an endogenous tone exerted by opioids from the enkephalin, dynorphin or the pro-opiomelanocortin family. The ability of narcotic antagonists such as naloxone to precipitate nausea or vomiting supports this hypothesis.

Cardiac glycosides such as digoxin can induce abdominal pains, nausea and vomiting. This probably relates to a central action on the CTZ and an irritant action within the gastrointestinal tract, which may be worsened by a cardiac arrhythmia.

Drugs enhancing 5-HT function (e.g. 5-hydroxytryptophan, the precursor of 5-HT, or selective serotonin reuptake inhibitors [SSRIs] such as fluoxetine and paroxetine; see Ch. 8) have been reported to induce nausea and occasionally vomiting. This may relate to increased 5-HT activity in both brain and intestine.

When administered orally, heavy metals such as copper sulfate, zinc sulfate, antimony and mercuric chloride have an irritant action in the gut, triggering the emetic reflex via vagal and splanchnic nerves. Some of these agents may also directly stimulate the central mechanisms. The ipecacuanha alkaloids also stimulate peripheral and central mechanisms, while *Veratrum* alkaloids stimulate the nodose ganglia of the vagus to trigger the emetic reflex.

POSTOPERATIVE NAUSEA AND VOMITING (PONV) provides one of the best examples of the multifactorial nature of nausea and vomiting. It may be triggered by:

- Inhalational agents, particularly nitrous oxide, which are variably associated with PONV.
- Intravenous anesthetics and spinal anesthesia.
- Certain types of surgery, particularly gynecologic, pediatric strabismus and abdominal surgery. The latter can cause stretching, distention or tissue damage (i.e. gastrointestinal irritation).
- Pain resulting from surgery or disease.
- Hypoxia, hypotension and carbon dioxide retention.
- Clumsy movement of the patient in the recovery room, ward or following day-case surgery, causing a labyrinthine disturbance.
- Certain pre- or postoperative drug treatments (e.g. opioid analgesics).
- Psychogenic factors such as anxiety.
- A high body weight.
- Sex and age. The risk of PONV is three times higher in adult females than in adult males, and children are twice as susceptible as adults.

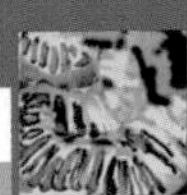

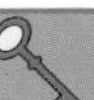

Major stimuli of nausea and vomiting

- Gastrointestinal irritation
- Motion sickness
- Hormone disturbance
- Intracranial pathology
- Metabolic disorders
- Psychogenic factors
- Pain
- Drugs and radiation
- Endogenous toxins

Individual responses to many emetic stimuli vary widely

Even the simple introduction of a spatula into the mouth to facilitate oral examination will immediately provoke a 'gagging' reflex in some people. Approximately 70% of women suffer PONV following gynecologic surgery, but it is not possible to identify those at risk. Patients who have had nausea and vomiting following previous surgery are likely to experience it again. Furthermore, women who experience pregnancy sickness are much more likely to develop nausea and vomiting in response to any hormonal disturbance (e.g. the contraceptive pill) or to traveling, and with migraine (Table 16.12). Also, people who have an emetic response to a first drug challenge are likely to show a similar response to subsequent challenge (i.e. individuals tend to have consistent responses). A simple enquiry may therefore identify people at greater risk (those who have a lower emetic threshold). These people are particularly likely to develop nausea and vomiting under emotional strain.

The frequency and intensity of episodes of nausea and vomiting vary enormously

A single short-lived bout of emesis induced by a single psychogenic stimulus is quite different from the intense, intractable and devastating nausea and vomiting caused by highly emetogenic chemotherapy. The first is unpredictable, and therefore untreatable by drugs, but the latter can now be efficiently managed in most patients.

The consequences of vomiting pose different problems to patient and clinician

To patients, a brief or persistent period of vomiting is always of concern. However, a brief period of vomiting in an otherwise healthy individual generally poses little medical risk, whereas, in the postoperative patient, even a brief but powerful period of retching or vomiting can cause tissue rupture. Not only will persistent nausea and vomiting incapacitate the patient, but the persistent vomiting may result in the loss of hydrochloric acid, leading to alkalosis and dehydration.

Persistent nausea or vomiting may be symptoms of an underlying disease

Persistent nausea or vomiting may be indicative of gastrointestinal, neurologic or metabolic disorders that require direct treatment, and it may be desirable to withhold antiemetic therapy until a diagnosis has been made.

Both central and peripheral systems mediate nausea and emesis

The causes of emesis provide vital clues to the stimuli influencing the emetic reflex, although the precise circuitry and transmitter mechanisms mediating the reflex remain largely unknown. However, key structures and pathways are now being identified, based on the results obtained almost exclusively from animals, of central and peripheral nerve lesions, intracerebral injection of drugs into discrete brain regions and electrophysiologic stimulation of discrete brain regions (Figs 16.8 and 16.9).

THE CHEMORECEPTOR TRIGGER ZONE (CTZ) is a key structure in mediating nausea and vomiting and is located within the area postrema, a circumventricular region located at the caudal end of the fourth ventricle. It lacks an effective blood–brain barrier and is therefore ideally suited for detecting emetic agents in both systemic circulation and the cerebrospinal fluid (CSF). A lesion of the CTZ abolishes the emetic response to many emetogens. The area postrema has numerous afferent and efferent connections with the underlying structures, the subnucleus gelatinosus and nucleus tractus solitarius. These brain regions are also important structures in the emetic reflex which, together with the area postrema,

Table 16.12 The number of women who reported sickness with oral contraceptives, travel, or migraine and the relationship to vomiting in pregnancy

Pregnancy sickness	Oral contraceptive sickness	Travel sickness	Migraine sickness
Vomiting	30 (70%)	77 (63%)	45 (65%)
No vomiting	13 (30%)	46 (37%)	24 (35%)

There was a higher than expected incidence of vomiting during pregnancy in these groups of women than in women who had no sickness.

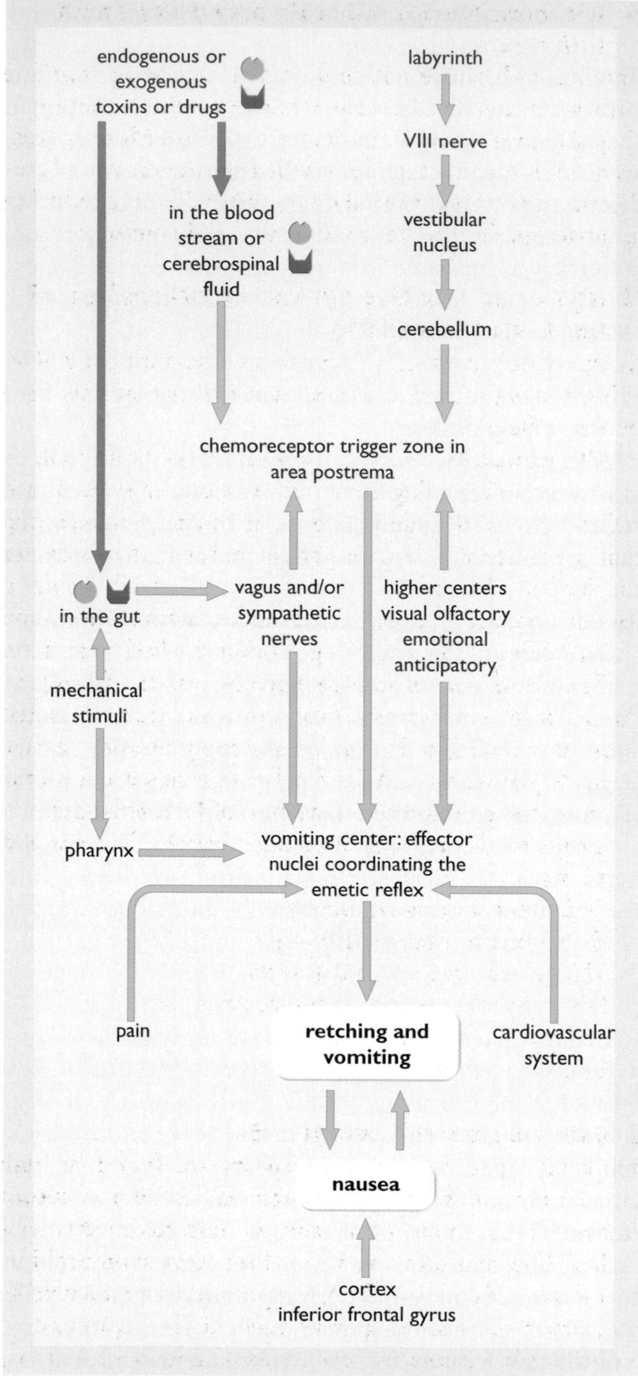

Fig. 16.8 The major emetic stimuli, pathways and structures mediating the emetic reflex and nausea.

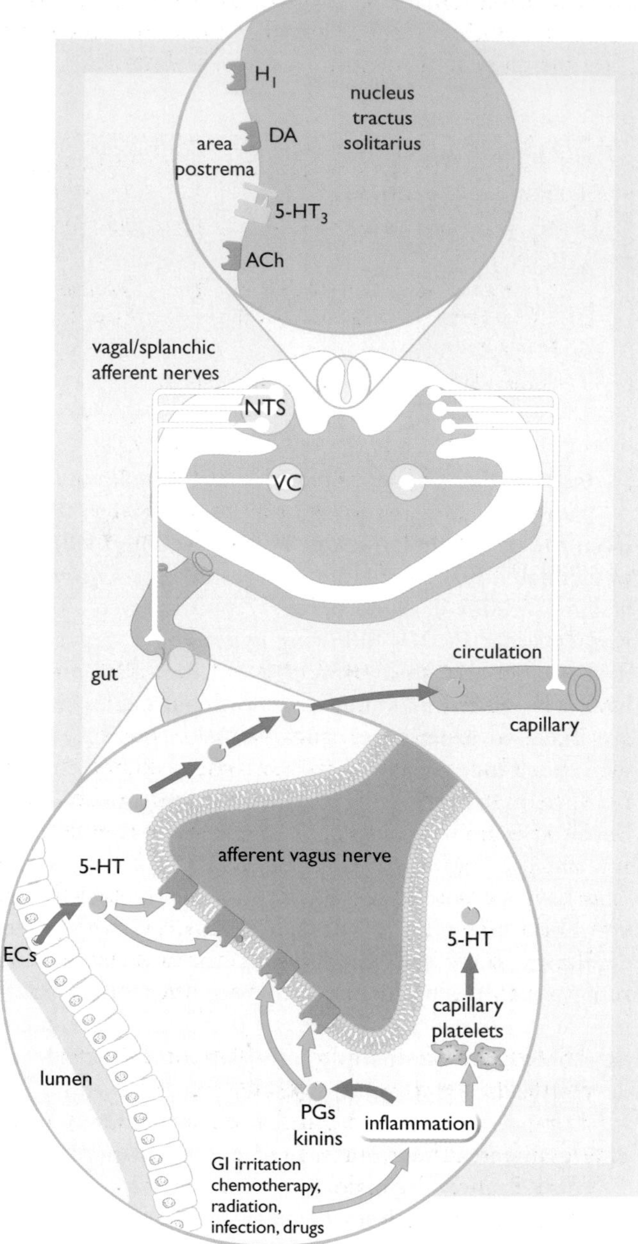

Fig. 16.9 Chemical transmitters mediating emetic stimuli. Stimuli in the gastrointestinal tract cause nausea and vomiting via neuronal (vagus nerve) and blood-borne influences on the central chemoreceptor trigger zone in the area postrema, nucleus tractus solitarius (NTS) and the 'vomiting center' (VC). 5-hydroxytryptamine (5-HT) released from the enterochromaffin cells (ECs), and possibly platelets acting on $5\text{-}HT_3$ receptors, may play a major role, along with inflammatory mediators released in the vicinity of afferent nerve endings (GI, gastrointestinal; PGs, prostaglandins).

receive vagal afferent fibers from the gastrointestinal tract, a major source of emetic stimuli.

THE 'VOMITING CENTER' is a second major 'structure' mediating nausea and vomiting and is more accurately described as a collection of effector nuclei rather than a discrete brain area. It receives major inputs from:

- The CTZ.
- The gut, of a vagal and sympathetic form.
- The cardiovascular system.
- A variety of limbic brain nuclei (e.g. the olfactory tubercle, amygdala, hypothalamus and ventral thalamic nucleus).

Electrical stimulation of all these structures can induce emesis. The latter nuclei may be involved in olfactory,

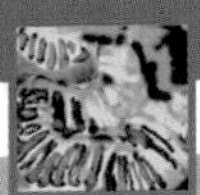

emotional/anticipatory, hormonal/stress and pain-induced vomiting, respectively. The location of the visual inputs to the emetic circuitry remains unknown.

Major systems mediating nausea and vomiting

- **The vagus and splanchnic nerves (stimuli from the gut)**
- **The cranial nerves (vestibular, olfactory, taste and visual stimuli, and touch from the oral cavity and pharynx)**
- **Forebrain systems (psychogenic stimuli)**
- **The chemoreceptor trigger zone (CTZ) in the area postrema (responds to circulating emetogenic neurotransmitters, hormones, toxins and drugs)**
- **The 'vomiting center' in the reticular formation (coordinates the visceral and somatic components of the emetic reflex)**

THE BRAIN REGIONS THAT PRODUCE THE SENSATION OF NAUSEA have been difficult to determine, since nausea is a subjective experience and animal models are not available. However, noninvasive magnetic source imaging revealed that there is neuronal activation in the cortex in the inferior frontal gyrus, in volunteers nauseated by ipecacuanha or vestibular stimulation. The activation caused by ipecacuanha, but not by vestibular stimulation, was inhibited by the 5-HT receptor antagonist ondansetron (see below). This brain area may therefore be important in the perception or sensation of nausea.

Retching, vomiting or regurgitation occasionally constitute a medical or surgical emergency

Retching, vomiting or regurgitation occasionally needs emergency treatment, for example:

- When induced by major intracranial pathology or intestinal obstruction.
- In infants, where fluid loss may cause dehydration.
- When the force of retching or vomiting tears esophageal tissue.
- In emergency surgery, when the patient has recently had a meal and therefore has a high risk of developing aspiration pneumonia. This is an important cause of death in pregnant women.
- In patients with a defective gag reflex, who have a high risk of developing aspiration pneumonia.
- When it is due to hyperemesis gravidarum.

The preferred treatment of nausea and vomiting is removal of the cause

Treatment of the cardiovascular pathology in migraine with the 5-HT_1 receptor agonist sumatriptan will relieve the neurologic manifestations, headache, gastrointestinal effects and nausea and vomiting, despite sumatriptan's having no direct effect on the emetic reflex (see Fig. 16.9).

Antiemetic therapy can be life-saving for patients with cancer

Patients with cancer will more readily accept or continue with what may be a curative course of chemotherapy if they are given effective antiemetic therapy. More aggressive chemotherapy regimens with a greater chance of eradicating the tumor can now be given without producing an unacceptable incidence of nausea and vomiting.

Drugs used for the symptomatic relief of nausea and vomiting

Symptomatic control of nausea and vomiting involves using drugs (Table 16.13) and procedures that affect the emetic reflex.

Although acute nausea itself poses no medical problem, it is a very distressing symptom and can cause as much suffering as pain. Indeed, a bout of retching or vomiting may be welcomed by the patient because it terminates the feeling of nausea. Persistent nausea usually leads to loss of appetite, reduced food intake, malnutrition, and serious debilitation, requiring prompt medical treatment.

There are now at least four major classes of drugs to control nausea and emesis. Procedures and treatments that alleviate retching and vomiting generally prevent nausea.

Inadequate control of the first bout of nausea and vomiting may compromise the treatment of later episodes.

Drugs used for the symptomatic relief of nausea and vomiting include:

- 5-HT_3 receptor antagonists.
- Dopamine receptor antagonists.
- Muscarinic receptor antagonists.
- Histamine H_1 receptor antagonists.
- Sedatives and hypnotics.
- Phenothiazines.

Dopamine receptor antagonists

Dopamine and dopamine receptors are found in high concentrations in the area postrema, the dorsal motor nucleus of the vagus nerve and the nucleus tractus solitarius. The traditional view has been that apomorphine, levodopa (via dopamine), lergotrile, bromocriptine and other dopamine agonists used in the treatment of Parkinson's disease induce nausea and vomiting by stimulating dopamine receptors in the CTZ. Dopamine receptor antagonists block such receptors and thereby prevent nausea and emesis.

SPECIFIC DOPAMINE RECEPTOR ANTAGONISTS (E.G. HALOPERIDOL AND FLUPHENAZINE) The use of these drugs is limited in two ways:

- First, they do not inhibit nausea and emesis induced by stimuli other than dopamine agonists (although droperidol is used in PONV, see below).
- Second, they have major adverse effects of motor impairment, severe akinesia and muscle rigidity, and dystonias (muscle spasm) caused by striatal dopamine receptor blockade, particularly in young people.

option. A potential treatment algorithm is shown in Figure 17.7.

The development of the symptoms of BPH is generally considered to arise from prostatic enlargement causing urethral restriction and bladder outflow obstruction. There are two components to the obstruction. There is the mechanical component arising from the physical obstruction induced by the enlarged prostatic mass, and a dynamic or fluctuating component related to the variations in smooth muscle tone in the prostate (see Fig. 17.5). Treatment modalities therefore aim either to reduce the mechanical obstruction or to induce relaxation of the periurethral prostate smooth muscle.

Drugs used in the treatment of BPH symptoms act either by reducing the tone in prostatic smooth muscle or by 'shrinking' the prostate

PROSTATE SHRINKERS Although many factors are involved in prostatic proliferation, the androgens, particularly dihydrotestosterone (DHT), have a prime role (see Fig. 17.4). A critical concentration of androgen is required to maintain the benign growth pattern and androgen deprivation results in significant involution of the glandular epithelial component of the prostate.

Finasteride is a drug specifically developed to inhibit the enzyme 5α-reductase that controls the production of DHT from testosterone. As anticipated, the drug has been shown to reduce circulating DHT concentrations to values almost as low as those found in castrated males. In several studies, consistent with the androgen dependency theory, a reduction in prostate size was observed in BPH patients treated with finasteride (5 mg) for periods of a year or more. In these long-term studies the need for surgery and incidence of urinary retention was reduced by up to 50%. Once again, this is consistent with an effect of finasteride on gland size and/or growth. Disappointingly, however, in most studies finasteride has little demonstrable effect on BPH symptoms, and certainly no effect over the first 6 months. The major adverse effect associated with the use of finasteride is a reduction in libido in up to 15% of patients. This is perhaps not surprising when considered in relation to the well-documented relationship between androgens and male sexual activity.

An alternative lower dose (1 mg) formulation of finasteride has been marketed for the treatment of male pattern baldness. The growth of certain types of hair is dependent on circulating and intrafollicular DHT levels. Although the prime form of the isozyme in the hair follicle is 5α-reductase 1, it is assumed that the generalized effect of finasteride on systemic androgens accounts for the benefit.

There are two isoforms of 5α-reductase, 5α-reductase 1 and 2. Finasteride inhibits only the latter, the major isoform in prostatic tissue. It has been argued that one of the limitations of finasteride is that circulating DHT

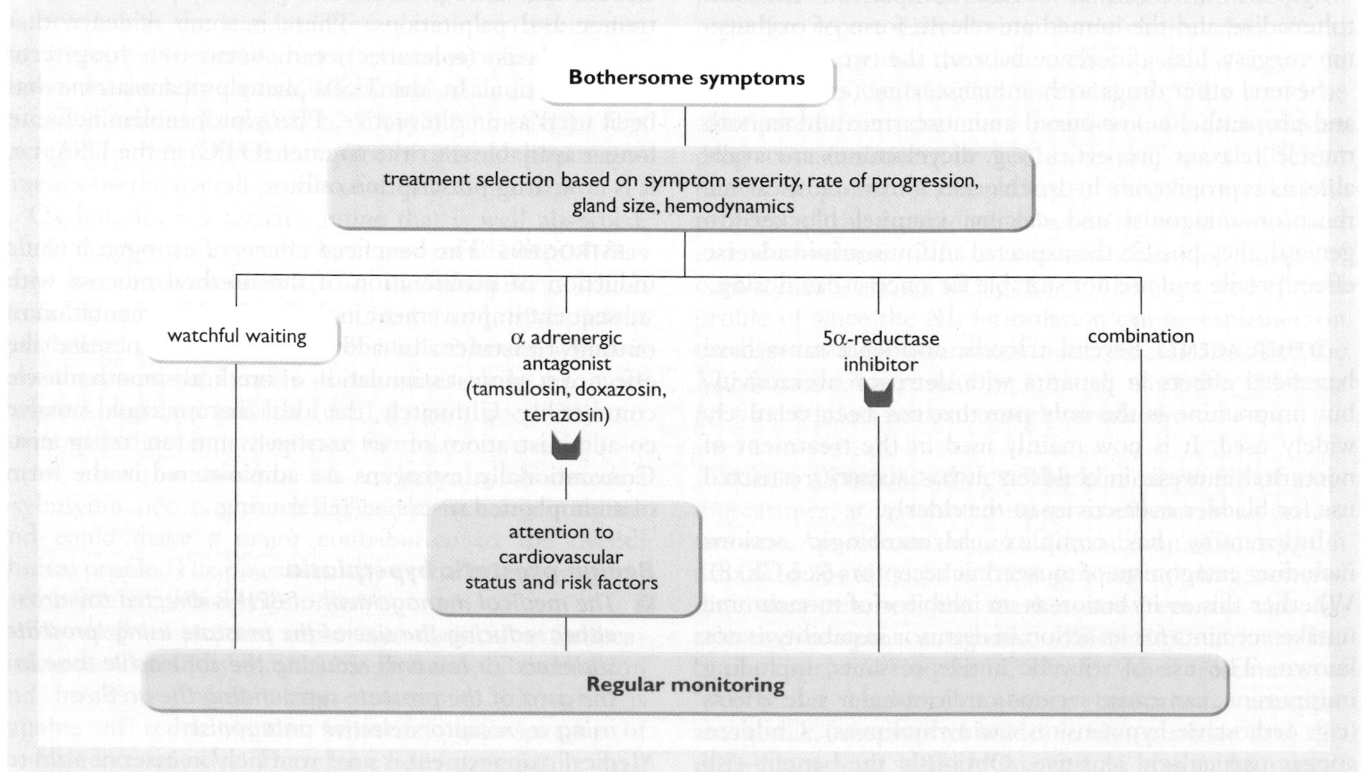

Fig. 17.7 Treatment options for the management of the lower urinary tract symptoms associated with benign prostatic hyperplasia.

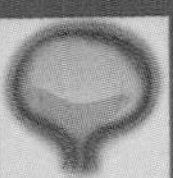

produced by extraprostatic 5α-reductase 1 (in e.g. skin, liver and fibroblasts) can maintain prostatic growth. On this basis several dual isozyme inhibitors are undergoing evaluation and dutasteride has recently been approved for the treatment of BPH. However, in the absence of long-term clinical data it is not known whether dual isozyme inhibitors offer any clinical advantage over finasteride and, indeed, with respect to androgen depletion-related side effects, whether they may be more problematic.

α_1 ADRENOCEPTOR SELECTIVE ANTAGONISTS (BLOCKERS)

In contrast to finasteride, patients taking α_1 receptor antagonists experience improvement in symptomatology that is almost immediate.

Since the initial use of phenoxybenzamine established the efficacy of a receptor antagonism in BPH, preferable drugs, initially prazosin, and then subsequently several other α_1 receptor selective antagonists (e.g. alfuzosin, doxazosin, indoramin, tamsulosin and terazosin) have become available. These now represent the mainstay of BPH therapy. The pharmacologic and clinical characteristics of this class of drugs are summarized in Table 17.5.

All data have been reviewed on several occasions by the α Receptor Antagonist Committee of the WHO International Consultation on BPH. This group has come to the conclusion that differences between α receptor antagonists are largely restricted to pharmacokinetic properties; i.e. at appropriate doses, all have equivalent efficacy and similar adverse effect profiles. On this basis the following summary of the key features of terazosin can be considered representative of the class, unless otherwise indicated. However, as indicated below, tamsulosin may differ to some extent from this profile.

Table 17.5 Summary of key features of α blockers

Alfuzosin. Has equal affinity for α_{1A}, α_{1B} and α_{1D} subtypes. It is available in immediate-release and sustained-release formulations with half-lifes of between 3 and 11 h, dependent on formulation. Tends to be used either q.d. or b.i.d.

Doxazosin. Longest half-life of all α blockers (16–22 h), with equal affinity for all 3 subtypes. It is used for comorbid treatment of hypertension

Prazosin. Although still widely used because of low generic cost, creates problems with patient compliance due to t.i.d. dosing and marked first dose orthostasis

Tamsulosin. Has been claimed to be 'uroselective' and has slightly higher affinity for prostatic α_{1A} receptor subtype than the α_{1B} and α_{1D} subtypes. Only available as one dose 0.4 mg, which can create problems for physicians. Marketed as once-daily dosing with $T_{1/2}$ of 16 h

Terazosin. Pharmacologic and clinical profile identical to doxazosin and also used as part of a treatment schedule for hypertension in several countries

Since the discovery of α_1 and α_2 receptors, our understanding of adrenoceptor pharmacology has increased substantially (Fig. 17.8). Three native α_1 adrenoceptor

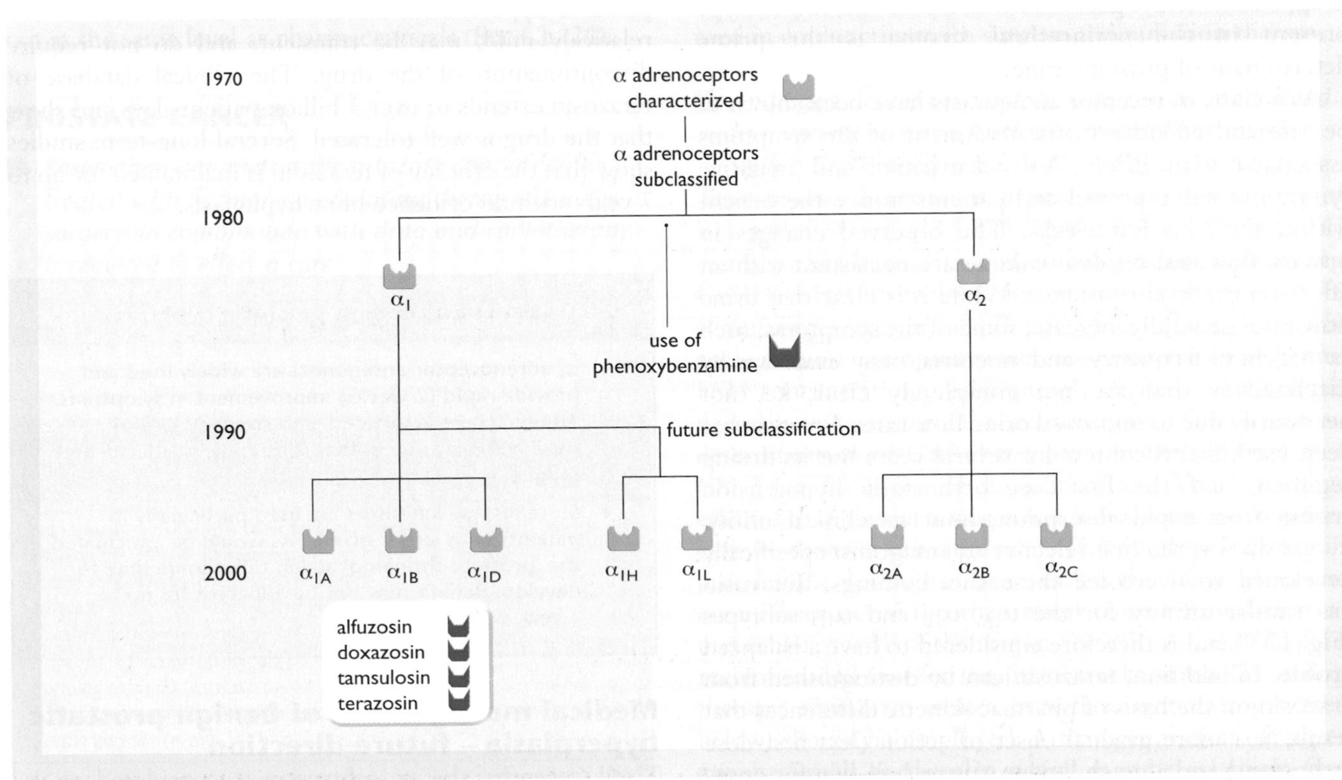

Fig. 17.8 Summary of adrenoceptor pharmacology.

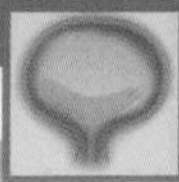

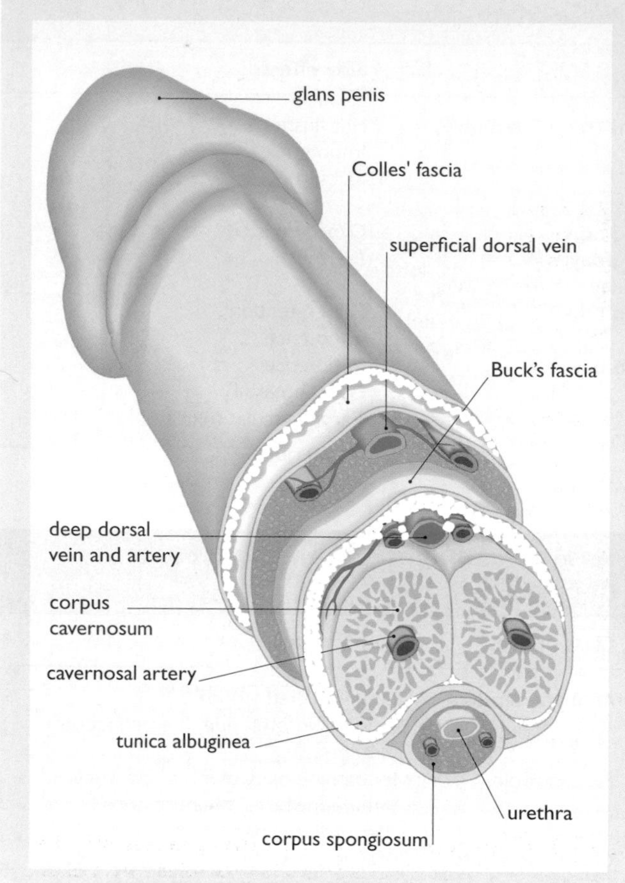

Fig. 17.12 Structure of the penis. The procreative function of the penis depends upon erection, which results from dilation of the cavernosal artery and filing of the corpora cavernosa and corpus spongiosum with arterial blood. The various fascias, particularly the tunica albuginea, prevent excessive dilation of the penis and limit venous drainage. Both arterial dilation, which increases flow, and reduction of venous outflow are important for maintaining erection.

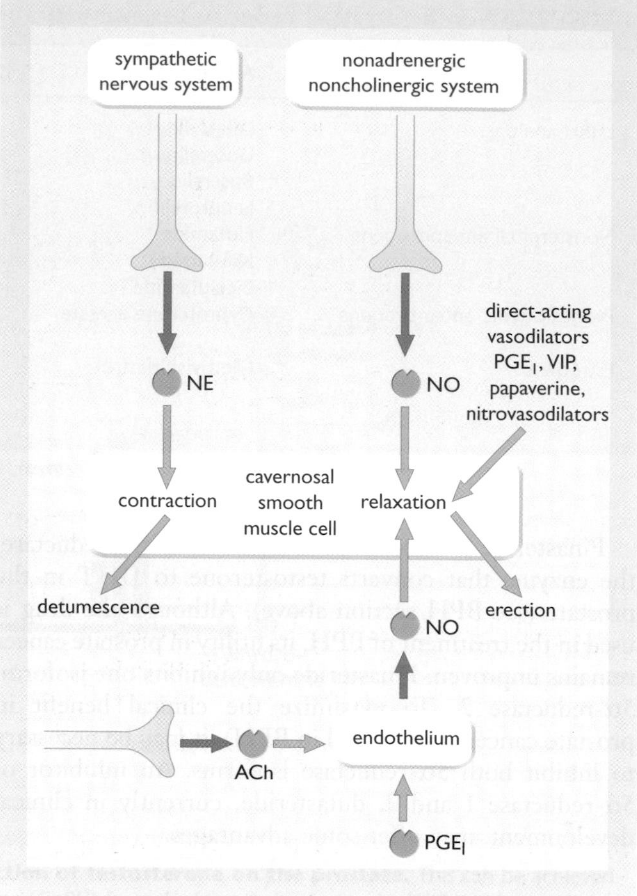

Fig. 17.13 Autonomic control of erection. The use of drugs to produce cavernosal smooth muscle relaxation. Smooth muscle tone is the prime determinant of the degree of erection (NO, nitric oxide; NE, norepinephrine; ACh, acetylcholine; PGE_1, prostaglandin E_1; VIP, vasoactive intestinal peptide).

local control systems and their various neuromodulator substances.

Almost certainly, ED occurs when an imbalance is created in the integrated response. Not surprisingly, the autonomic nervous system, i.e. the sympathetic noradrenergic and the nonadrenergic noncholinergic (NANC) nitric oxide (NO)-containing nerve fibers, provides the local neuromal control for normal erections. The neurotransmitters/neuromodulators controlling smooth muscle tone are shown in Table 17.11. However, the erectile process is unique among visceral functions in that there is an absolute requirement for central neural input to ensure normal function.

Of particular interest is the NANC system. Upon sexual stimulation, the neuromodulator nitric oxide (NO) is released and acts postjunctionally to activate an intracellular enzyme cascade (Fig. 17.14). NO is produced by the precursor L-arginine, which is converted by the enzyme nitric oxide synthase. Within the cavernosal smooth muscle cells, NO increases production of cyclic guanosine monophosphate (cGMP). cGMP which, in turn, decreases intracellular calcium concentrations, which leads to relaxation of the smooth muscle. Tissue engorgement and erection follow. cGMP is broken down, predominantly by an enzyme, phosphodiesterase type 5 (PDE5), which accounts in part for detumescence. However, detumescence is more directly controlled by activity in the sympathetic nervous system.

Table 17.11 Substances capable of modulating penile cavernosal smooth muscle contractility

Relaxation	Contraction
Acetylcholine	Norepinephrine
Nitric oxide	Endothelin-1
Vasoactive intestinal polypeptide	Neuropeptide Y
Prostaglandin E_1	ATP
Calcitonin gene-related peptide	

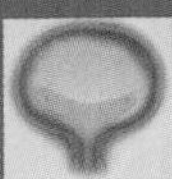

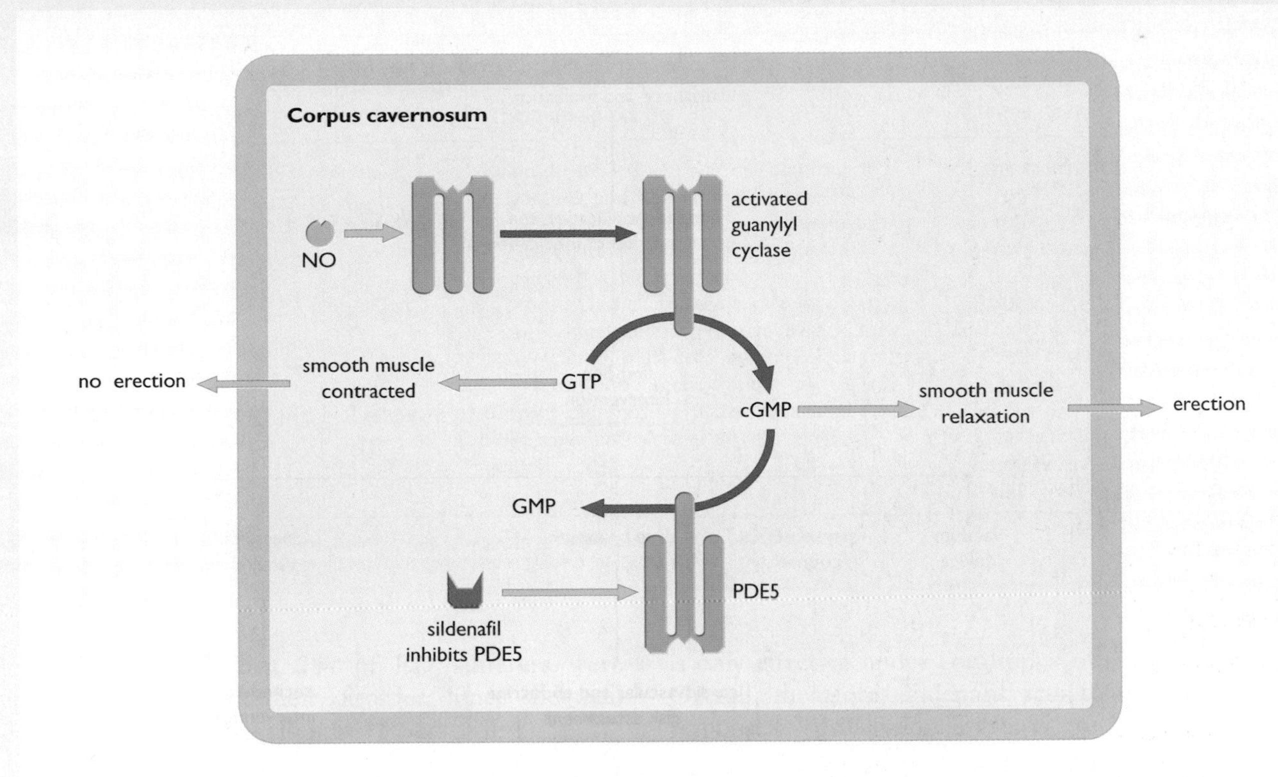

Fig. 17.14 The control of smooth muscle contraction and relaxation, and erection, in human corpus cavernosum. The effects of sildenafil are shown (cGMP, cyclic guanosine monophosphate; GMP, guanosine monophosphate; GTP, guanosine triphosphate; NO, nitric oxide; PDE5, phosphodiesterase type 5).

Released norepinephrine acts on postjunctional α_1 adrenoceptors, producing contraction of the corporal smooth muscle, leading to increased venous outflow and detumescence.

Drugs used for the treatment of erectile dysfunction

Prior to initiation of therapy a full diagnostic investigation must be completed

An algorithm for the management of patients with ED is shown in Figure 17.15. Subsequent to clinical evaluation and diagnosis of ED, a variety of management options are now available, dependent on patient preference. An obvious starting point is the modification of potentially reversible causes of the condition. In its simplest form, this can involve lifestyle modification, e.g. stress reduction, dietary changes, smoking cessation or establishing more effective control of blood glucose in diabetics. In other cases involving an iatrogenic basis for the ED (see Table 17.10), discontinuation or modification of ongoing therapy can achieve considerable success. More commonly, interventional therapy is needed. This can range from drugs, psychotherapy and minimally invasive procedures such as vacuum devices to more invasive procedures such as surgery.

Drugs can act peripherally, or centrally, to initiate or augment erections

Since the pioneering self-injection studies of Brindley in the 1970s, the use of drugs to produce cavernosal smooth muscle relaxation and thereby erection has increased dramatically. Traditionally, vasorelaxant substances such as papaverine and phenoxybenzamine have been administered by direct intracavernosal injection. As monotherapy, their use has been largely discontinued, owing largely to the relatively high incidence of penile fibrosis and penile fibrotic nodules. In several countries a Trimix strategy is widely used. This involves the injection of a combination of a mixture of phentolamine, papaverine and prostaglandin E_1 (PGE_1). The pharmacologic synergy (Table 17.12) of these drugs reduces the doses required for each drug separately and appears to result in a corresponding reduction in the incidence of penile fibrosis. However, the use of PGE_1 as monotherapy exceeds the use of all other injectables.

PGE_1 (alprostadil) is poorly absorbed orally and is broken down rapidly on entering the blood stream so that systemic concentrations are quite low. This necessitates the use of local delivery systems, usually intracavernosal. The response rate and magnitude of the response are excellent. Alprostadil (5–20 μg) is effective across a wide

Patients need careful evaluation prior to starting ciclosporin, particularly with regard to renal function. Ciclosporin blood levels are not routinely measured in patients with skin diseases as the doses used (maximum 5 mg/kg) are well below those typically used in organ transplantation. Patients taking ciclosporin are advised to avoid excess sun exposure, UVB or PUVA therapy, because of the well-established excess of skin cancers in patients who have had transplants. This increase is partly attributable to immunosuppressive therapy.

Ciclosporin is used for psoriasis more widely than for atopic eczema. It is indicated for severe psoriasis where conventional therapy is ineffective or inappropriate. Ciclosporin is also beneficial in psoriatic arthropathy (see Ch. 15) and can be used in conjunction with methotrexate to minimize the toxicity and cumulative dose of each agent.

The value of ciclosporin in a variety of rare and severe dermatoses, such as pyoderma gangrenosum, is being evaluated.

The second-generation T-cell inhibitor pimecrolimus has also been introduced for the treatment of atopic eczema.

Azathioprine

Azathioprine, a cytotoxic immunosuppressant is used in unresponsive atopic eczema both as a steroid sparing agent and alone. (See Chs 7 and 9 for more information about azathioprine.)

Emollients

Creams and ointments that improve skin hydration are called emollients. Ointments are generally greasy preparations which are insoluble in water and anhydrous, and are more occlusive than creams. Some newer ointments have both a hydrophilic and lipophilic component while others are water-soluble ointments. Emollients reduce the excess transepidermal water loss that is a feature of eczema, as evidenced by surface electrical capacitance, measurement of transepidermal water loss and molding of skin surface replicas. Thus, they help restore barrier function, but do not have an antiinflammatory effect. They can soothe itching by their cooling effect but this is a transient benefit. There is some evidence that they reduce the susceptibility of eczematous skin to irritants.

Emollients form the mainstay of treatment of ichthyosis. Preparations containing urea and propylene glycol, which improve penetration, have been shown to be superior to other emollients in lamellar ichthyosis. Emollients are also useful in the treatment of other dry scaly skin conditions such as psoriasis.

There is a wide selection of commercially available emollients, containing a variety of ointments and creams (see Table 18.1), some of which are very greasy and can be too occlusive. Others are more water soluble and creamy, but less hydrating and need more frequent application. A mixture of soft white paraffin and liquid paraffin in equal parts is a thick emollient, whereas many cream formulations are thin emollients. Patient preference is an important consideration since these agents need to be used regularly and persistently. In practice this is influenced by stinging on application, ease of application, appearance on the skin (is it obviously greasy?), smell, duration of action, effect on clothing and ease of removal.

Bath emollients are similar to emollients in action and are designed for addition to bath water to prevent skin drying while bathing.

Soap substitutes

Creamy cleansers are preferred to soaps in patients with atopic eczema, since the detergent in soaps can be both irritating and drying.

H_1 receptor antagonists

H_1 receptor antagonists (antihistamines, see Ch. 9) are widely used in the treatment of atopic dermatitis in an effort to alleviate itch. Although the results of clinical trials have suggested that the beneficial effect of H_1 receptor antagonists is due to their sedative effect (inhibiting scratching) some of the newer H_1 receptor antagonists, e.g. cetirizine, may have antiinflammatory properties (e.g. antieosinophilic activity) relevant to their effects in the treatment of atopic dermatitis.

H_1 receptor antagonists are the mainstay of treatment of urticaria and are also useful in the management of acute anaphylaxis and angioedema. In the treatment of urticaria, the choice of drug depends on the need for sedation, which is often desirable in acute urticaria but not in the chronic form.

H_1 receptor antagonists that are used to treat urticaria and pruritus are doxepin, desloratadine, fexofenadine and ebastine.

Histamine H_2 antagonists have sometimes been advocated in the treatment of urticaria but the evidence regarding their efficacy is conflicting. They have more recently been used at high dosage to treat viral warts but the results of clinical trials to date have been variable.

Approaches to the treatment of eczema are summarized in Figure 18.2.

Acne

Acne is a disease of the pilosebaceous unit

Acne is characterized by comedones (keratin plugs of the sebaceous duct openings), inflammatory papules, pustules, nodules, cysts and scars. The rash occurs where there is a high density of pilosebaceous glands (e.g. on the face, back and chest). Androgenic stimulation of the sebaceous glands accounts for the higher prevalence of acne at puberty. The active pilosebaceous follicles are heavily colonized by *Propionibacterium acnes*. The mechanism for keratin plug formation is poorly understood, but is

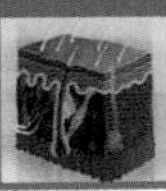

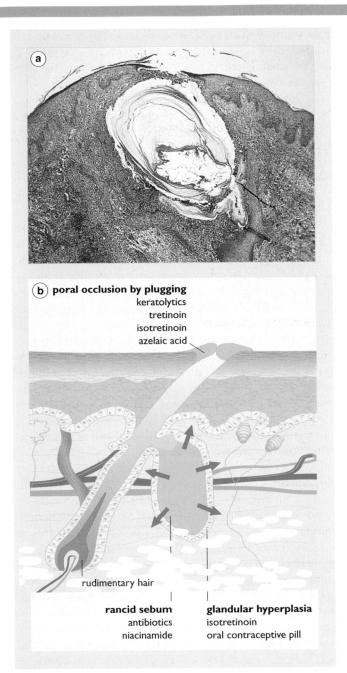

Fig. 18.3 Acne. (a) Histologically, acne is characterized by keratin plugs (comedones) which block the sebaceous follicles such that sebum cannot escape. In acne the sebaceous glands are often hyperplastic, and a site of an intense neutrophil influx. (Courtesy of Dr. P. McKee.) (b) Sites of drug action in acne.

thought to be pivotal in the disease process. Continued gland secretion in the presence of plugs results in swelling of the glands and ducts, with nodule and cyst formation and the induction of an inflammatory response producing inflammatory papules and pustules. Approaches to the treatment of acne are shown in Figure 18.3.

Keratolytics

Topical keratolytics (e.g. salicylic acid, sulfur) are used in acne to reduce the pore occlusion that is characteristic of acne.

SULFUR, although of proven efficacy, is rarely used because of its bad smell.

SALICYLIC ACID is soluble in alcohol, but only slightly soluble in water. It is thought to act by solubilizing the cell surface proteins that keep the stratum corneum intact, resulting in desquamation. It is keratolytic at a concentration of 3–6%, but higher concentrations can destroy skin.

Salicylic acid is absorbed percutaneously, and 1 g of 6% salicylic acid results in plasma concentrations of approximately 0.5 mg/dL (0.04 mmol/L). Salicylism and death have been recorded after topical application but the threshold for toxicity is 30–50 mg/dL (2.2–3.3 mmol/L). Such concentrations are unlikely to be achieved with keratolytic concentrations (3–6%), but safety issues should be borne in mind with higher, destructive concentrations, especially in children.

Adverse effects include urticarial and anaphylactic reactions in patients who are sensitive to salicylates.

Clinical uses of salicylic acid other than for acne include destruction of viral warts in concentrations of 16–40%, use in conjunction with topical glucocorticosteroids to increase skin penetration (concentrations of approx 10%). It is also used in conjunction with benzoic acid as Whitfield's ointment, which is fungicidal and used in the treatment of skin fungal infections.

AZELAIC ACID is a saturated nine-carbon-atom dicarboxylic acid. It was originally obtained by the oxidation of oleic acid by nitric acid but it can also be obtained by fermentation by a variety of microorganisms.

The observations that the *Pityrosporum* fungus can oxidize oleic acid to azelaic acid in culture, and that azelaic acid is a competitive inhibitor of tyrosinase, led to studies to test the hypothesis that this acid was responsible for the hypopigmentation which characterizes pityriasis versicolor and therefore might have a role in hyperpigmentation disorders.

In subsequent studies azelaic acid was shown to have a beneficial effect in melanosis due to hyperfunction of proliferative melanocytes, but no such depigmenting effect is seen on normal skin. In patients being treated for melasma those with coincident acne noticed improvement. Subsequent research has demonstrated that azelaic acid has:

- Antienzymatic and antimitochondrial activity: it is a reversible inhibitor of cytochrome P-450 reductase and 5α-reductase and can reversibly inhibit some enzymes of the respiratory chain as well as being a competitive inhibitor of tyrosine. It also has an inhibitory effect on anaerobic glycolysis.
- Antimicrobial and antiviral effect: in culture, azelaic acid inhibits both aerobic and anaerobic microorganisms including *P. acnes*. An inhibitory effect on vaccinia virus replication has been shown.

- Effect on tumoral cells in culture: a dose-dependent effect on proliferation and viability of melanoma cells, lymphoma and leukemia-derived cell lines while not affecting normal cells in culture.

In acne, inhibition of aerobic respiration and anaerobic glycolysis are thought to be important in its effects on microorganisms while the reduction of cellular energy production in keratinocytes may also be relevant. Azelaic acid is keratolytic and comedolytic. In part, it normalizes the disturbed terminal differentiation of keratinocytes in the follicle infundibulum. It is available as a topical cream for the treatment of acne.

Furthermore, anaerobic glycolysis is thought to be important in sebaceous glands, so that there may be an additional direct effect on sebaceous gland activity.

Azelaic acid is well tolerated. Benefit often occurs only after 4 weeks, while treatment should be continued for several months.

In pigmentary disorders the primary effect of azelaic acid is thought to be the reduction of cellular energy production. It has been shown to be as effective as hydroquinone (4%) in this regard.

BENZOYL PEROXIDE penetrates the stratum corneum and follicular openings unchanged, but converts to benzoic acid in the epidermis and dermis. Benzoic acid has several actions:

- Germicidal – reduction of facial microbial flora equal to that produced by systemic tetracycline.
- Keratolytic.
- Comedolytic.
- Antiinflammatory.
- Sebostatic? (this action is subject to some controversy).

Adverse effects of benzoyl peroxide include irritation with increasing concentrations and sensitizing properties. Up to 1% of patients develop a contact allergic dermatitis. Bleaching of hair, skin and clothing can be cosmetically unacceptable.

In addition to its use in acne, benzoyl peroxide has been used in combination with miconazole, where it is said to increase efficacy. A 20% lotion has been used to promote rapid re-epithelialization of wounds.

Mild keratolytics, e.g. urea, are also used to enhance the emollient effect of a cream or vehicle. Stronger keratolytic therapy is used for conditions such as viral warts.

Niacinamide

Niacinamide is the amide of vitamin B_3. Physiologically, it is converted to nicotinamide adenine dinucleotide (NAD) or the dinucleotide phosphate (NADP), both of which function as coenzymes (see Ch. 22). Niacinamide is thought to act by electron scavenging, inhibition of phosphodiesterase and/or increased tryptophan conversion to serotonin. It also has direct effects on inflammatory cells, inhibiting neutrophils, suppressing lymphocyte transformation and inhibiting mast cell histamine release. Niacinamide may be a useful treatment for acne. Clinical trials suggest that topical niacinamide gel is as effective as topical clindamycin in mild to moderate acne, and represents a nonantibiotic treatment that appears to be well tolerated. In acne its main effect seems to be inhibition of cyclic AMP phosphodiesterase and lymphocyte transformation, inhibiting epithelial proliferation in pilosebaceous units.

Antibiotics

TOPICAL ANTIBIOTICS (see Ch. 6) Topical administration of antibiotics for acne (Table 18.3) has been shown to be equieffective with benzoyl peroxide or tretinoin. However, long-term use of antibiotics risks the emergence of resistant organisms.

SYSTEMIC ANTIBIOTICS Oral antibiotics (Table 18.4) are more effective than topical antibiotics in the treatment of acne. Treatment should be continued for a minimum of

Table 18.3 Topical antibiotics – acne

Antibiotic	Efficacy	Other issues affecting choice
Clindamycin	1% clindamycin phosphate = oral minocycline and tetracycline = 5% benzoyl peroxide gel	
Erythromycin	Only lipid-soluble formulations (propionate or stearate) are effective 2% erythromycin gel = 1% clindamycin phosphate 1.5% erythromycin solution = 1% clindamycin phosphate solution	Erythromycin resistance common
Erythromycin with zinc castor oil in oily cream 1:9		May delay emergence of resistance
Erythromycin with benzoyl peroxide		May delay emergence of resistance
Tetracyclines	Effective and considered cosmetically acceptable by 90% of patients Topical tetracycline < topical niacinamide	Tetracycline resistance common Stains clothing and skin

'=', equi-effective; '<', less effective

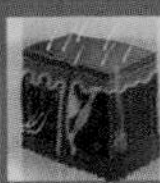

Table 18.4 Systemic antibiotics – acne

Antibiotic	Advantages	Disadvantages
Tetracyclines	Antibiotic of choice. Bacteriostatic at high doses; at low doses affect bacterial function	Not recommended under the age of 12 because of discoloration of teeth. Avoid in pregnancy and breast-feeding
Oxytetracycline		Chelates with calcium-containing food, so needs to be taken with water half an hour before food, otherwise there is reduced absorption
Minocycline	Compliance improved with once-daily dosing	Can cause hyperpigmentation due to deposition of drug in skin
Doxycycline	Compliance improved with once-daily dosing	Photosensitivity, which is dose-related
Erythromycin	Bacteriostatic Can be used in patients who may become pregnant or who are breastfeeding	
Trimethoprim	Equieffective to tetracycline Reserved as third-line treatment	
Clindamycin	Useful because of lipid solubility	Not to be used routinely because of risk of pseudomembranous colitis

6 months but some improvement should be evident at 3 months. If there is no improvement, a change is made in the antibiotic since resistant strains of *P. acnes* are increasingly common, particularly to erythromycin, tetracycline and doxycycline. Some of the therapeutic effect of these antibiotics is due to nonbacterial effects which include:

- Enzyme inhibition, e.g. *Corynebacterium acnes* lipase.
- Modulation of chemotaxis.
- Modulation of lymphocyte function.
- Modulation of cytokines, especially IL-1α expression.

Retinoids

Retinoids include vitamin A and its derivatives (Table 18.5) and have potent effects on:

- Cell differentiation, which they induce.
- Cell growth, inducing hyperplasia, hypergranulosis, and decreased numbers of tonofilaments and desmosomes in the epidermis. The latter effect is thought to account for the keratolytic effect.
- The immune response, stimulating cell-mediated cytotoxicity and acting as an adjuvant to stimulate antibody production to antigens that were not previously immunogenic.

They also reduce neutrophil migration, although the mechanism for this is not known.

Table 18.5 Retinoids

	Drug	Disease
1st generation	Retinol Tretinoin Isotretinoin	Acne
2nd generation	Etretinate Acitretin	Psoriasis (and other papulosquamous diseases)

Intracellularly, retinoids stabilize lysosomes, increase ribonucleic acid polymerase activity, increase incorporation of thymidine into DNA and increase prostaglandin (PG) E_2, cAMP and cGMP concentrations. These actions of retinoids are mediated by retinoic acid receptors (RARs), members of the thyroid/steroid superfamily of receptors. The RARs bind retinoids and DNA, and function as transcription factors initiating transcription (see Ch. 22).

TOPICAL RETINOIDS Tretinoin is the acid form of vitamin A (i.e. retinoic acid) (Table 18.6). It is formed by oxidation of the alcohol group in vitamin A, with all four double bonds in the side chain in the *trans* configuration. It is insoluble in water, but soluble in many organic

Table 18.6 Topical retinoids

Drug name	Advantages	Mode of action
Tretinoin Retinoic acid 0.01–0.05 in cream or gel		Binds to cytosolic retinoid acid-binding protein (RAR) with high affinity. Binds all nuclear receptors
Isotretinoin 0.05%	= Benzoyl peroxide and topical tretinoin	
Adapalene	More effective with less irritation than tretinoin. Only topical retinoid with significant anti-inflammatory effect	Does not bind cytosolic retinoid RAR and binds RAR β and α selectively in nucleus

'=' equi-effective

solvents. It is used topically in the treatment of acne, where its actions are attributed to decreased cohesion between epidermal cells and increased epidermal cell turnover. It is thought that this helps remove comedones, and convert closed comedones to open comedones.

The main adverse effect of topical retinoids is skin irritation. Patients should be warned to avoid exposure to ultraviolet light since tretinoin appears to increase the tumorigenic potential of ultraviolet light in animal studies.

A regular application of 0.05% tretinoin cream for a minimum of 4 months improves the appearance of photo-damaged skin, and is licensed for the treatment of mottled hyperpigmentation and fine wrinkling caused by chronic sun exposure. Recently, tazarotene has been introduced as a topical treatment for psoriasis; it is a vitamin A analog that acts as a retinoic acid receptor agonist. However, it is also very irritant.

ORAL RETINOIDS Isotretinoin is a synthetic retinoid available for systemic and topical use. Its main effect is to reduce the size and function of the sebaceous glands. A 4–6-month course is highly effective in the treatment of acne in the majority of patients.

Isotretinoin is well absorbed, extensively bound to plasma proteins, and eliminated. It is given at a dose of 0.5–1 mg/kg.

The adverse effects of isotretinoin resemble the effects of hypervitaminosis A, producing dry skin and mucous membranes, and epidermal fragility. Rarely, visual disturbances, hair thinning, myalgia and arthralgia, and raised liver enzymes have been reported. Cutaneous complications include photosensitivity, allergic vasculitis, granulomatous lesions and acne fulminans. Isotretinoin can cause benign intracranial hypertension (BIH), so frequent or unusual headaches are an indication to stop treatment and investigate. Since tetracyclines can also cause BIH, the two drugs should not be given together. Triglyceride concentrations increase during treatment, but this increase is rarely sufficient to stop therapy and is reversible on stopping treatment.

Isotretinoin is teratogenic and should be given to women of child-bearing age only after appropriate counseling and with adequate contraception

Treatment of acne

- Keratolytics should be used as first-line therapy
- If a systemic antibiotic is needed, tetracyclines are indicated in children over 12 years of age, but should not be given to children under 12 because of their effects on maturing teeth
- Oxytetracycline should be given before minocycline because of the rare reaction to minocycline involving liver, joints and fever
- In children under 12 years of age erythromycin is the systemic drug of choice
- In adults, tetracyclines should be given in preference to erythromycin, as erythromycin is used for life-threatening infections such as *Mycoplasma pneumoniae*
- Antibiotic resistance to *Propionibacterium acnes* is as high as 40% in patients with acne referred to hospital

Adverse effects of isotretinoin

- Teratogenicity
- Dry skin and mucous membranes
- Epidermal fragility
- Rarely, visual disturbances, hair thinning, myalgia and arthralgia, and raised liver enzymes
- Allergic vasculitis
- Granulomatous lesions
- Acne fulminans
- Benign intracranial hypertension
- Increased triglyceride concentrations

Psoriasis

Psoriasis is a genetically determined hyperproliferative disorder that can be triggered by infection, trauma, drugs, ultraviolet light and stress, and rarely by hypocalcemia. Psoriatic skin has a turnover rate of 7 days rather than the normal 56 days and is characterized by:

- Thickened skin plaques with superficial scales.
- Capillary dilation in the papillary dermis.
- An inflammatory infiltrate, predominantly of lymphocytes, in the dermis.
- A neutrophil infiltrate in the epidermis.

Capillary dilation may be an initiating event or an attempt to nourish the hyperproliferating skin. The precise contribution of inflammatory cells to the clinical disease is not clear.

Approaches to the treatment of psoriasis are shown in Figure 18.4.

Treatment regimens for psoriasis must be individualized. For localized disease, topical therapy is often sufficient. Vitamin D analogs are rapidly becoming first-line treatment not least because they are clean, nonstaining, nonsmelling preparations which afford a cosmetic advantage over tar and anthralin preparations. However, these preparations need to be applied accurately to affected sites and if the percentage of body area affected is large, the potential to disturb systemic calcium homeostasis needs to be considered. Anthralin (see below) is still the least toxic agent and offers the potential benefit of inducing remission. However, it is very messy to use and irritation can be a problem par-

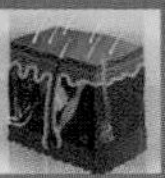

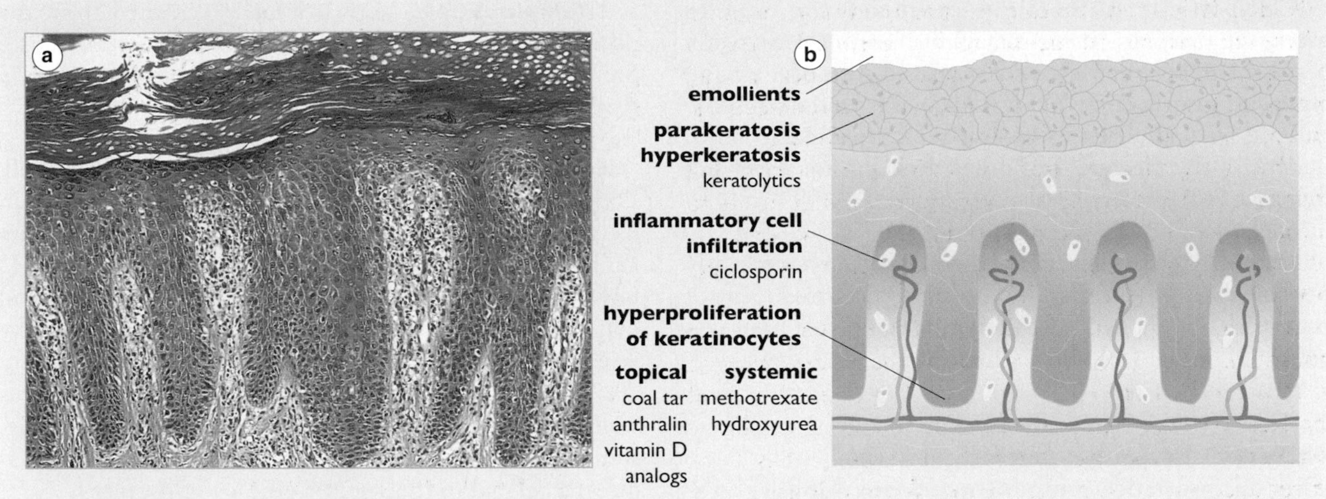

Fig. 18.4 Psoriasis. (a) Psoriasis is characterized by epidermal acanthosis, with clubbed papillae, suprapapillary thinning with dilation of the capillaries, and hyper- and parakeratosis. Lymphocytes predominate in the dermis, whereas neutrophils may form microabscesses in the epidermis. (Courtesy of Dr. P. McKee.) (b) Sites of drug action in psoriasis.

ticularly in those with fair skin. Most patients requiring anthralin are treated in daycare centers or as inpatients, so that a time commitment is required from the patients for the treatment to be worthwhile. Tar preparations often offer the best compromise between efficacy, ease of application, and tolerable mess and smell.

In patients with more widespread disease, combination therapy – in particular with light therapy – is often used. Again, to be effective, phototherapy demands committed patients, as treatment regimens involve hospital visits twice a week for 6–8 weeks.

In patients with associated psoriatic arthropathy, and in patients where the extent of the disease is causing great disability, systemic therapy may be used. All systemic agents used for psoriasis – methotrexate, hydroxycarbamide, ciclosporin and acitretin – have potentially serious adverse effects, and the decision to embark on such treatment needs to be reached after careful discussion with patients, and with well-defined clinical justification.

Vitamin D

- ***The naturally occurring active metabolite of vitamin D_3 – 1α, 25-dihydroxyvitamin D_3 (calcitriol), and two synthetic analogs – calcipotriol and tacalcitol – are effective when applied topically in patients with psoriasis***

Vitamin D analogs inhibit epidermal proliferation, induce terminal keratinocyte differentiation and have antiinflammatory properties.

Vitamin D receptors (VDRs) occur in keratinocytes, melanocytes, Langerhans' cells, dermal fibroblasts, monocytes and T lymphocytes in normal skin. They belong to the large family of structurally related ligand-inducible transcription factors, which includes the retinoid receptors and thyroid hormone receptors (see Chs 11 and 22).

In psoriasis, there is increased expression of VDRs in the basal and suprabasal layers of the epidermis, as well as a marked increase in the density of VDR positivity in intraepidermal and perivascular T cells and macrophages.

The effects of vitamin D analogs include:

- Inhibition of T-cell proliferation by blocking the transition of T cells from the early to the late G_1 phase of the cell cycle.
- Inhibition of the release of various cytokines, including interleukins (IL)-2, IL-6, IL-8, interferon (IFN)-γ, tumor necrosis factor (TNF)-β, and granulocyte–macrophage colony stimulating factor (GM-CSF).
- A reduction in the capacity of monocytes to stimulate T-cell proliferation and lymphokine release from T cells.
- Reduced neutrophil accumulation in psoriatic skin.

The mechanism of action of these analogs has not yet been elucidated. A goal is to develop analogs that induce the expression of the vitamin D-responding genes governing Ca^{2+} homeostasis, and analogs that induce expression of the vitamin D-responding genes influencing the keratinocyte cell cycle. Clearly, for the treatment of skin disease, such vitamin D analogs should optimally affect the cell cycle and have a minimal effect on systemic Ca^{2+} homeostasis.

CALCIPOTRIENE is a vitamin D_3 analog (a side-chain modification of 1α, 25-dihydroxyvitamin D_3), available for the topical treatment of psoriasis as a cream, ointment and scalp solution. It is effective alone, and has been shown to have a sparing effect when used with ultraviolet light treatment, ciclosporin, methotrexate and retinoids. Calcium metabolism is not affected at doses of less than 100 g/week.

Calcipotriene is the drug of choice for mild to moderate psoriasis. Its non-staining formulation greatly improves patient compliance compared with coal tar and anthralin preparations. It causes facial irritation in some patients. Calcipotriene has also been reported to be of benefit in the treatment of other dyskeratotic states and pityriasis rubra pilaris.

TACALCITOL (1α, 24-dihydroxyvitamin D_3) has recently become available in the UK for the topical treatment of psoriasis. It is applied once daily, and in clinical trials was tolerated on the face and in the flexures.

Anthralin

The antipsoriatic component of goa powder was identified as chrysarobin, an easily oxidizable reduction product of chrysophanic acid, in 1878. The synthetic chrysarobin substitute anthralin was introduced in 1915. Anthralin is unique because it can lead to remission of psoriasis.

A challenge with anthralin formulations is achieving a compound which is stable in the reduced active form over long periods, but which oxidizes rapidly within tissue. This has traditionally been achieved using zinc and salicylic acid paste, but newer cream and liposomal formulations have been developed.

One limitation of anthralin compounds is that they cause irritation and staining.

Anthralin is available as a cream (0.1–2%) and ointment (0.1–2%) for home use. The treatment is usually applied for 30–60 minutes (short-contact anthralin therapy) and then removed. Anthralin paste is largely confined to hospital use where it can be applied for 24 hours, or shorter time periods. Anthralin must be applied to a test area first before treating the whole body, as patient tolerance varies. The strength of anthralin is gradually increased (e.g. doubling concentration every 3–5 days) and is discontinued when the plaques have flattened. Anthralin inevitably stains the skin. This stain can be removed with a keratolytic agent. It also stains clothing. Anthralin can be used in combination with light therapy and coal tar baths (Ingram regimen).

No systemic toxicity has been reported with anthralin. However, it is irritant to normal skin, and therefore must be applied accurately to the plaques of psoriasis.

Tar preparations

Therapeutic tars are products of the destructive distillation of wood, coal or bitumen. They are highly complex mixtures with some 10 000 constituents. Petroleum tars have no therapeutic importance.

WOOD TARS (oil of cade, bee, birch and pine) are available as ointments, pastes and alcoholic paints. They may sensitize, but do not photosensitize.

BITUMINOUS TARS were originally obtained from the distillation of shale deposits containing fossilized fish. Some have a high sulfur content. They are less effective than coal tars and do not photosensitize.

COAL TAR is a black fluid with a characteristic smell. Different methods of distilling heated coal have been used to try to remove its color and odor. Coal tar modifies keratinization but its mechanism of action is poorly understood. The high boiling-point tar acids (phenolics) may be responsible for its therapeutic effect, possibly by releasing lysosomes in the granular layer. Coal tars are also antipruritic (and are therefore used for eczema as well as psoriasis), mildly antiseptic and photosensitizing. Refined tars are less phototoxic, but phototoxicity is directly related to therapeutic efficacy in psoriasis.

The carcinogenicity of pitch and heavy tar fractions is well established, but malignant tumors are extremely rare in relation to tar therapy. A few cases of genital cancer have been reported, but a recent 24-year follow-up has shown that the incidence of skin tumors in patients using coal tar is not increased.

The photosensitizing potential of coal tars is exploited in the Goeckerman regimen (i.e. combination therapy with ultraviolet light B) for psoriasis, which reduces epidermal DNA synthesis, possibly by forming cross-links between opposite strands on the DNA double helix.

The most common adverse effect is an irritant folliculitis. Phototoxicity and contact allergic dermatitis can also occur.

Acitretin

Acitretin is the main active metabolite of etretinate, an aromatic retinoid with a slow terminal elimination phase of several months.

Acitretin has a decreased lipophilicity and reduced elimination half-life (50 hours rather than 80 days for etretinate), a potential advantage, particularly in women of child-bearing potential as the retinoids are highly teratogenic. However, in some patients reversed metabolism of acitretin to etretinate has been demonstrated, so that pregnancy must be avoided for at least 2 years after the ingestion of acitretin, as with its predecessor, etretinate.

Acitretin is used in the treatment of psoriasis, particularly erythrodermic and generalized pustular psoriasis, at doses of 0.5–1 mg/kg. Higher doses are needed for chronic plaque psoriasis, but its use in combination therapy with psoralen plus ultraviolet light A (PUVA) or ultraviolet light B is increasing because it has an ultraviolet light-sparing effect.

Acitretin has a narrow therapeutic window and at doses of 1 mg/kg adverse effects are common. Dryness of the lips, eyes and mucous membranes are frequent as is desquamation of palms and soles and skin burning sensations. Hair loss, nose bleeds and paronychia are often a nuisance and may limit the dose. More serious

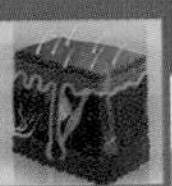

adverse effects include musculoskeletal effects resembling diffuse idiopathic skeletal hyperostosis. Prior and periodic radiographic screening is therefore advised for long-term use. As with isotretinoin, liver function and lipids should regularly be monitored.

In patients who cannot tolerate the usual therapeutic doses of acitretin, combination therapy can be considered. Acitretin has been used in combination with tar, dithranol, UVB and PUVA. Combination with methotrexate has been reported in difficult cases but these drugs pose potential interactions with increased blood levels of methotrexate and combined effects on liver toxicity. However, it is sometimes necessary to continue acitretin in a patient until the therapeutic effects of methotrexate are established since this takes 6 to 8 weeks.

It has been claimed that tumors, including solar keratoses, keratoacanthoma, epidermodysplasia verruciformis, basal cell epithelioma (BCE) and leukoplakia, sometimes disappear with isotretinoin or etretinate treatment. The use of retinoids in preventing skin tumors in high-risk patients, such as those with xeroderma pigmentosum and transplant patients, is currently being investigated in ongoing trials.

Methotrexate

Methotrexate exerts a strong antimitotic effect on keratinocytes by inhibiting DNA synthesis by competitive inhibition of dihydrofolate reductase (see Ch. 7). At doses used in the treatment of psoriasis, methotrexate also inhibits neutrophil chemotaxis. It is administered once a week for the treatment of psoriasis. Patients taking methotrexate must refrain totally from alcohol. Renal, hepatic and bone marrow function must be assessed prior to, and during, methotrexate treatment, and note should be taken of potential drug interactions.

Vitamin A analogs (see treatment of acne above)

Ciclosporin (see Eczema above)

Anti-TNF-α

Infliximab and eternacept, which both inhibit TNF-α (see Chs 9 and 15), have also been introduced for the treatment of psoriasis.

CD2 antagonists

Alefacept is an immunoglobulin G_1 dimer preparation that acts as an antagonist for CD2 or T cells. It is administered i.v. 7.5 mg with a half-life of 267 hours.

Photo(chemo)therapy

UVB therapy is effective in many patients with psoriasis. Other patients require stronger, PUVA photochemotherapy (psoralens + UVA). Psoralens are photoactivated chemicals that intercalate with DNA, forming cyclobutane adducts with pyrimidine in bases on subsequent exposure to ultraviolet light A. This forms the basis of PUVA photochemotherapy, an established treatment for psoriasis and mycosis fungoides, and possibly vitiligo.

Drugs acting on hair

Finasteride at 1 mg/mL has recently been launched for the treatment of male androgenic alopecia (see Ch. 17 for description of finasteride).

TOPICAL MINOXIDIL reverses androgenic alopecia in some patients. Its mechanism of action is unknown and its effect on androgenic alopecia is not permanent, with hair loss occurring within 4–6 months after it is stopped.

CYPROTERONE ACETATE plus ethinyl estradiol prevents the progression of androgenic alopecia in females.

Cyproterone acetate is the treatment of choice for female hirsutism. It is an antiandrogen and:

- Decreases adrenal androgen secretion.
- Competes with both testosterone and dihydrotestosterone for the androgen receptor.
- Inhibits the 5α-reductase enzyme.
- Inhibits luteinizing hormone secretion by its progestational effects.

A dose of 2 mg daily is sufficient, usually given in combination with an estrogen to ensure regular menstrual bleeding. An improvement may not be evident for 6–12 months. A male fetus can be feminized if a pregnancy occurs when cyproterone acetate is used alone.

LUTEINIZING HORMONE RELEASING HORMONE ANALOGS may improve hirsutism in patients with high androgen levels of ovarian origin.

DRUGS THAT MODIFY INFLAMMATORY RESPONSES IN THE SKIN

Glucocorticosteroids

Glucocorticosteroid effectiveness in skin diseases depends on:

- The skin disease (e.g. very effective in the treatment of lichen planus).
- The site to be treated (e.g. mild to moderate only for facial application).
- The age of the patient (e.g. the indications for a potent glucocorticosteroid in a child are limited).

In general, very potent glucocorticosteroids should be given to adults only under specialist supervision and should not be prescribed for children without consultation with a specialist.

Glucocorticosteroid penetration varies with:

- Body site. It is higher when applied to the genitals, face and scalp than when applied to the trunk and limbs.
- State of the skin. It is enhanced by the presence of erythema or skin erosion.
- Occlusion, which increases penetration at least tenfold.
- The vehicle used. Ointments produce greater penetration than creams.

- Drug concentrations. A high drug concentration produces higher penetration than a low concentration, but penetration is not proportional to concentration difference (e.g. increasing the concentration of hydrocortisone tenfold results in a fourfold increase in penetration).

Intralesional glucocorticosteroids are used for keloid and hypertrophic scars, chondrodermatitis nodularis helicis and acne cysts

Local injection is also sometimes helpful in alopecia areata and hypertrophic lichen planus that has not responded to topical glucocorticosteroids.

Intralesional administration of glucocorticosteroids overcomes the limited penetration of topical glucocorticosteroids and provides a high local concentration of glucocorticosteroid. Relatively insoluble glucocorticosteroids (e.g. triamcinolone acetonide, triamcinolone diacetate, triamcinolone hexacetonide, betamethasone acetate–phosphate) are used to achieve high local depots, which are gradually released for 3–4 weeks. The injections must be limited to 1 mg per site to avoid local skin atrophy.

Topical glucocorticosteroids are indicated for the treatment of inflammatory skin disorders and are a vital part of the acute treatment of most forms of dermatitis (eczema)

The potency of topical glucocorticosteroid used must be titrated to the disease severity and the minimum effective strength determined for each patient. In seborrheic dermatitis, a combination of glucocorticosteroids and antipityrosporal agents is useful to calm the eczema, but antipityrosporal agents used early in relapse should be sufficient.

Topical glucocorticosteroids are useful in the treatment of flexural psoriasis, but should not be used as a first-line treatment elsewhere, as a rebound exacerbation of the disease occurs on withdrawal. It is not uncommon for patients to require increasing doses of glucocorticosteroids to control the disease. If very potent glucocorticosteroids are then withdrawn, generalized pustular psoriasis can ensue, which is a medical emergency and often requires systemic treatment with agents such as methotrexate (see Ch. 7).

Potent topical glucocorticosteroids are used in the short term for treatment of vitiligo and alopecia areata, but are not continued for more than 4 weeks.

A trial of topical glucocorticosteroids is worthwhile for sarcoidosis, discoid lupus erythematosus and pemphigus, although systemic treatments are often necessary.

Systemic glucocorticosteroids are used for severe acute dermatoses, pemphigus, pemphigoid and lichen planus

Systemic glucocorticosteroids are used only for severe dermatologic diseases because the treatment benefits must outweigh the risks of long-term use (see Ch. 7). They are indicated for:

- Severe acute dermatoses such as anaphylaxis, acute contact allergic dermatitis, acute autoimmune connective tissue diseases and generalized vasculitis, and generalized drug eruptions.
- Chronic disabling disorders such as pemphigus and pemphigoid.
- Severe lichen planus.
- Pyoderma gangrenosum.
- Sarcoidosis.
- Various other unusual dermatoses.

All adverse effects of systemic glucocorticosteroids can be observed with significant systemic absorption of topical glucocorticosteroids

Local adverse reactions include worsening and spread of infection (viral, bacterial and fungal). Skin atrophy, striae, hirsutism, acne and depigmentation may occur with long-term use, and the application of potent glucocorticosteroids on the face induces a 'perioral dermatitis.'

Use of antimalarial drugs for the treatment of skin conditions

Hydroxychloroquine, chloroquine and mepacrine (see Ch. 6) have a beneficial effect on discoid and systemic lupus erythematosus, polymorphic light eruption and solar urticaria. There is evidence of a therapeutic response in cutaneous sarcoidosis and porphyria cutanea tarda. The mechanism of action of the drugs in these disorders is unknown, but they have been shown to:

- Inhibit prostaglandin synthesis, chemotaxis and hydrolytic enzymes.
- Stabilize membranes.
- Bind to DNA.

Sulfa drugs

Dapsone is the drug of choice in the treatment of leprosy. It is also used in the treatment of dermatitis herpetiformis, immunobullous disorders and numerous other rare dermatoses (see Ch. 6). Its mechanism of action is unclear, although neutrophils and immune complexes seem to be involved in the skin diseases influenced by the drug. Patients taking dapsone must be monitored for signs of hemolysis and methemoglobinemia. Hemolytic anemia is a common adverse reaction and, although rare, methemoglobinemia can be a rapidly fatal complication. Other sulfa drugs having some of the useful effects of dapsone are sulfapyridine and sulfamethoxypyridazine.

Other drugs modifying the immune response

Colchicine is an alkaloid derived from the autumn crocus (see Ch. 15) that:

- Inhibits neutrophil and monocyte chemotaxis, collagen synthesis and mast cell histamine release.

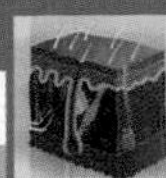

- Increases collagenolysis.
- Arrests mitosis in metaphase and is therefore antimitotic.

Colchicine has been used in the treatment of a variety of dermatologic diseases characterized by leukocyte infiltration of the skin, including Behçet's syndrome, psoriasis, palmoplantar pustulosis, dermatitis herpetiformis, Sweet's syndrome, necrotizing vasculitis, childhood dermatomyositis and systemic sclerosis.

Adverse effects include gastrointestinal disturbances, which are very frequent in patients taking relatively large doses of colchicine (see Ch. 15).

THALIDOMIDE is an immunomodulatory drug whose activities are not well characterized but may involve decreasing concentrations of TNF-α. It is used for the treatment of recalcitrant aphthous ulceration, especially in patients with HIV, and has been beneficial in the treatment of pyoderma gangrenosum and Behçet's syndrome. It is also efficacious in erythema nodosum leprosum.

Adverse effects include teratogenicity which may be profound. The drug is contraindicated in any woman who might become pregnant. Patients need to be closely monitored in order to detect neuropathy at an early stage, ideally while the problem is subclinical.

The kinetics of thalidomide are not well characterized; it has a half-life of 3–5 hours.

ORAL CONTRACEPTIVES Combination contraceptive pills containing cyproterone acetate, ethinyl estradiol and desogestrol are 'acne-friendly,' unlike most other contraceptive pills which tend to aggravate acne.

ALKYLATING AGENTS AND ANTIMETABOLITES Drugs such as alkylating agents and antimetabolites (see Ch. 6) are used in dermatology only if the disease is sufficiently disabling to justify the risk of their use (Table 18.7).

Table 18.7 Alkylating agents and antimetabolites used for the treatment of dermatologic diseases

Drug	Uses
Cyclophosphamide	Pemphigus, pemphigoid Wegener's granulomatosis Lupus erythematosus Polymyositis Mycosis fungoides Histiocytosis X
Chlorambucil	Mycosis fungoides Behçet's disease Lupus erythematosus Wegener's granulomatosis Glucocorticosteroid-resistant sarcoidosis
Mustine injection	Mycosis fungoides Sézary syndrome
Dacarbazine injection	Metastatic malignant melanoma
Methotrexate (given weekly; caution in the elderly and in patients with renal impairment)	Psoriasis Reiter's syndrome Pityriasis rubra pilaris Ichthyosiform erythroderma Sarcoidosis Pemphigus/pemphigoid Glucocorticosteroid-resistant dermatomyositis
Hydroxycarbamide (less effective than methotrexate)	Psoriasis
Azathioprine (glucocorticosteroid-sparing agent)	Pemphigus/pemphigoid Lupus erythematosus Dermatomyositis Wegener's granulomatosis Actinic reticuloid Pityriasis rubra pilaris Intractable eczema in adults
Bleomycin	Squamous cell carcinoma Mycosis fungoides and other lymphomas Viral warts (intralesional)
Melphalan	Scleromyxedema
Ciclosporin	Psoriasis Atopic dermatitis Pemphigus/pemphigoid Mycosis fungoides/Sézary syndrome
5-fluorouracil	Solar keratoses (topical) Keratoacanthoma (intralesional)

Their use is justified only if the disease is sufficiently disabling, since all of these drugs are potentially toxic, mutagenic and carcinogenic.

DRUGS THAT PROTECT THE SKIN FROM ENVIRONMENTAL DAMAGE

Sunscreens

The increasing occurrence of melanoma, nonmelanomatous skin cancers and skin aging has been associated with exposure to ultraviolet light. Sunburn before 10 years of age is a major risk factor for malignant melanoma. Photosensitivity can be a manifestation of some diseases and the use of certain drugs. These conditions are best prevented by sun avoidance or using physical barriers to solar penetration, such as clothing. If exposure is unavoidable, chemical sunscreens can be used to minimize exposure. The topical use of sunscreens reduces the risk of sunburn and probably prevents squamous cell carcinoma of the skin when used mainly during unintentional sun exposure. However, the use of sunscreens to extend the duration of intentional sun exposure may negate beneficial effects in preventing melanoma.

Sunscreens are classified as either absorbent or reflectant:

- Absorbent sunscreens are photo-absorbing chemicals and can be categorized according to the predominant active wavelength they filter (Table 18.8).
- Reflectant sunscreens are inert minerals such as titanium dioxide, zinc oxide, red petroleum and calamine. These are cosmetically less attractive because they are greasy and sticky and visible.

Table 18.8 Absorbent sunscreens and the predominant wavelength screened

Cinnamates	UVB
para-aminobenzoic acid	UVB
Salicylates	UVB
Benzophenones	UVA
Camphor	UVA
Dibenzoylmethane	UVA
Aminobenzoates (padimate O)	UVB
Anthralin	UVA

Ultraviolet (UV) A, 320–360 nm; UVB, 290–320nm.

Commercial preparations contain these ingredients in various proportions.

In practice, protection by sunscreens is about half that suggested by the skin protection factor

The efficacy of a sunscreen is expressed as the skin protection factor (SPF), which is the ratio of the time required to produce minimal erythema with a sunscreen to the time required without. The sun protection of a sunscreen is about half that suggested by the SPF in practice. This is because in laboratory tests to determine such protection, the amount of drug applied is much greater dose per unit area than the amount applied in practice. It is difficult to make allowances for loss of the sunscreen with sweating and swimming. Therefore:

- If the SPF is less than 10, the sunscreen is only mildly protective.
- If the SPF is 10–15, the sunscreen is moderately protective.
- If the SPF is higher than 15, the sunscreen will provide appreciable protection.
- If the SPF is higher than 25, the sunscreen will provide almost full protection, as required by patients with photosensitivity.

Sunscreen preparations have been refined to increase cosmetic acceptability, water resistance, durability and effectiveness. However, the active ingredients, the base, the fragrances and the stabilizer can all cause irritant, allergic, phototoxic or photoallergic adverse reactions.

Antiviral agents See also Chapter 6

Aciclovir cream can be used for primary or recurrent labial herpes simplex (cold sores) and for genital herpes simplex infections.

Penciclovir cream is a newer topical antiviral preparation which is licensed for labial herpes simplex infection. Both agents need to be used as early as possible in the outbreak and one study showed shortening of an attack by a mean of only 0.7 days using aciclovir cream.

Systemic therapy is recommended for vaginal or buccal infections, and for herpes zoster. In addition to reducing viral shedding and aiding healing, there is evidence that early antiviral treatment lessens the incidence of postherpetic neuralgia, which can be very disabling. Aciclovir is variably absorbed when orally administered. Consequently, in severe disease and in eczema herpeticum, parenteral administration is recommended. Prior to the development of antiviral agents, eczema herpeticum carried a significant mortality, and long-term eye damage caused considerable morbidity.

In adults, valaciclovir, a pro-drug with better bioavailability, has largely superseded aciclovir

Antiviral therapy can be life-saving for both chickenpox/shingles and herpes simplex infections in immunocompromised patients, and is sometimes used in this population for prophylaxis. It is generally inappropriate to treat immunocompetent patients with chickenpox, in whom the disease is milder.

Systemic aciclovir, valaciclovir and famciclovir decrease healing time and sometimes abort attacks of genital herpes. They are also useful in the treatment of varicella-zoster infections (i.e. chickenpox, shingles). In shingles, administration of antiviral therapy within 72 hours of onset of the rash shortens the duration of pain, as well as the rash, and reduces the incidence, severity and duration of chronic pain (postherpetic neuralgia). The risk of visual complications due to zoster affecting the ophthalmic branch of the fifth cranial nerve is also reduced by prompt treatment. Prophylactic aciclovir is indicated for immunocompromised patients and for patients who develop recurrent erythema multiforme after herpes infections.

Antibacterial agents

Topical antibiotics

Topical antibiotics (Table 18.9 and see Ch. 6) are used in the treatment of acne (see above).

Fusidic acid is active against *Staphylococcus aureus* on the skin and can be used to treat early superficial skin infections such as impetigo and folliculitis although systemic antibiotics are often necessary in these conditions. Fusidic acid resistance develops relatively rapidly, but, in the absence of the drug, re-colonization with fusidic acid-sensitive species occurs. Mupirocin is also active against *S. aureus*, including MRSA, but for this reason should probably be reserved for the treatment of MRSA. Linzinolid has also been introduced recently for the treatment of resistant organisms.

Nasal carriage of *S. aureus*, which can be the source of recurrent skin staphylococcal infection, is treated with neomycin and chlorhexidine. Nasal mupirocin can be used for resistant organisms. Silver sulfadiazine is often used in the prevention and treatment of infection in burn wounds. Sulfadiazine is a sulfonamide and some absorption occurs if extensive areas are treated (monitor for pancytopenia). Argyria has also been reported after prolonged use.

Topical metronidazole is used in the treatment of rosacea.

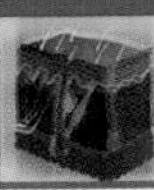

Table 18.9 Topical antibacterial drugs used in dermatology and their complications

Drug	Antibacterial spectrum	Uses	Complications
Bacitracin	Gram-positive organisms, anaerobic cocci, *Neisseria*, tetanus bacilli, diphtheria bacilli	Nasal staphylococcal carriers	Resistance with long-term use Contact allergic dermatitis Rarely contact urticaria
Gramicidin (available only in combination with neomycin, polymyxin, bacitracin, and nystatin)	As for bacitracin		Rarely contact allergic dermatitis
Mupirocin	Most Gram-positive aerobic bacteria including methicillin-resistant *Staphylococcus aureus* (MRSA)	Impetigo, nasal staphylococcal carriage	May cause irritation of nasal mucosa (contains propylene glycol)
Polymyxin B sulfate	Gram-negative organisms including *Pseudomonas*, *Escherichia coli*, *Enterobacter* and *Klebsiella*	Used in compound antibiotic preparations	Neurotoxic and nephrotoxic if systemically absorbed, therefore to be avoided in open wounds or denuded skin Contact dermatitis uncommon
Neomycin	Gram-negative organisms including *E. coli*, *Proteus*, *Klebsiella* and *Enterobacter*		Serum concentrations rarely detectable Contact dermatitis common with cross-sensitivity to streptomycin, kanamycin, paromomycin, gentamicin
Gentamicin	As for neomycin, but more effective against *Pseudomonas*, and active against staphylococci and group A hemolytic streptococci		Use of topical gentamicin should be limited because of concerns about the emergence of resistance Neurotoxic, nephrotoxic and ototoxic if absorbed Detected in plasma if applied to a large skin area, especially if denuded skin
Clindamycin	*Propionibacterium acnes*	Acne	10% absorption Rarely pseudomembranous colitis Skin irritation with alcohol vehicle, less with gel
Erythromycin	*P. acnes*	Acne	Resistance increasing Combinations are claimed to reduce emergence of resistant strains
Frythromycin in combination with benzoyl peroxide			
Erythromycin in combination with zinc acetate			
Metronidazole		Rosacea	Drying, burning, stinging
Tetracyclines (tetracycline, meclocycline)	*P. acnes*	Acne	Temporary yellow staining of skin Photosensitivity has not been a problem, but phototoxic Contraindicated in pregnancy, and in renal and hepatic disease

Systemic antibiotics

The majority of patients with cellulitis give the typical history of severe flu-like symptoms preceding, by 12–36 hours, any symptoms in the affected part, which then becomes red, warm and swollen, characteristics of streptococcal infection. The drug of choice is systemic penicillin. Rarely, staphylococcal infections cause cellulitis in debilitated, immunodeficient or diabetic patients. In these cases antistaphylococcal antibiotics should accompany the penicillin. Erythromycin should be used for patients who are penicillin allergic. Despite adequate antibiotic therapy, the signs may take several weeks to resolve. The temptation to change antibiotic therapy if the cellulitis is not spreading should be resisted. The time to resolution is least in patients who are treated adequately as soon as symptoms develop. Patients who have had one episode of cellulitis should be warned that they are at increased risk of a second attack and that antibiotic therapy should be sought immediately. Consideration should be given to continuing penicillin V longer term, e.g. 250 mg b.d. for 3–6 months, as second, and indeed, sequential attacks of streptococcal cellulitis are so common.

Antifungal agents

There are many topical and systemic antifungal agents for the treatment of skin, hair and nail infections with fungi and yeasts (see Ch. 6). Flutrimazole and sertaconazole are sterol demethylase inhibitors recently introduced for treatment of skin infections.

Antiseptic agents

Antiseptic agents (Table 18.10) may obviate the need for antibiotics.

Antiparasite preparations

Aqueous preparations of these drugs (Table 18.11) are preferred in the treatment of scabies as the alcoholic lotions used are irritant. A single application is usually sufficient, but an application on two or three consecutive days is needed for hyperkeratotic scabies. All members of the household must be treated at the same time. Applications are usually applied from the neck down, but treatment of the scalp, face and neck is recommended for children under 2 years of age, elderly patients,

Table 18.10 Antiseptic agents

Drug name	Uses	Comments
Chlorhexidine	Antiseptic skin cleanser	Alcoholic solutions not suitable before diathermy
Benzalkonium chloride	Antiseptic skin cleanser	
Triclosan	Antiseptic skin cleanser	
Potassium permanganate 1:10 000 solution	Antiseptic skin cleanser, astringent	
Cetrimide	Disinfectant and detergent properties	Occasional sensitizer
Hydrogen peroxide	Disinfectant used for deep wounds and ulcers	
Streptokinase–streptodornase and dextranomer preparations	Aid ulcer desloughing, which helps eradicate local infection	
Povidone-iodine	Disinfectant, less irritant	Caution in pregnancy, breast-feeding and renal impairment. Application to large wounds or severe burns may produce systemic effects such as metabolic acidosis, hypernatremia and renal impairment. Avoid regular use in patients with thyroid disease or those receiving lithium therapy. Rarely sensitivity
Hexachlorphene	Irritant	Avoid in neonates and large raw surfaces Avoid in pregnancy Can cause sensitivity and, rarely photosensitivity
Chlorinated solutions, e.g. dilute hypochlorite solution		No longer recommended because of irritancy, bleaches clothing

Table 18.11 Antiparasite preparations

Drug	Disease	Mechanism	Adverse effects
Lindane	Scabies (head lice resistance high so no longer recommended) Crab lice		Avoid in pregnancy, breast-feeding mothers, patients with low body weight, young children and those with a history of epilepsy
Malathion	Scabies: kills both adult lice and ova in vitro Head lice Crab lice	Organophosphate cholinesterase inhibitor	
Permethrin	Scabies Lice (but resistance increasing)	Neurotoxic	
Benzyl benzoate			Irritant, avoid in children
5% precipitate of sulfur in petrolatum			Rarely used because of odor and staining It is possible alternative for treating pregnant women and infants
Carbaryl	Head lice		

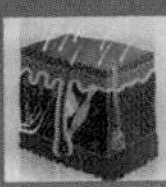

immunocompromised patients and those for whom a previous treatment has failed. Benzyl benzoate may require up to three applications on consecutive days.

Patients should be told that the itch of scabies can persist for several weeks and that itching does not necessarily indicate treatment failure.

For head lice, both malathion and carbaryl should be used as lotions rather than shampoos, and left in contact with the scalp for 12 hours. Aqueous formulations are preferred for asthmatic patients and small children to avoid alcoholic fumes. The treatment should be repeated after 7 days to kill lice emerging from any eggs that might have survived the first application.

For crab lice, treatment should be applied to the whole body for 12 hours, and repeated 7 days later.

Insect repellents

These agents repel insects primarily by vaporization of the active ingredients diethyltoluamide and dimethyl phthalate. The duration of action is limited by the rate of vaporization and washing and rubbing off. Few of the preparations currently available are effective for more than a few hours. Allergic reactions can develop, especially with prolonged use.

Barrier preparations

Barrier creams have been developed to protect the skin from irritants (e.g. in industry, for patients with dermatitis). They rely on:

- Water-repellent substances (e.g. silicones).
- Soaps.
- Impermeable deposits such as titanium, zinc and calamine.

Their efficacy is limited because they must be removable by washing and cannot be so occlusive that they block pores and follicles. They have a role in protecting skin from discharges and secretions and are used for diaper rash and colostomies.

Bandages and dressings

A variety of bandages and dressings are prescribable and play an important role in the management of skin problems. Medicated bandages impregnated with zinc paste, with or without coal tar/ichthammol are useful in the management of eczema, acting as an emollient, antipruritic and barrier to scratching. Bandages containing calamine and clioquinol and fabric dressings impregnated with povidone-iodine, chlorhexidine, framycetin, sodium fusidate and paraffin are also available.

Silicone gel sheets are clear, soft and semi-occlusive, and conform well to awkward contours of the body. They have a role in the treatment of hypertrophic scars. Their mechanism of action is not fully understood: pressure, temperature of the scar and oxygen tension within the scar are not involved, and it is currently believed that the gel may work by promoting scar hydration.

DRUGS ACTING ON SKIN CONSTITUENTS

Drugs acting on keratinocytes

Urea makes creams and lotions feel less greasy, increases the hydration of the stratum corneum (concentration, 2–20%) and is a keratolytic (20%). A concentration of 30–50% urea with occlusion can be used to soften the nail plate before nail avulsion.

Urea appears to act by modifying prekeratin and keratin, leading to increased solubilization. It may also cleave the hydrogen bonds that keep the stratum corneum intact. It is absorbed percutaneously, but is a natural product of metabolism, and is excreted in urine without systemic toxicity.

Adverse effects include irritation and stinging, especially with occlusion and in the perineal area. Hyaluronidase and diclofenac sodium (3%) are used in combination topically to treat solar keratosis. S-aminolevulinic acid and methyl aminolevulinate are used as part of photodynamic therapy to photosensitize the skin to treat premalignant keratosis. These drugs are thought to act as oxidizing agents.

SALICYLIC ACID Low concentrations (up to 2%) of salicylic acid are used in the treatment of acne (see above). Higher concentrations (up to 50%) can be used to eradicate warts and calluses, but are contraindicated in patients with diabetes mellitus or peripheral vascular disease because they can induce ulceration. Salicylic acid is absorbed percutaneously (see above).

PROPYLENE GLYCOL is keratolytic at a concentration of 40–70% and is useful in the treatment of hyperkeratotic conditions such as palmoplantar keratoderma, psoriasis, pityriasis rubra pilaris and hypertrophic lichen planus. Propylene glycol also increases the water content of the stratum corneum. This hygroscopic action encourages the development of an osmotic gradient through the stratum corneum, increasing the hydration of the outermost layers and drawing water out of the inner layers of the skin. Propylene glycol can be used alone or in a gel with 6% salicylic acid. It has the advantage of minimal absorption, and what is absorbed is oxidized in the liver to lactic acid and pyruvic acid, which are then used in general metabolism. Its major adverse effect is irritancy, and it can cause contact allergic dermatitis.

PODOPHYLLUM RESIN is an alcoholic extract of *Podophyllum peltatum*, used in the treatment of condyloma acuminatum and plantar warts. Podophyllotoxin and its derivatives are cytotoxic agents that act on the microtubule proteins of the mitotic spindle, preventing normal assembly of the spindle and arresting epidermal mitoses in metaphase. The tincture needs to be applied accurately on wart tissue so as to prevent severe erosion of the surrounding normal skin, allowing a contact time of 2–3 hours (possibly increasing to 6–8 hours if tolerated) for 3–5 applications only. If this is not successful, alternative treatment modalities should be considered as the resin is absorbed and distributed in lipids, including those in the central nervous system. If extensive areas need treatment they should be treated in sections to minimize absorption, particularly from intertriginous areas and large moist warts.

Adverse effects include nausea, vomiting, muscle weakness, neuropathy and even coma and death. Local irritation is common. Podophyllum resin is contraindicated during pregnancy because of its possible cytotoxic effects on the fetus. Imiquimod is a novel immunomodulator used for the treatment of genital warts. The precise mechanism of action of this drug has yet to be elucidated.

Drugs acting on nerves

Topical nonsteroidal antiinflammatory drugs and capsaicin can relieve pain

Local pain can be transiently relieved by topical nonsteroidal antiinflammatory drugs (NSAIDs) (see Ch. 6), while capsaicin (0.075%) cream is licensed for the treatment of postherpetic neuralgia. Capsaicin is a naturally occurring alkaloid found in fruits and capsicum. Crude extracts of capsicum or capsicum oleo-resin contain small amounts of capsaicin and a number of co-capsaicinoids, which are thought to cause the counter-irritant erythematous reaction that accompanies the application of these extracts. Capsaicin itself acts by depleting sensory C fibers of neuropeptides, particularly substance P. It is not a traditional counterirritant and does not induce vasodilation.

Recently, capsaicin has also been reported to activate vanilloid receptors on sensory nerves and it is possible that this activation renders the vanilloid receptor desensitized to endogenous activators which include low pH, heat and certain lipid mediators generated during the inflammatory process.

Topical applications relieve itch, partly by a cooling effect

Phenol, menthol and camphor are often added to topical applications to relieve itch and probably act as weak local anesthetics. Calamine, astringents such as aluminum acetate and tannic acid, and coal tar also have some topical antipruritic effect.

Itch may be relieved systemically by histamine H_1 antagonists (see eczema)

Hypnotics, chlorpromazine, trimeprazine and sedative antidepressants are sometimes helpful in the treatment of pruritus, possibly because they alter the perception of itch.

CAMOUFLAGE CREAMS

Camouflage creams contain titanium dioxide in an ointment base with a variety of color shades that can be matched to the site and skin color of the patient. The best results are achieved by camouflage consultants.

FURTHER READING

Beck LA. The efficacy and safety of tacrolimus ointment: A clinical review. *Journal of the American Academy of Dermatology* 2005; **53**: Supplement 2, S165–S170.

Carrasco DA, Vander Straten M, Tyring SK. A review of antibiotics in dermatology. *J Cutan Med Surg* 2002; **6**: 128–150.

Feldman SR, Kimball BA, Krueger GG et al. Etanercept improves the health-related quality of life of patients with psoriasis: results from a phase III randomized controlled trial. *Journal of the American Academy of Dermatology* 2005; **53**: 887–889.

Gottlieb AB. Therapeutic options in the treatment of psoriasis and atopic dermatitis. *Journal of the American Academy of Dermatology* 2005; **53**: Supplement 1, S3–S16.

Haider A, Shaw JC. Treatment of acne vulgaris, *JAMA* 2004; **292**: 726–735.

Krueger G, Ellis CN. Psoriasis—recent advances in understanding its pathogenesis and treatment. *Journal of the American Academy of Dermatology* 2005; **53**: Supplement 1, S94–S100.

Morison WL. Photosensitivity. *N Engl J Med* 2004; **350**: 1111–1117.

Schön MP, Boehncke WH. Medical Progress: Psoriasis. *N Engl J Med* 2005; **352**: 1899–1912, May 5, 2005.

Simons FER. Drug Therapy: Advances in H1-Antihistamines. *N Engl J Med* 2004; **351**: 2203–2217

Wellington K, Jarvis B. Topical pimecrolimus: A review of its clinical potential in the management of atopic dermatitis. *Drugs* 2002; **62**: 817–840.

Williams HC. Atopic Dermatitis. *N Engl J Med* 2005; **352**: 2314–2324.

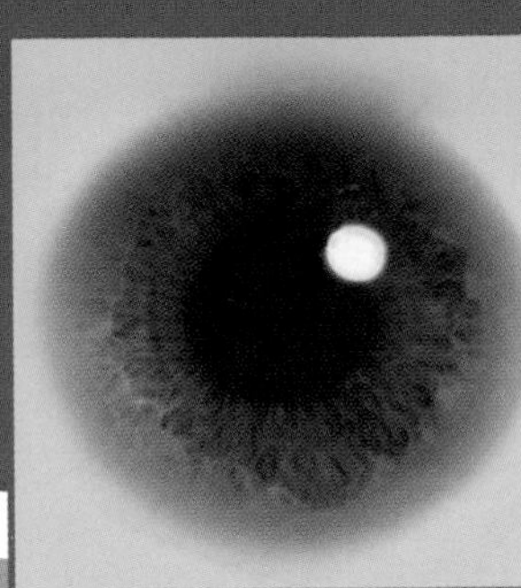

Chapter 19

Drugs and the Eye

BIOLOGY OF THE EYE AND PRINCIPLES OF DRUG USE FOR THE EYE

Structure and physiology of the eye

The eye focuses images from the external world onto the retina and converts them into electrical signals that are perceived by the brain. Since vision is a major sense, large areas of the brain are used for processing the information produced by the outposts of the central nervous system, the two retinae. The retinae are contained within the eyeballs and are connected to the rest of the central nervous system by the optic nerves.

The spherical eyeball is an organ of about 25 mm in diameter. It contains a lens and two fluid-filled chambers, and is enclosed by four layers of specialized tissue (Fig. 19.1):

- Cornea and sclera (an outer covering).
- Uveal tract containing the iris, ciliary body and choroid.

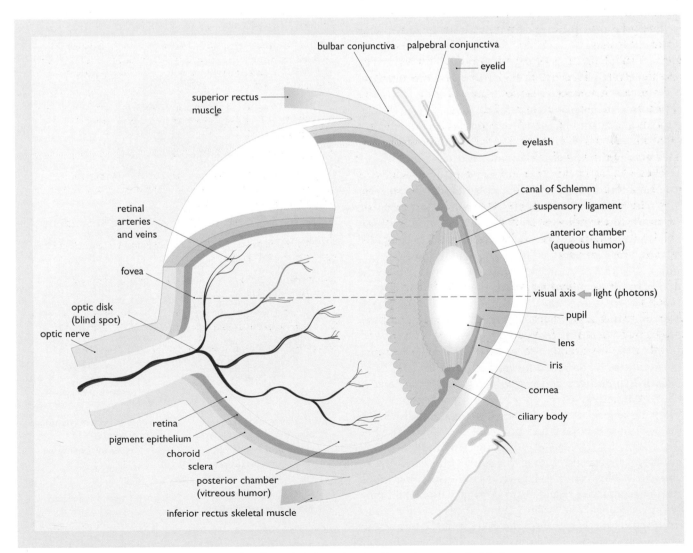

Fig. 19.1 Anatomy of the eye. A cross-section through the eye showing the major anatomical features.

- Pigment epithelium.
- Retina.

The most anterior part of the eye around the eyeball is the bulbar conjunctiva which also lines the inside of the eyelid where it becomes the palpebral conjunctiva.

The cornea is the transparent tissue at the front of the eye that allows light to enter the eyeball. It contains fine sensory fibers. The majority of the refractive power of the eye is at the air/corneal interface. The sclera, a continuation of the cornea, is the tough, protective coat of the eye (the white of the eye) while the uveal tract is a layer of tissue beneath the sclera. From the front of the eye to the back, the uveal tract forms the iris (a pigmented smooth muscle), the ciliary body and the choroid (a vascular bed beneath the retina). The retina is neural tissue and contains the photoreceptor cells (rods and cones). It forms the innermost layer of the eyeball. In order to reach the photoreceptor cells of the retina light must travel through the cornea, through the fluid-filled anterior chamber, the lens, the fluid-filled posterior chamber, and the cellular layers of the retina. Obviously, all the tissues in this pathway must be transparent in order to allow light to pass through. Any condition that reduces the transparency of one or more of such tissues will reduce vision.

The eye is moved within the orbit by six extraocular muscles

The six extraocular muscles are:

- The medial and lateral rectus muscles on either side of the eye.
- The superior rectus and oblique muscles above the eye.
- The inferior rectus and oblique muscles below the eye.

These striated (skeletal) muscles are under the control of motor (efferent) neurons in the oculomotor, trochlear and abducens nerves (the third, fourth and sixth cranial nerves, respectively). The extraocular muscles are unusual in that they are multiply innervated. Unlike the majority of mammalian striated fibers, which have between one and three neuromuscular end-plates, multiple innervated fibers, such as the rectus muscle, can have up to 80 end-plates per fiber.

Pupil size is controlled by light and reflex parasympathetic and sympathetic autonomic nerve system activity

High light levels reaching the retina cause constriction (miosis) of the pupil (the open center of the iris) while low light levels lead to dilation (mydriasis). Light entering one eye also causes the pupil of the other eye to constrict. This reflex is known as the consensual pupil response, and is a result of processing within the brain. It only occurs if the brain is able to process the visual information it receives from the two retinae. The consensual pupil response is therefore a useful diagnostic tool for assessing brain damage in comatose or unconscious patients. A small flashlight can be used to test for this reflex.

Activity in the parasympathetic nervous system maintains the tone of the iris such that, when it is increased, miosis results. Sympathetic stimulation (the 'fright, flight, and fight' response) causes mydriasis as does a reduced parasympathetic activity although the latter is predominant in controlling iris size.

The dilator pupillae (the radial smooth muscle of the iris) is innervated by sympathetic autonomic nerve system via fibers from the superior cervical ganglion. The neurotransmitter is norepinephrine and it acts upon α_1 adrenoceptors to produce limited pupil dilation. Drugs that are α_1 adrenoceptor agonists therefore contract the dilator pupillae and cause mydriasis (Fig. 19.2).

The constrictor pupillae (the sphincteric smooth muscle of the iris) is innervated by parasympathetic fibers arising from the ciliary ganglion. The parasympathetic nervous system neurotransmitter acetylcholine acts upon muscarinic receptors in the constrictor pupillae. Drugs that block muscarinic acetylcholine receptors are therefore also mydriatics (i.e. produce mydriasis).

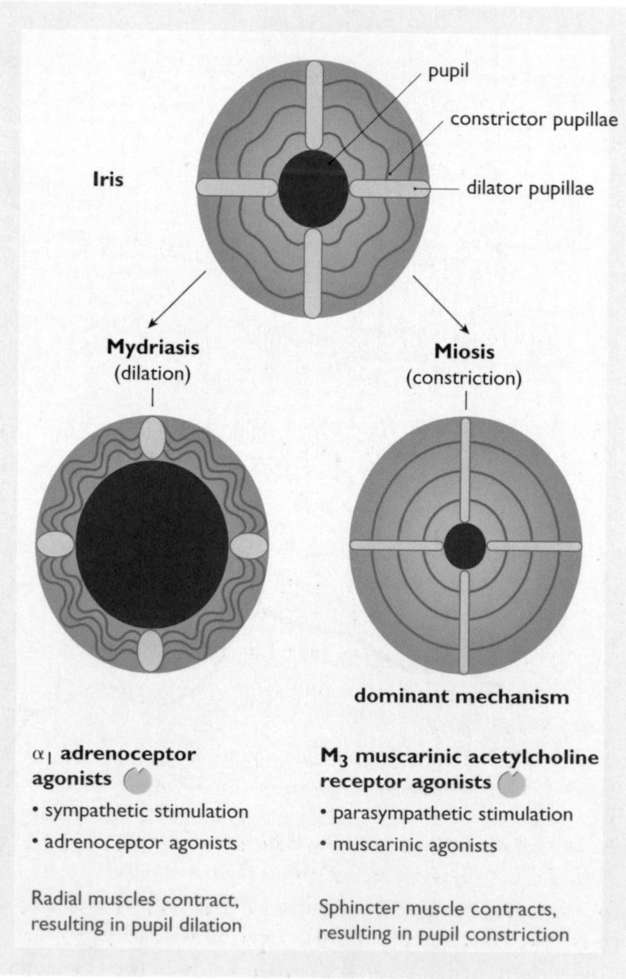

Fig. 19.2 Smooth muscle mechanisms involved in controlling pupil size.

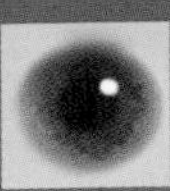

Drugs that are clinically useful in causing miosis are confined to muscarinic agonists and anticholinesterases and are known as miotics. Adrenoceptor antagonists such as phentolamine are miotics, but have little clinical value when used for such purposes in the eye because of the limited role of norepinephrine in controlling pupil iris size.

Some drugs acting within the central nervous system alter pupil size. For example, opioid receptor agonists, such as morphine, produce characteristic 'pinhole' pupils.

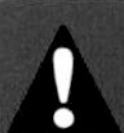

Effects of neuromuscular blocking drugs and the eye

- The multiply innervated muscle found in extraocular muscles contract in response to depolarizing neuromuscular blockers such as succinylcholine (see Chs 8 and 21), and intraocular pressure can increase as a result
- In the normal eye this may not be a problem because succinylcholine is normally very short acting
- If the eye has a penetrating injury, the ocular contents may prolapse as a result of extraocular muscle contracture

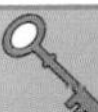

Causes of mydriasis (pupil dilation)

- Low light levels**
- Muscarinic receptor antagonists **
- Sympathetic stimulation*
- α_1 adrenoceptors agonists acting on the radial muscles of the iris

* Limited response
** Strong response

Causes of miosis (pupil constriction)

- High light levels**
- Parasympathetic stimulation**
- Directly or indirectly (anticholinesterases) acting muscarinic receptors agonists **
- Opiates acting in the central nervous system**
- α_1 adrenoceptor antagonists*

* Limited response
** Strong response

Accommodation is the mechanism whereby an image is focused upon the retina

Accommodation is the ability of the eye to change its refractive power and bend a path of light. Refractive power is usually measured in units of optical refraction known as diopters. The majority of the refractive power of the eye is located at the air/corneal interface and thus is fixed, and not adjustable. However, a small proportion of the refractive power can be varied as result of the ability of the lens to change its radius of curvature.

The lens is suspended in the eyeball from the ciliary muscle by suspensory ligaments. When the ciliary muscle relaxes, these suspensory ligaments are taut and stretch the lens into an ellipsoid shape. The low radius of curvature of the lens focuses distant objects onto the retina (for far, or distant vision). When the ciliary muscles contract, as a result of parasympathetic stimulation, and releasing acetylcholine to act upon muscarinic receptors, the suspensory ligaments relax and the lens takes on a more spherical shape. The curvature of the lens therefore increases and focuses near objects onto the retina (for near vision). The requirement of almost continuous contraction of ciliary muscles to accommodate for near vision explains why eyes get 'tired' after reading for long periods of time.

During accommodation for near vision, the pupils constrict, thereby confining light rays to the center of the lens, so reducing spherical aberration and thus improving the quality of the retinal image. This reflex is the accommodation pupil reflex. Drugs that block accommodation are often termed 'cycloplegics' and are exclusively muscarinic antagonists. There are no adrenergic receptors on ciliary muscle and therefore accommodation is not altered by sympatholytic nor sympathomimetic drugs.

The maximum ability to accommodate (of the order of 12 diopters) is seen in youth and young adulthood, and then it gradually decreases with age as the lens becomes less flexible. By age 50, the accommodative power of the lens reduces to 1 or 2 diopters. Thus, older people are generally 'long sighted' and need reading glasses, a natural condition of aging known as 'presbyopia.'

Aqueous humor production is a continuous process

The anterior chamber of the eyeball is filled with a watery fluid called aqueous humor. This is continually produced by blood vessels in the ciliary body at a rate of 3 mL/day. It flows first into the posterior chamber and then through the pupil into the anterior chamber (Fig. 19.3). Most of the aqueous humor drains into the episcleral veins via the trabecular meshwork, and the canal of Schlemm. Some 10% of the aqueous humor drains through the uveoscleral outflow tract into the circulation by a trans-scleral route.

The rate of production and subsequent drainage of aqueous humor is responsible for maintaining the intraocular pressure within its normal range of 12–20 mmHg. The production of aqueous humor is indirectly related to blood pressure and blood flow in the ciliary body. As occurs elsewhere in other vasculature, activation of α_1 adrenoceptors constricts blood vessels in the ciliary body. On the other hand, circulating epinephrine acting on β adrenoceptors in the ciliary body increases the production of aqueous humor. In addition, there may also be α_2 adrenoceptors located on the ciliary body that

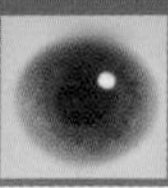

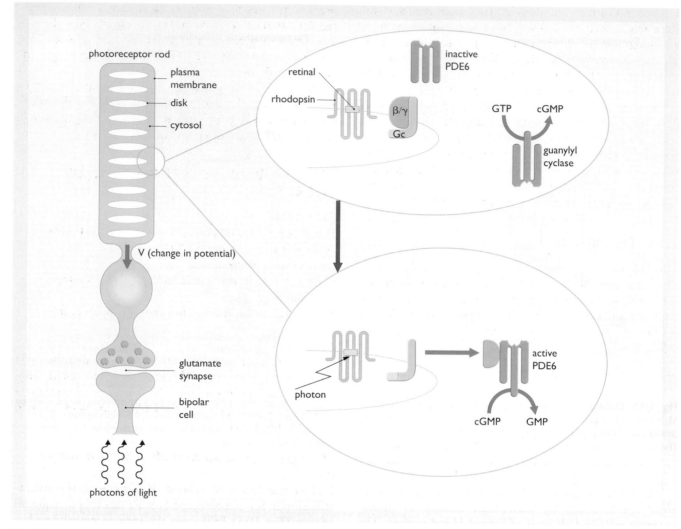

Fig. 19.5 Mechanisms of phototransduction in rod cells.

anchoring β/γ subunits, leading to activation of PDE6 and a consequent fall in cGMP concentrations.

In the plasma membranes of photoreceptor cells there is a special class of ion channels which are dependent upon cGMP binding for opening (so-called cGMP-gated channels). In the presence of cGMP, these channels allow the entry of cations into photoreceptor cells (so-called dark current), leading to depolarization. As with most neuronal cells, depolarization results in the opening of voltage-gated calcium channels located at presynaptic terminals, so releasing the neurotransmitter glutamate. Consequently, in the absence of light (i.e. dark, since photoreceptor cells contain relatively high concentrations of cGMP, the photoreceptor cells are depolarized and release neurotransmitter.

Conversely, in the presence of light, the PDE6 is activated, resulting in an increased conversion of cGMP to the inactive GMP molecule so that there is a fall in cGMP concentration. In consequence, the cGMP-gated ion channels carrying the dark current close. The photoreceptor cell hyperpolarizes, thereby closing the voltage-gated calcium channels on the presynatic terminal, so reducing glutamate release. Therefore, in the presence of light, photoreceptor cells have low cGMP concentrations, are hyperpolarized and are not releasing neurotransmitter. Therefore, at the first synapse of the visual system the presence of light is signaled by a decrease in glutamate release.

The next cells in the signaling chain, namely bipolar cells, fall broadly into two classes. ON-bipolar cells are those which respond to the cessation of neurotransmitter by depolarizing, whereas OFF-bipolar cells respond to the cessation of glutamate stimulation by hyperpolarizing. Therefore, the retina, at a very early stage in visual processing, actively codes both light and dark in parallel 'ON' and 'OFF' channels.

Different areas of the visual field have different functions

Although the image produced at the macula lutea and fovea is the most detailed, the visual field extends some 200° binocularly. Most of the peripheral retina functions

Table 19.7 Use of α adrenoreceptor agonists in the treatment of glaucoma

Drug	Receptor subtype	Adverse effects not expected from mechanism of action	Comments
Epinephrine	α and β	Black cornea	Endogenous neurohormone
Dipivefrin	α and β		Pro-drug of epinephrine (see Fig. 19.6)
Clonidine	α_2		Little used due to systemic adverse effects
Apraclonidine	α_2	Conjunctivitis Dermatitis	Less systemically active analog of clonidine
Brimonidine	α_2	Fatigue Drowsiness	

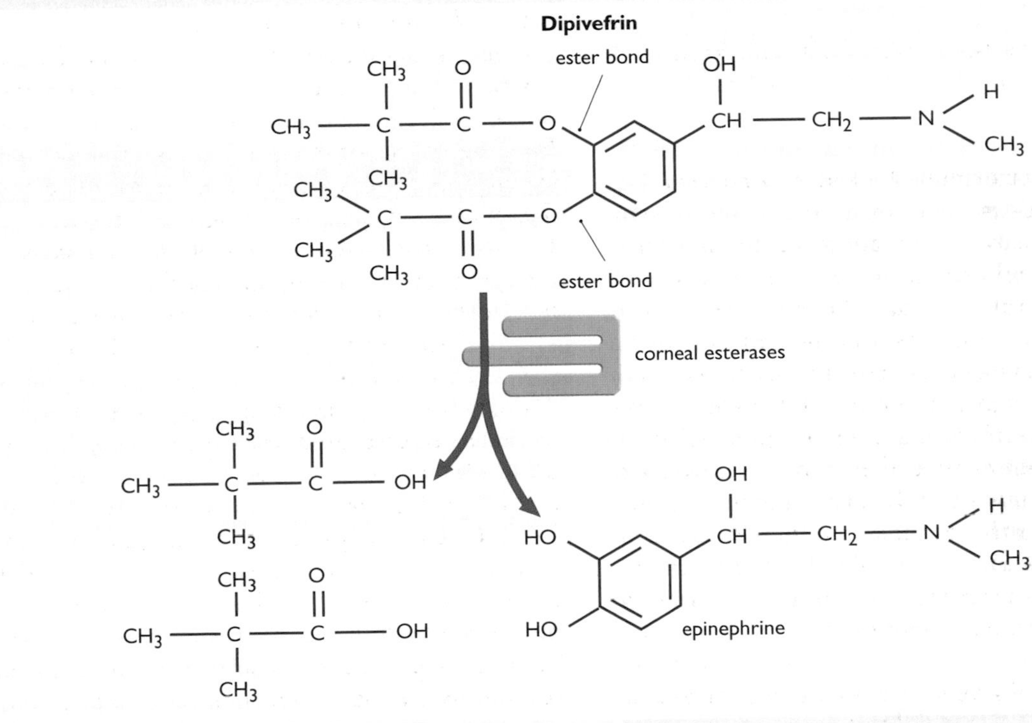

Fig. 19.6 The pro-drug dipivefrin, which is broken down to release epinephrine.

Ch. 13). The mechanism of action of apraclonidine, like that for epinephrine, in lowering IOP is unclear. A number of possibilities have been proposed:

- Activation of α_2 adrenoceptors in the ciliary body reduces aqueous humor formation directly.
- Activation of α_1 adrenoceptors reduces ciliary blood flow in a manner similar to epinephrine. Although apraclonidine is an α_2 selective agonist, it also activates α_1 receptors at high concentrations.
- Activation of presynaptic α_2 'autoreceptors' leads to decreased norepinephrine release and therefore reduced aqueous humor production following diminished postsynaptic β receptor stimulation.

The adverse effects of apraclonidine include those expected from an α receptor agonist: namely, hyperemia, eyelid retraction, vasoconstriction of the conjunctiva (blanching) and mydriasis.

Carbonic anhydrase inhibitors

Carbonic anhydrase inhibitors are drugs that are orally active in patients with glaucoma (Table 19.8). The conversion of carbon dioxide and water to carbonic acid (and therefore bicarbonate) is catalyzed by the enzyme carbonic anhydrase. Conversion, in the absence of carbonic anhydrase, is slow but it is up to 10 000-fold higher depending on the particular isoform of the enzyme. Since the production of aqueous humor depends on the active transport of bicarbonate and Na^+ ions, reducing the activity of carbonic anhydrase decreases aqueous humor production.

Acetazolamide, a sulfonamide derivative developed in the 1950s, is a carbonic anhydrase inhibitor that is effective in reducing IOP. However, because of its adverse effects, it is not well tolerated. Adverse effects, particularly in the elderly, include paresthesia, hypokalemia,

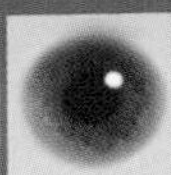

to detect movement and thereby trigger the eye to center on a new visual stimulus. For example, if something appears in the peripheral visual field of someone who is reading the reader may detect the movement but will only identify what has entered their visual field if they look up and center their fovea on that object.

Peripheral vision is also responsible for low light vision since most of the rod photoreceptors (responsible for night vision) are located outside the fovea. Loss of peripheral vision is termed 'tunnel vision' and is often associated with genetic retinal disease such as retinitis pigmentosa. Other diseases such as glaucoma and diabetes mellitus can also degrade the visual fields.

DISEASES OF THE EYE

Some of the many diseases of the eye are listed in Table 19.1. Only those that are treatable with drugs are discussed in this chapter. Despite claims to the contrary, there is no clear clinical evidence that drug treatment, or vitamin supplementation, prevents or cures cataracts, or genetic retinal dystrophy, although possible useful responses are seen in age-related macular degeneration where diet supplementation with vitamins C and E as well as β carotene has been claimed to reduce the risk of progression of the disease (AREDS trial) although the evidence is limited.

Drug therapy of glaucoma, inflammation of the eye, age-related macular degeneration, oculomotor disorders, tear deficiency and infections of the eye are varyingly effective and all are discussed in the chapter.

Table 19.1 Diseases of the eye and the various modes of treatment

Disease	Drugs	Surgery	None
Open-angle glaucoma	✓	–	–
Closed-angle glaucoma	✓	✓	–
Inflammation and allergic conditions	✓	–	–
Squints and oculomotor disorders	✓	✓	–
Tear deficiency	✓	–	–
Infections	✓	–	–
Detached retina	–	✓	–
Cataracts	–	✓	–
Retinitis pigmentosa	–	–	✓
Amblyopia	–	–	✓
Retinopathy	–	–	✓

PATHOPHYSIOLOGY OF DISEASES OF THE EYE

Glaucoma

■ *Glaucoma is caused by poor drainage of aqueous humor and can cause blindness*

Glaucoma is characterized by:

- An increase in intraocular pressure to more than 21 mmHg.
- Changes in the fundus, in particular optic disk 'cupping'.
- Visual field changes.

If untreated, glaucoma permanently damages the optic nerve and this can cause blindness. The two main types of glaucoma are open-angle (simple) and closed-angle glaucoma. The angle refers to the filtration angle formed between iris and cornea.

Characteristics of open-angle and closed-angle glaucoma

Open-angle glaucoma is a chronic disease that is primarily treated with drugs. The primary pathologic defect is reduced drainage of the aqueous humor into the canal of Schlemm. There is evidence that this reduced drainage can have congenital causes. Two rationales underlie the use of drugs to change the inadequate drainage. The first is to reduce the production of aqueous humor, the second is to increase its drainage (Table 19.2).

Closed-angle glaucoma results from forward ballooning of the peripheral iris (iris bombé) so that it touches the back of the cornea, thereby reducing flow of aqueous

Table 19.2 Drugs used to treat glaucoma

Type	Mechanism	Drug example	Comments
Decrease aqueous humor formation			
β adrenoceptor antagonists	Block β_1 receptor on ciliary body	Timolol maleate	First-line treatment
α adrenoceptor agonist	Agonist of prejunctional α_2 receptors and/or α_1 (vasoconstrictor) receptors on ciliary vessels	Apraclonidine	
Carbonic anhydrase inhibitors	Block carbonic anhydrase and reduce bicarbonate formation	Acetazolamide	
Increase drainage of aqueous humor			
Miotics	Activate muscarinic receptors on the iris and ciliary muscle causing pupil constriction and ciliary muscle contraction, which may improve uveoscleral outflow	Carbachol	
Prostaglandin analogs	A $PGF_{2\alpha}$ analog increases uveoscleral outflow	Latanoprost	Bimatoprost, Travoprost

Table 19.4 Corneal local anesthetics used in eye examinations and surgery

Drug	Duration of action	Use	Comments
Tetracaine	10 minutes	Minor surgery	Widely used
Benoxinate	10 minutes	Tonometry	Widely used and formulated with fluorescein
Proparacaine	11 minutes	Tonometry Minor surgery	Less stinging, useful in children
Lidocaine	50 minutes	Tonometry Minor surgery	Formulated with fluorescein

of visual function. In other words, IOP is a surrogate endpoint in treating patients so as to avoid loss of visual function.

Drugs that reduce aqueous humor production

The first drug used in glaucoma to reduce aqueous humor production is usually a β adrenoceptor antagonist (β blockers). Those selected for topical use on the eye are typically devoid of the local anesthetic properties seen with some members of this class of drugs. Propranolol is not used to treat glaucoma since it has local anesthetic effects at the locally high concentrations that are achieved with topical drug administration. Thus, propranolol would disadvantageously anesthetize the cornea. Examples of nonselective (block all types of β adrenceptors) β adrenoceptor antagonists used topically in the treatment of glaucoma include carteolol, levobunolol and timolol. These three are nonselective for receptor type, thus equally block β_1 and β_2 adrenoceptors (Table 19.6). (See Chs 8 and 13 for more information about β adrenoceptor antagonists.) The β blockers decrease the rate of aqueous humor formation by virtue of blocking β adrenoceptors in the ciliary body and thereby decreasing the action of circulating epinephrine from the adrenal medulla and norepinephrine released from the ciliary body's sympathetic nerves. Selective β_1 adrenoceptor antagonists such as betaxolol hydrochloride have also been shown to reduce intraocular pressure. Betaxolol may be better tolerated in patients with a history of reactive airways disease (e.g. asthma), presumably due to having a limited but useful degree of selectivity for β_1 receptors. However,

Table 19.6 Pharmacologic and pharmacokinetic characteristics of the of β adrenoceptor antagonists used in glaucoma

Drug	Relative potency	Half-life (h)	β_1 selective	Ocular discomfort
Timolol	5	4	No	++
Betaxolol	1	16	Yes	+++
Carteolol	10	5	No	0
Levobunolol	15	6	No	++
Metipranolol	2	2	No	+

caution and close monitoring is required if therapy with betaxolol is used in such patients.

Aqueous humor formation may also be decreased by a adrenoceptor agonists (Table 19.7). Epinephrine is not very effective for this purpose since it is poorly absorbed from the surface of the eye. It is also rapidly metabolized by enzymes such as monoamine oxidase. These problems do not occur with the pro-drug, dipivefrin hydrochloride. Dipivefrin hydrochloride is more lipophilic, and once in the eye it is converted to epinephrine, the active metabolite, by the action of corneal esterase enzymes (Fig. 19.6).

The mechanism of action by which epinephrine (dipivefrin) reduces intraocular pressure is controversial. One possibility is that it acts on β_2 receptors in the ciliary body to decrease production of aqueous humor. However, administration of epinephrine initially increases intraocular pressure as might be predicted by the fact that β adrenergic antagonists decrease IOP. It is only with chronic use that lowering of IOP occurs. This timecourse raises the possibility that epinephrine acts by desensitizing β adrenoceptor-mediated responses in the eye. (See Ch. 2 for discussion of desensitization.) A second hypothesis is that long-term use of epinephrine causes a reduction of the blood supply to the ciliary body via activation of α_1 adrenoceptors in arteries to cause vasoconstriction and a consequential decrease in the rate of formation of aqueous humor.

The use of apraclonidine, an α_2 adrenoceptor agonist, is generally confined to extreme or acute cases of elevated intraocular pressure since with chronic use it causes an allergic-type conjunctivitis or dermatitis in about 40% of patients. It is a derivative of the classic α_2 adrenoceptor agonist clonidine that is used to treat hypertension (see

Table 19.5 Fluorescent dyes used in eye examinations

Dye	Excitation	Emission	Use
Fluorescein sodium	480 nm (blue)	520 nm (yellow-green)	Tonometry Epithelial/corneal defects Aqueous leaks
Dichlorotetraiodofluorescein (rose bengal)	White light	Pink/magenta	Corneal damage Viral infections

Drugs used to treat otitis media

- **Frequent use of antibiotics in young children can result in gastrointestinal upset and oral *Candida* infection**
- **Aminoglycoside-containing eardrops can be ototoxic in the presence of middle ear inflammation**
- **Repeated use of antibacterial eardrops predisposes to secondary fungal infection**

Suppurative labyrinthitis

Bacterial infection of the spaces of the inner ear causes profound cochlear and vestibular destruction with the loss of both hearing and vestibular function in the affected ear. Intralabyrinthinal infection results from:

- The spreading of otitis media via the round or oval windows.
- A labyrinthinal fistula.
- Lateral extension of meningitis through the cochlear aqueduct and cribriform plate at the lateral end of the internal auditory canal.

When infection is due to otitis media, treatment includes surgical drainage and i.v. antibiotics (ceftriaxone for acute otitis media, nafcillin with ceftazidime plus metronidazole for chronic otitis media). If infection is due to meningitis, the appropriate i.v. antibiotic (see Ch. 6, Part 3) should be used. The use of concurrent i.v. glucocorticosteroids to try and reduce the incidence of postmeningitis hearing loss is controversial and is considered unproven by many.

Hearing loss

■ ***In addition to other causes, ototoxic drugs are a common cause of hearing loss***

Otosclerosis

Otosclerosis is characterized by an idiopathic circumscribed destruction of the endochondral otic capsule and its replacement with vascular bone followed by dense lamellar bone. A characteristic site for such changes is the anterior oval window niche, and when this occurs it results in stapes footplate becoming fixed with a resulting conductive hearing loss. Sensorineural hearing loss can result from a focus of otosclerosis adjacent to the endolymphatic space.

Epidemiologic studies indicate that there is a lower incidence of otosclerosis in regions with high fluoride concentrations in drinking water. However, the only widely recognized indication for prophylactically using fluoride in preventing the condition is where there is progressive sensorineural hearing loss and a high risk of otosclerosis. Calcium, 2–3 g daily, should be administered along with the fluoride.

Sudden sensorineural hearing loss

Sudden sensorineural hearing loss (SSHL) is usually unilateral and shows rapid progression within hours to days. It is associated with tinnitus and, less frequently, vertigo. There are a variety of causes (Table 20.4). If a specific cause cannot be identified, viral infection, vascular disorder or inner ear membrane rupture should be suspected.

SSHL is a medical emergency. When specific etiologies have been excluded, a moderate course of glucocorticosteroids, tapered over 10–14 days, is conventional treatment despite the fact that the effectiveness of such treatment has not been well established. The best responses appear to occur in patients with moderate hearing losses who start glucocorticosteroids within 10 days of diagnosis. Treatment is not required when there is mild hearing loss since this routinely recovers spontaneously, while there is no established benefit even with severe hearing loss. Other drugs used to treat SSHL include vasodilator drugs, plasma expanders and carbogen (5% CO_2, 95% O_2), but here again there is no unequivocal evidence as to their effectiveness.

Autoimmune hearing loss

Autoimmune sensorineural hearing loss typically affects young adults. It progresses slowly over months, and is not

Table 20.4 Various conditions that are a cause of sudden sensorineural hearing loss

Etiologic factors	Example
Congenital	Mondini's deformity
Acquired	
Physical factors	Barotrauma, electrical, concussion, temporal bone fracture, perilymph fistula
Chemical factors:	
Metabolic	Diabetes mellitus, hyperlipidemia, hypothyroidism (Pendred's syndrome)
Ototoxic medications	Antiinflammatory drugs, antibiotics, antineoplastics, loop diuretics
Infections and inflammation	Viral infection (measles, mumps, herpes zoster), bacterial infection (syphilis, mycoplasma, meningitis), chronic granulomatous disease (sarcoidosis)
Vascular	Vasculopathies, coagulopathies, emboli, migraine
Immunologic	Cogan's syndrome
Neoplastic	Acoustic neuroma, carcinoma
Idiopathic	Multiple sclerosis

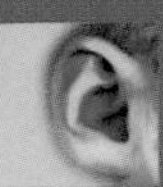

accompanied by another systemic disease, or by hereditary defects. Such hearing loss appears to involve an autoimmune reaction to a specific inner ear antigen. There is no vertigo, but in severe cases ataxia occurs when ambient light conditions are dim.

Treatment depends on the severity of the hearing loss, the likelihood of autoimmune dysfunction and the patient's general medical condition. For more severe and bilateral cases, prednisone for 2–4 weeks is the treatment of choice. A second immunosuppressive agent may be required if:

- There is a good response and hearing recovers, but the patient becomes chronically dependent on glucocorticosteroids in order to maintain hearing.
- There is a strong suspicion that autoimmunity is the cause. Cyclophosphamide, methotrexate or penicillamine can be effective, but when these immunosuppressants are used the patient must be closely monitored for adverse effects.

Tinnitus

Tinnitus is the perception of sound in the absence of an external source of sound. It can have a variety of origins which may be:

- Objective, and a result of sounds generated within the body such that these sound are audible to an observer.
- Subjective, and characterized by an auditory sensation in the absence of a physical sound.

The causes of objective tinnitus include musculoskeletal and vascular sounds, while disorders of the peripheral and central auditory systems are usually responsible for subjective tinnitus. The cause may be known (e.g. noise-induced, presbycusis).

The first symptom of drug-induced ototoxicity is often tinnitus. NSAIDs, antibiotics and antineoplastic agents are the most common cause of drug-induced ototoxicity. Most patients also have irreversible high-frequency sensorineural hearing loss.

Once an underlying disease has been excluded, the goal is to relieve the annoyance that the tinnitus causes. If it is mild, patients may simply need information about its cause and its benign nature. Masking, for example by use of a noise generator to 'cover' the subjective sound, is the prime treatment. Medication, and behavioral modification may be needed for intractable tinnitus. Medications that are used for tinnitus include:

- Local anesthetics (procaine, lidocaine, tocainide).
- Benzodiazepines (diazepam, alprazolam, clonazepam).
- Baclofen.
- Tricyclic antidepressants (amitriptyline).

Where local anesthetics are effective in alleviating or preventing tinnitus their action most probably involves blockade of sodium-dependent neuronal action potentials. The principal site of such actions is probably central and occurs at the level of the cochlear nerve and its brainstem connections. Lidocaine dramatically suppresses tinnitus in some patients, but must be given intravenously for this purpose.

Benzodiazepines improve a patient's emotional response to tinnitus, but are also thought to suppress tinnitus directly. In some patients this may be due to insufficient inhibitory activity in the ascending auditory system. As discussed in Chapter 8, benzodiazepines act by virtue of enhancing the activity of the inhibitory neurotransmitter γ-aminobutyric acid (GABA). Other medications which have been used with varying success in the treatment of tinnitus include tricyclic antidepressants such as amitriptyline.

Anti-tinnitus drugs

- **Tocainide is the only local anesthetic given orally, but it can have serious adverse cardiac effects**
- **Benzodiazepines should be used carefully in view of the habituation that they can induce**
- **Tricyclic antidepressants have antimuscarinic and cardiac adverse effects**

Vertigo

Vertigo is the hallucinatory perception of movement. It may be the result of disorders of the peripheral or central vestibular systems.

Peripherally induced vertigo is usually more severe and is associated with other aural symptoms such as hearing loss or tinnitus. The condition includes:

- Benign positional vertigo (either spontaneous or secondary to head trauma) which occurs with movements of the head. Episodes usually lasts less than 30 seconds. There is a sensation of rotary motion, either of the world moving, or of the sufferer moving in the world. Malpositioning of otoliths is presumed to trigger an attack of vertigo. The treatment involved using systematic head maneuvers and positioning to try and re-position the otoliths of the inner ear.
- Constant vertigo is often due to permanent hypofunction of the affected labyrinth as a result, for example, of acute vestibular neuronitis, suppurative labyrinthitis and vestibular trauma.
- Vertigo due to transient fluctuations in vestibular neuron activity as occurs with Ménière's disease and recurrent vestibulopathy.
- Centrally induced vertigo may be associated with signs of brainstem or cerebellar pathology.

Medical treatment of vertigo is aimed at stabilizing pathologic fluctuations in peripheral vestibular function and at promoting central compensation if there is a permanent decrease in vestibular function.

Vestibular neuronitis and vestibular trauma

Vestibular neuronitis results in an acute decrease in vestibular function, the results of which may be mild and reversible, or profound and permanent. Symptoms include a severe vertigo that can be accompanied by nausea. Its probable cause is an unknown virus. Vestibular trauma can induce vertigo with a similar range of severity depending upon whether there has been a brain concussion, total destruction of the vestibular structures or division of the vestibular nerve.

Adaptation to vertigo must begin in the first month after onset. Patients must remain active, since inactivity can predispose to incomplete adaptation and permanent ataxia. Antinauseants such as dimenhydrinate are useful for severe nausea while the vestibular suppressant drugs used in acute Ménière's disease (see next section) can be used sparingly. No drug specifically promotes central adaptation.

Ménière's disease and recurrent vestibulopathy

Ménière's disease is a peripheral vestibular disorder associated with intermittent excessive accumulation of endolymphatic fluid (endolymphatic hydrops). It causes episodes of severe rotary vertigo that continue for hours, as well as hearing loss, tinnitus and sensations of pressure within the ear. Initially these symptoms occur in 'attacks,' but eventually the condition 'burns out,' leaving the patient with a stable severe sensorineural hearing loss, and a permanent but usually well-compensated decrease in peripheral vestibular function.

Ménière's disease is treated with drugs and a restricted Na^+ intake to try and prevent the hydrops, as well as with physical therapy to adapt to the loss of vestibular function. Drugs that are used include:

- Diuretics (hydrochlorothiazide, furosemide) to limit endolymphatic fluid accumulation.
- Vestibular suppressants (sedatives, antihistamines, anticholinergics, narcotics).
- Vasodilating drugs.
- Aminoglycosides to ablate peripheral vestibular function.

Hydrochlorothiazide prevents recurrent vertigo in many patients. The usual dose is 10–50 mg daily. Doses greater than 25 mg can result in potassium depletion and the need for a diet high in potassium.

Meclizine moderates the severity of acute attacks, possibly due to pharmacologic antagonism at muscarinic cholinergic receptors, rather than at the expected H_1 histamine receptors. This is an example of H_1 receptor antagonists having a therapeutic benefit resulting from another type of pharmacologic action. If an attack becomes severe, a benzodiazepine such as diazepam or lorazepam not only provides sedation but also acts directly on the medial and lateral vestibular nuclei to suppress otolithic and semicircular canal activity. More selective anticholinergic drugs, such as scopolamine, are of limited use because their adverse antimuscarinic effects are more severe than those of meclizine. Some narcotics (e.g. fentanyl, droperidol) given parenterally are potent vestibular suppressants and are occasionally needed for an acute, incapacitating attack.

Chemical ablation of vestibular function can be used for recurrent incapacitating vertigo that cannot be controlled by drugs. Streptomycin can be given parenterally for active disease that is occurring in both ears. The dose is carefully titrated to a point of acceptable control of symptoms. However, complete ablation of all peripheral vestibular function is avoided since this can cause incapacitating oscillopsia and ataxia.

In unilateral Ménière's disease, gentamicin can be injected directly into the middle ear, from where it is actively transported across the round window into the labyrinthine fluids. Once within the fluid it probably acts on dark cells (thought to be important in the production of endolymph) and has a toxic effect on the vestibular hair cells. Most patients adapt well to unilateral destruction of vestibular function and have no further disabling spells of vertigo.

Recurrent vestibulopathy, also known as vestibular Ménière's disease, presents with similar recurrent vertigo, but with no auditory symptoms. The vertigo is typically more benign than that in Ménière's disease and is usually controlled by the drugs that are useful for treating Ménière's disease.

Drugs used in Ménière's disease and their possible actions

- Hydrochlorothiazide reduces endolymph production
- Meclizine has beneficial anticholinergic effects
- Benzodiazepines suppress vestibular activity and are sedatives
- Aminoglycosides induce a stable decrease in vestibular function

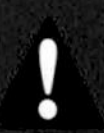

Drugs used for Ménière's disease

- Diuretic therapy can cause K^+ depletion, hyperglycemia and hyperlipidemia, and exacerbate gout
- Severe permanent ataxia and oscillopsia can follow streptomycin treatment of bilateral Ménière's disease if a total loss of vestibular function occurs
- Intratympanic gentamicin treatment is associated with a 10–20% incidence of hearing loss

Facial nerve palsy

Bell's palsy is an acute unilateral facial weakness or paralysis without an identifiable cause, although herpes simplex virus type I has been implicated. Herpes zoster oticus (HZO) is acute facial paralysis with pain and varicelliform lesions, which often involve the conchal bowl, the concave central portion of the external ear. It is probably due to varicella-zoster virus infection of the

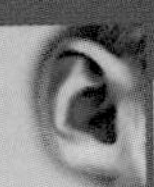

geniculate ganglion. Often there is an eighth cranial nerve involvement that produces profound sensorineural hearing loss as well as vestibular loss. Edema traps the facial nerve as it passes through the narrow fallopian canal, resulting in ischemia and neural dysfunction.

The use of glucocorticosteroids to treat acute facial paralysis is controversial. They are not indicated for incomplete facial paralysis since this usually recovers fully without medication. If used for complete facial paralysis in Bell's palsy or HZO, steroids should be given within the first 10 days of onset of symptoms and then at a moderate dose that is subsequently tapered.

Aciclovir (acycloguanosine) is a nucleoside analog that inhibits viral DNA replication (see Ch. 6, Part 2) and reduces functional deficits in immunocompromised patients with HZO. It has no proven benefit in the treatment of Bell's palsy. Ideally, treatment should be started as soon as possible after symptoms develop, up to about 72 hours after onset.

OTOTOXIC DRUGS

Four clinically important classes of drugs cause inner ear toxicity (Table 20.5). Both hearing and balance are usually affected. Tinnitus is an additional symptom that often accompanies drug-induced ototoxicity.

Analgesics and antipyretics

The tinnitus that is so characteristic of salicylate-induced ototoxicity is often accompanied by hearing loss. The mechanism of such salicylate ototoxicity is not fully understood. However, salicylates accumulate within extracellular fluid compartments and block prostaglandin synthesis within the stria vascularis by inhibiting cyclooxygenase. This results in vasoconstriction within the stria vascularis and, as a consequence, local ischemia and the inhibition of cochlear nerve action potentials. Salicylate ototoxicity occurs when serum concentrations exceed 0.35 mg/mL and is reversible within 48–72 hours of the salicylate being withdrawn.

Antimicrobials

Aminoglycoside antibiotics have adverse effects on both the kidneys and the inner ear. Streptomycin and gentamicin are the more vestibulotoxic whereas kanamycin, tobramycin and amikacin have greater effects on cochlear hair cells. Gentamicin-induced ototoxicity occurs in approximately 5% of patients. Netilmicin has a reported prevalence of hearing loss in 1 per 250 patients, and vestibular toxicity in 1 per 150 patients.

Aminoglycosides bind to the outer surface of the hair cell membrane and interfere with membrane Ca^{2+} channels. They also bind to phosphatidylinositol bisphosphate on the inner surface of the cell membrane. Interference with intracellular Ca^{2+} and polyamine-regulated processes causes additional membrane damage, eventually leading to cell death via apoptosis. The resulting ototoxicity can be reversible, but severe, irreversible and untreatable hearing deficits are common. Since some patients requiring aminoglycosides have debilitating conditions, their complaints of 'dizziness' and tinnitus may be overlooked, especially in bed-bound patients. Too often, permanent disabling vestibulotoxicity is only recognized with ambulatory patients when there are complaints of:

- Movement intolerance.
- Oscillopsia (difficulty in stabilizing gaze during head movements).
- Ataxia.

It is best to identify patients at an increased risk (Table 20.6) of aminoglycoside toxicity and limit their exposure to ototoxicity by monitoring serum concentrations and switching to non-ototoxic antibacterial drugs as soon as possible. Measurement of auditory function, for example by sequential audiometry, is a good way to detect ototoxicity. Hearing can be impaired even at blood concentrations considered within the normal range. The concentration of an aminoglycoside in the cochlear perilymph is both time- and plasma-dependent. As a result of such ototoxicity, aminoglycosides should given at the lowest effective dose for the briefest possible time.

The glycopeptide antibiotics, such as vancomycin, are increasingly used clinically as a result of the increasing problem of antibacterial resistance. The mechanism of ototoxicity of glycopeptide antibiotics is not well understood, but the pattern of outer hair cell loss preceding inner hair cell loss is similar to that seen with aminoglycosides.

Table 20.5 Different classes and examples of drugs that are ototoxic

Class	Examples
Analgesics and antipyretics	Salicylates, quinine
Antimicrobials:	
Aminoglycoside antibiotics	Gentamicin, neomycin
Glycopeptide antibiotics	Vancomycin
Macrolide antibiotics	Erythromycin
Antineoplastics	Cisplatin
Loop diuretics	Furosemide, ethacrynic acid

Table 20.6 Pathologic factors that increase the risk of ototoxicity with the use of aminoglycosides

Impaired renal function
Prolonged treatment (greater than 10 days)
Concomitant use of other nephrotoxic or ototoxic drugs (loop diuretics, high-dose erythromycin, vancomycin)
Advanced age
Previous aminoglycoside therapy
Pre-existing sensorineural hearing loss

High-frequency sensorineural hearing loss, 'blowing' tinnitus and vertigo can occur with large i.v. doses of erythromycin, a macrolide antibiotic. Patients at increased risk of such toxicity include those with hepatic or renal failure, legionnaires' disease and the elderly. The mechanism of macrolide ototoxicity is unknown, but it is reversible on withdrawal of the antibiotic.

Antineoplastics

Ototoxicity with cisplatin is probably due to the basic mechanism of action in causing labyrinthine hair cell degeneration. Cisplatin is primarily cochleotoxic and causes degeneration of the outer hair cells, spiral ganglion cells and cochlear neurons while sparing, to some extent, the vestibular system. The morphologic changes due to cisplatin that are found within the inner ear are similar to those seen in aminoglycoside ototoxicity. The outer hair cells of the basal turn of the cochlea are the most susceptible. Carboplatin also produces dose-dependent hearing loss. This is thought to result from generation of oxygen free radicals, and subsequent apoptosis of cochlear cells.

Diuretics

In the ear, the loop diuretics (furosemide and ethacrynic acid) inhibit cell membrane K^+ transport within the stria vascularis and are principally cochleotoxic. Like aminoglycosides, loop diuretics have adverse effects on both the kidney and inner ear while the toxic effects of the two classes of drugs can be synergistic. There is an increased risk of toxicity if furosemide is given as an i.v. bolus injection, or if the patient is elderly, or has renal failure. Tinnitus, hearing loss and vertigo may occur within minutes but can be reversible if the medication is promptly withdrawn.

FURTHER READING

Jackler R, Brackman D (eds). *Neurotology*. St. Louis: Mosby; 2002. [A recent text with excellent basic science and thorough clinical reviews.]

*http://www.merck.com/mrkshared/mmanual/*home.jsp [This site gives access to the *Merck Manual of Diagnosis and Therapy*. Section 7 deals with drugs used in the ear, nose and throat.]

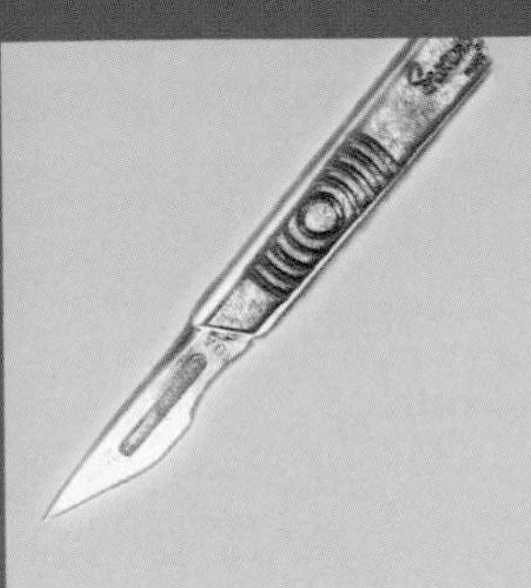

Chapter 21

Drugs Used in Anesthesia and Critical Care

PATHOPHYSIOLOGY OF SURGICAL INJURY AND CRITICAL ILLNESS

General and local anesthesia make surgery possible. The purpose of surgery is:

- To repair, remove or replace damaged or diseased tissues.
- To remove healthy tissue, as in organ donation for transplantation, or in the delivery of babies.

Modern surgery requires anesthesia (general or local).

The history of anesthesia offers lessons in drug discovery and drug use

Prior to the discovery and introduction of drugs that produced the state known as anesthesia, little could be done to alleviate the pain and fear of surgery. Surgery has been practiced for millennia, but all that could be done to reduce pain and fear was the use of ethanol, opium, mandragora (a herb) and cocaine. While some of these preparations reduce pain, anxiety and the level of consciousness, they do not produce general anesthesia, a word originally used by Dioscorides almost 2000 years ago but whose modern use is due to Oliver Wendell Holmes in 1847. He used it to describe the ability of ether and nitrous oxide to produce a reversible unconsciousness state in which surgery could be performed without pain and awareness (general anesthesia). Only 40 years later, with the introduction of local anesthetic drugs, was it realized that surgery could also be performed without pain if the surgical area was anesthetized by application of a local anesthetic drug while the patient remained conscious.

The actions of one of the first anesthetic drugs, nitrous oxide (synthesized by Priestly in 1776) were described by Davy who, with others in the 1790s, recognized that nitrous oxide, and later ether, altered consciousness. He also suggested that either could be used to produce unconsciousness as an aid in surgery. However, such prescience was 'an idea before its time' and was not acted upon. The use of either ether or nitrous oxide to purposefully induce anesthesia did not occur until 1846 despite the fact that both drugs were regularly used at parties ('ether frolics') to produce states of intoxication.

In the mid-1800s, as the intellectual medical climate changed, a desire to make surgery painless developed. Thus began a systematic effort to introduce nitrous oxide and ether into medicine as general anesthetics. Major steps forward were made in the USA in 1844–46 by Wells and Morton. Wells introduced nitrous oxide to dentistry while Morton introduced ether into surgery. The story of how these two innovators introduced anesthetics is a lesson in the trials and tribulations of medical innovators. In the UK, Simpson (1847), heartened by such studies, began a systematic search for new anesthetics. This search involved sniffing organic solvent vapors to test their effects on himself and his colleagues. Within a short period this extremely hazardous search led to the identification of chloroform, which became the anesthetic of choice in the UK for almost 100 years.

Well into the middle 1900s ether, nitrous oxide (available in steel cylinders in 1868) and chloroform were the mainstays of general anesthesia around the world. Their routine use led to a great deal of knowledge about anesthetics and the 'stages' of anesthesia while theories of anesthesia were promulgated. However, newer and better anesthetics were only slowly discovered. All of the above anesthetics are far from ideal. Nitrous oxide lacks potency and cannot be given at a concentration that produces complete anesthesia; ether has a slow onset of action and is irritating to the respiratory system as well as being flammable; chloroform is more potent, and not flammable, but can cause fatal cardiac arrhythmias and liver toxicity. The gas cyclopropane was discovered to be an anesthetic in 1929, and despite being explosive, was used for many years.

The above situation changed with the discovery of the hypnotic effects of barbiturates. This led to thiopental, a barbiturate that rapidly produces a brief anesthesia when injected intravenously providing a method for the fast induction of general anesthesia. A revolution occurred when Raventos and Suckling introduced halothane, the first of the new halogenated hydrocarbon anesthetics that was easy and safe to use by inhalation, and not explosive. The value of halothane was such that many of the newer drugs (see later) have been modeled upon it. Another significant step in anesthesia was the introduction of curare as a neuromuscular blocking drug. This allowed anesthesiologists to provide controlled muscle relaxation, thereby reducing the need for high concentrations of general anesthetics.

The ability to control anesthesia was helped by the recognition that patients given ether progressed through four stages of anesthesia. These were:

- A first stage of analgesia.
- A second stage of excitement, with loss or consciousness, but heightened reflexes.
- A third stage of surgical anesthesia, with all reflexes disappearing as the stage deepened.
- A final stage of medullary paralysis, with failure of respiration and vasomotor control, and ultimately death.

Other anesthetics do not show exactly the same stages, but the existence of such stages gives an idea of how anesthesia progresses through stages, especially stage two. Nowadays general anesthesia involves the use of drugs to produce loss of consciousness (hypnosis), analgesia, neuromuscular blockade, amnesia and blunting motor and autonomic nervous system reflexes. This generally requires a combination of drugs rather than a single anesthetic drug.

Regional (local) anesthetics have a different history. Koller early in the last century recognized that cocaine blocked the sensation of touch in the eye and as a result introduced it in ocular surgery. Cocaine blocks voltage- and time-dependent sodium channels in nerves, and as a result anesthetizes both sensory and motor nerves. With the synthesis of other local anesthetics (such as lidocaine in 1943) it became apparent that local anesthetics were useful for other types of surgery. Thus, a local area (e.g. skin) can be anesthetized if a local anesthetic drug is infiltrated into the area. Greater areas can be deprived of feeling if major nerves in the area are blocked. The largest areas of regional anesthesia occur if the drug is placed near the spinal cord as in spinal or epidural anesthesia. The use of local, versus general, anesthesia for surgery varies from country to country.

It is a paradox that surgeons seek to heal by first injuring. Of course, surgery is different from accidental trauma, because the nature and extent of injury are carefully controlled and the body's responses are partially attenuated by anesthesia. General anesthesia is accompanied by a depression of the respiratory and cardiovascular responses to surgery. This can sometimes be useful, but excessive depression of such responses can in turn lead to injury of critical organs, especially in those patients with limited respiratory and cardiovascular reserves. As a result, cardiorespiratory monitoring and treatment strategies during anesthesia parallel the 'ABC' approach used to resuscitate critically ill patients.

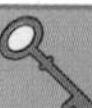

History of general anesthesia

- Nitrous oxide synthesized: 1776
- Nitrous oxide and ether used in surgery: 1844–1846
- Chloroform: 1847
- Cyclopropane: 1929
- Halothane: 1950s

ABC approach for the unconscious patient

- Airway: maintain patency
- Breathing: ventilate and oxygenate
- Circulation: compress chest to provide a pulse if one is not present, obtain intravenous access, administer fluids and drugs as required
- Defibrillate heart: if necessary; diagnose and treat reversible causes

Postoperative complications of surgery

- Circulation: bleeding, fluid loss, electrolyte imbalance, deep vein thrombosis, pulmonary embolism, pressure sores
- Surgical wound: infection, separation
- Gut: paralytic ileus, gastric ulceration, nutritional deficiency
- Major organ failure: brain, lungs, heart, kidneys, liver

The injury response to surgery

The suppression by anesthetics of physiologic responses to surgery is probably generally beneficial during the perioperative period. Responses to tissue injury involve local changes and stimulation of the neurologic pathways with respiratory, cardiovascular, endocrine, metabolic and inflammatory components which have evolved to increase the chance of survival following life-threatening injury. For example (Fig. 21.1):

- Local tissue factors lead to vasospasm and coagulation as a mechanism which reduces bleeding.
- Increased sympathetic nervous system activity compensates for reductions in circulating blood volume.

However, an accelerated clotting cascade results in a systemic hypercoagulable state while a large increase in catecholamine release from the sympathetic system results in tachycardia and hypertension, and an increasing risk of myocardial ischemia and congestive heart failure.

Anesthesia and control of postoperative acute pain decreases the above stress responses, and this in turn reduces cardiovascular risks.

Other than bleeding, surgical injury is associated with significant fluid shifts, especially when the abdomen is opened. Evaporation occurs from the large serosal surface area of the intestines while fluid accumulation develops in the interstitial compartment of the intestines – the so-called 'third space loss.' These fluid losses must be replaced perioperatively to avoid hypovolemia and hemodynamic instability. However, in the immediate days after surgery third space losses shift back, resulting in an expansion of the vascular compartment and predisposing patients with heart disease to angina and heart failure.

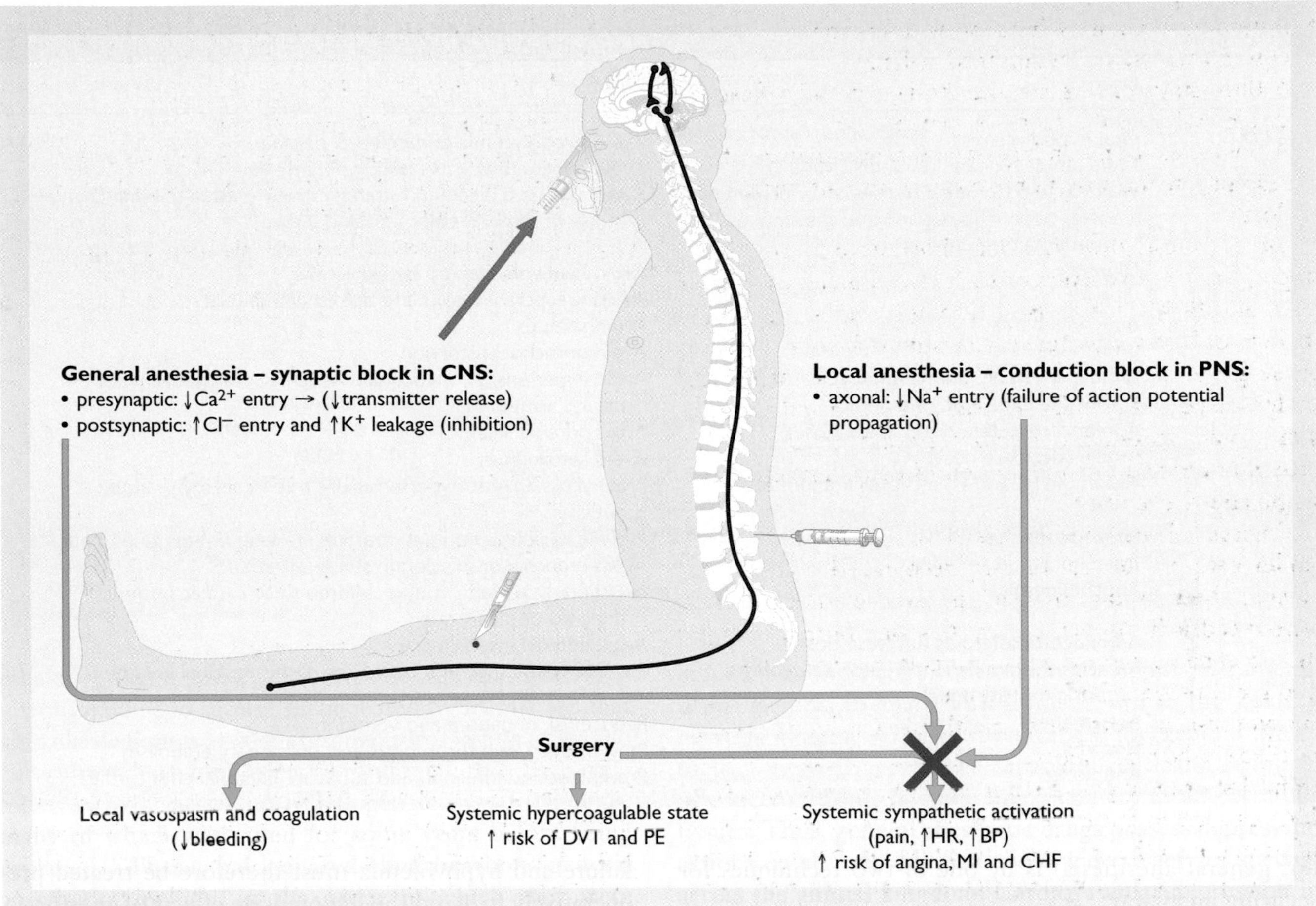

Fig. 21.1 Methods for suppressing physiologic responses to surgery by the drugs used in anesthesia.

The neurologic response to surgery is proportional to the magnitude of nociceptive stimuli (pain) and tissue injury. For example, the response to intra-abdominal surgery is greater than that to surgery of the extremities. Similarly, greater concentrations of anesthetics are required to suppress greater nociceptive stimuli.

Anesthetics and other perioperative drugs are used to suppress pain, anxiety and awareness, to maintain oxygenation, hemodynamic stability and fluid balance, and to prevent sepsis. Anesthesia is an insensitivity to pain that involves suppression of either:

- Central neural processing (general anesthesia).
- The afferent sensory reflex (local or regional anesthesia).

DRUGS AND PREMEDICATION PRIOR TO ANESTHESIA

Drugs are given before anesthesia for the following:

- Sedation.
- Analgesia.
- Muscarinic effects (Table 21.1).
- Prophylactic antibiotics given to prevent wound infection or bacterial endocarditis.
- Prophylactic anticoagulation given to prevent deep vein thrombosis. However, prophylactic anticoagulation is postponed if epidural or spinal anesthesia is used because of the risk of epidural hematoma and spinal cord compression.

Premedication and airway techniques prevent pulmonary aspiration

Anesthetics can cause regurgitation and vomiting with risk of aspiration because the normal protective airway reflexes are obtunded by anesthesia. Recent eating and drinking places patients at risk of pulmonary aspiration and death during anesthesia. Although the risk of pulmonary aspiration is reduced in elective surgery by preoperative fasting, postponing emergency surgery will not guarantee an empty stomach. Furthermore, both pain and opioids reduce gastric motility. To guard against aspiration of the stomach's acidic contents, antacids are given to neutralize acid. Histamine H_2 receptor antagonists and proton pump inhibitors both reduce acid production (see Ch. 16). Drugs that increase upper gastrointestinal tract motility, such as metoclopramide, aid stomach emptying. Such drugs have been given before anesthesia to fasting patients with a history of gastroesophageal reflux but this has not been very successful.

Prevention of pulmonary aspiration during emergency surgery (other than using regional local anesthesia and

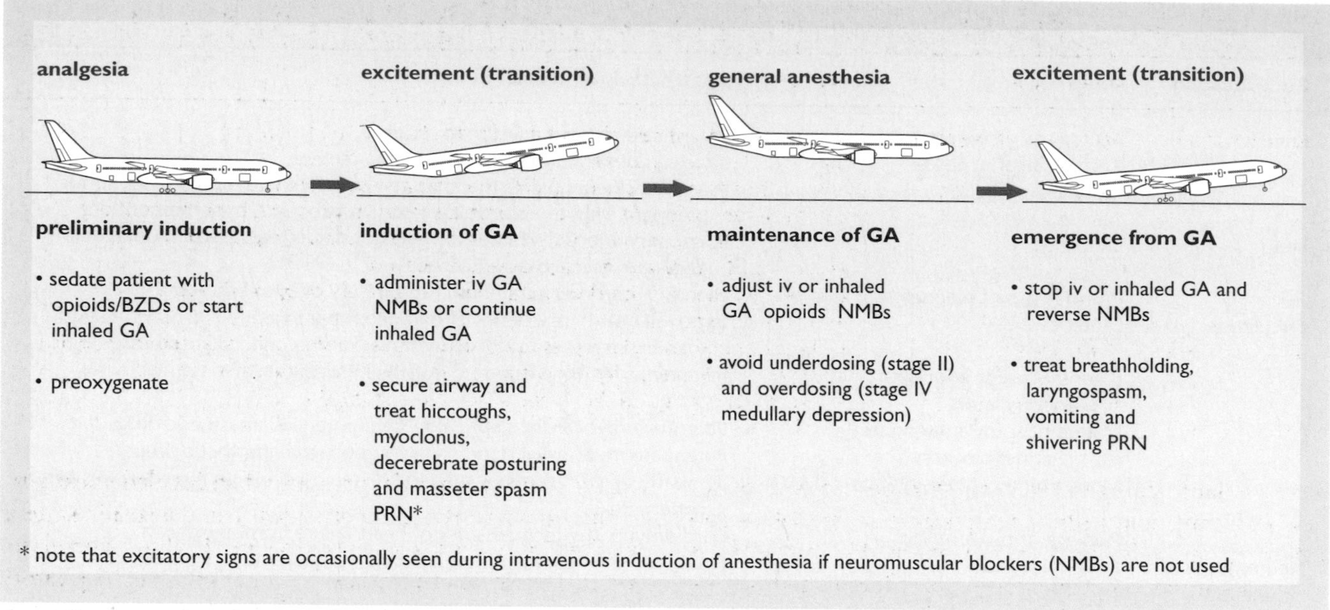

Fig. 21.2 The stages of general anesthesia. The choice of GA is described in the text. (GA, General Anesthetics), (BZD, benzodiazepines).

During the induction phase, airway, respiratory and circulatory reflexes are all progressively depressed in a dose-related manner by anesthetics. Respiratory effects include decreased ventilatory reflex responses to hypercarbia, and especially to hypoxemia. Circulatory effects include depression of myocardial contractility, vascular smooth muscle tone and autonomic nervous system control of the cardiovascular system. These ventilatory and cardiovascular depressant effects of anesthetics are offset in part by reflexes arising as a result of the nociceptive stimulation due to surgery.

A variety of electronic devices (for example BIS – bispectral index) are used in an attempt to monitor levels of anesthesia but their usefulness has not been completely validated. As a result of this, cardiorespiratory stability is used to infer the adequacy of depth of anesthesia.

Safe induction requires careful airway and ventilatory control, with frequent monitoring of pulse oximetry, capnometry and vital signs. Hemodynamic depression is managed firstly by ensuring adequate oxygenation and ventilation, and secondly by treating unrecognized hypovolemia, cardiac ischemia or excess anesthetic. Slow induction (using either an i.v. infusion or a volatile inhaled anesthetic), instead of fast induction (using an i.v. bolus), does not necessarily improve safety. For example, neuro-excitation with vomiting, laryngospasm, cough and apnea can occur with a slow transition during the passage from wakefulness to anesthesia. Although i.v. induction is preferred by adults, inhalation induction is still used in children where access to a vein can be limited as a result of poor patient cooperation.

Airway techniques determine the selection of anesthetic and this in turn affects the control of the airway and ventilation

Manual methods for maintaining a patent airway produce painful stimuli and reflex muscle activity and these must be suppressed so as to reduce patient injury. With respect to the intensity of stimulation produced by airway manipulation, an oropharyngeal and a laryngeal mask produce the least stimulation, whereas an endotracheal tube produces the most. As a result, higher doses of i.v. anesthetics and opioids are used for induction involving tracheal intubation. In addition, tracheal intubation generally requires the use of neuromuscular blockers (NMBs; see below) as is summarized in Table 21.3.

During the process of emergence from anesthesia, neither i.v. nor inhaled anesthetics provide residual analgesia

Opioids (e.g. morphine, meperidine, fentanyl, alfentanil, sufentanil, remifentanil – see Ch. 8) are administered perioperatively in part to help transition from the anesthetic to a pain-free, but awake, state. After surgery, an additional benefit of opioids during anesthesia is a reduced need for i.v. and inhaled anesthetics and, therefore, less circulatory depression. Emergence can be complicated by excessive doses of opioids producing dose-related respiratory depression (see Pain Management section on p. 583).

Inhaled anesthetics

Following the discoveries discussed previously, and the introduction of halothane, advances have included many

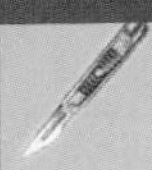

Table 21.3 Decisions that have to be made regarding airway and breathing during general anesthesia

Question	Alternatives	Rationale
Airway choice?	Face mask or laryngeal mask	Less invasive, but less reliable – best for procedures of short duration that do not require intubation
	Tracheal intubation	Requires neuromuscular blocker (NMB) and may cause trauma
		Ensures a secure airway (e.g. head and neck surgery, surgery in the prone position)
		Protects lungs from aspiration (e.g. bleeding airway, recently ingested food or swallowed blood, hiatus hernia, bowel obstruction)
		Facilitates mechanical ventilation (e.g. anesthetic-, NMB- or opioid-induced respiratory failure)
Breathing choice?	Spontaneous	Less invasive since inspiratory pressures are negative (versus positive during mechanical ventilation), but breathing may be inefficient. For short-duration procedure
	Mechanical	Treats respiratory failure and decreases oxygen consumption

newer volatile halogenated hydrocarbon vapor anesthetics. Enflurane and isoflurane appeared in the 1970s and 1980s, respectively. Further refinements led in the 1990s to two fluorinated hydrocarbons, sevoflurane and desflurane. These newer inhaled anesthetics are associated with significantly faster induction and emergence, as well as a lower risk of liver toxicity.

Pharmacokinetic and pharmacodynamic characteristics of inhaled anesthetics

Inhaled anesthetics differ pharmacokinetically from i.v. anesthetics since the lungs are the route for the administration and elimination of inhaled anesthetics. Inhaled anesthetics do not need to be metabolized in order to be eliminated by the lungs and therefore are preferred for maintaining anesthesia. The loss of drug in the expired air allows for a rapid washout of anesthetic from the brain and the heart, and therefore reversal of anesthesia.

Pharmacodynamically, inhaled anesthetics are administered at specific gas or vapor concentrations and not as a dose, since inspiration and expiration are inextricably linked. Since the partial pressure of an inhaled anesthetic in the lung and the brain are equal when a steady state is reached, the drug concentration in the lung correlates with the brain concentration. By monitoring end-expiratory anesthetic concentrations and hemodynamic responses, an anesthesiologist can assess graded 'dose'–response relationships during surgical procedures as the intensity of stimulation fluctuates. In contrast, with i.v. anesthetics the brain concentrations of anesthetic cannot be similarly estimated, although BIS monitoring can determine the effect on the brain.

The end-expiratory anesthetic concentration (minimum alveolar concentration or 'MAC' value) is a measure of the anesthetic potency for different inhaled anesthetics and different patients. It is, in a sense, analogous to an EC_{50} for a quantal concentration–response curve (see Ch. 2). MAC is the end-expiratory gas concentration that prevents movement in response to a surgical skin incision in 50% of subjects. MAC allows for a comparison of the potency of anesthetic with respect to the brain and cardiovascular systems (Table 21.4). For example, inhaled anesthetics given at 1.3 times their MAC prevent

Table 21.4 The comparative pharmacology and pharmacokinetics of various inhaled vapor anesthetics

	Halothane	Isoflurane	Sevoflurane	Desflurane
MAC	0.75%	1.2%	1.7%	6.0%
Respiratory irritation during inhaled induction	–	+	–	++
Heart rate	↓	↑↑	↑	↑↑
Blood pressure	↓	↓	↓	↓
Systemic vascular resistance	–	↓	↓	↓
Myocardial contractility	↓	–	–	–
Cardiac output	↓	–	–	–
Blood:gas partition coefficient*	2.3	1.4	0.6	0.4
Speed of onset (and recovery)	Slow	Medium	Rapid	Rapid
Metabolism	20%	0.2%	>2% (to fluoride)	<0.02%
Risk of 'hepatitis'	1:10 000?	Rare	Rare	Rare

* Blood:gas partition coefficient reflects solubility; higher numbers indicate higher solubility in blood relative to gas.
- no effect, + positive effect; ↑ increase, ↓ decrease.
The above values should be compared with nitrous oxide whose MAC is >100%, which increases heart rate, blood pressure and systemic vascular resistance but has no depressant effect on the heart. Its blood gas coefficient is 0.5, it has a rapid onset and recovery with 0% metabolism and there is no risk of producing hepatitis.

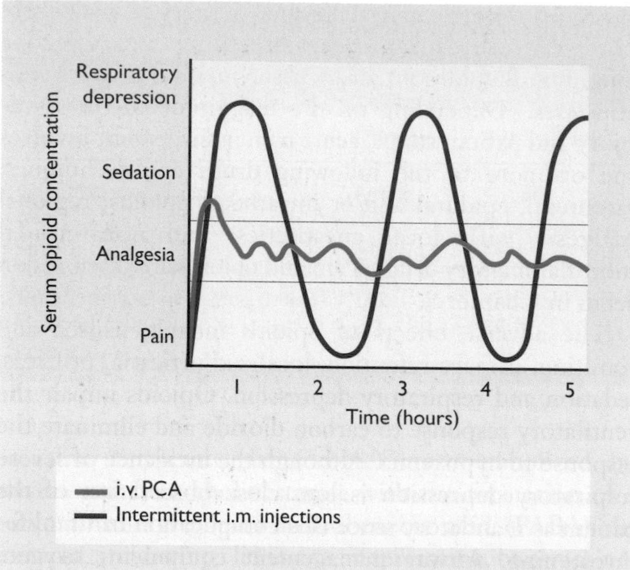

Fig. 21.3 Blood concentrations and effectiveness of morphine using i.v. patient-controlled analgesia (PCA) versus intramuscular (i.m.) morphine. (Adapted with permission of Dr. Pat Sullivan from *Anaesthesia for Medical Students*, Ottawa Civic Hospital, 1999.)

administration. In addition, a 4-hour dose limit can be programmed.

CRITICAL CARE

Prompt basic and advanced life support are critical for the unconscious patient. An unobstructed airway is of paramount importance. In addition to hypoxemia leading to brain damage, cardiac arrest or death, hypercarbia in patients with intracranial space-occupying lesions can produce cerebral vasodilation, increased intracranial pressure and further cerebral ischemia. Breathing must be maintained to ensure oxygen delivery and carbon dioxide elimination. If the patient remains unconscious, tracheal intubation is required to protect the airway from aspiration. Patients with multiple trauma, or with critical illness, typically have impaired oxygen delivery (Fig. 21.4). For example:

- Crush injuries to the chest, or pneumonia, cause atelectasis and 'hypoxic hypoxemia.'
- Bleeding decreases oxygen-carrying capacity and leads to 'anemic hypoxemia.'
- Inadequate blood flow due to circulatory failure produces 'ischemic hypoxemia.'

Removal of carbon dioxide can also be impaired, for example, as a result of depressed ventilatory drive due to head trauma, or ineffective respiration due to chest trauma. Initial management of critical illness includes routine oxygen therapy and close observation of vital signs.

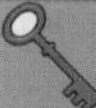

Monitoring for resuscitation and anesthesia

- **CNS: level of consciousness**
- **Airway and breathing: respiratory rate, pulse oximetry, expired capnometry, arterial blood gases**
- **Circulation: heart rate, blood pressure, EKG, urine output**

Oxygen therapy and mechanical ventilation

Oxygen supply devices provide a variable fraction of inspired oxygen (F_iO_2) mixed with room air. Supplemental oxygen can be administered via nasal prongs (F_iO_2 0.24–0.4 with oxygen flows 1–6 L/min) or via a vented mask (F_iO_2 0.4–0.6 with oxygen flows 5–8 L/min). Oxygen toxicity of the lung (and eye in premature neonates) may follow the use of a prolonged and high paO_2 (as with a F_iO_2 of 1.0 for 12 hours for lung; with the eyes being more sensitive).

When the essential purpose of a procedure is to provide oxygen, it is important to recognize that oxygen delivery to tissue (DO_2) is equal to the cardiac output times the oxygen-carrying capacity of the blood. The oxygen-carrying capacity of the blood in turn depends upon the partial pressure of arterial oxygen, hemoglobin content and its saturation characteristics, all of which can be determined. Cardiac output is the product of stroke volume and heart rate. Such equations allow one to clearly identify and correct causes of hypoxemia. Although the need for mechanical ventilation is often obvious in patients with severe head or chest trauma, a diagnosis of acute and progressive respiratory failure in patients with pre-existing cardiorespiratory disease can be difficult. An increasing respiratory rate, increasing pCO_2 and decreasing pO_2 in arterial blood may aid early diagnosis. Intubation and mechanical ventilation are not without risk in critically ill patients since anesthesia is often required with a resulting risk of cardiovascular depression. Although anesthesia, neuromuscular blockade and intubation may be required for adequate ventilation the use of opioids and benzodiazepines, rather than NMBs, can be sufficient to allow mechanical ventilation to be used.

Management of hemodynamic instability

Oxygen delivery depends on an intact circulation. Acute circulatory failure is due to either (Fig. 21.5):

- Hypovolemia (decreased preload).
- Compromised cardiac function (decreased heart rate, very high heart rate, decreased contractility, arrhythmias, heart valve malfunction). Septic shock from the release of vasoactive substances that cause hypovolemia via vasodilation and capillary leakage.

Management of hemodynamic instability requires monitoring heart rate, and arterial and central venous pressure. While most hypovolemias are hemorrhagic in

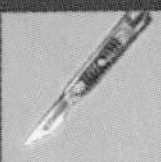

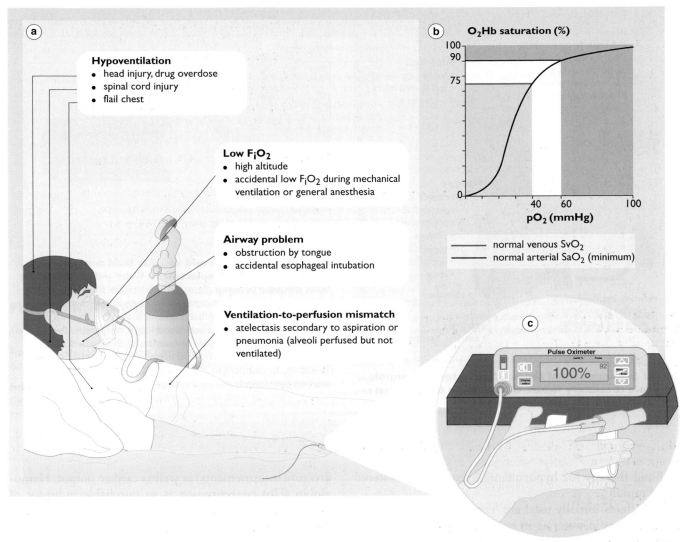

Fig. 21.4 Hypoxemia, oxygen saturation of hemoglobin and clinical monitoring. (a) Possible causes of hypoxemia. Normal oxygenation requires sufficient inspired oxygen, a patent airway, an intact respiratory center, an innervated and stable chest wall, ventilated and perfused alveoli plus an adequate cardiac output. (b) Oxyhemoglobin (O_2Hb) dissociation curve. The O_2Hb dissociation curve describes the relationship between the degree of saturation of Hb with oxygen and the partial pressure of oxygen (pO_2). The flat portion at the top of the sigmoid-shaped curve indicates near-maximal oxygen capacity for hemoglobin. Saturation of Hb with oxygen is about 90% when pO_2 is 60 mmHg and about 100% when pO_2 is 100 mmHg or greater. (c) Pulse oximetry can provide a noninvasive monitor of the oxygen content of arterial blood as well as the adequacy of pulsatile perfusion. However, pulse oximetry does not necessarily indicate circulatory adequacy (SaO_2, percentage saturation of arterial Hb; pO_2, partial pressure of oxygen; SvO_2, percentage saturation of venous Hb).

origin, nonhemorrhagic hypovolemia and cardiogenic circulatory failure can occur. For example, an elderly patient with a bowel obstruction can become hypovolemic as a result of gastrointestinal fluid accumulation and sepsis, and the associated circulatory failure can then lead to tachycardia and coronary hypoperfusion and eventually acute heart failure.

Healthy adults compensate for a hemorrhagic loss of up to 15% of their blood volume (i.e. 15% × 70 mL/kg) by means of increased cardiac output. However, the sympathetic reflexes necessary for such compensation are depressed by anesthesia and this can result in a precipitous fall in blood pressure and tissue perfusion. Thus, it is crucial to restore intravascular fluid volume prior to anesthesia. Most preoperative patients will develop signs of inadequate tissue perfusion once 30% of their blood volume is lost.

Fluid therapy and blood transfusions

The initial goal of treatment for acute circulatory failure (once an adequate airway and breathing have been ensured) is to ensure an adequate intravascular volume. Severe circulatory failure requires the temporary use of inotropic drugs and vasopressor drugs together with fluids (see below). Immediate surgical control of hemorrhage is the best treatment for bleeding.

monounsaturated (e.g. oleic acid) and polyunsaturated acids (e.g. linoleic acid, arachidonic acid). Linoleic acid is the only essential fatty acid, and must be provided in food. Fats of plant origin are usually composed largely of unsaturated fatty acids and as a result are liquids at room temperature. Catalytic hydrogenation during commercial food processing, a process known as 'hardening,' results in some of the double unsaturated bonds becoming saturated. This converts them from oils into solid fats.

Fats serve as a major source of energy as a result of their high energy content per unit weight compared with carbohydrates or proteins. Fats are stored as lipid droplets in special cells, adipocytes or fat cells. In addition to their energy value, fat content in the diet increases the palatability of food.

VITAMINS See below.

TRACE ELEMENTS See below.

INDIGESTIBLE FIBERS Indigestible fibers, consisting mainly of cellulose (non-starch polysaccharides) in the diet, help maintain appropriate motility in the gastrointestinal tract.

Expression of the energy content of food

Energy provided by carbohydrates, proteins and fats is expressed in terms of kilocalories (kcal). One calorie is defined as the amount of heat required to raise the temperature of 1 g of water by 1°C (from 14.5°C to 15.5°C). Fats provide the highest energy yield (Table 22.1). Carbohydrates and fats spare proteins from being utilized as an energy source. Nutritional proteins serve primarily for the synthesis of tissue proteins unless the intake of carbohydrates and fats is insufficient to provide adequate energy.

The average daily caloric requirement for a healthy adult with a light pattern of physical activity is about 2000 kcal but this can be tripled with severe physical activity. Several conditions influence the requirement for caloric intake. These include pregnancy, lactation, exercise, disease states, age and rate of growth. The elderly usually require a lower energy intake.

Table 22.1 Energy provided by carbohydrates, proteins and fats

Component	Average energy yield (kcal/g)
Carbohydrates	4
Proteins	4
Fats	9

Average values are given due to the large variation in the chemical composition of these nutrients.

Total parenteral nutrition (TPN)

Various clinical conditions can prevent patients from eating an adequate amounts of food. Such conditions include unconsciousness, inability to swallow, inflammatory bowel disease, surgery, trauma or malignant disease. As a result, patients may need nutritional support. This can be either by the enteral route (infusion of nutrient solutions into the upper gastrointestinal tract) or parenterally (i.v. infusion of nutrient solutions). The term total parenteral nutrition (TPN) is used when parenteral nutrition serves as the sole source of nutrition. TPN solutions are concentrated hypertonic solutions. Owing to their high osmolarity, it is not possible to use a peripheral venous line to give TPN because of the risk of thrombophlebitis. For this reason, TPN solutions are generally administered via a central venous line (superior vena cava, subclavian vein) since the greater flow in these veins adequately dilutes concentrated TPN solutions. TPN solutions provide the major components of nutrition:

- Source of nitrogen (essential and nonessential amino acids).
- Source of energy (dextrose) and fats (including the essential fatty acid linoleic acid).

With long-term TPN solutions, vitamins and trace elements are added in sufficient amounts to prevent deficiencies. Fat is given in the form of lipid emulsions. The most common complication of TPN solutions is infection around the intravenous line.

EXAMPLES OF EXCESSIVE AND INADEQUATE CALORIC INTAKE

Obesity

An imbalance in food intake can lead to obesity (excessive caloric intake compared with energy expended) or weight loss (inadequate caloric intake compared with energy expended). Obesity is a nutritional problem that has environmental, behavioral, socioeconomic and genetic components. It affects about a third of the adult population in the richer parts of the world and its prevalence is increasing. Obesity develops over years but obese children tend to remain obese in adulthood. Obesity may be defined in terms of body weight or, alternatively, as total body fat. The cosmetic standards for thinness, as well as for body weight (except for exceedingly high weight), are not of major concern. The most important problem is that obesity is associated with a three- to fourfold increase in morbidity due to medical complications such as cardiovascular diseases, hypertension, gallbladder disease, respiratory disease, osteoarthritis and some types of cancer.

A clinically useful quantitative measure is body mass index (BMI), which relates weight (in kilograms) and height (in meters) as weight/height^2. Overweight is arbitrarily defined as a BMI of greater than 25 and less than 30 kg/m^2. Obesity is a BMI equal to, or greater than

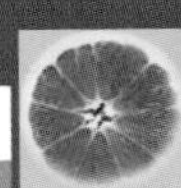

Table 22.2 Body mass index (BMI) as a measure of optimal body weight

Undernutrition	Normal weight	Overnutrition
Severe <15.9 kg/m^2 Moderate 16–16.9 kg/m^2 Mild 17.0–18.4 kg/m^2	18.5–24.9 kg/m^2	Overweight 25.0–29.9 kg/m^2 Obesity 30.0–39.9 kg/m^2 Morbid obesity >40.0 kg/m^2

30 kg/m^2 (Table 22.2). However, how body fat is distributed between central and peripheral compartments also correlates with increased risk. Morbidity and mortality is most associated with a central distribution of body fat (measured as the ratio of waist circumference to hip circumference), which is >0.9 in women and >1.0 in men. Acceptable values are <0.75 for women and <0.85 for men.

There are genetic determinants of obesity. The ab-gene and the protein leptin regulate food intake. Leptin, produced in adipose tissue, interacts with hypothalamic receptors to signal the filling of adipose tissue, and thereby regulates food intake and expenditure. Although increased levels of leptin have been detected in the obese, the structures of leptin and leptin receptor genes are normal in most obese patients. The potential role of leptins in the pathogenesis of obesity in humans is presently unclear.

Obesity increases the risk for:

- Cardiovascular system:
  - Workload on the heart
  - Sudden death due to cardiac arrhythmias
  - Atherosclerosis
- Diabetes mellitus:
  - Type II diabetes mellitus
- Cancer:
  - Endometrial and postmenopausal breast cancer in women
  - Prostate cancer in man
  - Colorectal cancer in men and women
- Pulmonary function:
  - Sleep apnea
- Joint problems:
  - Osteoporosis
  - Gout
- Skin problems:
  - Acanthosis nigricans
  - Skin turgor and friability
- Endocrine system:
  - Irregular and anovulatory cycles
  - Earlier menopause
  - Changes in thyroid hormone and its metabolism

Control of body weight

Essential or 'vital' organs, such as the brain, have a continuous demand for energy irrespective of food availability or frequency of meals. Since the necessary energy supply cannot be guaranteed on a meal-to-meal basis, there exist metabolic and hormonal pathways which store energy (for example, as glycogen in liver) and utilize it when food is unavailable.

A small imbalance in caloric intake over a long period, e.g. a daily excess of 50 kcal, will produce a 2 kg weight gain over a year. The hypothalmus is an important site from which energy intake and expenditure are regulated. Neural and endocrine signals originating from adipose tissue, neural and endocrine systems, and the gastrointestinal tract, are integrated in the hypothalamus from which afferent signals go to higher centers and produce feelings of hunger and satiety as well as to the autonomic nervous system and pituitary gland to control energy expenditure (Fig. 22.1). As a consequence, regulation of appetite and sensations of satiety are very complex processes controlled by both peripheral and central mechanisms.

Treatment of obesity

As a result of obesity being a multifactorial problem, various treatment strategies are used in treating the overweight. The importance of treatment strategies depends on several factors:

- The BMI value.
- The presence of central distribution of body fat.
- The presence of other coronary risk factors.

Individuals with associated risk factors are considered appropriate for treatment when the BMI value is 27 kg/m^2 or higher. For most people, an initial loss in body weight is relatively easy to achieve, but continuing weight loss and its long-term maintenance is more challenging. The average weight reduction with most of the available strategies does not exceed 10%. In fact, more than 90% of people who lose weight initially regain it subsequently. Therefore, combined strategies for treatment are recommended and followed on a regular basis.

BEHAVIORAL MODIFICATION is a way of changing eating behavior and increasing awareness of overeating. This may include:

- Daily recording food intake.
- Adjusting meal frequency.
- Adjusting speed of eating.
- Removing cues which result in overeating.
- Separating eating from other activities.

EXERCISE is individually adjusted for each patient based on motivation and the extent to which he or she is overweight. The primary purpose of exercise is to increase energy expenditure and improve cardiovascular fitness. It includes walking and cycling at fairly low levels of energy expenditure. Daily, long-term, low-

Table 23.1 The different classes of antibacterial drugs used in the treatment of oral infections

Penicillins	Penicillin V Amoxicillin Amoxicillin with clavulanate Ampicillin
Tetracyclines	Tetracycline Doxycycline Minocycline
Cephalosporins	Cefalexin Cefaclor
Macrolides	Erythromycin Azithromycin Clarithromycin
Clindamycin	
Metronidazole	

frequently encountered in acute oral infections. Amoxicillin is another first-choice antibacterial drug because of its oral bioavailability and effectiveness against Gram-negative organisms. Penicillin G or ampicillin is preferred for parenteral administration. Erythromycin and related macrolides are used as alternative drugs in patients with penicillin allergy or where infection is less severe. Clindamycin has a favorable spectrum that includes Gram-positive and anaerobic bacteria and is considered as the alternative choice to penicillin by some.

Cephalosporins are seldom drugs of first choice, but are used when staphylococcal organisms are involved as, for example, in cases of osteomyelitis or oral trauma.

Metronidazole, with its anaerobic spectrum of antibiotic activity, is rapidly becoming a drug of choice for selected periodontal infections. It is most often used in combination with a second antibiotic that has the desired spectrum of activity against aerobes.

Tetracyclines are generally limited in their dental use to those infections associated with the periodontium, but they are also used as an alternative to penicillin V in the treatment of actinomycosis.

The role of the quinolone antibiotics for common dental infections remains to be established. Recent information suggests that their use is appropriate in some oral infections where culture and sensitivity testing suggest a favorable outcome.

The drug interactions with the antibiotics used in dentistry are shown in Table 23.2.

Adverse effects of antibiotics

- **All antibiotics can cause gastrointestinal adverse effects and diarrhea**
- **Allergic reactions occur more frequently with the penicillins**
- **Antiinfectives alter the normal flora, causing a risk of opportunistic candidiasis, especially in immunosuppressed patients**
- **Tetracycline use in children causes permanent gray-yellow mottling of teeth**

Treatment of periodontal infections

Periodontitis (infection of the periodontium) can present in a variety of acute or chronic forms, and with different etiologies. In adults it is typically chronic with symptoms limited to an erythematous gingiva that bleeds on probing or brushing. The distinguishing feature of periodontal disease is a continuing infection of the supporting tissues of the teeth, resulting in a progressive loss of gingival attachment and alveolar bone. It is the most common cause of tooth loss in adults.

Periodontitis often remains undetected until a patient presents with loose teeth, or an acute exacerbation. People reporting bleeding gums or the presence of blood on the toothbrush should be referred for dental evaluation. In the younger age group it can present as a juvenile periodontitis.

Table 23.2 Drug interactions that occur with the antibiotics used in dentistry

All antibiotics	Reduced effectiveness of oral contraceptives Effectiveness of bactericidal drugs may be reduced when combined with bacteriostatic antibiotics
Penicillins and cephalosporins	Probenecid inhibits renal excretion and prolongs duration of action Allopurinol increases the risk of nonallergic skin rashes in patients taking ampicillin Bioavailability of atenolol may be decreased by ampicillin
Macrolides	May increase serum levels of theophylline, lithium, carbamazepine, valproic acid, ciclosporin and digoxin Compete with clindamycin for 50S ribosomal binding site in microorganisms Increase bioavailability of triazolam, enhancing the level of sedation Erythromycin may increase the effects of oral anticoagulants; therefore monitor blood clotting times
Tetracyclines	Absorption impaired when given concurrently with antacids, dairy products or iron salts Barbiturates, phenytoin, ethanol and carbamazepine may increase hepatic metabolism of doxycycline
Metronidazole	Avoid concurrent use with ethanol, ethanol-containing products, and disulfiram May potentiate warfarin oral anticoagulants, so monitor blood clotting times Barbiturates can decrease its effectiveness Can increase serum lithium levels

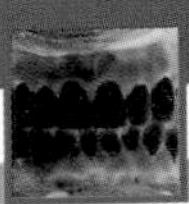

Management of periodontitis

Periodontal disease can be controlled by reducing the number of microorganisms that infect the periodontium

In order to control periodontal disease a variety of treatment modalities are required. All of these treatments are designed to reduce the number and types of microorganisms infecting the periodontium. The control of plaque and gingivitis is one way of reducing supragingival microorganisms and bacteria in plaque. However, if microbial invasion of the deeper tissues of the periodontium is involved, systemic antibacterial drugs, irrigation with antiinfectives and surgical debridement may be required to control the disease.

Systemic antibacterial drugs should include those that are effective against multiple anaerobic organisms. Selection depends on the causative organisms and their antibiotic sensitivity.

Tetracyclines and amoxicillin alone, or in combination with metronidazole or even ciprofloxacin, have been used. Recently, low-dose doxycycline (20 mg twice daily) has been introduced. It appears that this drug has no antimicrobial activity and may be effective by virtue of inhibition of the collagenase (released by bacteria in crevices) that is responsible for injury to the periodontium. A variety of special formulations of antibacterial drugs used in dentistry include:

- Tetracycline-containing monofilament fiber.
- Doxycycline polymer gel.
- Metronidazole gel.
- Minocycline powder.
- Chlorhexidine resorbable chip for adjunctive treatment in refractory periodontal disease.

The gels, fiber, powder or chips are placed into the periodontal pocket around the tooth where the drug is slowly released over several days. Contraindications to the use of these special dose forms include the presence of an acute, periodontal abscess or hypersensitivity to the individual drugs.

Prophylactic use of antiinfective drugs in dentistry

The prophylactic use of antibiotics in dentistry is not generally required in routine dental treatments of those without risk factors and with a normal immune system. However, patients with pre-existing myocardial or valvular pathology may be at risk for endocarditis secondary to bacteremia. Transient bacteremia (usually lasting less than 20 minutes) occurs with dental procedures including extractions, oral and maxillofacial surgery, periodontal therapy, deep scaling and other dental procedures. Specific microorganisms present in the oral cavity have been implicated as a cause of infective endocarditis in those patients recognized as being at risk.

Around the world, dental advisory groups have established guidelines for antibiotic prophylaxis for those patients at risk during dental surgery. Amoxicillin, penicillin V or a suitable alternative drug (clindamycin, a macrolide or cephalosporin) are usually recommended for prophylactic administration immediately prior to the dental procedure.

Prophylaxis guidelines to prevent bacterial endocarditis are not intended for prophylactic use in other 'at-risk' patients

There is considerable debate about the risk, benefits and antibacterial drug choice in patients who have joint prostheses. However, antibacterial prophylaxis may be considered for patients with a compromised immune system. Recommended guidelines are not available for every situation in every patient, so consultation between the patient's physician and dentist is advised. 'At-risk' patients with poor oral hygiene, extensive caries, gingivitis or periodontitis should be on a dental treatment program that includes elimination and prevention of dental disease (Table 23.3).

Common nonbacterial diseases of the oral mucosa

Candida *infection*

Candida albicans is the most common cause of oral yeast infections. The incidence of oral candidiasis has increased in recent years, and it is particularly common in those with human immunodeficiency virus (HIV) or other causes of immune deficiencies. A decreased flow of saliva in those with Sjögren's syndrome, or in those treated with certain drugs, contributes to the risk of candidiasis.

Table 23.3 The type of patients 'at risk' from invading bacterial infections that require antibiotic prophylaxis

Bacterial endocarditis can occur in patients with:
Prosthetic cardiac valves (bioprosthetic and homograft) A previous history of bacterial endocarditis Surgically constructed systemic–pulmonary shunts Complex congenital cyanotic cardiac malformations Rheumatic and other acquired valvular dysfunctions Hypertrophic cardiomyopathy Mitral valve prolapses with regurgitation
Other types of infection may develop in patients with:
A compromised immune system
The requirements for antibacterial drug prophylaxis and the drugs of choice are made after consultation between physician and dentist if a patient has:
Organ or tissue transplants Traumatic orofacial wounds Chemotherapy for cancer Vascular grafts A major joint prosthesis Renal dialysis Insulin-dependent diabetes mellitus

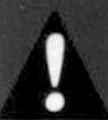

Systemic drugs used for oral mucosal diseases

- Suppression of adrenal cortical activity with systemic glucocorticosteroids
- Azathioprine can cause bone marrow depression, secondary infection and neoplasia
- Dapsone has been associated with severe cutaneous reactions and hematologic defects

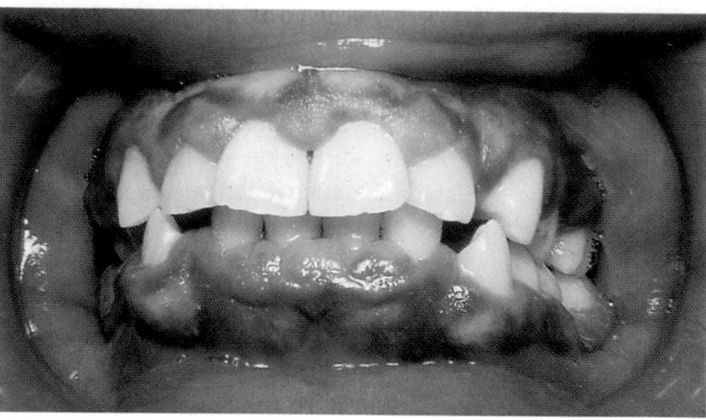

Fig. 23.6 Drug-induced gingival hyperplasia. The gingival papillae show mild hyperplasia associated with the use of phenytoin. Attention to dental hygiene and routine dental scaling to control local factors help to reduce the severity of the hyperplasia. Ciclosporin and Ca^{2+} antagonists produce a similar hyperplasia.

Drug-induced oral disease

Many dental patients take prescribed medications capable of inducing adverse effects manifest as painful oral mucosal reactions (stomatitis). Mucositis and oral ulcerations are associated with cancer chemotherapy. Other oral adverse reactions to drugs include lichenoid drug reactions, lupus erythematosus-like reactions, pemphigus-like drug reactions and erythema multiforme (Table 23.7).

Contact allergic reactions can occur in the mouth but are not common. Angioedema has been observed with some drugs and cinnamon-based ingredients in dentifrices. Dental materials, including metals and acrylic polymers, have also been implicated in soft-tissue allergic reactions.

Phenytoin, ciclosporin and the calcium channel blockers can cause a gingival hyperplasia (Fig. 23.6). This develops in approximately 40% of patients taking phenytoin. Among the calcium channel blockers, it is suggested that isradipine is less likely to cause gingival hyperplasia. In this condition the gingival mucosa begins to enlarge and cover the teeth. In severe cases this overgrowth almost entirely covers the teeth and has to be surgically reduced.

Drugs with anticholinergic effects frequently reduce saliva, leading to a drug-induced xerostomia. A dry mouth can also be due to systemic disease and must be considered in these cases.

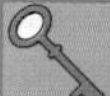

Xerostomia

- A common cause of a 'burning tongue'
- Carries a high risk for dental caries
- Carries a high risk for candidiasis
- May be caused by prescribed medications

Management of drug-induced adverse effects

The management of drug-induced oral adverse effects includes:

- Identifying the suspect drug.
- Working with physician and patient to seek alternative drugs where possible.

In addition, symptomatic treatment is used together with efforts to improve dental hygiene and control plaque. Acute inflammatory symptoms often respond to topical or systemic antiinflammatory glucocorticosteroids. Antifungal drugs such as nystatin or a chlorhexidine rinse

Table 23.7 Drug-induced adverse effects involving the mouth

Adverse effect	Causative drugs
Lichenoid-drug eruptions	Allopurinol, furosemide, chloroquine, chlorpropamide, gold salts, methyldopa, lithium salts, mercury, penicillamine, phenothiazines, propranolol, quinidine, spironolactone, thiazides, tetracyclines, tolbutamide
Lupus erythematosus-like eruptions	Gold salts, phenytoin, griseofulvin, isoniazid, penicillin, primidone, procainamide, thiouracil, hydralazine, streptomycin, methyldopa
Pemphigus-like drug eruptions	Penicillamine, phenobarbital, rifampin, captopril
Erythema multiforme	Antimalarials, barbiturates, carbamazepine, salicylates, chlorpropamide, sulfonamides, clindamycin, tetracyclines
Gingival hyperplasia	Phenytoin, ciclosporin, nifedipine (and other calcium channel blockers)
Xerostomia	Anorexiants, antidepressants, isotretinoin, anticholinergics, anticonvulsants, antihistamines, captopril, clonidine, prazosin, reserpine, diflunisal, piroxicam, antiparkinsonian drugs, antipsychotics, diuretics, cyclobenzaprine, opioids, albuterol

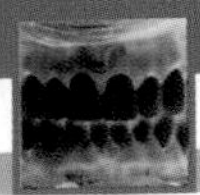

can be used for opportunistic candidiasis. Local anesthetic rinses may be beneficial for stomatitis due to cancer chemotherapy.

The symptom of having a dry mouth presents a significant challenge since there are no suitable artificial saliva substitutes, and drug-induced increases in salivary flow are unsatisfactory. Oral pilocarpine may give some benefit in patients who have received head and neck radiation. Cevimeline, a cholinergic agonist, was recently introduced for treatment of the dry mouth associated with Sjögren's syndrome.

FURTHER READING

Meecham JG, Seymour RA. *Drug Dictionary for Dentistry*. Oxford: Oxford University Press; 2002. [A handy guide to drugs used in dentistry.]

Rees TD. Drugs and oral disorders. *Periodontology 2000* 1998; **18**: 21–36. [An updated review of oral manifestations of drug reactions.]

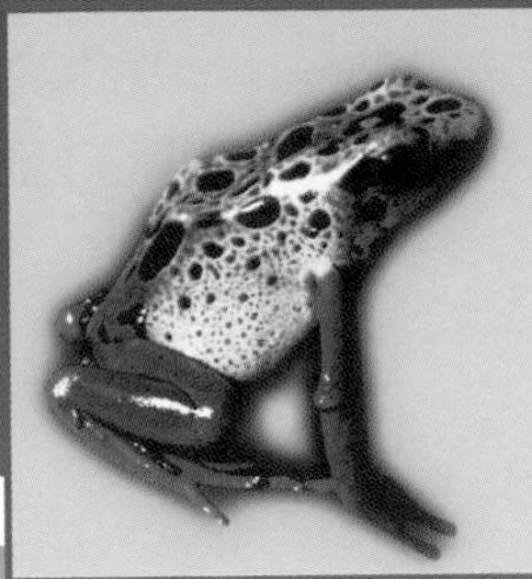

Chapter 24

Herbs, Toxins, Venoms and Poisons

This chapter discusses both the beneficial and adverse effects of a variety of chemicals derived from natural (herbs, toxins and poisons) and synthetic sources (many poisons). In the case of herbs, the intent behind their use is to derive a therapeutic effect. After all, many modern drugs have herbal origins or, in some cases (e.g. digoxin) are still obtained from plants. Other drugs (e.g. neuromuscular blocking drugs such as tubocurarine) arose from the investigation of the poisons found in plants. However, some herbal preparations are toxic to man, and the toxins and venoms present in plants and animals are generally recognized as being detrimental to human health. However, as with tetrodotoxin and botulinus toxin (see Ch. 2), therapeutic uses have been developed from such dangerous materials. While there are no simple semantic definitions for toxins, venoms and poisons, the latter term is often used to describe hazardous substances that are ingested or absorbed in some way from the environment, and may be natural or synthetic, organic or inorganic (e.g. toxic metals).

In this chapter herbs will be discussed first since they are used to try and achieve therapeutic effects. Their use is based upon ancient texts, cultural habits, inherited medicinal wisdom or other sources. The use of herbs and other substances for therapeutic and nefarious activities (poisoning one's enemies) stretches into distant antiquity.

Somewhat surprisingly, the use of herbs is still very widespread, even in countries where many modern pharmacologic discoveries and advances have been made. Reasons for this are many, but include irrational fear of 'science,' metaphysical belief systems, such as 'nature knows best,' unrestricted advertising by commercial or social mechanisms, and sheer perversity.

HERBS

Herbs as plants contain a multitude of molecules. Many of these molecules serve structural purposes, such as cellulose, and others are concerned with cellular metabolism, for example, multiple enzyme systems. Plants also produce organic molecules that help protect them against viruses, bacteria, fungi, insects, animals or even other plants that threaten their survival. Many of these chemicals are biologically active. Not surprisingly, therefore, plants are rich sources of chemicals with pharmacologic activity, many of which are potential drugs. When parts, or extracts, of plants are used for medicinal purposes they are called herbal medicines.

From antiquity to the present, plants and plant products have been used to treat disease (see Ch. 1).

The medical use of herbs is widespread and seems to be increasing. In a multi-ethnic group of patients attending an emergency department in New York, 22% reported that they used herbal medicines, with the highest percentage (37%) being Asians. In North America, most herbs are self-administered and provided by health food stores, herbalists or naturopaths. Prescription of herbal preparations by the medical profession is quite common in continental Europe and Asia. Germany and France have the highest per capita consumption of herbal medicines in Europe. Germans spent US$37 per capita on herbal preparations, a total of US$2.5 billion, in 1998.

The botanical name of a plant consists of its genus followed by its species designation. Table 24.1 lists important medicines that have been isolated and purified from plants, and illustrates several points in the complex relationship between plants and pharmacology:

- Many important drugs have been identified and purified from plants.
- Plants from quite different genuses can produce identical chemicals or drugs, e.g. *Atropa* and *Datura* spp., both of which produce atropine.
- Dissimilar chemicals with pharmacologically similar actions can be produced by plants from different genuses, e.g. *Hyoscyamus* and *Atropa* each produce antimuscarinic drugs (scopolamine and atropine). Similarly, plants from both *Digitalis* and *Strophanthus* genuses contain cardiac glycosides (digoxin and ouabain, respectively).
- Plants from different species of the same genus can produce different chemicals, e.g. *D. purpurea* and *D. lanata* respectively produce the cardiac glycosides digitoxin and digoxin.
- Traditional uses of a plant extract might or might not predict the pharmacology and subsequent use of pure compounds isolated from that plant, e.g. vincristine and vinblastine are used as anticancer drugs owing to their capacity to inhibit cell division. These drugs were isolated from the plant *Vinca rosa*, which had been claimed to have oral hypoglycemic

Table 24.1 Drugs obtained from plants traditionally used as herbal remedies or poisons

Botanical name of plant (common name)	Herbal products	Chemicals isolated: used as medicines
Atropa belladonna (deadly nightshade)	Belladonna leaf, belladonna tincture	Atropine, hyoscyamine
Datura stramonium (Jimson weed, thorn apple)	Stramonium, stramonium tincture	Atropine, hyoscyamine
Hyoscyamus niger (henbane)	Henbane tincture	Scopolamine (hyoscine)
Cinchona ledgeriana (cinchona tree)	Cinchona bark, jesuit bark, cardinal's bark, cortex peruanus	Quinine, quinidine
Colchicum autumnale (autumn crocus, meadow saffron)	Colchicum seed fluid extract, colchicum seed tincture	Colchicine
Digitalis purpurea (purple foxglove)	Digitalis folia (powdered leaf), tincture of digitalis	Digitoxin
Digitalis lanata (woolly foxglove)	Digitalis folia (powdered leaf), tincture of digitalis	Digoxin
Strophanthus gratus	Strophanthus seeds	Ouabain
Ephedra sinica	Ma huang	Ephedrine, pseudoephedrine, phenylpropanolamine
Papaver somniferum (opium poppy)	Powdered opium, laudanum (tincture of opium alkaloids)	Morphine, heroin, codeine, papaverine
Physostigma venenosum (Calabar or ordeal bean)	Whole beans	Physostigmine (eserine)
Pilocarpus jaborandi	Chewed leaves (induced sweating)	Pilocarpine
Rauwolfia serpentina	Rauwiloid, alseroxylon (raudixin)	Reserpine
Salix alba (white willow)	Extract of willow bark	Salicyclic acid
Strychnos toxifera, Chondrodendron tomentosum	Curare (arrow poison)	*d*-tubocurarine
Vinca rosa (periwinkle)	Alleged oral hypoglycemic	Vincristine, vinblastine

actions. In other words, pharmacologically active substances with unexpected actions can be isolated from herbs used for unrelated purposes.

Pharmacologists in the late nineteenth and early part of the twentieth centuries were active in the identification of pharmacologically active principles in plants, and in the standardization of herbal extracts. Their goal was to produce consistent and standardized medicines. Examples are belladonna leaf BP or digitalis leaf USP. The initials BP and USP, respectively, stood for British Pharmacopoeia and United States Pharmacopeia, and indicate that the medicine has been standardized according to officially approved methods. Bioassay procedures were extensively used for such purposes since there were no adequate chemical methods for assaying the constituents, or active ingredients, of herbs. Even with modern chemical techniques it is a formidable task to identify the dozens or more potentially active chemicals in any plant. When more than one plant is used in a herbal remedy, the problem increases more than proportionally.

Problems particular to herbal medicines

What is (are) the active ingredient(s)?

Herbal medicines contain many chemicals and there is often no agreement as to which of these chemicals are therapeutically active. An example is garlic (*Allium sativa*), which contains many sulfur compounds, several of which have possible therapeutic actions. Another is St. John's wort (*Hypericum perforatum*), which contains hypericins, but it is unlikely that these are responsible for the antidepressant effect claimed for the herb. Hyperforins are currently believed to be the therapeutically active constituents of St. John's wort.

Quality control for the herbal medicines – what do they really contain?

Herbal medicines are not required to pass any regulatory analysis in the USA prior to being sold as health food supplements. In the USA, herbs are governed under the Dietary Supplement Health and Education Act (DSHEA). Under this legislation, claims for treatment of disease cannot be made, but herbs can be claimed to be 'Health Modifiers.' The constituents of herbal remedies are not regulated unless there is an adverse report concerning a particular product, or sampling of a product shows it to be mislabeled, or to contain substances not mentioned on the label.

In Canada, all products intended for medicinal use, including natural health products, are issued a Drug Identification Number. These numbers are not required for raw materials such as bulk herbs or herbal preparations labeled as foods or nutrition supplements. In other jurisdictions around the world, rules are generally no tighter. In essence, herbal products are subject to much less regulation than conventional drugs.

Unfortunately, there are many examples of herbal medicines that have been adulterated with other (more toxic) herbs, potent synthetic drugs (e.g. phenylbutazone, synthetic corticosteroids or other prescription drugs) or heavy metals (mercury or lead).

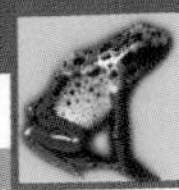

Table 24.2 Some direct adverse effects of herbs

Common names (botanical name)	Adverse effects	Putative constituents responsible	Putative mechanisms responsible
Aconite (*Aconitum carmichaelii*) Monkshood (*A. columbianum*)	Cardiac arrhythmias	Aconitine	Activation of sodium channels
Aristolochia fangchi	Renal toxicity and carcinogenesis	Aristolochic acid	Chromosomal damage
Chaparral (*Larrea tridentata*)	Liver toxicity		Cholestatis hepatitis
Comfrey (*Symphytum officinale*)	Jaundice, ascites, cirrhosis	Pyrrolizidines	Hepatic venous occlusion
Ephedra or ma huang (*Ephedra sinensis*)	Cardiac arrhythmias, CNS stimulation	Ephedrine, norephedrine and related compounds	Sympathomimetic activity
Germander (*Teucrium chamaedrys*)	Liver toxicity		
Licorice (*Glycyrrhiza glabra*)	Increases sodium retention and potassium excretion	Glycyrrhizins	Inhibition of cortisol metabolism in kidney leading to aldosterone-like effects
St John's wort (*Hypericum perforatum*)	Skin photosensitivity, drug interactions (increases ciclosporin metabolism)	Hypericins, hyperforins	Induction of cytochrome P-450 enzymes

The table is not inclusive of all herbs that have been shown to have adverse effects.

Occasionally, the plant constituents in herbal preparations are inadequately, or wrongly, named. For instance the term ginseng is applied to Siberian ginseng, but this plant is of the genus *Eleutherococcus*, not *Panax* as is American or Korean ginseng. Consequently, the term ginseng by itself has little botanical, or possibly pharmacologic meaning. Only the botanical name, consisting of genus and species, correctly identifies a plant.

How are herbal medicines standardized?

In general the chemical constituents of a plant vary in a manner that depends on the species, variety and part of the plant, conditions of growth (soil, water and temperature), season of the year and the age of the plant. These complexities and variations in chemical content should make standardization of active ingredients very important. In some cases standardization is attempted, but it is difficult and seldom accomplished. There are no regulations governing the standardization of chemical constituents for herbal medicines. Even if the label says 'Standardized' for some constituent, it usually is not known whether that constituent is the main contributor to any therapeutic effect. In other words, the potential for considerable variability to occur from one preparation to another is a concern for pharmacologically active herbal products.

Problems common to all herbs (as well as to prescription drugs)

How can effectiveness be determined?

To establish the therapeutic effectiveness of herbs as medicines, they should be tested in prospective, double-blind, randomized, controlled clinical trials (RCTs), preferably with a placebo arm as is done for official drugs. Very few herbs have been tested in this manner, though such is the generally expected standard of regulatory agencies for prescription drugs. Thus, at the present time there is no legal requirement that herbal preparations have to be demonstrated to be effective in the treatment of disease in any country. The explanations for this apparent discrepancy between the relatively unregulated availability of herbal medicines versus prescription drugs involve complex political, social and economic factors.

Adverse effects

There is a general belief amongst lay people that, because herbs are 'natural,' they are safe. This is not true, especially as many herbal preparations have pharmacologic activity – that is, they are not inert. Herbs and herbal preparations can cause direct adverse effects, produce serious allergic reactions and adverse drug interactions. An example is St. John's wort, which induces the enzymes involved in the metabolism of ciclosporin. This can lead to decreased steady-state concentrations of ciclosporin unless the dose is increased to compensate for this. St. John's wort also increases the action of antidepressant drugs that are modulators of serotonin uptake, such as the SSRIs. Herbs also can interfere with the function of some laboratory tests. For example, Siberian ginseng produces falsely high serum concentrations of digoxin when it is taken concomitantly with digoxin.

Examples of direct adverse effects of herbs are shown in Table 24.2.

Commonly used herbal medicines

Table 24.3 lists some common herbal medicines with their traditional indications for use. Current RCT evidence for effectiveness and some of their known adverse effects are included in the table. At the present time, none of the clinical trial-based evidence for effectiveness of herbal preparations can be considered conclusive. There are trials where some benefit over

Table 24.3 A compilation of some common herbal medicines with a brief summary of use and evidence of effectiveness obtained in randomized clinical trials (RCTs)

Common name (botanical name)	Traditional use	Therapeutic ingredients	Mechanism	Number of RCTs with placebo comparison (Result)	Adverse effects
Chamomile, German (*Chamomilla recutita*)	Tonic	Unknown	Unknown	0	Allergy
	Mouthwash, oral mucositis			1 (=)	
Devil's claw (*Harpagophytum procumbens*)	Antirheumatic for low back pain	Unknown		1 (=)	
Echinacea (*Echinacea purpurea*)	Immune stimulant for upper respiratory infections	Unknown	Immune stimulant	12 (?) 3 (+) 2 (=)	Allergy
Evening primrose (*Oenothera biennis*)	Atopic dermatitis	Unknown	Unknown	5 (2+, 3=)	
	Rheumatoid arthritis			3 (?)	
	Psoriatic arthritis			1 (=)	
	Premenstrual syndrome			2 (=)	
	Menopausal flushing			1 (=)	
	Obesity			1 (=)	
	Ulcerative colitis			1 (=)	
	Hyperactivity attention deficit			2 (=)	
	Raynaud's syndrome			1 (=)	
	Sjögren's syndrome			1 (=)	
	Psoriasis			2 (=)	
Feverfew (*Tanacetum parthenium*)	Migraine	Parthenolides	Unknown	2 (+)	Allergy
	Rheumatoid arthritis	Unknown		1 (=)	
Garlic (*Allium sativum*)	BP lowering	Unknown	Unknown	7 (?)	
	Cholesterol lowering	Unknown		13 (?)	
Ginger (*Zingiber officinale*)	Seasickness	Unknown	Unknown	1 (=)	
	Hyperemesis gravidarum	Unknown		1 (+)	
	Postoperative nausea/vomiting	Unknown		3 (2+, 1=)	
Ginkgo (Egb 761) (*Ginkgo biloba*)	Dementia progression	Ginkgolides, platelet activating factor (PAF) antagonists	Unknown	6 (5+, 1=)	Bleeding
	Tinnitus	Unknown			
Ginseng, American (*Panax quinquefolius*)	Exercise performance	Ginsenosides	Unknown	1 (=)	
Ginseng, Korean (*Panax ginseng*)	Exercise performance	Ginsenosides	Unknown	2 (=)	Gynecodynia
	Psychomotor performance	Ginsenosides		1 (=)	
	Flu vaccine immunization response	Ginsenosides		1 (+)	
Ginseng, Siberian (*Eleutherococcus senticossus*)	Exercise performance	Eleutherosides		1 (=)	Interferes with measurement of digitalis in blood
PC-SPES Eight herbs	Prostate cancer	Estrogenic compounds	Anti-testosterone	0	Gynecomastia, thrombosis
St John's wort (*Hypericum perforatum*)	Antidepressant	Hyperforins, hypericins	SSRI	2 (+)	Skin photo-sensitivity, drug interactions
Saw palmetto (Pemixon) (*serenoa repens*)	Prostatic hyperplasia	Unknown – antiadrenergic	Unknown	2 (+)	
Zemaphyte (ten herbs)	Atopic eczema	Unknown	Unknown	1 (+)	Liver toxicity

Following the number of RCTs reported is an indication of a therapeutic effect greater (+) than or equal (=) to placebo, (?) equivocal or unknown findings.

placebo has been shown but these trials require confirmation with larger trials of longer duration. There are very few data available for the long-term safety of any herbal preparations.

Summary

Plants are rich sources of biologically active chemicals and potential sources of effective medicines. However, more research, regulation and standardization are required

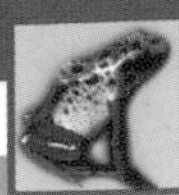

before herbal medicines can be recommended as effective and safe therapies by the criteria used for conventional drugs. At present, the rule is 'let the buyer beware.'

Healthcare providers should be aware that patients frequently take herbal products that may have powerful pharmacologic effects, cause adverse effects in their own right and have pharmacodynamic and pharmacokinetic interactions with prescribed drugs. Consequently, a careful history needs to be obtained from patients about their possible use of herbal preparations. This issue will likely grow in importance as herbal use continues to grow.

TOXINS, VENOMS AND POISONS

Every natural or synthetic chemical can cause injury if exposure is high enough

Exact definitions of terms such as toxin, venom and poison are not possible, chiefly because every chemical can cause injury if given in high enough doses (Table 24.4). Whether a chemical is considered a venom, toxin or poison depends mainly on its source, not its actions. Thus, for practical purposes:

- Toxins were originally described as the poisons produced by microorganisms, but the word is now used more broadly for other species (e.g. the ω conotoxins from coneshells).
- Venoms are substances injected by one species into another.
- Poisons are natural or synthetic chemicals that can injure, or impair, bodily functions. They may or may not have beneficial actions in addition to being poisonous.

Toxins and venoms are often proteins or polypeptides, particularly those produced by vertebrates, whereas poisons are often small molecules. Invertebrates and plants also produce a wide variety of toxins and poisons; many of the plant poisons are alkaloids (organic molecules containing nitrogen).

Table 24.4 Potency of potential toxins and poisons in terms their acute lethality

Lethal potency as lethal dose in mg/kg body weight	Potential poisonous substances
1 000 000	Water
10 000	Ethanol, other alcohols, general anesthetics
1000	Iron salts, vitamins
100	Barbiturates
10	Morphine, some snake venoms
1	Nicotine and many plant poisons
0.1	Curare, sea snake venoms, jellyfish toxins
0.01	Tetrodotoxin
0.001	Ciguatoxin, palytoxin
<0.0001	Botulinum toxin

Toxins, venoms and poisons have varying influences on our lives

Toxins, venoms and poisons influence and endanger human life in a variety of ways. Some examples include:

- Direct danger in the form of naturally occurring toxins and poisons that are ingested or inhaled (tobacco smoke).
- Danger from toxins generated by infectious organisms.
- Environmental poisons derived from natural sources.
- Environmental poisons due to industrial processes.
- Exposure to venomous organisms.
- Use of toxins and venoms as weapons of war and terrorism.

As has been noted by many, life is a toxic process. The oxygen that is so essential to aerobic life is potentially toxic to all tissue via its ability to form oxygen free radicals that are capable of damaging biological molecules. The world around us is replete with similar toxic elements and chemicals. The process of evolution results in continuous biological warfare between competing species. This has resulted in a huge variety of different toxic chemicals from relatively simple small molecules to very complex proteins. In addition, the chemical activities central to the industrialization process have resulted in a myriad of toxic chemicals, some of which were intentionally created as toxins for other species, or for our own species. Many of the chemicals produced by industry are incidental toxins whose potential danger is not recognized for years. A more sinister aspect is the use of poisons and toxins for purposes of warfare or other forms of human violence such as terrorism. Biological warfare is not a new development, since for centuries opposing armies have tried using infectious diseases against the opposition. Recent events have heightened our awareness of the large number of toxins and poisons that are available for violent purposes. The list is endless and includes, beside biological weapons, poison gases, anticholinesterase inhibitors and natural toxins. Some of these have already been used for terrorist purposes.

It appears that our world is full of potential chemical dangers but their importance should not be overrated since vigilance on the part of the medical profession and regulatory agencies relatively quickly recognizes potential dangers. For example, once the aflatoxins (hepatoxins) had been recognized to occur in contaminated peanuts steps were taken in richer countries to limit their danger. Similarly, in the richer countries with adequate infrastructure there is continuous monitoring and detection of other possible dangers, as is witnessed by removal of leaded gasoline. Unfortunately, fear of the unknown, a noisy media, and suspect political motives, can elevate what may be a very limited danger to the level of hysteria. In order to assess the extent of the real danger it is important that the degree of danger is properly identified and weighed against benefits. Thus, we use cars for transport on a daily basis but conveniently ignore the associated danger and willingly trade convenience for a danger over which, in reality, we have little control.

We should also remember that evolution has provided a number of protective biochemical and physiologic mechanisms. A classic example of the latter is the vomiting reflex whereby poisons ingested with food are detected by 'vomiting centers' in the area postrema in the medulla oblongata which, when activated, initiates vomiting that clears the stomach of its potentially poisonous contents. Despite the fact that such areas are anatomically within the CNS, they have no blood–brain barrier and thus are rapidly able to 'sense' poisons circulating in the blood. The liver, through the CYP enzymes, as well as such enzymes located in the gut and elsewhere, act as continuous detoxifiers of ingested and circulating poisons. Unfortunately, the above mechanisms readily come into play against potentially helpful exogenous molecules such as therapeutic drugs.

Toxins, venoms and poisons are potential sources of useful drugs

As illustrated by various examples given in this chapter and elsewhere, toxins, venoms and poisons have been a source of many drugs. Examples from plants include drugs such as atropine, tubocurarine, vinca alkaloids and eserine. Fungi have been the source of a host of antibiotics (e.g. penicillin, tetracyclines and ciclosporin) and anticancer drugs. Toxins from bacteria (streptokinase) and fractions from snake venoms (ancrod) are used to dissolve blood clots. In addition to therapeutic drugs, many pharmacologic tools have been isolated from venoms, toxins and poisons.

Acute toxicity results from brief exposure, chronic toxicity from months or years of exposure

Exposure to venoms involves direct contact with a venomous animal, whereas ingestion is a common route of exposure for toxins and poisons. Poisons continuously present in air, water and food (e.g. pesticides, heavy metals and chlorinated hydrocarbons) lead to chronic low-level exposure. Exposure by inhalation is a common route of poisoning in the workplace. The skin is an effective barrier to most water-soluble poisons, but not to markedly fat-soluble substances.

Toxins and poisons can be regarded as having direct or indirect mechanisms of action

Many toxins and poisons act in a relatively selective manner on target organs, often as the result of the particular physiologic and biochemical functions of those organs (Fig. 24.1). The kidneys are particularly vulnerable. However, metallothioneins, a unique protein class,

Organs that show increased susceptibility to poisons
Kidney
Kidney receives 25% of cardiac output
glomerulus
precipitates
damage filter
function
tubule
collecting duct
interstitial
damage
Poisons may be excreted or absorbed
Heavy metal damage tissue directly
Reactive intermediates are formed in the kidney
Lung
Huge surface area (a site for direct damage and good absorption)
epithelium
exposed to gases,
irritants,
metal vapors
trachea
bronchioles
alveolus
Alveoli trap particles
Blood-borne poisons cause direct damage to alveolar membrane and possibly pulmonary edema
Liver
Two blood supplies (portal vein and hepatic blood). Enterohepatic recirculation involves bile acids
extensive
metabolism
occurs in
liver cells
hepatic blood
supply
portal vein
Some poisons are detoxified, others are converted into toxic metabolites
Enterohepatic recirculation results in repeated exposure of the liver

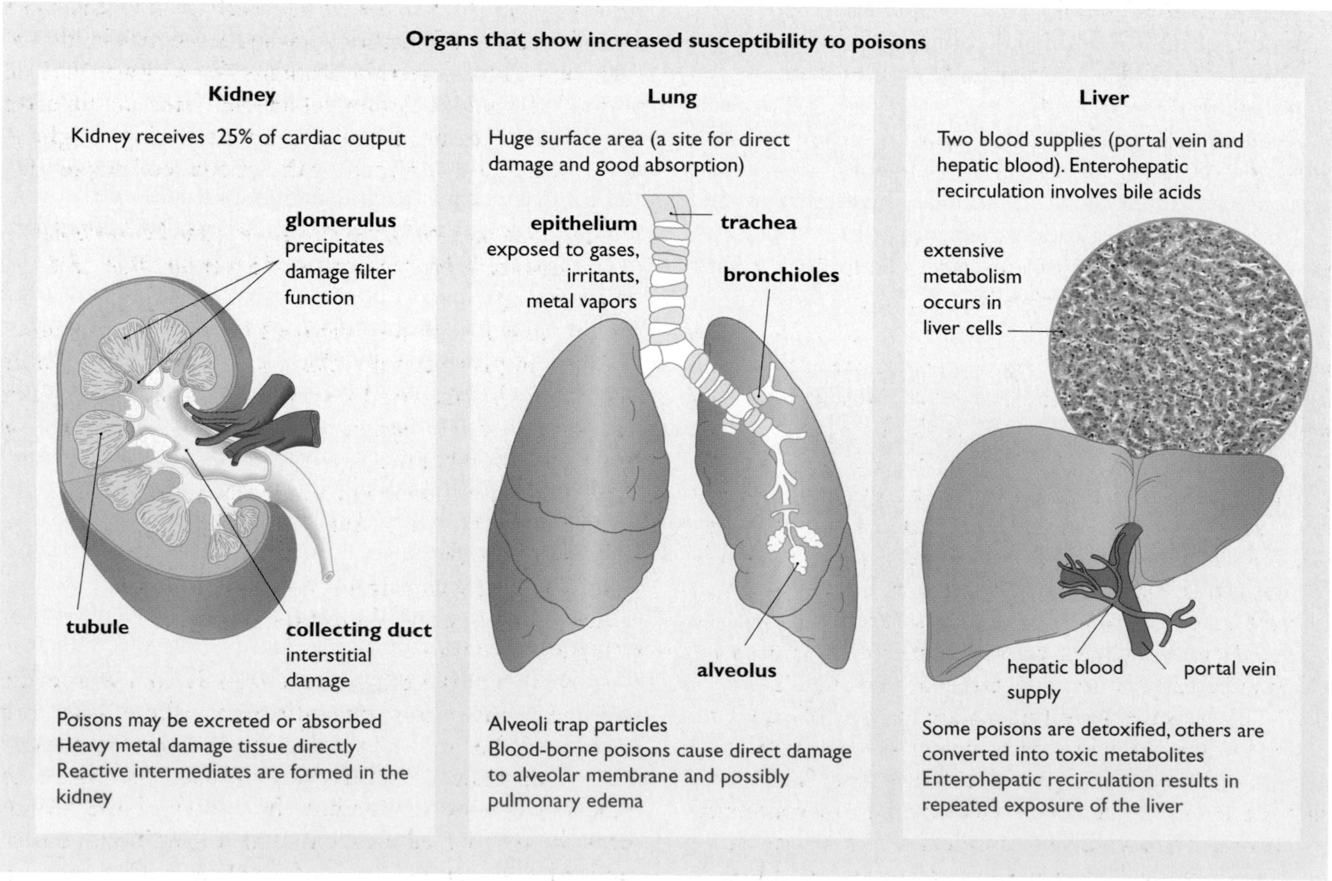

Fig. 24.1 The physiologic mechanisms influencing kidney, lung and liver responses to poisonous substances.

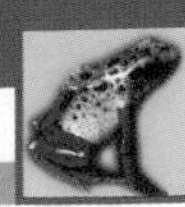

can help protect organs by avidly binding some poisons (e.g. cadmium).

Whether poison-induced damage is reversible, or irreversible, often depends upon the repair and regenerative capabilities of the target tissue. For example, liver damage is often reversible because the liver has a marked regenerative ability. However, damage to the central nervous system (CNS) is likely to be irreversible since neurons do not generally regenerate under normal conditions. The axons of neurons are particularly vulnerable since they have limited metabolic functions and rely on transport (often over long distances) of materials from the cell body. Furthermore, the normal age-related loss of neurons can result in neuropoisons reducing the age at which neurologic and behavioral deficits appear (e.g. drug-induced parkinsonism).

Poisons can act indirectly

Allergic reactions are immunologically mediated adverse reactions to repeated exposure and sensitization to allergens. Poisons can also act directly on the immune system to cause immunosuppression, thereby rendering a person liable to infection. The activation and recruitment of phagocytic cells to sites of chemically induced injury plays a role in the progression of tissue injury.

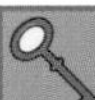

Chemicals hazardous to man

- Toxins from animals and plants
- Venoms from animals
- Poisons from natural and man-made sources

Approximately eight million people in the USA suffer an episode of acute poisoning each year

The hazards generated by exposure to poisons are monitored and limited by legal regulations resulting from recommendations made by the government committees and government agencies responsible for protecting the public from toxic hazards. A key measure in assessing the potential hazard to humans of a particular poison is its no-observed-adverse-effect level (NOAEL) of exposure. The NOAEL for a hazardous chemical is determined in laboratory animals by dosing them with the poison of interest and determining the largest dose that can be tolerated while producing an observable effect. For humans likely to be exposed to that particular poison, 1/100th of the NOAEL is the permitted maximum level of exposure. (The fraction is obtained by allowing 1/10 for individual differences, and 1/10 for species differences.) The use of such a measure relates to the fact that the Environmental Protection Agency (USA) considers a risk of one death per million individuals exposed to a poisonous substance as the maximum acceptable exposure level. To give this level of risk meaning in comparison with other hazards, consider that 20 000 people die each year in the USA from the effects of illicit drugs while acute toxicity due to drug or poison ingestion accounts for at least 10% of hospital admissions. Motor vehicle accidents and firearms are an even greater hazard. For an interesting insight as to how hazards are viewed by the public see Chapter 3.

Table 24.5 Principles for the treatment of envenomation and poisoning

Remove the source of poison or the victim from the source (e.g. rescue)
Remove and limit the absorption of the poison (e.g. fresh air, wash, emesis, limit contact)
Supportive therapy (e.g. ventilation, external cardiac massage, saline/oxygen, drugs)
Specific therapies:
Antivenins for animal venoms
Antitoxins for bacterial toxins
Chelators for heavy metals
Gases (e.g. oxygen for carbon monoxide)
Other drug therapies:
Ethanol for methanol
Digoxin antibodies for digoxin
Pyridoxine for isoniazid
Nitrite and thiosulfate for cyanide
N-acetylcysteine for acetaminophen
Specific antagonists:
Atropine and oximes for organophosphate anticholinesterase inhibitor poisoning
Flumazenil for benzodiazepine overdose
Opioid antagonists (naloxone) for opiate overdose
Anticholinesterases for neuromuscular blocking drugs

Standard medical procedures and specific therapies are available in many cases of envenomation and poisoning

The obvious first step in the treatment of envenomation or poisoning is to remove the source of exposure (Table 24.5). This is followed by procedures designed to limit absorption, and/or speed excretion of the venom or poison, for example by:

- Restricting dispersion of venom from the envenomation site by bandaging and immobilization.
- Removing poisons from the stomach or skin.
- Acidification, or alkalinization, of urine.
- Ingestion of water.

A very important treatment step is to use specific antidotes, antivenins or antitoxins, where they are available. Other steps can include hemodialysis to remove poisons or toxins by filtration, and hemoperfusion to remove them by circulating the blood of the victim through an activated charcoal filter. In addition, general supportive measures are used, such as giving oxygen, fluids and appropriate supportive drugs.

VENOMS, TOXINS AND POISONS FROM NATURAL SOURCES

Treatment of poisoning

- Remove the source of poison
- Minimize absorption of the poison
- Specific therapy, if available
- Supportive therapy

Venoms from animals

Venomous animals occur in all animal phyla (e.g. Fig. 24.2 and Table 24.6). Venoms are usually, but not always, proteins or polypeptides with complex three-dimensional structures, and many different mechanisms of action. Specialized venom glands and injection apparatus are required to inject the venom. In addition, fatal allergies can develop to venoms, particularly to those of bees, hornets and wasps. The venoms of such animals are not that lethal, with effects of their stings being mainly local skin reactions. Stinging is only fatal if there are many stings to an infant or other susceptible victims.

Snake venoms

Many snake venoms are complex mixtures of polypeptides and proteins: some of the latter are enzymes. Such enzymes can account for some of the systemic toxicity and much of the local toxicity that is seen following crotalid snake (rattlesnake and pit viper) bites. Crotalid venoms can affect blood coagulation and hemostasis, and cause tissue necrosis at envenomation sites. Enzymatic actions of such venoms include proteolysis, lipolysis and phospholipase activity. Such actions result in cell disruption, cell lysis, and generalized tissue damage.

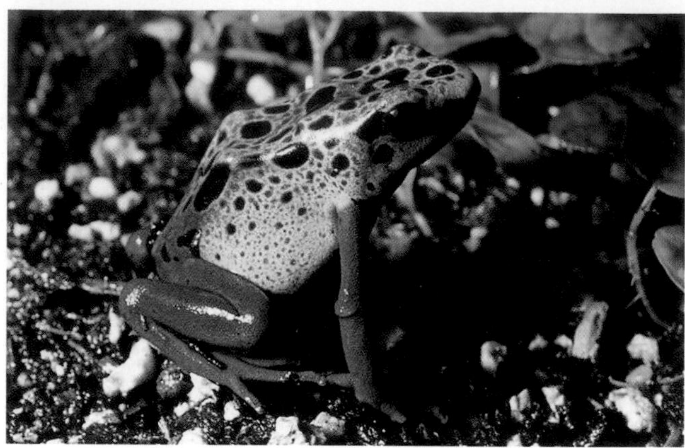

Fig. 24.2 A typical poisonous frog. Extracts from the skin of similar poisonous frogs (*Dendrobates* sp.) are painted on the tips of arrows and darts in Central and South America for hunting purposes. Many vertebrates are capable of injecting venoms, or contain poisons. (Photograph, Ron Kertesz, permission of the Vancouver Aquarium.)

Table 24.6 Source and mechanisms of action of a variety of animal venoms and toxins

Toxin	Source	Mechanisms of action
Small molecules		
Tetrodotoxin	Puffer fish, octopus, salamander	Na^+ channel blocker
Saxitoxin	Shellfish contaminated with dinoflagellates	Na^+ channel blocker
Ciguatoxin	Large tropical fish contaminated with dinoflagellates	Actions on Na^+ channel
Cardiac glycosides	Toad skin	ATPase inhibitor
Batrachotoxin	Frog skin	Na^+ channel activator
Domoic acid	Shellfish (mussels)	CNS toxin
Palytoxin	Sea anemone	Ionophore
Proteins and polypeptides		
α bungarotoxin	Elapid snakes (kraits)	Nicotinic receptor blocker
β bungarotoxin	Elapid snakes (kraits)	Presynaptic cholinergic nerves
α conotoxin	Coneshells	
μ conotoxin	Coneshells	Skeletal muscle Na^+ channel blocker
ω conotoxin	Coneshells	N-type Ca^{2+} antagonist
Cardiotoxin	Elapid snakes	Direct acting cardiotoxin
Phospholipases	Many snakes	Cell membrane destruction
Bacterial toxins		
Botulinum toxin	*Clostridium botulinum*	Synaptin in cholinergic nerve endings
Cholera toxin	*Cholera vibrio*	Activation of G_s protein
Pertussis toxin	*Bordetella pertussis*	Inactivates G_o/G_s protein
Endotoxin	Gram-negative bacteria	Cell membranes
Tetanus toxin	*Clostridium tetani*	Cell membrane ionophore
Staphylococcal toxin	*Staphylococcus* sp.	Enterotoxin

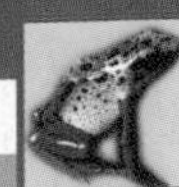

Nonenzymatic polypeptides and proteins in snake venoms can have selective molecular actions

Many elapid snake (e.g. cobra, krait) venoms contain neuromuscular-blocking polypeptides. Some of these block nicotinic cholinoceptors (see Chs 8 and 21) in such a selective manner that one such polypeptide (α bungarotoxin) was first used to identify and label nicotinic receptors in skeletal muscle. The related β bungarotoxin selectively blocks the release of acetylcholine at the neuromuscular junction of skeletal muscle.

The lethality of snake venoms varies widely

The danger posed by snake bites varies with the species and volume of venom injected. Many snakes have venom glands that contain enough venom to kill a number of humans, but snakes rarely inject all their venom when attacking humans. The lethality of particular snake venoms depends upon the toxicologic actions of their various components. Among the many venomous snakes, potentially the most dangerous are probably the tropical sea snakes (Hydrophiidae) which, despite having very small fangs, are able to inject lethal amounts of nicotinic cholinoceptor-blocking polypeptides. In addition, their venom also contains phospholipase enzymes that break down skeletal muscle membranes to cause myoglobinuria and potential kidney failure.

Antivenins (antibodies) are produced as treatment for many snake venoms as well as for those from spiders and scorpions. Treatment with antivenins combined with local procedures using bandaging and immobilization are used to limit the escape of venom from the wound site. The treatments can be very effective in treating snake bite and other forms of envenomation. It is increasingly recognized that systemic effects following envenomation can be limited by reducing the lymphatic spread of venom from the envenomation site.

Studies into the actions of snake venoms have led to pharmacologic developments

A bradykinin-potentiating polypeptide isolated from a Brazilian snake venom led to the development of captopril, the first clinically useful angiotensin-converting enzyme inhibitor (see Ch. 13). Ancrod is a fibrinolytic factor from the Malayan pit viper (*Agkistrodon rhodostoma*) that breaks down fibrinogen into fragments of fibrin and thereby produces afibrinogenemia. The highly selective molecular actions of other components of snake venoms have led to their use as pharmacologic tools and potential therapeutic agents.

Other venoms

Other well-studied venoms include those from scorpions. Scorpion venoms can be lethal for children, but are not so lethal to adults. These venoms target a variety of cellular constituent macromolecules, including K^+ channels. Many marine animals contain venoms, including vertebrates such as fishes (e.g. stingrays, scorpion and lion fish) which have venomous spines. Their venoms can inflict severe pain and injury, but are not usually lethal. Such venoms are usually mixtures of proteins and polypeptides. On the other hand, tetrodotoxin is a small molecular weight poison found in puffer fish. It is a highly selective sodium channel blocker that has been used as a local anesthetic and as a pharmacologic tool. Interestingly, puffer fish are eaten after very careful preparation to remove their most poisonous parts (liver and intestine) as a delicacy (fugu) in Japan.

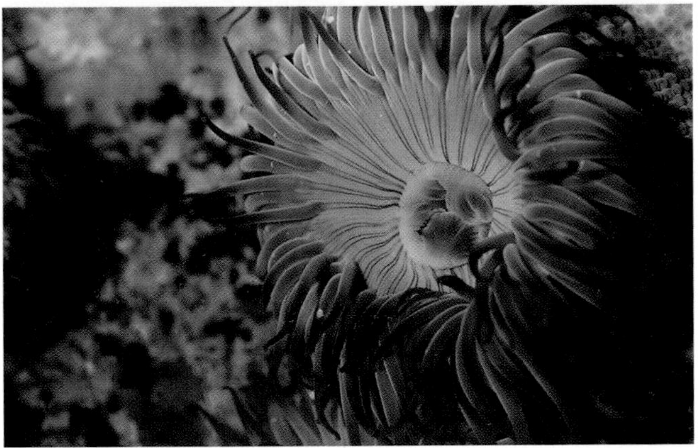

Fig. 24.3 Many marine invertebrates contain venoms and poisons. Venoms in corals, anemones and jellyfish are contained within special cellular stinging organelles called nematocysts. Nematocysts contain a stinging thread that penetrates the skin and injects venom. Many of these invertebrates are very attractive and children are particularly liable to be stung. (Photograph, Ron Kertesz, permission of the Vancouver Aquarium.)

Nonvertebrate species also possess dangerous venoms:

- The venoms of jellyfish (coelenterates) and corals (Fig. 24.3) are found within special organelles known as nematocysts. The amount of venom that can be injected by nematocysts is limited unless large areas of the skin are involved. Some of the box jellyfish found in tropical Australian waters can cause fatal stings in children, while many coastal areas around the world are subject to invasions by jellyfish such as the Portuguese man-of-war (not a true jellyfish but a hydroid, *Physalia* sp.)
- Some species of octopus inject tetrodotoxin, a selective blocker of Na^+ channels, into their prey. In Australia such species have killed children.
- Venoms of various tropical shellfish, the coneshells, show remarkable selectivity for various molecular targets. Depending upon the species concerned (Fig. 24.4), coneshells are predators of fish, worms or other coneshells. Coneshells inject their venoms via a specialized hollow harpoon. Each prey-specific species of coneshell has its own special conotoxins that target in a very selective manner such specific molecular sites as ion channels and receptors. For example, certain conotoxins are specific blockers of neuronal (N) type calcium channels. One such conotoxin is currently used by local injection for treatment of severe pain.

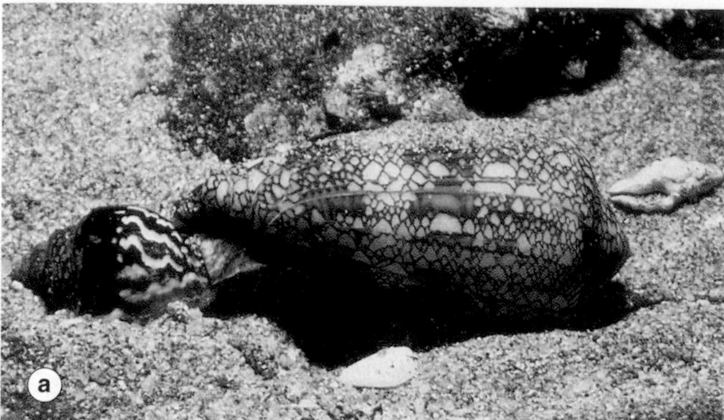

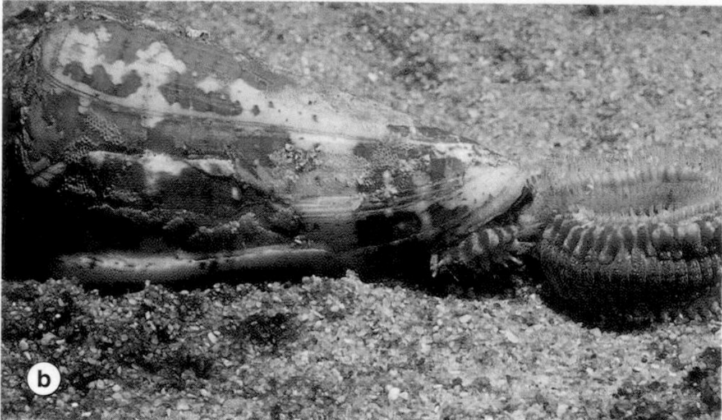

Fig. 24.4 Different coneshells have evolved venoms that are relatively specific for their prey species, whether other snails, worms or even fish. Conotoxins are often highly selective in their actions on specific ion channels in cell membranes. (Photographs, Alex Kerstitch.)

Various other phyla contain toxins whose actions relate to the role such venoms play in the ecology of the species. Examples include the stings of various insects such as bees and hornets. Other fascinating examples include ticks which produce venomous saliva which has anticoagulant, antiinflammatory and analgesic properties. The latter peptides help the tick avoid detection by their host for 7–10 days. Leeches are able to attach themselves to their hosts and draw blood without being detected. Leeches inject hirudin, a thrombin antagonist, to ensure a continuous flow of blood that they ingest. Hirudin is used clinically (see Ch. 13) as an anticoagulant.

Toxins and poisons from other species

Vertebrate species, apart from those with venoms, contain few substances that are poisonous to other species. Invertebrate species (e.g. fungi and bacteria), on the other hand often, contain toxins. Bacterial toxins are produced by many different bacterial species and probably serve purposes other than killing the species that serves as hosts for the bacteria. Many antibacterial polypeptides isolated from bacteria are presumably used for defense purposes. Fungi also use a large variety of complex non-protein molecules as deterrents to competitors and predators. Fungal poisons have adverse effects on many species, especially bacteria. Thus, the source of most antibiotics used therapeutically is still fungi, although they are often used in the form of semi-synthetic derivatives of the parent compound. On the other hand, fungal contamination of food, and eating the wrong type of what are erroneously thought to be edible fungi, are the cause of many cases of poisoning. Examples of the former include aflatoxin, a liver toxin and carcinogen, produced by *Aspergillus flavus*, a contaminant of peanuts. Various large poisonous fungi are often ingested in mistake for the edible species. These poisonous fungi contain a wide variety of toxic molecules which produce damage, particularly to the liver and the kidneys.

Bacterial toxins vary in their chemical nature and actions

Botulinum toxin is one of a group of bacterial endotoxins that includes tetanus and diphtheria toxins. Botulinum toxin itself is an orally absorbed protein from *Clostridium* sp. (an anaerobe) that is responsible for potentially fatal botulism. Poisoning typically occurs by ingesting preformed botulinum toxin formed in inadequately canned foods, or via contamination of wounds with live organisms. The latter is a much rarer cause of botulism. Symptoms of botulism are the result of the failure of acetylcholine release from all peripheral cholinergic nerve endings (see Chs 8 and 9). This results in disruption of cholinergic transmission in autonomic nervous system ganglia, as well as parasympathetic and motor neurons. In the latter, the loss of acetylcholine release from motor nerve endings results in muscle weakness, diplopia and respiratory failure, while the loss in the former lead to autonomic dysfunction. Therapy for botulism is supportive, although the use of antitoxin may be of value. Recovery depends on recovery of nerve endings with acetylcholine. Botulinum toxin is so potent that a single molecule can disable a single nerve ending. Botulinum toxin is used therapeutically to treat various dystonias involving muscle spasm such as around the eyes, in the neck or in the anus in the presence of an anal fissure. It is even used to disperse wrinkles.

Cholera toxin from the *Cholera vibrio* causes intense diarrhea. The molecular mechanism involves ADP ribosylation of the adenylyl cyclase stimulatory G_s protein, causing irreversible inactivation of GTPase and therefore permanent activation of G_s protein (see Ch. 2). cAMP accumulates and causes salt and water hypersecretion from gut epithelium. In contrast, pertussis toxin inactivates G_i/G_o proteins.

Other exotoxins released from bacteria, as well as endotoxins released by bacterial breakdown, are often responsible for many of the adverse consequences of bacterial infection. Complex polysaccharide endotoxins have a variety of actions including causing cardiovascular collapse (endotoxic shock) and fever.

Poisons from plants

Plants use chemicals for defense, and as a result produce many poisons, and even venoms (stinging plants), to deter

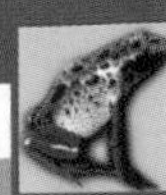

Table 24.7 Sources and toxic actions of a variety of plant and fungal poisons

Poison	Source	Mechanism of action
Plant poisons		
Atropine, scopolamine	Solanaceae (jimson weed, deadly nightshade)	Muscarinic receptor antagonists
Cardiac glycosides	Digitalis, strophanthus, oleander, convallaria	ATPase inhibitors
Aconitine	Hellebores	Cardiac Na^+ channel activator
Capsaicin	*Capsicum* sp. (peppers)	Substance P depleter
Ricin	Castor bean	Protoplasmic poison
Myristicin	Nutmeg and mace	Hallucinogenic
Emetine	*Ipecacuana* sp.	Vomiting center stimulant
Pennyroyal oil	*Mentha* sp.	Hepatotoxic and oxytoxic
Safrole	Sassafras tree	Animal carcinogen
Pyrrolizidines	Heliotropium, comfrey (herbal tea)	Hepatotoxic
Fungal toxins		
Muscarine	*Clitocybe, Amanita* sp., *Inocybe* sp.	Muscarinic agonist
Phallotoxins, amatoxins	*Amanita* sp. (death cap, destroying angel)	Hepatotoxic
Coprine	*Coprinus* sp.	Blocks aldehyde dehydrogenase
Ibotenic acid	*Amanita* sp.	Hallucinogenic
Psilocybin	*Psilocybe* sp.	Hallucinogenic
Aflatoxins	*Aspergillus* sp.	Hepatocarcinogenic
Ergot alkaloids	*Claviceps* sp.	Multiple actions
Orelline	*Cortinarius* sp.	Nephrotoxic

or kill predators (Table 24.7). Plant toxins and poisons are usually small organic nitrogen-containing molecules. The diversity, availability and ease of ingestion of plant poisons led to the discovery of many drugs (e.g. atropine, tubocurarine, digoxin, reserpine, morphine, caffeine, nicotine, paclitaxel, aspirin, quinidine, quinine and vincristine).

Plant poisons are particularly dangerous to domestic animals and children. Information about the nature of the common plant poisons and their treatment is readily obtained from Poison Control Centers. Not all cases of such poisoning are recognized and the physician should be aware of possible plant poisoning when faced with a patient exhibiting perplexing symptoms. It should be noted that herbal concoctions can contain plant poisons. Many cases of liver and kidney damage have been caused by folklore medicines.

INDUSTRIAL AND ENVIRONMENTAL POISONS

Industrial poisons are either intentional products of industry, or byproducts of industrial processes (e.g. air or water pollution). Environmental poisons can reach the environment to cause acute or chronic poisoning. Some are carcinogenic and/or mutagenic. While the concentration of industrial poisons can be high enough in the workplace to produce acute poisoning, concentrations in the general environment are usually not high enough to constitute an acute toxic hazard. However, low concentrations in the general environment can be sufficient to produce chronic poisoning.

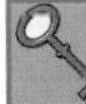

Industrial poisoning

- **The major industrial poisons are metals (in elemental, salt and organic forms), air pollutants and gases, aromatic and aliphatic hydrocarbons (liquids and vapors), insecticides, pesticides and herbicides**
- **All produce both acute and chronic toxicity**
- **Their low-level mutagenic and carcinogenic actions can be difficult to detect**

Metals

Heavy metals such as mercury, cadmium and lead are toxic both in the form of salts or as the elemental metal particularly when they are present as vapors or dust. The mechanism of toxicity for heavy metals often involves their combination with specific chemical groups on essential macromolecules (Table 24.8). Heavy metals such as arsenic tend to react with oxygen/sulfur groups on essential molecules, such as enzymes, to form inactive metal complexes (coordination compounds).

Mercury

Mercury has extensive industrial uses and is a common cause of accidental poisoning. Paints, mercury thermometers and laboratories are less common sources. Toxic amounts of mercury vapor can be absorbed from the lungs. Ingestion of inorganic and organic mercurial salts is mainly responsible for oral poisoning. Methylmercury-contaminated food led to hundreds of deaths in Iraq,

Table 24.8 Cellular mechanisms involved in producing heavy metal toxicity

Metal	Site and mechanism of molecular actions	Tissue and organ target responses
Mercury	Direct toxicity Sulfhydryl binding and disruption of important macromolecules (enzymes, pumps, receptors) Also binds phosphoryl, amino and other groups	Corrosive damage to lungs and gastrointestinal tract CNS, lung and renal damage
Lead	Sulfhydryl group binding Impaired heme synthesis	CNS and peripheral nervous system, cardiovascular, blood, kidney and skin
Cadmium	Binds to macromolecules and disrupts function	Lung and renal damage
Arsenic	Sulfhydryl groups and oxidative metabolism uncoupling	Peripheral nervous system, CNS, gastrointestinal tract, liver and cardiovascular system

while its environmental accumulation in seafoods poisoned residents of Minamata Bay, Japan.

Elemental (liquid) mercury is poorly absorbed in the gut, but the vapor is well absorbed from the lungs. Acute poisoning affects the respiratory tract, producing cough, dyspnea and interstitial pneumonitis. Ingestion of inorganic mercury compounds results in acute corrosive damage to the gastrointestinal tract, as well as renal damage. Symptoms of chronic poisoning are insidious in presentation and are often neurologic (visual disturbances, ataxia, paresthesias and neurasthenias) in origin. The diagnosis of mercury poisoning is based upon symptoms, history and mercury concentrations of >40 μg/L in blood and >5 μg/L in urine (Fig. 24.5).

The amount of oral absorption of mercury compounds depends upon the ionic form of the element. Inorganic salts of mercury are absorbed as Hg^{2+} (approximately 10% of ingested dose). Organic mercurial molecules are well absorbed orally, and distributed fairly uniformly throughout the body. Mercury readily forms covalent bonds with sulfur (in the form of -S- bonds or -SH groups). This formation of covalent bonds is the ultimate mechanism responsible for poisoning. Mercury also binds to phosphoryl, carboxyl, amide and amine groups, disrupting the functioning of enzymes, receptors and other important cellular macromolecules.

Specific treatment of elemental mercury poisoning includes the use of chelators such as intramuscular dimercaprol for those with severe intoxication, or oral penicillamine for a less severe exposure.

Oral succimer is a useful replacement for penicillamine. Dimercaprol is contraindicated for organic mercurial poisoning since its administration can elevate mercury concentrations in the brain. The enterohepatic recirculation of mercury allows for the rational oral use of non-absorbable polythiol resins which irreversibly bind intestinal mercury so that it is subsequently lost in feces. L-cysteine, infused intra-arterially, forms a dialyzable complex with methylmercury. Organic mercurial poisoning is harder to treat since organic mercury does not chelate well (see below). In the past, organic mercurial drugs were used to treat syphilis and various parasitic infections. Their therapeutic effects were limited by mercurial toxicity.

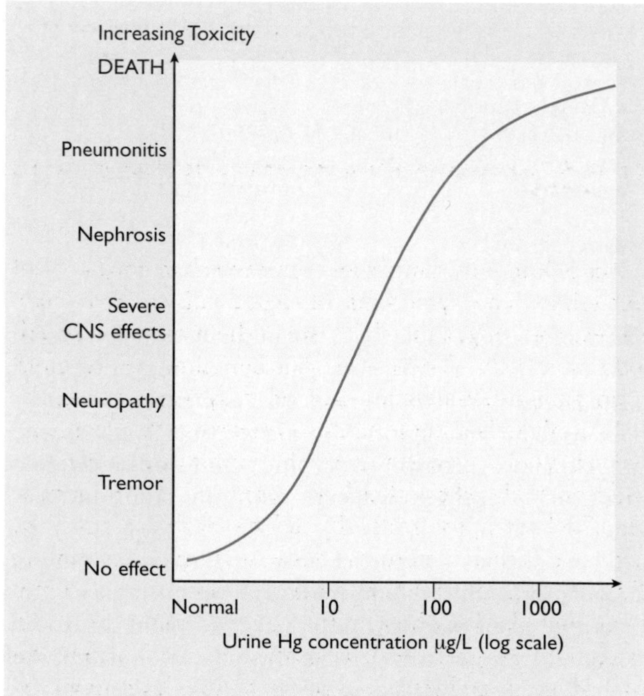

Fig. 24.5 The concentration–toxic response relationship which relates the concentration of mercury found in urine and the corresponding symptoms of mercury poisoning.

Lead

Lead was formerly used routinely over the centuries in the manufacture of water pipes, glazes and paints. In some countries organic lead compounds are still added to gasoline to prevent its premature ignition in the engine ('antiknock' additive). Older paints have a lead content of up to 40% of their dry weight. For such reasons, environmental and occupational exposure used to be common, and still is in some countries. Chronic lead poisoning, particularly in urban regions, has led to government restrictions on lead use, especially in paint and gasoline (Fig. 24.6).

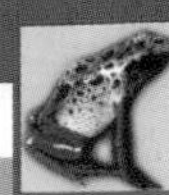

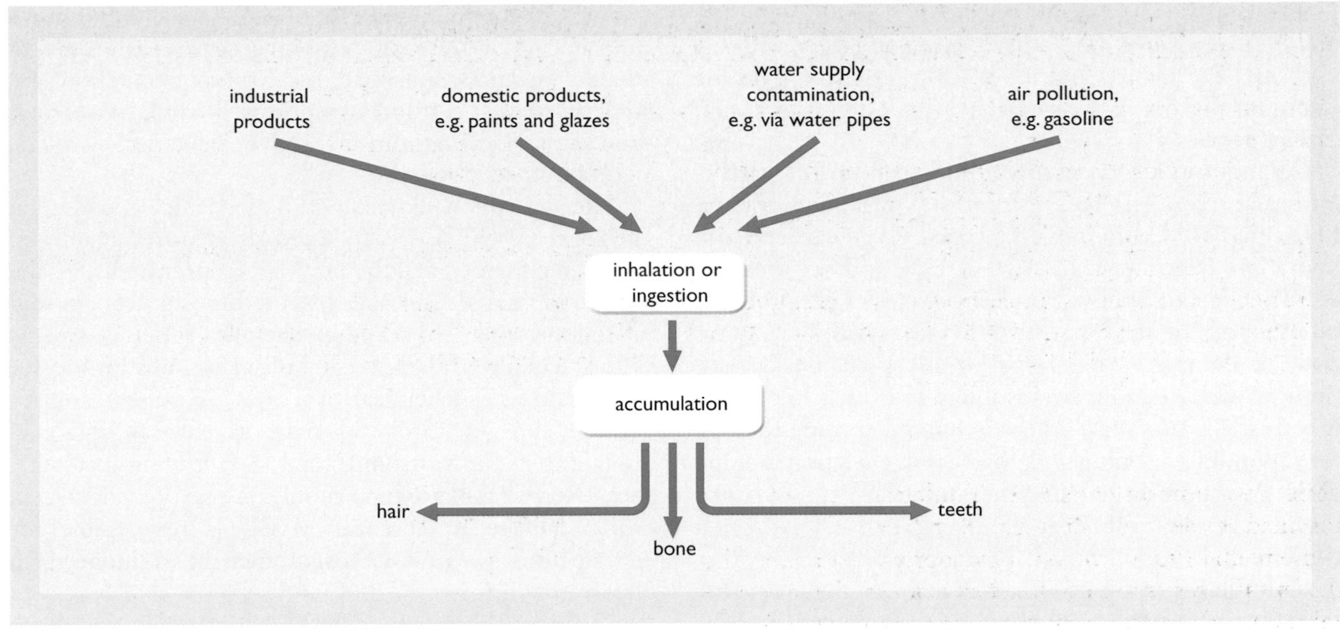

Fig. 24.6 Sources of the lead responsible for lead poisoning, and how lead is distributed within the body.

Acute lead poisoning is less common than chronic lead poisoning. The symptoms of acute poisoning include nausea, vomiting, a metallic taste in the mouth and severe abdominal pain. There can also be acute severe CNS symptoms, a hemolytic crisis, kidney damage and shock.

Chronic poisoning (plumbism) causes gastrointestinal, neuromuscular, renal and CNS symptoms, as well as symptoms related to other body systems. Neuromuscular and CNS symptoms usually follow severe poisoning. Gastrointestinal symptoms follow less severe poisoning (Fig. 24.7). CNS symptoms are more common in children. They include disturbed motor control, restlessness and irritability. Progressive deterioration of mental function may occur in children as a result of low-level environmental exposure to lead. It is difficult to diagnose and detect low levels of lead toxicity.

Lead is absorbed from both the gastrointestinal and respiratory tracts, and gastrointestinal absorption is greater in children. Lead is distributed throughout the body, and deposited in bones, teeth and hair. Chelation therapy that is guided by the blood concentrations of lead is useful. In order of priority the drugs used are:

- $CaNa_2$ ethylenediaminetetra-acetic acid (EDTA) (i.m. or i.v.).
- Dimercaprol (i.m.).
- D-penicillamine (orally).
- Succimer.

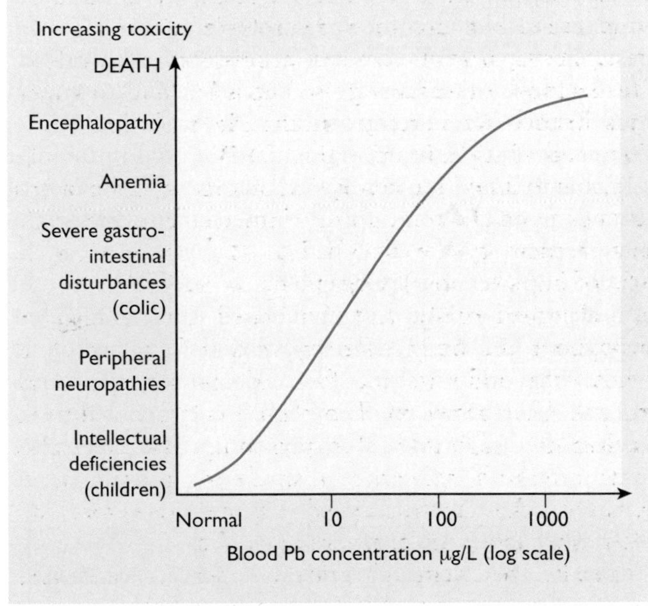

Fig. 24.7 The concentration–toxic response relationship for the concentration of lead in blood and the corresponding symptoms of lead poisoning.

Cadmium

Perhaps surprisingly, cadmium poisoning can be as common as mercury or lead poisoning. This poisoning is due in part to the widespread and increasing industrial use of cadmium in plastics, paints and batteries. Cadmium accumulates in foods such as animal livers and kidneys, food grains, and particularly shellfish. Exposure as a result of food contamination is important, but industrial workers can also be exposed to cadmium vapors in the air.

Acute poisoning is generally due to airborne exposure. It is associated with initial lung irritation followed by pneumonitis, chest pains, residual emphysema and possibly fatal pulmonary edema. Oral ingestion results in vomiting, diarrhea and abdominal cramps.

The outcome of chronic poisoning depends upon the mode of exposure. The lung is a major target with air exposure, the kidney and lungs with ingestion. Chronic cadmium poisoning is associated with osteomalacia and carcinogenesis.

Cadmium (Cd^{2+}) is poorly absorbed from the gastrointestinal tract. Absorption from the lungs is up to four times higher. Cadmium distributes slowly around the body, but concentrates in the kidney and, as a result, kidney damage follows oral ingestion. The proximal tubules are damaged first, and the glomeruli later. Lung tissue is damaged directly by an unknown mechanism. 'Itai-itai' disease in Japan was found to be due to chronic ingestion of cadmium. There is limited specific therapy for cadmium poisoning and, in general, chelation therapy does not appear to be beneficial.

Arsenic

Arsenic has been used extensively in the past for therapeutic purposes, including the treatment of syphilis and parasitic infections. Indeed, some arsenical drugs are still in use for the latter. Most arsenic poisoning arises from industrial and environmental exposure. High concentrations of arsenic occur naturally in some water supplies, including some in the western USA. Certain pesticides and herbicides are also a source of arsenic (Table 24.9). Arsenicals are sometimes added to animal food stock to promote growth, or in excess amounts as vermin poisons. Arsenic was commonly used in the past as a cosmetic and for murderous purposes. In the case of the former use it was applied to the skin to lighten the complexion.

Acute arsenical poisoning is now rare because the availability of arsenical compounds is strictly regulated. Symptoms following acute ingestion develop within 12 hours. They include severe gastric pain, projectile vomiting and severe diarrhea. Renal collapse, anuria and shock can rapidly lead to death. Neuropathies and encephalopathies are common sequelae of acute poisoning if death does not occur. Chronic poisoning causes early signs of muscle weakness and myalgias, hyperpigmentation and hyperkeratosis. Other symptoms include sweating, stomatitis, lacrimation, excessive salivation, coryza, dermatitis and alopecia.

The absorption characteristics of arsenic depend upon the form in which it is ingested. It is stored mainly in heart, lung, liver and kidney, but concentrates in the keratin of the hair and nails (useful forensic facts), as well as in bones and teeth. The biochemical action of arsenic is to uncouple oxidative metabolism by substituting for phosphate in biochemical processes. It causes capillary leakage and myocardial damage as well as epithelial sloughing in the gastrointestinal tract leading to bloody feces. Renal capillaries and tubules are severely damaged, while damage to cerebral vessels is responsible for neuropathies. Central necrosis and cirrhosis can occur in the liver.

Arsenic is also carcinogenic and teratogenic. It induces squamous and basal cell skin carcinomas, and possibly lung and liver cancers. Specific treatments for arsenic poisoning include chelation therapy with intramuscular dimercaprol, followed by oral penicillamine or succimer.

Table 24.9 Arsenical drugs and poisons

Type of arsenic	Poison/drug
Inorganic	
Elemental Trivalent arsenite Pentavalent arsenate	Insecticides, rat poisons, fungicides (source of most arsenical poisoning via food contamination)
Arsine gas	Released by acids
Organic	
Antiparasitic drugs	Carbarsone, tryparsamide, melarsoprol (rarely used)

Arsenic is a common cause of acute heavy metal poisoning, and is the second most common source (after lead) of chronic heavy metal poisoning.

Chelators

Chelators are molecules that complex with, and thereby 'hold,' metal ions in inactive forms that are suitable for mobilization and subsequent excretion. The chelators used medically for this purpose include EDTA, diethylenetriaminepenta-acetic acid (DTPA), dimercaprol, succimer (Fig. 24.8), penicillamine and deferoxamine. The principal therapeutic use of chelators is to treat heavy metal poisoning. However, chelators have also been promoted for use in such diseases as atherosclerosis (chelation therapy). However, controlled clinical trials of such therapies have failed to show that they have any therapeutic benefit.

EDTA is usually given as its calcium disodium salt. The sodium ions are easily displaced from EDTA by heavier toxic metals such as manganese, zinc and iron. Administration of EDTA is by intravenous or intramuscular routes, although the latter route of administration is painful. Treatment schedules must be followed carefully since rapid infusion of EDTA in other than as the calcium disodium salt form can cause transient hypocalcemia. However, since the body has a huge excess of calcium over EDTA ions, calcium concentrations quickly return to normal.

DIMERCAPROL is a dithiol analog of glycerol. Since the chelate formed with thiol groups of dimercaprol is not very stable, dimercaprol therapies include maximization of chelate excretion. Dimercaprol is given intramuscularly and is more effective when given early after exposure. Adverse effects of dimercaprol include reversible hyper-

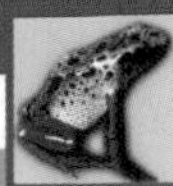

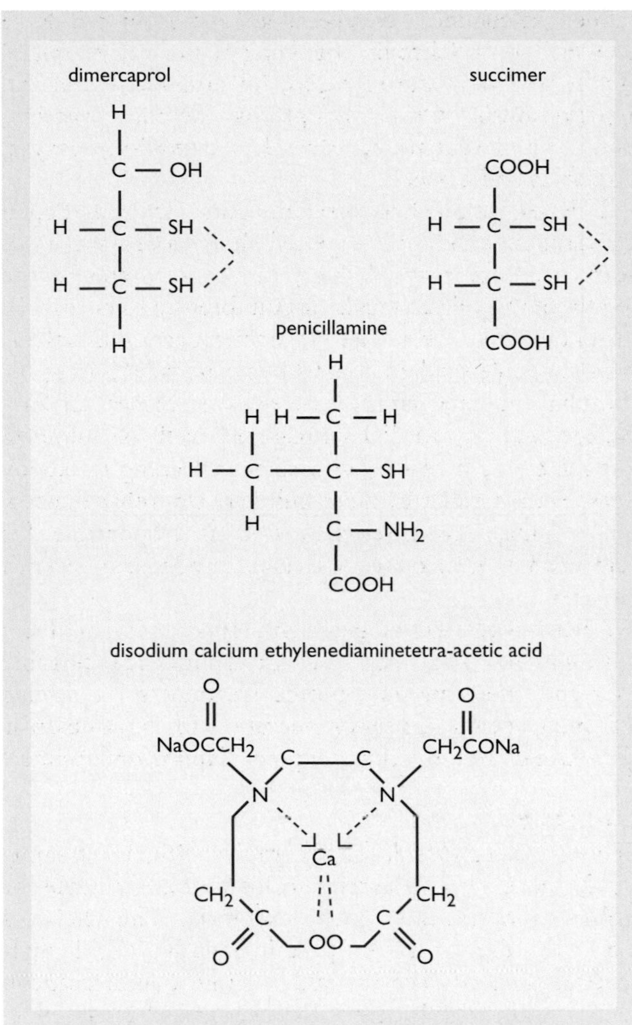

Fig. 24.8 Molecular structures of important chelator drugs.

tension, tachycardia, nausea, vomiting, burning sensations, salivation, pain and feelings of anxiety and unrest.

SUCCIMER, a thiol derivative of succinic acid, combines with cysteine to form a mixed disulfide. It chelates arsenic, lead and mercury, as well as other heavy metals, and is less toxic than dimercaprol.

PENICILLAMINE (D-β-β-dimethylcysteine), another thiol-containing chelator, is well absorbed when given orally and is metabolized slowly.

Air pollutants

Most urban air pollution is due to carbon monoxide (CO), sulfur oxides, hydrocarbons and nitrogen oxides. These come from burning coal and its products, as well as oil and gasoline and their products. Photochemical pollution (smog) contains hydrocarbons, oxides of nitrogen and photochemical oxidants. Airborne particles account for 10% of all air pollution (Fig. 24.9).

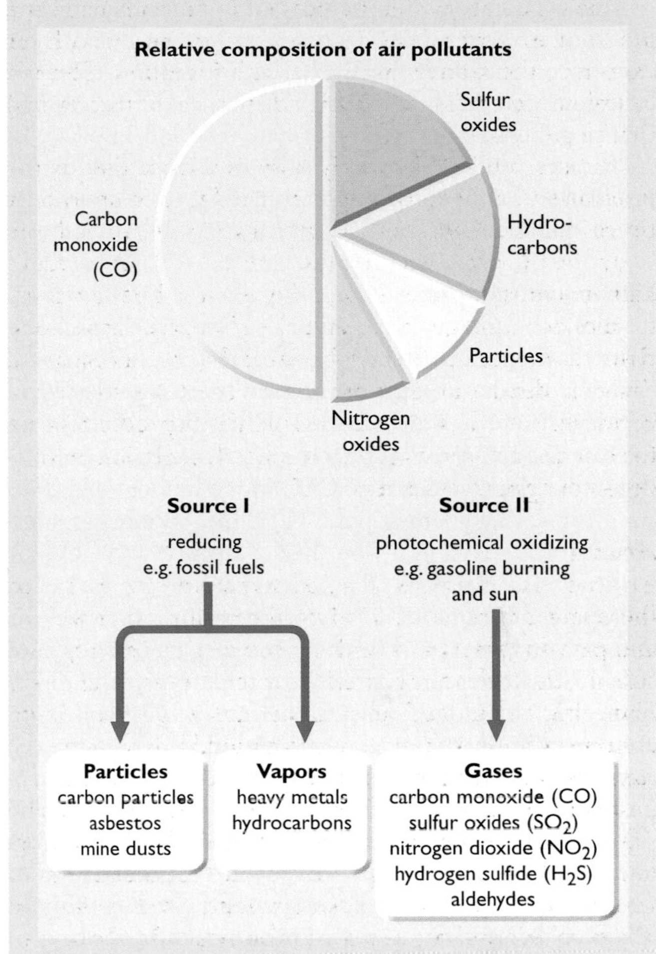

Fig. 24.9 Type and relative abundance of air pollutants.

Airborne particles

Airborne particles >5 µm in diameter are usually deposited in the upper airways, whereas those of 1–5 µm in diameter can reach the terminal airways and alveoli. A mucus blanket, propelled by the coordinated movement of cilia (the mucociliary escalator) carries larger insoluble particles upwards to the pharynx from whence they can be expectorated, or swallowed. Silica particles larger than 1 µm reach the alveoli where they are expelled, phagocytized or absorbed into the lymphatic system. Pneumoconiosis is caused by inhalation of small dust particles which are phagocytized. These phagocytized particles subsequently form fibrotic silicotic nodules throughout the lungs. Symptomatic pneumoconiosis usually takes years to develop. However, as pneumoconiosis develops it increases the susceptibility of lungs to infection.

Asbestos (fibrous hydrated silicates) was widely used in industry until it was recognized that bronchial cancer can occur 20–30 years after initial exposure to asbestos. Concomitant smoking increases the chance of developing such a cancer. Mesoepithelioma (in the pleura or peritoneum) is a rapidly fatal malignancy that appears related to exposure to chrysolite asbestos fiber, and occurs 25–40 years after initial exposure. The wave of litigation following the recognition and publicity of the carcinogenic risk of asbestos bankrupted many manufacturers and their insurance companies. It also led to a massive removal of asbestos, and possibly greater exposure of the public than would have occurred if it had been left in place. In such cases the correct calculation of a toxic risk to the population can be difficult and sometimes can be severely overestimated.

Carbon monoxide

Carbon monoxide is a colorless, odorless, tasteless nonirritating gas formed by incomplete combustion of carbon compounds, e.g. car exhaust. It is a major cause of accidental and suicidal deaths. When fire occurs in an enclosed space, most victims die from acute CO poisoning rather than from burns. CO bind to hemoglobin (Hb) to form carboxyhemoglobin (COHb), which has high affinity for oxygen. The high affinity of CO for hemoglobin (220 times that of oxygen) means that even low concentrations of CO 'lock-up' Hb and can cause dangerous hypoxia. The oxygen-carrying capacity of blood is inversely proportional to the amount of COHb present in the blood. Thus, the effects of CO poisoning are due entirely to hypoxia. In addition to decreasing the oxygen-carrying capacity of blood ('functional anemia'), CO also impairs the capacity of Hb to deliver oxygen to tissue. This is due to a shift in the oxygen dissociation curve to the left (Fig. 24.10). Moderate concentrations of COHb have little effect on vital functions (blood pressure, heart rate) at rest in healthy subjects owing to the considerable reserve in oxygen-carrying capacity of blood, and to the reserve in the cardiovascular system.

COHb will fully dissociate from Hb and the free CO is excreted easily by the lungs. Treatment of CO poisoning therefore involves immediate transfer to fresh air, with artificial respiration if required. Rapid administration of 100% oxygen is often the only therapy required. It is important to note that some transcutaneous oximeters used clinically do not distinguish well between carboxy- and oxyhemoglobin, and therefore do not properly assess the degree of CO poisoning. The cardiovascular system, particularly the heart, is susceptible to low concentrations of CO because the heart normally extracts a large fraction of oxygen delivered to it.

Experimental and clinical studies suggest that long-term exposure to CO facilitates the development of arteriosclerosis. The fetus is especially susceptible to CO and the persistent low levels of COHb produced by smoking during pregnancy may adversely affect fetal development.

In addition to CO being formed during a fire, the burning of plastic materials can release halogenated compounds that are acutely toxic to the lung and cause massive tissue and capillary damage resulting in death from acute respiratory distress syndrome (ARDS). Fires in aircraft and factories are particularly dangerous in this respect since they often contain large amounts of flammable plastic materials. Fatal lung damage can occur in victims that have been apparently safely rescued from fires and are not excessively burned.

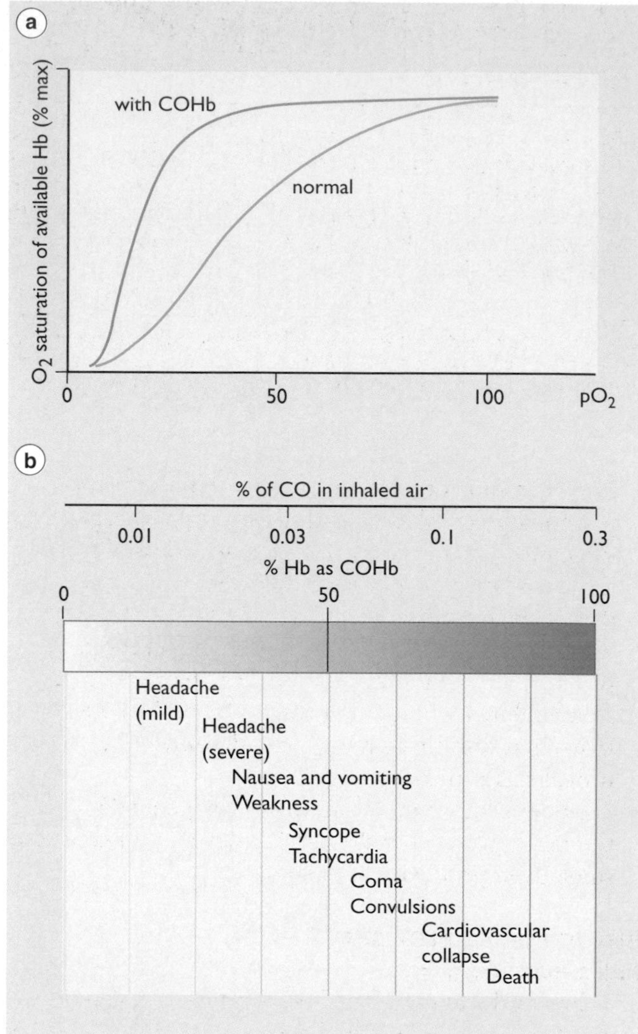

Fig. 24.10 Effects of carboxyhemoglobin (COHb) on oxygen dissociation from hemoglobin (a), and the symptoms associated with CO poisoning (b). The affinity of carbon monoxide (CO) for hemoglobin (Hb) is 220 times higher than for oxygen, thereby decreasing the oxygen-carrying capacity of blood. In addition, COHb shifts the oxyhemoglobin (O_2Hb)–oxygen saturation curve to the left, making oxygen release during hypoxia more difficult. This is illustrated in the upper panel which is normalized to 100% maximum. If the data were expressed as absolute oxygen content, the values in the presence of COHb would be decreased compared with normal.

Other air pollutants

Other air pollutants include sulfur oxides, nitrogen oxides and aldehydes:

- Inhaled sulfur dioxide causes moderate parasympathetic-dependent bronchoconstriction in normal people. However, this can be very severe in asthmatics. Asthmatics are sensitive to sulfur dioxide concentrations as low as 0.25 parts per million.

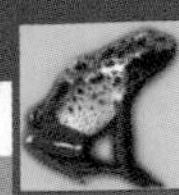

Table 24.10 Dangerous industrial chemicals

Solvents and vapors	Poisons (varying selectivity)
Gasoline, kerosene and their derivatives	Pesticides (many synthetic and a few natural compounds)
Hydrocarbons (e.g. butane, ethane)	Insecticides (organophosphates, organochlorines, pyrethrins)
Halogenated hydrocarbons	Vermin poisons
Aromatics (e.g. benzene, toluene)	Many rodenticides and general fumigants
Alcohols (ethanol, methanol, propanol)	Herbicides
Higher alcohols (glycols)	
Ethers	

Most of these are varyingly toxic to humans. Solvents and vapors sometimes have similar CNS toxic effects and produce similar symptoms. There are many solvents and vapors whose chemical nature makes them ideal fuels and solvents. Herbicides and insecticides have relatively selective actions, but vermin poisons are not so selective. Industrial chemicals generally cause acute toxicity.

- Nitrogen dioxide is a lung irritant that can cause pulmonary edema. It is a particular risk to farmers since nitrogen dioxide is formed and released from silage and may be a cause of pulmonary damage ('silo-filler's lung').
- Aldehydes are formed by sunlight acting on the products of incomplete combustion, or are released from aldehyde-containing resins. Formaldehyde irritates respiratory mucous membranes and can provoke skin reactions.
- Acrolein is more irritating than formaldehyde. It is the major reason for the irritating quality of cigarette smoke and photochemical smog.

Industrial chemicals

Petroleum distillates

Gasoline and kerosene are hydrocarbon distillates from mineral oil. They contain aliphatic, aromatic and other potentially toxic hydrocarbons. Most gasoline products contain benzene, and chronic exposure to benzene can cause leukemia. Intoxication following ingestion, or inhalation, of gasoline and kerosene (Table 24.10) resembles that due to ethanol. Inhalation of vapors of gasoline can cause ventricular fibrillation or chemical pneumonitis complicated by bacterial pneumonia and pulmonary edema. Death due to hemorrhagic pulmonary edema can occur within 24 hours of inhalation. The medical management of such poisoning is symptomatic and supportive.

Gasoline-contaminated drinking water can unknowingly result in chronic gasoline exposure, and possible toxicity. The higher molecular weight constituents of gasoline, like many organic solvents, depress the CNS and cause dizziness and incoordination. Neuropathy is an important toxic effect of *n*-hexane.

Halogenated hydrocarbons and other toxic solvents

Halogenated hydrocarbons are widely used industrial solvents (Fig. 24.11). Several small chlorinated hydrocarbons are formed in drinking water as a result of the chlorination process used to destroy bacterial contaminants. In addition, other halogenated hydrocarbons can accidentally contaminate water supplies. Since there are epidemiologic correlations (whether casual or causal is not really known) between water chlorination and cancer of the colon, rectum and bladder, there is concern about the exposure of large populations to chlorinated drinking water. At the moment it seems that the benefits of chlorination seem to outweigh its disadvantages and so there has been only limited shifts to using ozone rather than chlorine to make water safe for drinking.

Transient exposure to carbon tetrachloride vapor causes ocular and nasal irritation, nausea, vomiting, dizziness and headache. Death may result from ventricular fibrillation, or respiratory depression. Serious and delayed toxic effects include liver and kidney damage. Hepatotoxicity is a frequent toxicity due to halogenated hydrocarbons in general. However, this does not occur with the halogenated hydrocarbons that are used as inhalational anesthetics (see Ch. 21).

Alcohols

Methanol (wood alcohol) is another common industrial solvent. In some countries it is added as a contaminant to ethanol in order to justify lower taxes on the latter. The absorption, distribution and metabolism of methanol and ethanol are similar, and for both, their metabolism is by a zero-order kinetic process (see Ch. 2). Methanol inebriates less than ethanol, and produces headache, vertigo, vomiting, upper abdominal pain and hyperventilation. Retinal damage may be severe and lead to blindness (see Ch. 19). The other major problem with methanol is metabolic acidosis, which can be severe.

Ethanol has a 100-fold greater affinity for the alcohol dehydrogenase enzyme than methanol. The enzyme is responsible for the intermediate formation of aldehydes which are tissue toxins. As a result, a specific treatment for methanol poisoning is to maintain blood ethanol concentrations at >100 mg/100 mL, thereby preventing formation of the toxic metabolites of methanol, namely formaldehyde and formic acid (acidosis). Dialysis may be required to lower methanol concentrations to try to avoid methanol-induced blindness. Maintaining appropriate

Toxic solvents

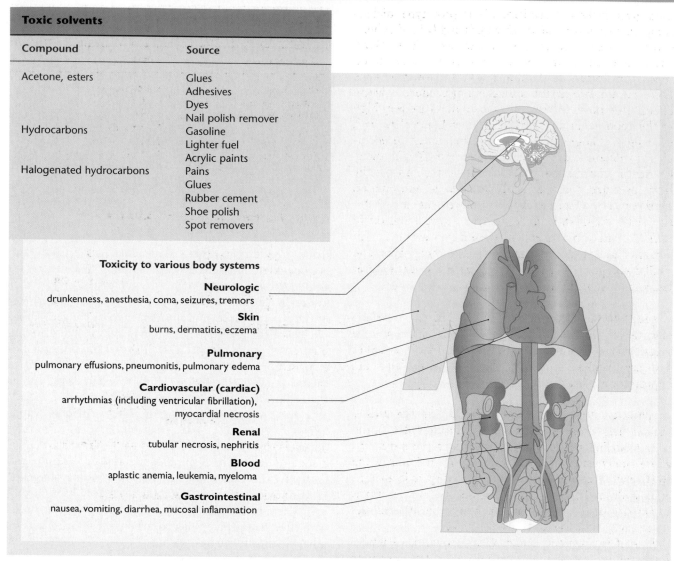

Compound	Source
Acetone, esters	Glues Adhesives Dyes Nail polish remover
Hydrocarbons	Gasoline Lighter fuel Acrylic paints
Halogenated hydrocarbons	Pains Glues Rubber cement Shoe polish Spot removers

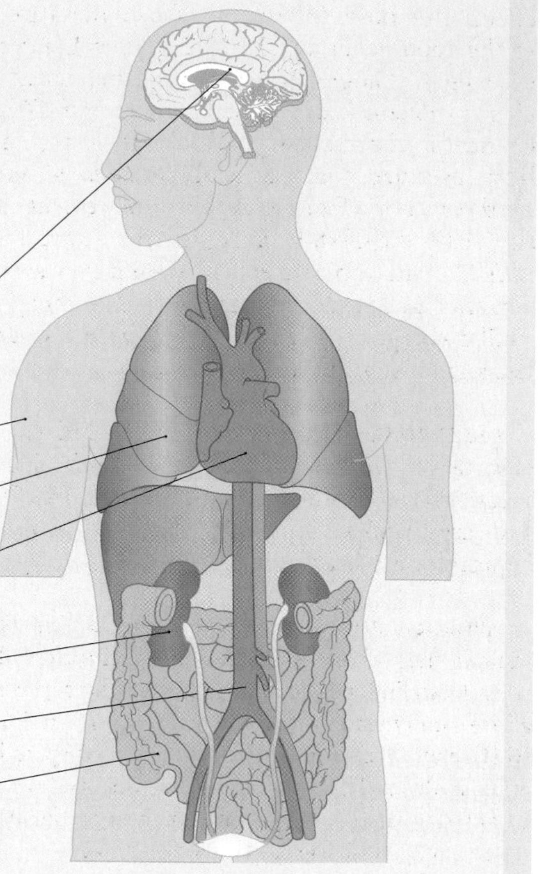

Fig. 24.11 Toxic solvents and the toxic effects of halogenated hydrocarbons on various body systems.

ethanol concentrations in blood while conducting hemodialysis may present a pharmacokinetic challenge. Methylpyrazole (fomepizole), an alcohol dehydrogenase inhibitor, can be of benefit in the therapy of methanol poisoning.

Other alcohols (isopropanol, ethylene and ethylene glycol (antifreeze), and propylene alcohol) are also toxic. Fomepizole is effective in the treatment of ethylene glycol poisoning.

Aromatic hydrocarbons

Benzene is an excellent solvent, but is highly toxic and carcinogenic. Toxic effects following acute and limited exposure to benzene include blurred vision, tremors, disturbed respiration, cardiac arrhythmias, paralysis and unconsciousness. Chronic intoxication can cause aplastic anemia and leukemia.

Toluene is a CNS depressant and in low concentrations produces fatigue, weakness and confusion, but it probably does not cause aplastic anemia or leukemia. 'Glue sniffers' inhale toluene vapors released from glue.

PESTICIDES

Over 0.5 billion kilograms of pesticides are used in the USA every year while 2.0 billion are used worldwide. Herbicides are the most commonly used, followed by insecticides and fungicides.

Insecticides

The insecticide residues that contaminate food result in low-level exposures of the general population to these toxic substances. Normally, acute poisoning only results from eating heavily contaminated foods, during agricultural spraying or with intentional poisoning.

Organochlorine insecticides

Chlorinated ethane derivatives, such as DDT, have been

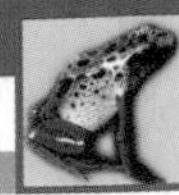

used extensively as insecticides. The prototype, dichlorodiphenyltrichloroethane (DDT), is highly lipid-soluble and therefore is only slowly eliminated from tissue. DDT has a wide margin of safety to humans and there are no reports of human deaths due to DDT. However, since DDT accumulates in the food chain, it produces adverse effects on raptors. These birds (as hunters) are very high in the food chain and high DDT levels interfere with their eggs. These and analogous other potential ecological problems led to the banning of DDT in many countries. Unfortunately, DDT was, and is, one of the best insecticides for controlling malarial mosquitoes. Methoxychlor (Fig. 24.12a), a replacement for DDT, stimulates the CNS by antagonizing γ aminobutyric acid (GABA) ionotropic receptors, resulting in decreased Cl^- currents and reduced inhibition. Methoxychlor and similar compounds can induce convulsions before other less serious signs of toxicity are seen.

CHLORINATED CYCLODIENES, unlike DDT, are readily absorbed from intact skin. Aldrin and dieldrin have the greatest carcinogenic potential among the insecticides and are banned in the USA, while chlordane and heptachlor are banned for use on crops.

HYDROCARBONS that have been used as insecticides include the γ isomer of benzene hexachloride (BHC), and the related lindane. Poisoning with lindane causes tremors, ataxia, convulsions and prostration. Both lindane and BHC have been implicated as causes of aplastic anemia. The hydrocarbon toxaphene causes tumors in mice. Other chlorinated hydrocarbon insecticides concentrate several thousand-fold in the food chain.

It is of interest that some plants grown in pesticide-free conditions (so-called organic vegetables) are found to contain much greater amounts of natural toxic chemicals than those grown in the presence of synthetic pesticides. This suggests an evolutionary response to increased pest predation in the absence of synthetic pesticides. The implications of such findings are not known but they do serve as a cautionary note against overly simplistic answers to the complex problems associated with human activities.

Organophosphate insecticides

Organophosphate insecticides (irreversible cholinesterase inhibitors) are alternatives to organochlorine insecticides (Fig. 24.12b). One of them, parathion, is the most frequent cause of fatal poisoning. Cholinesterase inhibition, due to phosphorylation of the enzyme, results in acetylcholine accumulation in humans, excessive muscarinic (parasympathetic) receptor stimulation (hypersecretion, diarrhea, sweating), confusion, agitation and coma. In addition, cholinesterase inhibition leads to excess accumulation of acetylcholine at neuromuscular junctions, leading to tetany and muscle weakness. Respiratory failure due to weakness of respiratory muscles may

a. The four major organochlorines. and their analogs

Compound	Analogs
DDT	Methoxychlor
Benzene chloride	Lindane
Cyclodienes	Aldrin Chlordane Dieldrin
Toxaphenes	Toxaphene

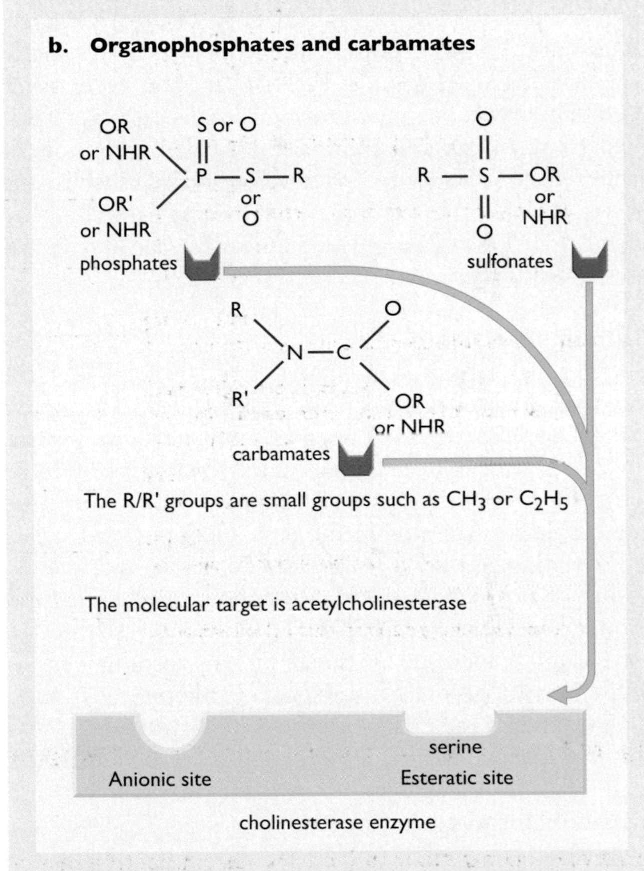

c. Pyrethrins

Pyrethrins are plant extracts, while pyrethroids are semi-synthesized analogs
Metabolized rapidly by man
Allergenic

Fig. 24.12 Poisonous organochlorine insecticides, pesticides and herbicides. (a) The four major organochlorine insecticides and their analogs. All contain multiple chlorines on a hydrocarbon, but vary in their toxicity. Their MWs range from 300 to 500; all are lipid soluble and therefore easily penetrate the CNS and also induce liver CYP enzymes. (b) These organophosphates and carbamates are anticholinesterase inhibitors and have chemical structures based upon phosphate, sulfonate or carbonate groups that target the esteratic binding site on cholinesterase enzymes. Over 35 phosphate and 20 carbamate anticholinesterases have been used commercially. (c) The pyrethrins are based on natural insecticides.

occur. Treatment of organophosphate insecticide poisoning includes the use of atropine as a muscarinic receptor antagonist in both the periphery and the CNS (see Chs 2 and 8) as well as artificial ventilation to support respiration if necessary. If organophosphate poisoning is detected early, pralidoxime can be used to reactivate the cholinesterase which has been inactivated by phosphorylation. Once reactivated, the accumulated acetylcholine can be hydrolyzed. Pralidoxime is most effective when used early after poisoning. The phosphorylated cholinesterase is thought to 'age' with time, presumably owing to conformational changes, that make it less susceptible to reactivation. (See Ch. 8 for more details.) Organophosphate cholinesterase inhibitors were originally developed as nerve gases in World War II but were never used. They have been used for murderous purposes since then by terrorists and some armies. Currently, modern armies attempt to protect themselves against such toxins by using injectable atropine and oximes as well as by taking orally reversible anticholinesterases – a controversial use of such drugs.

Botanic insecticides

Botanic insecticides such as pyrethrin (Fig. 24.12c) are increasingly used as less toxic insecticides. The crude extract, pyrethrum, is obtained from the pyrethrum plant (related to chrysanthemums) and is considered safe in terms of direct toxicity, but can cause contact dermatitis and respiratory allergy. In the past, nicotine was used as an insecticide, but it is extremely toxic and readily absorbed through the skin. Rotenone, another natural product previously used in Malaysian jungle streams to catch fish for food, rarely causes human poisoning and is used to treat head lice, scabies and other ectoparasites. Local effects include conjunctivitis, dermatitis and rhinitis. Other insecticides are used as ectoparasiticides (e.g. lindane is used as a miticide for scabies, and malathion for nits, see Ch. 18).

General pesticides

Fumigants

Fumigants, as their name suggests, are used to control insects, rodents and soil nematodes using a fumigation process. Such fumigants include hydrogen cyanide (HCN), acrylonitrile, carbon disulfide, carbon tetrachloride, ethylene dibromide, ethylene oxide and methyl bromide. All of these chemicals are very poisonous to all living things as well as to humans.

HCN is a rapidly acting poison that kills rapidly after fatal exposure. Its most horrific intentional use was as a poison in the mass murders of World War II and in legal constituted gas chambers. HCN is released incidentally during fires in which nitrogen-containing plastics are burned.

HCN has a high affinity for ferric iron, particularly in mitochondrial cytochrome oxidase where it inhibits cellular respiration. HCN victims usually either die quickly from cellular hypoxia or recover fully. However, chronic neurologic sequelae can occur as result of cellular hypoxia before subsequent recovery.

Treatment of cyanide poisoning has to be immediate, and involves certain specific steps. One of the first steps is to giving nitrites. The administration of nitrates result in the formation of methemoglobin, which has a greater affinity for HCN than hemoglobin, thus in effect reducing CN levels. This initial step is followed by the administration of sodium thiosulfate, which reacts with the CN radical to form nontoxic thiocyanate, which is subsequently excreted. Supportive therapies, such as the administration of oxygen, are also initiated. Such antidotes are life saving in cases of cyanide posioning providing they are initiated rapidly enough. It is important to know that cyanide salts are equal in their toxicity to HCN.

Rodenticides

The toxicity of rodenticides varies. For example, the anticoagulant warfarin is relatively safe to nonrodent species since toxicity depends upon its repeated ingestion. However, sodium fluoroacetate and fluoracetamide, which are among the most effective rodenticides, are very poisonous to man.

Strychnine, a poisonous alkaloid, is still used occasionally as a pesticide, and it is a source of accidental poisoning. Its acts to increase neuronal excitability. This excitability leads to severe seizures resulting from selective blockade of the neuronal inhibition that is mediated by glycine.

Other rodenticides include white or yellow elemental phosphorus spread onto bait. Zinc phosphide reacts with water and acid in the stomach to produce the extremely poisonous phosphine. Thallium sulfate is a very hazardous chemical that is not in the least selective for rodents. As a result its use is now strictly regulated in many countries.

Herbicides

Most herbicides have low toxicity to humans, but have caused human fatalities. Dioxin (plus its byproducts, CDD and TCDD) is a minor impurity in herbicides, and a byproduct of manufacturing processes that use chlorine (e.g. paper making). Several epidemiologic studies of people exposed to high concentrations of dioxin suggest low toxicity, but other studies suggest that TCDD might be carcinogenic and teratogenic.

Several substituted dinitrophenols are used to kill weeds and, as a result, human poisoning with dinitro-orthocresol (DNOC) has occurred. The short-term toxicity of dinitrophenols is due to uncoupling of oxidative phosphorylation. Death or recovery occurs within 24–48 hours.

Paraquat is responsible for many accidental or suicidal poisonings. It damages the lungs, liver and kidneys. The serious nature of its delayed pulmonary toxicity makes prompt treatment mandatory. Many other herbicides have relatively low acute toxicities.

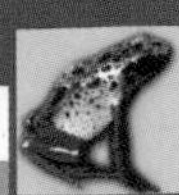

Fungicides

Fungicides are a heterogeneous group of chemical compounds, but few have been extensively investigated for toxicity. Dithiocarbamates have teratogenic and/or carcinogenic potential.

CARCINOGENESIS AND MUTAGENESIS

Chemicals known to cause cancer in humans after prolonged exposure include vinyl chloride, benzene and naphthylamine. The US government has listed about 250 potential carcinogens that are either synthetic or accidentally produced. These chemicals should be avoided.

Common activities expose whole populations to carcinogens. Obvious examples include cigarette smoke that contains many cancer-causing chemicals. The chronic consumption of ethanol increases the risk of esophageal and liver cancer. Charcoal broiling contaminates food with carcinogenic polycyclic aromatic hydrocarbons (the carcinogenic hydrocarbons found in coal tars). Some foods contain natural carcinogens (from plant and fungal origins) and these probably account in part for the regional differences found in the incidence of various cancers worldwide. Many occupations have been found over the last 150 years to be associated with quite specific cancers. These identified and obvious dangers are now avoided in the workplace where adequate protection is provided. In other situations there appear to be causal relationships between occupation and cancer risk, but proof of the presence of carcinogens has still to be formally proven. One example is the excess incidence of cancer in firemen.

Many steps are involved in chemical carcinogenesis. The nature of exposure to carcinogens is important in that duration, dose and frequency are all important. The chemical induction of cancer involves processes of initiation, promotion and progression.

Initiation (by initiating agents) is the conversion of normal cells into neoplastic cells via actions on DNA. However, additional events convert transformed cells to malignant cells. In animals, promoter chemicals increase the incidence of cancers, or decrease the latency to tumor growth, although they do not themselves act directly on DNA or produce mutations.

A mutation is an alteration in DNA sequence that may change the cellular phenotype. Spontaneous mutagenesis is always occurring and is due mostly to unknown mechanisms. Cells have inherent protective and repair mechanisms that normally prevent such mutations from becoming significant. However, this natural rate can be increased 10-1000-fold by mutagens and overwhelm the natural defenses. Mutations are more likely to cause cancer in cells that have deficient DNA repair enzymes, or in situations in which cellular division is so rapid that DNA repair is incomplete. Many cancers are thought to begin as a routine mutation, or are a hereditary trait.

Table 24.11 Carcinogens, cocarcinogens and promoters

Genotoxic agents (mutagenic)	Chemical alkylating agents Ionizing and ultraviolet (skin) radiation Nickel, cadmium Hydrocarbons (polycyclics) and polyamines (arylamines, nitrosamines)
Epigenetic agents	Hormones such as estrogens Promoters such as phorbol esters Trauma Alcohol ingestion

The actions of chemical carcinogens are either genotoxic or epigenetic

Genotoxic carcinogens (Table 24.11) react covalently with DNA to produce genetic mutations. Mutagenic potential can be detected by tests such as the Ames test for bacterial mutagenicity. Genotoxic carcinogens can be further subclassified on the basis of whether they require biotransformation before they become active. Most genotoxic agents are procarcinogens or activation-dependent genotoxic agents. Nitrosamines are typical procarcinogens.

Epigenetic agents enhance the effects of genotoxic carcinogens. They act by:

- Increasing the effector concentration of a genotoxin.
- Enhancing the metabolic activation of a genotoxin.
- Decreasing the detoxification of a genotoxin.
- Inhibiting DNA repair.
- Increasing the proliferation of DNA-damaged cells.

Tumor promoters enhance carcinogenic activity when given after a genotoxin. Phorbol esters are tumor-promoting agents that act by binding to protein kinase C. TCDD (dioxin) is also a potent tumor promoter. Immunosuppressive drugs are epigenetic agents that suppress the immune system and thereby ‘allow’ carcinogenesis to occur.

Asbestos is an example of an epigenetic carcinogen

Asbestos fibers are centers of mitotic activity and these add to tobacco smoke as a carcinogenic mechanism. Smokers have a 10-fold greater risk of developing lung cancer than nonsmokers. Asbestos increases this risk to 50-fold.

Mechanisms of action of chemical mutagens and carcinogens

- Genotoxins cause genetic damage, which may lead to cancer
- Epigenetic compounds amplify the cancer-forming actions of genotoxins
- Promoters (chemical, physical and biologic) amplify the adverse effects of mutagens and carcinogens

FURTHER READING

Braun L, Cohen M (eds). *Herbs and Natural Supplements: an Evidence-Based Guide*. New York: Elsevier Mosby; 2005. [A useful compendium of the evidence for the effectiveness, or otherwise, of herbs.]

Brin MF, Jankovic J, Hallet M. *Scientific and Therapeutic Aspects of Botulinum Toxin*. Philadelphia: Lippincott, Williams and Wilkins; 2002. [Covers all aspects of botulism.]

Ernst E, Pittler MH, Stevinson C, White A (eds). *The Desktop Guide to Complementary and Alternative Medicine: an Evidence-Based Approach*. London: Harcourt; 2001.

Hendriks AJ, Maas-Diepeveen JL, Heugens EH, Van Straalen NM. Meta-analysis of intrinsic rates of increase and carrying capacity of populations affected by toxic and other stressors. *Environ Toxicol Chem* 2005; **24**: 2267–2277. [Modelling procedures used to try and predict the actual dangers posed to society by toxins.]

Horowitz BZ. Botulinum toxin. *Crit Care Clin* 2005; **21**: 825–839. [An overview of botulinus toxins, actons, mechanisms and uses.]

Klaassen CD (ed.). *Casarett and Doull's Toxicology: the Basic Science of Poisons*, 6th edn. New York: McGraw-Hill; 2001. [A standard toxicological reference book.]

Krenzelok EP. The Pittsburgh Poison Center profile of an American poison information center. *Przegl Lek* 2005; **62**: 538–542. [An example of the range of activities and services provided by a US poison center.]

Nash RA. Metals in medicine. *Altern Ther Health Med* 2005; **11**: 18–25. [An overview of metal poisoning including chelation therapy.]

Sullivan JB, Krieger GR. *Clinical Environmental Health and Toxic Exposures*, 2nd edn. Baltimore: Lippincott, Williams and Wilkins; 2001. [Source for material on toxicological hazards in the environment.]

WEBSITES

http://www.herbalgram.org/default.asp?c=-herb_info [This website is made by American Botanical Council and it provides general information about herbs.]

http://toxnet.nlm.nih.gov/ [This website provides detailed information about various toxins and poisonings.]

http://www.merck.com/mrkshared/mmanual/sections.jsp [Merck Manual.]

Index

Illustrations are in italics. Indexed items mentioned in both text and illustration on the same page have been given just a single reference in plain type.

B

C

D

F

G

H

M

N

O

P

Q

R

T

W

X

Y

Z